DESK ENCYCLOPEDIA OF
HUMAN AND
MEDICAL VIROLOGY

DESK ENCYCLOPEDIA OF HUMAN AND MEDICAL VIROLOGY

EDITOR-IN-CHIEF

Dr BRIAN W J MAHY

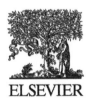

AMSTERDAM • BOSTON • HEIDELBERG • LONDON • NEW YORK • OXFORD
PARIS • SAN DIEGO • SAN FRANCISCO • SINGAPORE • SYDNEY • TOKYO
Academic Press is an imprint of Elsevier

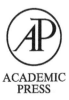

ACADEMIC
PRESS

ELSEVIER

Academic Press is an imprint of Elsevier
Linacre House, Jordan Hill, Oxford, OX2 8DP, UK
525 B Street, Suite 1900, San Diego, CA 92101-4495, USA

British Library Cataloguing in Publication Data
A catalogue record for this book is available from the British Library

Library of Congress Cataloguing in Publication Data
A catalogue record for this book is available from the Library of Congress

ISBN: 978-0-12-375147-8

For information on all Elsevier publications
visit our website at books.elsevier.com

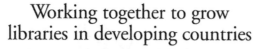

EDITOR-IN-CHIEF

Brian W J Mahy MA PhD ScD DSc
Senior Scientific Advisor,
Division of Emerging Infections and Surveillance Services,
Centers for Disease Control and Prevention,
Atlanta GA, USA

ASSOCIATE EDITORS

Dennis H Bamford, Ph.D.
Department of Biological and Environmental Sciences
and Institute of Biotechnology, Biocenter 2,
P.O. Box 56 (Viikinkaari 5),
00014 University of Helsinki,
Finland

Charles Calisher, B.S., M.S., Ph.D.
Arthropod-borne and Infectious Diseases Laboratory
Department of Microbiology, Immunology and Pathology
College of Veterinary Medicine and Biomedical Sciences
Colorado State University
Fort Collins
CO 80523
USA

Andrew J Davison, M.A., Ph.D.
MRC Virology Unit
Institute of Virology
University of Glasgow
Church Street
Glasgow G11 5JR
UK

Claude Fauquet
ILTAB/Donald Danforth Plant Science Center
975 North Warson Road
St. Louis, MO 63132

Said Ghabrial, B.S., M.S., Ph.D.
Plant Pathology Department
University of Kentucky
201F Plant Science Building
1405 Veterans Drive
Lexington
KY 4050546-0312
USA

Eric Hunter, B.Sc., Ph.D.
Department of Pathology and Laboratory Medicine, and
Emory Vaccine Center
Emory University
954 Gatewood Road NE
Atlanta Georgia 30329
USA

Robert A Lamb, Ph.D., Sc.D.
Department of Biochemistry,
Molecular Biology and Cell Biology
Howard Hughes Medical Institute
Northwestern University
2205 Tech Dr.
Evanston
IL 60208-3500
USA

Olivier Le Gall
IPV, UMR GDPP, IBVM,
INRA Bordeaux-Aquitaine, BP 81,
F-33883 Villenave d'Ornon Cedex
FRANCE

Vincent Racaniello, Ph.D.
Department of Microbiology
Columbia University
New York, NY 10032
USA

David A Theilmann, Ph.D., B.Sc., M.Sc
Pacific Agri-Food Research Centre
Agriculture and Agri-Food Canada
Box 5000, 4200 Highway 97
Summerland
BC V0H 1Z0
Canada

H Josef Vetten, Ph.D.
Julius Kuehn Institute, Federal Research Centre for
Cultivated Plants (JKI)
Messeweg 11-12
38104 Braunschweig
Germany

Peter J Walker, B.Sc., Ph.D.
CSIRO Livestock Industries
Australian Animal Health Laboratory (AAHL)
Private Bag 24
Geelong
VIC 3220
Australia

PREFACE

The *Desk Encyclopedia of Human and Medical Virology* is the second in a series of four volumes that reproduce many of the chapters in the third edition of the *Encyclopedia of Virology*, edited by Brian W J Mahy and Marc H V van Regenmortel, published by Academic Press/Elsevier 2008. It contains 81 chapters that relate to human/medical virology. The first section includes 42 chapters that describe general features of common human viruses, and this is followed in Section 2 by five more specialized chapters related to HIV/AIDS. In Section 3, there are 23 chapters describing exotic virus infections, including one now-eradicated virus (smallpox) and some now controlled by vaccination, such as yellow fever. Section 4 includes seven chapters describing some viruses that have been associated with oncogenesis, and Section 5 contains four general chapters of interest to medical virology.

In bringing all these topics under one cover, it is hoped that the book will provide a convenient reference source and an up-to-date introduction to recent advances in medical virology. In combination with the first volume, the *Desk Encyclopedia of General Virology*, this book could provide excellent material for a teaching course in virology for medical students.

Brian W J Mahy

CONTRIBUTORS

C Adams
University of Duisburg–Essen, Essen, Germany

E Adderson
St. Jude Children's Research Hospital, Memphis, TN, USA

J Angel
Pontificia Universidad Javeriana, Bogota, Republic of Colombia

H Attoui
Institute for Animal Health, Pirbright, UK

A G Bader
The Scripps Research Institute, La Jolla, CA, USA

A D T Barrett
University of Texas Medical Branch, Galveston, TX, USA

R Bartenschlager
University of Heidelberg, Heidelberg, Germany

N W Bartlett
Imperial College London, London, UK

D Baxby
University of Liverpool, Liverpool, UK

P Beard
Imperial College London, London, UK

E D Belay
Centers for Disease Control and Prevention, Atlanta, GA, USA

M Benkö
Veterinary Medical Research Institute, Hungarian Academy of Sciences, Budapest, Hungary

M Bennett
University of Liverpool, Liverpool, UK

P Biagini
Etablissement Français du Sang Alpes-Méditerranée, Marseilles, France

R F Bishop
Murdoch Childrens Research Institute Royal Children's Hospital, Melbourne, VIC, Australia

P Britton
Institute for Animal Health, Compton, UK

K S Brown
University of Manitoba, Winnipeg, MB, Canada

J J Bugert
Wales College of Medicine, Heath Park, Cardiff, UK

R M Buller
Saint Louis University School of Medicine, St. Louis, MO, USA

J S Butel
Baylor College of Medicine, Houston, TX, USA

S Bühler
University of Heidelberg, Heidelberg, Germany

C H Calisher
Colorado State University, Fort Collins, CO, USA

R Cattaneo
Mayo Clinic College of Medicine, Rochester, MN, USA

D Cavanagh
Institute for Animal Health, Compton, UK

A Chahroudi
University of Pennsylvania School of Medicine, Philadelphia, PA, USA

T J Chambers
Saint Louis University School of Medicine, St. Louis, MO, USA

Y Chang
University of Pittsburgh Cancer Institute, Pittsburgh, PA, USA

A V Chintakuntlawar
University of Oklahoma Health Sciences Center, Oklahoma City, OK, USA

J Chodosh
University of Oklahoma Health Sciences Center, Oklahoma City, OK, USA

P Clarke
University of Colorado Health Sciences, Denver, CO, USA

J I Cohen
National Institutes of Health, Bethesda, MD, USA

P L Collins
National Institute of Allergy and Infectious Diseases, Bethesda, MD, USA

J E Crowe Jr.
Vanderbilt University Medical Center, Nashville, TN, USA

A J Davison
MRC Virology Unit, Glasgow, UK

A Dotzauer
University of Bremen, Bremen, Germany

S Dreschers
University of Duisburg–Essen, Essen, Germany

W P Duprex
The Queen's University of Belfast, Belfast, UK

J East
University of Texas Medical Branch – Galveston, Galveston, TX, USA

B T Eaton
Australian Animal Health Laboratory, Geelong, VIC, Australia

R M Elliott
University of St. Andrews, St. Andrews, UK

D Falzarano
University of Manitoba, Winnipeg, MB, Canada

H Feldmann
National Microbiology Laboratory, Public Health Agency of Canada, Winnipeg, MB, Canada

B Fleckenstein
University of Erlangen – Nürnberg, Erlangen, Germany

M A Franco
Pontificia Universidad Javeriana, Bogota, Republic of Colombia

T K Frey
Georgia State University, Atlanta, GA, USA

T W Geisbert
National Emerging Infectious Diseases Laboratories, Boston, MA, USA

A Gessain
Pasteur Institute, CNRS URA 3015, Paris, France

U A Gompels
University of London, London, UK

E A Gould
University of Reading, Reading, UK

R Grassmann
University of Erlangen – Nürnberg, Erlangen, Germany

M Gravell
National Institutes of Health, Bethesda, MD, USA

K Y Green
National Institutes of Health, Bethesda, MD, USA

H B Greenberg
Stanford University School of Medicine and Veterans Affairs Palo Alto Health Care System, Palo Alto, CA, USA

T S Gritsun
University of Reading, Reading, UK

D J Gubler
John A. Burns School of Medicine, Honolulu, HI, USA

B Harrach
Veterinary Medical Research Institute, Budapest, Hungary

T J Harrison
University College London, London, UK

L E Hensley
USAMRIID, Fort Detrick, MD, USA

F van Heuverswyn
University of Montpellier 1, Montpellier, France

E Hunter
Emory University Vaccine Center, Atlanta, GA, USA

T Hyypiä
University of Turku, Turku, Finland

S L Johnston
Imperial College London, London, UK

P Karayiannis
Imperial College London, London, UK

K Khalili
Temple University School of Medicine, Philadelphia, PA, USA

P H Kilmarx
Centers for Disease Control and Prevention, Atlanta, GA, USA

C D Kirkwood
Murdoch Childrens Research Institute Royal Children's Hospital, Melbourne, VIC, Australia

N R Klatt
University of Pennsylvania School of Medicine, Philadelphia, PA, USA

W B Klimstra
Louisiana State University Health Sciences Center, Shreveport, LA, USA

L D Kramer
Wadsworth Center, New York State Department of Health, Albany, NY, USA

I V Kuzmin
Centers for Disease Control and Prevention, Atlanta, GA, USA

R A Lamb
Howard Hughes Medical Institute at Northwestern University, Evanston, IL, USA

M D A Lindsay
Western Australian Department of Health, Mount Claremont, WA, Australia

D C Liotta
Emory University, Atlanta, GA, USA

J S Mackenzie
Curtin University of Technology, Shenton Park, WA, Australia

R Mahieux
Pasteur Institute, CNRS URA 3015, Paris, France

B W J Mahy
Centers for Disease Control and Prevention, Atlanta, GA, USA

E O Major
National Institutes of Health, Bethesda, MD, USA

A A Marfin
Centers for Disease Control and Prevention, Atlanta, GA, USA

T D Mastro
Centers for Disease Control and Prevention, Atlanta, GA, USA

M McChesney
University of California, Davis, Davis, CA, USA

J B McCormick
University of Texas, School of Public Health, Brownsville, TX, USA

A L McNees
Baylor College of Medicine, Houston, TX, USA

P S Mellor
Institute for Animal Health, Pirbright, UK

X J Meng
Virginia Polytechnic Institute and State University, Blacksburg, VA, USA

P P C Mertens
Institute for Animal Health, Pirbright, UK

H Meyer
Bundeswehr Institute of Microbiology, Munich, Germany

P de Micco
Etablissement Français du Sang Alpes-Méditerranée, Marseilles, France

B R Miller
Centers for Disease Control and Prevention (CDC), Fort Collins, CO, USA

P D Minor
NIBSC, Potters Bar, UK

E S Mocarski Jr.
Emory University School of Medicine, Emory, GA, USA

T P Monath
Kleiner Perkins Caufield and Byers, Menlo Park, CA, USA

P S Moore
University of Pittsburgh Cancer Institute, Pittsburgh, PA, USA

L Moser
University of Wisconsin – Madison, Madison, WI, USA

A W Neuman
Emory University, Atlanta, GA, USA

M S Oberste
Centers for Disease Control and Prevention, Atlanta, GA, USA

W A O'Brien
University of Texas Medical Branch – Galveston, Galveston, TX, USA

G Olinger
USAMRIID, Fort Detrick, MD, USA

J E Osorio
University of Wisconsin, Madison, WI, USA

M A Pallansch
Centers for Disease Control and Prevention, Atlanta, GA, USA

S Parker
Saint Louis University School of Medicine, St. Louis, MO, USA

R F Pass
University of Alabama School of Medicine, Birmingham, AL, USA

M Peeters
University of Montpellier 1, Montpellier, France

J S M Peiris
The University of Hong Kong, Hong Kong, People's Republic of China

P J Peters
Centers for Disease Control and Prevention, Atlanta, GA, USA

H Pfister
University of Köln, Cologne, Germany

L L M Poon
The University of Hong Kong, Hong Kong, People's Republic of China

A Portner
St. Jude Children's Research Hospital, Memphis, TN, USA

C M Preston
Medical Research Council Virology Unit, Glasgow, UK

A Rapose
University of Texas Medical Branch – Galveston, Galveston, TX, USA

W K Reisen
University of California, Davis, CA, USA

B K Rima
The Queen's University of Belfast, Belfast, UK

C M Robinson
University of Oklahoma Health Sciences Center,
Oklahoma City, OK, USA

C E Rupprecht
Centers for Disease Control and Prevention, Atlanta,
GA, USA

K D Ryman
Louisiana State University Health Sciences Center,
Shreveport, LA, USA

M Safak
Temple University School of Medicine, Philadelphia,
PA, USA

L B Schonberger
Centers for Disease Control and Prevention, Atlanta,
GA, USA

D A Schultz
Johns Hopkins University School of Medicine, Baltimore,
MD, USA

S Schultz-Cherry
University of Wisconsin – Madison, Madison, WI, USA

A Silaghi
University of Manitoba, Winnipeg, MB, Canada

G Silvestri
University of Pennsylvania School of Medicine,
Philadelphia, PA, USA

M A Skinner
Imperial College London, London, UK

D W Smith
PathWest Laboratory Medicine WA, Nedlands,
WA, Australia

G L Smith
Imperial College London, London, UK

M Sova
University of Texas Medical Branch – Galveston,
Galveston, TX, USA

P Tattersall
Yale University Medical School, New Haven, CT, USA

J M Taylor
Fox Chase Cancer Center, Philadelphia, PA, USA

H C Thomas
Imperial College London, London, UK

A S Turnell
The University of Birmingham, Birmingham, UK

K L Tyler
University of Colorado Health Sciences, Denver, CO, USA

A Vaheri
University of Helsinki, Helsinki, Finland

P K Vogt
The Scripps Research Institute, La Jolla, CA, USA

L-F Wang
Australian Animal Health Laboratory, Geelong,
VIC, Australia

S C Weaver
University of Texas Medical Branch, Galveston, TX, USA

R M Welsh
University of Massachusetts Medical School, Worcester,
MA, USA

C A Whitehouse
United States Army Medical Research Institute of
Infectious Diseases, Frederick, MD, USA

M Yoshida
University of Tokyo, Chiba, Japan

L S Young
University of Birmingham, Birmingham, UK

T M Yuill
University of Wisconsin, Madison, WI, USA

CONTENTS

GENERAL FEATURES OF COMMON HUMAN VIRUSES

Adenoviruses: General Features

B Harrach, Veterinary Medical Research Institute, Budapest, Hungary

Introduction

Adenoviruses are middle-sized, nonenveloped, icosahedral, double-stranded DNA viruses of animals. The prefix adeno comes from the Greek word ἀδήν (gland), reflecting the first isolation of a virus of this type from human adenoid tissue half a century ago. Adenoviruses have since been isolated from a large variety of hosts, including representatives of every major vertebrate class from fish to mammals. Using polymerase chain reaction (PCR) technology, a large variety of putative novel adenoviruses have been detected, but isolation of such viruses and *in vitro* propagation is hampered in most cases by the lack of appropriate permissive cell cultures. Some human and animal adenoviruses can cause diseases or even death, but most are not pathogenic in non-immuno-compromised, healthy individuals. Adenoviruses have been used as model organisms in molecular biology, and important findings of general relevance have emerged from such studies, including splicing in eukaryotes. Adenoviruses have become one of the most popular vector systems for virus-based gene therapy and vaccination and have potential as antitumor tools. Wide prevalence in diverse host species and a substantially conserved genome organization make adenoviruses an ideal model for studying virus evolution.

Taxonomy

Adenoviruses belong to the family *Adenoviridae*. No higher taxonomical level has yet been established, despite the fact that certain bacteriophages (*Tectiviridae*), the green alga virus *Paramecium bursaria Chlorella virus 1* (*Phycodnaviridae*), and a virus of Archaea living in hot springs (sulfolobus turreted icosahedral virus) seem to have common evolutionary roots with adenoviruses.

There are four official genera in the family. Two genera (*Mastadenovirus* and *Aviadenovirus*) comprise adenoviruses that have probably co-evolved with mammals and birds, respectively. The other two genera (*Atadenovirus* and *Siadenovirus*) have a broader range of hosts. Atadenoviruses were named after a bias toward high A+T content in the genomes of the initial representatives, which infect various ruminant and avian hosts, as well as a marsupial. Every known reptilian adenovirus also belongs to the atadenoviruses, although their genomes do not show the same bias toward high A+T content. The very few known siadenoviruses were isolated from or detected by PCR in birds and a frog. This genus was named in recognition of the presence of a gene encoding a potential sialidase in the viruses concerned. The single confirmed fish adenovirus falls into a separate group that may eventually found a fifth genus; adenovirus-like particles have been described in additional fish species.

Within each genus, the viruses are grouped into species, which are named according to the host first described and supplemented with letters of the alphabet (**Table 1**). Host origin is only one of several criteria that are used to demarcate the species. Phylogenetic distance is the most significant criterion, with species defined as separated by more than 5–10% amino acid sequence divergence of hexon and DNA polymerase (pol), respectively. Further important characteristics come into play, especially if DNA sequence data are not available: DNA hybridization, restriction fragment length polymorphism, nucleotide composition, oncogenicity in rodents, growth characteristics, host range, cross-neutralization, ability to recombine, number of virus-associated (VA) RNA genes, hemagglutination properties, and organization of the genome. However, all of these ancillary data are expected to accord with the results of phylogenetic calculations. Thus, for example, chimpanzee adenoviruses are classified into human adenovirus species. Adenoviruses of humans have been studied far more intensively than those of other animals, and the six species (*Human adenovirus A* to *Human adenovirus F*; abbreviated informally to HAdV-A to HAdV-F) correspond to substantial 'groups' or 'subgenera' defined previously. Each human adenovirus serotype is abbreviated to HAdV hyphenated to a number.

To illustrate the need to proceed carefully in developing adenovirus taxonomy, the case of the newest adenovirus isolated from human samples (HAdV-52) is illuminating. This virus seems to be sufficiently different from other human adenoviruses to merit the erection of a new species. However, it is very similar to some previously characterized Old World monkey adenoviruses (simian adenoviruses 1 and 7 (SAdV-1, SAdV-7) plus others). One taxonomical proposal would be to establish a new species, *Human adenovirus G*, containing HAdV-52 and the related monkey adenoviruses. Clearly, this would depend on epidemiological data demonstrating that HAdV-52 is properly a human virus and not an occasional, opportunistic transfer from monkeys. For similar reasons and others, classification of many nonhuman adenoviruses into species is not yet resolved.

Virion Morphology and Properties

The icosahedral capsid is 70–90 nm in diameter and consists of 240 nonvertex capsomers (called hexons), each

Table 1   The taxonomy of family *Adenoviridae*[a]

Genus/species	Serotype	Strain	Genome
Mastadenovirus			
Bovine adenovirus A	BAdV-1		G
Bovine adenovirus B	BAdV-3		G
Bovine adenovirus C	BAdV-10		
Canine adenovirus	CAdV-1, 2		G
Equine adenovirus A	EAdV-1		
Equine adenovirus B	EAdV-2		
Human adenovirus A	HAdV-12, 18, 31		12
Human adenovirus B	HAdV-3, 7, 11, 14, 16, 21, 34, 35, 50		G
	Simian adenovirus 21 (SAdV-21)		G
Human adenovirus C	BAdV-9, HAdV-1, 2, 5, 6		1, 2, 5
Human adenovirus D	HAdV-8–10, 13, 15, 17, 19, 20,		9, 17
	22–30, 32, 33, 36–39, 42–49, 51		26, 46, 48, 49
Human adenovirus E	HAdV-4, SAdV-22–25		G
Human adenovirus F	HAdV-40, 41		G
Murine adenovirus A	MAdV-1		G
Ovine adenovirus A	BAdV-2, OAdV-2–5		BAdV-2
Ovine adenovirus B	OAdV-1		
Porcine adenovirus A	PAdV-1, 2, 3		3
Porcine adenovirus B	PAdV-4		
Porcine adenovirus C	PAdV-5		G
Tree shrew adenovirus	TSAdV-1		G
Goat adenovirus (ts)	GAdV-2		
Guinea pig adenovirus (ts)	GPAdV-1		
Murine adenovirus B (ts)	MAdV-2		
Ovine adenovirus C (ts)	OAdV-6		
Simian adenovirus A (ts)	SAdV-3		G
Squirrel adenovirus (ts)	SqAdV-1		
?	HAdV-52		G
?	SAdV-1–2, 4–20		1, 6, 7, 20
Aviadenovirus			
Fowl adenovirus A	FAdV-1	CELO	G
Fowl adenovirus B	FAdV-5	340	
Fowl adenovirus C	FAdV-4, 10	KR95, CFA20	
Fowl adenovirus D	FAdV-2, 3, 9, 11	P7-A, 75, A2-A, 380	9
Fowl adenovirus E	FAdV-6, 7, 8a, 8b	CR119, YR36, TR59, 764	
Goose adenovirus	GoAdV-1–3		
Duck adenovirus B (ts)	DAdV-2		
Pigeon adenovirus (ts)	PiAdV-1		
Turkey adenovirus B (ts)	TAdV-1, 2		
Psittacine adenovirus?	Psittacine adenovirus 1		
Falcon adenovirus?	Falcon adenovirus 1		
Atadenovirus			
Bovine adenovirus D	BAdV-4, 5, 8, strain Rus		4
Duck adenovirus A	DAdV-1		G
Ovine adenovirus D	GAdV-1, OAdV-7		7
Possum adenovirus	PoAdV-1		
Bearded dragon adenovirus (ts)	BDAdV-1		
Bovine adenovirus E (ts)	BAdV-6		
Bovine adenovirus F (ts)	BAdV-7		
Cervine adenovirus (ts)	Odocoileus adenovirus 1 (OdAdV-1)		
Chameleon adenovirus (ts)	ChAdV-1		
Gecko adenovirus (ts)	GeAdV-1	Fat-tailed gecko	
Snake adenovirus (ts)	SnAdV-1	Corn snake, python	G
Gekkonid adenovirus(?)	Tokay gecko adenovirus		
Helodermatid adenovirus(?)	Gila monster adenovirus		
Scincid adenovirus(?)	Blue-tongued skink adenovirus		
Genus Siadenovirus			
Frog adenovirus	FrAdV-1		G
Turkey adenovirus A	TAdV-3		G
?	Raptor adenovirus 1	Harris hawk	

Continued

Table 1   Continued

Genus/species	Serotype	Strain	Genome
Unassigned Viruses in the Family			
?	White sturgeon adenovirus 1 (WSAdV-1)		
?	Crocodile adenovirus		

[a]Official genus and species names as published in the Eighth Report of the ICTV are in italics, and tentative species (ts), proposed species (marked by a query) or single isolates are not. Because of confusion in the serotype numbering in some cases (e.g. among fowl adenoviruses), certain characteristic strains are shown for easier identification. Available full genome sequences are noted by G or by the number of the sequenced serotype(s) if those listed are not all available.

8–10 nm in diameter, and 12 vertex capsomers (pentons), each with a protruding fiber 9–77.5 nm in length. The members of genus *Aviadenovirus* that have been studied have two fiber proteins per vertex. Fowl adenovirus 1 (FAdV-1) even has two, tandem fiber genes of different lengths, resulting in two fibers of different sizes at each vertex. Members of species *Human adenovirus F* (and HAdV-52 and the related monkey viruses) also have two fiber genes of different lengths, but the fibers are distributed in single copies alternately on the vertices. The main capsomers (hexons) are formed by the interaction of three identical polypeptides (designated hexon, and also as polypeptide II, after a Roman numeral system based on the relative mobilities of structural proteins under reducing conditions in sodium dodecyl sulfate-polyacrylamide gel electrophoresis). Each hexon has two characteristic parts: a triangular top with three 'towers', and a pseudohexagonal base with a central cavity. Hexons, or more exactly their bases, are packed tightly to form a protein shell that protects the inner components of the virion.

In members of the genus *Mastadenovirus* 12 copies of polypeptide IX are found between the nine hexons in the center of each facet. However, polypeptide IX is not present in the members of any other genus. Two monomers of polypeptide IIIa penetrate the hexon shell at the edge of each facet, and multiple copies of polypeptide VI form a ring underneath the peripentonal hexons. Penton bases are formed at the vertices by the interaction of five copies of polypeptide III, and are tightly associated with one (or, in the aviadenoviruses, two) fibers, each consisting of three copies of polypeptide IV in the form of a shaft of characteristic length with a distal knob. Polypeptide VIII is situated at the inner surface of the hexon shell. Polypeptides VI and VIII appear to link the capsid to the virion core, which consists of a single copy of the DNA genome complexed with four polypeptides (V, VII, X, TP). Polypeptide V exists only in mastadenoviruses.

Adenoviruses are stable on storage in the frozen state. They are stable to mild acid and insensitive to lipid solvents. Heat sensitivity varies among the genera.

Nucleic Acid, Genome Organization, and Replication

The adenovirus genome is a linear molecule of double-stranded DNA (26 163–45 063 bp) containing an inverted terminal repeat (ITR) of 36–368 bp at its termini, with the 5′ ends of the genome linked covalently to a terminal protein (TP). The nucleotide composition is 33.7–63.8% G+C. The genetic organization of the central part of the genome is conserved throughout the family, whereas the terminal parts show large variations in length and gene content (**Figure 1**). Splicing was first discovered in adenoviruses, and is a common means of expressing mRNAs in this virus family. In the conserved region, most late genes are expressed by splicing from the rightward-oriented major late promoter located in the pol gene. The early genes encoding pol, the precursor of TP (pTP), and the DNA-binding protein (DBP) are spliced from leftward-oriented promoters. Where it has been examined, splicing is also a common feature of genes in the nonconserved regions.

Replication of various human adenoviruses has been studied in detail, in particular with HAdV-2. Virus entry takes place via interactions of the fiber knob with specific receptors on the surface of a susceptible cell followed by internalization via interactions between the penton base and cellular α_v integrins. After uncoating, the virus core is delivered to the nucleus, which is the site of virus transcription, DNA replication, and assembly. Virus infection mediates the shutdown of host DNA synthesis and later RNA and protein synthesis. Transcription of the adenovirus genome by host RNA polymerase II involves both DNA strands of the genome and initiates (in HAdV-2) from five early (E1A, E1B, E2, E3, and E4), two intermediate, and the major late (L) promoter. All primary transcripts are capped and polyadenylated, with complex splicing patterns producing families of mRNAs. In primate adenoviruses, one or two VA RNA genes are usually present upstream from the main pTP coding region. These are transcribed by cellular RNA polymerase III and facilitate translation of late mRNAs and blocking of the cellular interferon response. Corresponding VA RNA genes have not been identified in nonprimate adenoviruses, although a nonhomologous VA

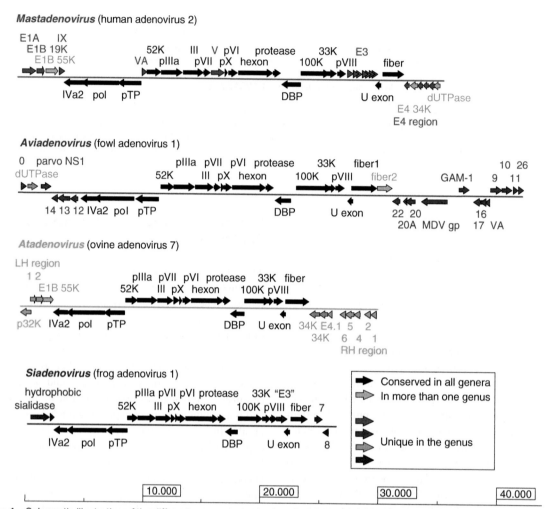

Figure 1 Schematic illustration of the different genome organizations found in representative members of the four adenovirus genera. Black arrows depict genes conserved in every genus, gray arrows show genes present in more than one genus, and colored arrows show genus-specific genes. Reprinted from Benkö M, Harrach B, Both GW, *et al.* (2005) Family *Adenoviridae* In: Fauquet CM, Mayo MA, Maniloff J, Desselberger U, and Ball LA (eds.) *Virus Taxonomy: Eighth Report of the International Committee on Taxonomy of Viruses*, pp. 213–228. San Diego, CA: Elsevier Academic Press, with permission from Elsevier.

RNA gene has been mapped in some aviadenoviruses near the right end of the genome. More generally, the replication of aviadenoviruses has been shown to involve significantly different pathways from those characterized in human adenoviruses. This is not unexpected, given the considerable differences in gene layout between nonconserved regions of the genome.

Proteins

About 40 different polypeptides (the largest number being in fowl adenoviruses and the smallest in siadenoviruses) are produced. Almost a third of these compose the virion, including a virus-encoded cysteine protease, which processes a number of precursor proteins (these are prefixed with p). With the exception of polypeptides V and IX, the other structural proteins are conserved in every genus. Products of the four early regions of mastadenoviruses modulate the host cell's transcriptional machinery (E1 and E4), assemble the virus DNA replication complex (E2), and subvert host defense mechanisms (E3). The E2 region (encoding DBP, pol, and pTP) is well conserved throughout the family, while the E3 and E4 regions show great variation in length and gene content among the mastadenoviruses. E1A, E1B 19K, and the E3 and E4 regions (with the exception of 34K) occur only in mastadenoviruses. Genes encoding proteins related to 34K are also present in atadenoviruses, sometimes in duplicate. Intermediate (IX, only in mastadenoviruses, and IVa2) and late gene products (in some mastadenoviruses expressed from five transcription units, L1–L5) are concerned with assembly and maturation of the virion. Late proteins include: 52K (scaffolding protein) and pIIIa (L1); III (penton base), pVII (major core protein), V (minor core protein, only in mastadenoviruses) and pX (L2); pVI, hexon (II) and protease (L3); 100K, 33K (and an unspliced version, 22K) and pVIII (L4); and fiber (IV) (L5). Seemingly, there are no lipids in adenovirus particles. However, the fiber proteins and some of the nonstructural proteins are glycosylated.

Antigenic Properties

Adenovirus serotypes are differentiated on the basis of neutralization assays. A serotype is defined as either exhibiting no cross-reaction with others or showing a homologous/heterologous titer ratio of greater than 16 (in both directions). For homologous/heterologous titer ratios of 8 or 16, a serotype assignment is made either if the viral hemagglutinins are unrelated (as shown by lack of cross-reaction in hemagglutination-inhibition tests), or if substantial biophysical, biochemical, or phylogenetic differences exist. Antigens at the surface of the virion are mainly type specific. Hexons are involved in neutralization, and fibers in neutralization and hemagglutination inhibition. Soluble antigens associated with virus infection include surplus capsid proteins that have not been assembled. The genus-specific antigen is located on the basal surface of the hexon, whereas serotype-specific antigens are located mainly on the tower region. Practical problems may arise during serotyping (and in phylogenetic calculations) from the occasional occurrence of homologous recombination in the hexon gene (e.g., HAdV-16 and SAdV-23). Under natural circumstances, recombination occurs only between members of the same species.

Biological Properties

The natural host range of adenovirus types is usually confined to one animal species or to closely related species. This also applies for cell cultures. Some human adenoviruses (mainly in species *Human adenovirus C*) cause productive infection in various animal (rodent or ruminant) cells. Several viruses cause tumors in newborn rodents. Subclinical infections are frequent in various virus–host systems. Transmission occurs from the throat, feces, the eye, or urine, depending on the virus serotype. Certain human adenovirus types (given in parentheses below) are predominantly associated with a specific pathology, such as adenoidal–pharyngeal conjunctivitis (3, 4, 7, and 14), acute respiratory outbreaks (4, 7, 14, and 21), epidemic kerato-conjunctivitis (8, 19, and 37), or venereal disease (3). HAdV-40 and HAdV-41 can be isolated from the feces of young children with acute gastroenteritis, and only the rotaviruses are known to cause more cases of infantile viral diarrhea. HAdV-11 is associated with hemorrhagic cystitis (mostly in immuno-suppressed patients after organ transplantation). The newer types of human adenovirus (42–51) were isolated from acquired immune deficiency syndrome patients. In mammals, mastadenovirus infection is common, but disease is usually manifested only if predisposing factors (such as management problems, crowding, shipping, or concurrent bacterial infections) are also present. Canine adenovirus, which can cause hepatitis or respiratory disease in dogs, seems to be an exception and has caused epizootics in foxes, bears, wolves, coyotes, and skunks.

Certain siadenoviruses and atadenoviruses that may have undergone host switches during their evolution seem to be more pathogenic in general in their new hosts: birds, ruminants, and a marsupial. Egg drop syndrome virus (duck adenovirus 1, DAdV-1) or turkey hemorrhagic enteritis virus (turkey adenovirus 3, TAdV-3) can cause serious economical losses for the poultry industry. An atadenovirus (Odocoileus adenovirus) caused a hemorrhagic epizooty and killed thousands of mule deers in California.

Adenoviruses infecting susceptible cells cause similar cytopathology consisting of early rounding of cells, aggregation or lysis of chromatin, followed by the later appearance of characteristic eosinophilic or basophilic nuclear inclusions.

HAdV-5 has been engineered and used extensively as a gene delivery vector. Other human adenoviruses such as HAdV-35, or even nonhuman serotypes (ovine adenovirus 7 and canine adenovirus 1), are being tested as a means of overcoming the problem posed by preexisting neutralizing antibodies in the human population, and also to achieve targeting to specific organs and tissues. Bovine, porcine, canine, and fowl adenovirus types have also been tested as novel antigen delivery vectors for immunizing the cognate animal species.

Mastadenoviruses

Mastadenoviruses occur only in mammals, and in general, mammals are host to only mastadenoviruses. However, half of the adenoviruses found in ruminant species are atadenoviruses and the only marsupial adenovirus identified so far is also an atadenovirus. Mastadenoviruses were originally distinguished from aviadenoviruses on the basis of different genus-specific complement-fixing antigens. Virus infectivity is inactivated by heating at 56 °C for more than 10 min.

The mastadenovirus genomes that have been sequenced range in size between 30 288 bp and 37 741 bp, and in nucleotide composition from 40.8% to 63.8% G+C. The ITR is considerably longer (93–368 bp) and more complex (containing a variety of cellular factor-binding sites) than in members of the other genera. Proteins encoded only by the mastadenoviruses are polypeptides V and IX, and most of those from the E1A, E1B, E3, and E4 regions. Polypeptide IX, besides cementing the hexons on the outer surface of the capsid, has been demonstrated to act as a transcriptional activator, and also takes part in nuclear reorganization during infection. Polypeptide V is a core protein that, in association with cellular protein p32, seems to be involved in the transport of viral DNA into the nucleus of the infected cell. The E3 and E4 regions can differ markedly even among different mastadenovirus species. The E3 region is considerably shorter and simpler in nonprimate adenoviruses than in monkey, ape, and human adenoviruses. The simplest layout is found in murine adenovirus 1, where it consists of a single 12.5K gene. In the E4 region, only the 34K gene seems to be conserved in all mastadenoviruses. This gene is duplicated in bovine adenovirus 3 and porcine adenovirus 5.

The entry processes of human mastadenoviruses into the cell are well characterized. The coxsackievirus and adenovirus receptor (CAR) is the most common, but not the only, receptor for the attachment to the cell.

Aviadenoviruses

Members of the genus *Aviadenovirus* occur only in birds and possess a common genus-specific complement-fixing antigen. However, birds can also harbor siadenoviruses and atadenoviruses. Aviadenovirus virions contain two fibers per vertex. Fowl adenovirus 1 (FAdV-1) has two fiber genes, and two projections of considerably different lengths from each penton base. Other fowl adenoviruses also have two fibers per vertex, but apparently only one fiber gene, and the projections are therefore of similar lengths. For attachment of FAdV-1 to the cell, the long, but not the short, fiber utilizes CAR. The aviadenovirus genomes are considerably larger (20–45%) than those of mastadenoviruses. FAdV-1 and FAdV-9, with genomes of 43 804 and 45 063 bp, respectively, represent the longest adenovirus DNA molecules known to date. The nucleotide composition of the partial or full genome sequences characterized so far is between 53.8% and 59% G+C. The length of the ITR is 51–72 bp.

The genes encoding polypeptides V and IX are absent from aviadenovirus genomes, as well as the genes in the mastadenovirus E1 and E3 regions (**Figure 1**). A dUTP pyrophosphatase (dUTPase) gene is situated next to the left end of the genome in the aviadenoviruses studied to date; a dUTPase gene is also present in some mastadenoviruses, but it is at the right genome end. The right end of aviadenovirus genomes contains a large number of transcription units that are confined to this genus. The majority of genes and proteins from this region have not yet been characterized in detail. The GAM-1 protein of FAdV-1 has been demonstrated to have an anti-apoptotic effect, and to activate the heat-shock response in the infected cell. GAM-1, in synergy with the protein encoded by ORF22, binds the retinoblastoma protein and can activate the E2F pathway. Some as yet uncharacterized aviadenovirus gene products are similar to proteins of other viruses, such as the nonstructural protein NS1 (Rep protein) of parvoviruses, or triacylglycerol lipase, a homolog of which occurs in an avian herpesvirus (Marek's disease virus).

Aviadenoviruses have been isolated from various poultry species including turkey, goose, and Muscovy duck, as well as a number of wild birds, such as falcon and parrots. However, chicken adenoviruses have been studied in most detail. Twelve fowl adenovirus serotypes have been classified into species *Fowl adenovirus A* to *Fowl adenovirus E* (FAdV-A to FAdV-E). Unfortunately, the type numbering of fowl adenoviruses became inconsistent when different systems were adopted in Europe and North America. The resulting confusion was partially resolved by the introduction of FAdV-8a and FAdV-8b types, though their distinctness could not be fully confirmed because of the ambiguous results of serum neutralization tests.

Avian adenoviruses have been associated with diverse disease patterns, including body hepatitis, bronchitis, pulmonary congestion, edema, and gizzard erosion in various bird species, but they generally seem to be less pathogenic than siadenoviruses and atadenoviruses in birds. An exception to this is FAdV-4, the causative agent of hydro-pericardium syndrome in chickens, which causes considerable losses mainly in Asia. FAdV-1 (chick embryo lethal orphan virus), FAdV-9, and FAdV-10 are studied extensively for their potential feasibility as gene delivery vectors.

Atadenoviruses

As opposed to the mastadenoviruses and aviadenoviruses, which have clear host origins, the members of genus *Atadenovirus* represent a much broader host range spanning several vertebrate classes. This genus was originally established to cope with the classification of certain exceptional bovine and ovine adenoviruses with unusual characteristics. The name refers to the nucleotide composition of the first members of this genus, which is biased toward high A+T content. The large phylogenetic distance between the ruminant atadenoviruses and the mastadenoviruses and aviadenoviruses (**Figure 2**) inspired a hypothesis that they may have originated via tranfers of adenoviruses with lower vertebrate hosts. Indeed, recent studies have confirmed that every reptilian adenovirus for which data are available belongs to this genus. However, atadenoviruses found in reptiles seem to have a balanced nucleotide content. Additional atadenovirus types have been detected in various species of birds and mammals, including duck, domestic and wild ruminants, as well as a marsupial, the brushtail possum. DAdV-1, which was originally isolated from flocks of laying hens that showed a sharp decrease in egg production, was moved to the genus *Atadenovirus* from the genus *Aviadenovirus*.

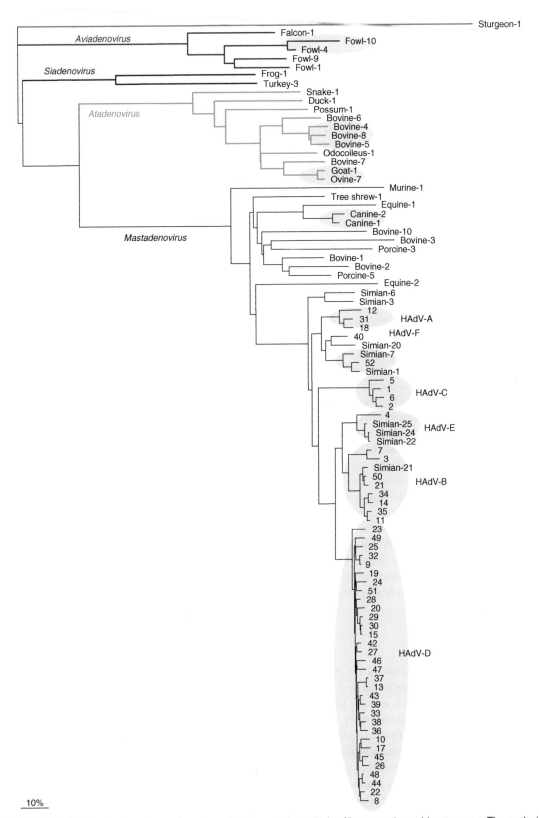

Figure 2 Phylogenetic tree of adenoviruses based on distance matrix analysis of hexon amino acid sequences. The analysis was performed using the Protdist and Fitch programs of the PHYLIP 3.65 package. The unrooted tree was visualized with white sturgeon adenovirus as the outgroup. Adenoviruses are denoted by the name of the host and the serotype number, or only by the serotype number for human adenoviruses. Viruses that belong to the same species are grouped by light-blue ovals, and human adenovirus species are indicated by their informal abbreviations. Data for HAdV-16, HAdV-41, and SAdV-23 were excluded, as evolution of their hexon genes may have involved homologous recombination events. The bar indicates 10% difference between two neighboring sequences.

The virions of bovine atadenoviruses are more heat stable than those of mastadenoviruses. They retain substantial infectivity after treatment for 30 min at 56 °C.

The size of sequenced atadenovirus genomes ranges from 27 751 bp (snake adenovirus 1, SnAdV-1) to 33 213 bp (DAdV-1) with an ITR of 46 (OAdV-7) to 118 bp (SnAdV-1). For ruminant, marsupial, and avian atadenoviruses, the nucleotide composition ranges between 33.7% (OAdV-7) and 43% G+C (DAdV-1).

The common ancestry of the atadenoviruses is supported by their shared genomic organization. Putative early regions (LH and RH) on the genome ends occupy the places of the mastadenovirus E1 and E4 regions (**Figure 1**). The functions of the novel genes in these regions have been elucidated only partially. The LH region includes a gene encoding a novel structural protein (p32K), and genes LH1 (not present in DAdV-1), LH2, and LH3. LH3 seems to be weakly related to the E1B 55K gene of mastadenoviruses, and its product has also been shown to be a structural protein. In the RH region, E4.3 and E4.2 seem to be homologs of the E4 34K gene of mastadenoviruses. E4.1 is absent from DAdV-1. Closer to the right end, different numbers of RH genes are found in different viruses. Many genes seem to be the result of duplication events, with one family encoding putative F-box proteins. There is only one copy of an F-box gene in SnAdV−1, whereas five are present in ovine adenovirus 4. Surprisingly, SnAdV−1 also encodes a protein that is homologous to the gene 105R product found in tree shrew adenovirus, a mastadenovirus. The DAdV-1 genome has an extension at the right end containing seven additional genes, which are so far unique to this virus. These genes are likely to be host specific in their function. This region of the DAdV-1 genome also encodes a VA RNA gene that is seemingly homologous to that of FAdV-1. In atadenoviruses, no immuno-modulatory genes such as those in the mastadenovirus E3 region have yet been identified, though it is likely that they exist.

Siadenoviruses

The fourth genus has been established for two adenoviruses that are of very distant host origin and yet share a similar genome organization and are phylogenetically closely related. These are frog adenovirus 1 (FrAdV-1), which was isolated from the renal tumor of a leopard frog, and TAdV-3, which was isolated from birds. Additional strains of TAdV-3, originating from turkey, pheasant and chicken, as well as avirulent (vaccine) strains, show little or no diversity in terms of nucleotide sequence or serology, respectively. The genomes of FrAdV-1 and TAdV-3 are collinear and represent the minimal gene content recognized among adenoviruses to date (**Figure 1**). In addition to the set of genes occupying the central genome region and conserved throughout the whole family, only five additional genes have been identified. The protein encoded next to the left ITR seems to be related to bacterial sialidases. Adjacent to this is a gene predicted to code for a highly hydrophobic protein. The E3 gene takes this name solely because of its position between the pVIII and fiber genes; it is not homologous to any of the mastadenovirus E3 genes, or to any other known genes. Similarly, ORF7 and ORF8, which are situated at the right end of the genome, have no recognizable homologs elsewhere. The genes encoding polypeptides V and IX are absent, as well as those in the mastadenovirus E1, E3 and E4 regions. FrAdV-1 and TAdV-3 have the shortest adenovirus genomes, 26 163 and 26 263 bp in size, respectively, with ITRs of 36 and 39 bp and nucleotide compositions of 38% and 35% G+C.

The evolutionary history of siadenoviruses awaits elucidation. In the same way that it is possible that atadenoviruses originated with reptiles (see above), the siadenoviruses may represent adenoviruses that have co-evolved with amphibians, with TAdV-3 the result of an interclass host switch.

FrAdV-1 is supposedly nonpathogenic, whereas TAdV-3 is associated with serious diseases in various hosts, including hemorrhagic enteritis in turkeys, marble spleen disease in pheasants, and splenomegaly in chickens. Recently, a putative novel siadenovirus has been detected in fatally diseased birds of prey.

Phylogeny

The five clusters of adenoviruses defined by gene organization and sequence-based phylogenetic calculations correspond to the four recognized genera (*Mastadenovirus, Aviadenovirus, Atadenovirus,* and *Siadenovirus*) plus one proposed genus for fish adenoviruses (**Figure 2**). The evolutionary distances among the adenoviruses seem to be generally proportional to those among their hosts, supporting co-evolution of virus and host. However, there are some exceptions where very distantly related viruses infect the same host, for example, the bovine mastadenoviruses and atadenoviruses. Thus, in addition to co-evolution, several host switches might have occurred. According to this hypothesis, the mastadenoviruses and aviadenoviruses represent co-evolution, whereas reptilian adenoviruses may have switched to ruminants, birds, and marsupials. Indeed, genome organization and phylogenetic analysis indicate that SnAdV-1 most closely represents the most ancient common ancestor of the atadenoviruses. Siadenoviruses may have an amphibian origin, though the small number of viruses in this group limits analyses of this possibility. More recent host switches can also be identified within genera, for example between humans and other primates, or vice versa.

See also: Adenoviruses: Malignant Transformation and Oncology; Adenoviruses: Pathogenesis.

Further Reading

Benkö M, Harrach B, Both GW, et al. (2005) Family *Adenoviridae*. In: Fauquet CM, Mayo MA, Maniloff J, Desselberger U, and Ball LA (eds.) *Virus Taxonomy: Eighth Report of the International Committee on Taxonomy of Viruses*, pp. 213–228. San Diego, CA: Elsevier Academic Press.

Burnett RM (1997) The structure of adenovirus. In: Chiu W, Burnett RM, and Garcea RL (eds.) *Structural Biology of Viruses*, pp. 209–238. Oxford: Oxford University Press.

Davison AJ, Benkö M, and Harrach B (2003) Genetic content and evolution of adenoviruses. *Journal of General Virology* 84: 2895–2908.

Doerfler W and Böhm P (eds.) (2003) Adenoviruses: Model and vectors in virus host interactions. In: *Current Topics of Microbiology and Immunology*, vol. 272. Berlin: Springer.

Farkas SL, Benkö M, Élö P, et al. (2002) Genomic and phylogenetic analyses of an adenovirus isolated from a corn snake (*Flaphe guttata*) imply common origin with the members of the proposed new genus *Atadenovirus*. *Journal of General Virology* 83: 2403–2410.

Kovács GM, LaPatra SE, D'Halluin JC, and Benkö M (2003) Phylogenetic analysis of the hexon and protease genes of a fish adenovirus isolated from white sturgeon (*Acipenser transmontanus*) supports the proposal for a new adenovirus genus. *Virus Research* 98: 27–34.

Russell WC (2000) Update on adenovirus and its vectors. *Journal of General Virology* 81: 2573–2604.

Wold WSM and Tollefson A (eds.) (2006) Methods in molecular medicine. In: *Adenovirus Methods and Protocols*, 2nd edn., vol. 131, pp. 299–334. Totowa, NJ: Humana Press.

Zsivanovits P, Monks DJ, Forbes NA, et al. (2006) Presumptive identification of a novel adenovirus in a Harris hawk (*Parabuteo unicinctus*), a Bengal eagle owl (*Bubo bengalensis*), and a Verreaux's eagle owl (*Bubo lacteus*). *Journal of Avian Medicine and Surgery* 20: 105–112.

Adenoviruses: Pathogenesis

M Benkő, Veterinary Medical Research Institute, Hungarian Academy of Sciences, Budapest, Hungary

History

Adenoviruses were first recognized as distinct agents in 1953, although certain disease conditions that were later clarified as being caused by adenoviruses had been described previously in humans as well as in animals. These include epidemic keratoconjunctivitis, the viral etiology of which had been suggested as early as 1930. It had also been recognized before the discovery of adenoviruses that the so-called fox encephalitis and dog hepatitis were caused by the same virus. Also, the first avian adenovirus (chicken embryo lethal orphan (CELO) virus) isolate had erroneously been obtained when bovine samples of lumpy skin disease were examined for an infectious etiological agent by inoculation into embryonated eggs.

The actual discovery of human adenoviruses was the result of targeted investigations into the etiology of an acute, respiratory illness frequently affecting young military recruits in the USA. The first isolates (those assigned low type numbers) were obtained either from diseased soldiers or from adenoid tissues removed by tonsillectomy (hence the name adenovirus). Morphologically indistinguishable viruses were classified as new serotypes on the basis of the results of cross-neutralization tests. The number of human adenovirus serotypes grew rapidly during the 1960s and 1970s. There are 51 human adenovirus serotypes known to date, and an additional candidate has been discovered recently. Nonhuman animal adenoviruses were initially described largely in domesticated species of economic importance. Although a considerable number of new human or animal adenoviruses were isolated from diseased individuals, many were recovered from primary tissue cultures, such as simian adenoviruses from Vero cells and bovine adenoviruses from calf kidney or testicle cell cultures.

The striking diversity of human adenoviruses was recognized early on, and various biological properties, most of which have obvious influences on pathogenicity, were used to establish a basis for subclassification (**Table 1**). The criteria used for grouping human adenoviruses included differences in hemagglutination properties, nucleotide composition of the genomic DNA (i.e., G+C content), and oncogenicity *in vivo* and *in vitro* (the latter indicated by malignant transformation in tissue culture). Four hemagglutination groups (I–IV) and six human adenovirus subgroups (A–F) were established. In the most recent taxonomy, the latter groups, which were often referred to as subgroups or subgenera, are now correctly termed species *Human adenovirus A* (abbreviated informally to HAdV-A) through *Human adenovirus F* (HAdV-F). Phylogenetic analyses of nucleotide and protein sequences and characteristic features of genome organization fully support this classification. Each species consists of a collection of serotypes; for example, human adenovirus 12 (HAdV-12) is a member of species HAdV-A. Species are also being erected for animal adenoviruses in a similar manner.

Table 1 Features of human adenoviruses

Species Serotype	Hemagglutination group	Tumors in animals	Transformation in tissue culture	G+C content in DNA[a]	Associated disease and affected organs
Human adenovirus A HAdV-12, 18, 31	IV (no or weak hemagglutination)	High	Positive	45–47 (48–49)	Cryptic enteric infection
Human adenovirus B HAdV-3, 7, 11, 14, 16, 21, 34, 35, 50	I (complete agglutination of monkey erythrocytes)	Moderate	Positive	48–52 (50–52)	Conjunctivitis Acute respiratory disease Hemorrhagic cystitis Central nervous system
Human adenovirus C HAdV-1, 2, 5, 6	III (partial agglutination of rat erythrocytes)	Low or negative	Positive	55–56 (57–59)	Endemic infection Respiratory symptoms
Human adenovirus D HAdV-8–10, 13, 15, 17, 19, 20, 22–30, 32, 33, 36–39, 42–49, 51	II (complete agglutination of rat erythrocytes)	Low or negative (mammary tumors)	Positive	48–57 (57–61)	Keratoconjunctivitis In immunocompromised and AIDS patients
Human adenovirus E HAdV-4	III	Low or negative	Positive	57 (57–59)	Conjunctivitis Acute respiratory disease
Human adenovirus F HAdV-40, 41	IV	Negative	Negative	51	Infantile diarrhea

[a]Values are based on complete genome sequences. Estimates made previously using other methods are shown in parentheses.

Prevalence and Spread

Adenoviruses are abundant and widespread, and in principle every vertebrate species could host at least one species. Endemic or enzootic infections that are frequently inapparent seem to be very common. In contrast, epidemic or epizootic occurrence is relatively rare and normally has much more significant consequences. The nonenveloped virions shed by infected individuals are rather stable in the environment and can survive for long periods. Virions are not only able to tolerate adverse environmental effects, such as drought and moderate temperature or pH changes, but are also resistant to lipid solvents and simple disinfectants. There is evidence that human adenoviruses can persist and perhaps even retain infectivity in natural or communal water sources. Moreover, freshwater and marine bivalves have also been found to accumulate adenoviruses. Because of their stability, adenoviruses have become a major indicator of viral pollution in the environment. Vertical transmission has also been documented in several host species, including birds and cattle.

Although different species or types of adenovirus have different affinities for various organs and tissues, primary virus shedding is likely through the intestines. Adenoviruses are often transmitted by person-to-person contact, particularly among young children where fecal–oral spread is common. Aerosol transmission is also possible and is probably not rare in crowded populations. Adenovirus DNA may be found in tonsillar tissue, peripheral blood lymphocytes, and lung epithelial cells long after clinical disease has abated. Swimming pool-related outbreaks, particularly of strains causing keratoconjunctivitis or pharyngitis, are not uncommon. In poultry and other farm animals, transportation, crowding, and mixing of different populations can lead to mass infections.

Epidemiology

The tropism and pathogenicity of human adenoviruses are largely type- and species-dependent. Respiratory pathogens are common, although infections of a large variety of different organs have been described. The fiber protein is likely to mediate primary tissue tropism, but the specific determinants, epitopes, and receptors have been mapped only preliminarily. The most common clinical manifestations connected to each human adenovirus species are listed below (also see **Table 1**). HAdV-B contains two phylogenetic lineages, which are informally termed subspecies HAdV-B1 and HAdV-B2.

HAdV-A

HAdV-12, HAdV-18, and HAdV-31 can replicate efficiently in the intestines, and, based on serological surveys, are common in the population, especially in children with gastrointestinal disease. However, their role in the etiology of infant diarrhea is yet to be determined. Serotypes belonging to this species are generally difficult to isolate and culture.

HAdV-B1

Respiratory pathogens HAdV-3, HAdV-7, HAdV-16, and HAdV-21 belong here. Seasonal outbreaks of febrile respiratory diseases, mainly during winter, can be caused in infants by HAdV-7 in most parts of the world. Similar diseases, usually with a less severe outcome, can be seen among school children. In some countries, HAdV-3 is the dominant serotype, whereas HAdV-7 seems to have a number of different genotypes that shift occasionally in certain geographic areas. HAdV-4 (from species HAdV-E) and HAdV-14 (from subspecies HAdV-B2) are most often implicated in the etiology of acute respiratory outbreaks among freshly enlisted military recruits in the USA, in addition to HAdV-7 and HAdV-21.

HAdV-B2

HAdV-11, HAdV-34, and HAdV-35 cause persistent interstitial infection in the kidney and hemorrhagic cystitis. These, along with one of the most recently described human adenoviruses (HAdV-50), are most often shed in the feces or urine of acquired immune deficiency syndrome (AIDS) patients and organ or tissue transplantation recipients. Severe respiratory infections caused by a novel variant of HAdV-14 with seemingly elevated pathogenicity have emerged in the USA during 2006 and 2007.

HAdV-C

The low serotype designations (HAdV-1, HAdV-2, HAdV-5, and HAdV-6) of viruses in this group reflect the relative ubiquity of the species. They can easily be isolated and, indeed, comprise approximately half of all human adenovirus serotypes reported to the World Health Organization. HAdV-1, HAdV-2, and HAdV-5 are known to maintain endemic infections, and most teenagers will have had infections with more than one serotype. The site of persistence is lymphoid tissue, and shedding can last for a couple of years after primary infection.

HAdV-D

This species contains 32 serotypes and therefore encompasses well over one half of all known human adenoviruses. HAdV-8, HAdV-19, and HAdV-37 cause epidemic keratoconjunctivitis, especially in dry climates or densely populated areas. Other serotypes are rarely isolated except from immunocompromised patients.

HAdV-E

This is the only species that has a single serotype, namely HAdV-4, although different genotypes of this virus have been described. HAdV-4 strains have been most often implicated in respiratory diseases among military recruits in the USA. In Japan, HAdV-4 is the second most important cause of adenovirus-associated eye disease after HAdV-8.

HAdV-F

The so-called enteric or fastidious HAdV-40 and HAdV-41 are classified here. The genetic distance between these two serotypes comes close to meriting separation into different species, but, for practical reasons including indistinguishable pathology, they remain in a single species.

These viruses are a major cause of infantile diarrhea all over the world. In Europe, a shift in dominance from HAdV-40 in the 1970s to HAdV-41 after 1992 has been observed. Because of a deletion in the E1 region near the left end of the genome, HAdV-40 and HAdV-41 can be isolated and cultured only in complementing, transformed cell lines such as 293 or A547. The most recently described human adenovirus serotype, namely HAdV-52, was also recovered from patients with diarrhea. HAdV-52 has not yet been classified into a species.

Epizootiology

Simian Adenoviruses

A series of simian viruses (termed SVs) were isolated from various tissue cultures prepared from apes and monkeys. These were numbered serially, irrespective of the virus family to which they belong, since identification and allocation to a family were performed later. A considerable number of the SV isolates have been identified as adenoviruses. In many cases, unfortunately, the original SV numbers have been retained as the numbers of the adenovirus type, and thus a somewhat confusing system of SAdV numbering can still be encountered in publications as well as in the records of the American Type Culture Collection. To date, there are 25 simian adenoviruses (SAdV-1 through SAdV-25). SAdV-1 to SAdV-20 originate from Old World monkeys, whereas SAdV-21 to SAdV-25 are from chimpanzees. There are no known examples of New World monkey adenoviruses, though it is likely that they exist.

There are few data concerning prevalence or pathogenicity of simian adenoviruses in their natural hosts. An interesting mixing and grouping can be observed among the primate adenoviruses, suggesting that they can sometimes be less host specific, apparently readily infecting closely related hosts.

Canine Adenoviruses

Only two serotypes of adenovirus have been isolated from carnivores, both termed canine adenoviruses. CAdV-1 is the causative agent of infectious canine hepatitis, a life-threatening disease of puppies. Regular vaccination worldwide has decreased the number of clinical cases. Serologically indistinguishable viruses have been shown to cause encephalitis in numerous other carnivore species such as foxes, raccoons, bears, and skunks. The disease caused by a genetically closely related but serologically distinct virus, CAdV-2, is called kennel cough and is common among breeder stocks.

Interestingly, in spite of a limited number of inclusion-body-hepatitis-like conditions in felids, focused attempts to find a distinct feline adenovirus remain unsuccessful. It is likely, however, that cats living in close proximity with humans can harbor HAdV-1 or HAdV-5 from species HAdV-C.

Porcine Adenoviruses

At least five porcine adenovirus types (PAdV-1 to PAdV-5) are recognized. These represent three different species. Species PAdV-A contains three serotypes (PAdV-1 to PAdV-3) that are fairly similar to each other and cause no specific diseases. PAdV-4 (in species PAdV-B) has been described as associated with neurological disease, and PAdV-5 (in species PAdV-C) is most distantly related to PAdV-A. The pathogenic roles of porcine adenoviruses need further investigation.

Equine Adenoviruses

Two equine adenovirus serotypes (EAdV-1 and EAdV-2) were described several decades ago, but their genetic characterization has lagged behind that of other adenoviruses. Only very short, partial sequences from the hexon gene are available, and apparently these contain poorly resolved areas that will need thorough revisiting. Certain Arabian horse lineages carry a genetic defect that, when present in the homozygous state, causes severe combined immunodeficiency disease. Affected animals are incapable of mounting an immune response, and foals usually die of pneumonia due to equine adenovirus, which is harmless in immunocompetent animals.

Bovine, Ovine, Caprine, and Other Ruminant Adenoviruses

There is an amazing diversity of adenoviruses that can infect ruminant hosts. The adenoviruses described above all belong to various species in genus *Mastadenovirus*, as do a number of ruminant adenoviruses. Unusual bovine adenoviruses that are substantially different from mastadenoviruses, as judged for example by the absence of the genus-specific antigen, were described almost four decades ago. Out of the roughly one dozen bovine adenovirus serotypes (in the BAdV series) recognized to date, six are now classified in a separate genus, *Atadenovirus*. One ovine (OAdV-7) and one goat (GAdV-1) adenovirus are also classified as atadenoviruses.

Bovine mastadenoviruses were recognized early on, and were found occasionally to cause enzootic broncho-pneumonia or calf pneumo-enteritis. Oddly enough,

experimental infection of young calves with the isolated adenoviruses seldom, if at all, resulted in convincing reproduction of disease. BAdV-10 is one of the most interesting ruminant mastadenoviruses in that all five isolates originated from diseased or dead animals. Genomic analysis of these isolates, one from New Zealand and four from Northern Ireland, revealed genetic variations in and around the fiber gene, suggesting that the virus might be undergoing some kind of adaptation process. Propagation of BAdV-10 strains has been difficult, with most success achieved on either primary testicle cells or a pulmonary alveolar cell line. It is noteworthy that BAdV-10 not only clusters together with mouse adenovirus (MAdV-1) on phylogenetic trees but also that it has a very simple E3 region. BAdV-10 has been proposed as an example of an adenovirus that may be in the process of switching from one host to another. Crossing the host barrier has also been suggested for BAdV-2, with two subtypes, one of which is capable of infecting calves and the other sheep. Based on evolutionary relationships, BAdV-2 is presently classified into species OAdV-A together with OAdV-2 to OAdV-5.

Bovine atadenoviruses have been found more often in the intestines, and disease reproduction was more frequently successful. Serological evidence is available for the occurrence of mastadenoviruses and atadenoviruses in a large number of free living and wild ruminant hosts. A novel atadenovirus was recently recovered from mule deer during an epizootic in California causing high mortality.

Avian Adenoviruses

Adenoviruses isolated from poultry and waterfowl were initially classified into genus *Aviadenovirus*. In addition to the criterion of host origin, aviadenoviruses can be distinguished from mastadenoviruses on the basis of a lack of the genus-common complement-fixing antigen. A large number of serotypes have been described from chicken. Some of these viruses have been isolated from other species as well. For example, strains serologically identical to CELO virus have also been found to cause bronchitis in quails. The pathologic roles of aviadenoviruses are not fully understood. The results of experimental infections have been ambiguous in the majority of cases. A specific condition referred to as hydro-pericardium syndrome has been clearly associated with fowl adenovirus 4 (FAdV-4) from species FAdV-C. Another specific disease called gizzard erosion, however, could not be linked to a definite aviadenovirus type, and experimental infections gave contradictory results.

Duck adenovirus 1 (DAdV-1) is the causative agent of egg drop syndrome (EDS), which results in depressed egg production accompanied by the production of abnormal (soft-shelled or deformed) eggs. The disease was first experienced in Europe in 1976, and soon became known worldwide. Retrospective serological studies confirmed the presence of hemagglutination inhibitory antibodies to EDS virus in archive sera originating from a large number of wild and domestic bird species, with a predominance in waterfowl, which are now considered as the main reservoir. The virus was initially assigned to genus *Aviadenovirus*, but was recorded as an exception because of its lack of common complement-fixing antigens with other fowl adenoviruses. Genome analysis of the EDS virus revealed its relatedness to atadenoviruses, and DAdV-1 has consequently been moved into this genus, which is hypothesized to be the adenovirus lineage of reptilian hosts.

Turkey adenovirus 3 (TAdV-3), better known as turkey hemorrhagic enteritis virus, shows cross-reactivity with neither aviadenoviruses nor DAdV-1, and used to be viewed as another exception among the aviadenoviruses. Serologically indistinguishable strains have been associated with various pathological entities in turkey, pheasant, and chicken. Based on genome analyses and phylogenetic calculations, TAdV-3 is a member of genus *Siadenovirus*, along with the single known adenovirus from an amphibian host, frog adenovirus 1 (FrAdV-1). This lineage has been tentatively proposed to represent adenoviruses that have coevolved with amphibians. Interestingly, a recently described sensitive polymerase chain reaction (PCR) method led to the detection of a novel type (and likely new species) of siadenovirus in diseased birds of prey. A novel avian adenovirus has also been isolated from falcons.

Reptilian Adenoviruses

Every adenovirus found in reptiles thus far is an atadenovirus. Adenovirus infections in various snake and lizard species have been described repeatedly, but the number of virus strains isolated is very limited. In Germany, captive boid snakes from multiple collections and breeders seem to be infected with the same type of adenovirus, and also frequently by a parvovirus. Neutralizing antibodies to the adenovirus have been found in 13% of more than 100 serum samples originating from free-living and captive snakes of miscellaneous species. Bearded dragons, a reptile pet of growing popularity in North America and Europe, seem frequently to have an adenovirus infection. Partial sequence analyses have revealed that identical viruses are present on both continents. At least six additional atadenovirus types have been detected by PCR in various lizard species.

Frog and Fish Adenoviruses

Data concerning adenovirus infection of aquatic vertebrates are scarce. In fact, only a single adenovirus has been isolated from each of the two host classes, amphibians and fish. Interestingly, FrAdV-1 was isolated from a renal tumor of a leopard frog on a reptilian cell line (TH1) prepared from turtle heart tissue. FrAdV-1 has a genome organization similar to that of TAdV-3, and the common evolutionary origin of these two viruses in genus *Siadenovirus* is supported by phylogenetic calculations. The only adenovirus isolate available from fish was obtained from an ancient chondrostei species, the white sturgeon. Partial genomic characterization implies a likely new genus. Nuclear inclusion bodies typical of adenoviruses and adenovirus-like particles have been observed by light and electron microscopy, respectively, in damaged tissues of a couple of other fish species, but molecular confirmation of adenovirus infection has not yet been successful.

Pathogenesis

Adenovirus infections of man generally occur in childhood, and the outcome varies in severity from asymptomatic to explosive outbreaks of upper or lower respiratory tract manifestations. Less commonly, adenoviruses cause gastrointestinal, ophthalmic, urinary, and neurological diseases. The vast majority of adenovirus-caused diseases are self-limiting. However, immunocompromised patients, above all organ transplant recipients, individuals infected with human immunodeficiency virus (HIV) developing AIDS, and those receiving radiation and chemotherapy against tumors, represent special populations that are prone to experience grave, frequently fatal consequences of adenovirus infection. In numerous cases, the organ to be transplanted itself proves to be the source of invasive adenoviruses. Sporadic fatal infections may occasionally occur in healthy, immunocompetent individuals. In such cases, the presence of certain predisposing immunogenetic factors cannot be excluded. Cellular immune responses are also important for the recovery from acute adenovirus infection. Peripheral blood mononuclear cells have been found to exhibit proliferative responses to HAdV-2 antigen. This function is mediated by CD4+ T cells, which seem to recognize conserved antigens among different human adenovirus serotypes.

The incubation period from infection to clinical symptoms is estimated to be 1–7 days and may be dose dependent. Clinical symptoms during the initial viremia are dominated by fever and general malaise. Recovery from infection is associated with the development of serotype-specific neutralizing antibodies that protect against disease or reinfection with the same serotype of the virus but do not cross-react with other serotypes.

Pathology by adenoviruses is partially the consequence of viral replication and cell lysis. Correspondingly, in various tissues and organs, such as bronchial epithelium, liver, kidney, and spleen, disseminated necrotic foci can be observed upon necropsy or histopathological examination. Characteristic intranuclear inclusion bodies and so-called smudge cells contain large amounts of adenovirus capsid proteins. Besides the lesions caused by virus replication, direct toxic effects of high doses of structural proteins, as well as the host's inflammatory respond, may contribute to the aggravation of pathology. Experimental infection of animals with various adenovirus types seldom results in a pathology similar to that experienced with the same virus under natural circumstances. One of the few exceptions is turkey hemorrhagic enteritis, the pathogenesis of which has been studied in detail and is due to TAdV-3, which causes intestinal hemorrhages and immunosuppression. By *in situ* DNA hybridization and PCR, the presence of virus-specific DNA as evidence for virus replication has been demonstrated in the immunoglobulin M-bearing B lymphocytes and macrophage-like cells, but not in CD4+ or CD8+ T lymphocytes. Interestingly, fewer virions were present in the intestines, which are the principal site of pathology, than in the neighboring lymphoid organs including spleen and cecal tonsils. This finding strongly suggests that the intestinal lesions induced by TAdV-3 are mediated by the immune system. Systemic or intestinal hemorrhagic disease of ruminants seems to be related to virus replication in endothelial cells.

Detection and Identification

With the development of modern techniques, especially PCR and direct DNA sequencing, the number of adenoviruses detected in various organ samples of human or animal origin has increased rapidly. However, there is no official agreement or convention on the criteria that would be prerequisites for the approval of new serotypes. The conventional methods, including virus isolation in tissue culture, raising antisera, and performing a large set of cross-neutralization tests, are cumbersome, and the majority of medical and veterinary diagnostic laboratories do not possess appropriate prototype strain and serum collections. Full genomic sequences should validate new types even in the absence of isolated virus strains. However, the value of short sequences from PCR fragments is still a topic of debate. In principle, PCR and sequencing should be able to replace serotyping if appropriate targets are identified.

Human medical laboratories use commercially available tests, such as complement fixation and enzyme immunoassay, to detect adenovirus-specific antibodies that cross-react with all serotypes. Nearly all adults have serologic evidence of past infection with one or more adenoviruses. For the detection of human or animal adenovirus-specific DNA, the most common target in PCR methods was initially the gene encoding the major capsid protein, the hexon. With subsequent restriction enzyme digestion, typing systems for human adenoviruses

have also been elaborated. Recently, a novel nested PCR method targeting the most conserved region of the adenovirus DNA polymerase gene has been published. The highly degenerate consensus primers seem to be capable of facilitating amplification of DNA from every adenovirus known, irrespective of genus affiliation. A major drawback of this exceptionally sensitive method is the relaxed specificity required. Although its application cannot be recommended for routine diagnostic purposes, it may come in handy for finding novel adenoviruses, especially in cases where adenovirus involvement is strongly suspected from other evidence, such as electron microscopy.

Prevention and Therapy

In the USA, orally administrable, live, enteric-coated vaccines against HAdV-4, HAdV-7, and HAdV-21 were used in military units for a couple of decades. After the cessation of vaccine production in 1996, the impact of adenovirus infection among military recruits increased, and re-emergence of HAdV-7 and especially HAdV-4 has been verified. Since 1999, 12% of all recruits were affected by adenovirus disease. Efforts to resume vaccination are in progress.

In the veterinary practice, dog vaccination schedules all over the world invariably include a live or killed CAdV-1 component against dog hepatitis. Inactivated vaccine for horses against equine adenoviruses has been prepared in Australia. In farm animals, inactivated bivalent vaccines (containing one mastadenovirus and one atadenovirus) have been in use in several countries for controlling enzootic calf pneumonia or pneumo-enteritis. In poultry practice, commercially available or experimental vaccines for the prevention of EDS or turkey hemorrhagic enteritis are applied occasionally. There are several attempts ongoing for the production of recombinant subunit vaccines, which should be safer than vaccines derived from infected birds or tissue culture.

No specific anti-adenovirus therapy has yet been established. Recent advances in understanding the pathophysiology of fulminant adenovirus diseases in immunocompromised patients have prompted the consideration of applying donor lymphocyte infusions after transplantation.

Cidofovir is a monophosphate nucleotide analog that, after undergoing cellular phosphorylation, competitively inhibits incorporation of dCTP into virus DNA by the virus DNA polymerase. Incorporation of the compound disrupts further chain elongation. Cidofovir demonstrates activity *in vitro* against a number of DNA viruses, including adenoviruses. There are a limited number of experiences with using this drug against adenovirus infections, and its clinical utility remains to be determined.

See also: Adenoviruses: General Features; Adenoviruses: Malignant Transformation and Oncology.

Further Reading

Barker JH, Luby JP, Sean Dalley A, *et al.* (2003) Fatal type 3 adenoviral pneumonia in immunocompetent adult identical twins. *Clinical Infectious Diseases* 37: 142–146.

Jones MS, Harrach B, Ganac RD, *et al.* (2007) New adenovirus species found in a patient presenting with gastroenteritis. *Journal of Virology* 81: 5978–5984.

Kojaoghlanian T, Flomenberg P, and Horwitz MS (2003) The impact of adenovirus infection on the immunocompromised host. *Reviews in Medical Virology* 13: 155–171.

Leen AM, Bollard CM, Myers GD, and Rooney CM (2006) Adenoviral infections in hematopoietic stem cell transplantation. *Biology of Blood and Marrow Transplantation* 12: 243–251.

Leen AM, Myers GD, Bollard CM, *et al.* (2005) T-cell immunotherapy for adenoviral infections of stem-cell transplant recipients. *Annals of the New York Academy of Sciences* 1062: 104–115.

Neofytos D, Ojha A, Mookerjee B, *et al.* (2007) Treatment of adenovirus disease in stem cell transplant recipients with cidofovir. *Biology of Blood and Marrow Transplantation* 13: 74–81.

Schrenzel M, Oaks JL, Rotstein D, *et al.* (2005) Characterization of a new species of adenovirus in falcons. *Journal of Clinical Microbiology* 43: 3402–3413.

Tang J, Olive M, Pulmanausahakul R, *et al.* (2006) Human CD8+ cytotoxic T cell responses to adenovirus capsid proteins. *Virology* 350: 312–322.

Wellehan JFX, Johnson AJ, Harrach B, *et al.* (2004) Detection and analysis of six lizard adenoviruses by consensus primer PCR provides further evidence of a reptilian origin for the atadenoviruses. *Journal of Virology* 78: 13366–13369.

Anellovirus

P Biagini and P de Micco, Etablissement Français du Sang Alpes-Méditerranée, Marseilles, France

Glossary

Apoptosis Mechanism that allows cells to self-destruct when stimulated by the appropriate trigger.

Hepatitis Disease or condition marked by inflammation of the liver.

Rhinitis Inflammation of the mucous membrane of the nose.

Tamarin American monkey that is related to the marmoset.

Tupaia Small mammal native to the tropical forests of Southeast Asia, also known as the tree shrew.

Unassigned genus Genus that is not assigned taxonomically to any existing virus family.

Introduction

In 2004, the International Committee on Taxonomy of Viruses (ICTV) officially created the genus *Anellovirus* (from latin 'Anello', the ring) to accommodate circular single-stranded DNA viruses isolated from humans and some other animal species. The genus *Anellovirus* is an unassigned genus and its members are thereby distinguished from viruses belonging to other families with circular single-stranded DNA genomes that infect bacteria, plants, and vertebrates, such as circoviruses, nanoviruses, and geminiviruses.

The genus *Anellovirus* officially includes one species *Torque teno virus* (TTV), one tentative species Torque teno mini virus (TTMV) and several yet unclassified animal viruses. Recently, a third group of anelloviruses infecting humans was further identified and called 'small anellovirus' in anticipation of its official designation.

This group of viruses is characterized by a very high genomic variability, a high prevalence in human populations, a still unknown significance for host health and the absence of well-defined mode(s) of transmission.

Historical Overview of Anelloviruses

TTV was the first virus with circular single-stranded DNA genome identified in humans. It was initially discovered in 1997 by means of a subtractive technique (representational difference analysis, RDA) in the serum of a Japanese patient (initials T.T.) with post-transfusion non-A–G hepatitis. The short nucleotide sequence obtained (~500 nt) was initially extended to ~3700 nt; subsequently, the resolution of an additional GC-rich region of about 120 nt permitted to complete the TTV genome sequence and highlighted the circular nature of the viral genome.

TTMV was discovered at the end of 1999 during a study of TTV prevalence in blood donors. Some unexpected amplification products were sequenced and identified as highly divergent when compared to known TTV sequences. A circular genome of about 2900 nt was further characterized and initially designated TTV-like mini virus (TLMV) by analogy with TTV. Following a taxonomic re-evaluation of the status of this virus, it has been officially named TTMV by ICTV.

A putative third member of the genus *Anellovirus*, the 'small anellovirus', has been identified in 2005 using a sequence-independent polymerase chain reaction (PCR) amplification method. Two highly divergent circular sequences (~2200 and ~2600 nt) were initially characterized in human plasma samples by this approach.

Using a primer system located on a relatively well-conserved region of the genome, extremely divergent anellovirus sequences were also characterized in several animal species: examples were found in cats (~2100 nt), in dogs (~2800 nt), in pigs (~2900 nt), and in tupaia (~2200 nt). Circular genomes, highly divergent or similar to those identified in humans, were also identified in nonhuman primates.

Virion Properties, Genome, and Replication

Members of the genus *Anellovirus* are nonenveloped viruses, with an estimated diameter of about 30–32 nm for TTV and slightly less than 30 nm for TTMV. The buoyant density of virions in CsCl is 1.31–1.33 g cm^{-3} for TTV and 1.27–1.28 g cm^{-3} for TTMV. The genomes of anelloviruses are negative stranded. This has been demonstrated by hybridization studies using sense or reverse nucleic acid probes. They are hydrolyzed by DNase I and Mung Bean nuclease as well.

The genome organization shows: (1) a coding region with at least two main open reading frames (ORF1 (long) and ORF2 (short)) deduced directly from the nucleotide sequence, generally overlapping, and (2) a noncoding region containing a GC-rich zone that forms a stem–loop structure (**Figure 1**). Respective sizes differ widely depending on the isolates studied. On the basis of the TTV prototype 1a, the coding region is about 2600 nt long, with the ORF1 and ORF2 composed of 770 and

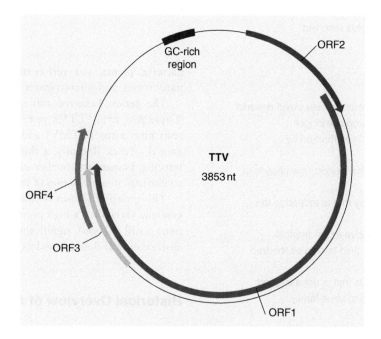

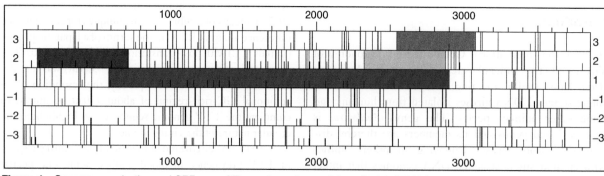

Figure 1   Genome organization and ORF map of *Torque teno virus* prototype (isolate TTV1a).

202 amino acids respectively, while the noncoding region is composed of about 1200 nt with a short zone (~110 nt) of high GC content (~90%). Sequences analysis reveals a variable G+C content for anelloviruses: calculated values from full-length sequences are ~52%, ~38%, and ~39% for TTV, TTMV, and the 'small anellovirus', respectively.

The replication mechanism of anelloviruses is not well known. However, some studies highlighted the presence of TTV mRNA forms and double-stranded DNA in bone marrow and in various human tissues and organs (including the liver), suggesting an active replication in these locations. The presence of double-stranded DNA forms would suggest, as for other circular single-stranded DNA viruses, a rolling-circle mechanism for replication. Three types of TTV mRNAs (2.9, 1.2, and 1.0 kbp), generated by an alternative splicing, have been detected in bone marrow cells and were also obtained following transfection of a permuted whole-genome into African green monkey COS cells. Identification of these mRNAs permitted to establish the functionality of both ORF1 and ORF2 and confirmed the implication of additional ORFs. Transfection into the 293 cell line (human embryonic kidney cells) of a full-length TTV clone not only confirmed the existence of the three mRNA classes but also further demonstrated the expression of six different proteins following an alternative translation strategy. Importance of the untranslated region (UTR) of TTV was highlighted by the identification of a basal promoter ~110 nt upstream the transcription initiation site, and by the presence of enhancer elements in a ~490 nt region upstream this promoter.

The absence of a tissue culture system that would support efficient replication of anelloviruses hindered for a long time the studies of virus–host cell interactions. Interestingly, a human liver cell line (the Chang Liver cell line) does support TTV replication following infection with contaminated sera, and releases significant and persistent levels of infectious viral particles into culture fluid supernatants.

Information concerning the functions of the various proteins expressed during the anellovirus cell-cycle infection is fragmentary. The ORF1 might encode a single polypeptide combining structural and functional roles, that is, the capsid and replication functions of the virus. The presence of conserved motifs related to the Rep protein in the ORF1 would confirm the involvement of a rolling-circle mechanism for the anellovirus replication. Expression studies identified TTMV ORF2 as a dual-specificity protein phosphatase which could be involved in mechanisms of immune evasion and virus persistence. The TTV ORF3 gene would also generate two variants of a protein with a different serine-phosphorylation state which could be involved in the virus-replication cycle. Finally, a putative TTV protein located upstream the ORF1 was shown to induce apoptosis in hepatocellular carcinoma-derived cells.

Phylogenetic and Taxonomic Aspects

The genetic diversity among anelloviruses is far larger than within any other defined group of ssDNA viruses. The considerable genetic heterogeneity is exemplified by the large number of highly divergent full-length sequences progressively identified as TTV, TTMV, and 'small anellovirus' genomes.

Historically, primer extension of the initial sequence (~500 nt, N22 clone) to about 3700 nt (TA278 clone) primarily suggested a distant resemblance of TTV to parvoviruses, based on the apparent linear nature of the characterized genome. The circular nature of the genome was subsequently elucidated (TTV-1a clone), leading to the possible assignment of TTV members to the families of viruses possessing a circular single-stranded DNA genome. This initiated studies on circular single-stranded DNA viruses infecting humans.

Concomitant comparisons of short nucleotide sequences obtained by PCR in the N22 region allowed to identify three distinct genotypes (differing by 27–30% nucleotide divergence) describing TTV genetic diversity in early 1999. The progressive characterization of partial and complete nucleotide sequences had not only demonstrated the existence of a large number of genotypes but has also allowed to classify these genotypes into five distinct clusters (~50% nucleotide divergence) representing the TTV major phylogenetic groups, as defined in 2002 (**Figure 2**). The creation of the genus *Anellovirus* by ICTV in 2004 has officially presented such classification, but it is possible that the next ICTV report will bring significant changes to the taxonomic status of anelloviruses, such as the creation of a specific family hosting several genera accommodating many species, and modify phylogenetic clusters due to the description of new genomic sequences.

Despite the fact that genomic sequences from TTMV and 'small anellovirus' are not as well described as those of TTV, they revealed a high genetic heterogeneity, at least of the same magnitude of that identified for TTV or greater. In 2005, the available full-length TTMV sequences clustered in four major phylogenetic groups (~40% nucleotide divergence), whereas the only two 'small anellovirus' complete sequences described exhibited a nucleotide divergence reaching 46%. Extremely divergent isolates (as compared to human TTV, TTMV, and 'small anellovirus') have been also identified in nonhuman primates and low-order mammals.

A low degree of sequence homology exists between TTV, TTMV, the 'small anellovirus', and animal isolates. However, there is a ~130 nt long sequence that is relatively well conserved between the viral groups, which is located within the UTR downstream of the GC-rich region (**Figure 3**). Moreover, the genome organization of anelloviruses globally appears similar. It includes a coding region containing at least two main ORFs, and a

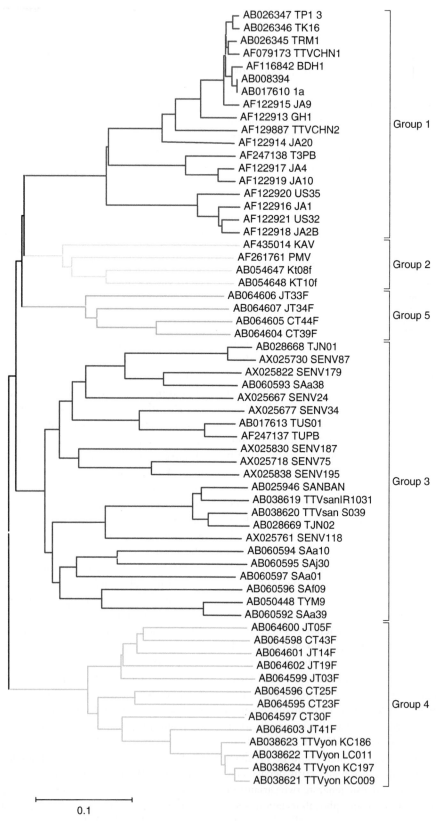

Figure 2 Phylogenetic relations among members of species *Torque teno virus* (neighbor-joining tree built with full-length nucleotide sequences).

```
yonKC197   ...CGAATGGTACACTTTTTTGCTGGCCCGTC--CGCGGCG-AGAGCGCGAGCGAAGCGA-GCGATCGA
JT33F      ..........CT.......CTAC.-.............A....G-A..C.-..GCA-.G..GATC...
TTV1a      ..........CT.......CCAC.-.............A....GTGAA..C.-..G..-.-..A....TC
PMV        ..........CT.......CCAC.-.............A.A.C.-..G..-.-..GAG..CG
TUS01      ..........CT.......CCAC.-.............A....A...C.-..G..-.-..GAG..CG
TGP96      ..........CT......A...C.-..A.A...-.GA.AC.--G.GATC.CTTC..---.-T..CTCC
NLC026     ..........CT......A...C.-..A.A...-.GA.AC.--T.GAAC.C.AC...-.-T..CTCC
PB4TL      ..........CT......A...C.-.TA.A...-.GA.AC.--GAA.ACG.-AC.A---.-...CTTC
CBD279     ..........CT......A.CAC.-..A.A...-.GA.AC.--G..ATC.AAG.C---.-T..CT.C
SAV1       ..........CT......ACC.C.-.TA.A.GGT..A.G.ACCG.AT......C....G.A.G..CC
```

```
yonKC197   --GCGTCCCGTGGGCGGGTGCCGTAGGTGAGTT-TACACACCGAAGTCAAGGGGCAATT-CGGGC....
JT33F        A.......A.............A................C..................................
TTV1a      C.........A.............A........................................
PMV        C..................A..............................................
TUS01      C.........A............G................C..................................
TGP96      AG..TGAA.T.........A....A.......G.A.AC.....T....T..........................
NLC026     AG..TGA.TTA.........A.........G.A.AC.....T..........................
PB4TL      .G..TGAT.T...........T.A.......GTA.AC.........A..........................
CBD279     CG..TGAT.T.........A....A.......G.A.AC...........T..........................
SAV1       CG..TG...........A...CG.......G.A.AC......G...T..........................
```

Figure 3   Alignment of the nucleotide sequence of TTV, TTMV, and 'small anellovirus' representative isolates identified in humans (conserved zone, UTR region).

UTR generally having a GC-rich stretch. The respective sizes of each of these components is however variable between isolates.

Accurate phylogenetic analyses inside each viral group are feasible by comparing full-length ORF1, and to a lesser extent ORF2 nucleotide sequences. By contrast, phylogenetic analysis of short nucleotide sequences located in the N22 region or on the UTR proved to be unreliable. The latter approach is also biased by the occurrence of recombination events which are statistically more frequent in this location than in the rest of the genome.

The amino acid sequence comparisons of translated ORF1 or ORF2 proved to be reliable for phylogenetic analyses, and is the only approach for taxonomic studies combining all *Anellovirus* members which markedly differ in sequence and size. Such comparisons at the amino acids level have also highlighted that most, if not all, of the anelloviruses possess an ORF1 with an arginine-rich N-terminal part and motifs related to the Rep protein, while the ORF2 exhibits the well-conserved motif $WX_7HX_3CX_1CX_5H$. Interestingly, the same features are found in the chicken anemia virus (CAV), the type species of the genus *Gyrovirus* of the family *Circoviridae*. CAV possesses a negative-sense genome, a similar genome organization to anelloviruses, with overlapping ORFs, and several viral proteins with functions supposedly similar to their counterparts in members of the genus *Anellovirus*.

Distribution, Epidemiology, and Transmission

In 1997, the identification of TTV DNA in the blood of Japanese patients with hepatitis of unknown etiology was the starting point of the research on this new group of viruses. Despite its initial identification in populations with liver disorders, further epidemiological studies not only identified the virus in populations with parenteral risk exposure, including intravenous drug users, hemophiliacs, or HIV infected patients, but also in populations without proven pathology like blood donors. It was also clearly demonstrated that TTV is distributed worldwide, as the virus was detected in rural or urban populations in Africa, Americas, Asia, Europe, and Oceania.

Due to the enormous genetic variability characterizing anelloviruses, the choice of the viral DNA target for PCR amplification proved to be highly important for the sensitivity of PCR assays. It was in direct correlation with the progressive determination of full-length genomic sequences and the identification of highly conserved regions between viral isolates. So, early estimated prevalence values for TTV DNA ranged from 1% to 5% in the general population but increased dramatically within 1 year to ~80% in blood donor cohorts, revealing a wide and intriguing dispersion of anelloviruses in human populations without any apparent disease. Higher prevalence values (~90%) are generally identifiable in cohort of patients with health disorders, such as cancer, diabetes mellitus, HIV infection, or under hemodialysis treatment. It was also shown that the prevalence of viremia increased slightly with age. Data relating to TTMV and the 'small anellovirus' tend to reveal similar features concerning their prevalence in human populations.

Subsequent information concerning anellovirus infection in humans has been obtained by the analysis of the distribution of the five major TTV phylogenetic groups in blood donors: interestingly, it revealed a nonrandom pattern of group distribution and a predominant prevalence of phylogenetic groups 1, 3, and 5 in Brazilian and French cohorts. For the latter, the first study of TTMV distribution revealed a predominance of phylogenetic group 1 over the three other groups considered.

Mixed infections appeared as an important characteristic of the *Anellovirus*–host relationship. The possible co-infection of an individual by multiple viral strains of TTV, TTMV, or 'small anellovirus', even highly divergent, is frequent. As demonstrated for TTMV with the analysis of multiples clones of a single PCR, intraindividual viral genetic diversity could reach values above 40%.

Initially described in plasma and serum samples, TTV, TTMV, and 'small anellovirus' DNA have been subsequently isolated in various biological specimens such as peripheral blood mononuclear cells (PBMCs), saliva and nasal secretions, feces, and in other body fluids including semen and tears. Identification of anelloviruses in breast milk, in cord blood samples, and in the blood of newborns, was also described.

These data would suggest that the high rates of prevalence of anelloviruses in various body fluids of healthy subjects might be due to a possible transfusion, fecal–oral, saliva droplet, sexual, or mother-to-child route(s) of transmission.

The presence of anelloviruses members is not limited to human hosts since they were also detected in nonhuman primates such as chimpanzees and tamarins, in tupaias, in popular pets like cats and dogs, and in domesticated farm animals such as pigs and cows. Viral genomic sequences identified in these hosts were either highly divergent or very similar when compared to those obtained from humans. The fact that TTV partial sequences already identified in human blood were found in the blood of farm animals suggests that interspecies transmission could occur. In the same way, intravenous inoculation of TTV-positive human serum or infected fecal supernatant into chimpanzees demonstrated that TTV can be transmitted to primates.

Detection Approaches/Viral Load

Genomic DNA detection has been the mostly developed approach for the identification of anelloviruses in biologic samples. Historically, due to the limited knowledge of TTV genomic sequences, initial PCR systems were restricted to a short portion of the genome in the center of the ORF1. This region was extensively targeted in nested or hemi-nested PCR protocols, but despite improvements in the design of degenerate primers or optimization of the PCR protocols, detection of TTV DNA appeared restricted to certain genotypes and revealed reduced sensitivity when the virus content in samples was low. Extension of the TTV genomic sequence allowed the design of alternative PCR systems located in different parts of the viral genome and their use

in combined detection approaches; such strategy permitted to significantly improve the estimated TTV prevalence in the general population. The growing knowledge of virus genome diversity, as revealed by the characterization of highly divergent full-length genomic sequences, permitted to identify a short and relatively well-conserved zone suitable for optimum primer design. The current 'gold' method for viral DNA detection is based on the use of highly conserved primers, genotype-independent, located in the UTR of the genome upstream the ORF1. This PCR system increased the positive detection rates of samples for TTV DNA and also proved to be applicable to the efficient detection of TTMV, 'small anellovirus' DNA, and highly divergent genomes identified in animals as well.

Real-time PCR assays were developed using such conserved PCR systems in order to gain insights on quantitative aspects of viral infection; such an approach demonstrated that plasma viral loads vary widely, ranging generally between $\sim 10^3$ and $\sim 10^8$ genomes ml^{-1} in individuals.

Distinct amplification systems, designed using a representative dataset of nucleotide sequences specific to the major phylogenetic groups of TTV and TTMV, have also been used for the analysis of the genetic distribution of members of the genus *Anellovirus* in some human cohorts, including blood donors.

Alternative strategies in the diagnosis of viral infection were proposed in a few studies describing serologic (IgG and IgM detection tests, Western blot test using partial ORF1 recombinant protein) and *in situ* hybridization approaches.

Clinical Significance

Since their discovery, the question of a possible implication of anelloviruses in a particular disease is still a matter to debate.

Historical presentation of TTV as associated with elevated transaminase levels in post-transfusion hepatitis of unknown etiology suggested that the virus was able to induce non-A–G hepatitis. Therefore, TTV was suspected as a possible cause of some forms of acute and chronic hepatitis and fulminant liver failure, and could be involved in liver diseases. The identification of TTV in the general population seems to refute this interpretation and led to the suggestion that the virus may cause only occasional liver injury, either by the implication of hepatotropic variants or by the presence of host determinants enhancing the pathogenicity of TTV.

The further identification of TTMV and 'small anellovirus' DNA in humans has increased the number of hypotheses concerning the impact of anelloviruses in human health. Hence, based on studies involving patient cohorts with well-defined health disorders, it has been suggested that this class of viruses may also be implicated in various diseases such as pancreatic cancer, systemic lupus eythematosus, idiopathic inflammatory myopathies, or chromosomal translocations. The implication of anelloviruses in respiratory diseases has also been proposed following studies involving cohorts of children suffering from asthma or rhinitis. It has also been suggested that the respiratory tract could be a site of primary infection in young children and a site of continual replication of TTV and related viruses.

Other studies suggested a possible link between the viral load and the immune status of the host because of high TTV or TTMV titers in plasma samples from immuno-compromised patients, but this remains hypothetical since the loads of TTV and TTMV can differ extensively among individuals in the general population.

To overcome the limitations of a diagnosis of anellovirus infection based only on highly conserved amplification systems, it has been suggested that it would be useful to compare individuals with specific diseases with a reference population such as blood donors. Such an approach may lead to the recognition of a possible pathogenic role of these viruses.

Alternatively, anelloviruses may be considered as part of the 'normal' human flora.

Further Reading

Bendinelli M, Pistello M, Maggi F, et al. (2001) Molecular properties, biology, and clinical implications of TT virus, a recently identified widespread infectious agent of humans. Clinical Microbiology Reviews 14: 98–113.

Biagini P, Charrel RN, de Micco P, and de Lamballerie X (2003) Association of TT virus primary infection with rhinitis in a newborn. Clinical Infectious Diseases 36: 128–129.

Biagini P, Gallian P, Attoui H, et al. (2001) Genetic analysis of full-length genomes and subgenomic sequences of TT virus-like mini virus human isolates. Journal of General Virology 82: 379–383.

Biagini P, Gallian P, Cantaloube JF, et al. (2006) Distribution and genetic analysis of TTV and TT MV major phylogenetic groups in French blood donors. Journal of Medical Virology 78: 298–304.

Biagini P, Todd D, Bendinelli M, et al. (2005) Anellovirus. In: Fauquet CM, Mayo MA, Maniloff J, Desselberger U, and Ball LA (eds.) Virus Taxonomy: Eighth Report of the International Committee on Taxonomy of Viruses. San Diego, CA: Elsevier Academic Press.

Hino S and Miyata H (2007) Torque teno virus (TTV): Current status. Reviews in Medical Virology 17: 45–57.

Jones MS, Kapoor A, Lukashov V V, et al. (2005) New DNA viruses identified in patients with acute viral infection syndrome. Journal of Virology 79: 8230–8236.

Maggi F, Pifferi M, Fornai C, et al. (2003) TT virus in the nasal secretions of children with acute respiratory diseases: Relations to viremia and disease severity. Journal of Virology 77: 2418–2425.

Nishizawa T, Okamoto H, Konishi K, et al. (1997) A novel DNA virus (TTV) associated with elevated transaminase levels in posttransfusion hepatitis of unknown etiology. Biochemical and Biophysical Research Communications 241: 92–97.

Okamoto H, Nishizawa T, Kato N, et al. (1998) Molecular cloning and characterization of a novel DNA virus (TTV) associated with posttransfusion hepatitis of unknown etiology. Hepatology Research 10: 1–16.

Okamoto H, Nishizawa T, Takahashi M, et al. (2001) Heterogeneous distribution of TT virus of distinct genotypes in multiple tissues from infected humans. Virology 288: 358–368.

Okamoto H, Takahashi M, Nishizawa T, et al. (2002) Genomic characterization of TT viruses (TTVs) in pigs, cats and dogs and their relatedness with species-specific TTVs in primates and tupaias. Journal of General Virology 83: 1291–1297.

Pifferi M, Maggi F, Caramella D, et al. (2006) High torquetenovirus loads are correlated with bronchiectasis and peripheral airflow limitation in children. Pediatric Infectious Disease Journal 25: 804–808.

Takahashi K, Hoshino H, Ohta Y, Yoshida N, and Mishiro S (1998) Very high prevalence of TT virus (TTV) infection in general population of Japan revealed by a new set of PCR primers. Hepatology Research 12: 233–239.

Takahashi K, Iwasa Y, Hijikata M, and Mishiro S (2000) Identification of a new human DNA virus (TTV-like mini virus, TLMV) intermediately related to TT virus and chicken anemia virus. Archives of Virology 145: 979–993.

Arboviruses

B R Miller, Centers for Disease Control and Prevention (CDC), Fort Collins, CO, USA

Glossary

Arbovirus A virus that is biologically transmitted to vertebrates by infected hematophagous arthropods.

Hematophagous arthropods Arthropods, including mosquitoes, ticks, sandflies, blackflies, biting-midges, etc., that gain nourishment by feeding on vertebrate blood.

M_r The relative molar mass of a virion.

Transovarial transmission Transmission of an arbovirus from an infected arthropod female to her progeny via viral infected ovaries.

Vertical transmission Transmission of an arbovirus from an infected female vector to her progeny.

Zoonoses An infectious disease transmissible from vertebrate animals to humans under natural conditions.

Introduction

The term 'arbovirus' is used to define viruses transmitted by blood-feeding arthropods. The word was coined by virologists investigating taxonomically diverse viruses that shared this biological feature. These agents are maintained in nature in various transmission cycles, from simple to complex, by replicating in blood-feeding arthropods that transmit the virus in their saliva to vertebrates. The virus then replicates or is 'amplified' in the vertebrate where it becomes accessible in peripheral blood to other blood-feeding arthropods, completing the cycle. These viruses thus are, 'arthropod-borne viruses', or arboviruses.

The *International Catalog of Arboviruses Including Certain Viruses of Vertebrates* lists 545 viruses that are known or suspected to be arthropod-borne as well as viruses with 'no known vector'. Many of the viruses in the catalog infect and replicate in vertebrates other than humans and livestock. Arboviruses circulate in nature, going largely unnoticed until they produce disease in humans and/or domestic animals or wildlife. Of the 545 viruses listed in the catalog, 134 are known to cause human disease. Arboviruses including *Yellow fever virus* (genus *Flavivirus*, family *Flaviviridae*), *Crimean-Congo hemorrhagic fever virus* (genus *Nairovirus*, family *Bunyaviridae*), and *Japanese encephalitis virus* (genus *Flavivirus*, family *Flaviviridae*) are capable of producing severe disease in humans; while other arboviruses including *Rift Valley fever virus* (genus *Phlebovirus*, family *Bunyaviridae*), *Venezuelan equine encephalitis virus* (genus *Alphavirus*, family *Togaviridae*), and *West Nile virus* (genus *Flavivirus*, family *Flaviviridae*) can cause clinical disease in humans and domestic animals.

Although arboviruses are found throughout the world, the majority is found in the tropics, where arbovirus transmission can occur without interruption, thus increasing opportunities for these viruses to evolve. The biological characteristic of arthropod transmission has evolved independently in diverse virus lineages; for instance, in the virus family, *Flaviviridae*, some members are transmitted by ticks, others by mosquitoes, others have no known vector and may be exclusively viruses of vertebrates, and still others appear to have been transmitted by vectors but secondarily have lost this ability over evolutionary time. Viruses in another primitive lineage in the family only replicate in mosquitoes.

Taxonomy and Classification

The most important human and veterinary arboviral pathogens listed in the catalog are found primarily in select genera of three virus families: the *Bunyaviridae* (three of five genera), the *Flaviviridae* (one of three genera), and the *Togaviridae* (one of two genera). Arboviruses also belong to other virus families: the *Rhabdoviridae* (two of six genera), the *Reoviridae* (two of 12 genera), and the *Orthomyxoviridae*

(one of five genera) (**Table 1**). The viruses in these families all have genomes consisting of RNA molecules in various configurations; there is only a single arbovirus, *African swine fever virus* (genus *Asfivirus*), in the family *Asfarviridae* that has a DNA genome. Viruses have been classified by using serological and molecular methodologies.

Virion: Physical Properties, Composition, and Genome Organization

African swine fever virus has a sedimentation coefficient $S_{20,W}$ of about 3500 S and a buoyant density of 1.095 g cm^{-3} in Percoll and 1.19–1.24 g cm^{-3} in CsCl. Virions are susceptible to irradiation, ether, deoxycholate, and chloroform, and they are inactivated at 60 °C for 30 min. Virions can survive for years at 4 °C and they are stable over a wide range of pH. The asfivirus particle consists of a nucleoprotein core that is 70–100 nm in diameter, surrounded by two internal lipid layers, and a 170–190 nm icosahedral capsid ($T = 189$–217) with an external, lipid-containing envelope. The mature virion has 1892–2172 capsomers and a diameter of 175–215 nm. The genome of African swine fever virus is a single molecule of double-stranded DNA that is covalently close-ended and ranges from 170 to 190 kbp in size. Mature virions contain more than 50 proteins, including an inhibitor of apoptosis homolog protein, guanyltransferase, poly A polymerase, protein kinase, and RNA polymerase. There are 150 open reading frames (ORFs) that are read from both strands. Early mRNA synthesis begins in the cytoplasm of the infected cell using enzymes in the virus core; viral DNA replication and assembly take place in perinuclear areas. Viral transcripts are capped at the 5′-end, and the 3′-end is polyadenylated. Formation of the capsid takes place on two layers of membranes derived from the endoplasmic reticulum (ER); extracellular virus acquires a membrane by budding through the cellular plasma membrane.

In the *Bunyaviridae*, virion M_r is $(3$–$4) \times 10^8$ with sedimentation coefficients (S_{20W}) in the range of 350–500 S. Buoyant densities in sucrose and CsCl are 1.16–1.18 and 1.20–1.21 g cm^{-3}, respectively. Virions contain 50% protein, 20–30% lipid, and they are sensitive to heat, irradiation, formaldehyde, and lipid solvents. Bunyavirus virions are spherical with a diameter of 80–120 nm and have a lipid bilayer that contains glycoprotein projections (5–10 nm). Virion envelopes are obtained from Golgi membranes and the ribonucleocapsids exhibit helical symmetry. The three arboviral genera in the family *Bunyaviridae* (*Nairovirus, Orthobunyavirus,* and *Phlebovirus*) have slightly different genome organizations; however, all have segmented, single-stranded, negative-sense RNA genomes with an L-segment that codes for the viral polymerase, an M-segment that codes for two envelope glycoproteins, and an S-segment that codes for the viral nucleocapsid protein. Synthesis of viral mRNA

Table 1 Representative arboviruses associated with human and livestock illnesses

Virus	Genus	Family	Host/associated illness	Arthropod vector	Primary host	Distribution
African swine fever	*Asfivirus*	Asfarviridae	Swine, bush pigs/hemorrhagic fever	Soft ticks, *Ornithodoros*	Wild boar	Africa, Spain, Portugal
Crimean–Congo hemorrhagic fever	*Nairovirus*	Bunyaviridae	Human/hemorrhagic fever	Hard ticks, *Hyalomma*	Wild and domestic animals	Africa, Asia, Europe
La Crosse	*Orthobunyavirus*	Bunyaviridae	Human/encephalitis	Mosquitoes, *Aedes triseriatus*	Chipmunks, squirrels	North America
Rift Valley fever	*Phlebovirus*	Bunyaviridae	Human/hemorrhagic fever, hepatitis, retinitis, encephalitis Livestock/abortion, fever, hepatitis	Mosquitoes, *Culex* and *Aedes*	Cattle and sheep	Africa, Arabian Peninsula
Dengue 1–4	*Flavivirus*	Flaviviridae	Human/fever, hemorrhagic fever	Mosquitoes, *Aedes aegypti*, *Aedes albopictus*	Humans, primates	Worldwide in tropics
Japanese encephalitis	*Flavivirus*	Flaviviridae	Human/fever, encephalitis	Mosquitoes, *Culex*	Wading birds, pigs	Asia, Pacific Islands
Kyasanur Forest disease	*Flavivirus*	Flaviviridae	Humans, primates/fever, encephalitis, hemorrhagic fever	Hard ticks, *Hemaphysalis*	Camels, rodents	India, Saudi Arabia
Murray Valley encephalitis	*Flavivirus*	Flaviviridae	Humans/fever, encephalitis	Mosquitoes, *Culex*	Birds	Australia
Rocio	*Flavivirus*	Flaviviridae	Humans/fever, encephalitis	Mosquitoes, *Culex*	Birds	South America
West Nile	*Flavivirus*	Flaviviridae	Humans/fever, encephalitis	Mosquitoes, *Culex*	Birds	Africa, Asia, Europe, Americas
Yellow fever	*Flavivirus*	Flaviviridae	Humans, New World primates/fever, hemorrhagic fever, hepatitis	Mosquitoes, *Aedes*, *Hemagogus*, *Sabethes*	Primates	Africa, South America
Thogoto	*Thogotovirus*	Orthomyxoviridae	Humans/fever, optic neuritis, encephalitis	Hard ticks	Wild and domestic vertebrates	Africa, Europe
Colorado tick fever	*Coltivirus*	Reoviridae	Humans/fever, myalgia, encephalitis	Ticks, *Dermacentor*	Ground squirrels	Western North America
Banna	*Seadornavirus*	Reoviridae	Humans/fever, myalgia, encephalitis	Mosquitoes, *Culex*, *Aedes*, *Anopheles*	Pigs, cattle	Asia
Vesicular stomatitis Indiana	*Vesiculovirus*	Rhabdoviridae	Humans/fever Domestic animals/ fever, vesicles in the mucosa	Sandflies, blackflies, mosquitoes	Wild and domestic vertebrates	Americas
Chikungunya	*Alphavirus*	Togaviridae	Humans/fever, arthralgias, rarely encephalitis	Mosquitoes, *Aedes*	Humans, primates	Africa, Asia
O'nyong-nyong	*Alphavirus*	Togaviridae	Humans/fever, arthralgias, lymphadenopathy	Mosquitoes, *Anopheles*	Unknown	Africa
Ross River	*Alphavirus*	Togaviridae	Humans/fever, arthralgia	Mosquitoes, *Aedes*, *Culex*	Macropods	Australia, Pacific Islands
Sindbis	*Alphavirus*	Togaviridae	Humans/fever, arthralgia	Mosquitoes, *Culex*, *Culiseta*, *Aedes*	Passerine birds	Europe, Africa, Asia, Australia
Mayaro	*Alphavirus*	Togaviridae	Humans/fever, arthralgia	Mosquitoes, *Haemagogus*	Primates	Americas
Eastern equine encephalitis	*Alphavirus*	Togaviridae	Humans, equines, pheasants /fever, encephalitis	Mosquitoes, *Culiseta*, *Culex*	Birds	Americas
Western equine encephalitis	*Alphavirus*	Togaviridae	Humans, equines/fever, encephalitis	Mosquitoes, *Culex*	Birds	Americas
Venezuelan equine encephalitis	*Alphavirus*	Togaviridae	Humans, equines/fever, encephalitis	Mosquitoes, *Culex* (*Melanoconion*)	Rodents	Americas

takes place in the cytoplasm using host cellular capped primers ('cap-stealing' or 'cap-snatching'). Mature virions are produced by budding into the Golgi cisternae, although *Rift Valley fever virus* has been observed to bud at the cell surface.

Flavivirus virion M_r is about 6×10^7; virions have sedimentation coefficients of approximately 200 S and have buoyant densities of about 1.19 g cm^{-3} in sucrose. Virions are stable at weakly alkaline pH but they are inactivated at acidic pH values, at heat above 40 °C, in organic solvents, and on irradiation. Virions are spherical with icosahedral symmetry and about 50 nm in diameter. There are two glycoproteins in the lipid bilayer: M and E in mature, extracellular virions and prM and E in immature virions; prM is cleaved to M by host-cell enzymes during maturation. The E-glycoprotein is a rod-shaped, dimeric structure that does not form spike-like projections; rather, it lies parallel to the viral membrane in a neutral pH environment. The flavivirus genome is capped and consists of single-stranded, positive-sense RNA that codes ($5' \rightarrow 3'$) for three structural proteins and seven non-structural proteins contained in a single ORF; the 5'- and 3'-ends are noncoding regions (NCRs) necessary for viral replication and translation. A nascent polyprotein is transcribed and cleaved co- and post-translationally by cellular and viral proteases. Viral RNA synthesis, virion assembly, and acquisition of a lipid envelope take place in the ER; mature virions are released by exocytosis.

Orthomyxovirus virion M_r is 250×10^6 and buoyant density is 1.19 g cm^{-3} in sucrose. $S_{20,w}$ is 700–800 S and virions are sensitive to irradiation, solvents, heat, and detergents. Virions are spherical (80–120 nm) and sometimes pleomorphic with surface glycoproteins projecting 10–14 nm from the surface. The nucleocapsid is segmented and has helical symmetry. Within the genus, *Thogotovirus*, the negative-sense, single-stranded, segmented RNA genome is comprised of six segments for *Thogoto virus* (family *Orthomyxoviridae*) and seven segments for *Dhori virus* (family *Orthomyxoviridae*); the genome is about 10 kb in size. Interestingly, the glycoprotein, coded by the fourth segment, shares sequence similarity with a surface glycoprotein of insect baculoviruses. Thogoto virus nulceocapsids are transported to the nucleus where viral enzymes synthesize 5'-capped mRNA that are polyadenylated. Protein synthesis occurs in the cytoplasm, although early on in infection certain proteins are found in the nucleus and later transported to the cytoplasm. Viral membrane proteins are transported through the Golgi cisternae to the cellular plasma membrane; nulceocapsids bud through the plasma membrane in regions populated by viral membrane proteins.

In the *Reoviridae*, coltiviruses and orbiviruses have a buoyant density of 1.38 and 1.36 g cm^{-3}, respectively, in CsCl. Viruses are sensitive to low pH, heat, and detergent but are stable for long periods at 4 °C in the presence 50% fetal bovine serum. Coltivirus virions are 60–80 nm in diameter consisting of two concentric capsid shells with a core structure that is about 50 nm in diameter while the orbivirus, bluetongue virus is 90 nm in diameter with core particles 73 nm in diameter. Virus particles have icosahedral symmetry and are closely associated with granular matrices and filamentous formations in the cytoplasm. The mosquito-borne seadornaviruses and tick-borne coltiviruses have genomes composed of 12 double-stranded (dsRNA) segments that are, respectively, 21 000 and 29 000 bp in size; each genome segment is flanked 5' and 3' by similar noncoding sequences. Coltivirus VP1 (the largest segment) encodes the viral RNA-dependent RNA polymerase. There is no indication of virus release prior to cell death; more than 95% of coltivirus progeny virions and 60% of seadornavirus progeny virions remain cell associated. Orbivirus core particles are arranged as hexameric rings composed of capsomeres. The viral genome is composed of ten segments of dsRNA surrounded by the inner capsid shell. Inclusion bodies and tubules are produced during viral replication. Flat hexagonal crystals formed from the major outer core protein may also be produced during orbivirus replication. Unpurified virus is associated with cellular membranes although mature virus lacks a lipid envelope. Virions can leave the host cell by budding through the plasma membrane and transiently acquiring an envelope that is unstable and is rapidly lost.

Rhabdovirus virion M_r is 3–10×10^8 and $S_{20,w}$ is 550–1045 S. Buoyant density in sucrose is 1.7–1.9 g cm^{-3} and 1.19–1.20 g cm^{-3} in CsCl. Heat above 56 °C, lipid solvents, and irradiation will inactivate virions. Rhabdoviruses are 'bullet-shaped' or 'cone-shaped', 100–430 nm in length, and 45–100 nm in diameter. Trimers of the viral glycoprotein (G), 10 nm long and 3 nm in diameter, known as 'peplomers' cover the outer surface of the virus. The nucleocapsid is 30–70 nm in diameter and shows helical symmetry. It is composed of RNA and N (nucleocapsid proteins) collectively with the L-(transcription and replication factors) and P-(polymerase cofactor) proteins that interact with the envelope G-protein via the M-(binds to N and G) protein. The genomes are negative-sense, single-stranded RNA molecules that encode five major polypeptides. Viral genes are transcribed as monocistronic mRNAs that are capped and polyadenylated. After the nucleocapsid is released into the cytoplasm, the viral genomic RNA is transcribed by the virion transcriptase. Genome replication occurs in the cytoplasm by full-length positive-strand RNA synthesis followed by full-length negative-strand RNA synthesis. Nucleocapsids are synthesized in the cytoplasm and viral membranes are acquired as viruses bud from the host-cell plasma membranes.

Togavirus virion M_r is approximately 52×10^6. Virions have a buoyant density of 1.22 g cm^{-3} in sucrose and an $S_{20,w}$ is of 280 S. Virions are sensitive to heat, acidic pH, solvents, and irradiation. Togavirus viruses are spherical, 70 nm in diameter, and they have heterodimer spikes in the envelope consisting of two virus glycoproteins, E1 and E2. The envelope surrounds a 40 nm nucleocapsid that has icosahedral symmetry ($T = 4$). Togaviruses have a genome that is positive-sense, single-stranded RNA; the mRNA is capped and polyadenylated. There are four genes coding for nonstructural proteins situated at the 5'-end of the genome and five genes coding for structural proteins located at the 3'-end of the genome. Negative-sense RNA, synthesized during RNA replication, is utilized as the template for production of genome-length, positive-sense RNA as well as for creation of a 'subgenomic' 26S mRNA that is capped and polyadenylated and is translated to make the viral structural proteins. The polyprotein is cleaved by a combination of cellular and viral proteases. Noncoding sequences located at the 5'- and 3'-termini of the genome are required for both negative and positive RNA synthesis. The nucleocapsids are assembled in the cytoplasm; viral surface glycoproteins are processed in the ER and translocated through the Golgi apparatus to the cellular plasma membrane where they are acquired as the nucleocapsids bud through the membrane.

Evolutionary Relationships Among Arboviruses

The biological characteristic of viral replication in arthropods followed by transmission to vertebrates in the course of blood feeding has arisen independently in seven families of viruses. Taxonomic relationships within the arboviruses were originally based on analyses of antigenic cross-reactivity data obtained from neutralization, complement fixation, and hemagglutination tests. Virion morphology, determined by electron microscopy, was also important in taxonomic classification.

The availability of viral, genomic, nucleic acid sequences and sophisticated nucleic acid analyses and phylogenetic software has enabled hypothesis testing of arboviral evolution. Defining the deeper nodes in evolutionary trees has been difficult because of the limited number of sequences from different virus species in each virus family. Predictably, the arboviruses that are most well-characterized are those associated with disease. It will be difficult to formulate an accurate and robust theory of arboviral evolution until this sampling bias is resolved by obtaining data from other viruses, those not necessarily associated with disease. Brief summaries of the best-studied arbovirus groups are presented below.

Evolutionary Relationships of the Flaviviruses

The genus, *Flavivirus* is currently composed of about 70 different viruses that infect a wide variety of vertebrate hosts from birds to bats, transmitted by ticks and mosquitoes; some have no known vector associations and others are found only in mosquitoes.

Flavivirus-related sequences have been detected in the genomes of *Aedes* mosquitoes suggesting flavivirus sequence integration into an eukaryotic genome. Another curious finding is the discovery of defective Dengue virus 1 (genus *Flavivirus*, family *Flaviviridae*) virions that are transmitted by *Aedes aegypti* to humans over long periods of time. The defective genomes have acquired a stop codon in the envelope glycoprotein gene resulting in a truncated E-protein. This defective lineage persists through complementation by co-infection of host cells with functional viruses. The relevance of these findings on virulence and pathogen transmission are unknown.

The detection of diverse quasispecies populations of Dengue virus 3 in *Aedes aegypti* mosquitoes and in humans suggests that flaviviral mutation frequencies are similar to those of other RNA viruses. Estimates of flavivirus evolutionary rates suggest they are generally less than those for single-host RNA viruses, reflecting the evolutionary constraints of obligatory replication in vertebrate and invertebrate hosts. Approximation of the degree of amino acid divergence between mosquito-borne and tick-borne viruses indicates that flaviviruses in the tick-borne group evolve two to three times more slowly than do the mosquito-borne viruses. This is probably the result of limited virus replication and the lengthy tick life cycle, which can be measured in years. Ixodid (hard) ticks feed only three times during their life cycle (larva→nymph→adult) with months passing between ecdysis (molting) and feeding on a subsequent vertebrate host, thus allowing virus lineages to persist for long periods of time in a quiescent arthropod. Also, an infected tick can directly infect another tick co-feeding on the same uninfected animal host, eliminating the need for a viremic vertebrate as had been demonstrated for tick-borne encephalitis virus and *Ixodes ricinus* ticks. This 'nonviremic' transmission may result in viruses persisting for long periods of time in the tick, further constraining rates of evolutionary change. This is in marked contrast to mosquitoes where viral replication occurs rapidly and to high titers over a life span measured in days. The increased amount of RNA replication in mosquitoes generates more virus variation, thereby increasing opportunities for viral evolution.

Data sets from alignments of sequences from the nonstructural genes NS3 and NS5 and whole-genome alignments have been examined for phylogenetic signal in determining evolutionary relationships among most viruses in the family. In general, data alignments from the NS3 genes and from the full-length genomes have proven to be the most useful in elucidating the basal divergence of derived lineages. Hypotheses based on recent studies suggest that the absence of a vector is the ancestral condition for the family as a whole (genera *Hepacivirus*, *Pestivirus*, and *Flavivirus*); within this family, arboviruses occur only in the *Flavivirus* genus.

Within the genus *Flavivirus*, determination of the divergence of the three main groups (no known vector, mosquito-borne, and tick-borne) is equivocal. Phylogenetic analysis of the NS5 data set suggests that the no-known vector group diverged before the arthropod-borne viruses while analysis of the NS3 and full-genome data sets imply that the mosquito-borne flaviviruses diverged first and form a sister clade to the no-known vector and tick-borne viruses. If the mosquito-borne viruses were the first divergent group, we would expect the existence of a lineage of unknown flaviviruses occurring in mosquitoes. The recent discovery of the flavivirus, *Kamiti River virus*, which replicates in mosquitoes exclusively, adds support to the speculation that there may be a large number of unidentified flaviviruses existing in nature that are the descendants of a primitive, mosquito–host lineage.

Attempts have been made to associate epidemiology, disease pattern, and biogeography with the major virus clades using either partial sequences of the NS5 gene or of the E-gene. The mosquito-borne flaviviruses partition into two groups: viruses that cause neuroinvasive disease (Japanese encephalitis virus and West Nile virus) and are transmitted by *Culex* vectors to bird amplification reservoirs, and viruses that cause hemorrhagic disease (Yellow fever virus and dengue viruses) and are transmitted by *Aedes* vectors to primate amplification reservoirs. The tick-borne viruses also formed two groups, one associated with seabird hosts and another associated with rodents. The no-known vector viruses split into three groups, two associated with bats and one with rodents. The above associations undoubtedly reflect the complex interactions and selection pressures between arboviruses, arthropod vectors, and vertebrate hosts over evolutionary time.

Regardless of which group diverged first, the flaviviruses probably originated in the Old World. Within the *Aedes* mosquito-borne clade, only Yellow fever virus, the four dengue viruses, and West Nile virus are established in the Americas; the presence of these viruses represents relatively recent introductions from Africa or Asia. With the exception of the *Powassan virus* (family *Flaviviridae*), all the tick-borne flaviviruses occur in the Old World. Evidence for the Old World origin of the no-known vector group is less convincing. The rodent-borne viruses are only found in the New World with the exception of *Apoi virus* (family *Flaviviridae*); the bat-borne group has representatives that occur worldwide. These observations could be explained by a single dispersion event of an ancestral virus from the Old World into the New World that resulted in infection of resident rodents. Rodents generally occupy a small geographic range and are less likely to widely disperse viruses, increasing the likelihood of founder effects, genetic drift, and viral allopatric speciation. Migratory bats on the other hand are capable of transporting viruses over long distances.

Evolutionary Relationships of the Alphaviruses

The genus *Alphavirus* in the family *Togaviridae* is comprised of 29 described species. Within the genus, viruses have been grouped into eight antigenic complexes by classic serological techniques. Phylogenetic relationships in the genus have been estimated using nucleic acid and amino acid alignments from the E1, nsP1, and nsP4 codons. Phylogenetic trees produced from analyses of alignments of nucleic acids and amino acids generally support the antigenic groups as monophyletic clades. The antigenic complexes are also associated with disease syndromes, as described for the flaviviruses with the exception of hemorrhagic fevers. For example, members of the Eastern equine encephalitis and Venezuelan equine encephalitis complexes produce neuroinvasive disease in humans and equines, while members of the *Semliki Forest virus* complex commonly cause mild to severe arthralgias. Interestingly, the Western encephalitis virus complex contains viruses capable of causing both disease syndromes; arthralgias in the *Sindbis virus* clade and neuroinvasive disease caused by Highlands J and Western equine encephalitis viruses. This dichotomy in disease associations is the probable result of an ancient, genomic recombination event. Two of the viruses in this complex, Highlands J and Western equine encephalitis, are descendents of a recombinant ancestral alphavirus; presumably, the genetic material responsible for the potential to cause encephalitis came from an Eastern equine encephalitis virus-like ancestor and a Sindbis-like virus.

Molecular studies using phylogenetic analyses of alphaviruses have shown that the majority of genome sequence divergence results in synonymous substitutions, indicating that rates of evolutionary change are constrained by purifying selection. This conservation is revealed in the 26S subgenomic promoter sequences; they are functionally interchangeable between Sindbis virus and other alphaviruses. Again, the hypothesis to explain the lower rates of evolution in these viruses in contrast to nonarboviral RNA viruses is the restraint imposed by required replication in hosts with and hosts without a backbone.

An examination of alphavirus phylogenetic divergence demonstrates the importance of host switching and host mobility. An intriguing example is the relationship between the closely related Chikungunya and O'nyong-nyong viruses. *Chikungunya virus* is thought to have originated in Africa in a sylvan, *Aedes*–primate transmission cycle. *O'nyong-nyong virus* (family *Togaviridae*) is genetically very similar to Chikungunya virus yet it has become adapted to *Anopheles funestus* and *Anopheles gambiae* moquitoes. Molecular studies with chimeric Chikungunya–O'nyong-nyong viruses indicate that an ancestor of Chikungunya virus became adapted to replication in anopheline mosquitoes. This is significant because *Anopheles* species as arboviral vectors are the exception, rather than the rule.

In general, alphavirus divergence is highest when virus transmission occurs focally, usually in small vertebrate hosts, such as rodents which have restricted geographic ranges. Virus transmission in these isolated foci can produce new genotypes as has been elegantly demonstrated for viruses in the Venezuelan equine encephalitis complex. Conversely, genomic divergence is less for viruses that are amplified in wide-ranging vertebrates like birds where genotypic mixing and selection maintains a dominant genotype.

Disease Associations

Although arboviruses are represented in diverse viral taxa, the disease syndromes they produce in humans can be arbitrarily classified into three major groups: systemic febrile illness, meningitis and/or encephalitis, and hemorrhagic fever. It is important to note that these syndromes represent a spectrum of disease severity: from sub-clinical infections to fatal outcomes. The factors responsible for differential disease severity are unknown but age and the immune status of the host are important as well as the amount of virus inoculated (dose) and the relative pathogenicity of the infecting arbovirus strain. Disease is most often correlated with infection of dead-end hosts including humans and their domestic animals; there is little evidence of these viruses causing harm in their natural hosts.

Febrile illness caused by infection with dengue viruses (serotypes 1–4), West Nile, Chikungunya, and other viruses consists of fever, headache, muscle and joint pain, and sometimes with rash. In a certain subset of cases, infection with West Nile virus progresses to encephalitis, resulting in fatalities or neurological sequelae in survivors, whereas infection with the dengue viruses rarely results in encephalitis or a hemorrhagic syndrome. Age-associated disease syndromes have been noted with West Nile virus infection: inapparent infection in children, typical fever syndrome in adults, and neuroinvasive disease in the elderly. Other arboviruses that can produce a febrile illness associated with polyarthritis are the alphaviruses, Chikungunya, O'nyong-nyong, Sindbis, Ross River, Barmah, and Mayaro. These febrile illnesses are impossible to differentiate on a clinical basis and are often confused with malaria and other common viral infections, including influenza. No fatalities are associated with uncomplicated febrile illnesses although recovery time can be prolonged and sequelae are commonly observed.

More serious illnesses are caused by arboviruses that have a tropism for the central nervous system, including Japanese encephalitis, Saint Louis encephalitis, West Nile, Eastern equine encephalitis, Western equine encephalitis, Venezuelan equine encephalitis, and *LaCrosse* (genus *Orthobunyavirus*, family *Bunyaviridae*) viruses. Illness begins with fever, chills, headache, malaise, drowsiness, anorexia, myalgia, and nausea. The syndrome can progress to confusion, stupor, and coma. These infections can be life-threatening and survivors may suffer from severe neurological sequelae.

Another serious manifestation of infection by some arboviral pathogens is hemorrhagic fever. Infection with the flavivirus Yellow fever virus can produce a clinical spectrum ranging from a mild febrile illness to fulminating fatal disease. Flaviviruses in the mammalian tick-borne virus group that can cause hemorrhagic fevers include Kyasanur Forest disease and Omsk hemorrhagic fever viruses. Infection with Rift Valley fever and Crimean-Congo hemorrhagic fever viruses can also result in hemorrhagic fever.

The above-mentioned examples are all for human infections. As might be expected, domestic animals may exhibit similar disease syndromes following arboviral infection. Infections that can produce febrile illness in animals include the alphavirus *Getah* in horses, *Bovine ephemeral fever virus* (genus *Ephemerovirus*, family *Rhabdoviridae*) in cattle, and Crimean-Congo hemorrhagic fever virus in cattle, sheep, and goats. More severe disease with encephalitis results from infection with West Nile, Eastern equine encephalitis, Western equine encephalitis, and Venezuelan equine encephalitis viruses in horses. Infection with the flavivirus *Wesselsbron virus*, *Bluetongue virus* (genus *Orbivirus*, family *Reoviridae*) and Nairobi sheep disease virus (genus *Nairovirus*, family *Bunyaviridae*) in sheep, and African swine fever virus in pigs can result in hemorrhages. Infection of sheep, goats, and cattle with Rift Valley fever virus can result in abortions while infection with the orthobunyavirus *Akabane virus* (family *Bunyaviridae*) can result in congenital malformations.

Transmission Cycles

Human and livestock encroachment into natural transmission cycles is the most common means of exposure to arboviral infections. This virus transmission scenario is sometimes termed 'spillover' because the principal enzootic vector(s) has a wide host feeding range not limited to the natural, amplifying, vertebrate hosts. Arboviruses in this category of transmission include, but are not limited to, West Nile, sylvan Yellow fever, Western equine encephalitis and La Crosse viruses. African swine fever virus is maintained in sub-Saharan Africa in a cycle involving *Ornithodoros* ticks and warthogs. Infected ticks infesting warthog burrows can also transmit the virus to their progeny by transovarial transmission. Infected warthogs do not show signs of the disease; however, domestic swine are severely affected with mortality rates approaching 100%. In addition to tick bite, transmission between domestic pigs can occur through direct contact and the ingestion of infected offal.

Domestication of animals for human use has provided arboviruses with new and abundant hosts. For example, Rift Valley fever virus circulates in extensive areas of

Africa and is transmitted by certain species of *Aedes* and *Culex* mosquitoes to various native vertebrates. The virus is thus maintained by horizontal transmission in the vertebrates and by transovarial and/or vertical transmission of the virus in mosquito eggs during periods of drought. El Nino events can lead to sustained rainfall and flooding, resulting in the production of massive numbers of other species of *Aedes* and *Culex* mosquitoes that enter into the existing, endemic transmission cycle. Infected vectors disperse and bloodfeed on livestock, initiating a secondary amplification cycle. Viremic livestock become the source for a dramatic increase in the numbers of infected vectors, which in turn engenders human epidemics and livestock epizootics.

The third pattern of arboviral transmission is one in which humans serve as both the reservoir and amplification hosts. Arboviruses maintained in human→vector→human cycles are generally transmitted by domestic mosquito vectors, most importantly, *Aedes aegypti*. The dengue viruses, the most important arboviruses in terms of human disease, are the classic example of an arbovirus that has adapted to the human host. Other examples include Chikungunya and Yellow fever viruses which can cause spectacular outbreaks in areas infested with *Aedes aegypti* vectors. These latter viruses generally disappear after a sufficient numbers of humans become immune, but persist in sylvan transmission cycles until nonimmune human hosts become available or when human herd immunity wanes.

See also: Crimean-Congo Hemorrhagic Fever Virus and Other Nairoviruses.

Further Reading

Calisher C (2005) A very brief history of arbovirology focusing on contributions by workers of the Rockefeller Foundation. *Vector Borne and Zoonotic Diseases* 5: 202.

Cook S and Gould E (2006) A multigene analysis of the phylogenetic relationships among the flaviviruses (Family: *Flaviviridae*) and the evolution of vector transmission. *Archives of Virology* 151: 309.

Karabatsos N (1985) *International Catalog of Arboviruses Including Certain Other Viruses of Vertebrates*, 3rd edn. San Antonio: American Society of Tropical Medicine and Hygiene.

Knipe DM and Howley PM (eds.) (2001) *Fields Virology*, 4th edn. 2 vols. Philadelphia: Lippincott.

Monath TP (ed.) (1988) *The Arboviruses: Epidemiology and Ecology*. 5 vols. Boca Raton: CRC.

Theiler M and Downs WG (1973) *The Arthropod-Borne Viruses of Vertebrates*. New Haven, CT: Yale University Press.

Weaver SC and Barrett ADT (2004) Transmission cycles, host range, evolution and emergence of arboviral disease. *Nature Reviews Microbiology* 2: 789.

Astroviruses

L Moser and S Schultz-Cherry, University of Wisconsin – Madison, Madison, WI, USA

Glossary

Enterocytes Epithelial cells lining the intestines.
Intussusception Obstruction of the intestine.
Interstitial nephritis Inflammation of the kidney.
Poult Young turkey.
Villi Finger-like intestinal projections lined with enterocytes.

Introduction

Astroviruses are enteric viruses first identified in the feces of children with diarrhea. Detection was originally based on a five- to six-pointed star morphology of virions by electron microscopy (EM). However, only about 10% of viral particles display these structures; the remaining 90% of particles have a smooth surface and a size similar to other small, round-structured viruses like picornaviruses and caliciviruses. Thus, accurate diagnostics were difficult to obtain and the true prevalence of astrovirus within a population was difficult to assess. Development of much more sensitive detection techniques like real time reverse transcription-polymerase chain reaction (RT-PCR), cell culture RT-PCR, and astrovirus-specific enzyme-linked immunosorbent assays (ELISAs) have made detection more accurate and specific, even allowing diagnosis of specific serotypes. Utilizing these techniques, astroviruses have been found in approximately 3–8% of children with diarrhea. Astroviruses can also be isolated in a subset of asymptomatic individuals, suggesting that a proportion of infected individuals shed the virus asymptomatically or for some time after the resolution of other symptoms of infection. Asymptomatic carriers may be a major reservoir for astroviruses in the environment and could contribute to dissemination of the virus.

The release of astroviruses into the environment is a concern due to the extreme stability of the virus.

Astroviruses are resistant to inactivation by alcohols (propanol, butane, and ethanol), bleach, a variety of detergents, heat treatment including 50 °C for an hour or 60 °C for 5 min, and UV treatment up to 100 mJ cm^{-2}. Human astroviruses are known to survive up to 90 days in both marine and tap water, with survival potential increasing in colder temperatures. Studies have described the isolation of infectious virus from water treatment facilities. Furthermore, astroviruses can be concentrated by filter-feeding shellfish like oysters and mussels in marine environments. Astroviruses are transmitted fecal–orally, and contaminated food and water have been linked to astrovirus outbreaks.

History and Classification

Astroviruses were originally observed by Appleton and Higgins in 1975 as a small round virus in stools. Later that year, Madeley and Cosgrove identified the virus in association with diarrhea in children and bestowed the name astrovirus (from the Greek *astron*, meaning star) for the star-like morphology of a proportion of viral particles seen by EM (**Figure 1(a)**). Because of genomic similarities, astroviruses were originally thought to belong to either the families *Picornaviridae* or *Caliciviridae*. However, the lack of a helicase and use of a frameshifting event during replication (discussed below) distinguish astroviruses so completely that, in 1993, the International Committee on Taxonomy of Viruses (ICTV) classified astroviruses as a unique family, *Astroviridae*, composed of a single genus *Astrovirus*. Continued investigation into newly discovered astroviruses led to the division of the family into two genera, *Mamastrovirus* and *Avastrovirus*, by the ICTV in 2005. ICTV nomenclature abbreviates astrovirus AstV, with a single-letter abbreviation for the species type (i.e., human astrovirus; HAstV; turkey astrovirus; TAstV, etc.). Successive, serologically distinct isolates of astroviruses are named sequentially within that species (i.e., HAstV-1 through HAstV-8).

Epidemiology

Humans

Astroviruses have been detected throughout the world. While the exact incidences of infection vary from study to study, community-acquired astroviruses are found in 3–6% of children with infectious gastroenteritis. In some developing countries, infection rates as high as 20% have been observed. In many cases, astroviruses are the second most commonly detected viral pathogen in young children after rotavirus. Astrovirus infections are identified in up to 2% of asymptomatic individuals. These data may underrepresent actual astrovirus infections, as studies generally survey individuals visiting medical care centers.

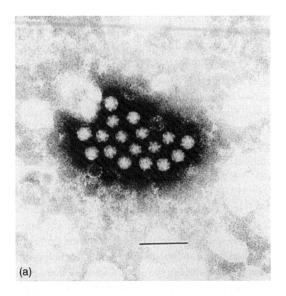

(a)

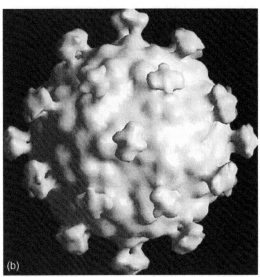

(b)

Figure 1   (a) Astroviruses have historically been identified by the five- to six-pointed star morphology visible by electron microscopy. Scale = 100 nm. (b) A reconstruction of the astrovirus virion, based on cytoelectron microscopy, along the twofold axis of symmetry. Reprinted from Matsui SM and Greenberg HB (1996) Astroviruses. In: Fields BN, Knipe DM, and Howley PM (eds.) *Fields Virology*, 3rd edn., pp. 875–893. Philadelphia: Lippencott-Raven.

Because astrovirus disease is generally mild in humans (see the section discussing pathogenesis), hospital cases may represent only a slight proportion of actual infections in the community. In support of this, serological studies have demonstrated that up to 90% of children have been exposed to at least one strain of astrovirus by age 9.

Eight serotypes of human astrovirus have been identified to date, with all eight circulating within the global population to various levels. HAstV-1 is by far the most prevalent serotype, comprising 25–100% of astroviruses in a region, and the most prevalent reactivity of antibodies detected, although serological surveys of all serotypes have not been undertaken. HAstV-6, -7, and -8 are the least frequently detected, although three to four serotypes of HAstV are often detected in a region at any given time. The differing prevalence of serotypes could be a reflection of severity; perhaps HAstV-1 infection results in a higher frequency of hospital visits than other serotypes and is therefore overrepresented in hospital-based epidemiological studies. Alternatively, serotypes may be restricted by region. For example, one Mexican study identified HAstV-1 as the predominant serotype throughout the country, but HAstV-3 and -8 were prominent in select regions.

Viral infection occurs with equal frequency in boys and girls and predominantly in children under the age of 2. Infection is not restricted to young children, however, and has been noted in individuals of all ages, including immunocompetent adults and the elderly. Immunodeficient individuals, particularly those that are HIV-positive, appear to be at an increased risk of astrovirus infection.

Astrovirus infection occurs year-round, but with the highest frequency during the autumn and early winter months. In tropical climates, infection correlates with the rainy season. These seasonal correlations likely reflect the indoor confinement of the population as well as the increased stability of astroviruses in cold, damp conditions. Astrovirus outbreaks have also been associated with high-density environments, including childcare centers, primary and junior high schools, military recruiting centers, elderly care centers, and swimming pools. Astrovirus as a cause of hospital-acquired viral diarrhea in young children is second only to rotavirus, occurring at rates of 4.5–6%, and, in some studies, surpasses rotavirus in rates of nosocomial infections.

Interestingly, astrovirus infection occurs quite frequently (up to 50%) as a co-infection with other enteric pathogens. The most frequent co-pathogens are noroviruses and rotaviruses, but infections with adenoviruses, parasites, and enteric bacteria are often detected as well. The importance of this in humans is not entirely clear. In a study specifically examining co-infections, astrovirus co-infection with rotavirus increased the duration of diarrhea and vomiting over either virus alone, although whether this difference was statistically significant is unknown.

Animals

Most animals are not routinely screened for astrovirus infection, so our knowledge of the prevalence of infection is limited to surveillance studies. Astroviruses have been found in association with most animals examined, although the effect of infection varies with species (see below). While astroviruses were originally identified in humans, they have since been identified in both mammalian and avian species, including rabbits, mice, calves, sheep, piglets, dogs, red-tailed deer, kittens, mink, turkeys, ducklings, chicken, and guinea fowl. At least three serotypes of bovine astroviruses are postulated to exist based on distinct neutralizing antibodies (one in the United States and two in the United Kingdom). In addition, astroviruses have been isolated from mink across Scandinavia, and serological studies have demonstrated that astroviruses were prevalent in chicken flocks in the 1980s as well as in 2001. Interestingly, two very different manifestations of chicken astrovirus infection have been described (see the section on pathogenesis), suggesting that distinct chicken astroviruses may circulate; however, this is yet to be proven. The best epidemiologically characterized animal astroviruses are the turkey astroviruses. Surveillance of turkey flocks in the 1980s isolated astrovirus from 78% of diseased flocks, but only 29% of normal flocks. Astroviruses were the first pathogen detected in many flocks and were most commonly detected in birds less than 4 weeks of age. Similar to human infections, turkey astrovirus was frequently isolated with other pathogens, most commonly rotavirus-like viruses. The early age of infection and the prevalence of co-infections led one group to postulate that astrovirus infection may predispose birds to infection by other viruses.

Virus Propagation

Attempts at *in vitro* propagation of astroviruses have been met with varying degrees of success. The most successful techniques utilize cultured cells from the host species and provide exogenous trypsin in the culture. Successful propagation of human astroviruses was originally achieved by repeated passage through primary human embryonic kidney cells; it was later discovered that direct passage through the human intestinal cell line Caco-2 would also yield infectious virus. Propagation of porcine, bovine, and chicken astroviruses has been successful in their respective host cells *in vitro*. However, many astroviruses still have not been adapted to propagation *in vitro* for unknown reasons, while others lose infectivity with subsequent passages and therefore cannot be maintained continuously. This problem has been circumvented in some systems by passing the virus through an animal system, as is the case for the turkey astrovirus, in which highly concentrated virus can be obtained from infected turkey embryos *in ovo*.

Molecular Virology and Protein Expression

Astroviruses contain one copy of positive-sense, single-stranded RNA. The genome is approximately 6.8 kb long and contains three open reading frames (ORFs), ORF1a, -1b, and -2, as well as 5' and 3' untranslated regions (UTRs) (**Figure 2**). The RNA is polyadenylated, but lacks a 5' cap structure. The 5' and 3' UTRs are highly conserved and are believed to contain signals important for genome replication.

Astroviruses initiate infection by binding to an unknown receptor and entering the cell via receptor-mediated endocytosis. The plus-strand genome is released into the cytoplasm by unknown mechanisms and ORF1a and -1b are immediately translated by the host machinery. ORF1a is 2.8 kb and encodes a polypeptide of approximately 110 kDa. This polypeptide contains a variety of conserved motifs, including several putative transmembrane domains, a bipartite nuclear localization sequence (NLS), and a serine protease motif. The translated polypeptide is cleaved by both cellular protease(s) and the viral protease into at least five peptides. The actual function of each protein remains largely unknown. The transmembrane domains may localize to the endoplasmic reticulum (ER) membrane to facilitate replication, as all plus-strand RNA viruses have been shown to replicate in association with a membrane. One peptide, NSP1a/4, colocalizes with the viral RNA at the ER membrane; mutations in NSP1a correlate with increased viral titers *in vitro* and *in vivo*, suggesting a role for this protein in viral replication. The role for the NLS remains unclear; some reports suggest viral antigen is observed in the nucleus, while others find that it is excluded.

The second reading frame, ORF1b, overlaps ORF1a by 70 nucleotides and has no detectable start codon. Intensive research has determined that ORF1b is translated by a frameshift into the −1 frame. This frameshifting event is unique among plus-strand animal RNA viruses and requires a highly conserved shifty heptameric sequence (A_6C) as well as a downstream hairpin structure. This event, which occurs with frequencies up to 25% in cells, results in an ORF1a/1b fusion peptide. Cleavage near the 1a/1b border releases the ORF1b gene product: the viral RNA-dependent RNA polymerase (RdRp). Astrovirus polymerase is a supergroup 1 RdRp, a group which generally utilizes a VPg to initiate transcription. Although a VPg is postulated to exist and a putative VPg genomic linkage site has been identified, its existence is yet to be empirically proven.

Expression of the RdRp results in production of a minus-strand viral template. This generates multiple copies of the plus-strand genome as well as a polyadenylated subgenomic RNA (sgRNA) containing short 5' and 3' UTRs and ORF2. ORF2 is in the 0 frame and overlaps ORF1b slightly (four nucleotides) in human astroviruses. Production of the capsid protein from a sgRNA not only temporally restricts capsid production to later in the viral replication cycle, but also allows for massive capsid protein expression; it is estimated that sgRNA is produced in tenfold excess of the viral genome by 12 h post infection (hpi). The sgRNA is about 2.4 kb and encodes the single structural protein of approximately 87 kDa. This peptide is cleaved by an intracellular protease to approximately 79 kDa; mutational analyses suggest that this 8 kDa stretch is required for efficient expression of the capsid protein. Individual capsid proteins multimerize spontaneously to form icosahedral structures of about 32 nm (**Figure 1(b)**). Positive-sense genomes are packaged into these viral-like particles (VLPs), possibly through interactions with the first 70 amino acids of the capsid protein. The virions are released by an unknown mechanism, which may involve cellular caspases, after which the capsid undergoes an extracellular trypsin-mediated maturational cleavage. This increases infectivity up to 10^5 fold, condenses the

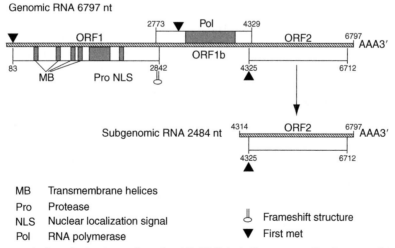

Figure 2 The genomic organization of astroviruses (based on HAstV-1), including open reading frames and encoded protein features, is shown. Reprinted from *Virus Taxonomy: Sixth Report of the International Committee on Taxonomy of Viruses*, 1995, p. 365, *Astroviridae*, Murphy FA, Fauquet CM, Bishop DHL, *et al.* (eds.), copyright 1995, with kind permission of Springer Science and Business Media.

virion to approximately 28 nm, and transforms the 79 kDa capsid protein into at least three smaller peptides of approximately 34, 29, and 26 kDa. Computational predictions suggest that VP34 may comprise the core of the virion while VP29 and VP26 form spike-like projections that may be important for viral tropism and receptor binding. This is corroborated by studies suggesting that VP26 is only loosely associated with the virion. These spikes are also thought to be responsible for the star morphology visible by EM (**Figure 1(a)**).

Evolution

Examination of nucleotide changes and nonsynonymous amino acid changes from the whole genome and across species suggests that an ancient divergence between avian and mammalian astroviruses occurred approximately 310 million years ago. Mammalian astroviruses split more recently into two distinct clades: human astroviruses and feline/mink-associated astroviruses. Phylogenetic clustering of the human astroviruses together argues against continual human–animal interspecies transmission. It is hypothesized that at least two interspecies transmission events (avian to porcine, porcine to feline) led to the current division of viruses. Further comparison of synonymous mutations by codon usage generates an astrovirus evolutionary pattern which mirrors the evolution of respective hosts, suggesting that recent evolution of the virus may have been in adaptation to the host. As RNA viruses, astroviruses are expected to undergo frequent genetic changes. However, nucleotide changes occur at rates of approximately 5% in human viruses over time, despite the co-circulation of muptiple serotypes within a region. Nucleotide and amino acid comparisons of ORF1a of human astroviruses demonstrate two distinct lineages, known as genogroup I (HAstV-1 to -5) and genogroup II (HAstV-6 and -7). Comparisons of ORF1b or ORF2 lack these distinct groups, leading investigators to postulate that a recombination event at the ORF1a/1b junction occurred before HAstV-6 or -7 diverged.

Clinical Features, Pathology, and Pathogenesis

Mammalian Astroviruses

Astrovirus infection in mammals presents clinically as gastroenteritis. Disease has been most closely studied in humans and, in volunteer studies, astrovirus-infected individuals develop diarrhea, the most prominent symptom, as well as vomiting, nausea, anxiety, headache, malaise, abdominal discomfort, and fever. Onset of symptoms at 2–3 days post infection (dpi) correlates with shedding of the virus in feces, although shedding can continue after resolution of other symptoms. Astrovirus infection has also

been associated with intussusception, although a causative role has not been established.

The earliest studies of astrovirus pathogenesis utilized gnotobiotic sheep and calves as models. In calves, astrovirus infection was localized to the dome epithelial cells overlying Peyer's patches. These cells appeared flat or rounded and released cells were identified in the intestinal lumen. Astrovirus infection in calves was shown to be specifically targeted to M cells and led to the sloughing of necrotic M cells into the intestinal lumen. Enterocytes were never observed to be infected. Specific tropism of the virus for immune cells suggests that astrovirus may have an immunomodulatory role in calves. While the virus replicated in these animals and could be detected in their feces, the calves displayed no clinical signs. In most bovine studies, viral infection is asymptomatic, although changes in the feces from solid and brown to soft and yellow were noted in one study. Mild villus atrophy and slight changes in villus-to-crypt ratios have been noted but no changes in xylose absorption were observed. Despite the lack of symptoms, viral shedding continued until the termination of the experiment.

Studies in sheep have shed more light on histological changes associated with infection. Astrovirus-infected sheep developed a transient diarrhea as early as 2 dpi, but virus was detected at early as 14 hpi and initially confined to the lumenal tips of the intestinal villi. By 23 hpi, virus was observed coating the microvilli and infection had spread to the apical two-thirds of the villi. This correlated with sloughing of degenerate cells from the apical portion of the villi, which continued through 38 hpi. At this time, villus blunting was apparent in the ileum and midgut. Furthermore, normal epithelial cells lining the villi were replaced with immature, cuboidal cells reminiscent of crypt cells. Neither these immature cells nor crypt cells were ever observed to be infected, suggesting that only mature enterocytes are susceptible to infection. By 5 dpi, viral infection had cleared and intestinal histology had returned to normal.

Volunteer studies in humans have not explored the underlying causes of astrovirus pathogenesis; our knowledge is therefore limited to intestinal biopsies taken for other reasons, but generally support the observations described above. In a biopsy from a child shedding large quantities of astrovirus, slight histological changes, including mild villous blunting and irregular epithelial cells, were observed. Infection increased distally through the small intestine. Similarly to animal models, astrovirus infection was restricted to the apical two-thirds of intestinal villi and could be identified in infected cells.

Avian Astroviruses

In avian species, astrovirus infection has a much broader range of disease than in mammals. While astrovirus does cause gastroenteritis in turkeys and chickens, it can also cause nephritis in chickens and a severe, often fatal, hepatitis in young ducklings.

Turkey astrovirus was the first discovered avian astrovirus and remains the best characterized in terms of pathogenesis, due in part to the development of the turkey as a small animal model. In these animals, virus could be detected from 1 to 12 dpi in the intestines. Viral replication was limited to the enterocytes on the apical portion of the villi, but the virus could be detected throughout the body, including the blood. The development of viremia is rare among enteric viruses and its function remains unclear. Infected turkeys developed a yellow, frothy, gas-filled diarrhea from 1 to 12 dpi. Diarrhea occasionally contained undigested food, but never blood. The intestines of infected birds became thin walled, flaccid, and distended. Despite these changes, histological examination suggested that only mild changes occur during infection. A mild crypt hyperplasia and shortening of the villi were noted from 4 or 5 to 9 dpi, and single degrading enterocytes could be identified. However, TUNEL staining suggested that the amount of cell death in infected intestines is similar to control birds. D-xylose absorption, a measure of intestinal absorption, was significantly decreased from 2 to 5 dpi in one study and up to 13 dpi in another. This effect was exacerbated in the presence of another enteric pathogen, turkey coronavirus. Astrovirus infection also caused a significant growth depression in turkey poults by 5 dpi; infected birds never recovered from this, leading to flock unevenness. Infected birds also demonstrated a transient (3–9 dpi) reduction of the thymus, which returned to normal by 12 dpi.

Avian infection by astroviruses can present with nonenteric symptoms as well. Infection of ducklings with duck astrovirus causes a severe hepatitis. Infected birds develop liver hemorrhage, swollen kidneys, and hepatocyte necrosis. On farms, infection leads to mortality rates of 10–25% in adult (4–6-week-old) ducks, but can reach 50% in ducklings under 14 days of age. In chickens, infection with the astrovirus avian nephritis virus (ANV) results in discoloration of the kidney, development of renal lesions, and interstitial nephritis by 3 dpi. Pathogenesis is age dependent, with 1-day-old chicks the most susceptible and adult birds the least. ANV infection can result in mortality rates of up to 33%, although rates appear to be strain specific.

Immune Response

The immunological response to astrovirus infection is poorly defined; however, observations in humans and animal models suggest that both the adaptive and innate responses play important roles in controlling and eliminating the virus.

The humoral immune response likely plays a major role in astrovirus immunity. The biphasic infection pattern of young children and the elderly suggests that antibodies are protective during the middle of life. Indeed, serological studies have indicated that approximately 50% of neonates have maternally acquired antibody to HAstV, which wane by 4–6 months of age. Children then acquire anti-HAstV antibodies rapidly due to astrovirus exposure. By the age of 9, up to 90% of the population has been exposed to HAstV-1. Furthermore, volunteer experiments demonstrate that astrovirus exposure generally leads to an increase in anti-astrovirus antibody titer. While astrovirus antibodies protected individuals from symptoms associated with infection, virus was identified in the feces, suggesting that such antibodies do not necessarily prevent viral replication. Additionally, immunoglobulin treatment has been attempted as a treatment for severe or chronic astrovirus infection. The results have been mixed and difficult to interpret, as the presence of astrovirus-specific antibodies in the immunoglobulin treatment was not always confirmed.

Cellular immunity may also play a role in controlling and/or preventing astrovirus infection. Studies have demonstrated that most individuals possess HLA-restricted, astrovirus-specific T cells. When stimulated with astrovirus in vitro, these cells produce tumor necrosis factor, interferon gamma, and occasionally interleukin (IL)-5 but not IL-2 or IL-4. These cytokines are typical of the T-helper-type response thought to be important in controlling viral infections. Individuals deficient in T and B-cell functions are unable to control infection, shedding virus to very high titers ($\geq 10^{14}$ particles ml^{-1}) and for extended periods of time (up to 18 months), further supporting the importance of cellular immunity.

Experiments in a turkey model demonstrate that the adaptive response is not the only important immunological response. In this model, no increase in T cells (CD4$^+$ or CD8$^+$) could be demonstrated after TAstV-2 infection. Moreover, while infected turkeys produced a slight increase in antibody production, these antibodies were not neutralizing and did not prevent against future infection. However, it was noted that macrophages from TAstV-2 infected turkeys produced significantly higher levels of nitric oxide (NO) both in vivo and upon stimulation ex vivo. Inhibition of NO in vivo led to a significant increase in viral production, while addition of exogenous NO decreased viral production to below the detection limit, suggesting that NO is an important factor in controlling astrovirus infection. The importance of macrophages and their role in astrovirus infection has been corroborated by observations in astrovirus-infected lambs, where EM showed virions within macrophages. Furthermore, it is possible that astroviruses have a mechanism to combat this response, as macrophages in astrovirus-infected turkeys demonstrate a reduced ability to phagocytose.

Treatment, Prevention, and Control

Because astrovirus infection is generally mild and self-limiting in humans, treatment is generally restricted to fluid rehydration therapy. This can often be accomplished at home; thus, hospital admittance is rare. No vaccine is yet available for humans, and as noted above, immunoglobulin treatment for immunocompromised individuals has been met with varying degrees of success. Additionally, no treatment for astrovirus-infected animals exists. The best solution, therefore, is prevention of transmission, which is best done in humans by conscientious hand and food washing. The stability of astroviruses and their resistance to inactivation make them difficult to eliminate after introduction. This is a significant problem in hospitals, where individuals are generally immunocompromised and therefore more susceptible to infection. One outbreak in a bone marrow transplant ward prompted the hospital to scrub the entire ward with warm, soapy water. However, surveillance of the subsequent inhabitants demonstrated fecal shedding of astroviruses, underscoring the difficulty in removing the virus. This is also a significant problem in commercial farming, where astrovirus infection of animals significantly decreases productivity. Its introduction and maintenance in this environment can mean drastic financial losses. In each of these environments, early detection and thorough disinfection are keys to limiting transmission and controlling infection.

See also: Enteric Viruses; Rotaviruses.

Further Reading

Koci MD (2005) Immunity and resistance to astrovirus infection. *Viral Immunology* 18: 11–16.

Koci MD and Schultz-Cherry S (2002) Avian astroviruses. *Avian Pathology* 31: 213–227.

Matsui SM and Greenberg HB (1996) Astroviruses. In: Fields BN, Knipe DM, and Howley PM (eds.) *Fields Virology,* 3rd edn., pp. 875–893. Philadelphia: Lippincott-Raven.

Monroe SS, Carter MJ, Herrmann JE, Kurtz JB, and Matsui SM (1995) *Astroviridae.* In: Murphy FA, Fauquet CM, Bishop DHL, *et al.* (eds.) *Virus Taxonomy: Sixth Report of the International Committee on Taxonomy of Viruses,* pp. 364–367. Vienna: Springer.

Monroe SS, Jiang B, Stine SE, Koopmans M, and Glass RI (1993) Subgenomic RNA sequence of human astrovirus supports classification of *Astroviridae* as a new family of RNA viruses. *Journal of Virology* 67: 3611–3614.

Bunyaviruses: General Features

R M Elliott, University of St. Andrews, St. Andrews, UK

Glossary

Ambisense Coding strategy used by some bunyaviruses in which a genome segment encodes proteins in both positive and negative sense orientations. This strategy also is employed by arenaviruses.

Bunyavirus Any member of the family *Bunyaviridae.*

Cap snatching Cleavage of the capped 5′-end of a cellular mRNA to produce short oligonucleotides that are used to prime viral mRNA transcription. The cellular sequences are incorporated into the viral mRNAs.

Reassortment Exchange of genome segments during the course of a mixed infection; generates new viruses.

Reverse genetics Rescue of infectious virus from cloned cDNA copies of the viral genome.

Vector competence Ability of an arthropod to transmit a pathogen.

Introduction

Currently more than 300 mainly arthropod-transmitted viruses are classified within the family *Bunyaviridae.* The majority of these viruses are classified into one of five genera: *Orthobunyavirus, Hantavirus, Nairovirus, Phlebovirus,* and *Tospovirus,* though more than 40 remain unassigned. The basic features that unite these viruses are similar virion morphology, negative-sense tripartite single-stranded RNA genome, and cytoplasmic site of viral replication with intracellular maturation in the Golgi. However, considering the large number of viruses within this one taxonomic grouping, it is not surprising that considerable diversity occurs in terms of biological behavior, and in genome coding and replication strategies. In this article, genus-specific traits are indicated with the terms orthobunyavirus, hantavirus, etc., while the term bunyavirus is reserved for familial traits. Bunyaviruses in all five genera impinge on human health and well-being (**Table 1**), either directly in causing diseases ranging from encephalitis (e.g., La Crosse virus) to hemorrhagic

Table 1 Selected important pathogens in the family *Bunyaviridae*

Genus/ virus	Disease	Vector	Distribution
Orthobunyavirus			
Akabane	Cattle: abortion and congenital defects	Midge	Africa, Asia, Australia
Cache Valley	Sheep, cattle: congenital defects	Mosquito	N. America
La Crosse	Human: encephalitis	Mosquito	N. America
Oropouche	Human: fever	Midge	S. America
Tahyna	Human: fever	Mosquito	Europe
Hantavirus			
Hantaan	Human: severe hemorrhagic fever with renal syndrome (HFRS), fatality 5–15%	Field mouse	Eastern Europe, Asia
Seoul	Human: moderate HFRS, fatality 1%	Rat	Worldwide
Puumala	Human: mild HFRS, fatality 0.1%	Bank vole	Western Europe
Sin Nombre	Human: hantavirus cardiopulmonary syndrome, fatality 50%	Deer mouse	N. America
Nairovirus			
Crimean–Congo hemorrhagic fever	Human: hemorrhagic fever, fatality 20–80%	Tick, culicoid fly	Eastern Europe, Africa, Asia
Nairobi sheep disease	Sheep, goat: fever, hemorrhagic gastroenteritis, abortion	Tick, culicoid fly, mosquito	Africa, Asia
Phlebovirus			
Rift Valley fever	Human: encephalitis, hemorrhagic fever, retinitis, fatality 1–10% Domestic ruminants: necrotic hepatitis, hemorrhage, abortion	Mosquito	Africa
Sandfly fever	Human: fever	Sandfly	Europe, Africa
Tospovirus			
Tomato-spotted wilt	Plants: over 650 species, various symptoms	Thrips	Worldwide

fever (e.g., Crimean-Congo hemorrhagic fever virus), or indirectly by causing disease in animals (e.g., Cache Valley and Akabane viruses) or crop plants (e.g., tomato spotted wilt virus). Furthermore, this family contains prime examples of emerging viruses such as Sin Nombre and related hantaviruses that have been identified in the Americas since 1993.

Bunyavirus Biology

Viruses in each genus are associated with a principal arthropod vector, with the exception of hantaviruses, which have no arthropod involvement in their life cycle. Gross generalizations can be made that orthobunyaviruses are mainly transmitted by mosquitoes, nairoviruses primarily by ticks, and phleboviruses by phlebotomine flies, ticks, and, notably for Rift Valley fever virus, mosquitoes as well. Tospoviruses are plant-infecting bunyaviruses that are transmitted by thrips. In all cases, the virus can replicate efficiently in the vector without doing overt damage to it, though behavioral changes to mosquito feeding patterns have been noted with some of them. Hantaviruses cause persistent infections in rodents and usually one particular

hantavirus is associated with rodents of one particular species. Humans are infected by inhaling aerosolized rodent excretions. Human-to-human transmission is rare but has been reported for Andes hantavirus.

The maintenance and transmission cycles of orthobunyaviruses have been studied in more detail than for other bunyaviruses, and involve both horizontal and vertical transmission between a restricted number of mosquito and vertebrate hosts (**Figure 1**). The integrity of the cycles is maintained even when the geographic distributions of the different hosts overlap in nature. Horizontal transmission usually refers to transmission to susceptible vertebrate hosts via the biting arthropod, with the resulting vertebrate viremia a source for infection for another feeding arthropod. Humans are often dead end hosts in that they rarely function as a source for further vector infection. Horizontal transmission can also refer to venereal transmission between mosquitoes, and has been reported for orthobunyaviruses. Vertical transmission is a major maintenance mechanism, particularly in periods of unfavorable climatic conditions. Virus can be maintained in mosquito eggs over winter or during periods of drought for months if not years, and when conditions allow, mosquito larvae emerge infected with the virus.

Vector competence is the term used to describe the ability of a particular arthropod species to transmit a virus, and is governed by both host and viral factors. After ingestion of virus in a blood meal, the virus infects the midgut cells, and then escapes into the hemocoel to allow disseminated infection of all organs. High level replication in the salivary glands provides the viral inoculum for transmission at the next feeding occasion. For orthobunyaviruses in the California serogroup, experiments with reassortant viruses (see later) determined that the viral factors associated with efficient infection of midgut cells and subsequent transmission mapped to the medium (M) RNA genome segment.

Virion Proteins and RNA Segments

The spherical bunyavirus particle is about 100 nm in diameter and electron microscopy reveals a fringe of spikes on the surface (**Figure 2**). The virion consists of four structural proteins: two internal proteins (N and L) and two external glycoproteins, termed Gn and Gc, which are inserted in the Golgi-derived viral membrane (**Figure 3**). The N protein (2100 copies per particle) encapsidates the RNA genome segments to form ribonucleoprotein complexes termed RNPs or nucleocapsids, to which the L protein (25 copies per particle) associates. There is no equivalent of a matrix protein to stabilize the virion

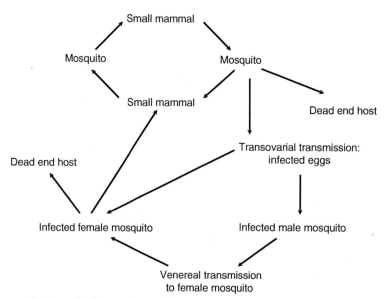

Figure 1   Life cycle of mosquito-transmitted bunyaviruses. From Elliott RM and Koul A (2004) *Bunyavirus/Mosquito Interactions*, symposium 63, pp. 91–102. Society for General Microbiology.

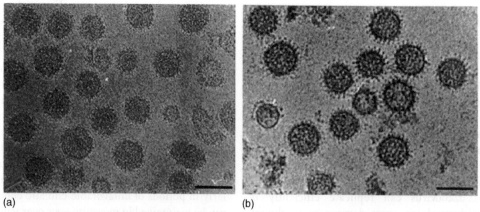

(a)   (b)

Figure 2   Electron micrographs of vitrified-hydrated La Crosse orthobunyavirus virions. (a) Small defocus value which demonstrates the membrane bilayer; (b) large defocus value which demonstrates the glycoprotein spikes (see Elliott (1990) for further details). Scale = 100 nm. The photographs were generously provided by Dr. B. V. V. Prasad. From Elliott RM (1990) Molecular biology of *Bunyaviridae*. *Journal of General Virology* 71(Pt. 3): 501–522.

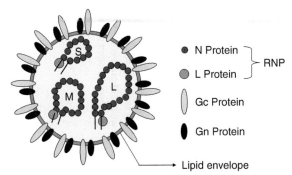

Figure 3   Schematic of bunyavirus particle.

Table 2   Consensus 3′ and 5′ terminal nucleotide sequences of bunyaviral genome RNAs

Orthobunyavirus	3′ UCAUCACAUGA...UCGUGUGAUGA 5′
Hantavirus	3′ AUCAUCAUCUG.........AUGAUGAU 5′
Nairovirus	3′ AGAGUUUCU...........AGAAACUCU 5′
Phlebovirus	3′ UGUGUUUC...............GAAACACA 5′
Tospovirus	3′ UCUCGUUAG............CUAACGAGA 5′

structure, and it is presumed that interaction between the cytoplasmic tail(s) of either or both of the glycoproteins and the N protein in the RNP is important for structural integrity of the virion.

The three genomic RNA segments, which are designated L (large), M (medium), and S (small), characteristically have complementary terminal sequences that are similar for the three segments of viruses within a genus, but differ between genera; the genus-specific consensus sequences are shown in **Table 2**. A consequence of the terminal complementarity is that the ends of the RNAs may base-pair, and circular or panhandle bunyavirus RNAs have been seen in the electron microscope. Bunyavirus nucleocapsids are also circular, and the ends of the RNA segments are base-paired within the RNP. It is probable that the encapsidation signal for the N protein is at the 5′-end of the RNA.

Coding Strategies of the Viral Genomes

Complete nucleotide sequences have been determined for at least one representative of each genus in the *Bunyaviridae* which has allowed the coding strategies of the individual genome segments to be elucidated. These are shown schematically in **Figure 4**.

The L RNA encodes the L protein using a conventional negative-strand strategy, that is, in a complementary positive-sense mRNA. The L protein contains motifs found in all RNA polymerases, and expression of recombinant L proteins, via a variety of systems, demonstrated the L

had RNA synthesis activity. The L protein is therefore at least a component of the virion-associated transcriptase.

The M segment encodes in the complementary sense mRNA the virion glycoproteins in the form of a precursor polyprotein. The M segment gene products have been implicated in many biological attributes of the virus including hemagglutination, virulence, tissue tropism, neutralization, and cell fusion. By convention, the glycoprotein of greater molecular weight (or slower electrophoretic mobility in sodium dodecyl sulfate–polyacrylamide gels) was termed G1, and the smaller glycoprotein G2. However, functional analyses of glycoproteins of viruses in different genera have revealed some commonality between the glycoproteins according to whether they are encoded at the N- or C-terminal region on the polyprotein. Therefore, the glycoproteins are now referred to as Gn or Gc. In the case of orthobunyaviruses, hantaviruses, and phleboviruses, the precursor is co-translationally cleaved to yield the mature proteins, which are characteristically rich in cysteine residues.

Orthobunyaviruses encode an additional, nonstructural protein called NSm between Gn and Gc, while some phleboviruses encode an NSm protein upstream of the glycoproteins, also as part of the precursor. Only the N-terminal domain of NSm is required for orthobunyaviruses to replicate in cell cultures, while the entire NSm region of Rift Vally fever phlebovirus can be deleted without compromising replication in cultured cells. However, the function of these NSm proteins remains unknown.

Tospoviruses encode an NSm protein, using an ambisense strategy. The NSm coding region is contained in the 5′ terminal part of the viral genomic RNA, but is translated from a subgenomic mRNA. This mRNA is transcribed from the full-length complement of the genomic RNA. The tospovirus NSm functions as a movement protein by forming tubular structures that penetrate through plasmadesmata and allow cell-to-cell transport of viral nucleocapsids.

Processing of the nairovirus M segment-encoded polyprotein is more complex, occurs over a period of several hours and involves the production of a number of intermediate proteins. Upstream of Gn are two domains, a highly variable region at the N-terminus (resembling the mucin-like domain observed in other viral glycoproteins) followed by a second domain (connector domain), both of which are cleaved in separate events from Gn, while a further domain is cleaved from between mature Gn and Gc (**Figure 3**). The function(s) of the released domains awaits further investigation.

The NSs protein of orthobunyaviruses and phleboviruses is dispensable for replication and is regarded as an accessory virulence factor. Although these NSs proteins are of different sizes, show no obvious sequence similarity, and are encoded by different mechanisms, they appear to

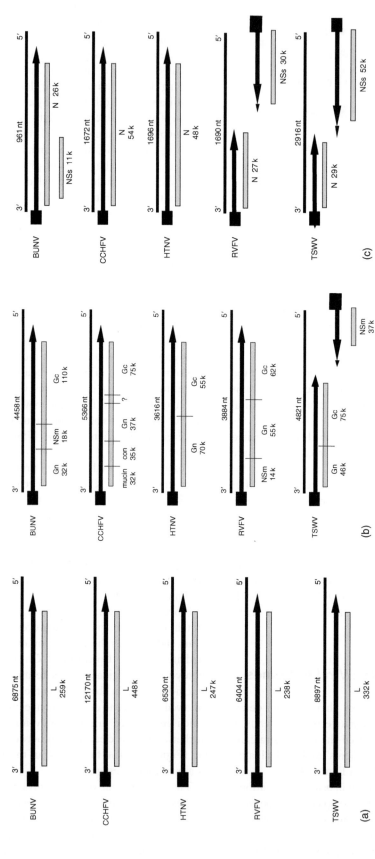

Figure 4 Coding strategies of bunyavirus genome segments. (a) L segment; (b) M segment; (c) S segment. Genomic RNAs are represented by thin lines (the length in nucleotides is given above each segment) and the mRNAs are shown as arrows (filled square indicates host-derived sequences at 5′-end). Gene products, with their apparent M_r, are represented by light colored boxes. Abbreviations: BUNV, Bunyamwera orthobunyavirus; CCHFV, Crimean-Congo hemorrhagic fever nairovirus; HTNV, Hantaan hantavirus; k, mole weight of protein 2; RVFV, Rift Valley fever phlebovirus; TSWV, tomato spotted wilt tospovirus. In (b), CCHFV M segment, mucin represents mucin-like region; con the connector region; and ? unidentified protein product.

have a similar function in antagonizing the host interferon (IFN) response. Studies on Bunyamwera and La Crosse orthobunyaviruses, engineered by reverse genetics (see below) to ablate the NSs open reading frame, and on an attenuated variant of Rift Valley fever phlebovirus that expresses a truncated NSs protein, showed that these mutant viruses induce IFN, whereas wild-type viruses do not. Further work revealed that the NSs proteins inhibited RNA polymerase II-mediated host transcription, thus preventing synthesis of IFN mRNA.

The S RNA segments also show great diversity in their coding strategies. The bunyavirus S segment encodes two proteins, N, and a nonstructural protein, NSs, in different overlapping reading frames in the complementary-sense RNA. The two proteins are translated from the same mRNA species, the result of alternative initiation at different AUG codons. For hantaviruses and nairoviruses, a single open reading frame, encoding the N protein, is found in the S segment complementary-sense RNA. The S segments of phleboviruses and tospoviruses employ an ambisense coding strategy; the N protein is encoded in the complementary-sense RNA corresponding to the 3' half of the genomic S segment, whereas the coding sequence for the NSs protein is contained in the 5' half of the genomic RNA. The proteins are translated from separate subgenomic mRNAs.

Genome Segment Reassortment

In common with other viruses with segmented genomes, bunyaviruses can reassort their genome segments during co-infection (**Figure 5**), and this phenomenon has been extensively studied for orthobunyaviruses in both cell cultures and in mosquitoes. There are barriers to the extent to which reassortment occurs in that it is restricted to antigenically closely related viruses within a genus, and certain segment combinations seem favored over others. In mosquitoes, reassortment of orthobunyavirus RNA segments occurs following ingestion of two viruses in a single blood meal or in separate feedings (mimicking interrupted feeding due to the host's physical reaction to the mosquito) provided the two events are temporally close. If the time between the infections is greater than 2 or 3 days, there is resistance to infection with the second virus. Reassortant viruses were used to map viral proteins and biological functions to these proteins with individual genome segments before the advent of nucleotide sequencing. Reassortment has been detected in nature, for instance, among various orthobunyaviruses, and of significance is the discovery that Ngari (originally called Garrissa) virus, an orthobunyavirus associated with human hemorrhagic fever, is a reassortant between the relatively innocuous viruses Bunyamwera and Batai.

Viral Replication Cycle

Attachment, Entry, and Uncoating

Infection of the target cell is mediated by one or both of the virion glycoproteins interacting with the cellular receptor. Receptors have not been formally identified for any bunyavirus, though cellular entry of hantaviruses involves $\beta 1$-integrins (apathogenic hantaviruses) or $\beta 3$-integrins (pathogenic hantaviruses). The relative importance of either of the glycoproteins in attachment

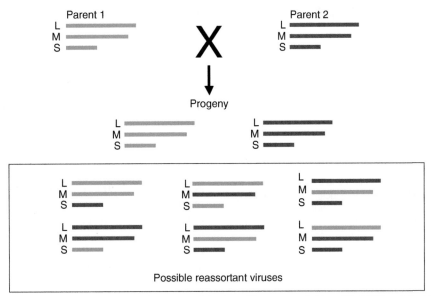

Figure 5 Generation of reassortant bunyaviruses following coinfection of the same cell. From Elliott RM and Koul A (2004) *Bunyavirus/Mosquito Interactions*, symposium 63, pp. 91–102. Society for General Microbiology.

has not been fully elucidated and may differ between the genera. For orthobunyaviruses, it has been suggested that Gc is the major attachment protein for vertebrate cells, whereas Gn may contain the major determinants for attachment to mosquito cells. Neutralization and hemagglutination-inhibition sites have been mapped to both glycoproteins encoded by hantaviruses and phleboviruses, suggesting that for these viruses both Gn and Gc may be involved in attachment. In common with many other enveloped viruses bunyaviruses can fuse cells at acidic pH; at least for orthobunyaviruses, this is accompanied by a conformational change in Gc. Based on electron microscopic studies of phleboviruses, entry into cells is by endocytosis. It is probable that uncoating occurs when endosomes become acidified, thus initiating fusion of the viral membrane and endosomal membrane, followed by release of the nucleocapsids into the cytoplasm.

Transcription

The classical scheme for replication of a negative-strand RNA virus is that the infecting genome is first transcribed into mRNAs by the virion-associated RNA polymerase or transcriptase (**Figure 6**). This process, termed primary transcription, is independent of ongoing protein synthesis. Following translation of the primary transcripts into viral proteins, the genome is replicated via a complementary full-length positive-strand RNA, the antigenome, and then further mRNA synthesis (secondary transcription) ensues.

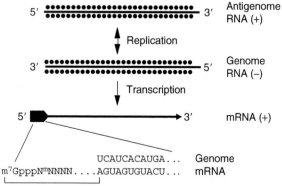

Host mRNA-derived primer

Figure 6 Transcription and replication scheme of negative-sense bunyavirus genome segments. The genome RNA and the positive-sense complementary RNA known as the antigenome RNA are only found as ribonucleoprotein complexes and are encapsidated by N protein (filled square). The mRNA species contain host-derived primer sequences at their 5'-ends (filled square) and are truncated at the 3'-end relative to the vRNA template; the mRNAs are neither polyadenylated nor encapsidated by N protein. The sequence at the 5'-end of an orthobunyavirus mRNA is shown. From Elliott RM (2005) Negative strand RNA virus replication. In: Mahy B and ter Meulen V (eds.) *Topley and Wilson's Microbiology and Microbial Infections*, 10th edn., vol. 1, pp. 127–134. London: Hodder Arnold.

Transcriptase activity has been detected in detergent-disrupted virion preparations of representatives of most *Bunyaviridae* genera. The enzymatic activity was weak compared to, for example, the transcriptase of vesicular stomatitis virus, which has hampered extensive biochemical characterization of the enzyme. However, the bunyavirus transcriptase was shown to be stimulated by oligonucleotides of the (A)nG series, cap analogs (e.g., mGpppAm) and natural mRNAs, such as alfalfa mosaic virus RNA 4. These appeared to act as primers for transcription. Further support for this notion was provided by sequencing studies of the 5'-ends of both *in vivo* and *in vitro* synthesized mRNAs, which showed they contained an additional 10–18 nontemplated nucleotides; a cap structure was present at the 5' terminus. *In vitro*, an endonuclease activity which specifically cleaved methylated capped mRNAs was detected. Taken together, these data indicate that bunyavirus transcription is markedly similar to that of influenza viruses in using a cap-snatch mechanism to prime transcription. In contrast to influenza viruses, bunyavirus transcription is not sensitive to actinomycin D or α-amanitin, and occurs in the cytoplasm of infected cells. The apparent reiteration of viral terminal sequences at the junction between the primer and viral sequence itself suggests that the polymerase may slip during transcription; further analysis of hantavirus RNAs suggests that this may occur during replication as well, and has been dubbed prime-and-realign.

Analysis of bunyavirus primary transcription *in vivo*, however, appeared initially to produce results incompatible with the presence of a virion transcriptase, in that no mRNA synthesis could be detected in the presence of protein synthesis inhibitors in certain virus-cell systems. Further work showed that only short transcripts were produced in the absence of protein synthesis *in vivo*; subsequent gel electrophoresis analyses of the *in vitro* transcriptase products showed that these too were short transcripts. If the *in vitro* reaction was supplemented with rabbit reticulocyte lysate, however, full-length RNAs were synthesized. The translational requirement was not at the level of mRNA initiation, but rather during elongation or, more precisely, to prevent the transcriptase from terminating prematurely. A model to account for these observations proposes that in the absence of ribosome binding and protein translation the nascent mRNA chain and its template can base-pair, thereby preventing progression of the transcriptase enzyme. This translational requirement is not ubiquitous, however, since concurrent translation is not needed for efficient readthrough of premature termination sites in some strains of BHK cells or in C6/36 mosquito cells. Reconstitution and mixing experiments suggest that the translational requirement is mediated by a host cell factor, present in some BHK cells, which may promote interaction between the nascent mRNA and its template.

The 3'-ends of the bunyavirus mRNAs are not co-terminal with their genome templates. For the nonambisense segments, mRNAs terminate 50–100 nucleotides before the end of the template, though there does not appear to be a universal termination signal in the bunyaviruses. The pentanucleotide sequence UGUCG has been mapped as the transcription-termination signal in the Bunyamwera orthobunyavirus S segment, and the same or highly related motifs have been identified in the Bunyamwera virus L segment and in the S segments of other orthobunyaviruses. However, the motif is not present in orthobunyavirus M segments nor in the genomes of viruses in other genera. The subgenomic mRNAs transcribed from ambisense S segments terminate within the noncoding intergenic sequences in the RNA (**Figure 7**); for some but not all viruses, the intergenic region has the potential to form a stable hairpin structure, though the role of secondary structure in transcription termination is unclear. Bunyavirus mRNAs are not demonstrably 3' polyadenylated, but many have the potential to form stem–loop structures which may confer stability.

Genome Replication

In order to replicate the negative-sense genome RNA, a full-length complementary, positive-sense RNA, the antigenome, must be synthesized (**Figures 6** and **7**). This molecule differs from the positive-sense mRNA in that it does not have the 5' primer sequences and the 3'-end extends to the 5' terminus of the genomic RNA template. Experiments with minigenome systems show that only the viral L and N proteins are required for replication,

but it is not known what controls the switch from transcriptive to replicative mode of the polymerase. Two events differ between transcription and replication: initiation, which does not require a primer, and readthrough of the mRNA termination signal. The difference in initiation may be because the RNA polymerase is modified by a cellular protein. In the infected cell antigenomes are only found assembled into nucleocapsids; therefore, encapsidation of the nascent antigenome RNA may prevent its interaction with the template, thereby overcoming the mRNA termination signal.

Assembly and Release

Maturation of bunyaviruses characteristically occurs at the smooth membranes in the Golgi apparatus, and hence is inhibited by monensin, a monovalent ionophore. The viral glycoproteins accumulate in the Golgi complex and cause a progressive vacuolization. However, the morphologically altered Golgi complex remains functionally active in its ability to glycosylate and transport glycoproteins destined for the plasma membrane. Using recombinant expression systems, it has been shown that the targeting of the bunyavirus glycoproteins to the Golgi is a property of the glycoproteins alone, and does not require other viral proteins or virus assembly. Electron microscopic studies revealed that viral nucleocapsids condense on the cytoplasmic side of areas of the Golgi vesicles, whereas viral glycoproteins are present on the luminal side. The absence of a matrix-like protein in bunyaviruses, which for other viruses may function as a bridge between the nucleocapsid and the glycoproteins,

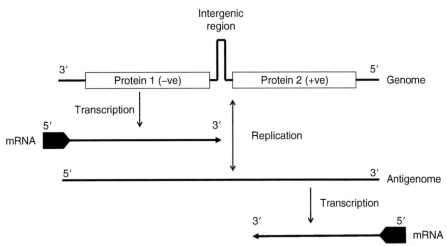

Figure 7 Transcription and replication scheme of ambisense-sense bunyavirus genome segments. The genome RNA encodes proteins in both negative- and positive-sense orientations, separated by an intergenic region that can form a hairpin structure. The proteins are translated from subgenomic mRNAs, with the mRNA encoding protein 2 transcribed from the antigenome RNA after the onset of genome replication. From Elliott RM (2005) Negative strand RNA virus replication. In: Mahy B and ter Meulen V (eds.) *Topley and Wilson's Microbiology and Microbial Infections*, 10th edn., vol. 1, pp. 127–134. London: Hodder Arnold.

suggests that direct transmembrane interactions between the bunyavirus nucleocapsid and the glycoproteins may be a prerequisite for budding. After budding into the Golgi cisternae, vesicles containing viral particles are transported to the cell surface via the exocytic pathway, eventually releasing their contents to the exterior.

There are important exceptions, however, to the above maturation scheme; Rift Valley fever phlebovirus has been observed to bud at the surface of infected rat hepatocytes, and it appears that a characteristic of the newly described American hantaviruses which cause hantavirus pulmonary syndrome is assembly and maturation occurring at the plasma membrane.

Persistent Infections

Arboviruses share a common biological property in their capacity to replicate in both vertebrate and invertebrate cells. The outcomes of these infections can be markedly different; whereas infection of vertebrate cells is often lytic, leading to cell death, infection of invertebrate cells is often asymptomatic, self-limiting, and leads to a persistent infection. For bunyaviruses this has been demonstrated both at the organismic level and in cultured cells. Studies of persistent infections of mosquito cells with orthobunyaviruses showed no inhibition of host cell protein synthesis, in sharp contrast to replication in mammalian cells. A feature of the persistently infected cells was the excess amount of S segment RNA they contained, but although the level of S mRNA remained high the amount of N protein translated declined. Blockage of N protein synthesis was shown to be because N was able to encapsidate its own mRNA, thereby preventing its translation. Defective L segment RNAs were also found in the persistently infected cells, but these were not packaged into virions. In contrast, a novel type of defective interfering particle was produced which contained only S segment RNA. It is highly probable that host cell factors contribute to these events, but the identity of these factors awaits further investigation.

Reverse Genetics

Reverse genetic approaches to the study of bunyavirus RNA synthesis have been described, in which transiently expressed recombinant N and L proteins transcribe and replicate synthetic RNA transcripts containing a reporter gene. A system to recover infectious Bunyamwera orthobunyavirus entirely from cloned cDNA copies of the three genome segments was developed in 1996, and improvements to this system paved the way for the subsequent recovery of La Crosse virus and Rift Valley fever viruses. These represent significant accomplishments in bunyavirology and will allow future in-depth studies of the functions of all the viral proteins as well as detailed investigation of biological properties such as virulence, tissue tropism, and vector competence. It is expected that similar systems will be developed for viruses in the other *Bunyaviridae* genera. In the longer term, the design and recovery of specifically modified viruses having potential as vaccines may be feasible. For instance, a recombinant Bunyamwera virus containing a modified L RNA segment (L coding region flanked by M segment noncoding sequences) was found to be attenuated for replication in cell cultures and in mice.

See also: Crimean-Congo Hemorrhagic Fever Virus and Other Nairoviruses; Hantaviruses.

Further Reading

Billecocq A, Spiegel M, Vialat P, *et al.* (2004) NSs protein of Rift Valley fever virus blocks interferon production by inhibiting host gene transcription. *Journal of Virology* 78: 9798–9806.

Bridgen A and Elliott RM (1996) Rescue of a segmented negative-strand RNA virus entirely from cloned complementary DNAs. *Proceedings of the National Academy of Sciences USA* 93: 15400–15404.

Bridgen A, Weber F, Fazakerley JK, and Elliott RM (2001) Bunyamwera bunyavirus nonstructural protein NSs is a non-essential gene product that contributes to viral pathogenesis. *Proceedings of the National Academy of Sciences USA* 98: 664–669.

Elliott RM (ed.) (1996) *The Bunyaviridae*, 337pp. New York: Plenum Press.

Elliott RM (1990) Molecular biology of *Bunyaviridae*. *Journal of General Virology* 71: 501–522.

Elliott RM (2005) Negative strand RNA virus replication. In: Mahy BWJ and ter Meulen V (eds.) *Topley and Wilson's Microbiology and Microbial Infections*, 10th edn., vol. 1, pp. 127–134. London: Hodder Arnold.

Elliott RM and Koul A (2004) *Bunyavirus/Mosquito Interactions*, symposium 63, pp. 91–102. Society for General Microbiology.

Lowen AC, Boyd A, Fazakerley JK, and Elliott RM (2005) Attenuation of bunyavirus replication by rearrangement of viral coding and non-coding sequences. *Journal of Virology* 79: 6940–6946.

Lowen AC, Noonan C, McLees A, and Elliott RM (2004) Efficient bunyavirus rescue from cloned cDNA. *Virology* 330: 493–500.

Nichol ST, Beaty BJ, Elliott RM, *et al.* (2005) *Bunyaviridae*. In: Fauquet CM, Mayo MA, Maniloff J, Desselberger U,, and Ball LA (eds.) *Virus Taxonomy: Eighth Report of the International Committee on Taxonomy of Viruses*, pp. 695–716. San Diego, CA: Elsevier Academic Press.

Nichol ST, Spiropoulou CF, Morzunov S, *et al.* (1993) Genetic identification of a hantavirus associated with an outbreak of acute respiratory illness. *Science* 262: 914–917.

Sanchez AJ, Vincent MJ, Erickson BR, and Nichol ST (2006) Crimean-Congo hemorrhagic fever virus glycoprotein precursor is cleaved by Furin-like and SKI-1 proteases to generate a novel 38-kilodalton glycoprotein. *Journal of Virology* 80: 514–525.

Schmaljohn C and Hooper JW (2001) *Bunyaviridae*: The viruses and their replication. In: Knipe DM and Howley PM (eds.) *Fields Virology* 4th edn., pp. 1581–1602. Philadelphia: Lippincott Williams and Wilkins.

Weber F, Bridgen A, Fazakerley JK, *et al.* (2002) Bunyamwera bunyavirus non-structural protein NSs counteracts the induction of type I interferon. *Journal of Virology* 76: 7949–7955.

Won S, Ikegami T, Peters CJ, and Makino S (2006) NSm and 78-kilodalton proteins of Rift Valley fever virus are nonessential for viral replication in cell culture. *Journal of Virology* 80: 8274–8278.

Common Cold Viruses

S Dreschers and C Adams, University of Duisburg–Essen, Essen, Germany

Glossary

ASM Acid sphingomyelinase (EC 3.1.4.12), enzyme cleaving sphingomyelin to ceramide and phosphatidylcholine under low pH conditions.
ICAM-1 Intercellular adhesion molecule-1, belongs to the immunoglobulin superfamily.
IRES Internal ribosomal entry site; the sequence enables ribosomes to start translation within a mRNA.
ITAM Immunoreceptor-tyrosine based activation motif; enables proteins to bind to non-receptor tyrosine kinases.
NPDA Niemann–Pick disease type A; patients lack a functional ASM gene and suffer from a malfunctioning lipid storage due to the accumulation of sphingomyelin.
MBCD Methyl-β-cyclodextrin; drug depleting cholesterol out of membranes.

Introduction

Everyone knows the first signs of a common cold. Symptoms usually begin 2–3 days after infection and often include obstruction of nasal breathing, swelling of the sinus membranes, sneezing, cough, and headache. Although the symptoms are usually mild, this (probably the most common illness known to man) exhibits an enormous economic impact due to required medical attention or restriction of activity. According to estimations of the National Center for Health Statistics (NCHS), the common cold caused 157 million days of restricted activity and 15 million days lost from work in 1992. The progress of molecular biology in the twentieth century allowed the isolation and *in vitro* culture of rhinoviruses as well as their ultrastructural and molecular analysis. From the beginning of recorded history to our time people have been interested in how the common cold is spread. Famous ancient investigators, among them Hippocrates and Benjamin Franklin to name two, were the first to suggest inhalation of contaminated air as the origin of infection. This observation still holds its validity, but touching infectious respiratory secretions on skin and on environmental surfaces (desktops, doorknob, etc.) and subsequently touching the eyes or nose is now believed the most common mode of transmission. This article aims to summarize the knowledge about rhinoviral infections and discusses mechanisms of internalization, activation of host-cell receptor molecules, and details of possible therapeutic strategies.

Taxonomic Identification, Genome Organization, and Replication Cycle of Rhinoviruses

The establishment of cell and tissue culture techniques as well as nucleotide sequencing methods allowed for taxonomic classification of rhinoviruses. An overall RNA sequence compilation revealed a close genetic similarity to polio- and coxsackiviruses; hence, rhinoviruses were identified as members of the family *Picornaviridae*.

Genome Organization

The genomic organization is similar in all genera of *Picornaviridae* (**Figure 1**). The 5′ end of the RNA is joined to a small viral protein called VPg, which is a prerequisite for the synthesis of the negative RNA strand as a template for replication. The genomes of *aphtho-, erbo-, kobu-, tescho-, cardioviruses* (e.g., the foot and mouth disease virus) contain an additional gene (leader) at the 5′ end of the RNA. The 5′ end also contains the internal ribosomal entry site (IRES) sequence and allows binding to the ribosomal subunits of the host translational machinery. Following the IRES sequence is a single long open reading frame (ORF) encoding the structural (or capsid forming) proteins designated as the P1 precursor and nonstructural proteins (proteases and RNA-dependent RNA polymerase) designated as the P2/P3 precursors(s) (see **Figure 1**). The RNA genome is completed by the 3′ nontranslated region and a poly-A tail.

Translation of the Polyprotein, Processing, and Capsid Maturation

The protease 2A^{pro} coded by the P2 precursor was found to have multiple functions. It is required for the inital proteolytic separation of the P1 and P2/P3 precursors in the nascent rhinoviral polyprotein, but also inactivates the cellular *eLF-4F* complex, thereby inhibiting the translation of the cellular mRNA and initiating the virus host shutoff (VHS – the translational machinery of the host cell is producing viral proteins only). Further steps of the post-translational maturation are catalyzed by the protease 3C^{pro}/3CD^{pro} (see below). Products of the latter proteolytic activity are the VPg protein and the RNA

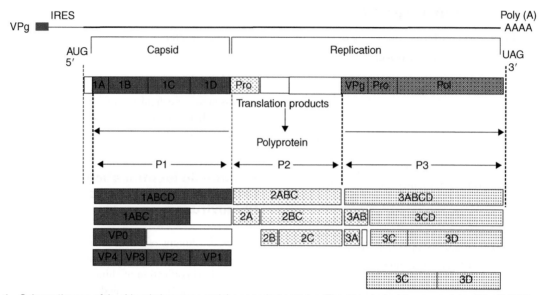

Figure 1   Schematic map of the rhinoviral genome and the encoded proteins. The rhinoviral genome consists of the 5′ IRES sequence (thin black line), followed by one open reading frame (bold black line) and the polyadenylation site. At the 5′ end the VPg protein is linked covalently to the RNA. Below, the regions representing the rhinoviral polyprotein are given. Compounds forming the capsid (structural proteins P1, blue boxes) and nonstructural proteins (P2–P3) such as proteases and the polymerase (light-blue dotted boxes and red dotted boxes, respectively) are translated into one polyprotein. The polyprotein becomes (auto-) proteolytically cleaved until the mature proteins are ready to form new viral particles.

polymerase. The capsid is composed of four proteins (viral proteins, VP1–VP4, see **Figure 1**), which arise from a single polyprotein generated from the viral RNA genome functioning as an mRNA. The very first cleavage occurs while translation is still in process. This first proteolytic maturation *in cis* is carried out by the protease 2A^{pro}, which separates structural proteins from those necessary for the replication (designated as P1 and P2/P3, see **Figure 1**). A series of further cleavages form VP1, VP3, and VP0; the latter is finally processed to result in VP2 and VP4. Many picornaviruses undergo VP0 cleavage during virion maturation. Apparently, intact VP0 is necessary for correct assembly of the protomers, whereas processing of VP0 is necessary for the final maturation of the virion. Both viral proteases are targets for an inhibitor screen (see below).

Genome Replication

The following steps of rhinoviral reproduction probably do not differ from other members of the *Picornaviridae*. The RNA genome can be instantly translated; however, for replication of the genome a complementary (−) strand must be synthesized first. Essential for this step is a priming reaction, which is started by the VPg precursor 3AB. The hydrophobic portion of this protein is anchored in endomembranes and is linked to a poly-U tail. After formation of an RNA:RNA duplex at the 3′ end of the (+) strand, the polymerase synthesizes new (−) RNA strands. Only 5–10% of all rhinoviral RNAs are (−) strands.

The synthesis of a complete genome takes 45 s to a minute, underlining that the reproduction cyle of picornaviruses in general and of rhinoviruses in particular is a fast process.

Synthesis of rhinoviral RNA in nasal washings could be detected 12 h post infection by quantitative reverse transcription-polymerase chain reaction (RT-PCR). The production of viral RNA and viral particles peaks within 48–72 h and declines thereafter.

Attachment and Entry

Studying any viral reproduction prompts the question of how viruses attach and invade cells. Therefore, the identification of cellular receptors binding to rhinoviruses was a landmark in examining how the infection cycle works. Intercellular adhesion molecule-1 (ICAM-1; CD54) was first detected as the receptor for major group rhinoviruses and later very low density lipoprotein (V)LDL as the receptor for minor group rhinoviruses (**Figure 2**). The receptors were isolated by using monoclonal antibodies directed against cellular surface proteins (see below). The receptors for the minor and major group rhinoviruses are structurally nonrelated, and the molecular reason why rhinoviruses as well as other members of the *Picornaviridae* (e.g., coxsackieviruses) use different receptors is not well understood. One strain (CAV-A21) of the rhinovirus-related family of coxsackieviruses needs to engage both ICAM-1 and decay-accelerating factor (DAF; CD55), whereas other

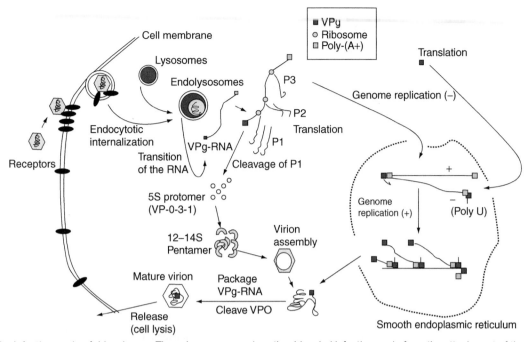

Figure 2 Infection cycle of rhinoviruses. The scheme summarizes the rhinoviral infection cycle from the attachment of the capsid to the release of newly synthesized capsids. Shown are the internalization of the capsids via endocytosis, the transport to the endolysosmal compartment, transition of the RNA to the cytoplasm, synthesis of viral RNA within the smooth endoplasmic reticulum, maturation of the capsid proteins, and self-assembly.

coxsackieviruses require DAF or integrins for binding. HRV binding to ICAM-1 allows a conformational change of the rhinoviral capsid and is a prerequisite for the uncoating of viral RNA. Although binding to (V)LDL receptors is also important for the internalization, the acidification of the endosome seems to be indispensable for proper entry, in particular for minor group rhinoviruses. (V)LDL receptors are well-described molecules, and the uptake of their natural ligands via clathrin-coated vesicles suggested that minor group rhinoviruses enter the host cell via the same pathway. Microscopical studies have detailed the uptake of the minor group rhinovirus HRV2. This viral serotype was shown to cluster to membrane domains positive for clathrin, supporting the notion of an uptake mechanism depending on clathrin-coated vesicles. In line with this finding is the blockade of HRV2 uptake by overexpression of dynamin-K44, a transdominant negative isoform of dynamin, which is required for pinching off clathrin-coated vesicles from the plasma membrane. Uptake of rhinoviruses via clathrin-coated vesicles is very fast and does not take longer than 30 min. Moreover, preincubation with methyl-β-cyclodextrin (MBCD) interrupts the uptake of HRV2 at an early stage. Rhinoviral capsids pile up close to the plasma membrane and are not transported to the endolysosomal compartment in cells treated with MBCD. MBCD depletes cholesterol from cellular membranes and leads to destabilization of membrane domains which are thought to play a central

role in signal transduction and endocytosis. Recent work indicates that another subgroup of membrane domains termed ceramide-enriched membrane platforms plays a crucial role in the infection cycle of rhinoviruses. These studies demonstrate that pharmacological or genetic inhibition of ceramide-enriched platforms reduces rhinoviral titers in epithelial cells. Membrane domains may not only be involved in the first steps of internalization, but also play a role in transport of vesicles and fusion of transport vesicles, endosomes, and endolysosomal vesicles, finally triggering acidification of the vesicle which is required for uncoating of rhinoviruses and transition of the RNA to the cytoplasm (see below).

Virion/Particle Structure and Phylogenetic Considerations

Human rhinoviruses (HRVs) represent the serologically most diverse group of picornaviruses (over 100 serotypes have already been identified). The reason for this diversity is not known.

The Canyon Hypothesis

Ultrastructural analysis of rhinoviruses by X-ray crystallography resulted in a structural model of rhinoviruses

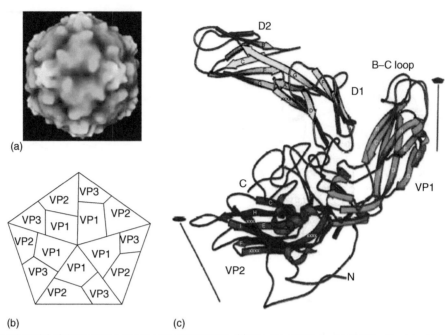

(a)

(b)   (c)

Figure 3 Structural model of rhinoviruses and receptor interaction. (a) The structural model of rhinoviruses was evaluated from cryo-electron microscopic data, the schematic drawing (b) represents the position of the capsid proteins VP1–VP3 in the rhinoviral capsid. (c) Schematic drawing of the viral canyon structure (represented by the capsid compounds VP1 and VP2 given in blue and green, respectively) and the D1 and D2 domains of the receptor ICAM-1. The antiparallel β-strand structures of VP1, VP2, and ICAM-1 are listed in alphabetical order.

(**Figure 3**). Along the fivefold icosahedral axis of the virion a 2.5 nm depression, the so-called 'canyon', was detected. The genomic region encoding the peptide residues that form this structure is more conserved than regions encoding any other structure on the virion surface. Studies using mutated viral strains showed that point mutations in the genomic region covering the capsid protein VP1 changed the affinity of radiolabeled mutant viruses to purified host cell membranes (**Figure 4** and **Table 1**). Alterations of amino acids at position 103 (Lys), 155 (Pro), 220 (His), or 223 (Ser), had the strongest effect regarding the binding affinity of rhinoviral capsids. The structural analysis revealed a juxtaposition of these amino acids at the 'bottom of the canyon'. It is noteworthy that most of the substitutions reduced the binding of capsids to host cell membranes; however, the biochemical property of one amino acid (Pro 155) is of special importance because a change to glycine led to a higher binding affinity and an enhanced yield of mutated virus. Most publications concerning rhinoviral structure described members of the major group rhinoviruses, while only few publications dealt with the structure of minor group rhinoviruses. It was possible to define structural differences between HRV2 (representing minor group rhinoviruses) and HRV14 (representing major group viruses) by analyzing a special subportion of the 'canyon', the 'pocket' region within the VP1 protein. This region binds in particular to hydrophobic compounds – for example, fatty acids supplemented by membranes of the

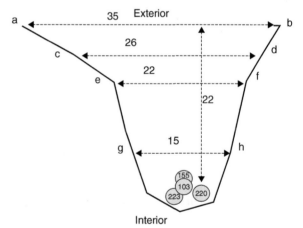

Figure 4 Mutations in the rhinoviral protein VP1 interfere with attachment and growth. The figure displays a scheme of the HRV-14 canyon. Distances are shown in angstrom and circled numbers represent the four amino acids targeted in the studies. Coordinate points used in determining distances are as follows: a, O^{81} of Asp-91; b, O^{e2} of Glu-210; c, O^{81} Asn-92; d, O Glu-210; e, O^{e2} Glu-95; f, N^{e2} Gln-212; g, O^{11} Asp-101; h, C^{81} Ile-215. Modified from Colonno RJ, Condra JH, Mizutani S, Callahan PL, Davies ME, and Murcko MA (1988) Evidence for the direct involvement of the rhinovirus canyon in receptor binding. *Proceedings of the National Academy of Sciences, USA* 85(15): 5449–5453.

host cell. The interaction of the virus with the fatty acid seems to stabilize the virus during its spread from cell to cell, but it must be removed prior to the uncoating process. For major group viruses the fatty acid is displaced

Table 1 Mutations in the rhinoviral protein VP1 interfere with attachment and growth

Position of wt amino acids	Substitutions	Virus yield (pfu/cell)
103 Lys	—	160
	Ile	84
	Arg	54
	Asn	140
155 Pro	—	160
	Gly	1
220 His	—	160
	Ile	10
	Trp	14
223 Ser	—	160
	Ala	8
	Thr	70
	Asn	88

by ICAM-1. The minor group viruses exhibit a higher affinity for the fatty acids and binding of LDL-R is insufficient to expel the fatty acid in the 'pocket' of VP1. The conformational change of the viral capsid is obligatory for the transition of the viral RNA into the cytoplasm. Acidification of the endolysosomal compartment transfers the native virus to a so-called C-antigenic subviral particle in which VP1 forms a channel with a diameter around 10 A – large enough for the RNA to escape. Concomitantly, the N-terminus of VP1 and the entire VP4 are extruded and interact with the endolysosomal membrane. Studies with rhinovirus-related poliovirus identified a 3 kDa peptide from the N-terminus of VP1 capable of integrating into artificial liposomes.

Rhinoviral Antigenicity

Antibodies that neutralize rhinoviruses *in vitro* and *in vivo* permitted the identification of the epitopes in the viral capsid critically important for binding to the receptors and/or release of the RNA into the cytoplasm. Antigenicity in HRVs has been extensively studied in serotypes HRV2 and HRV14. In HRV14 four antigenic sites were identified, designated NIm-IA, NIm-IB, NIm-II, and NIm-III. The sites could be accurately located at the external surface of the virus. In HRV2 three antigenic sites, called A, B, and C could also be mapped. Antigenic site A is located within the B–C loop of VP1 that flanks the rim of the canyon structure, thus, corresponding to the NIm-IA, NIm-IB site of HRV14. Site B encompasses residues from VP1, VP2, and VP3. VP2 residues of site B comprise a continuous epitope that is equivalent to the NIm-II site of HRV14 and mainly defined by the VP2 loop between the β-barrel strands E and F. Antigenic site C includes two amino acids of VP2 which do not correspond to any of the immunogenic sites of major group rhinoviruses.

Phylogenetic Considerations

In addition to the classification based on serotyping, rhinoviruses can be grouped in different ways, on the basis of shared structural and biological properties (e.g., receptor specificity), sensitivity to antiviral agents or at least genetic similarity. The phylogenetic analysis of the genomic VP4/VP2 interval of 97 different rhinoviral serotypes resulted in two phylogenetic clades, A and B. Surprisingly, some of the 76 serotypes of class A were identified as minor group rhinoviruses such as HRV 1A, 2, etc., whereas class B consists of 25 serotypes, among them major group HRV 14. According to the phylogenetic analysis, two rhinoviral serotypes (HRV 23 and HRV25) which bind to ICAM-1 (major group) constitute an 'intermediate' class between A and B, respectively. Further studies showed that soluble ICAM-1 could not compete with viral binding to cellular ICAM-1. Furthermore, the phylogenetic analysis identified one serotype, namely HRV 87, as closely related to another *Picornaviridae* genus the enteroviruses, namely enterovirus 70. HRV87 does not bind to either ICAM-1 or (V)LDL receptors, but to sialoproteins, which also bind enterovirus 70. Although HRV 87 is acid-labile like all other rhinovirus serotypes, it appears to belong to the enterovirus species D. In general, the analysis shows a greater phylogenetic heterogeneity for minor group rhinoviruses than for major group rhinoviruses, which may indicate that minor group serotypes evolved more recently.

Rhinovirus Infection Models

Rhinoviruses show an almost strict specificity for human cells. Most studies, therefore, have to be carried out in human volunteers or, alternatively, in primates, which necessitates special requirements regarding biosafety of the rhinoviral stock preparations, and raises ethical questions. Some publications reported that host restriction could be overcome by using a method to select rhinovirus strains which are able to infect murine cells. Another possible technique to overcome the host range problem is by expression of human/murine chimeric rhinoviral receptors. Engineered ICAM-1 molecules, stably expressed in murine cell lines, bind rhinoviruses and permit the uptake in murine respiratory cells and L-cells. The latter study underlined that mutations in noncapsid proteins (genomic region P2) are necessary to adapt viral proteins to the new host cell and finally allow an appropriate replication in murine cells. Other researchers developed human ICAM-1 transgenic mice that were recently used in infection studies with coxsackiviruses, and might also be utilized to study rhinoviral infections. Interestingly, a common finding of the field is noteworthy: receptors such as ICAM-1, VCAM-1, and also the (V) LDL play a predominant role in rhinovirus binding, uptake, and associated signal transduction processes. However, these data were determined from infection experiments employing poorly differentiated epithelial cells in culture. In contrast, these molecules are only infrequently expressed *in vivo* on the apical surface, leading to the question of how viruses access these receptors *in vivo*. In addition, the issue whether epithelial cell layers are the primary targets of rhinoviruses remains to be determined, since infections do not result in cytopathic effects in the ciliated epithelial cells as shown for many other respiratory viruses. Many studies focused primarily on the detection of rhinovirus RNA in rhinopharyngeal tissues by means of RT-PCR or *in situ* hybridization showed that cells and tissues (e.g., the germinal layer in the adenoid tissue below the epithelial layer) are positive for rhinoviral RNA. Rhinoviruses can be cultured in WI-38 fibroblasts suggesting that fibroblasts in the rhinopharyngeal tissue can be targets for rhinoviral infection. It is also possible that rhinoviruses attach to and invade the epithelial layer by a mechanism different from that observed in cultured epithelial cells, that is, binding to ICAM-1 and (V) LDL receptors. Further studies are required to address these questions.

Host Cell Reactions upon Rhinoviral Infections – The Molecular Origin of Symptoms

Infection of the upper respiratory tract by HRV16 has been demonstrated to occur at localized portions of the epithelia and does not cause widespread lysis of the infected epithelia. This observation has suggested that the pathology induced by rhinovirus may be due in part to cytokine dysregulation rather than extensive epithelial necrosis observed in other viral infections.

HRV, as well as other respiratory pathogens, have been shown to induce production of many cytokines and chemokines, among them IL-4, IL-6, IL-8, and granulocyte macrophage colony stimulating factor (GMCSF), to name the most frequently published. The induction of chemokines triggers the inflammatory response, which is considered to enhance exacerbations like asthma and chronic obstructive pulmonary disease (COPD). A common feature of asthma and COPD exacerbations is a high level of IL-8 and an increased number of neutrophils in the sputum and nasal secretions of patients suffering an HRV infection.

Little is known, however, about the primary signaling pathways initiated by the rhinoviral infection cycle. Because signal transduction pathways of the LDL receptor family are difficult to understand, the experimental design concentrated on ICAM-1, the receptor for major group rhinoviruses. ICAM-1-inhibiting antibodies abrogated IL-8 production, but infection with UV-inactivated rhinovirus failed to do so, indicating that binding and entry events induced the chemokine response rather than causing effects resulting from viral replication. HRV ligation to ICAM-1 provokes recruitment of the tyrosine kinase syk to membrane domains in human airway epithelial cells. The tyrosine kinase syk belongs to the family of src receptor tyrosine kinases. The immunoreceptor tyrosine-based activation motif (ITAM) of syk recruits another protein, ezrin, and the syk–ezrin complex finally binds to ICAM-1. Autophosphorylation of syk activates the MAP-kinase p38-K in a biphasic manner, that is, after 1 h and 8–12 h after infection with major group rhinovirus HRV14. This finding is especially interesting because the induction of chemokines is temporally correlating with the second p38-K activation peak. The PI-3 kinase is related to the family of MAP kinases. Again, subsequent studies concentrated on very early phases (5–60 min post infection) of rhinoviral infection. Active PI-3 kinase could be precipitated from lysates of infected cells and isolated plasma membranes showed the presence of metabolic products (i.e., PI $(3,4,5)P_3$) of the PI-3 kinase. The same studies identified Akt and nuclear factor kappa B (NF-κB) as downstream targets of PI-3 kinase and thus completing this signal transduction pathway showed the binding of NF-κB to the IL-8 promoters.

Interestingly, the activation of PI-3 kinase is functionally connected to the HRV entry. Inhibition of PI-3 kinase by application of the drug Wortmannin reduced the uptake of radiolabeled HRV, due to the retention of HRV2 in endosomal compartments, which results in a reduced transition of the RNA and, therefore, a reduced viral titer.

Inflammatory reactions require effector cells such as macrophages and monocytes. A recent publication addressed the question if the production of chemokines is restricted to the nasal epithelial tissues or if chemokines are synthesized and secreted by lymphocytes. Therefore, alveolar macrophages and monocytes were infected with rhinovirus. After infection with HRV16 the production of the macrophage attractive protein-1 (MCP-1) was shown to be increased in monocytes and macrophages. Surprisingly, HRV16 induces the same signal transduction pathways in lymphocytes as in epithelial cells. Again, the p38-K is activated and engages the nuclear factor ATF-2 involving NF-κB. The signal transduction could be attenuated by preincubation of the lymphocytes with ICAM-1, suggesting that HRV can bind to and enter lymphocytes. However, propagation of rhinoviruses in lymphocytes was not an aim of this study. Finally, these results present the novel idea that cell types other than epithelial cells contribute to viral exacerbations of asthma as well as causing the symptoms of the common cold.

Antirhinoviral Strategies

Although the common cold is usually mild, with symptoms lasting a week or less, it is a leading cause of physician visits and of school/job absence in addition to several more severe exacerbations like asthma (see above). Initial studies that employed monoclonal antibodies to define candidates of viral receptors demonstrated a surprising 'immunological resistance' of rhinoviruses. On the one hand this is due to the fact that over 100 different rhinoviral serotypes have been isolated and antibodies raised against one serotype after immunization are not necessarily protective against a different serotype. However, the identification of the so-called 'canyon' allowed an additional explanation: if this 'canyon' represents the predominant site of receptor interactions, it is difficult to block with antibodies since the canyon is too narrow to enable interactions with the antigen. Both findings seem to rule out vaccination as a standard antirhinoviral treatment. Hence, the canyon structure dominated the development of therapeutic strategies (**Table 2**). Researchers were able to design chemical structures designated as 'pocket factors', interacting with amino acid residues in the canyon. Because of their chemical similarity to the primarily described drug WIN51711, an isoxazole derivative, such chemicals are generally termed WIN compounds. WIN compounds seem to function both as competitors for binding to the receptor and in a steric blockage interfering with the conformational change of the capsid necessary for the release of the genomic RNA. While WIN compounds have a significant effect in reducing the viral titer *in vitro*, the *in vivo* application was difficult. Structurally related substances like flavinoids, for example 4–6 Dichlorflavane, exhibited a better feasibility regarding application, but caused only little reduction of rhinovirus titers. The chemokines interferon-α/β are produced after viral infection. Host cells detect the presence of double-stranded RNA via activation of the toll-like receptor 3 (TLR-3),

and the main function of interferons is to induce IFN-stimulated genes, which attenuate viral replication. Some groups tested the application of interferons and interferon-inducers, respectively, and their interference with rhinoviral replication and production. Although high doses of interferons applied intranasally exhibited a prophylactic effect, these high doses of interferons required for the protective effect caused local erosions and nasal stuffiness.

Therefore, the interest shifted to alternative methods to attenuate or even to block rhinoviral infections and their symptoms. Even though vaccination seemed to be impossible (as pointed out before), some studies dealt with the question of how the human immune system responds to a rhinoviral infection. Rhinovirus inoculation induced both IgG and IgA presence in the serum and the airway, respectively, which neutralized the identical serotype upon reinfection. In studies using several different rhinovirus serotypes the generation of cross-reacting antibodies could be observed. Individuals with preexisting cross-reacting antibodies or cross-reacting antibodies derived from rabbits exhibited a partial immunity when challenged with any new rhinovirus serotype. However, a complete immunity is barely to be expected, because many studies showed that antirhinovirus-protecting IgA titers decreased already 2 months after infection. Nevertheless, a vaccination could attenuate the exacerbations of the infection, that is, reduce asthma and COPD.

Recent work indicates that lipid domains in the plasma membrane of infected cells are functional in signal transduction events caused by rhinoviral infections. Moreover, the lipid composition could influence the interaction of viral proteins with vesicular membranes during the transition of the RNA and replication. For example, rhinovirus uptake is sensitive to treatment with MBCD and blocks p38-K signaling, thus interrupting the release of chemokines and attenuate symptoms. The acid sphingomyelinase (ASM), which was shown to be crucial

Table 2 Substances interfering with the rhinoviral propagation

Tested compound	Functions in or interferes with
WIN factors	Interaction with the canyon structure, viral adhesion is suppressed
AG 7088	Blocks protease 3 C irreversibly and stops capsid maturation
Soluble ICAM-1	Competition with ICAM-1
Cytochalasin B	Interference with microfilaments and inhibition of vesicle maturation
Bafilomycin	Blocking endosomal acidification
Erythromycin	Reduction of ICAM-1 receptor, blocking endosomal acidification
Impramine	Blocking ASM and inhibiting ceramide-enriched platforms
Desipramine	Blocking ASM and inhibiting ceramide-enriched platforms
Nocodazole	Interference with macrofilaments and inhibiting vesicle maturation
zVAD	Antiapoptotic agent blocking caspases and release of new viruses
Wortmannin	PI-3-kinase inhibitor, blocks vesicle maturation
MBCD	Depletes cholesterol, destroys functional membrane domains, transport of virus is blocked

for generation of ceramide-enriched platforms, a subentity of lipid domains, might be an additional target to prevent HRV infections. Fibroblasts isolated from NPDA patients (Niemann-Pick disease type 1) lacking functional ASM were shown to be resistant to HRV infections. The ASM can be inactivated pharmaceutically by tricyclic antidepressants such as amitryptiline and imipramine. Studies in which the ASM was inhibited by these substances showed a dramatic decrease of viral reproduction, suggesting that the ASM is critically involved in the propagation of rhinoviruses in human cells. Drugs derived from the structure of tricyclic antidepressants might therefore be effective against rhinovirus infections.

Aside from antiviral drugs targeting the attachment and entry processes, antirhinovirus therapy could benefit from the identification of chemicals inhibiting viral maturation. As pointed out earlier, activation of protease 3C is a crucial step in the assembly of the capsid. Tripeptidyl alpha-ketoamides were identified as human rhinovirus protease 3C inhibitors. The protease 3C-inhibiting drug AG7088 (*ruprintivir*) showed a 100-fold reduction of rhinoviral titers and abrogated inflammatory responses as well. Clinical trials indicated that AG7088 could be administered to volunteers without adverse reactions. Subsequent studies are in progress, aiming at another rhinoviral protease (i.e., 2A) as a target for antirhinoviral therapy.

Further Reading

Colonno RJ, Condra JH, Mizutani S, Callahan PL, Davies ME, and Murcko MA (1988) Evidence for the direct involvement of the rhinovirus canyon in receptor binding. *Proceedings of the National Academy of Sciences, USA* 85(15): 5449–5453.

Olson NH, Kolatkar PR, Oliveira MA, *et al.* (1993) Structure of human rhinovirus complexed with its receptor molecule. *Proceedings of the National Academy of Sciences USA* 90: 86–93.

Rossman MG (1989) The canyon hypothesis. Hiding the cell receptor attachment site on a viral surface from immune surveillance. *Journal of Biological Chemistry* 264: 14587–14590.

Rossman MG, Arnold E, Erickson JW, *et al.* (1985) Structure of human common cold virus and functional relationship to other picornaviruses. *Nature* 317: 145–153.

Rossman MG, Bella J, Kolatkar PR, *et al.* (2000) Cell recognition and entry by rhino- and enteroviruses. *Virology* 269: 239–247.

Verdaguer N, Blaas D, and Fita I (2000) Structure of human rhinovirus serotype 2 (HRV2). *Journal of Molecular Biology* 300: 1179–1194.

Wang X, Lau C, Wiehler S, Erickson S, *et al.* (2006) Syk is downstream of intercellular adhesion molecule-1 and mediates human rhinovirus activationof p38 MAPK in airway epithelial cells. *Journal of Immunology* 177: 6859–6870.

Coronaviruses: General Features

D Cavanagh and P Britton, Institute for Animal Health, Compton, UK

Glossary

Infectious clone A full-length DNA copy of an RNA virus genome from which full-length viral RNA can be generated, leading to production of infectious virus.

Nidovirales (nidoviruses) An order comprising positive-sense RNA coronaviruses, toroviruses, arteriviruses, and roniviruses that have a common genome organization and expression, similar replication/transcription strategies, and form a nested set of 3′ co-terminal subgenomic mRNAs (*nidus*, Latin for nest).

Ribosomal frameshifting Movement (shift) backward by one nucleotide of a ribosome that is on an RNA, caused by particular RNA structures and sequences. Subsequent continuation of the progress of the ribosome is in a different open reading frame.

Introduction

Coronaviruses are known to cause disease in humans, other mammals, and birds. They cause major economic loss, sometimes associated with high mortality, in neonates of some domestic species (e.g., chickens, pigs). In humans, they are responsible for respiratory and enteric diseases. Coronaviruses do not necessarily observe species barriers, as illustrated most graphically by the spread of severe acute respiratory syndrome (SARS) coronavirus among wild animals and to man, with lethal consequences. As a group, coronaviruses are not limited to particular organs; target tissues include the nervous system, immune system, kidney, and reproductive tract in addition to many parts of the respiratory and enteric systems. A great advance in recent years has been the development of systems ('infectious clones') for modifying the genomes of coronaviruses to study all aspects of coronavirus replication, and for the development of new vaccines.

Taxonomy and Classification

The genus *Coronavirus* together with the genus *Torovirus* form the family *Coronaviridae*; members of these two genera are similar morphologically. The *Coronaviridae*, *Arteriviridae*, and *Roniviridae* are within the order *Nidovirales*. Members of this order have a similar genome organization and produce a nested set of subgenomic mRNAs (*nidus*, Latin for nest). To date, coronaviruses have been placed into one of three groups (**Table 1**). Initially, this was on the basis of serological relationships which subsequently have been supported by gene sequencing.

Virion Properties

Virions have a buoyant density of approximately $1.18 \, \mathrm{g \, ml^{-1}}$ in sucrose. Being enveloped viruses (**Figure 1(a)**), they are destroyed by organic solvents such as ether and chloroform.

Virion Structure and Composition

All coronaviruses have four structural proteins in common (**Figure 1(b)**): a large surface glycoprotein (S; *c.* 1150–1450 amino acids); a small envelope protein (E; *c.* 100 amino acids, present in very small amounts in virions); integral membrane glycoprotein (M; *c.* 250 amino acids); and a phosphorylated nucleocapsid protein (N; *c.* 500 amino acids). Group 2a viruses have an additional structural glycoprotein, the hemagglutinin-esterase protein (HE; *c.* 425 amino acids). This is not essential for replication *in vitro* and may affect tropism *in vivo*.

Virions are *c.* 120 nm in diameter, although they can be up to twice that size, and the ring of S protein spikes is approximately 20 nm deep. When present, the HE protein forms a layer 5–10 nm deep. In some species, the S protein is cleaved into two subunits, the N-terminal S1 fragment being slightly smaller than the C-terminal S2 sequence. The S protein is anchored in the envelope by a transmembrane region near the C-terminus of S2. The functional S protein is highly glycosylated and exists as a trimer. The bulbous outer part of the mature S protein is formed largely by S1 while the stalk is formed largely by S2, having a coiled-coil structure. S1 is the most variable part of the S protein; some serotypes of IBV differ from one another by 40% of S1 amino acids. S1 is the major inducer of protective immune responses. Variation in the S1 protein enables one strain of virus to avoid immunity induced by another strain of the same species.

The M glycoprotein is the most abundant protein in virions. In most cases, only a small part (~20 amino acids) at the N-terminus protrudes at the surface of the virus. There are three membrane-spanning segments and the

Table 1 Species of coronavirus[a]

Group 1	Group 2	Group 3
Subgroup 1a	*Subgroup 2a*	
Transmissible gastroenteritis virus (TGEV)	*Murine hepatitis virus* (MHV)	*Infectious bronchitis virus* (IBV)
Feline coronavirus (FCoV)	*Bovine coronavirus* (BCoV)	*Turkey coronavirus* (TCoV)
Canine coronavirus (CCoV)	*Porcine haemagglutinating encephalomyelitis virus* (HEV)	*Pheasant coronavirus* (PhCoV)
	Equine coronavirus (EqCoV)	
Ferret coronavirus (FeCoV)	Canine respiratory coronavirus (CRCoV)	
	Human coronavirus HKU1	
Subgroup 1b		*Duck coronavirus[b]* (DCoV)
Human coronavirus (HCoV) 229E	*Human coronavirus* (HCoV) OC43	*Goose coronavirus* (GCoV)
Porcine epidemic diarrhoea virus (PEDV)	*Human enteric coronavirus* (HECoV)	*Pigeon coronavirus* (PiCoV)
	Rat coronavirus (RCoV)	
	Puffinosis coronavirus	
Bat coronavirus-61		
Bat coronavirus-HKU2		
Human coronavirus NL63	*Subgroup 2b*	
	Severe acute respiratory syndrome coronavirus (SARS-CoV)	
	Bat-CoV-HKU3-1	

[a]Recognized virus species.
[b]The viruses duck coronavirus, goose coronavirus, and pigeon coronavirus have been recommended by the Coronavirus Study Group for recognition as species by the ICTV.
Official virus species names are in italics. Coronaviruses that have not yet been recognized as distinct species have names that are not italicized. Rabbit coronavirus is considered as a tentative member of the genus. A coronavirus has been isolated from a parrot. On the basis of very limited sequence data, it is not clear in which, if any, of the three groups that this virus would be placed.

C-terminal half of the M protein is within the lumen of the virus. In transmissible gastroenteritis virus (TGEV), a proportion of M molecules have four membrane-spanning segments, resulting in the C-terminus also being exposed on the outer surface of the virus (M' in **Figure 1(b)**). The E protein is anchored in the membrane by a sequence near its N-terminus.

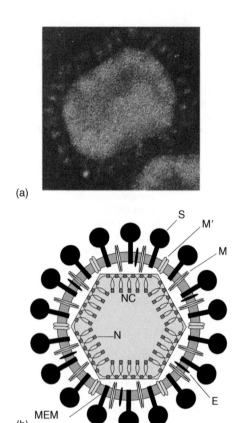

(a)

(b)

Figure 1 (a) Electron micrograph of an IBV virion, showing the bulbous S protein. (b) Diagrammatic representation of the composition and structure of a coronavirus virion: S, spike glycoprotein; M, M′, integral membrane glycoprotein; E, small envelope protein; N, nucleocapsid protein; NC, nucleocapsid (nucleoprotein) comprising the RNA genome and N protein. Cryoelectron microscopy of TGEV has indicated a core structure comprising the NC and the M protein. Two forms of M protein (M, M′) have been observed for TGEV (see main text). The coronavirus membrane proteins, S, E, M, and M′, are inserted into a lipid bilayer (MEM) derived from internal cell membranes. (b) Reproduced from González JM, Gomez-Puertas P, Cavanagh D, Gorbalenya AE, and Enjuanes L (2003) A comparative sequence analysis to revise the current taxonomy of the family *Coronaviridae. Archives of Virology* 148: 2207–2235, with permission from Springer-Verlag.

Genome Organization and Expression

Coronaviruses have the largest known RNA genomes, which comprise 28–32 kb of positive sense, single-stranded RNA. The overall genome organization is being 5′ UTR–polymerase gene–structural protein genes–3′ UTR, where the UTRs are untranslated regions (**Figure 2**). The first 60–90 nucleotides at the 5′ end form a leader sequence. The structural protein genes are in the same order in all coronaviruses: (HE)–S–E–M–N. Interspersed among these genes are one or more gene (depending on the species; SARS-CoV has four) that encode small proteins of unknown function. Some of these genes encode two or three proteins. In some cases (e.g., gene 3 of IBV and gene 5 of murine hepatitis virus (MHV)), translation of the third and second open reading frame (ORF), respectively, is effected by the preceding ORFs acting as internal ribosome entry sites. The proteins encoded by these small ORFs are mostly not required for replication *in vitro*; some of them might function as antagonists of innate immune responses, though this has not yet been demonstrated.

Following entry into a cell and the release of the virus ribonucleoprotein (genome surrounded by the N protein) into the cytoplasm, ribosomes translate gene 1, which is approximately 20 kb, into two polyproteins (pp1a and pp1ab). These are cleaved by gene 1-encoded proteases, to generate 15 or 16 proteins (**Figure 3**). Translation of ORF 1b involves ribosomal frameshifting, which has two elements, a slippery site followed by an RNA pseudoknot. At the slippery site (UUUAAAC in IBV), the ribosome slips one nucleotide backward and then moves forward, this time in a −1 frame compared with translation ORF 1a, resulting in the synthesis polyprotein 1ab.

Proteins, including the RNA-dependent RNA polymerase, from gene 1 associate to form the replicase complex, which is membrane associated. Coronavirus subgenomic mRNAs are generated by a discontinuous process. At the beginning of each gene is a common sequence (CUUAACAA in the case of IBV) called a transcription regulatory sequence (TRS). It is believed that when the polymerase producing the nascent negative sense RNA, reaches a TRS, RNA synthesis is attenuated, followed by continuation at the 5′ end of genomic RNA. This results in the addition of a negative copy of the leader sequence to the negative-sense RNA, resulting in a negative-sense copy of an sg mRNA. Of course, progress of the polymerase is not always halted at a TRS. Rather, it sometimes continues, producing a nested set of negative-sense sg mRNAs. These are the templates for the generation of the positive-sense sg mRNAs (**Figure 2**). The amount of each sg mRNA does not necessarily decrease in a linear fashion; the efficiency of termination by a TRS is dependent on adjacent sequences, which are different for each gene. The leader sequence is found at the very 5′ end of the genomic RNA and at the 5′ ends of each sg mRNA.

Replication Cycle

The N-terminal (S1) part of the S protein mediates that mediates attachment to cells. It is a determinant of host species specificity and, in some cases, pathogenicity, by

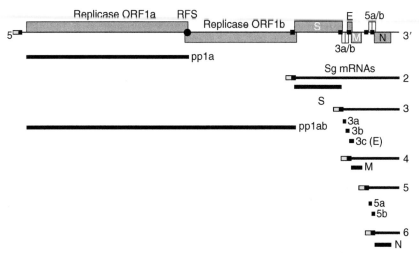

Figure 2 Schematic diagram representing the genomic expression of the avian coronavirus IBV. The upper part of the diagram shows the IBV genomic RNA, with the various genes highlighted as boxed regions. The black boxes represent the transcription regulatory sequences (TRSs) found upstream of each gene and direct the synthesis, via negative-sense counterparts, of the sg mRNAs (2–6 for IBV). The leader sequence, represented by a gray box, is at the 5′ end of the genomic RNA and at the 5′ ends of the sg mRNAs. The genomic RNA is translated to produce two polyproteins, pp1a and pp1ab, that are cleaved by virus-encoded proteases to produce the replicase proteins. The structural proteins, S, E, M, and E, and the accessory proteins, 3a, 3b, 5a, and 5b, produced from IBV genes 3 and 5, respectively, are translated from the sg mRNAs. The proteins produced by the sg mRNAs are represented by lines below the corresponding sg mRNA. All of the sg mRNAs, except the smallest species, are polycistronic but only produce a protein from the 5′-most gene. The ribosome frameshift (RFS) region, denoted as a black circle on the genomic RNA, directs the −1 frameshift event for the synthesis of pp1ab. Translation of the genomic RNA results in the production of pp1a. However, the translating ribosomes undergo the −1 frameshift about 30% of the time resulting in pp1ab. The 5′ and 3′ UTR sequences are represented as single lines downstream of the leader and N gene sequences, respectively.

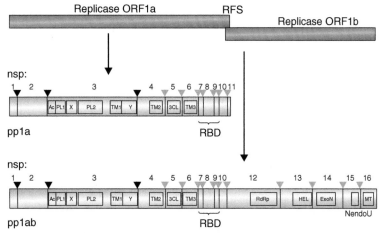

Figure 3 Organization of the coronavirus replicase gene products. Translation of the coronavirus replicase ORF 1a and ORF 1b sequences results in pp1a and pp1ab; the latter is a C-terminal extension of pp1a, following a programmed −1 frameshift event (see legend to **Figure 2**). The two polyproteins are proteolytically cleaved into 10 (pp1a; nsp1–11) and 16 (pp1ab; nsp1–16) products by the papain-like proteinases (PL1^{pro} and PL2^{pro}) and the 3C-like (3CL^{pro}) proteinase. The PL^{pro} proteinases cleave at the sites indicated with a black triangle and the 3CL^{pro} proteinase cleaves at the sites indicated with a gray triangle. The nsp11 product of pp1a is produced as a result of the ribosomes terminating at the ORF 1a translational termination codon, a −1 frameshift results in the generation of nsp12, part of the pp1ab replicase gene product. Various domains have been identified within some of the replicase products: Ac is a conserved acidic domain; X = ADP-ribose 1′-phosphatase (ADRP) domain; PL1 and PL2 the two papain-like proteinases; Y is a conserved domain; TM1, TM2, and TM3 are conserved putative transmembrane domains; 3CL = 3CL^{pro} domain; RdRp, RNA-dependent RNA polymerase domain; HEL, helicase domain; ExoN, exonuclease domain; NendoU, uridylate-specific endoribonuclease domain; MT, 2′-O-ribose methyltransferase domain. nsp's 7–9 contain RNA-binding domains (RBDs).

determining susceptible cell range (tissue tropism) within a host. The C-terminal S2 part triggers fusion of the virus envelope with cell membranes (plasma membrane or endosomal membranes), which can occur at neutral or slightly acidic pH, depending on species or even strain. The virus glycoproteins (S, M, and HE, when present) are synthesized at the endoplasmic reticulum. Both subunits of the S protein are multiply glycosylated, while the M protein has one or two glycans close to its N-terminus. Interestingly, glycosylation of the M protein can be either N- or O-linked, depending on the type of coronavirus, although experiments using reverse genetics showed that conversion of an O-linked glycosylated M protein to an N-linked version had no effect on virus growth.

Early and late in infection, formation of virus particles can occur in the endoplasmic reticulum–Golgi intermediate compartment (ERGIC) and endoplasmic reticulum, but most assembly occurs in the Golgi membranes. The M protein is not transported to the plasma membrane; its location at internal membranes determines the sites of virus particle formation. It interacts with the N protein (as part of the RNP) and C-terminal part of the S protein, retaining some, though not all, of the S protein at internal membranes. The E protein is essential for virus particle formation, though it is not known how it functions. It has a sequence that determines its accumulation at internal membranes, and its interaction with the M protein. The latter interacts with the C-terminus of the S protein, retaining some of it at internal membranes, and with the N protein (itself part of the ribonucleoprotein structure), enabling the formation of virus particles with spikes.

Genome Replication and Recombination

Following infection of a susceptible cell, the coronavirus genomic RNA is released from the virion into the cytoplasm and immediately recognized as an mRNA for the translation of the replicase pp1a and pp1ab proteins. These proteins are cleaved by ORF1a-encoded proteases, after which they become part of replicase complexes for the synthesis of either complete negative-sense copies of the genomic RNA or negative-sense copies of the sg mRNAs. The negative-sense RNAs are used as templates for the synthesis of genomic RNA and sg mRNAs (**Figure 2**). Following synthesis of the sg mRNAs, the structural proteins are produced for the assembly and encapsidation of the *de novo*-synthesized genomic RNA, resulting in the release of new infectious coronavirus virions. The release of new virions starts 3–4 h after the initial infection. As indicated above, the synthesis of the sg mRNAs is the result of a discontinuous

process in which the synthesis of a negative-sense copy of an sg mRNA is completed by the addition of the negative-sense leader sequence by a recombination mechanism. If a cell is infected with two related coronaviruses, the polymerase may swap between two RNA templates, in a similar way to addition of the leader sequence. This 'copy-choice' mechanism of genetic recombination results in a chimeric RNA. Such RNAs may give rise to new viruses with modified genomes with a capacity to infect a different cell and, in some cases, new host species.

Evolutionary Relationships among Coronaviruses

Phylogenetic analyses of the structural proteins have resulted in the grouping of coronavirus species in accordance with earlier antigenic groups (**Table 1** and **Figure 4**).

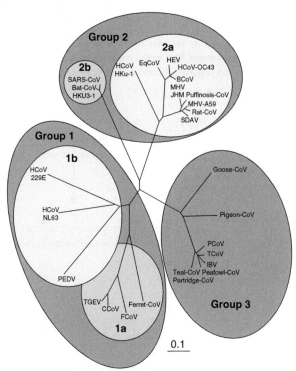

Figure 4 Phylogenetic relationship of aligned coronavirus-derived nucleoprotein amino acid sequences. The complete N protein sequences represent coronaviruses from each of the three groups (**Table 1**). The tree is unrooted and the three main coronavirus groups, 1–3, are highlighted as dark gray ellipsoids. Groups 1 and 2 are divided into two subgroups, a and b, representing some divergence of the sequences within their corresponding groups. Similar relationships are observed when comparing other structural proteins and replicase-derived proteins.

Members of subgroups have higher amino acid sequence identities to each other (≥60%) than to members of another group in the same group (with which they share ≤40% identity). Comparing one group with another, protein sequence identities are generally in the range 25–35%. Unlike other members of group 2, SARS-CoV does not have an HE glycoprotein. Phylogenetic analysis using all the encoded proteins indicates that recombination has been a feature of coronavirus evolution. For example, some group 1a viruses are clearly recombinants between a feline and canine group 1 coronavirus.

Diseases and Host Range

Probably all coronaviruses replicate in epithelial cells of the respiratory and/or enteric tracts, though not necessarily producing clinical damage at those sites. Avian IBV not only causes respiratory disease but can also damage gonads in both females and males, and causes serious kidney disease (dependent on the strain of virus, and to some extent on the breed of chicken). IBV is able to replicate at virtually every epithelial surface in the host. Some coronaviruses have their most profound effect in the alimentary tract (e.g., porcine TGEV causes ≥90% mortality in neonatal pigs). Human coronaviruses are known to be associated with enteric and respiratory diseases (e.g., diarrhea), in addition to respiratory disease. SARS-CoV was also associated with diarrhea in humans, in addition to serious lung disease. Other coronaviruses, for example, MHV and porcine HEV, spread to cells of the central nervous system, producing disease, for example, acute or chronic demyelination in the case of MHV.

Coronavirus replication and disease are not necessarily restricted to a single host species. Canine enteric CoV and feline CoV can replicate and cause disease in pigs; these two viruses have proteins with very high amino acid identity to those of porcine TGEV. Canine respiratory CoV has proteins, including the S protein (which is the attachment protein and a determinant of host range), with very high amino acid identity (≥95%) to other group 2 viruses Hu CoV-OC43 and BCoV. This raises the possibility of co-infection in these hosts. Bovine CoV causes enteritis in turkeys following experimental oral infection. There is evidence that pheasant CoV can infect chickens, and IBV infect teal (a duck), though without causing disease. The most dramatic demonstration that coronaviruses can have a wide host range was provided by SARS-CoV. This may have had its origin in bats, was transferred to various other species (e.g., civet cat) that were captured for trade, and then caused lethal disease in humans.

Persistent infections *in vivo* are well known for MHV, and less well known for other coronaviruses (e.g., IBV). Following infection of very young chickens, IBV is re-excreted when hens start to lay eggs. The trigger for release is probably the stress of coming into lay.

The S protein is a determinant of both tissue tropism within a host and host range. This has been elegantly demonstrated by genetic manipulation of the genome of MHV, which is unable to attach to feline cells. Replacement of the MHV S protein gene with that of CoV from feline coronavirus resulted in a recombinant virus that was able to attach, and subsequently replicate in, feline cells. However, other proteins can also affect pathogenicity. Research with genetically modified coronaviruses, using targeted recombination or 'infectious clones', has shown that modifications to proteins encoded in ORF1 and the small genes interspersed among the structural protein genes, result in attenuation of pathogenicity. Although the roles of these 'accessory proteins' are not known, this may offer a route to the development of a new generation of live vaccines. Currently, the most widely used prophylactics for control of IBV in chickens include killed vaccines and live vaccines attenuated by passage in embryonated eggs. However, disease control is complicated by extensive variation in the S1 protein which is the inducer of protective immunity.

Further Reading

Britton P and Cavanagh D (2007) Avian coronavirus diseases and infectious bronchitis vaccine development. In: Thiel V (ed.) *Coronaviruses: Molecular and Cellular Biology* pp. 161–181. Norfolk, UK: Caister Academic Press.

Britton P and Cavanagh D (2007) Nidovirus genome organization and expression mechanisms. In: Perlman S Gallagher T,, and Snijder EJ (eds.) *Nidoviruses*, pp. 29–46. Washington, DC: ASM Press.

Cavanagh D (2003) SARS vaccine development: Experiences of vaccination against avian infectious bronchitis coronavirus. *Avian Pathology* 32: 567–582.

Cavanagh D (2005) *Coronaviridae*: A review of coronaviruses and toroviruses. In: Schmidt A and Wolff MH (eds.) *Coronaviruses with Special Emphasis on First Insights Concerning SARS*, pp. 1–54. Basel: Birkhäuser.

Cavanagh D (2005) Coronaviruses in poultry and other birds. *Avian Pathology* 34: 439–448.

Enjuanes L, Almazán F, Sola I, and Zuñiga S (2006) Biochemical aspects of coronavirus replication: A virus–host interaction. *Annual Reviews in Microbiology* 60: 211–230.

González JM, Gomez-Puertas P, Cavanagh D, Gorbalenya AE, and Enjuanes L (2003) A comparative sequence analysis to revise the current taxonomy of the family *Coronaviridae*. *Archives of Virology* 148: 2207–2235.

Masters PS (2006) The molecular biology of coronaviruses. *Advances in Virus Research* 66: 193–292.

Siddell S, Ziebuhr J, and Snijder E (2005) Coronaviruses, toroviruses and arteriviruses. In: Mahy BWJ and ter Meulen V (eds.) *Topley and Wilson's Microbiology and Microbial Infections, Virology*, pp. 823–856. London: Hodder Arnold.

Coxsackieviruses

M S Oberste and M A Pallansch, Centers for Disease Control and Prevention, Atlanta, GA, USA

Published by Elsevier Ltd.

Glossary

Chemosis Edema of the bulbar conjunctiva.
Conjunctival hyperemia Increased blood flow to the conjunctiva.
Cytopathic effect Degeneration of cultured cells due to virus infection and replication, often characteristic of a given virus.
Exanthem Illness characterized by skin eruption (rash).
Myalgia Nonspecific muscle pain or tenderness.
Nuclear pyknosis Condensation and reduction in size of the nucleus, often the result of a pathogenic process.
Pleurodynia Illness characterized by chest pain due to inflammation of the pleura, the membrane surrounding the lungs and chest cavity.
Protomer Basic unit of a virus capsid, containing one or more viral proteins.

History

The coxsackieviruses (genus *Enterovirus*, family *Picornaviridae*) were discovered in the late 1940s, as a result of intense efforts to develop better systems to propagate and study poliovirus. At the time, nonhuman primates were the model system for poliovirus and poliomyelitis, as cell culture and inoculation of suckling mice were just being introduced. Investigators at the New York State Department of Health inoculated suckling mice with fecal suspensions from two suspected poliomyelitis cases. The mice became paralyzed, but the viruses were not polioviruses – the virus was later named 'coxsackievirus' (CV) for the patient's home town, Coxsackie, New York. Subsequent studies identified related viruses, some causing spastic paralysis rather than the flaccid paralysis observed with the initial isolates. Based on these differences in pathogenicity, the viruses were classified as group A coxsackieviruses (flaccid paralysis) or group B coxsackieviruses (spastic paralysis), with the individual virus types being numbered sequentially within each group (e.g., coxsackievirus A2 or coxsackievirus B5). Once cell culture became established as a standard laboratory technique, additional viruses were discovered that were able to replicate in culture but caused no disease in mice. Since many of these were derived from stools of healthy individuals and they were not yet known to cause disease in humans, they were termed enteric cytopathic human orphan viruses or 'echoviruses' – these were also named using consecutive numbers (e.g., echovirus 9). The early coxsackieviruses had been isolated from cases of 'nonparalytic poliomyelitis' (aseptic meningitis), showing that this disease was not necessarily caused by polioviruses. Other illnesses, including herpangina, rash, pleurodynia, and myocarditis, were also shown to be associated with coxsackievirus infection; later, the echoviruses were later shown to be associated with many of these same illnesses.

Taxonomy and Classification

As mentioned, the term 'coxsackievirus' was applied to enteroviruses that caused paralysis upon intracerebral inoculation in suckling mice, with the type of paralysis – flaccid versus spastic – being used to place strains in group A or group B. When it was discovered that antigenically related viruses could have varying degrees of pathogenicity in mice, the original naming convention was abandoned and since 1967 all new enteroviruses (whether coxsackievirus-like or echovirus-like) have been named 'enterovirus' followed by a sequential number, starting with enterovirus 68. Enteroviruses have traditionally been classified antigenically, using well-characterized, standardized antisera in a neutralization assay, either in cell culture or in suckling mice (for viruses that replicate poorly in culture). Using this approach, 30 coxsackievirus serotypes were defined, with 24 in group A and six in group B. Coxsackievirus A23 was later discovered to be antigenically identical to echovirus 9, so CVA23 was dropped as a distinct serotype.

It was recognized early on that there were many limitations to the antigenic typing approach. In addition to the labor-intensive nature of the neutralization assay and the requirement for extensive characterization of new antisera, different serotypes may cross-react in complex combinations and individual strains of a given type may react differently with different preparations of homotypic antisera. Once nucleotide sequences became available for a large number of serotypes, it became clear that the sequences of certain parts of the capsid-coding region could serve as a surrogate for antigenic type. In the late 1990s and early 2000s, several investigators developed typing systems based on polymerase chain reaction (PCR) amplification of a portion of the capsid region, followed by sequencing and analysis of the sequence to

Table 1 Coxsackievirus taxonomy

Species	Serotype
Human enterovirus A[a]	CVA2–8, CVA10, CVA12, CVA14, CVA16
Human enterovirus B[b]	CVA9, CVB1–6
Human enterovirus C[c]	CVA1, CVA11, CVA13, CVA17, CVA19–22, CVA24

[a]Also includes EV71, EV76, EV89–92.
[b]Also includes all echoviruses, EV69, EV73–75, EV77–88, EV93, EV97–98, EV100–101.
[c]Also includes polioviruses, EV95–96, EV99, and EV102.

determine type. Eventually, VP1 was settled upon as the most reliable region for molecular virus typing. Sequence comparisons have shown that CVA15 is a strain of CVA11 and CVA18 is a strain of CVA13.

Sequence relationships are now recognized as a primary discriminating characteristic in enterovirus taxonomy. There are currently eight species in the genus *Enterovirus*: *human enterovirus* (HEV) A–D, *Poliovirus, Bovine enterovirus, Porcine enterovirus*, and *Simian enterovirus A*. There are current proposals to merge *Poliovirus* with HEV-C and to move the two human rhinovirus species from their own genus into *Enterovirus*. The coxsackieviruses are distributed among three species: HEV-A (CVA2–8, CVA10, CVA12, CVA14, and CVA16), HEV-B (CVA9, CVB1–6), and HEV-C (CVA1, CVA11, CVA13, CVA17, CVA19–22, and CVA24) (**Table 1**).

Host Range and Virus Propagation

Coxsackieviruses are primarily human pathogens but many can also infect certain nonhuman primate species and all serotypes are able to infect and cause disease in mice (by definition), though there is some variability among strains of any given type. Infection of nonhuman primates often fails to induce clinical disease, but CVA7 can induce polio-like paralysis in monkeys. Swine vesicular disease virus, an important livestock pathogen because symptoms of illness are similar to those of foot and mouth disease, is closely related genetically and antigenically to CVB5. Genetic and epidemiologic studies strongly suggest that human CVB5 was introduced into swine decades ago, with subsequent adaptation and diversification in the new host species.

The best specimens for virus isolation are stool specimens or rectal swabs, throat swabs or washings, and cerebrospinal fluid, in that order. Isolation from stool is most sensitive because virus is usually present at higher titer and it is present in stool longer than in any other specimen. Nonfecal specimens are most likely to yield virus isolates if they are obtained early in the acute phase

of illness. For cases of acute hemorrhagic conjunctivitis, the best specimens are conjunctival swabs and tears. A number of different primary cell cultures and continuous cell lines, both generally of human or monkey origin, have been used for isolation and propagation of coxsackieviruses. These cell systems include primary monkey kidney cells; monkey kidney cell lines such as BGM, Vero, and LLC-MK2; and human cell lines such as HeLa, Hep2, KB, and RD. Virus infection and replication results in a characteristic cytopathic effect which is observed microscopically 1–7 days after inoculation. The cells become rounded and refractile, with nuclear pyknosis and cell degeneration. Ultimately, the cells are lysed and become detached from the surface of the culture vessel.

Attempts at virus isolation in cell culture may sometimes be unsuccessful, necessitating the inoculation of suckling mice. For example, CVA1, CVA19, and CVA22 are rarely, if ever, isolated in culture, but grow readily in suckling mice. If the virus titer is extremely low, blind passage in mice may be necessary; blind passage may also be needed to allow the virus to adapt to growth in mice. The two groups of coxsackieviruses can be distinguished by the distinct pathology that they cause in mice. With CVA infection, newborn mice develop flaccid paralysis and severe, extensive degeneration of skeletal muscle (sparing the tongue, heart, and CNS), and they may have renal lesions. Death usually occurs within a week. CVB infection proceeds more slowly and is characterized by spastic paralysis and tremors associated with encephalomyelitis, focal myositis, brown fat necrosis, myocarditis, hepatitis, and acinar cell pancreatitis.

Epidemiology, Geographic Distribution, and Seasonality

The coxsackieviruses are distributed worldwide, but there can be significant geographic and temporal variation in prevalence of individual serotypes. These differences are attributed to differences in climate and public hygiene, overall population immunity (e.g., an increase in the number of susceptible individuals in the years following an outbreak), and other factors. In the United States, for example, CVA9 is among the most commonly reported enteroviruses, but circulation tends to peak every 3–5 years. CVB2, CVB4, and CVB5 are also common, with cyclic peaks of activity, and CVB5 has been associated with large outbreaks, while CVB1 and CVB3 circulate at low, relatively constant levels, and CVB6 is rarely reported. Like the other enteroviruses, most coxsackievirus infections tend to occur during the warmer months in areas with a temperate climate, peaking in late summer or fall. In the tropics, peak activity generally correlates with the rainy season.

Coxsackieviruses are isolated in the highest titer and for the longest time in stool specimens but can also be isolated from respiratory secretions. Fecal-oral transmission and spread by contact with respiratory secretions (person-to-person, fomites, and possibly large particle aerosol) are the most important modes of transmission. The relative importance of the different mode probably varies with the virus and the environmental setting. Viruses that cause a vesicular exanthem are also presumably spread by direct or indirect contact with vesicular fluid, which contains infectious virus. Exceptions to the usual modes of enterovirus transmission are the agents of acute hemorrhagic conjunctivitis, coxsackievirus A24 variant (CA24v), and enterovirus 70 (a member of HEV-D). These two viruses are seldom isolated from respiratory or fecal specimens and are probably transmitted primarily by direct or indirect contact with eye secretions.

Virion Structure and Host Cell Receptors

Coxsackievirus virions, like those of other picornaviruses, are approximately 30 nm in diameter, with little discernable fine-scale structure (**Figure 1**). Sixty copies of each of the mature virion proteins, VP1–VP4, form an icosahedral virion particle with pseudo $T = 3$ symmetry. The proteins VP1–VP3 combine to form the virion protomer, with VP4 internal to the particle.

Virus infection is dependent on the presence of specific receptors. At least four distinct receptors are used by coxsackieviruses for entry into human cells. CVA9 uses integrin $\alpha_v\beta_3$, CVB1–6 use the 'coxsackievirus–adenovirus receptor' (CAR) and some may also use decay-accelerating factor (DAF), and some of the HEV-C coxsackieviruses use intracellular adhesion molecule 1 (ICAM-1). The receptor (s) used by most viruses in HEV-A, and by many of the viruses in HEV-C remain unknown.

Genetics, Genetic Diversity, and Evolution

Like the other enteroviruses, the coxsackievirus genome is a single-stranded, polyadenylated, positive-sense RNA of approximately 7.4 kbp, with a 22-amino-acid virus-encoded protein ($3B^{VPg}$) covalently linked to the $5'$ end. Flanked by $5'$- and $3'$-nontranslated regions (NTRs), the single long open reading frame encodes a polyprotein of approximately 2200 amino acids that is processed during and following translation by viral proteases to yield the mature viral polypeptides (**Figure 2**). The P1 region encodes the capsid proteins 1A-1D (VP4, VP2, VP3, and VP1, respectively). The P2 and P3 regions encode proteins involved in polyprotein processing, RNA replication, and shutdown of host cell protein synthesis.

Coxsackieviruses, like other picornaviruses, evolve extremely rapidly, because the viral RNA-dependent

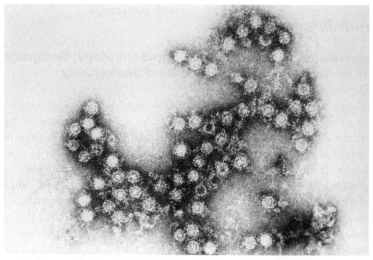

Figure 1   Electron micrograph of coxsackievirus B4 virions. Image courtesy of CDC Public Health Image Library.

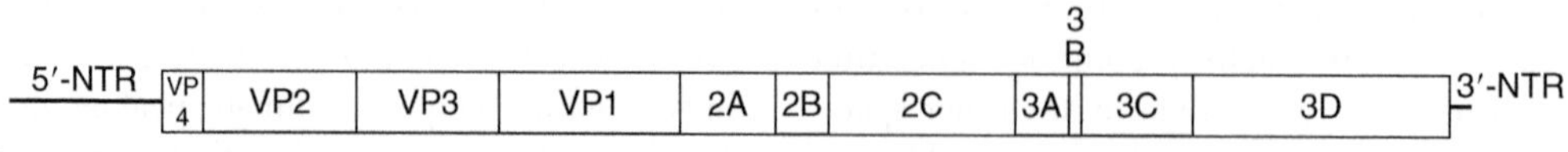

| 5′-NTR | VP4 | VP2 | VP3 | VP1 | 2A | 2B | 2C | 3A | 3B | 3C | 3D | 3′-NTR |

Figure 2   Coxsackievirus genome, indicating the locations of the mature viral proteins, 1A-1D (VP4, VP2, VP3, and VP1, respectively), 2A–2C, and 3A–3D, flanked by the 5′- and 3′-nontranslated regions (NTRs).

RNA polymerase is error-prone and lacks a proofreading function (like other RNA virus replicases). Most of the nucleotide substitutions are translationally silent, because most substitutions that become fixed in a virus population are in the third ('wobble') position of codons. This phenomenon is likely due to intense selection against amino acid substitutions, especially in the proteins that are required for replication, protein processing, and shutdown of host cell synthesis. Most viable amino acid substitutions occur in surface loops of the external capsid proteins, VP1, VP2, and VP3, while residues that contribute to the proteins' beta-barrel structure tend to be highly conserved within a serotype and, to a large extent, within a species. Within a serotype, VP1 nucleotide sequence can vary by up to 25%, representing near-saturation of synonymous sites, as well as multiple nonsynonymous substitutions – the amino acid sequence can vary by as much as 15% with a type.

The different enterovirus species each form a distinct phylogenetic group throughout the coding region, as well as in the 3'-NTR. In the 5'-NTR, the human enteroviruses form only two clusters: cluster I contains HEV-C and HEV-D, while cluster II contains HEV-A and HEV-B. The nonhuman species each form distinct 5'-NTR clusters. The coxsackie B virus capsid sequences cluster together as a group, probably reflecting their shared, but unique, use of CAR as a receptor. In other parts of the coding region, the CVB are not phylogenetically coherent; rather, they interdigitate with other viruses in HEV-B, due to the high frequency of RNA recombination within any given enterovirus species.

Pathogenesis and Immunity

Much of the disease associated with coxsackievirus infection is thought to be a direct result of tissue-specific cell destruction, analogous to the cytopathic effect in cultured cells (**Figure 3**). For the most part, the detailed mechanisms of virus-induced disease have not been well-characterized. The primary site of infection is typically the respiratory or gastrointestinal epithelium, leading to viremia that may result in a secondary site of tissue infection. Such secondary spread of virus to the CNS can result in aseptic meningitis or, rarely, encephalitis or paralysis. Other tissue-specific infection can result in pleurodynia or myocarditis. Disseminated infection can lead to exanthems, nonspecific myalgias, or severe multiple-organ disease in neonates. Some disease manifestations, enteroviral exanthems and myocarditis, for example, are thought to result from the host immune response to the infection.

Enterovirus infection elicits a strong humoral immune response. Often the response is heterotypic; that is, infection with one serotype induces a broad immune response that cross-reacts with several other serotypes. Young children develop a more homotypic response, whereas older children and adults tend to develop a more heterotypic response. This age difference in the specificity of the

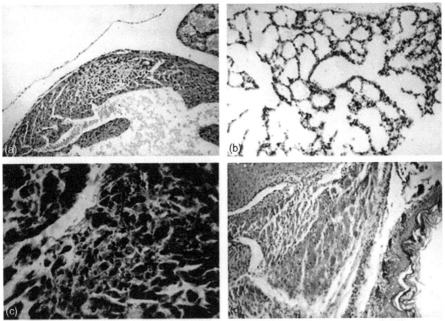

Figure 3 Tissue damage caused in baby mice by a freshly isolated strain of coxsackievirus B (a–c) or coxsackievirus A (d). (a) A large necrotic focus in the atrial myocardium ($\times$ 100); (b) steatitis in the interscapular brown fat pad ($\times$ 250); (c) a ventricular focus of necrotic cardiomyocytes ($\times$ 450); (d) intercostal muscles with diffuse hyalinization of myocytes and mild inflammatory infiltrate ($\times$250). Reproduced from Pozzetto B and Gaudin OG (1999) Coxsackieviruses (*Picornaviridae*). In: Granoff A and Webster R (eds) *Encyclopedia of Virology*, 2nd edn. San Diego: Academic Press, with permission from Elsevier.

antibody response probably reflects exposure to a greater number of serotypes with increasing age. The heterotypic response may reflect the presence of epitopes that are shared among multiple serotypes, but the actual mechanism is unknown. The presence of antibody does not prevent infection or primary virus replication, but it is sufficient to protect from disease, probably by limiting spread of the virus to secondary sites such as the CNS. Infection also elicits a T-cell response which helps clear the virus, but the cell-mediated immune response is not required for protection from disease.

Clinical Manifestations

Coxsackievirus infections can result in a wide variety of disease syndromes (**Table 2**). Most infections are asymptomatic or result in only mild upper respiratory tract symptoms (common cold). Other mild enteroviral illness, such as fever, headache, malaise, and mild gastrointestinal symptoms, may also occur. Serious illness that brings the patient to the attention of a physician is much less frequent. Inapparent infections and prolonged excretion of virus, especially in stools, are common. These properties of enterovirus infection, and the fact that enterovirus infection is extremely common, make it difficult to establish a definitive link between infection and specific disease unless the virus can be isolated from a nonsterile site that is linked to the observed pathology (e.g., isolation from cerebrospinal fluid in the case of aseptic meningitis). Often, the association between infection and disease is based on studies of outbreaks in which a large number of persons with the same clinical signs and symptoms have evidence of infection with the same serotype. Such studies have clearly demonstrated that enterovirus infection can cause aseptic meningitis, pericarditis, pleurodynia, myocarditis, and encephalitis.

Central Nervous System Disease

The most commonly recognized serious manifestation of enterovirus infection is CNS disease, usually aseptic meningitis, but sometimes, encephalitis or paralysis. Aseptic meningitis is the most common CNS infection in the United States, and enteroviruses are the main recognized cause of aseptic meningitis in both children and adults in developed countries. Other than poliovirus, echoviruses and group B coxsackieviruses are most commonly isolated from cases of enterovirus-associated CNS disease, but this may be largely an artifact of low-efficiency isolation of group A coxsackieviruses in culture.

Febrile Rash Illnesses

Herpangina is a common illness in school-age children, characterized by vesicular inflammation of the oral mucosa, including throat, tonsils, soft palate, and tongue. Herpangina has commonly been associated with CVA2–6, CVA8, and CVA10, as well as with some of the echoviruses. Hand, foot, and mouth disease (HFMD) is characterized by vesicular rash on the palms, soles, and oral mucosa, with frequent involvement of the limbs and trunk. CVA 16 and EV71 are the most common viruses isolated from HFMD cases, but CVA4, CVA6, and CVA10 are also frequent causes. Many of the coxsackieviruses (both groups A and B) may also be associated with undifferentiated rash, often in connection with other symptoms such as meningitis.

Prenatal, Perinatal, and Neonatal Infection

A number of enterovirus serotypes have been associated with severe illness in neonates, including generalized disseminated infection that can mimic some aspects of bacterial sepsis. CVB4 infection is associated with a higher risk for severe disease in infants less than 1 month old, but other CVB serotypes and other enteroviruses can also cause similarly severe disease in this age group. Neonatal disease can also include other typical enterovirus syndromes, such as meningitis, encephalitis, pneumonia, hepatitis, myocarditis, and pancreatitis. One systematic study in Nassau County, New York, estimated that one of every 2000 infants in that area was hospitalized during the first 3 months of life for CVB sepsis-like disease, with significant mortality. This probably underestimates the true rate, since virus isolation studies may be insensitive and other enteroviruses were not included in the estimate.

Table 2 Diseases commonly associated with coxsackievirus infection

Illness or syndrome	Group A	Group B
Acute hemorrhagic conjunctivitis	X[a]	
Aseptic meningitis	X	X
Encephalitis[b]	X	X
Exanthema	X	X
Hand, foot, and mouth disease	X[c]	
Hepatitis	X	X
Herpangina	X	
Infantile diarrhea	X	
Myocarditis/pericarditis		X
Paralysis[b]	X	X
Pleurodynia		X
Respiratory illness	X	X
Severe systemic infection in infants		X
Undifferentiated febrile illness	X	X

[a]CVA24 variant.
[b]Rare.
[c]Primarily CVA16 and EV71; also CVA6, CVA10.

Although there are few studies that examine the relationship between enterovirus infection and adverse effects on the fetus, one study found serologic evidence of CNS infection with CVB in ventricular fluid from 4 of 28 newborns with congenital neural tube defects. The infants had neutralizing antibody to only one CVB serotype in the ventricular fluid, but to several in serum. The unique distribution of antibodies in the ventricular fluid compared to that in serum supports the purported association. The mothers had antibodies to the same serotype as well as some other CVB serotypes. No virus was isolated from infants or mothers. Two other studies have documented an association between enterovirus infection and miscarriages and stillbirths. Further studies are needed to assess the possibility of enterovirus infection of the fetus.

Acute Hemorrhagic Conjunctivitis

Coxsackievirus A24 variant and enterovirus 70 are associated with acute hemorrhagic conjunctivitis. This disease is different from other enteroviral illnesses, having occurred in global pandemics since its introduction around 1969. The incubation period for these agents is shorter than for other enteroviruses (24–72 h); systemic illness is much less common and conjunctival replication the rule. The disease is characterized by acute onset of lacrimation, severe pain, chemosis and periorbital edema, photophobia, conjunctival hyperemia, and mild-to-severe subconjunctival hemorrhages. The disease is usually bilateral. It is generally self-limiting, but may lead to secondary bacterial infection.

Other Acute Illnesses

Group B viruses have been associated with pleurodynia, also known as 'Bornholm disease' or 'epidemic myalgia'. Pleurodynia is characterized by sudden onset of chest pain, due to inflammation of the diaphragm, accompanied by general malaise, headache, fever, and sore throat. Enteroviruses, primarily the coxsackieviruses, are also a common cause of respiratory illness. Most of these infections are relatively mild – even subclinical – and restricted to the upper respiratory tract (e.g., common cold, croup, and epiglottitis). Occasionally, the lower respiratory tract becomes infected, resulting in more serious illness, such as bronchiolitis or pneumonia, especially in very young children.

Cardiac Disease

Although the association between myocarditis and pericarditis and enterovirus infection is clearly established, it is not yet clear how often enterovirus infections are responsible for the disease syndromes. One study has shown that CVB IgM in a group of patients with acute myocarditis is significantly higher than in controls.

Enterovirus RNA has also been detected in myocardial biopsy specimens from patients with myocarditis. These and other studies suggest, but do not clearly show, that CVB infection may be associated with a large fraction of cases of acute myocarditis. By contrast, different studies have failed to show conclusive evidence for the involvement of enterovirus infection in idiopathic dilated cardiomyopathies.

Diabetes

As with myocarditis, numerous studies have suggested a link between enterovirus infection and the onset of type I diabetes mellitus. In some cases, enteroviruses, such as CVB4, have been isolated from pancreas of fulminant diabetes cases, but most of the evidence is indirect, through serologic studies. Several mechanisms have been hypothesized to explain the possible link between infection and diabetes onset, including direct, lytic destruction of insulin-producing beta cells in the pancreas; molecular mimicry of self-antigens, resulting in induction of prediabetic autoimmunity that eventually leads to beta-cell destruction; and indirect damage mediated through activation of a nonspecific inflammatory response in the pancreas ('bystander effect'). A number of studies are attempting to address various steps in virus-induced diabetes pathogenesis, in human patients and in animal model systems.

Treatment and Prevention

Antiviral therapy is not presently available for enterovirus infections, so treatment is directed toward ameliorating symptoms. Drugs have been identified that exhibit antiviral activity against several enteroviruses in tissue culture and experimental animals, and some have been tested in human clinical trials; however, no enterovirus drugs are currently licensed in the United States or elsewhere. Interferon has been proposed for treatment of acute hemorrhagic conjunctivitis, but further studies are needed to evaluate its effectiveness. Chronic enterovirus infections in patients with agammaglobulinemia have been treated with γ-globulin, and in some cases this has controlled the infection.

No vaccines are available to prevent coxsackievirus infection or disease. General preventive measures include enteric precautions and good personal hygiene. Nosocomial infections are most serious in newborns and persons with compromised immune systems, but others may also be affected. Hospital staff can inadvertently carry the virus between patients or become infected themselves and spread the virus. The main strategy to prevent nosocomial infections is to manage patients with suspected enterovirus infection using enteric precautions. During outbreaks, patients and staff can be cohorted. In some cases, neonatal nurseries were closed to new admissions during newborn outbreaks to prevent further spread of the virus.

See also: Echoviruses; Human Eye Infections; Poliomyelitis; Rhinoviruses.

Further Reading

Bergelson JM, Cunningham JA, Droguett G, et al. (1997) Isolation of a common receptor for coxsackie B viruses and adenoviruses 2 and 5. *Science* 275(5304): 1320–1323.

He Y, Bowman VD, Mueller S, et al. (2000) Interaction of the poliovirus receptor with poliovirus. *Proceedings of the National Academy of Sciences, USA* 97(1): 79–84.

Huber S and Ramsingh AI (2004) Coxsackievirus-induced pancreatitis. *Viral Immunology* 17: 358–369.

Hyöty H and Taylor KW (2002) The role of viruses in human diabetes. *Diabetologia* 45: 1353–1361.

Hyypiä T and Stanway G (1993) Biology of coxsackie A viruses. *Advances in Virus Research* 42: 343–373.

Khetsuriani N, LaMonte A, Oberste MS, and Pallansch MA (2006) Enterovirus Surveillance – United States, 1970–2005. *Morbidity and Mortality Weekly Report Surveillance Summaries* 55(SS-8): 1–20.

Kim K-S, Hufnagel G, Chapman N, and Tracy S (2001) The group B coxsackieviruses and myocarditis. *Reviews in Medical Virology* 11: 355–368.

Muckelbauer JK, Kremer M, Minor I, et al. (1995) The structure of coxsackievirus B3 at 3.5 Å resolution. *Structure* 3: 653–667.

Pallansch MA and Oberste MS (2004) Coxsackievirus, echovirus, and other enteroviruses. In: Gorbach SL, Bartlett JG,, and Blacklow NR (eds.) *Infectious Diseases,* 3rd edn, pp. 2047–2051. Philadelphia, PA: Lippincott Williams and Wilkins.

Pallansch MA and Roos R (2006) Enteroviruses: Polioviruses, coxsackieviruses, echoviruses, and newer enteroviruses. In: Knipe DM, Howley PM, Griffin DE, et al. (eds.) *Fields Virology*, 5th edn Philadelphia, PA: Lippincott Williams and Wilkins.

Pozzetto B and Gaudin OG (1999) Coxsackieviruses (*Picornaviridae*). In: Granoff A and Webster R (eds.) *Encyclopedia of Virology,*, 2nd edn San Diego: Academic Press.

Rossmann MG, He Y, and Kuhn RJ (2002) Picornavirus–receptor interactions. *Trends in Microbiology* 10(7): 324–331.

Semler BL and Wimmer E (eds.) (2002) *Molecular Biology of Picornaviruses.* Washington, DC: ASM Press.

Stanway G, Brown F, Christian P, et al. (2005) Picornaviridae. In: Fauquet CM, Mayo MA, Maniloff J, Desselberger U,, and Ball LA (eds.) *Virus Taxonomy: Eighth Report of the International Committee on Taxonomy of Viruses*, pp. 757–778. San Diego, CA: Elsevier Academic Press.

Tracy S, Oberste MS,, and Drescher K (eds.) (2008) *Coxsackie B viruses. Current Topics in Microbiology and Immunology.* Berlin: Springer.

Echoviruses

T Hyypiä, University of Turku, Turku, Finland

History and Classification

Echoviruses belong to the species *Human enterovirus B* (HEV-B), in the genus *Enterovirus* of the family *Picornaviridae*. Original classification of picornaviruses was based mainly on physicochemical properties and pathogenesis in experimental animals. At the beginning of the twentieth century, poliomyelitis was transmitted to monkeys using a filterable agent from clinical patients and 40 years later, new related human picornaviruses (coxsackieviruses), that characteristically caused disease in newborn mice, were isolated. Based on the disease signs observed in mice they were classified into A and B subgroups. After introduction of tissue cultures for virus propagation, a number of new viruses were isolated that exhibited similar physicochemical characteristics (resistance to organic solvents and low pH) with polio- and coxsackieviruses, but grew exclusively in cell culture. Since the disease association of these viruses was at that time unclear, they were grouped among ECHO viruses, which stands for enteric (isolated mainly from stool samples), cytopathogenic (cytopathic effect observed in tissue culture), human (no disease in monkeys or in newborn mice), orphan (disease association not confirmed). There

are 28 distinct echovirus serotypes (EV1–33); EV1 and EV8 represent the same serotype, serotype 10 was identified to be a reovirus, serotype 28 was reclassified as a rhinovirus, and serotypes 22 and 23 were reclassified as members of a separate picornavirus genus, *Parechoviridae* (**Table 1**). Polioviruses, coxsackieviruses, and echoviruses formed human enteroviruses. Later, new enterovirus serotypes were not classified into the subgroups but were given successive numbers in the order of their identification (enteroviruses 68–71).

When sequence analysis became available, it was possible to determine the genetic relatedness of individual virus serotypes and strains. It was shown that echoviruses form a genetically rather coherent cluster and they are closely related to certain other enteroviruses. Molecular criteria replaced the previous enterovirus subgroup division in classification and currently echoviruses belong to the HEV-B species together with coxsackie B virus 1–6, coxsackievirus A9, and enterovirus 69 serotypes. More recently, identification of new enterovirus types has been exclusively based on comparison of the VP1 gene sequences, which correlate well with the previous serotype division. Currently, there are approximately 100 distinct enterovirus types, 63 of which have been assigned

Table 1 Summary of the molecular and clinical characteristics of echoviruses

Family	*Picornaviridae*
Genus	*Enterovirus*
Species	*Human enterovirus B*
Serotypes	1–7, 9, 11–21, 24–27, 29–33
Virus capsid	Nonenveloped, icosahedral, contains 60 copies of each of the capsid proteins VP1–4
Genome	Single-stranded, infectious RNA, approximately 7400 nt
Viral proteins	Cap-independent translation utilizing the internal ribosome entry site; translated as a polyprotein (2200 amino acids); the capsid proteins are at the N-terminus and the C-terminal part of the polyprotein contains the nonstructural proteins (2A, 2B, 2C, 3A, 3B, 3C, and 3D)
Receptors	
Most echoviruses	Decay-accelerating factor (CD55)
Echovirus 1	$\alpha 2\beta 1$ integrin
Echovirus 9 (Barty)	αV integrins
Entry route	Endocytosis
Replication	Viral RNA synthesis takes place on cytoplasmic membranes
Clinical manifestations	Meningitis, encephalitis, generalized infections of newborns, myocarditis, rashes, respiratory infections, severe infections in immunocompromised patients
Diagnosis	RT-PCR, virus isolation, serology

to serotypes. Further studies of the new members of the genus will show how many of them share biological properties with the classical echovirus serotypes.

Molecular Characteristics and Replication

Virus Particle

In general, echoviruses share the basic properties of other representatives of the enterovirus genus, where polioviruses are considered as the type members. Enteroviruses are composed of a protein capsid consisting of 60 copies of each of the four structural proteins (VP1–4) and enclosing a single-stranded infectious RNA genome, approximately 7400 nt in length. The diameter of the icosahedral virus particle is around 30 nm and the RNA genome represents about 30% of the molecular mass of the virion. VP1–3 are exposed on the surface of the virus particle and they all share the eight-stranded antiparallel β-barrel structure. These capsid proteins are responsible for the recognition of the cellular receptors and they contain the neutralizing B-cell epitopes, located in the variable loops connecting the β-strands and in the C-termini of the proteins. VP4 is located inside the virion

and it contains a myristic acid, covalently linked to the N-terminus. Five VP1 molecules form a star-shaped structure around the fivefold symmetry axis that is surrounded by a surface depression (a canyon), while VP2 and VP3 molecules alternate around the threefold axis. The structural subunits are a protomer, composed of one copy of each of the capsid proteins and a pentamer including five protomers. The three-dimensional structure of at least two echovirus serotypes (EV1 and EV11) have been determined by X-ray crystallography and some additional serotypes have also been studied by cryoelectron microscopy. In general, the detailed architecture of these echoviruses closely resembles that of other enteroviruses. Structural, immunological, and other biological reasons for the existence of almost 30 distinct echovirus serotypes in contrast to three polioviruses are currently not known.

The organization of the echovirus genome is analogous to other enteroviruses and the functions of the proteins have been mainly predicted on the basis of the findings reported for polioviruses. The capsid proteins are located at the N-terminal part (P1 region) of the polyprotein encoded by the viral RNA and the nonstructural proteins, necessary for replication, are at the C-terminal part (P2 and P3 regions). The 5′ noncoding region (NCR) contains around 750 nt, and it includes the structured elements important in translation (internal ribosome entry site, IRES) and genome replication. A small viral protein (3B, also known as VPg) is covalently linked to the 5′ terminus of the genome. The length of the 3′ NCR, also containing predicted secondary structures, is approximately 100 nt and it is followed by a poly(A) tract. The variation in the lengths of all echovirus genomes is in the range of 100 nt. The maximum difference between the 5′ NCR sequences is less than 25%; the capsid protein genes are rather variable (around 60–80% identity between the amino acid sequences of VP1), and less diversity is found at the nonstructural region (80–100% amino acid identity).

Replication Cycle

In most picornaviruses, the interaction with a specific cellular receptor takes place through structures located on the bottom of the canyon with the terminal domains of immunoglobulin (Ig) superfamily molecules. This interaction leads to conformational changes which give rise to further uncoating and release of the genome into the cytoplasm. Instead, many echoviruses attach to decay-accelerating factor (DAF, CD55) that belongs to a family of regulatory proteins protecting the cells from autologous complement-mediated lysis. DAF contains four short consensus repeat domains and is anchored to the surface of the plasma membrane. DAF-binding echoviruses interact mainly with the consensus repeat domain 3 but may also recognize binding sites in domains 2 or 4.

Interaction of DAF with echoviruses does not lead to similar alterations in the conformation of the virus particle that are observed after interaction of the Ig superfamily member receptors. Structural studies have revealed that the binding site of DAF in echovirus 7 is located in the VP2 protein close to the twofold symmetry axis in contrast to the binding site of the Ig superfamily molecules in the canyon. DAF is also recognized by certain coxsackie A and B viruses but the binding mechanisms are different and the conformational changes in these viruses are induced by subsequent interaction with members of the Ig superfamily molecules. Therefore, it is thought that additional cellular factors are also needed for successful internalization and uncoating of the DAF-binding echoviruses. Candidate molecules include β2-microglobulin, complement control protein CD59, and heparan sulfate.

Sequence analysis of the mouse-pathogenic echovirus 9 Barty strain revealed that there was a 10-amino-acid-long insert to the C-terminal end of the VP1 protein when compared to the Hill strain of the same serotype which does not cause disease in mice. This insert contains an arginine-glycine-aspartic acid (RGD) motif, known to interact with αV integrins, and this sequence has also been found in clinical isolates. Interestingly, coxsackievirus A9, another mouse-pathogenic member of the HEV-B species, contains a functional RGD motif in a similar position and recognizes αV integrins.

Echovirus 1 is the only picornavirus that is known to interact with α2β1 integrin (a collagen receptor) on the cell surface. The virus binds to the I (inserted) domain in the α2 subunit which is also recognized by collagen but there are remarkable differences between these interactions. The binding site has been localized to the outer wall of the canyon. As in the case of DAF interaction with other echoviruses, binding of the α2I-domain to EV1 does not bring about the conformational changes needed for uncoating *in vitro*. Attachment of the virus to the integrin gives rise to clustering of the receptor molecules which is known to be able to induce signaling events which may play an important role in the subsequent internalization processes.

Entry of echoviruses has been studied in serotypes 1 and 11. The integrin interaction of EV1 is followed by endocytosis of the virus–receptor complex into cytoplasmic structures which are rich in caveolin-1. This internalization process is initiated in lipid rafts and, subsequently, the virus entry can occur either in caveolae or through a faster route into caveosomes, which are preexisting intracellular organelles. How the EV1 genome is released from the caveosomes to the cytoplasm, is currently not known. Echovirus 11 appears to use similar mechanisms during entry. In the plasma membrane, DAF is present in lipid rafts, which are cholesterol-rich domains, and it has been shown that cholesterol depletion inhibits DAF-mediated echovirus infection. The virus can also be copurified with components found in lipid rafts.

When released to the cytoplasm, the picornavirus genome is infectious and it can act directly as an mRNA encoding a large polyprotein that is subsequently processed to the mature viral polypeptides. Based on similarity echovirus nonstructural proteins with those of poliovirus, viral replication cycles are evidently very similar. The proteolytic cleavages take place as a cascade and some of the intermediate products (2BC, 3AB, and 3CD) exhibit also specific activities. 2A is a protease responsible for the cleavage between the VP1 and 2A proteins and, in addition, it causes shut-off of host-cell protein synthesis by cleaving a cellular factor needed for cap-dependent translation. Proteases 3C and 3CD are responsible for other proteolytic processing events except the cleavage between VP4 and VP2 which may be autocatalytic.

In the infected cells, the viral nonstructural proteins associate with host-cell membrane compartments and modify these to establish a specialized complex for viral RNA synthesis. In these replication complexes, containing almost all the nonstructural proteins with multiple interactions with each other and viral RNA, the genome is copied through a complementary template to new genomic strands. 3D is an RNA-dependent RNA polymerase responsible for the synthesis of the positive and negative strands. Due to the deficient proof-reading activity of the viral RNA-dependent RNA polymerases, errors are frequently generated during the replication and in picornaviruses every new genome contains approximately one mutation. 3B (VPg), found at the 5′ termini of the RNA strands during replication but not during translation, plays a role in the priming of the RNA synthesis. The role of the 3AB protein is thought to be anchoring of VPg to the membranes for priming. The exact role of the 2B protein in the replication cycle is not known. It increases membrane permeability that may facilitate release of the mature viruses from the cells and it also interferes with cellular protein secretion. The 2C protein contains three motifs found in NTPases/helicases. Moreover, 2C and some other nonstructural proteins are involved in rearrangements of intracellular vesicles during formation of the replication complexes. In the assembly of infectious virions, the protomers form pentamers which can associate to form empty capsids. It is not clear whether the viral genome can be inserted into these particles or if they represent a reservoir of the structural units, finally assembling around viral RNA. The mature viruses are released as a result of the lysis of the cells.

Viral replication has dramatic effects in the host cell, including inhibition of cellular protein synthesis and secretion, interference with RNA synthesis and transport, and activation of other processes that together induce the cytopathic effect. Both apoptotic and anti-apoptotic effects, caused by enterovirus replication in cells, have been reported and also more detailed alterations can be detected. In EV1-infected cells, approximately 2% of the studied genes were induced whereas around 0.5% were downregulated. The activated genes included immediate-early response genes as well as genes involved in apoptotic pathways and cell growth regulation. Viral macromolecule synthesis was also observed to activate protein kinases known to control expression of several cellular genes. Further studies on the events during the infection may reveal cellular activities that are necessary for the infection or play a crucial role in the pathogenesis and they can become new potential targets of chemotherapy.

Clinical Manifestations

In general, the disease pattern caused by echoviruses is highly variable and most of the infections are evidently subclinical like those caused by other human enteroviruses. No specific disease condition can be directly associated with a certain echovirus and different serotypes cause identical clinical illnesses, while the same serotype can have a different clinical outcome in patients during the same epidemic.

Members of HEV-B species are among the most common causes of meningitis that may occur as sporadic cases as well as large epidemics. Typically, the symptoms and signs include fever, headache, nausea, stiffness of the neck, and may be associated with respiratory illness, rash, or myalgia. The manifestations may also exhibit signs of meningoencephalitis. Paralysis is a rare consequence of echovirus infection although some cases have been reported.

In neonates, a severe generalized infection, often clinically indistinguishable from bacterial sepsis, can include meningitis or meningoencephalitis, myocarditis, and hepatitis. A similar syndrome is caused by echoviruses and coxsackie B viruses. The transmission occurs transplacentally or soon after delivery from the mother but can also originate from other infected infants. Immunocompromised patients may develop serious chronic echovirus infections, like meningoencephalitis, occasionally with fatal outcome. These complications occur in individuals with B-cell deficiencies and gammaglobulin has been used for the prevention and treatment of the infections.

Echoviruses are associated with mild respiratory infections (e.g., common cold, bronchiolitis, and herpangina) that cannot be clinically distinguished from illnesses caused by other viral respiratory pathogens. Entroviruses cause maculopapular rashes with similar manifestations caused by other infections. Roseola-like skin manifestations can also occur during enterovirus infections and the 'Boston exanthem', caused by echovirus 16, was the first one of these infections recognized. Although echoviruses and other enteroviruses replicate in the gastrointestinal tract and nausea as well as diarrhea can be associated with the infection, they are not considered as major causative agents of acute viral gastroenteritis. Echoviruses have been isolated from individual cases of conjunctivitis but their role in the disease compared to enteroviruses causing epidemics (coxsackievirus A24 and enterovirus 70) is not important. Epidemics of uveitis, a severe eye infection, caused by echoviruses 11 and 19, have been described in Russia.

Myocarditis is often associated with coxsackie B viruses but other enteroviruses are evidently also responsible for this disease where specific diagnosis is usually difficult. Although neonatal myocarditis can be fatal, the manifestations of the disease in older age groups are often nonspecific, and the cardiac involvement is usually suspected on the basis of ECG findings and severe symptoms are uncommon. There is also evidence that enteroviruses could have an etiological role in the development of dilated cardiomyopathy.

Members of the HEV-B species have also been associated with the development of type 1 diabetes. This is based largely on seroepidemiological studies but, for instance, echoviruses have also been isolated from prediabetic and diabetic individuals and enterovirus genomes have been detected in the blood of patients with recent onset of diabetes. However, the role of enteroviruses in the process leading to type 1 diabetes remains unknown today. Echoviruses and other enteroviruses have also been suspected to have a role in amyotrophic lateral sclerosis, a chronic progressive neurological disorder, but further studies are required to clarify this association. Involvement of viruses, including enteroviruses, in the chronic fatigue syndrome has also been suspected, but this disease is still poorly characterized and the pathogenesis is not understood. It is known that echoviruses can cause chronic infections in cell culture models and availability of new animal models will further clarify their pathogenesis in the future. Sensitive and specific molecular methods will also cast light in the occurrence of echoviruses in diseases where the etiology is presently unknown.

Based on the observations about the protective effects of the inactivated poliovirus vaccine and appearance of severe chronic enterovirus infections in agammaglobulinemic patients, it is thought that protective immunity in enterovirus infections is mainly antibody mediated. It seems that the response is largely serotype specific and systemic infections may result in life-long immunity. Cell-mediated immunity against enterovirus infections is still rather poorly understood but there is evidence that cross-reactive epitopes between virus serotypes may exist.

Laboratory Diagnosis

Echoviruses can be detected from the cerebrospinal fluid (CSF) and respiratory tract samples during the acute phase of infection, but they may be excreted in stool samples for weeks or even months after the infection. Identification of enteroviruses has been classically based on isolation in cell culture followed by neutralization typing using antiserum pools. Although the advantage of the methods is that it gives information about the serotypes, the problem is the time and labor required. In spite of accelerated protocols, based on immunological staining of the infected cells, the isolation method is of limited use when specific diagnosis is required at the acute phase of the illness.

Introduction of the reverse transcription-polymerase chain reaction (RT-PCR) methods for the molecular detection of human picornaviruses revolutionized rapid diagnosis of the enterovirus infections, in particular those affecting the central nervous system. By this means, it is possible to obtain the results in a few hours which has an important impact in the differential diagnosis and treatment of the illness. Currently used RT-PCR methods take advantage of the conserved regions in the 5' noncoding region of the genome and do not therefore allow further typing of the detected enteroviruses. However, it has been shown that sequences of the VP1 gene correlate well with the current enterovirus serotypes which makes it possible to obtain more detailed information about the individual virus types. Often amplification of the VP1 sequences, utilizing less well-conserved primers, is not possible directly from the clinical material and requires a cell culture enrichment step. In the future, multiplex RT-PCR and microarray methods may provide us with new tools where the high sensitivity of the molecular methods can be combined with an informative collection of data about the pathogen.

There are no highly sensitive and specific standardized serological assays available for enteroviruses. Neutralization assays are serotype specific, but due to the large number of different viruses, the usage of this method is restricted to epidemiological studies. In-house methods, based on enzyme immonoassays or complement fixation tests, are widely used in diagnostic laboratories. The antigens are usually heat-treated to increase cross-reactivity and synthetic peptides containing conserved sequences are also in use. The presence of enterovirus-specific IgM antibodies or an increase in antibody titers between samples collected at the acute and convalescent phase of the illness are considered as a sign of acute infection.

Epidemiology

Transmission of echoviruses occurs through the respiratory and gastrointestinal routes and the epithelial tissue at these sites is the primary location of replication. This can be followed by viremia and infection of secondary target organs. It is possible that respiratory transmission may predominate in areas with improved hygiene. Several nosocomial outbreaks have been described in neonatal units. In addition to direct contact with infected individuals, the infection can be obtained from contaminated water and food. There is no evidence of animal reservoir for these viruses.

In many studies, echoviruses have been the most commonly isolated enteroviruses and there is an extensive number of reports of outbreaks from different geographical areas during several decades in the literature. Most frequently, the echoviruses have been isolated from children of less than 5 years of age that can be understood for immunological reasons and because of the increased risk of transmission. The occurrence of the infections in this age group does not necessarily correlate with the appearance of disease, since, for instance, meningitis may be detected more frequently in older children. Approximately half of the isolations originate from infections of the central nervous system and isolation from respiratory and gastrointestinal infections are more rarely used. One of the reasons for this is most probably that in mild infections specific diagnostic procedures are more rare. EV4, EV6, EV7, EV9, EV11, and EV30 have been among the predominating serotypes.

Enterovirus infections occur typically during the late summer and early autumn months in temperate climates while elsewhere, the viruses often appear to circulate through the year. The infections are more common in males and in individuals with lower socioeconomic status. Due to the high number of serotypes and the population immunity, there are considerable differences between the epidemiological periods, and variation from small local outbreaks to widespread epidemics is seen. There is also extensive fluctuation in the occurrence of the serotypes during the years and, for instance, echovirus 30 that has been responsible for large meningitis epidemics worldwide may sometimes represent almost half of the isolations but be absent during another epidemic season.

The epidemiological studies during the twentieth century were based on virus isolation and subsequent typing which provided information about the circulating serotypes. Since the RT-PCR assays only can give information about the presence or absence of enteroviruses in clinical samples, this epidemiological surveillance is significantly changing its character. However, introduction of molecular epidemiological analysis, based on the comparison of genomic sequences, has given new information about the circulation and evolution of the virus strains. The approach has been used in studies of, for example, echovirus 30 and the investigations have shown that there has been one predominant genotype with several distinct lineages circulating in Europe and in Northern America since 1978. These strains are clearly different from those isolated some decades ago and some genetic lineages seem to have completely disappeared during this time.

It has become clear that recombination is a frequent phenomenon in the evolution of enteroviruses. It has been mostly found to occur among the members of the species and in particular in the genome region encoding nonstructural proteins. Since the virus isolates are identified primarily on the basis of the serotype, based on the capsid region sequences, this heterogeneity of the genomes has not previously been observed in the epidemiological studies. Therefore, future studies may give a new picture about the circulating and reemerging genetic lineages. Although it is clear that the nonstructural gene region is evolving rapidly, the rules for the appearance of genetically mosaic strains which become predominant by their superior fitness and other properties remain still unclear. The importance of these events in the generation of new pathogenic strains would be highly important to understand and molecular epidemiological approaches and studies on picornavirus evolution in general will hopefully be able to cast new light on these questions.

Future Perspectives

There are currently no vaccines available against other human picornaviruses except polioviruses and hepatitis A virus. The number of echovirus and other enterovirus serotypes makes vaccine development particularly challenging, since the protection from infection is primarily thought to be mediated by serotype-specific neutralizing antibodies. The most promising chemotherapeutic agent developed against clinical picornavirus infections so far has been pleconaril, a capsid-stabilizing small molecule. It has been successfully used in severe enterovirus infections but due to side effects observed in a treatment study against common cold it is not in general use. Other molecules, based on a similar principle, as well as inhibitors of the virus-specific proteases have also been developed, and they are likely to become tools for the treatment of enterovirus infections in the near future. Since echoviruses, with a few exceptions, do not replicate in experimental animals, testing of antiviral drugs is problematic. However, there are promising results showing that the infection can be successfully transmitted to transgenic mice expressing human receptors for an echovirus.

An interesting application in cancer therapy is the use of naturally occurring or modified viruses. For instance, adenovirus-based systems have been used for this purpose. There are also enteroviruses that have been reported to have such an effect. An example is EV1 shown to exhibit tropism for human ovarian cancer cells.

As illustrated by these few examples, increasing knowledge of echoviruses and their replication is likely to provide us with new tools for the treatment of these infections in the future. New disease associations may also be found by using the improved diagnostic methods. Development of an enterovirus vaccine is a particularly important and demanding goal. Understanding of the cell tropism and detailed multiplication mechanisms of these viruses in the body may also provide us with new tools for the development of tools against clinical illnesses.

Acknowledgments

The original studies carried out in our laboratory were supported by grants from the Academy of Finland and the Sigrid Juselius Foundation.

See also: Coxsackieviruses; Enteric Viruses.

Further Reading

Minor PD and Muir PA (2004) Enteroviruses. In: Zuckerman AJ, Banatwala JE, Pattison JR, Griffiths PD,, and Schoub BD (eds.) *Principles and Practice of Clinical Virology*, pp. 467–489. New York: Wiley.

Pallansch MA and Roos RP (2001) Enteroviruses: Polioviruses, coxsackievirus, echoviruses, and newer enteroviruses. In: Knipe DM and Howley PM (eds.) *Fields Virology,* 4th edn., pp. 723–775. Baltimore, MD: Lippincott Williams and Wilkins.

Racaniello VR (2001) *Picornaviridae:*The viruses and their replication. In: Knipe DM and Howley PM (eds.) *Fields Virology,* 4th edn., pp. 685–722. Lippincott Wiliams & Wilkins.

Rotbart H (2002) Enteroviruses. In: Richman DD, Whitley RJ,, and Hayden FG (eds.) *Clinical Virology*, pp. 971–994. Washington, DC: ASM Press.

Semler B and Wimmer E (eds.) (2002) *Molecular Biology of Picornaviruses.* Washington, DC: ASM Press.

Enteric Viruses

R F Bishop and C D Kirkwood, Murdoch Childrens Research Institute Royal Children's Hospital, Melbourne, VIC, Australia

Introduction

The intestinal tract, lined by replicating epithelial cells, bathed in nutrient fluids and maintained at optimal temperature provides an ideal milieu for growth of many viruses. 'Enteric viruses' represent a wide spectrum of viral genera that invade and replicate in the mucosa of the intestinal tract, and that can be grouped as follows:

- viruses causing localized inflammation at any level of the intestinal tract, predominantly in small intestinal mucosa, resulting in acute gastroenteritis, for example, rotaviruses, caliciviruses, adenoviruses, astroviruses;

- viruses that multiply at any level of the intestinal tract, causing few enteric symptoms prior to producing clinical disease at a distant site, for example, measles virus, reoviruses (in mice), enteroviruses (including polioviruses, coxsackieviruses, enteroviruses, hepatitis A and E); and
- viruses that spread to the intestinal tract during the later stages of systemic disease, generally in an immunocompromised host, for example, human immunodeficiency virus (HIV), cytomegalovirus.

This article focuses upon the first category of viruses that cause enteric disease associated with primary replication in the intestinal tract.

Viruses Associated with Acute Gastroenteritis

Acute gastroenteritis is one of the most common health problems worldwide. More than 700 million cases are estimated to occur annually in children less than 5 years of age, resulting in few deaths in developed countries, but more than 2 million deaths in developing countries.

Worldwide, a diverse group of viral, bacterial, and parasitic pathogens cause acute enteric symptoms including nausea, vomiting, abdominal pain, fever, and acute diarrhea. Infections with viral agents, unlike those with bacterial or parasitic pathogens, cannot be treated with antibiotics, and many cannot be prevented by improvements in quality of drinking water, food, or sanitation.

Until the early 1970s most viral agents causing gastroenteritis in humans were largely unknown. Studies using electron microscopy of intestinal contents resulted in the discovery of numerous viral enteropathogens now classified as caliciviruses, rotaviruses, astroviruses, or 'enteric' adenoviruses. Caliciviruses are now recognized as the most important cause worldwide of outbreaks of viral gastroenteritis in humans of all age groups. Rotaviruses are the single most important cause of life-threatening diarrhea in children <5 years old. Astroviruses and adenoviruses also cause severe diarrhea in children. **Table 1** lists the characteristics of the major viruses associated with acute gastroenteritis. Other viruses linked to gastroenteritis in humans include coronaviruses, toroviruses, picornaviruses, and picobirnaviruses. Understanding many features of these 'enteric viruses' has been based on parallel studies of related viruses infecting animals.

Caliciviruses

History

The family *Caliciviridae* contain small RNA viruses that cause enteric disease in a wide variety of hosts including cattle, pigs, rabbits, and humans. Infections in other hosts, for example, sea lions, cats, and primates, appear to cause predominantly systemic and respiratory symptoms. Caliciviruses are small nonenveloped viruses of 27–35 nm diameter (**Figure 1**) with a genome comprising a single-stranded positive-sense polyadenylated RNA genome of 7400–7700 nucleotides (nt). Typical calicivirus particles show cup-like hollows (calices) on the virus surface. Some caliciviruses have an indistinct appearance described as 'feathery'.

The 'Norwalk agent' (now classified as a calicivirus) was identified in 1972 by Kapikian and colleagues, using immune-electron microscopy (IEM) to search for the causa-

Table 1 Characteristics of major enteric viruses causing acute gastroenteritis in humans

Characteristic Family	Norovirus/ Sapovirus Caliciviridae	Rotavirus Reoviridae	Adenovirus Adenoviridae	Astrovirus Astroviridae
	Divided into genogroups, each with distinct genetic clusters	Six groups (A–F) Group A-multiple serotypes based on outer capsid proteins.	Six subgenera, more than 50 serotypes Enteric serotypes (Ad40–41)	Eight serotypes
Virion size (nm)	28–35	70	80	28
Capsid organization	Two structural proteins (orf2–56–62 kDa, orf3–22 kDa)	Two outer capsid proteins (VP7–38 kDa, VP4–88 kDa) Two inner protein layers (VP6–41 kDa, VP2–88 kDa)	Capsomer – composed of three proteins: hexon, penton, and fiber.	Precursor cleaved into several proteins (e.g., 20 kDa, 29 kDa and 31 kDa)
Nucleic acid	ssRNA (plus sense)	dsRNA	dsDNA	ssRNA (plus sense)
Genome organization	Three open reading frames (1, 2, and 3)	11 segments which encode specific protein.	Linear chromosome with multiple transcription/ translation units	2 open reading frames (1a, 1b, and 2)

ss, single-stranded; ds, double-stranded; kDa, kilodalton.

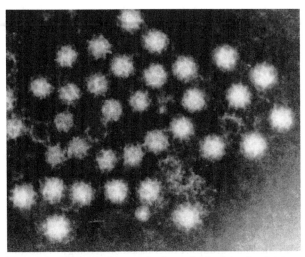

Figure 1 Electron micrograph of negatively stained calicivirus particles (NoV) in fecal extract.

tive agent of an 1968 outbreak of gastroenteritis in humans in Norwalk, Ohio, USA. Many related viruses have been implicated as causes of gastroenteritis, and given names identifying the geographical location of the outbreak (e.g., Marin County, Snow Mountain, Hawaii, Sapporo).

Classification

Classification of caliciviruses was hampered for many years by the inability to culture these viruses, and study their genetic and protein structure. Caliciviruses causing enteric infections (in humans and other animals) are classified as belonging to the family *Caliciviridae*, which is divided into four genera. The genus *Norovirus* (NoV), and genus *Sapovirus* (SaV) cause human and animal infections. Other genera infect rabbits (*Lagovirus*) or sealions, cats, and primates (*Vesivirus*). The genome organization and reading frame usage differs between the four genera. For noroviruses, the genome contains three open reading frames (ORFs). The largest (ORF1) encodes a polyprotein which undergoes proteolytic cleavage to produce an NTPase, a 3c-like protease, and an RNA-dependent RNA polymerase (RdRp). ORF2 encodes the major capsid protein and ORF3 a putative minor capsid protein.

Noroviruses are subdivided into five genogroups (GI–GV). Genogroups GI, GII, and GIV infect humans, GIII infects cattle and GV infects mice. GI and GII contain at least 10 and 20 distinct genetic clusters, respectively. Sapoviruses are divided into genogroups (GI–GV), of which GI, GII, GIV, and GV infect humans. GI and GII are further divided into four and three genetic clusters.

The inability to culture human caliciviruses delayed the introduction of diagnostic tests, resulting in an under-appreciation of the significance of these agents for many years. Currently, over 20 different reverse

transcription-polymerase chain reaction (RT-PCR) assays targeting regions on the RdRp gene and the capsid gene have been described and utilized in epidemiological studies. This large genetic diversity of human caliciviruses makes routine detection difficult.

Geographic and Seasonal Distribution

Human NoV are the leading causes of 'nonbacterial gastroenteritis' outbreaks in all age groups worldwide. Outbreaks frequently occur in communities such as nursing homes, hospitals, schools, and cruise ships. No consistent seasonal variation has been observed. Infection involves transmission via person-to-person contact or ingestion of contaminated food and water.

Epidemiological studies have identified caliciviruses in 60–95% of outbreaks in many countries. Estimates of disease burden in USA suggest that caliciviruses are responsible annually for 23 million illnesses and 50 000 hospitalizations. Strains of NoV GII cluster 4 (GII-4) have been the most common type identified worldwide in the past 5 years (2001–2005) in both adults and children. Prevalence rates of calicivirus (predominantly NoV) in young children admitted to hospital with acute gastroenteritis in many countries range from 3.5% to 20% annually. Strains of SaV, while playing a minor role overall, are more generally associated with childhood gastroenteritis than with disease in older children and adults. Caliciviruses may be important enteric pathogens in patients with hereditary or acquired immunodeficiency.

Genetics

The genera *Norovirus* and *Sapovirus* are genetically diverse, and multiple strains co-circulate in human populations. Individual dominant strains emerge every 2–5 years, and often have a global impact, such as the GII-4 strains identified in USA, Europe, Japan, and Australia in 1995/ 1996 and again in 2004. NoV recombinant strains, with polymerase and capsid genes derived from different ancestral clusters, have been identified in Thailand and Australia. Repeated attempts to adapt NoV and SaV to growth in cell culture have failed. Diagnostic techniques and analysis of antigenic variation rely predominantly on molecular biological techniques. Cloning and expression of the major viral capsid protein (VP1) in baculovirus expression systems has led to the formation of virus-like particles (VLPs) morphologically similar to native virus and their incorporation into enzyme immunoassay (EIA) assays.

Pathogenesis

Pathogenesis of NoV and SaV infection is poorly understood as a result of the long-standing inability to adapt these viruses to cell culture, and the absence of a small animal model. Symptomatic enteritis in human volunteers infected with 'Norwalk agent' showed changes in jejunal biopsies (mucosal inflammation, absorptive cell abnormalities, villus shortening, and crypt hypertrophy) that persisted for at least 4 days after remission of clinical symptoms and reverted to normal after 2 weeks. No identifiable viral particles were detected by electron microscopy in any affected intestinal tissue. The recent demonstration that human noroviruses can infect and replicate in a three-dimensional cell culture model of human intestinal epithelium, should improve our understanding of the pathogenesis, and antigenic diversity of this important group of enteric viruses. These studies will also be enhanced by discovery of a norovirus that infects mice, and that replicates after transfection of cultured kidney cells.

Immune Responses, Prevention and Control

Mechanisms of immunity to NoV are unclear. Infection results in formation of IgG and IgM serum antibody that are broadly reactive within, but not between, genogroups. The role of these antibodies in immune protection is unknown. Infected individuals can develop short-term immunity to homologous viruses but the molecular diversity of NoV circulating in communities makes it difficult to predict whether long-term immunity can develop. It is unclear why a proportion of exposed individuals remain uninfected during outbreaks. Recent studies suggest that histo-blood group antigens and the secretor status may be genetic susceptibility markers for infection. At present the major control strategies for prevention of human calicivirus infection rely on prevention of contamination of food and water supplies.

Rotaviruses

History

Virus particles, later classified in the genus *Rotavirus*, were first described in 1963 by Adams and Kraft as a cause of epidemic diarrhea in infant mice (EDIM). Similar particles (NCDV) were recognized in 1969 by Mebus and colleagues as a cause of severe diarrhea in newborn calves in Nebraska, USA. Neither virus was considered relevant as a causative agent of severe diarrhea in young children until 1973 when Bishop, Davidson, Holmes, and Ruck described a 'new virus' (later shown to be antigenically related to EDIM and NCDV) in duodenal biopsies and diarrheal feces from young children admitted to hospital in Melbourne, Australia with severe acute diarrhea. Named because of their wheel-like appearance in negatively stained extracts examined by electron microscopy (rota = Latin for wheel) rotaviruses have

since become established as causes of severe acute diarrhea in the young of many mammalian and avian species worldwide. Rotavirus enteritis affects all children regardless of socioeconomic status, and results in over 600 000 deaths annually in young children in developing countries.

Classification

Rotaviruses are nonenveloped icosahedral viruses of 70 nm (**Figure 2**) diameter that belong to the genus *Rotavirus* within the family *Reoviridae*. The double-stranded RNA genome is contained within a triple-layer of viral proteins (VPs) comprising a core (VP1, VP2, VP3), an inner capsid (VP6), and an outer capsid (VP4, VP7). Rotaviruses are classified into groups A to G based on serology of the VP6 protein. The majority of human and mammalian infections, due to group A viruses, are further classified into serotypes by antigenic differences on VP7 (G-serotypes) and into genotypes by genetic differences on VP4 (P-genotypes). To date there are at least 11 of 15 G-serotypes and 15 of 26 P-genotypes identified in humans. Groups B and C have been identified infrequently in humans. Groups D to G have been identified only in nonhuman mammalian or avian species.

Geographic and Seasonal Distribution

Five rotavirus serotypes G1P[8], G3P[8], G4P[8], G2P[4], and G9P[8] have been the most common serotypes causing severe human disease globally during the past 30 years. G1P [8] strains have been consistently present worldwide. Yearly winter epidemics of rotavirus disease are regularly observed

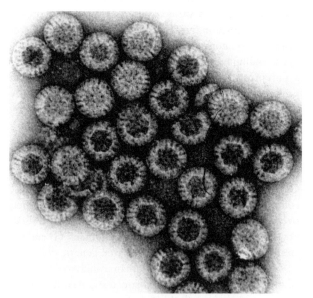

Figure 2 Electron micrograph of negatively stained triple-shelled rotavirus particles in fecal extract.

in countries with temperate climates, whereas rotavirus disease is prevalent year-round in tropical climates lacking defined winter seasons.

Host Range

Group A rotaviruses infect humans and other mammals repeatedly throughout life. Most primary rotavirus infections in animals occur during the neonatal period. Most primary rotavirus infections in humans occur during the first 24 months of life. Children worldwide will experience at least one rotavirus infection by 5 years of age.

In general, group A rotaviruses are species specific. However, rotavirus strains with gene segments of feline, bovine, or porcine origin have been isolated from children, suggesting the occurrence of cross-species infection in nature. Cross-species infections can be established experimentally, and comprise one of the strategies for human vaccine development.

Genetics

The rotavirus genome consists of 11 segments of double-stranded RNA that can be separated by polyacrylamide gel electrophoresis, allowing epidemiological studies mapping the genetic diversity of strains within and between serotypes. Each gene segment encodes a separate protein, with the exception of gene segment 11 which encodes two proteins. Reassortment of genes between human strains and human and animal strains occurs *in vivo* and *in vitro*.

Pathogenesis

Rotaviruses are transmitted from person to person by the fecal–oral route, or via aerosols. Rotaviruses replicate in the cytoplasm of mature nonreplicating enterocytes lining the upper portions of the small intestinal villi, eventually causing cytolysis. Profuse watery diarrhea results from a combination of mechanisms including malabsorption secondary to loss of enterocytes responsible for absorption and digestion, activation of the enteric nervous system, and stimulation of intestinal secretion by the rotavirus nonstructural protein NSP4. Rotavirus antigenemia and viremia occur during the acute phase of severe primary rotavirus disease. As a result, complete rotavirus particles have been found in liver, lung, spleen, pancreas, thymus, and kidneys of experimental animals. It is not clear if the virus is replicating at these sites.

Clinical Features

Clinical symptoms in children are strongly influenced by age, with severe often life-threatening diarrhea occurring after primary infection in young children, and in aged people in nursing homes. Excretion of rotavirus particles in detectable numbers (by EIA, RT/PCR) continues for 5–10 days, and occasionally up to 50 days. Excretion can continue for months in immunodeficient children and animals. Reinfections occur throughout life, and are usually asymptomatic or associated with mild symptoms. Symptoms of primary infection require medical attention in 1:5 children, result in hospitalization in 1:65 children and death in 1:293 (almost all in young children in developing countries). Treatment is based upon replacement of fluid and electrolyte loss, usually achieved by oral administration of fluids containing glucose and electrolytes. Occasionally, delayed repair of the small intestinal mucosa is associated with disaccharide or monosaccharide malabsorption leading to malnutrition.

Immune Response/Prevention and Control

Primary rotavirus infection protects against severe symptomatic disease on reinfection, and is associated with humoral and cellular immune responses to individual rotavirus proteins. Neutralizing antibody to VP4 and VP7 outer capsid proteins contribute to protection, possibly by interfering with viral replication and limiting the extent of intestinal damage. The role of immune responses to other proteins is uncertain. Virus-specific cytotoxic T cells are not essential for protection.

The importance of rotavirus disease worldwide and its contribution to childhood mortality in developing countries has resulted in strong initiatives, supported by the World Health Organization, to develop live oral rotavirus vaccines to be administered to infants before 3 months of age. Two contrasting vaccines, a single attenuated G1P[8] human rotavirus and a pentavalent human–bovine G1-G4,P[8] reassortant vaccine, have been proved to be safe and effective in preventing severe rotavirus disease. Both have the potential to radically change global childhood mortality and morbidity.

Adenovirus

History and Classification

Adenoviruses were first detected in 1953 in cultured fragments of tonsillar and adenoidal tissue from children. They are nonenveloped icosahedral viruses approximately 80 nm in diameter (**Figure 3**). The genome is composed of double-stranded DNA. The family *Adenoviridae* comprises three genera: *Mastadenovirus* (mammalian) classified into subgenera A–F representing more than 50 serotypes, *Aviadenovirus* (birds), and a newly recognized genus *Atadenovirus* identified in sheep and reptiles. Most are readily cultivatable. Adenovirus infections occur worldwide in many mammalian species, are species specific, usually

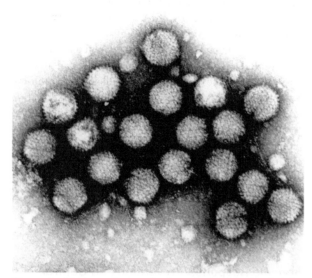

Figure 3 Electron micrograph of negatively stained 'enteric' adenovirus particles (showing characteristic hexagonal shape) in fecal extract. Courtesy of professor M. Studdert.

associated with disease in the respiratory, urinary, and ocular systems, and are frequently shed in feces in the absence of any gastrointestinal symptoms.

In 1975, Flewett and colleagues in Birmingham, UK, noticed the presence of large numbers of adenovirus particles in negatively stained extracts of diarrheal stools examined by EM. These proved difficult to culture, were designated 'enteric' adenoviruses (EAd), and are now classified as serotypes EAd40 and EAd41 within subgenus group F. Cultivation of EAd remains difficult. The most reliable growth has been achieved in human embryonic kidney cells (293 cells) immortalized by transfection with regions of Ad5.

Geographic and Seasonal Distribution

EAd40 and EAd41 occur worldwide, causing severe acute enteritis in 5–15% of hospitalized young children. Outbreaks occur at unpredictable intervals year-round with no seasonal prevalence. Nosocomial epidemics occur in day-care nurseries and in hospital wards for children and adults. Group A adenoviruses (serotypes 12, 18, 31) have also been implicated in epidemics, usually in older age groups.

Genetics/Evolution

The adenovirus virion is composed of at least 10 different structural polypeptides and contains a linear 33–45 kbp DNA. Virus capsomers are arranged as hexons, the corners of which have antenna-like (fiber) projections presumed involved in cell attachment. The DNA genomes of groups A–F are genetically diverse, and differences

can be illustrated by analysis using genome restriction endonucleases. The heterogenous genome in groups A–F makes recombination between subgenera unlikely, with exception of groups A and F which show a close evolutionary relationship.

Diagnoses of EAd infection rely on EIA that detects the hexon antigen common to groups A–F, followed by determination of restriction enzyme patterns and/or reactions in EIA incorporating neutralizing, monoclonal antibodies specific for Ed40 and 41.

Pathogenesis

EAd replicate within the epithelial cells of the small intestine. Group A adenoviruses have also been grown from mesenteric lymph nodes and appendices. The mechanisms causing diarrhea are not clear, but destruction of infected epithelial cells has a role.

Clinical Features

Adenovirus diarrhea is more common in infants <12 months old than in older children, and can be protracted with a mean duration of 12 days. Adenovirus diarrhea occurs in immunocompromised patients. Nonseasonal epidemics of EAd diarrhea occur in hospital wards, orphanages, and day-care nurseries. Occasional fatal cases have been reported in children. Evidence from animal models (with non-EAd) suggests that viremia occurs, and can lead to infection of other tissues. The natural history of disease and development of immunity is unknown.

Astroviruses

History and Classification

Astroviruses were first described in the UK in 1975 by Madeley and Cosgrove studying an outbreak of diarrhea in newborn babies in an obstetric hospital nursery. Astroviruses are small, round nonenveloped plus-stranded RNA viruses 28–30 nm diameter (**Figure 4**) occasionally exhibiting virions with a superficial star shape. They are members of the genus *Astrovirus* in the family *Astroviridae*. They have been detected in humans (children and adults) and a range of mammalian (sheep, cattle, pigs, dogs, cats, and mice) and avian (turkeys, ducks) species, usually associated with diarrhea. There are currently eight serotypes of human astrovirus, designated HAstV 1–8, based on reactivity with polyclonal antisera. HAstV 1 is most common worldwide.

Prevalence rates as a cause of diarrhea vary from 2% to 16% (hospital-based studies), and 5% to 17% (community-based studies). Most astrovirus infections have been recorded during colder months in temperate climates and year-round in tropical countries. A longitudinal study in Mayan children in a poor community in Mexico found a high prevalence (61%) of astrovirus infection in a birth cohort of 271 children followed for 3 years. Infection occurred primarily in infants <12 months old, and showed a high rate of asymptomatic infection and prolonged shedding (2–17 weeks) in many infants. Astrovirus infection has also been associated with persistent diarrhea (lasting for 14 days or more) in children in Bangladesh. Astroviruses are widespread in developed countries, causing outbreaks in day-care centers, hospitals, and nursing homes for the elderly. They are an important cause of enteritis in immunocompromised patients.

Genetics and Evolution

The HAst genome is a polyadenylated plus-stranded RNA molecule of approximately 7 kbp. The genome contains two open reading frames (ORFs), ORF1a and -1b, code for nonstructural proteins and ORF2 encodes for the capsid protein. Genetic diversity in all serotypes exists, but no association has been shown between serotypes and ability to cause severe gastroenteritis. Astrovirus diagnostic assays include commercially available EIA kits, electron microscopy and RT-PCR detection and genotyping of diarrheal feces.

Pathogenesis

Acute astrovirus infection induces a mild watery diarrhea in young children that lasts for 2–3 days and may be associated with vomiting, fever, and anorexia. The lack of a small animal model has hampered studies of the mechanism of astrovirus-induced diarrhea. Experimental models of astrovirus enteritis in turkeys and in gnotobiotic

lambs show mild histopathological changes in the intestine (despite high mortality from severe osmotic diarrhea) together with viremia. Experimental astrovirus infection in calves is asymptomatic, with viral replication apparently targeted to M cells. It is possible that none of these animal models illuminate pathogenesis of HAstV infection in humans. Cultivation of HAstV was initially difficult, but can now regularly be achieved using a human colon cancer derived epithelial cell line (CaCo2 cells).

Coronaviruses/Toroviruses

Members of the genera *Coronavirus* and *Torovirus* are enveloped plus-strand single-stranded RNA viruses belonging to the family *Coronaviridae*. Electron microscopy shows them to be pleomorphic fringed particles 100–140 nm at maximum dimension (**Figure 5**). Coronaviruses and toroviruses can be distinguished by differences in peplomer structure and reaction in IEM using specific antisera.

Coronaviruses and toroviruses cause diarrhea, respiratory, and/or hepatic disease in many animal species, including cattle, mice, swine, cats, and dogs. In general, most of these viruses are species specific and disease is most severe in infant animals. Transmission is fecal–oral and due to virus lability may require close contact. Coronaviruses and toroviruses have been implicated in human diarrheal disease but there is still no consensus about their importance. Similar particles have been seen frequently in children without diarrhea, particularly in children in developing countries. Morphological similarities between these viruses and fragments of intestinal brush border make diagnosis difficult. Several studies

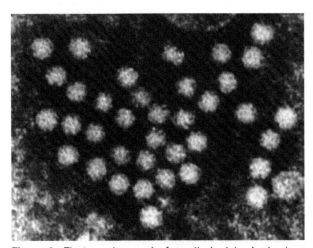

Figure 4 Electron micrograph of negatively stained astrovirus particles (showing star-shape) in fecal extract.

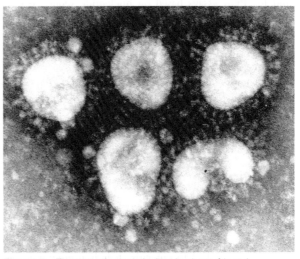

Figure 5 Electron micrograph showing large fringed pleomorphic coronavirus particles (with adherent antibody) in fecal extract.

have implicated coronaviruses as causative agents of necrotizing enterocolitis outbreaks in newborn babies.

Toroviruses were first described as a cause of diarrhea by Woode and colleagues in 1979 when Breda virus was identified in a severe outbreak of neonatal calf diarrhea in USA. Toroviruses are now also known to infect horses (Berne virus) and swine. Human infections were first described by Flewett *et al.* in Birmingham UK in 1984, but have rarely been reported since then.

The pathogenesis of diarrhea has been studied in animal models using infection with coronavirus (TGE) in piglets, and with Breda viruses in calves. Both replicate in epithelial cells of small intestine and descending colon causing diarrhea 24–72 h later. Breda virus also replicates in crypt cells.

Many animal coronaviruses can be propagated in cell culture. Isolation of human enteric coronaviruses is difficult and serological studies can be confounded by antibody resulting from repeated respiratory coronavirus infection. Enteric infection can be confirmed in feces by detection of viral RNA by RT-PCR, or IEM using antibodies to the viral envelope glycoproteins.

Picornaviruses

Picornaviruses are 24–30 nm featureless spherical particles containing single-stranded positive-sense RNA. They have been found in diarrheal feces from humans but their etiological role is often not clear. The first clear evidence implicating a picornavirus as an enteric pathogen identified Aichi virus, as a cause of oyster-associated epidemics of gastroenteritis in Japan in 1989. Aichi viruses are now classified as a new genus *Kobuvirus* within the family *Picornaviridae* (kobu = Japanese for knob). Isolation of Aichi virus in Vero cells has permitted development of EIA and RT-PCR assays based on nucleotide sequence data. Serological assays show seroconversion resulting from infection and a prevalence rate for antibody of 7.2% in Japanese children aged 7 months to 4 years and rising to 80% in adults by age 35.

The new genus *Parechovirus* within the family *Picornavirideae* contains at least one serotype (previously echovirus 22) that has been implicated as an enteric pathogen in humans.

Parvoviruses

Parvoviruses are small 22–26 nm single-stranded DNA viruses comprising a genus *Parvovirus* in the family *Parvoviridae*. Some animal parvoviruses have been clearly linked to enteritis including bovine, feline, mink, and canine strains. Canine parvovirus infection emerged after 1977. This lethal neonatal enteric infection,

accompanied by viremia and widespread systemic infection, shows a pathogenesis distinct from most enteropathogenic viruses. The virus infects and destroys crypt epithelial cells resulting in flat mucosa with fused and stunted villi. Damage has been likened to that caused by radiation.

Other small viruses, resembling parvoviruses, have been seen by EM in diarrheal feces in humans. Evidence linking them to causation of disease is not convincing. They have often been present as dual infections with known enteric pathogens. In addition, their resemblance to some phages makes diagnosis uncertain.

Picobirnaviruses

These are a group of currently unclassified small viruses detected in the feces of humans and animals without diarrhea. Picobirnaviruses are 35–41 nm particles with a bi- or tri-segmented dsRNA genome and have been detected in Europe, South America, and Australia. They are found significantly more often in patients with HIV-related diarrhea than those without diarrhea. Their role in gastroenteritis in healthy individuals remains unknown.

See also: Astroviruses.

Further Reading

Atmar RL and Estes MK (2001) Diagnosis of noncultivable gastroenteritis viruses, the human caliciviruses. *Clinical Microbiology Reviews* 14: 15–37.
Bresee JS, Widdowson M-A, Monroe SS, and Glass RI (2002) Foodborne viral gastroenteritis: Challenges and opportunities. *Clinical Infectious Diseases* 35: 748–753.
Chadwick D and Goode JA (2001) *Gastroenteritis Viruses. Novartis Foundation Symposium*, 2nd edn.. New York: Wiley.
Chiba S, Estes MK, Nakata S, and Calisher CH (eds.) (1996) *Viral gastroenteritis. Archives of Virology* 5th edn.: 119–128.
Duckmanton L, Luan B, Devenish J, Tellier R, and Petric M (1997) Characterisation of torovirus from human faecal specimens. *Virology* 239: 158–168.
Franco MA, Angel J, and Greenberg HB (2006) Immunity and correlates of protection for rotavirus vaccines. *Vaccine* 24: 2718–2731.
Glass RI (2006) New hope for defeating rotavirus. *Scientific American* 294: 33–39.
Hall GA (1987) Comparative pathology of infection by novel diarrhoea viruses. In: Bock G and Whelan J (eds.) *Novel Diarrhoea Viruses. Ciba Foundation Symposium*, vol. 128, pp. 192–217. Chichester: Wiley.
Hansman GS, Oka T, Katayami K, and Takeda N (2007) Human Sapovirus: Genetic diversity, recombination and classification. *Reviews in Medical Virology* 17: 133–141.
Mendez-Toss M, Griffin DD, Calva J, *et al.* (2004) Prevalence and genetic diversity of human astroviruses in Mexican children with symptomatic and asymptomatic infections. *Journal of Clinical Microbiology* 42: 151–157.
Ramig RF (1997) Genetics of the rotaviruses. *Annual Reviews of Microbiology* 51: 225–255.
Ramig RF (2004) Pathogenesis of intestinal and systemic rotavirus infection. *Journal of Virology* 78: 10213–10220.
Schwab KJ, Estes MK, and Atmar RL (2000) Norwalk and other human caliciviruses: Molecular characterization, epidemiology and

pathogenesis. In: Cary JW, Linz JE, and Bhatnagar D (eds.) *Microbial Foodborne Diseases: Mechanisms of Pathogenesis and Toxin Synthesis*, pp. 469–493. Lancaster, USA: Technomic Publishing Company.

Straub TM, Honer zu Bentrup K, Orosz-Coghlan P, *et al.* (2007) *In vitro* cell culture infectivity assay for human noroviruses. *Emerging Infectious Diseases* 13: 396–403.

Tiemessen CT and Kidd AH (1995) The subgroup F adenoviruses. *Journal of General Virology* 76. 481–497.

Yamashita T, Sugiyama M, Tsuzuki H, *et al.* (2000) Application of a reverse transcription-PCR for identification and differentiation of Aichi virus, a new member of the picornavirus family associated with gastroenteritis in humans. *Journal of Clinical Microbiology* 38: 2955–2961.

Flaviviruses: General Features

T J Chambers, Saint Louis University School of Medicine, St. Louis, MO, USA

Glossary

Cirrhosis Disease of the liver, with fibrosis and distortion of the cellular architecture.

Enzootic A disease or maintenance transmission cycle which occurs in a continuous manner among nonhuman animals within a certain geographic zone.

Epizootic Above average activity or occurrence of disease or pathogenic agent among nonhuman animals.

Sylvatic Located in forested regions.

Thrombocytopenia A reduction in the normal quantity of circulating blood platelets.

Zoonosis A disease of animals communicable to man.

General Features

The family *Flaviviridae* includes three genera, *Flavivirus*, *Pestivirus*, and *Hepacivirus*, that together comprise approximately 80 known viruses (**Table 1**), many of which cause diseases in human or animal hosts. Viruses in these genera are antigenically distinct from viruses in other genera and overall sequence homology is approximately 20%. The flaviviruses constitute the largest genera within the family, including arthropod-borne viruses that cause encephalitis and hemorrhagic fever. Pestiviruses exhibit a host range that includes pigs and ruminants. Hepaciviruses cause chronic liver disease in humans. Flaviviruses were originally classified as the 'group A' members of the family *Togaviridae*, distinguished serologically from 'group A' arboviruses (e.g., equine encephalitis viruses) but later assigned as constituting a unique family of viruses. Although vector associations together with antigenic properties previously served to classify the *Flaviviridae*, modern taxonomy based

on nucleotide sequencing has been used to establish their phylogenetic and evolutionary relationships.

Members of the *Flaviviridae* are enveloped viruses which share a common genome organization and replication strategy. Their virions are small, spherical particles containing the capsid–genome complex and membrane-associated envelope proteins, which confer antigenic properties. The genomes are small, single-stranded, plus-sense RNA molecules ranging in size from 9.6 to 12.3 kbp. Viral proteins are encoded within a single long open reading frame that contains the structural proteins, followed by nonstructural proteins (protease(s), RNA helicase, RNA-dependent RNA polymerase (RdRp), other enzymatic activities involved in RNA replication, and several small hydrophobic membrane proteins).

Flaviviruses and pestiviruses exhibit generally broad cellular host range *in vitro*, whereas growth of hepaciviruses is very restricted. Entry of viruses into host cells occurs by receptor-mediated endocytosis, requiring a low pH-dependent fusion activity of the major envelope proteins. Cellular receptors involved in the entry process have been difficult to definitively identify. Viral replication occurs in association with intracellular membranes via a negative-strand RNA intermediate. Characteristic ultrastructural changes are induced in the membranes. Mature viruses are generated by budding through host intracellular membranes followed by release at the cell surface. Further details of these processes and unique features of each genus are described below.

Flaviviruses

History and Classification

The genus includes >70 viruses, approximately 40 of which are mosquito-borne, 16 tick-borne, and 18 without a known vector. The prototypic flavivirus, yellow fever virus (from the Latin *flavus* for 'yellow'), is recognized as a human

Table 1   Taxonomy of viruses of the family *Flaviviridae*

Genus *Flavivirus* (12 complexes[a]; 1 tentative species/
  subspecies)
  Tick-borne viruses
    Mammalian tick-borne virus complex (10 members)
    Seabird tick-borne virus complex (3 members)
  Mosquito-borne viruses
    Aroa virus complex (4 members)
    Dengue virus complex (5 members)
    Japanese encephalitis virus complex (10 members)
    Kokobera virus complex (2 members)
    Ntaya virus complex (6 members)
    Spondweni virus complex (2 members)
    Yellow fever virus complex (10 members)
  Viruses with no known arthropod vector
    Entebbe bat virus complex (3 members)
    Modoc virus complex (6 members)
    Rio Bravo complex (7 members)
  Tentative members of the genus
    Alkhurma virus (1 member)
Genus *Pestivirus* (4 species plus 1 tentative species)
  Border disease virus (2 serotypes)
  Bovine viral diarrhea virus-1 (4 serotypes)
  Bovine viral diarrhea virus-2 (2 serotypes)
  Classical swine fever virus (*Hog cholera virus*), (4 serotypes)
  Tentative species in the genus
    Pestivirus of giraffe
Genus *Hepacivirus* (1 species)
  Hepatitis C virus (6 genotypes)
  Unassigned viruses in the family
    Tamana bat virus
    Cell-fusing agent
    GB virus A
    GBV A-like agents
    GB virus B
    GB virus C/Hepatitis G virus

[a]Complex refers to closely related viruses, representing genetic
and antigenic clusters, and viral species in the complexes are
enumerated in parentheses, or otherwise indicated. All others
represent virus strains or serotypes.
Reproduced in revised form from Calisher CH and Gould EA
(2003) Taxonomy of the virus family Flaviviridae. *Advances in
Virus Research* 59: 1–19, with permission from Elsevier.

disease agent for at least the past 300 years. In the early
twentieth century, the virus was isolated and characterized
as an arthropod-transmitted agent, and a live-attenuated
vaccine (yellow fever strain 17D) was developed. Other
flaviviruses causing a range of human diseases were identified
within the nineteenth and twentieth centuries. The most
important of these are Japanese encephalitis (JEV), West
Nile virus (WNV), the tick-borne encephalitis (TBEV),
and the dengue (DENV) viruses, which cause outbreaks
of human disease on a large scale. Many other flaviviruses
not listed in **Table 1** are causes of acute fever, meningoencephalitis, or hemorrhagic fever in humans on a regional
basis throughout the world.

Based on comparative genomic sequence analysis, it
is hypothesized that flaviviruses evolved as separate
tick-borne, mosquito-borne, and no-known-arthropod
vector lineages, which diverged at an early point after

the origin of the genus *Flavivirus* from a common ancestor
whose identity remains unknown. This ancestral virus is
assumed to have originated in central Africa as long ago as
10 000 years. There has been a general agreement between
the phylogenetic clustering of flaviviruses and classification on the basis of serological relationships. Viruses such
as the cell-fusing agent (CFA) and Tamana bat virus display homology that is distant enough to suggest a possible
link among the three genera, but exact relationships
remain unclear. According to this scheme, tick-borne
viruses diverge first, followed by the mosquito-borne
viruses. Yellow fever virus is representative of so-called
Old World mosquito-borne (species *Aedes*) viruses. Additional clades, such as the dengue viruses and those of
the JEV antigenic complex, vectored primarily by *Culex*
mosquitoes, are believed to have diverged subsequently.

Epidemiology and Clinical Disease

The epidemiologic situation for flaviviruses involves both
the appearance of new viruses, with several described in
recent years, as well the emergence and re-emergence
of established viruses. A number of contributing factors,
such as human activities (urbanization, transportation, and
land-use practices) and also natural phenomena (bird
migration, host–vector relationships, and climate change),
drive this process. Flaviviruses exhibit both global and
regional distribution based on these various factors.
Dengue has become the most significant cause of viral
hemorrhagic fever globally, with a dramatic increase in
prevalence of dengue involving up to 2.5 billion persons
at risk and an annual infection rate of 50 million cases. JEV
is regarded as the most important cause of epidemic viral
encephalitis worldwide, causing up to 50 000 cases annually, and has spread from Southeast Asia to the south and
west in recent years. West Nile virus, originally recognized
as a cause of febrile illness primarily in Africa, the Middle
East, and India, caused outbreaks of severe encephalitis in
Eastern Europe and the former Soviet Union in the 1990s
prior to its due appearance in the US in 1999. Since 1999, it
has become distributed across North America and parts
of Central and South America. In North America, it has
caused annual outbreaks of encephalitic disease involving
thousands of cases. Yellow fever is currently restricted to
tropical Africa and South America, where it regularly
causes endemic and periodic epidemic disease involving
thousands of cases on a regular basis. The true incidence is
believed to be underreported and may be as high as
200 000 cases per year, mainly in Africa.

Most flaviviruses are zoonotic viruses maintained
in enzootic transmission cycles which depend on birds,
rodents, or nonhuman primates as reservoirs, with humans
usually dead-end hosts. However, dengue viruses are
exceptions, due to their adaptation to humans and maintenance in urban-based areas in transmission cycles that do

not require animal reservoirs as they seem to exist in sylvatic cycles in Africa and Asia.

Structure and Replication

The structure and replication of the flaviviruses have served for many years as a model for the entire family, since the first report of the genomic sequence for yellow fever virus in 1985. The use of molecular clones, together with the ease of propagating most of these viruses in cell lines *in vitro*, and the advent of modern expression systems for production and purification of viral proteins, have facilitated progress for understanding the molecular biology of the family. A number of different molecules in different cell types have been characterized as candidate receptors, including glycosaminoglycans. The best characterized receptor interaction is between dengue virus and dendritic cell (DC)-specific intercellular adhesion molecule 3 (ICAM-3)-grabbing nonintegrin (DC-SIGN), present on human dendritic cells. Fc and complement receptors can also mediate entry of the dengue viruses and several other viruses through the process of antibody-dependent enhancement occurring in the presence of subneutralizing antibody levels.

The virions contain a lipid envelope, have a buoyant density of 1.19–1.3 g ml^{-1}, and are sensitive to inactivation by heat, acid pH, organic solvents, and detergents. Currently the virion structure is best understood for dengue

viruses and TBEVs. Dengue viruses, as reconstructed from cryoelectron microscopy (cryo-EM) images at 24 Å resolution, exist as a smooth particle comprised of dimeric units of the envelope (E) protein arranged in a head-to-tail fashion on its surface with icosahedral symmetry, encasing a nucleocapsid composed of capsid protein and genomic RNA (**Figure 1**). These genomes are on the order of 11 kbp (42 S sedimentation) and differ from other flavivirus genera in having a 5′ cap. The 5′ untranslated region (UTR) encodes a unique secondary RNA structure. The 3′ UTR contains conserved sequences and secondary structures, including a unique terminal stem–loop structure required for viral RNA replication (**Figure 2**). Such structures are found among both mosquito and tick-borne viruses despite differences in nucleotide sequence, arguing for conserved mechanisms relating to viral replication.

The flavivirus polyprotein undergoes co- and post-translational processing to produce the mature viral proteins. Structural proteins (capsid, prM (precursor to M), and E (envelope)) are generated by cleavage by host signalase in association with membranes of the endoplasmic reticulum, whereas nonstructural proteins (NS1, -2A, -2B, -3, -4A, -4B, and -5) are generated primarily by cleavage reactions mediated by the viral NS3 serine protease together with its NS2B cofactor. NS1 is a soluble, cell surface, and intracellular protein which is involved in viral RNA synthesis, together with NS3 (protease, helicase, and NTPase activities), NS5 (methyltransferase and

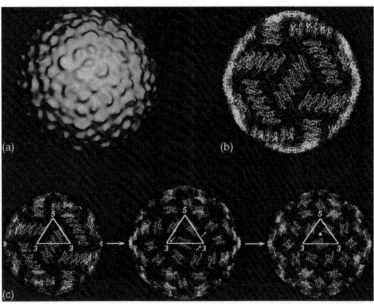

Figure 1 Structure of the dengue-2 virion as determined by cryo-EM. (a) An image reconstruction model of the virion in which the smooth surface is shown. (b) E protein dimers are displayed in the 'herringbone' arrangement, as fitted into the electron density map. (c) Acid-catalyzed rearrangement of the E protein dimers into the fusion-active state. Triangle represents the icosahedral asymmetric unit with three- and fivefold symmetry axes shown. The small arrows indicate the rotation of the E protein according to the proposed model. Reproduced from Lindenbach BD and Rice CM (2003) Molecular biology of the flaviviruses. *Advances in Virus Research* 59: 23–61, with permission from Elsevier, and adapted from Kuhn RJ, Zhang W, Rossmann MG, *et al.* (2002) Structure of dengue virus: Implications for flavivirus organization, maturation, and fusion. *Cell* 8: 717–725.

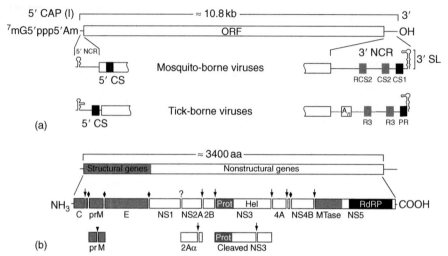

Figure 2 Organization and expression of the flavivirus genome. (a) RNA elements of the 5′ and 3′ noncoding regions (NCRs) flanking the open reading frame (ORF) for mosquito- and tick-borne viruses are indicated. The 5′ CAP structure and 5′ and 3′ stem–loop (SL) structure are shown. Conserved sequence elements for mosquito- and tick-borne viruses are denoted by CS, RCS, and CS, R, PR, respectively. A_n indicates a polyadenylate sequence contained within the variable region (dotted line) of some tick-borne isolates. (b) Expression and processing of the polyprotein. Cleavage events mediated by host signalase and furin-like enzyme are depicted by solid diamonds and triangle, respectively. Question mark indicates processing of NS1-2A by an unknown host enzyme. Downward arrows indicate cleaveage by the viral NS3 protease (PROT). HEL, helicase; MTase, methyltransferase. Reproduced from Lindenbach BD and Rice CM (2003) Molecular biology of the flaviviruses. *Advances in Virus Research* 59: 23–61, with permission from Elsevier.

RdRP activities), and the hydrophobic proteins of the NS2 and NS4 regions. Viral replication occurs in association with intracellular membranes that are reorganized into packets of vesicles, convoluted membranes, and paracrystalline arrays. The capsid protein is responsible for formation of the viral nucleocapsid. During subsequent virus maturation, prM acts as a molecular chaperone for the E protein, and undergoes a furin-like cleavage to form the fusion-competent heterodimer prM–E complex. The E protein is the major virion surface protein that harbors receptor binding and fusion activity. Structural characterization of the TBEV E protein has revealed that this protein resembles the E1 protein of the alphaviruses, both of which are designated as 'class II' viral fusion proteins, distinguished from the class I proteins typified by the influenza hemagglutin by major differences in overall fold, and a flat elongated orientation on the virion surface rather than an extended spike.

Pathogenesis

Flaviviruses are readily propagated in a variety of cell lines in culture, including cells of mammalian origin, in which cytopathic effects and plaque formation are common, as well as in mosquito-derived cells. Many of these infected cell types exhibit cell fusion and syncytia formation and are capable of supporting persistent infection. *In vivo*, flaviviruses cause syndromes in humans ranging from febrile illness to acute meningoencephalitis and hemorrhagic fever. Flaviviruses are inherently

neurotropic viruses, possibly reflecting the propensity of viruses of the early phylogenetic branches to propagate in the central nervous system of arthropod vectors, and in turn, in vertebrate hosts, in which disease manifestations occur. Arthropod vectors undergo chronic infections that serve to deliver virus into enzootic and zoonotic transmission cycles that lead to infections of humans and animals. Whereas many of the encephalitic flaviviruses which typically depend on avian species as reservoirs and for amplification cycles, dengue and yellow fever viruses have adapted to primate hosts, and cause hemorrhagic fever as a primary disease manifestation. Nonhuman primates have been used for characterization of yellow fever and dengue viral infections and for evaluation of experimental vaccines for dengue viruses. Most flaviviruses are pathogenic for laboratory rodents, particularly mice, which have been used as models for experimental studies of acute flavivirus encephalitis.

Flavivirus resistance is a phenomenon observed in certain inbred strains of mice, in which markedly reduced susceptibility to encephalitic strains, such as of WNV, have been observed. The genetic basis of this resistance has been mapped to a single autosomal dominant locus which encodes the Oas1B gene. It is not known yet if there is an analogous resistance mechanism that operates in humans to explain variability in susceptibility to these viruses. A recent study has also suggested a link between CCR5D32 (a common mutant allele of the chemokine and human immunodeficiency virus (HIV) receptor CCR5) and fatal WNV infection.

Flaviviruses are transmitted via feeding by chronically infected arthropod vectors. Following local replication at the site of inoculation and in regional lymph nodes, virus disseminates by viremia, with distribution to target organs in the periphery, including primarily visceral organs in the case of hemorrhagic fever viruses, and meninges, brain, and spinal cord in the case of encephalitic agents. Skin Langerhans (dendritic) cells are implicated as sites of initial virus replication as well as early spread of virus to lymphatic tissues. Monocytes and macrophages are also major targets of infection by dengue viruses. Flaviviruses also interact with many other cell types *in vivo* and elicit changes in cell surface molecules that are believed to influence pathogenesis of encephalitis and hemorrhagic fevers. Upregulation of surface molecules such as major histocompatibility complex (MHC) I and ICAM-1 has been observed.

Pathogenesis of both hemorrhagic fever due to yellow fever virus and acute encephalitis due to JEV complex and TBEV complex members are generally associated with cytopathic effects of the virus in target organs, although many viruses have been shown to induce apoptotic cell death as well. Flavivirus infections of the central nervous system, as typified by members of JEV complex or TBEV complex viruses, range from mild meningitis to severe destructive encephalitis, in which neurons of the brain and spinal cord are targeted. Mortality rates are as high as 40% and permanent neurologic effects may occur in survivors. Persistent and congenital infections have been described for some of the encephalitic viruses. Primary infection with dengue viruses either is generally characterized by flu-like illness or is asymptomatic. However, some secondary infections with heterologous serotypes result in a distinct form of hemorrhagic disease. This involves an immunopathogenic process of antibody-dependent enhancement of infection mediated by heterologous antibodies, in concert with activation of cross-reactive memory T-cells, cytokine release, and diffuse capillary leakage. This is referred to as dengue hemorrhagic fever and may be accompanied by a shock syndrome. Yellow fever causes a unique form of acute hemorrhagic fever with characteristic cytopathology in the liver and kidneys, and is fatal in up to 50% of severe cases.

Diagnosis and Prevention

Because flaviviruses may cause many different disease syndromes, disease manifestations are variable. Although diagnosis is often suspected on the basis of clinical findings, case history, and geographical distribution, a range of laboratory tests are available for determining infection with specific viruses, including virus isolation, serologic techniques (enzyme immunoassay, hemagglutination inhibition, immunofluorescence, complement fixation, dot blot immunoassays, and plaque neutralization), antigen

detection, and reverse transcriptase/polymerase chain reaction (RT/PCR) amplification. Detection of immunoglobulin M (IgM) by immunoassay is a common diagnostic test for flaviviruses, but in some cases persistence of high IgM levels from previous infections with other flaviviruses can complicate the diagnosis of recent infections. Detection of IgM antibody in cerebrospinal fluid is of use in cases of flavivirus encephalitis. RT/PCR of serum is a sensitive and rapid technique that has increasing application for flaviviruses, but must be carried out during the viremic stage, which can differ from one flavivirus infection to another. For instance, RT/PCR for dengue viruses loses sensitivity after the first week of infection due to clearance of viremia.

Outside of mosquito control measures, vaccination is the only available means of preventing flavivirus infections in humans. The live-attenuated yellow fever 17D vaccine has been used since its original development in 1936 for prevention of yellow fever and is one of the safest and most effective vaccines ever developed for human use. Inactivated vaccines are available for prevention of diseases caused by JEV and TBEV. Development of vaccines for dengue viruses and WNVs have been pursued because of the increasing public health burdens associated with these agents, but are still in investigational stages. At this time, there are no antiviral agents or other therapies licensed for treatment of flavivirus infections.

Pestiviruses

History and Classification

The genus *Pestivirus* includes four accepted species that are important causes of veterinary disease in farm animals which are of great economic consequence worldwide: *Classical swine fever virus, Bovine viral diarrhea virus 1* and *2,* and *Border disease virus.* The host range of pestiviruses is restricted to 'artiodactyles' (cloven-hoofed ruminants and pigs). Classical swine fever virus (CSFV) infects members of the Suidae as the natural hosts. Bovine viral diarrhea virus (BVDV) is a pathogen primarily of cattle. Classical swine fever was characterized (e.g., 'hog cholera') in the 1800s, but the viral cause not established until *c.* 1904. The diseases caused by BVDV in cattle were described in the 1940s and 1950s. Border disease virus (BDV) was discovered in 1959 in the border region of England and Wales, as a congenital viral infection affecting sheep and goats. Pestiviruses exhibit great genetic diversity, and characterization of new isolates, including those from wildlife species, about which understanding is limited, will have future impact on the classification of viruses of this genus.

Prior to use of genomic sequencing, pestiviruses were differentiated by host species of origin, and antigenic cross-reactivity prevented assignments to different serogroups, even though differences among groups could be demonstrated with monoclonal antibodies. Comparison of genomic sequences later revealed the existence of two genotypes of bovine viral diarrhea virus (BVDV-1 and BVDV-2), which became significant after it was recognized during the 1980s that BVDV-2 strains could cause a severe acute hemorrhagic syndrome, with some of the first isolations of BVDV-2 arising during BVDV1 vaccine breaks. The two genotypes are distinguishable antigenically, but not to a level which allows classification into different serotypes. Subtypes (BVDV-1a, -1b, -2a, -2b) also exist. BVDVs also display pronounced heterogeneity in phenotype (e.g., biotype and virulence type). Biotypes (cytopathic vs. noncytopathic) are defined on the basis of cytopathic effects in cultured epithelial cells. However, virulence phenotype *in vivo* correlates with the noncytopathic rather than the cytopathic biotype.

The authentic form of BDV is predominantly an ovine pathogen, although pigs are also affected. Three major genotypes have recently been identified within the BDV species, referred to as BDV-1, BDV-2, and BDV-3.

Epidemiology and Clinical Disease

BVDVs cause infections throughout the world. In the US, both BVDV-1a and BVDV-1b isolates are common, with BVDV-1b more prevalent. The prevalence of BVDV-2 appears to be greater in North America than elsewhere, and is relatively rare in Europe and Asia. However, a number of isolates have been made in South America. BVDV-2a isolates also are more predominant than BVDV-2b, which are rare. BVDV is endemic in many cattle populations, with maximum rates of persistent infection sometimes reaching 1–2%, and seropositivity as high as 65%. BVDVs also cross species barriers among animal hosts, with or without evidence of disease.

Ruminant pestiviruses frequently cause persistent infections in cattle and sheep, which serve as reservoirs for maintenance of virus, resulting in transmission from asymptomatic viremic animals to naive animals upon introduction into new herds; transmission by acutely infected animals can also occur. Contact with waste products as well as with contaminated animal feed and farm equipment may also spread infection. Animals acquire pestiviruses through the nasal and oropharyngeal tracts. Direct contact is the most efficient means of transmission. Other transmission routes may apply, as in the case of closed, nonpasturing herds which sometimes develop BVDV infections. A number of factors including the density of cattle populations and regional practices of cattle trading affect the introduction of BVDV into naive herds.

Manifestations of illnesses caused by BVDV are diverse, ranging from mild transient infections to severe acute disease involving the enteric, respiratory, and hematologic systems. Postnatally acquired infections may cause fever, diarrhea, and cough associated with virus shedding, but seroconversion and clearance of infection leads to lifelong

immunity. Persistent infections (PIs) occur after virus crosses the placenta in nonimmune animals to cause intrauterine infection early in fetal life. PI animals continuously excrete large amounts of virus and remain BVDV-antibody-negative due to immune tolerance. These animals may develop mucosal disease (MD), a fatal disease with profuse bloody diarrhea due to extensive ulceration of the gastrointestinal tract.

CSFV is the cause of a highly contagious and serious disease of pigs, and is of worldwide importance. Classical swine fever (CSF) is endemic in large portions of Asia, and has been reported in parts of Central and South America. CSF has been progressively eradicated from Western Europe, but periodic reintroduction has occurred. Eradication efforts have also generally led to control of CSF in North America and Australia. CSF can also be spread through pig products, with swill-feeding of pigs a particularly efficient means of transmission, in many regions now outlawed. Spread by semen of infected boars can also occur. CSF is an acute illness with significant mortality, but has become less common now than milder chronic forms of CSF and persistent infections following intrauterine transmission. The latter can result in stillbirth or yield piglets which develop late-onset disease.

BDV is an economically important cause of congenital infection in sheep and goats with a probable worldwide distribution; prevalence in sheep may be up to 50%. Vertical transmission results principally in abortion and stillbirth. Surviving animals are small and weak, and exhibit tremor and hairy fleece ('hairy shaker syndrome'). Infections are spread by these persistently infected animals, and can cause acute postnatal infections. Border disease can also be caused by bovine viral diarrhea disease types.

Structure and Replication

Pestivirus virions are 40–60 nm in size, contain three glycoproteins in the virion envelope complexed as disulfide-linked homo- and heterodimers, and have a buoyant density of $1.134 \, \text{g ml}^{-1}$ in sucrose. They are sensitive to heat, organic solvents, and detergents, but in contrast to flaviviruses, BVDV and CSFV are highly stable in acidic environments, although virus entry is through a low-pH endosome compartment. CD46 has been identified as a receptor for BVDV; however, glycosaminoglycans, such as heparan sulfate, may act as a receptor for cell culture-adapted BVDV and CSFV. It is believed that pestiviruses invade host cells after binding by envelope glycoproteins E^{rns} and E2. Low-density-lipoprotein receptor has also been proposed as a BVDV receptor.

The pestivirus genome is *c.* 12.3 kbp, with variant genomes of larger and smaller size generated by recombination events (**Figure 3**). Pestivirus genomes lack a 5′ cap structure, and translation is mediated by a 5′ internal ribosome entry site (IRES) element that has similarities

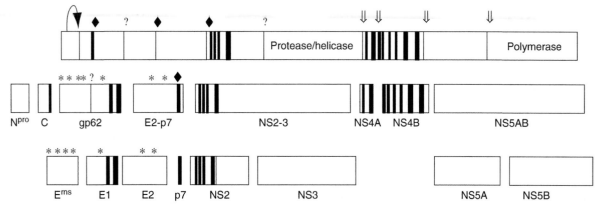

Figure 3 Pestivirus genome organization and processing, based on the cytopathic NADL strain of BVDV. Open boxes indicate mature proteins, with shaded regions representing stretches of hydrophobic amino acids. Diamonds and question marks indicate proteolytic processing by signalase and an unknown host enzyme, respectively. Downward arrows mark cleavages by the viral serine protease. The autoproteolytic cleavage by N^{pro} is shown as a curved arrow. Asterisks indicate proteins which undergo glycosylation. Reproduced from Lindenbach BD and Rice CM (2001) *Flaviviridae*: The viruses and their replication. In: Knipe DM and Howley PM (eds.) *Fields Virology,* 4th edn., vol. 1. Baltimore, MD: Lippincott Williams and Wilkins, with permission.

to the hepatitis C virus (HCV) IRES. The 3′ UTR contains a short polyC tract, as well as variable and conserved regions, the latter of which encodes hairpin structures. The open reading frame codes for 4000 amino acids, and is processed into at least 12 mature proteins: N^{pro}, C, E^{rns}, E1, E2, p7, NS2, NS3, NS4A, NS4B, NS5A, and NS5B. N^{pro} is a unique N-terminal leader autoprotease, which is followed by the four structural proteins C, E^{rns}, E1, and E2. E^{rns}, which is not found in other viruses of the family, is a heavily glycosylated protein that is secreted from cells and exhibits a ribonuclease activity and a lymphocytotoxic activity that is involved in pathogenesis. E1 and E2 are integral membrane proteins that form the heterodimeric complex which mediates virus entry. Antibodies directed against E^{rns} and E2 confer protective immunity. The p7 protein serves as a membrane leader sequence for NS2. NS2, together with the N-terminus of NS3, is an autoprotease with specificity for the NS2–NS3 junction. This cleavage is necessary for RNA replication and pathogenesis of BVDV disease, but, paradoxically, the uncleaved NS2–NS3 precursor is required for virion formation. NS3 also has multiple functions, including protease (together with the NS4A cofactor), helicase, and nucleoside triphosphatase activities. By analogy with the hepaciviruses, NS4B is involved in cellular membrane reorganization and scaffolding for the replicase complex, which includes NS5B (RdRp). NS5A is a large, hydrophilic phosphorylated zinc metalloprotein analogous to the hepacivirus NS5A, and likely to function in the regulation of viral RNA synthesis.

Pathogenesis

Growth of pestiviruses in cell culture generates virus yields that are not robust, due to intracellular sequestration of the viral progeny and association with serum components that also cause difficulties with virus purification. Whereas susceptible cell culture systems are mainly derived from cells from the natural host species, lack of cytopathogenicity (e.g., 'noncp' biotypes) is common, in contrast to the cytopathic variants ('cp' biotypes), which arise spontaneously during infections in animal hosts.

In vivo, pestiviruses cause acute and persistent infections. BVDV causes a complex pathogenesis involving broad tissue tropism, and a propensity for high cytopathogenicity through mechanisms that remain poorly defined. There is evidence that cytopathic strains cause cell death by activating apoptosis through a double-stranded RNA (dsRNA)-dependent pathway, as well as by mechanisms related to oxidative stress. This process may underlie the development of MD associated with superinfection by a cytopathic strain.

Infection of cows by noncytopathic BVDV during the first 4 months of pregnancy can lead to birth of persistently infected calves immunologically tolerant to BVDV. Subsequently, the calves develop MD after superinfection by cp BVDV. Cytopathic strains associated with such cases are generated by mutations occurring in the genomes of noncytopathic strains, and require the production of NS3 which is cleaved from its NS2-3 precursor. This phenomenon is often a consequence of recombination events which introduce sequences allowing cleavage by host ubiquitin C-terminal hydrolase, or in other cases, by the N^{pro} autoprotease itself. Point mutations can also result in cytopathic variants. Production of NS3 is believed to be the basis for both BVDV cytopathogenicity in cell culture and pathogenesis of MD in immunologically tolerant PI calves.

Following inoculation of the mucosal surface, BVDV gains access to and replicates in lymphatic tissue, in many cases associated with leukopenia. Viremia has been experimentally demonstrated within 2–4 days. In severe cases, as in MD supervening in persistently infected calves, there is disseminated infection, mucosal ulceration, and hemorrhagic disease associated with platelet deficiency and dysfunction. Persistent viral infection is typically found in lymphoid tissue of the intestine, circulating mononuclear cells, and neurons in the central nervous system.

CSF is a disseminated infection that in its most severe form involves extensive thrombosis, endothelial damage, and severe thrombocytopenia resulting in hemorrhagic disease, necrosis, and multiorgan dysfunction. Viral infection of lymphoid tissue causes depletion of lymphocytes and germinal follicles and induces an immunosuppressive state with delayed appearance of CSF-specific antibodies. Superinfection with other pathogens can complicate the disease course.

BDV typically causes a less inflammatory disease, although a variant type of disease with necrosis of central nervous system has been described. Persistent infection of newborn lambs commonly involves widespread lymphoid infection and teratogenic lesions in multiple organs, with endocrine and neurologic abnormalities.

Diagnosis, Control, and Prevention

In the context of control programs for BVDV, diagnostic assays are employed for both surveillance at the herd and population levels, and also at the level of individual animals for identification of persistently infected animals that require elimination. Tests to determine immunity (antibody in serum or milk) as well as presence of virus are commonly done. Detection of antibodies by virus neutralization test or by antibody ELISAs are both used for diagnosis. Presence of virus can be demonstrated by virus isolation, antigen detection, or RT-PCR. Use of these assays depends on a variety of considerations, including age of animals to be tested, the epidemiological situation, and vaccination history.

Laboratory confirmation of CSFV infection has traditionally depended on virus isolation and detection of antigen in organ tissue, although more rapid techniques, such as antigen ELISA and RT-PCR, have been developed. Early diagnosis of infection based on antibody detection is limited by the slow appearance of virus-specific antibodies and lack of specificity of some antibody ELISA tests.

Vaccines have been developed against both CSFV and BVDV. However, control programs based on detection and eradication of persistently infected animals, as well as on quarantining and maintaining closed herds, have been employed to reduce the economic losses caused by these viruses. National eradication campaigns conducted in Scandinavia in the 1990s were particularly successful, facilitated by development of ELISA for detection of BVDV antibodies. Due to the high effectiveness of these programs, the threat of reintroduction of virus into uninfected herds became apparent, and vaccination was recommended in some regions as a prophylactic measure against a resurgence of infections. Although some questions remain about the duration of protection and its efficacy in preventing fetal infection, newer vaccine regimens combined with comprehensive BVDV control programs are probably the best approach to lowering the incidence of PI in calves and reducing the problem of BVDV outbreaks. Commercial BVDV vaccines include either inactivated or modified live vaccines. Although there are some data to indicate that both antibody and cellular immune mechanisms are important for protection against BVDV infection, more studies are needed to define the protective mechanisms associated with these vaccines.

Live-attenuated vaccines for CSF have been available since the 1960s, but are not universally employed because of interference with traditional serologic methods to demonstrate absence of disease. Stamping-out policies are therefore employed as control efforts. Research into the use of marker vaccines, which do not exhibit interference in detection of infection, is ongoing, together with modeling studies to assess the impact of vaccine and eradication policies on control of disease.

Hepaciviruses

History and Classification

After serologic screening tests for the detection of hepatitis B and hepatitis A viruses were introduced in the 1970s to eliminate these viruses from human blood supplies, the role of HCVs in causing up to 90% of transfusion-associated hepatitis was recognized. The term hepatitis C virus (HCV) was coined in 1989 after identification of an RNA genome of this virus from cDNA libraries of human serum containing the infectious agent. In humans, infection with HCV commonly evolves into a chronic persistent hepatitis which can lead to progressive hepatic cirrhosis and hepatocellular carcinoma. Lack of a suitable cell culture system for propagating HCV had until only recently been a major impediment to progress in understanding the details of its replication. In addition, studies of HCV pathogenesis have been hampered by the lack of animal model systems, and progress has depended on use of clinical data from human cases, or from the use of a chimpanzee model.

Hepaciviruses display great genetic heterogeneity on a worldwide basis and are classified into six genotypes based on nucleotide sequence similarity, and further classified into multiple subtypes (identified by lowercase letters: e.g., 1a, 1b, 2a) as well as quasispecies for a given viral isolate. These divisions correspond to sequence divergence rates of c. 30–35%, 20–25%, and 1–10%, respectively. This level of genetic diversity has implications for the epidemiology of

HCV transmission, clinical manifestations of liver disease caused by HCV, response to treatment, and development of a prophylactic vaccine.

Epidemiology and Clinical Disease

It is estimated that there are at least 170 million chronically infected HCV subjects worldwide, with prevalence varying from 0.1% to as high as 18% (Egypt). In areas where HCV has been eliminated from blood supplies by donor screening, use of illicit injectable drugs remains the most important mode of transmission. Various other forms of exposure, including occupational and sexual exposures, are involved in some cases of transmission. HCV is a primary cause of cirrhosis, a significant cause of hepatocellular carcinoma, and in the United States is the leading reason for liver transplantation. There is great variability in the spectrum of disease. Acceleration of disease is observed in persons who are older at the time of infection, and in the setting of continuous alcohol exposure, and co-infection with HIV or hepatitis B virus (HBV). Individuals who sustain infection at a younger age tend to have slower progression.

Genotypes 1, 2, and 3 are found worldwide, but with regional differences with respect to distribution. Genotypes 1a and 1b are predominant in the United States and Europe, 2a and 2b are relatively common in North America and Europe, and type 3a common in the United States and Europe among intravenous drug abusers. Genotype 4 is notable in the Middle East/North Africa region, whereas 5 is found in South Africa, and 6 in Hong Kong. Additional genotypes (e.g., 7–11) have been identified but have been proposed as variants of genotype 6. Genotypes are useful in establishing genetic markers of HCV in epidemiologic investigations and for determining modes of transmission. Differences in terms of disease potential and treatment response among genotypes also have been described, such as the relative resistance of genotype 1 to interferon alpha (IFN-α) therapy. This genotype has been associated with more aggressive liver disease as well, but it is unclear if this results from a longer duration of infection among people infected with this genotype. Genotypic differences may affect usefulness of diagnostic immunoassays for HCV antibody which are based on various portions of the HCV genome.

Structure and Replication

In contrast to those of flaviviruses and pestiviruses, hepacivirus virions have been difficult to visualize, and exhibit larger size and lower buoyant density (1.03–1.1 $g\,ml^{-1}$) as a result of association with immunoglobulins and low-density lipoproteins. HCV genomes contain a 9.6 kb RNA which differs in some structural features from flaviviruses and pestiviruses (**Figure 4**). The 5′ UTR is the most highly conserved region of the genome and contains an IRES which mediates cap-independent translation of viral RNA. The structure of the IRES has been resolved, including studies of complexes with the ribosomal 40S subunit and the human translation factor eIF3. These efforts may facilitate the design of small molecules capable of inhibiting this critical viral factor. Because of its high sequence conservation, the 5′ UTR has also been used for development of sensitive detection assays for HCV infection. The 3′ UTR exhibits a tripartite structure, containing several unique elements, including a short variable region, a poly(U/UC) tract, and a highly conserved RNA sequence (the X-tail). A unique RNA structure, the *cis*-acting replication element (CRE) within the NS5 region, has also been identified.

The HCV polyprotein (*c.* 3000 amino acids) is processed by cellular (signalase) and viral proteases into mature viral proteins, consisting of the core, E1 and E2, the hydrophobic p7 peptide, and six nonstructural proteins (NS2, NS3, NS4A, NS4B, NS5A, and NS5B). Unique properties of several of these proteins have been characterized. The RNA-binding core protein has been associated with a range of effects on host cells, including transactivation, but the relevance to HCV pathogenesis *in vivo* is unknown. Alternative forms of core, produced by frameshifting, have been described. The E1 and E2 proteins form the heterodimeric complex of the virion that serves receptor binding, membrane fusion, and entry. These proteins exhibit the highest mutation rate at both the nucleotide and amino acid level. E2 in particular contains a hypervariable region (HVR-1) which undergoes an extremely high mutation rate and, because antibody epitopes are found within this region, it is believed that the mutations provide a mechanism for HCV to escape antibody responses involved in controlling virus infection. The small membrane-associated p7 protein forms an amantadine-sensitive ion channel which may function in the secretory pathway during virus maturation.

HCV encodes two known proteases involved in polyprotein processing, the NS2-3 autoprotease, and the NS3 serine protease, that with its NS4A cofactor mediates cleavage of the remainder of the nonstructural region. The structure of the NS3-4A protease has been solved, promoting interest in a new class of antiviral agents that target its protease activity. NS3 can also cleave adaptor proteins (Toll-like receptor-3 adaptor TRIF (TICAM-1) and Cardiff (IPS-1, VISA, or MAVS)) required for activation of interferon regulatory factor 3, indicating a role for NS3 in downregulating the dsRNA signaling pathway that leads to induction of interferon beta and other genes involved in antiviral defense.

The NS4B protein is a mediator of the reorganization of intracellular membranes that together with other viral and host proteins generates the 'membranous web' scaffold for formation of RNA replication complexes. NS5A is a

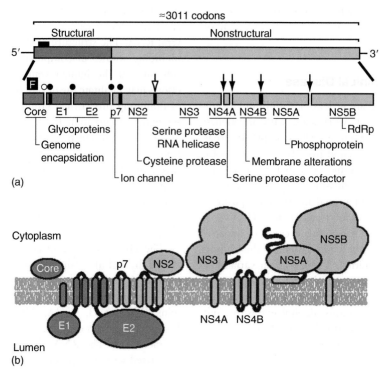

Figure 4 HCV genome organization and processing. (a) The HCV genome and polyprotein encoding structural and nonstructural genes and known functions. Closed and open circles indicate signal peptidase cleavage sites and signal peptide peptidase cleavage sites, respectively. F represents an alternative open reading frame protein produced by ribosomal frameshifting within the core region. Open and closed arrows indicate cleavage by the NS2 autoprotease and the NS3/4A serine protease, respectively. (b) Proposed topology of the HCV proteins with respect to the intracellular membrane. Reprinted by permission from Macmillan Publishers Ltd; *Nature* (Lindenbach BD and Rice CM (2005) Unravelling hepatitis C virus replication from genome to function. *Nature* 436(7053): 933–938), Copyright (2005).

multidomain protein containing an RNA-binding activity. Differential phosphorylation of NS5A appears to have a role in regulation of HCV RNA synthesis, as a molecular switch for critical steps in the transition from RNA synthesis to virus packaging. NS5A also interacts with interferon-induced dsRNA-activated protein kinase PKR. Mutations in the domain of NS5A which affect this interaction (interferon sensitivity-determining region (ISDR) have been reported to influence the response of HCV to interferon alpha. The NS5B protein contains the RdRp activity that forms the core of the replication complex, and together with other NS3, NS5A, and cellular factors, synthesizes the genome-length plus- and minus-strand RNAs involved in the replication of the virus. NTPase and helicase activities participating in this process are encoded in the NS3 protein. Cellular proteins that have been implicated in function of the replication complex by interacting with NS5A and NS5B include VAP-A and -B (vesicle-associated membrane protein-associated proteins A and B), geranylgeranylated protein FBL-2, and cyclophilin B. These proteins appear to affect the assembly and function of the replication through such interactions such as membrane localization and RNA binding.

Recent progress in understanding HCV genome replication has been achieved through the use of HCV replicon systems. Initially established for genotype 1b, these were subgenomic constructs that encoded only the 5′ and 3′ structures and the nonstructural proteins required for viral RNA replication. Studies with additional iterations of replicons, including those for other genotypes, as well as full-length versions that exhibit efficient replicative functions *in vitro*, are excellent tools for studying the virus life cycle, in the absence of robust propagation of infectious HCV viruses in cultured cells. Crystal structures of several HCV proteins harboring key enzymatic functions, including NS3 protease, helicase, NS5A, and NS5B are known and are being applied to the development of HCV-specific antiviral agents.

The exact cell entry process for HCV has not been definitively characterized. It is believed that CD81, a tetraspanin family protein widely found on cell substrates, is involved in HCV entry, but requirements for other cell surface molecules on hepatocytes probably exist. Other proposed receptors include the LDL receptor, the class B type I scavenger receptor, mannose-binding lectins DC-SIGN and L-SIGN, heparan sulfate proteoglycans, and the asialoglycoprotein receptor. Further studies are needed to demonstrate the role of such molecules in HCV infections, and will be facilitated with new model systems such as retrovirus pseudoparticles that express HCV glycoproteins and exhibit low-pH-dependent infectivity for hepatic cell lines.

Pathogenesis and Clinical Disease

HCV causes acute and chronic forms of viral hepatitis. Acute hepatitis resembles that caused by other agents of viral hepatitis, but overt symptoms are not as frequent, despite biochemical evidence of liver disease in most subjects and appearance of HCV RNA in the serum. HCV causes persistent infection in most infected individuals, who then have chronic hepatitis throughout their lives in the absence of treatment and who remain at risk for cirrhosis and hepatocellular carcinoma. The infection is often diagnosed by screening of asymptomatic blood donors, or by the appearance of either chronic fatigue or features otherwise typical of viral hepatitis. Such individuals have persistent viremia and evidence of chronic inflammatory disease on liver biopsy.

Currently HCV is believed to cause persistent infection because primary and secondary immune responses are inadequate in breadth and magnitude to control the infection. Underlying mechanisms include the inherent difficulty in optimizing an immune response within the liver, and HCV-specific factors which suppress the host immune response, including effects of the core protein on host gene expression, inhibition of the interferon-induced protein kinase PKR by E2 and NS5A proteins, and NS3 inhibition of the dsRNA signaling pathway. The high genetic variability of HCV results in viral variants that may contribute to virus persistence through escape from antibody and from cytotoxic lymphocyte responses directed at specific epitopes.

The mechanism of liver injury associated with persistent HCV infection is believed to be immune-mediated and initiated by virus-specific T-lymphocytes which infiltrate the liver. Such cells are predominantly of a T_H-1 phenotype and produce interferon gamma and tumor necrosis factor alpha (TNF-α). Because these cytokines have been implicated in noncytolytic clearance of other viral agents in the liver, other mechanisms of hepatocyte injury and death associated with HCV have been proposed, including Fas-Fas ligand-mediated apoptosis, perforin-dependent killing by cytolytic T-cells, or TNF-α itself. HCV is not highly cytopathic for hepatocytes; however, fat deposits and eosinophilic inclusions are often seen in liver cells. In the absence of virus clearance, repeated episodes of hepatocellular injury and regeneration trigger development of hepatic fibrosis, cirrhosis, and eventual hepatocellular carcinoma. Additional factors that promote this process include coexistent infection with other agents of viral hepatitis, alcohol intake, and iron overload. Extrahepatic manifestations can also occur in association with HCV infection, typically manifesting as skin and renal disease caused by a systemic vasculitis involving immune complexes with viral proteins.

Diagnosis and Treatment

Diagnosis of chronic hepatitis C infection is established by screening enzyme immunoassay to detect circulating antibodies to HCV proteins, followed by confirmatory determination of HCV RNA in serum, using qualitative and quantitative tests based on target (RT-PCR and transcription-mediated amplification) and signal amplification (branched DNA (bDNA)) techniques. Quantitation of serum HCV RNA helps to identify patients likely to benefit from treatment and undergo virus clearance as defined by a sustained viral response (SVR). Determination of the HCV genotype guides treatment decisions, as genotypes 1 and 4–6 are less amenable to treatment than are genotypes 2 or 3. Therapeutic trials have shown that combinations of interferons and ribavirin are more effective than is interferon alone and pegylated (long-acting) interferons have yielded improved SVR rates. An SVR is less common in patients with genotype 1 infections, high pretreatment HCV RNA levels, or advanced stages of fibrosis. Liver biopsy is used to establish the pre-treatment stage of liver disease and to facilitate decisions concerning the need for therapy. Advances in the future diagnosis and management of HCV will require close monitoring of the transmission of this infection, as well as extending treatment to populations not usually evaluated in clinical trials, and the development of new therapies, including antiviral agents targeting the viral protease and RNA polymerase.

GB Viruses

GB viruses are unassigned members of the family that include GB-A and -B, which are marmoset viruses, and GB-C, which was detected in the serum of human chronic hepatitis cases. GB-C and hepatitis G were discovered coincidentally and currently given the taxonomic assignment GBV-C/HGV. Currently there are five genotypes of this virus.

GBV-C/HGV is related to HCV, sharing 29% amino acid homology, and similarities in genome organization and structure, including a 5' IRES, and a 3000 amino acid polyprotein but there are notable differences. GBV-C/HGV contains a capsid protein in the nucleocapsid; but this protein has not been identified. The E2 protein lacks both the extensive glycosylation and the hypervariable region found in the HCV E2 protein, which may in part explain the less frequent occurrence of persistent infection by GBV-C/HGV.

The 3' UTR also differs from that of HCV. GBV-C/HGV is not hepatotropic, but rather replicates in mononuclear cells and bone marrow. Infection of humans is common, but no disease association has yet been identified. Instead, a beneficial effect of GBV-C/HGV infection on the outcome of HIV infection has been observed, presumably as a result of altered cellular immune responses caused by persistent infection.

See also: Tick-Borne Encephalitis Viruses; Yellow Fever Virus.

Further Reading

Chambers TJ and Monath TP (eds.) (2003) *The Flaviviruses: Advances in Virus Research,* vols. 59–61. San Diego, CA: Academic Press.

Chang KM (2003) Immunopathogenesis of hepatitis C virus infection. *Clinics in Liver Disease* 7: 89–105.

Cocquerel L, Voisset C, and Dubuisson J (2006) Hepatitis C virus entry: Potential receptors and their biological functions. *Journal of General Virology* 87: 1075–1084.

Calisher CH and Gould EA (2003) Taxonomy of the virus family Flaviviridae. *Advances in Virus Research* 59: 1–19, with permission from Elsevier.

Gubler DJ and Kuno G (eds.) (1997) *Dengue and Dengue Hemorrhagic Fever.* London: CABI.

Heinz FX, Collett MS, Purcell RH, *et al.* (2000) Family *Flaviviridae.* In: Van Regenmortel MHV, Fauquet CM Bishop DHL, *et al.* (eds.) *Virus Taxonomy: Seventh International Committee for the Taxonomy of Viruses,* pp. 859–878. San Diego, CA: Academic Press.

Houe H (1999) Epidemiological features and economical importance of bovine virus diarrhoea virus (BVDV) infections. *Veterinary Microbiology* 64: 89–107.

Kovács F, Magyar T, Rinehart C, *et al.* (2003) The live attenuated bovine viral diarrhea virus components of a multi-valent vaccine confer protection against fetal infection. *Veterinary Microbiology* 96: 117–131.

Kuhn RJ, Zhang W, Rossmann MG, *et al.* (2002) Structure of dengue virus: Implications for flavivirus organization, maturation, and fusion. *Cell* 8: 717–725.

Lindenbach BD, Evans MJ, Syder AJ, *et al.* (2005) Complete replication of hepatitis C virus in cell culture. *Science* 309: 623–626.

Lindenbach BD and Rice CM (2001) *Flaviviridae:* The viruses and their replication. In: Knipe DM and Howley PM (eds.) *Fields Virology,* 4th edn., vol. 1. Baltimore, MD: Lippincott Williams and Wilkins.

Lindenbach BD and Rice CM (2003) Molecular biology of the flaviviruses. *Advances in Virus Research* 59: 23–61.

Lindenbach BD and Rice CM (2005) Unravelling hepatitis C virus replication from genome to function. *Nature* 436(7053): 933–938), Copyright (2005).

Radostits OM, Gay CC, Blood DC, and Hinchcliff KW (eds.) (2000) Bovine virus diarrhoea, mucosal disease, bovine pestivirus complex. In: *Veterinary Medicine, A Textbook of the Diseases of Cattle, Sheep, Pigs, Goats, Horses,* 9th edn., pp. 1085–1105. New York: WB Saunders.

Ridpath JF (2003) BVDV genotypes and biotypes: Practical implications for diagnosis and control. *Biologicals* 2: 127–133.

Tassaneetrithep B, Burgess TH, Granelli-Piperno A, *et al.* (2003) DC-SIGN (CD209) mediates dengue virus infection of human dendritic cells. *Journal of Experimental Medicine* 197: 823–829.

Tautz N, Meyers G, and Thiel HJ (1998) Pathogenesis of mucosal disease, a deadly disease of cattle caused by a pestivirus. *Clinical and Diagnostic Virology* 10: 121–127.

Hepadnaviruses: General Features

T J Harrison, University College London, London, UK

Introduction

The infectious nature of viral hepatitis has been recognized throughout human history, including by documentation of epidemics of jaundice (campaign jaundice) associated with warfare. Parenteral transmission of hepatitis (serum hepatitis) was recognized from the end of the nineteenth century following transmission by routes such as tattooing, the reuse of syringes and needles, and contamination of vaccines by 'stabilization' with human 'lymph' or serum. The viral etiology of infectious and serum hepatitis was recognized in studies involving transmission to volunteers, during and after World War II. In addition, these studies established different incubation times for infectious (short incubation) and serum (long incubation) hepatitis. The terms hepatitis A and hepatitis B were coined and became accepted for infectious (or epidemic) and serum hepatitis, respectively.

Progress with hepatitis B began with the serendipitous discovery of the envelope protein of the virus, hepatitis B surface antigen (HBsAg), originally termed Australia antigen. This was discovered in 1965 by Blumberg, who precipitated an antigen–antibody complex by immunodiffusion of sera from a multiply transfused patient and an Australian aboriginal, during a study of blood and leukocyte antigens. The protein was later recognized to be associated with transmission of hepatitis and could be detected in the sera of a proportion of patients with viral hepatitis. Electron microscopic studies in the late 1960s led to the discovery of particles of around 20 nm diameter that are now known to be composed of membrane-embedded HBsAg, secreted from the hepatocytes as non-infectious, subviral particles. In 1970, Dane visualized larger, 42 nm particles with electron dense cores. Originally termed 'Dane particles', these are the hepatitis B virions and were shown later to contain a small circular

DNA genome that was partially single-stranded and associated with a DNA polymerase activity that could render the molecule fully double-stranded.

The development of tests for HBsAg, and for antibodies to hepatitis A virus, led to the recognition of transmission of hepatitis, termed non-A, non-B hepatitis (NANBH), potentially by other viruses. Post-transfusion (or parenterally transmitted), PT-NANBH is caused principally by hepatitis C virus and enterically transmitted, ET-NANBH, by hepatitis E virus. The genomes of these viruses were cloned in 1989. Earlier, in 1977, Rizzetto had described a novel antigen–antibody system, termed delta/anti-delta, in patients with hepatitis B. The delta antigen is now known to be the nucleocapsid protein of hepatitis D virus (HDV), a defective virus that requires HBsAg to form its envelope.

The Hepadnaviruses

Hepatitis B virus (HBV) is now recognized as the prototype of a family of viruses that infect mammals and birds. The *Hepadnaviridae* (named for *hepa*totropic *DNA* viruses) are divided into mammalian (*Orthohepadnavirus*) and avian (*Avihepadnavirus*) genera.

In the 1960s, it was noted by Snyder that eastern woodchucks (*Marmota monax*) in a colony in the Philadelphia Zoo were highly susceptible to the development of chronic hepatitis and hepatocellular carcinoma, and he proposed a viral etiology. The sera of animals with chronic hepatitis proved to contain a virus with similar biochemical properties to HBV and this was named woodchuck hepatitis virus (WHV). A search for similar viruses in relatives of the woodchuck turned up a closely related virus, ground squirrel hepatitis virus (GSHV) in the Beechey ground squirrel (*Spermophilus beecheyi*; *Spermophilus* and *Marmota* are genera of the family *Sciuridae*). Other related viruses are endemic in Richardson ground squirrels (*Spermophilus richardsonii*) in Canada (Richardson ground squirrel hepatitis virus, RGSHV) and arctic ground squirrels (*Spermophilus parryi kennicotti*) in Alaska (arctic squirrel hepatitis virus, ASHV).

Reports of hepatocellular carcinoma in farmed ducks in China led to the discovery of duck hepatitis B virus (DHBV; the 'B' is included to avoid confusion with the picornavirus, duck hepatitis virus, and is retained in the names of the other avian hepadnaviruses) in flocks of Pekin ducks (*Anas domesticus*) in China and the USA. In the USA, up to 10% of ducks in some commercial flocks are persistently infected. The discovery of DHBV was followed by the identification of related viruses in grey herons (*Ardea cinerea*) in Germany (heron hepatitis B virus, HHBV), in Ross's geese (*Anser rossii*; Ross's goose HBV, RGHBV) and snow geese (*Anser caerulescens*; snow goose HBV, SGHBV), in white storks (*Ciconia ciconia*;

STHBV) and in grey crowned cranes (*Balearica regulorum*; CHBV). Recently, other hepadnaviruses have been isolated from a variety of exotic ducks and geese, including teal, widgeon, and sheldgeese. However, because these birds were kept in captivity, it is not clear that these novel viruses are native to the species from which they were first isolated. Indeed, RGHBV and SGHBV also were isolated from captive birds and are quite distinct viruses (**Figure 1**), despite the fact that the two avian species mix and may interbreed in the wild.

Biology of the Viruses

As noted above, hepadnavirus particles consist of a DNA-containing nucleocapsid enveloped with the surface proteins embedded in a lipid bilayer derived from the internal membranes of the host cell. Excess surface proteins are secreted as subviral particles, which may serve to subvert the immune response to the surface proteins. The surface open reading frame (ORF) in the mammalian viruses contains three, in-frame initiation codons leading to the synthesis of large (L, pre-S1+pre-S2+S), middle (M, preS2+S), and small (or major, S) surface proteins (**Figure 2(a)**). The pre-S1 region contains an endoplasmic reticulum-retention signal involved in virion assembly; its incorporation into subviral particles leads to the formation of tubular, rather than spherical, forms. The avian viruses have only large (pre-S+S) and small (S) surface proteins, the middle protein being absent (variants of HBV with small deletions that abrogate synthesis of the middle protein also seem to be viable). For both classes of virus, the ligand that interacts with the major cellular receptor seems to reside within the domain unique to the large surface protein and it is this interaction that seems to be responsible for the high degree of species specificity of this virus family. The primary receptor for DHBV is carboxypeptidase D but the receptors and co-receptors of the mammalian viruses remain to be identified.

Within the nucleocapsid, the genome (around 3.2 kbp for HBV, 3.3 kbp for the rodent viruses, and 3.0 kbp for the avian viruses) is composed of two linear strands of DNA held in a circular configuration by base-pairing of a short region where the 5′ ends overlap. As noted above, one strand (the plus strand) of the HBV genome is incomplete, usually being approximately 60–80% full length. On the other hand, the genome of DHBV tends to be almost completely double-stranded, while it has been reported that SGHBV produces a significant proportion of virions containing single-stranded DNA.

With its small size, the HBV genome was one of the first viral genomes to be cloned and sequenced completely. Four overlapping ORFs are conserved among the mammalian viruses (**Figure 2(a)**). These encode the surface

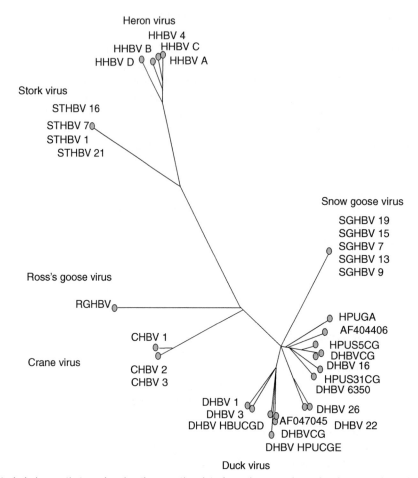

Figure 1 An unrooted phylogenetic tree showing the genetic relatedness between hepadnaviruses isolated from ducks, geese, herons, storks, and cranes. Reproduced from Prassolov A, Hohenberg H, Kalinina T, *et al.* (2003) New hepatitis B virus of cranes that has an unexpected broad host range. *Journal of Virology* 77: 1964–1976, with permission from American Society for Microbiology.

and nucleocapsid proteins, the polymerase, and a small protein called x (HBxAg) for its unknown function. HBxAg is now known to be a transactivator of transcription and is presumed to act by upregulating the activity of the viral promoters and may be important in 'kick-starting' a new infection. The X ORF is absent from the genomes of the avian viruses (**Figure 2(b)**). However, the avian viruses do encode an ORF that resembles X but lacks an initiation codon; it is not know whether this is expressed during infection.

The hepadnaviruses replicate by reverse transcription of a pregenomic RNA and have been termed 'pararetroviruses'. The replication of HBV, many features of which were elucidated using as a model DHBV in its natural host, is discussed elsewhere in this encyclopedia. Briefly, the viruses are believed to enter the host cell via endosomes with delivery of the genomes to the nucleus, where they are converted to a covalently closed circular (ccc) form that is the template for transcription. The

pregenomic RNA, which is also the mRNA for the nucleocapsid protein and polymerase, has a stem–loop structure near to the 5′ end. This is recognized by the polymerase, which also acts as a protein primer, and DNA synthesis begins, also signaling encapsidation. Reverse transcription and second-strand synthesis take place in immature cores in the cytoplasm; completion of the cores being followed by envelopment and exocytosis. Early in infection, some nascent cores cycle back to the nucleus to build up a pool of ccc DNA templates.

Genetic Variation and Epidemiology

HBV originally was typed serologically on the basis of the reactivity of HBsAg. All types share a common determinant known as *a*; this has been mapped to a hydrophilic region, roughly between amino acid residues (aa) 111 and 156 of the (226 aa) small surface protein, S. This highly

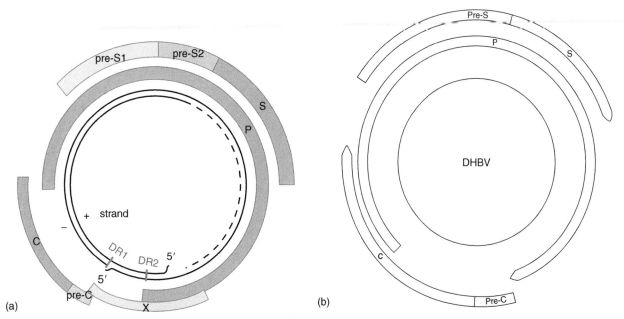

Figure 2 (a) Organization of the HBV genome. The inner circles depict the complete minus strand and incomplete plus strand and the positions of the direct repeats (DR) are indicated. The blocks surrounding the genome show the locations of the four overlapping ORFs; C and S contain two and three in-frame initiation codons, respectively. (b) Organization of the DHBV genome. A simplified view illustrating the single pre-S region and lack of an X ORF. (a) Reproduced from Kidd-Ljunggren K, Miyakawa Y, and Kidd AH, *et al.* (2002) Genetic variability in hepatitis B viruses. *Journal of General Virology* 83: 1267–1280, with permission from Society for General Microbiology.

conformational region, comprising a number of overlapping epitopes, is the main target of the humoral response, and antibodies synthesized during convalescence or in response to the hepatitis B vaccine are protective. Two pairs of mutually exclusive subdeterminants, *d* or *y* and *w* or *r*, correlate with variation (in both cases between lysine and arginine) at aa 122 and aa 160, respectively. Thus, four principal subtypes are recognized (*adw, adr, ayw,* and (rarely) *ayr*) and these show varying geographical distribution.

The error-prone nature of HBV DNA replication, via an RNA intermediate and without proofreading, is balanced by constraints on variation imposed by overlapping ORFs and the various *cis*-acting elements all being embedded in ORFs. Nonetheless, individual isolates of HBV vary by up to 10–14% of nucleotide positions and genotypes have been defined on the basis of >8% nucleotide sequence divergence. Currently, eight genotypes (A–H) are recognized and most of these have been divided further into subgenotypes. Genotype A is found in northern Europe and North America, B and C in east and Southeast Asia, D in a wide area though southern Europe and North Africa to India, E in western Africa, and F in South and Central America. Arguably, too few of the most recently described genotypes have been isolated to establish an epidemiological pattern, but G has been

found in the USA and Europe, and H in the USA and Central America.

HBV has also been isolated from a variety of nonhuman primates. The first such complete sequence was derived from HBV from a captive chimpanzee and, at the time, it was not possible to determine whether this represented a divergent human isolate (i.e., the result of an unintentional human-to-chimpanzee transmission) or a genuine chimpanzee virus. Some years later, a related virus was isolated from a white-handed gibbon (*Hybolates lar*) and complete sequences now are available from a considerable number of chimpanzees, gorillas, orangutans, and gibbons. The most divergent of the primate hepadnaviruses sequenced at the time of writing is from the woolly monkey (*Lagothrix lagotricha*), a New World monkey. Woolly monkey HBV (WMHBV) shows around 20% nucleotide sequence divergence from HBV.

Figure 3 shows a dendrogram of the eight human HBV genotypes along with the primate viruses and rooted using WMHBV as an outgroup. Fewer genome sequences are available for the rodent hepadnaviruses. Isolates of WHV vary in fewer than 4% of nucleotide positions and differ from GSHV and ASHV in around 15% (no sequence is available for RGSHV). **Figure 4** shows a dendrogram of the primate and rodent hepadnavirus sequences, rooted using DHBV as an outgroup.

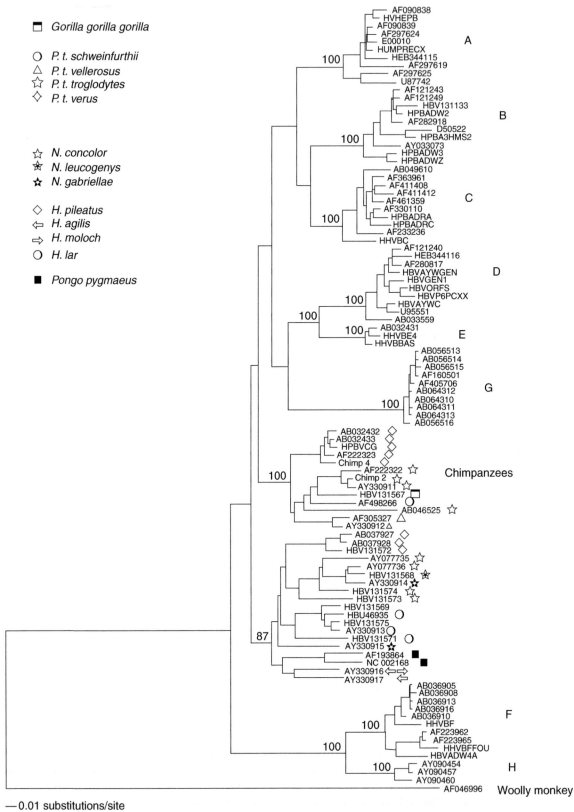

— 0.01 substitutions/site

Figure 3 Dendrogram showing the relatedness of the eight genotypes of HBV and hepatitis B viruses isolated from nonhuman primates. The tree is rooted using the woolly monkey HBV sequence as an outgroup. Reproduced from Starkman SE, MacDonald DM, Lewis JCM, Holmes EC, and Simmonds P (2003) Geographic and species association of hepatitis B virus genotypes in non-human primates. *Virology* 314: 381–393, with permission from Elsevier.

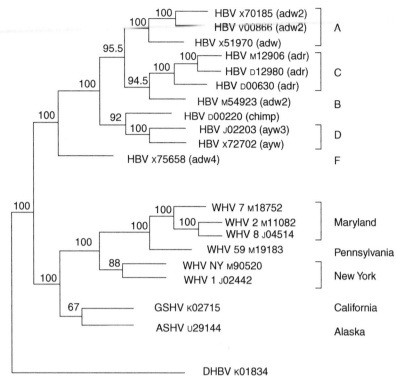

Figure 4 Dendrogram showing the relatedness of HBV and the rodent hepadnaviruses, rooted using DHBV as an outgroup. Reproduced from Testut P, Renard CA, Terradillos O, *et al.* (1996) A new hepadnavirus endemic in arctic ground squirrels in Alaska. *Journal of Virology* 70: 4210–4219, with permission from American Society for Microbiology.

As noted above, the avian hepadnaviruses show somewhat less-restricted host specificity than those infecting mammals. **Figure 1** shows a phylogenetic tree of viruses isolated from ducks, geese, herons, storks, and cranes. Some of these viruses may originate from species of birds other than those from which they were first isolated, and it seems quite possible that many other varieties of avian hepadnaviruses remain to be described.

Clinical Features and Pathology

The clinical features of acute viral hepatitis in humans are nonspecific and are not dependent on the etiology of the infection; they include fatigue, anorexia, myalgia, and malaise. Jaundice may be evident in the more severe cases, but often the infections may be anicteric (without jaundice) or even asymptomatic. In hepatitis B, these clinical features are evidence of a robust immune response to the virus and a sign that the infection will be cleared by the immune system. In a minority of cases, less than 5% of immune competent adults, asymptomatic infections persist in individuals who do not mount a vigorous immune response. Such persistent infections, originally termed the chronic carrier state, are defined formally by the persistence of HBsAg in serum for more than 6 months.

When a persistently infected woman gives birth, she will almost invariably pass on the virus to her infant. HBV normally does not cross the placenta and transmission is believed to occur during or immediately after the birth process. Infants who are infected perinatally have a very high probability (>90%) of becoming persistently infected – they are extremely immune tolerant of the virus and the infection may persist even for life. A soluble protein, HBeAg, which is related to the nucleocapsid protein, is secreted from the infected hepatocytes and may cross the placenta and induce tolerance in the foetus. A protein equivalent to HBeAg is made by all of the hepadnaviruses, including the avian viruses.

HBV infections of children up to the age of 5 also are much more likely to progress to chronicity than those in adults. Thus, in regions of the world where HBV is highly endemic, and more than 8% of individuals are persistently infected, the virus is maintained in the population by mother-to-infant transmission and horizontal transmission from persistently infected young children to their peers. These regions include sub-Saharan Africa, China, and Southeast Asia (**Figure 5**). Areas of intermediate endemicity (2–7% of individuals persistently infected) include North Africa, Eastern Europe, and northern Asia. In areas of low endemicity, such as North America and Western Europe, important routes of transmission include sexual contact and parenteral exposure.

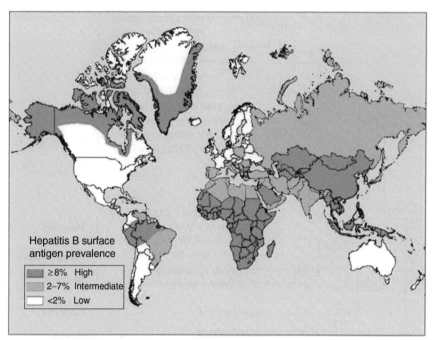

Hepatitis B surface
antigen prevalence

≥8% High
2–7% Intermediate
<2% Low

Figure 5 Global prevalence of persistent HBV infection (HBsAg in serum). Reproduced from http://www.cdc.gov/ncidod/diseases/hepatitis/slideset/hep_b/slide_9.htm, with permission from Central Food Technological Research Institute.

HBV seems not to be cytopathic and, in immune tolerant individuals, massive amounts of virus may be produced over long periods of time with little damage to the liver. However, such replication leads to the accumulation of hepatocytes with integrated (partial) copies of the viral genome and these seem to be at high risk of becoming neoplastic. Integration is not part of the HBV life cycle and seems to be a dead-end for the virus, but may be detected in almost all HBV-associated primary liver tumors.

In persistent infections, tolerance may break down over time, particularly with a cell-mediated immune response to the virus. Liver damage is attributable especially to the lysis of infected hepatocytes by cytotoxic T cells and peptides derived from the core (C) ORF seem to be a major target. In the long term, chronic active hepatitis may lead to the development of fibrosis, cirrhosis, and ultimately, end-stage liver failure. Cirrhosis also is a high risk for the development of primary liver cancer (hepatocellular carcinoma, HCC). However, almost all HCCs arising in HBV-infected livers contain chromosomally integrated HBV DNA and, in contrast to hepatitis C, in hepatitis B HCC may develop in the absence of cirrhosis and even on a background of almost normal liver histology.

The rodent hepadnaviruses can also become persistent in their natural hosts and chronic hepatitis, cirrhosis, and HCC may ensue. On the other hand, DHBV infection of ducks results in very little pathology, the infection may be passed vertically through the egg, and hatchlings are extremely immune tolerant of the virus. The avian and rodent systems have been studied experimentally. DHBV in its natural host has been especially useful. As noted above, the DHBV system had an important role in the elucidation of the mode of replication of the viral DNA. It has also been valuable for testing nucleoside and nucleotide analogs for potential therapeutic use. Despite their closer relatedness to humans, woodchucks are not best suited to experimentation; they are large, hibernate in the winter, and wild-caught animals have many parasites. Nevertheless, these animals have been used in various studies, including investigations of the actions of antiviral agents, the immune response in chronic infection, and the development of HCC.

Prevention and Treatment of Infection

HBV infection can be prevented by immunization, intramuscular administration of HBsAg leading to a protective anti-HBs response. The first vaccine (so-called plasma-derived vaccine) was produced by purifying HBsAg from the plasma of hepatitis B carriers. Second-generation vaccines contain HBsAg produced from yeast or (less commonly) mammalian cells by recombinant DNA technology. The World Health Organization recommends universal immunization of infants and this is now carried out in many countries. The key is to break the chain of transmission from infected mothers to their infants, and giving the vaccine within 24 h of birth protects 70–90% of such babies. Protective efficacy may be increased by giving passive protection with hepatitis B immune globulin (HBIG) at a contralateral site. In Taiwan, one of the first countries with a high prevalence of HBsAg to introduce universal immunization of infants, that prevalence has been reduced from more than 10% to less than 1% in the immunized cohort. Furthermore, although HCC is very rare in children, the incidence of childhood HCC has been reduced and all indications are that universal immunization against hepatitis B will, in time, lead to a marked decrease the incidence of HCC worldwide.

Prior to the introduction of nucleoside and nucleotide analogs, persistent HBV infection was treated most often by the administration of interferon. Up to 30% of individuals so treated cleared the virus. Interferon seemed to work by upregulating the cytotoxic T-cell response to the virus, rather than by a direct antiviral action. Responses were notably poor in patients from China and the Far East, presumably because these individuals had been infected early in life and were very immune tolerant.

As noted above, HBV replicates via reverse transcription of an RNA pregenome, and some of the nucleoside and nucleotide analogs introduced for the treatment of human immunodeficiency virus (HIV) infection are also active against HBV. The first to be licensed for such use was lamivudine (3TC); monotherapy reduces the viral load considerably but resistance develops in around 15% of treated patients per year. Resistance parallels that seen in HIV, with mutations affecting the 'YMDD' motif in the active site of the polymerase. Resistance to adefovir dipivoxil arises less frequently and the drug is active against lamivudine-resistant HBV. Other drugs also have been licensed but regimens of combined therapy are less well developed than those used for HIV. It should be noted also that, while such treatments reduce the viral load considerably, they rarely result in complete clearance of the infection.

Hepatitis D Virus

HDV merits a brief mention because of its particular association with HBV. As noted above, a novel antigen, termed delta, was discovered in patients with hepatitis B and this turned out to be the nucleocapsid protein of HDV. The HDV genome is a single-stranded circle of RNA that resembles the viroids and virusoids of plants; it is believed to be replicated by the host RNA polymerase II,

with cleavage and rejoining of the circle mediated by a ribozyme activity. Unlike the viroids and virusoids, the RNA contains (in the antigenomic sense) an ORF, encoding the delta antigen. HDV requires HBsAg for envelopment and exocytosis, and for subsequent binding and entry to the target hepatocyte. HDV has been transmitted experimentally to WHV-infected woodchucks and is there enveloped by WHsAg.

HDV was first discovered in Italy and is found in the Mediterranean area, reportedly with a declining prevalence, and also in the Far East and South America. The virus may be acquired as a coinfection with HBV or by super-infection of someone already HBsAg-positive. In both cases, disease may be more severe than with HBV alone, and chronic delta hepatitis may progress to cirrhosis more frequently, and more rapidly, than chronic hepatitis B. The hepatitis B vaccine also protects against coinfection but there is no licensed vaccine to protect hepatitis B carriers against HDV infection.

See also: Hepatitis B Virus: General Features.

Further Reading

Cougot D, Neuveut C, and Buendia MA (2005) HBV induced carcinogenesis. *Journal of Clinical Virology* 34(supplement 1): S75–S78.

Harrison TJ (2006) Hepatitis B virus: Molecular virology and common mutants. *Seminars in Liver Disease* 26: 87–96.

Kidd-Ljunggren K, Miyakawa Y, Kidd AH, et al. (2002) Genetic variability in hepatitis B viruses. *Journal of General Virology* 83: 1267–1280.

Lavanchy D (2005) Worldwide epidemiology of HBV infection, disease burden, and vaccine prevention. *Journal of Clinical Virology* 34(supplement 1): S1–S3.

McMahon BJ (2005) Epidemiology and natural history of hepatitis B. *Seminars in Liver Disease* 25(supplement 1): 3–8.

Norder H, Courouce A-M, Coursaget P, et al. (2004) Genetic diversity of hepatitis B virus strains derived worldwide: Genotypes, subgenotypes, and HBsAg subtypes. *Intervirology* 47: 289–309.

Prassolov A, Hohenberg H, Kalinina T, et al. (2003) New hepatitis B virus of cranes that has an unexpected broad host range. *Journal of Virology* 77: 1964–1976.

Schultz U, Grgacic E, and Nassal M (2004) Duck hepatitis B virus: An invaluable model system for HBV infection. *Advances in Virus Research* 63: 1–70.

Starkman SE, MacDonald DM, Lewis JCM, Holmes EC, and Simmonds P (2003) Geographic and species association of hepatitis B virus genotypes in non-human primates. *Virology* 314: 381–393.

Taylor JM (2006) Hepatitis delta virus. *Virology* 344: 71–76.

Tennant BC, Toshkov IA, Peek SF, et al. (2004) Hepatocellular carcinoma in the woodchuck model of hepatitis B virus infection. *Gastroenterology* 127: S283–S293.

Testut P, Renard CA, Terradillos O, et al. (1996) A new hepadnavirus endemic in arctic ground squirrels in Alaska. *Journal of Virology* 70: 4210–4219.

Zoulim F (2006) Antiviral therapy of chronic hepatitis B. *Antiviral Research* 71: 206–215.

Hepatitis B virus, Division of Viral Hepatitis, Centers for Disease Control and Prevention. http://www.cdc.gov/ncidod/diseases/hepatitis/slideset/hep_b/slide_9.htm (accessed August 2007).

Hepatitis A Virus

A Dotzauer, University of Bremen, Bremen, Germany

Glossary

Antibody prevalence The percentage of a population with antibodies against a certain disease at a given time.

Aplastic anemia Disease characterized by a decrease in blood cells resulting from underproduction due to bone marrow failure; also called hypoplastic anemia.

Incidence The rate of occurrence of new cases of a particular disease in a population in a certain period of time.

Polyprotein processing Cascade of proteolytic cleavage events resulting in release of mature proteins from the polyprotein.

Serine-like protease Proteolytic enzyme characterized by a catalytic triad similar to that in serine-type proteases with Ser, His, and Asp.

History

Jaundice has been known as an epidemic disease for centuries, but the earliest outbreaks of what was almost certainly hepatitis A were documented by Rayger, occurring in Preßburg, now Slovakia, in 1674 and 1697. Besides sporadic occurrence of the disease, characterized by a slow increase and slow decrease of the number of infected persons in the course of months (spread by person-to-person contact), with an overall small number of infections, larger vehement epidemics (spread by contaminated water and food) were reported in later times. The first pandemic wave occurred in the 1860s and the first considerable record of the disease was registered during the American Civil War.

In the second half of the nineteenth century, the disease became known as 'icterus catarrhalis' (catarrhal jaundice; inflammation of the biliary tract was supposed) or 'icterus epidemicus' (epidemic jaundice) as well as campaign jaundice, as epidemics are common in military medical history.

At the turn of the nineteenth to the twentieth century, the disease was recognized as infectious and transmissible by person-to-person contact. The terms 'hepatitis epidemica' (epidemic hepatitis) and 'hepatitis infectiosa' (infectious hepatitis) were introduced as synonyms for catarrhal jaundice.

Detailed epidemiologic recordings have been conducted since the beginning of the twentieth century.

Two large pandemic waves were observed during the twentieth century, the first one originating during World War I and reaching its summit between 1918 and 1922, and the second one originating in the early 1930s reaching its widest distribution with the beginning of World War II.

During World War II, hepatitis had been demonstrated to be caused by at least two separate filterable agents, and the resulting diseases were called hepatitis A (infectious hepatitis) and B (serum hepatitis), and the etiological agents hepatitis A virus (HAV) and hepatitis B virus (HBV), respectively.

After World War II, epidemiologic studies in human volunteers showed that hepatitis A is spread by the fecal–oral route, and provided information on the duration of viremia and shedding of virus in feces. In the late 1960s and early 1970s, it was shown that marmoset monkeys and chimpanzees could serve as animal models for human hepatitis A, and replication of HAV in cell cultures was established between 1979 and 1981.

The etiologic agent was identified through immune electron microscopy by Feinstone *et al.* in 1973.

The molecular cloning of the HAV genome in the 1980s revealed that the genomic organization of HAV is similar to that of picornaviruses, and the first infectious cDNA clone of HAV was reported by Cohen *et al.* in 1987.

The disease manifestations by hepatocellular destruction could be attributed to an immunopathogenic mechanism in the late 1980s by Vallbracht *et al.*

An inactivated vaccine has been available since 1992.

Taxonomy

HAV is the only member of the genus *Hepatovirus* within the family *Picornaviridae*.

All human HAV strains known belong to only one serological group, but phylogenetic analysis of the VP1–2A junction region and the VP1 coding region, respectively, revealed that several distinct HAV genotypes (seven in the case of VP1–2A junction analysis, five in the case of VP1 region analysis), which include several subgenotypes, can be distinguished by the degree in their genetic heterogeneity. These genotypes correlate with the geographic origin of the virus isolates. Genotype I is the most common type worldwide, particularly genotype IA. The cell culture-adapted viruses most commonly used are variants of the Australian strain HM175 (genotype IB) and the German strain GBM (genotype IA).

Morphology and Physicochemical Properties

The infectious spherical virion is a nonenveloped particle with a diameter of c. 27 nm. The icosahedral capsid, which embodies the viral RNA genome, contains 60 copies of each of the three major proteins, VP1 (also known as 1D), VP2 (1B), and VP3 (1C) (see **Table 1**). It is not known whether the small protein VP4 (1A) is integrated into the capsid. The mature HAV virion seems to have a different structure than other picornaviruses, as a usually prominent feature of picornaviruses and one which represents the viral attachment site to cellular receptors, the canyon surrounding the fivefold symmetry axes, is obviously missing.

The HAV particle has a buoyant density of c. 1.33 g cm^{-3} in CsCl and a sedimentation coefficient of c. 160S. Empty capsids found in feces have a sedimentation constant of about 70S. HAV is extremely resistant to acid (pH 1.0 for 2 h at room temperature) and thermal inactivation (60 °C for 1 h).

Genome Organization and Expression, Replication, Morphogenesis

The linear, single-stranded, positive-sense RNA genome of HAV is ~7500 nt in length and is not capped but covalently linked by a tyrosine-O^4-phosphodiester bond to the 2.5 kDa viral protein 3B (also known as VPg; see **Table 1**). It encompasses a structurally complex 5′ non-translated region (NTR) of ~740 bases, followed by a single open reading frame encoding a polyprotein (c. 250 kDa; ~2230 amino acids) and a 3′ NTR of ~60 bases which terminates with a poly(A) tail of about 60 nt. In the polyprotein, the capsid proteins and those with functions during virion assembly represent the N-terminal third (VP4, VP2, VP3, VP1, also known as P1 region, and 2A) (see **Table 1** and **Figure 1**) with the remainder of the polyprotein comprising a series of proteins required for RNA replication (2B and 2C followed by 3A to 3D) (see **Table 1** and **Figure 1**).

The viral polyprotein is translated directly from the messenger-sense genomic RNA, which is released into the cellular cytoplasm after uncoating of the virion. An internal ribosomal entry site (IRES) located within the 5′ NTR (see **Table 1**) is involved in the cap-independent initiation of protein synthesis. The IRES of HAV differs from that of other picornaviruses and forms its own group (type III picornavirus IRES). Translation from the HAV IRES requires all of the initiation proteins, including eIF4E and intact eIF4G, and infection with HAV does not result in cleavage of the translation initiation factor eIF4G to block cap-dependent host protein synthesis, as featured by other picornaviruses. The HAV IRES directed initiation of translation, which depends on the entire 5′ NTR, is enhanced by sequences of the 5′ terminal coding region and by the cellular protein poly(A) binding protein (PABP), which mediates circularization of the template RNA and seems to be necessary for HAV protein translation. Involvement of the host cells poly(C) binding protein 2 (PCBP2), polypyrimidine tract binding protein (PTB), and glyceraldehyde 3-phosphate dehydrogenase (GAPDH) is described, but the functional significance of these interactions is uncertain.

Proteolytic processing of the primary polyprotein (see **Figure 1**) occurs simultaneously with translation and is largely carried out by the viral 3C protease, which is a serine-like protease in which cysteine replaces the nucleophilic serine in the catalytic triad of the active center and for which, in contrast to other picornaviruses, no additional cellular substrate has been described so far.

Synthesis of viral RNA by the viral 3D polymerase follows the accumulation of the nonstructural proteins spanning 2B to 3D, which induce the assembly of a macromolecular replication complex on membranes that are recruited from the endoplasmatic reticulum. The proteins 2B, 2C, and 3A may be involved in the structural rearrangements of the intracellular membranes. RNA transcription is most likely protein-primed, with the uridylylated VPg protein 3B representing the primer for the negative-sense RNA replication intermediate and the subsequent positve-sense genomic RNA synthesis. A participation of the 5′ terminal NTR structures in the switch from translation to replication on the same viral RNA is suggested.

HAV morphogenesis is poorly understood. The primary polyprotein cleavage event occurs at the 2A/2B junction mediated by the 3C protease resulting in the structural precursor P1–2A. The steps then resulting in particle formation are not entirely clear, but the following model is suggested (see **Figure 1**). The P1–2A structural precursors assemble to a pentameric structure and are further cleaved by the 3C protease to generate the precursors VP4–VP2 (also known as VP0) and VP1–2A, as well as VP3 resulting in the structural building block (VP0, VP3, VP1–2A)$_5$. The 2A C-terminal extension of VP1 is a critical structural intermediate in virion morphogenesis, maybe clamping the pentamer at the fivefold symmetry axis. After assembly of 12 such pentamers with the genomic RNA to provirions (12 × (VP0, VP3, VP1–2A)$_5$-RNA), two subsequent maturation cleavage events occur. First, the cleavage at the VP1/2A junction leading to the removal of 2A seems to result from the action of an unknown host protease and, second, VP0 is cleaved into VP4 and VP2 by an unknown mechanism. 2A has never been identified in infected cells, which may indicate an extracellular cleavage event for the VP1–2A processing, and the role of VP4 in virion morphogenesis is mysterious. While the HAV polyprotein appears to

Table 1   HAV regulatory genomic regions and HAV proteins; all numbering refers to HAV strain HM175 (accession no. NC_001489)

Regions/proteins	Nucleotide position	Length in amino acids	Proposed or known function	Remarks
5′ nontranslated region (5′ NTR)	1–734		5′ stem–loop region (nucleotides 1–94): required for RNA replication	Mechanisms regulating switch from translation to replication are not clear
			Polypyrimidine tract pY1 (nucleotides 99–138): unknown function Internal ribosomal entry site (IRES) (nucleotides 152–734): directs cap-independent initiation of translation	Picornaviral type III IRES
3′ nontranslated region (3′ NTR)	7416–7478		Involved in regulation of RNA replication Extended by 40–80 adenylates, which are structurally involved in translation (closed-loop model)	
1A	735–803	23	VP4	Not myristoylated So far not identified in mature virions
1B	804–1469	222	Capsid protein VP2	During morphogenesis, precursor VP4–VP2 (VP0), presumably cleaved autocatalytically
1C	1470–2207	246	Capsid protein VP3	
1D	2208–3023/ 3026/ 3029	272 273 274	Capsid protein VP1	Heterogeneous C-terminus, presumably depending on HAV strain and host cell During morphogenesis, precursor VP1–2A, presumably cleaved by cellular protease
2A	3024/3027/ 3030–3242	71/72/73	Morphogenesis	So far not identified in infected cells
2B	3243–3995	251	Structural rearrangements of intracellular membranes for replication	Peripheral association with membranes Influence on membrane permeability Mutations accompany adaptation to growth in cell culture
2C	3996–5000	335	Structural rearrangements of intracellular membranes for replication	Integral association with membranes Mutations accompany adaptation to growth in cell culture
3A	5001–5222	74	As 3AB VPg precursor (pre-VPg)	Interacts with membranes, may anchor pre-VPg to cellular membranes through a central region of 21 hydrophobic amino acids
3B	5223–5291	23	VPg (virus protein genomic) Supposed protein primer for RNA replication	Tyr[3] attached to 5′ terminus of genomic RNA
3C	5292–5948	219	Sole protease	Serine-like protease, with replacement of Ser by Cys in catalytic triad: Cys[172], His[44], Asp[84]
3D	5949–7415	489	RNA-dependent RNA polymerase	

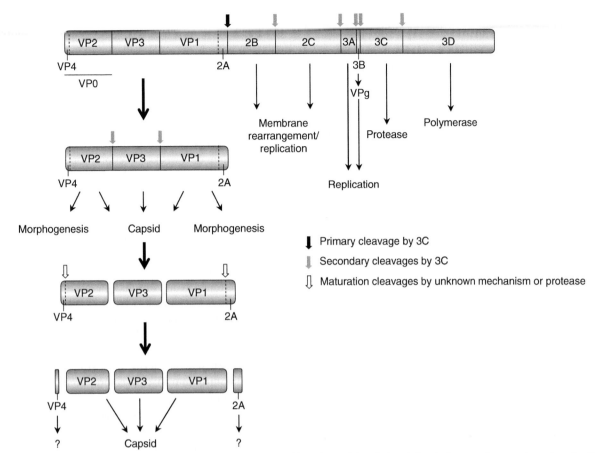

Figure 1 HAV polyprotein processing and known or supposed functions of the viral proteins during morphogenesis and replication. The polyprotein that results from IRES-directed translation is cleaved by the viral protease 3C to release certain precursor proteins with biologically relevant functions as well as the mature nonstructural proteins. Primary cleavage results in release of the structural precursor VP4–VP2–VP3–VP1–2A, which associate to assembly intermediates (pentamers), which are stabilized by 3C cleavage of the VP3 junctions (VP4–VP2 (VP0), VP3, VP1–2A)$_5$. After assembly of the intermediate protein building blocks and the viral genome to provirions, maturation cleavages occur through an unknown proteolytic activity to release VP4 from VP2 and by a so far unknown cellular protease to release 2A from VP1, resulting in the infective virion with 60 copies of each of the main structural proteins VP1, VP2, and VP3.

possess the short VP4 segment at its N-terminus, this putative VP4 moiety has never been identified in virions. Moreover, the HAV-VP4 sequence does not contain a myristoylation signal, which is important for the morphogenesis of other picornaviruses.

Host Range, Transmission, and Tissue Tropism

Under natural conditions, only humans and certain species of nonhuman primates seem to be susceptible to HAV. These primates, which are also used as animal models, include chimpanzees, marmosets, and owl monkeys.

HAV is transmitted via the fecal–oral route. As the virus is excreted in feces, it is typically acquired by ingestion of feces-contaminated food or water. Direct person-to-person spread occurs under poor hygienic conditions.

The site of replication is the liver. The events that occur during the passage of HAV across the intestinal epithelium into blood, in which the virus reaches the liver, are not clearly understood. Although HAV antigen and the T-cell immunoglobulin mucin 1 (TIM1; function so far unknown) protein, which has been identified as a cell surface protein binding HAV (HAV$_{cr1}$), could be detected in different organs, such as kidney, spleen, and gastrointestinal tract, no extrahepatic sites of HAV replication have been clearly identified. Furthermore, it was demonstrated that infection of polarized intestinal cells does not result in penetration of the epithelium. A functional cellular receptor, whose selective expression in the liver is assumed, could not be identified so far. Some studies suggest that the hepatotropism of HAV may be supported by immunoglobulin A (IgA)-virus complexes (HAV/IgA), as HAV/IgA uptake via the hepatocellular asialoglycoprotein receptor (ASGPR) results in infection of hepatocytes (IgA-carrier hypothesis).

The virus progeny produced in the liver is then released back into the intestinal tract via bile.

Cell Culture and Growth Characteristics

HAV can infect a variety of primate and nonprimate cell lines, including nonhepatic cells, *in vitro*. The virus exhibits a protracted replication cycle and normally establishes a noncytolytic, persistent infection with low virus yields, and there is no evidence that HAV notably interferes with the macromolecular synthesis of its host cell. After infection of cultivated cells with wild-type virus, a minimum of 8 weeks elapses before HAV can be isolated. Although a more rapid replication and higher virus titers are obtained after serial virus passages in cultivated cells resulting in cell culture-adapted viruses, even the replication of these virus variants is not detectable within the first few days after infection. Adaptation of HAV to growth in cultivated cells seems to be achieved by varying sets of multiple interacting mutations, with adaptive mutations within the IRES enhancing viral translation in a cell-type-specific fashion, and mutations clustering in the 2B and 2C proteins (see **Table 1**) increasing replication regardless of the cell line used.

The virus apparently downregulates its own replication and this may, for example by supporting the ability of HAV to inhibit innate cellular antiviral defense mechanisms, be important for the establishment of persistent infections. A large proportion of the virus progeny remain cell associated, but extensive release of HAV from the cells also occurs, caused by an unknown mechanism.

Several cytopathogenic variants of HAV have been isolated which induce apoptosis resulting in cell death. These variants are highly cell culture adapted and characterized by a rapid replication phenotype and high virus yields. In these variants, both the downregulation of viral replication and the ability to inhibit the innate defense mechanisms are less effective. The molecular mechanisms resulting in apoptosis are not known.

Clinical Features and Pathology

Infections with HAV may produce a wide spectrum of manifestations ranging from silent infections, over icteric courses to fatal fulminant hepatitis. The acute icteric course of infection varies between common, over prolonged to relapsing hepatitis A. Persistent infections or chronic disease have not been described.

The clinical presentation of the disease depends on the age of infection. The likelihood of having symptoms and the severity of the disease increases with the age of the patient. Inapparent infections (asymptomatic or at least anicteric) are normally observed in very young children, under the age of 2. However, clinically obvious disease can occur even in infancy (aged 2 weeks to 8 months) and may be characterized by prolonged courses. In children under 5 years of age *c.* 3%, in children 5–15 years old *c.* 30%, and in individuals over the age of 18 years as many as 70% may develop a clinically apparent disease.

Common Course of Infection

The incubation period ranges from 2 to 6 weeks with a mean duration of 4 weeks. The prodromal (preicteric) period of normally 4–6 days (which may vary from 1 day to more than 2 weeks) is characterized by nonspecific symptoms, like anorexia, nausea with vomiting, malaise, abdominal pain, loss of appetite, accelerated pulse, rash, headache, and fever (38–39 °C) as well as by gastrointestinal symptoms, normally in form of obstipation, but diarrhea is also observed.

The prodromal symptoms disappear with the onset of jaundice, which is seldom abrupt (in 15% of the cases no obvious prodrome is observed before appearance of jaundice). The icteric phase, which ranges from 2 to >22 days (mean duration 3 weeks), is marked by jaundice, which may start with scleral icterus, dark beer-colored urine (conjugated bilirubinuria), clay-colored stool, and clearly decelerated pulse.

The reconvalescence period ranges from 3 to 6 weeks, but fatigue, dullness, right upper quadrant tenderness, and fast exhaustion may remain for 2–4 months. In almost all cases the liver is enlarged.

The clinical symptoms are accompanied by several biochemical parameters (see **Figure 2**). Elevation of aminotransferase levels in serum (alanine aminotransferse (ALT) and to a lesser degree aspartate aminotransferase (AST)), which reflect hepatocellular damage with release of the liver enzymes into the circulation, roughly correlate with the severity of the disease. Elevation of serum alkaline phosphatase activity and in the serum bilirubin level relate to intrahepatic cholestasis.

At the onset of symptoms, seroconversion to anti-HAV occurs.

Large amounts of HAV, which are produced in the liver and released into the gastrointestinal tract via bile, already occur in the feces during the late incubation period when no clinical symptoms are observable and are shed for approximately three weeks until a few days after the onset of elevated levels of liver enzymes in the serum. Fecal shedding of HAV reaches its maximum just before the onset of hepatocellular injury.

Viremia occurs a few days before and during the early acute stage of the clinical and biochemical hepatitis, in which it roughly parallels the shedding of virus in feces, but at a lower magnitude.

More sensitive methods (especially nucleic acid amplification technologies) demonstrated that low levels of viral RNA may be present in feces and blood for many weeks.

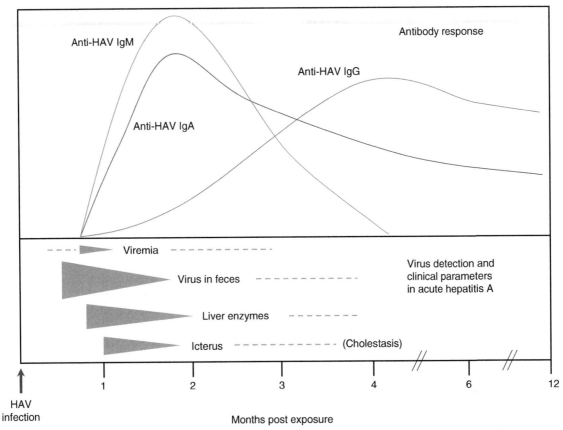

Figure 2 Course of clinically relevant events in acute hepatitis A. This figure schematically shows the mean duration and intensity of certain parameters. The dotted lines indicate that the duration and intensity of the events may vary.

Prolonged Hepatitis A

In 8.5–15% of the cases, jaundice lasts for up to 17 weeks. The biochemical abnormalities are resolved by 5 months. Occasionally, prolonged courses are accompanied by high serum bilirubin levels persisting for months (cholestatic hepatitis A). The cholestatic form is marked by extensive itching of the skin.

Relapsing Hepatitis A

After initial improvement in symptoms and liver test values (serum aminotransferase levels), one or more relapses of the disease (mostly biphasic) are described for up to 20% of the patients. These relapses occur between 30 and 90 days after the primary episode, when high titers of neutralizing antibodies are already present. The severity of symptoms, the biochemical abnormalities, and the immunoglobulin M (IgM) response are essentially the same as observed during the initial phase, with a tendency to greater cholestasis. The pathogenesis of relapsing hepatitis is not understood and basically two hypotheses are suggested: that the disease is a manifestation of a persistent viral infection, or, alternatively, that the relapse may represent a manifestation of an enterohepatic

cycling of HAV, which may be supported by anti-HAV IgA (IgA-carrier hypothesis). But none of these hypotheses is currently supported by *in vivo* data.

Fulminant Hepatitis A

In rare cases, acute hepatitis A results in a fatal deterioration in liver function with massive destruction of liver cells. Surprisingly, no vigorous inflammatory response is observed. The fatality rate is below 1.5% of all hospitalized icteric cases. This course of the disease is accompanied with fever over 40 °C. This outcome is more frequent in adults, especially in patients over 50 years of age, than in children, and the risk is increased in patients with underlying chronic liver disease.

Extrahepatic Manifestations

Extrahepatic manifestations of the disease are rare and the etiology is uncertain. Besides frequently observed transient suppression of hematopoiesis, rare cases of aplastic anemia (pancytopenia) with a lethality rate of over 90% are described, and it was demonstrated that HAV infects monocytes and inhibits their further differentiation. In some patients, interstitial nephritis was observed. In connection with the finding that the HAV-binding receptor HAV_{cr1} is identical with the T-cell immunoglobulin mucin 1 (TIM1), a protein suggested to play a role in asthma susceptibility, and by statistical evaluation of medical records, it was suggested that HAV exposure may leave a protective effect on the development of asthma and allergic diseases.

Pathology

The pathology of the liver in acute hepatitis A has been studied in humans and several animal models. The pathological lesions, which are caused by an immunopathogenic mechanism, are characterized by hepatocellular necrosis, which is most prominent in periportal regions, accompanied with large inflammatory infiltrates of mononuclear cells.

Innate and Adaptive Immune Response

Innate Immune Response

HAV, which does not interfere with the replication of other viruses, prevents the synthesis of beta-interferon (IFN-β), but is not resistant to alpha- and beta-interferon (IFN-α/β) exogenously added to persistently infected cells. It could be demonstrated that HAV does inhibit dsRNA-induced transcription of IFN-β by blocking effectively interferon regulatory factor 3 (IRF-3) activation due to an interaction of HAV with the mitochondrial antiviral signaling protein MAVS (also known as IPS-1, VISA, or Cardif), which is a component of the retinoic acid-inducible gene I (RIG-I) and melanoma differentiation-associated gene 5 (MDA-5) signaling pathway. Signaling through the Toll-like receptor 3 (TLR-3) pathway may also be partially impaired.

HAV also has the ability to prevent apoptosis induced by accumulating dsRNA, but the underlying mechanism is not clear.

Gamma interferon (IFN-γ) produced by HAV-specific HLA-dependent cytotoxic T lymphocytes (CTLs) may contribute to the elimination of HAV infections by inducing an antiviral state in the later course of the infection.

Adaptive Immune Response

Neutralizing anti-HAV IgM antibodies are present in almost all patients at the onset of the symptoms (see **Figure 2**). These antibodies disappear in the course of 3 months, but in the case of prolonged courses IgM can be detected up to 1 year after onset of icterus. Anti-HAV IgA antibodies are also detectable at the onset of the symptoms (see **Figure 2**). This response reaches its peak titer 50 days post infection and may last for >5 years. The majority of the IgA remains as serum IgA in circulation and is not secreted into the intestinal tract as secretory IgA by the polymeric immunoglobulin receptor (pIgR) pathway. But a significant fraction of this serum IgA is released into the gastrointestinal lumen via bile by liver functions under participation of the hepatocellular IgA-specific asialoglycoprotein receptor (ASGPR). The role of IgA antibodies in the protection against HAV infections appears to be limited, and studies suggest that HAV-specific IgA may serve as a carrier molecule for a liver-directed transport of the virus, supporting the hepatotropic infection by uptake of HAV/IgA immunocomplexes via the ASGPR (IgA-carrier hypothesis). Neutralizing anti-HAV immunoglobulin G (IgG) antibodies are also detectable 3 weeks post infection for the first time, but this response develops slowly, reaching its peak titer 4 months post infection (see **Figure 2**). Anti-HAV IgG persists lifelong, although the titer may fall to undetectable levels after several decades. Neutralizing antibodies, which are effective in eliminating the virus from the blood, do recognize a conformational epitope clustered into a major, immunodominant antigenic site involving residues contributed by VP3 and VP1.

HAV-specific, HLA-restricted cytotoxic $CD8^+$ T lymphocytes (CTLs) have been detected within the liver during acute HAV infection and play prominent roles both in eliminating the virus and in causing liver injury (immunopathogenesis). Gamma interferon (IFN-γ), released by these CTLs, may stimulate HLA class I expression on hepatocytes and in the following promote upregulation of the normally low level display of antigen on liver cells. Specific T-cell epitopes have not been identified so far.

Diagnosis

Since the clinical presentation of hepatitis A cannot be distinguished from hepatitis due to the other hepatitis viruses, serologic tests or nucleic acid amplification techniques are necessary for a virus-specific diagnosis.

The routine diagnosis of acute hepatitis A is made by detection of anti-HAV IgM in the serum of patients (see **Figure 2**). A further option is the detection of virus in the feces.

In order to improve the safety of blood and blood products, blood screening with HAV-specific polymerase chain reaction (PCR) is performed, which reduces the window period of up to 3 weeks post infection during which HAV infection fails to be diagnosed by serologic assays.

Epidemiology

HAV occurs worldwide and accounts for over 1.5 million clinical cases reported annually. The seroprevalence pattern ranges from high endemicity, such as in Africa, South Asia, and Latin America, where infection normally occurs in childhood, over intermediate endemicity, such as in Eastern Europe and the northern parts of Asia, to low endemicity, such as in Western Europe and North

America, where the majority of the population remains susceptible to HAV infection. However, the epidemiology pattern is complex and continuously changing, with considerable heterogeneity among different countries. In general, the anti-HAV antibody prevalence inversely correlates with the quality of the hygienic standards, and the incidence declines in many populations through improvements in public sanitation and living conditions. These improvements result in an increase of the pool of susceptible adults, with a shift in the age of infection to older age groups, in which a more severe disease is observed, leading to an increased morbidity.

A minor seasonal distribution of HAV infections is observed, with a peak occurring during fall and winter, mentioned in almost all earlier and contemporary reports, nowadays possibly as a result of exposure during summer vacation spent in endemic countries.

At special risk for acquisition of hepatitis A are international travelers from areas of low endemicity to endemic areas, employees of child-care centers and sewage plants, gully workers, injecting drug users, homosexually active men, and persons with an increased risk of developing a fulminant disease, such as persons with chronic hepatitis C virus (HCV) infections.

The high physical stability of HAV provides a good opportunity for common-source transmission. Community-wide outbreaks are reported in association with infections of food handlers, and linked to contaminated food and drink, or uncooked clams from contaminated water. Hepatitis A is most commonly acquired by sharing the household with an infected person.

Prevention and Control

There is no specific treatment for hepatitis A. As almost all HAV infections are spread by the fecal–oral route, good personal hygiene, high-quality standards for public water supplies, and proper disposal of sanitary waste are important measures to reduce virus transmission.

Until the availability of an active prophylaxis, the disease could be prevented for up to 5 months with a certainty of 80–90% by passive immunization with pooled IgG of at least 100 IU anti-HAV. IgG is still used for postexposure prophylaxis. If administered within 2 weeks after exposure, either development of the disease is prevented or the severity of the disease as well as virus shedding is reduced.

Since 1992, inactivated vaccines for active immunization have been available. These vaccines contain purified, formalin-inactivated virions produced in cell culture, which are absorbed to an aluminum hydroxide adjuvant. They are highly immunogenic and protect against both infection and disease caused by all strains of HAV with 100% efficacy for at least 10 years, which is consistent with the finding that all human HAV strains belong to one single serotype.

Candidate live, attenuated HAV vaccines have been developed using virus adapted to growth in cell culture, but were poorly immunogenic. Nonetheless, such a vaccine has been widely used in China and appears to be capable of inducing protective levels of antibody.

See also: Hepatitis B Virus: General Features; Hepatitis C Virus; Hepatitis E Virus.

Further Reading

Bell BP (2002) Global epidemiology of hepatitis A: Implications for control strategies. In: Margolis HS, Alter MJ, Liang JT, and Dienstag JL (eds.) *Viral Hepatitis and Liver Disease*, pp. 9–14. Atlanta: International Medical Press.
Cuthbert JA (2001) Hepatitis A: Old and new. *Clinical Microbiology Reviews* 14: 38–58.
Gerety RJ (ed.) (1984) *Hepatitis A*. London: Academic Press.
Gust ID and Feinstone SM (1988) *Hepatitis A*. Boca Raton, FL: CRC Press.

Hepatitis B Virus: General Features

P Karayiannis and H C Thomas, Imperial College London, London, UK

Glossary

Icterus Jaundice, or yellowing of the skin and particularly the whites of the eyes, due to failure to excrete bilirubin, a bile pigment.

History

It was not until the mid-1960s that hepatitis A (HAV) and B (HBV) viruses were recognized as the causative agents for infectious and serum hepatitis, respectively. These studies, performed by Krugman and colleagues at the

Willowbrook State School for mentally handicapped children, were preceded a few years earlier by the description of the Australia antigen in the sera of patients with leukemia. The connection between Australia antigen, or hepatitis B surface antigen (HBsAg) as it is now known, and HBV became apparent in later studies performed by the teams of Prince and Blumberg. These studies set the groundwork for the subsequent serological tests for the diagnosis of HBV and allowed detailed investigations into the epidemiological and virological aspects of infection.

Electron microscopic studies in 1970 by Dane and Almeida and their colleagues led to the visualization of the infectious virion or Dane particle, and the nucleocapsid core, respectively. This was followed in the early 1970s by the characterization of the virus genome, the virion-associated proteins, and the detailed definition of the serological profiles in acute and chronic HBV infection, performed primarily by Robinson's group at Stanford. The connection between the virus and the development of hepatocellular carcinoma (HCC) followed soon after, but the absence of a cell culture system for propagation of the virus impeded the study of its molecular biology. This changed in the early 1980s with the development of genetic engineering techniques that allowed the cloning of the viral genome, the study of its protein funtions, and the unravelling of the fascinating mechanism of its replication strategy. The polymerase chain reaction (PCR) allowed the speedy amplification and sequencing of virus isolates that led to the identification of quasispecies, virus mutants, and genotypes by bioinformatic approaches. In 1987, Carman and colleagues described the molecular basis of HBe antigen negative viremia (precore stop mutation – see below) and described the first, and most common, vaccine escape variant (arginine 145) in vaccinated children born to HBV-infected mothers (see below).

The introduction of a plasma-derived vaccine, following its extensive evaluation by Smuzness and colleagues in chimpanzees, constitutes another historical landmark in HBV research. This was soon followed by the production of a recombinant vaccine, which has effectively reduced the prevalence of the infection in many countries of the world where the virus was endemic. Almost concurrently, interferons were used for the first time in the treatment of chronic hepatitis B. These remain, with the subsequently introduced nucleos(t)ide analogs, the main treatment options in order to prevent progression of chronic liver disease to cirrhosis and HCC.

Taxonomy and Classification

Hepatitis B is the prototype virus of the family *Hepadnaviridae*, a name that signifies the hepatotropism and DNA nature of the genome of its members. There are two genera within the family. The genus *Orthohepadnavirus* contains members that infect mammals, and, other than HBV, includes hepadnaviruses that infect rodents such as woodchucks (woodchuck hepatitis virus, WHV) and squirrels (70% nucleotide identity). In recent years, HBV-like isolates have also been obtained from primates such as chimpanzees, gibbons, gorillas, orangutans, and woolly monkeys. These are more closely related to HBV and may in fact represent progenitors of the human viruses (**Figure 1**). The *Avihepadnavirus* genus on the other hand contains members that infect birds such as ducks (duck hepatitis B virus, DHBV), herons, storks, and geese. Over the years, the woodchuck and duck animal models, as well as chimpanzees, which are susceptible to infection with human HBV isolates, have proved invaluable in the study of the replication of these viruses, the natural history of

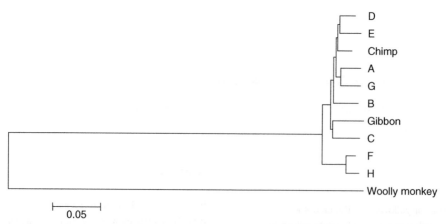

Figure 1 Phylogenetic tree based on the nucleotide sequences from the HBsAg region of all known human HBV genotypes and isolates from a chimp, gibbon, and woolly monkey. The tree was constructed using the Mega 2 software and rooted to the woolly monkey sequence.

infection, and the testing for efficacy of vaccines and antiviral drugs.

Distribution and Epidemiology

Conservative estimates place the number of persons chronically infected with HBV at over 350 million worldwide. The prevalence of HBV infection varies by geographical region, so that in northwestern Europe, North America, and Australia it is 0.1–2%. In the Mediterranean region, Eastern Europe, Middle East, Indian subcontinent, and Central and South America, it is 3–7%, while in Africa and the Far East it is 10–20%. This geographical distribution of HBV infection is mirrored by the incidence of HCC in the same regions. In areas of high endemicity, the virus is transmitted perinatally from carrier mothers to their infants, or horizontally from infected siblings and other children in early childhood. In areas of intermediate endemicity apart from perinatal transmission, household and sexual contact, as well as percutaneous exposure, are likely routes of infection. Finally, in Western countries, transmission is nowadays through sexual contact or intravenous drug use.

Virion Structure and Genome Organization

The infectious virion or Dane particle measures about 42 nm in diameter and consists of an outer envelope containing hepatitis B surface proteins (HBsAg) in a lipid bilayer (**Figure 2**). This in turn encloses the nucleocapsid core of the virus, within which lies the viral genome and a copy of its polymerase. Apart from virions, liver hepatocytes release into the circulation subviral particles devoid of nucleic acid and consisting entirely of HBsAg. These are the 22 nm spheres and the filamentous

forms of similar diameter, which outnumber the virions by 100–10 000-fold.

The viral genome is a relaxed circular, partially double-stranded DNA molecule of 3.2 kbp in length, and contains four wholly or partially overlapping open reading frames (ORFs) (**Figure 3**). In addition, all regulatory elements such as enhancers, promoters, and encapsidation and replication signals lie within these ORFs. The Pre-S/S ORF encodes the three envelope glycoproteins, which are known as the large (L), middle (M), and small (S) HBsAgs, produced by differential initiation of translation at each of three in-frame initiation codons. The proteins are therefore co-terminal and the sequence of the more abundant small protein is shared by the other two. The M protein has an additional 55 amino acid residues at its N-terminus encoded by the Pre-S2 region, while the L protein includes in addition another 125 residues from the Pre-S1 region. The Pre-S1 protein is thought to contain the region responsible for the virus interaction with the hepatocyte receptor. All three proteins are glycosylated, while the L and S proteins may also be present in an unglycosylated form in particles.

The precore/core ORF contains two in-frame initiation codons and therefore yields two translation products. Initiation of translation from the first results in synthesis of the precore polypeptide, which forms the precursor of the soluble hepatitis B e antigen (HBeAg). This protein contains a signal peptide at its N-terminus that anchors the protein in the endoplasmic reticulum membrane. Cleavage by signal peptidase in the lumen is followed by further processing of the C-terminus. The resulting protein is the HBeAg, a nonstructural protein and marker of active virus replication. Moreover, the protein is thought to have a tolerogenic effect on the immune response to the virus. The nucleocapsid or core protein is synthesized following initiation of translation at the second initiation codon. The HBeAg and core proteins are translated from two separate transcripts known as the precore mRNA and the pregenomic RNA (pgRNA), respectively. The

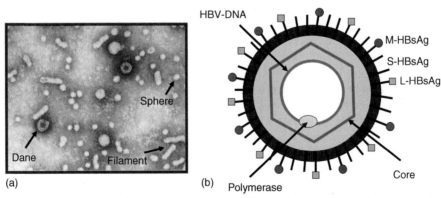

Figure 2 Structure of the hepatitis B virion. (a) Electron micrograph of HBV purified from plasma showing the infectious Dane particle and the spherical and filamentous subviral particles. (b) Cartoon of the virion and its components.

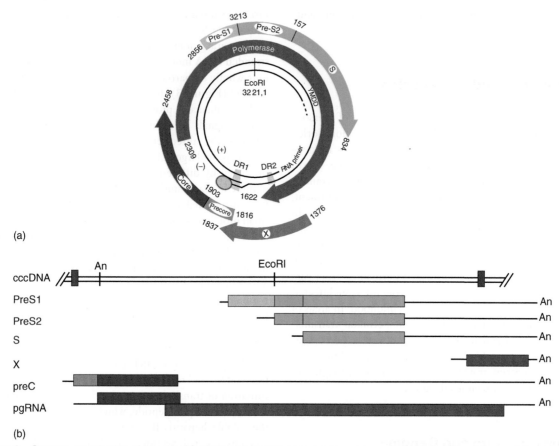

Figure 3   Genome organization of the virus (a) and the transcripts encoding the various viral proteins (b), synthesized from cccDNA. All of them terminate at the common polyadenylation site. Reproduced from Hunt CM, Mc Gill JM, Allen MI, *et al.* (2000) Clinical relevance of hepatitis B viral mutations. *Hepatology* 31: 1037–1044. American Association for Liver Diseases. Reprinted with permission of Wiley-Liss, Inc., a subsidiary of John Wiley & Sons, Inc.

latter also encodes the polymerase ORF of the virus, which covers almost all of the genome. The polymerase has multifunctional enzymatic actions as described below. Finally, the fourth ORF encodes for the X protein, which modulates host cell signal transduction and acts as a gene transactivator under experimental conditions.

Replication Strategy

The life cycle of the virus begins with its attachment to the appropriate hepatocyte receptor, which still remains unknown. In contrast, the region between residues 21 and 47 of Pre-S1 has long been known to be involved in virus binding to the hepatocyte membrane (**Figure 4**). The virion is internalized and uncoated in the cytosol, whence the genome translocates to the nucleus, where it is converted into a double-stranded covalently closed circular DNA (cccDNA) molecule, following completion of the shorter positive (+)-strand and repair of the nick in the negative (−)-DNA strand. The cccDNA constitutes the template for viral transcript synthesis by the host RNA

polymerase II. All the transcripts terminate at a common polyadenylation signal situated within the proximal end of the core ORF, and their synthesis is controlled by individual promoters and the two enhancer elements, Enh 1 and 2.

The pgRNA is longer than genome length (3.5 kbp) and, apart from encoding the core and polymerase proteins, also forms the template for (−)-DNA strand synthesis (**Figure 5**). The polymerase has three functional domains, each one in turn involved in DNA priming (terminal protein), reverse transcription (rt), and pgRNA degradation (RNase H). There is also a spacer region of unknown function between the terminal protein and the rt domain. Once synthesized, the polymerase engages epsilon (ε), a secondary RNA structure at the 5′ end of the pgRNA, triggering encapsidation of the complex by the core protein. The subsequent steps in virus nucleic acid synthesis then take place within the nucleocapsid. Host cell factors including chaperones from the heat shock protein family are thought to be instrumental in aiding encapsidation, stabilization, and activation of the polymerase.

As pgRNA is longer than genome length, its terminal sequence duplicates the elements contained in its 5′ end

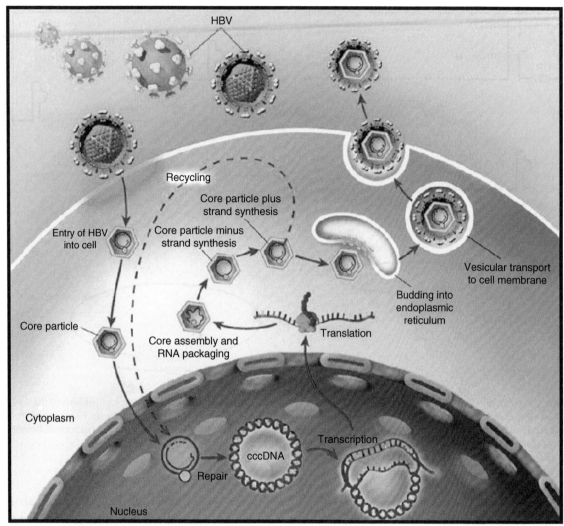

Figure 4 Diagrammatic representation of the life cycle of the virus. Reproduced from Ganem D and Prince AM (2004) Hepatitis B virus infection – Natural history and clinical consequences. *New England Journal of Medicine* 350: 1118–1129, with permission from Massachusetts Medical Society.

and includes the direct repeat 1 (DR1) and ε (**Figure 5**). The bulge of the ε structure serves as a template for the synthesis of a 3–4-nt-long DNA primer, which is covalently attached to the polymerase through a phosphodiester linkage between dGTP and the hydroxyl group of a tyrosine residue in the terminal protein (96). This event involves the ε structure at the 5′ end of the pgRNA, and is then followed by the translocation of the polymerase–primer complex to the 3′ end, where it hybridizes with the DR1 region with which it shares similarity. How this translocation occurs remains unknown. As the complex proceeds toward the 5′ end of the pgRNA, the (−)-DNA strand is synthesized by reverse transcription and the RNA template is concurrently degraded by the RNase H activity of the polymerase, except for the final 18 or so ribonucleotides. A second translocation event then occurs during which the ribonucleotide primer hybridizes with the DR1 region at the 5′ end of the newly synthesized

(−)-DNA strand. A template exchange occurs that allows the (+)-DNA strand synthesis to proceed along the 5′ end of the complete (−)-DNA strand, effectively circularizing the genome. (−)- and (+)-DNA strand synthesis occurs within the nucleocapsid as already mentioned, and this is facilitated through pores allowing entry of nucleotides. Once the maturing nucleocapsid is enveloped by budding through the endoplasmic reticulum membrane, the nucleotide pool within the capsid cannot be replenished, hence the incomplete nature of the (+)-DNA strand.

Subtypes

The S protein sequence shared by all three envelope proteins contains the major immunogenic epitope of the virus referred to as the '*a*' determinant. This epitope, shared by all isolates of the virus, is recognized by

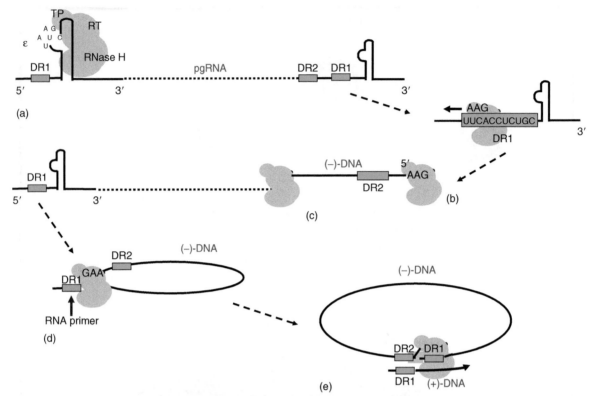

Figure 5 Replication strategy of the virus. (a) Primer synthesis; (b) translocation and binding to DR1; (c) synthesis of the (–)-DNA strand; (d) RNA primer fragment preserved from the degradation of the pgRNA; (e) (+)-DNA strand synthesis. Reproduced from Karayiannis P (2003) Hepatitis B virus: Old, new and future approaches to antiviral treatment. *Jouranl of Antimicrobial Chemotherapy*. 51: 761–785, with permission from Oxford University Press.

neutralizing antibodies and is conformational in nature, probably encompassing residues 110–160. In addition, there are subtypic specificities originally detected by antibodies. The presence of lysine (K) or arginine (R) at position 122 confers *d* or *y* specificity, respectively. Similarly, specificities *w* and *r* are conferred by the presence of K or R at position 160. Moreover, the *w* subdeterminant can be further divided into *w1–w4* specificities. There are nine subtypes of the virus (**Table 1**) depending on the presence of other subtype-determining residues elsewhere in the '*a*' determinant region.

Genotypes

Nucleotide sequencing studies soon established that the virus could be divided into genotypes based on sequence divergence of >8% (**Table 1**). There are currently eight genotypes, designated A–H, with characteristic geographical distribution. Genotypes A and D occur frequently in Africa, Europe, and India, while genotypes B and C are prevalent in Asia. Genotype E is restricted to West Africa, and genotype F is found in Central and South America. The distribution of genotypes G and H is less clear, but

these have been described from isolates in central America and Southern Europe. These genotypes can be further subdivided into a total of 21 subgenotypes; A1–3, B1–5, C1–5, D1–4, and F1–4. Subgenotypes of B and C differ in their geographical distribution, with B1 dominating in Japan and B2 in China and Vietnam, while B3 and B4 are confined to Indonesia and Vietnam, respectively. Subgenotype C1 is common in Japan, Korea, and China, C2 in China, Southeast Asia, and Bangladesh, C3 in Oceania, and C4 in Australian aborigines. Recombinants between genotypes A and D, as well as between B and C, have also been described.

Likely differences between genotypes in relation to pathogenesis and response to antiviral treatment are beginning to emerge. Genotype C is more frequently associated than B with abnormal liver function tests, lower rates of seroconversion to anti-HBe, higher levels of serum HBV-DNA, cirrhosis, and HCC. Moreover, there is a better sustained response to interferon treatment in patients with genotype B than those with C, and in patients with genotype A than those with D. Genotype A infection appears to be associated with biochemical remission and clearance of HBV-DNA more frequently than genotype D, and has a higher rate of HBsAg clearance compared with genotype D.

Table 1　Genotype determining amino acid variation over the 'a' determinant region of HBsAg, and relationship between genotypes and subtypes

Genotype	Subtype	Amino acid sequence of 'a' determinant (positions 122–160)																																				
		K	T	C	T	T	P	A	Q	G	N	S	M	F	P	S	C	C	C	T	K	P	T	D	G	N	C	T	C	I	P	S	S	W	A	F	A	K
A	Adw	a	–	–	–	–	–	–	–	–	–	–	–	–	–	–	–	–	–	–	–	–	–	–	–	–	–	–	–	–	–	–	–	–	–	–	–	–
	adw2/ayw1	a	–	–	–	–	–	–	–	–	–	–	–	–	–	–	–	–	–	–	–	–	–	–	–	–	–	–	–	–	–	–	–	–	–	–	–	–
B	adw1/ayw1	a	–	–	–	–	–	–	–	–	T	–	–	–	–	–	–	–	–	–	–	–	–	S	–	–	–	–	–	–	–	–	–	–	–	–	–	R
C	ayr/adrq+/adrq-/adr	–	–	–	–	I	–	–	–	–	T	–	–	–	–	–	–	–	–	–	–	–	–	S	–	–	–	–	–	–	–	–	–	–	V	–	–	R
D	ayw2/ayw3/ayw4	R	–	M	–	–	–	T	–	–	T	–	–	–	–	–	–	–	–	–	–	–	–	S	–	–	–	–	–	–	–	–	–	–	G	–	–	–
	ayw4	R	–	–	–	–	–	T	–	–	T	–	–	–	–	–	–	–	–	–	–	–	–	S	–	–	–	–	–	–	–	–	–	–	G	–	–	–
E	ayw4	R	–	–	–	–	–	L	–	–	T	–	–	–	–	–	–	–	–	–	S	–	–	S	–	–	–	–	–	–	–	–	–	–	G	–	–	–
F	adw4q-/adw2/ayw4	a	–	–	–	–	–	L	–	–	T	–	–	–	–	–	–	–	–	–	S	–	–	S	–	–	–	–	–	–	–	–	–	–	G	L	–	–
G	adw2	–	–	–	–	–	–	–	–	–	–	–	–	Y	–	–	–	–	–	–	–	–	–	S	–	–	–	–	–	–	–	–	–	–	G	–	–	–
H	adw4	–	–	–	–	T	V	–	–	–	T	–	–	Y	–	–	–	–	–	–	–	–	–	S	–	–	–	–	–	–	–	–	–	–	G	–	–	–

[a] R or K.

In contrast to the differences observed in response to interferon therapy, treatment with nucleos(t)ide analogs does not show differential responses between genotypes.

Variants

The HBV genome is not as invariant as originally thought. As HBV replicates through an RNA intermediate that is reverse-transcribed, this step in the replication cycle of the virus is prone to errors made by the viral reverse transcriptase. It is estimated that the HBV genome evolves at a rate of $1.4–3.2 \times 10^{-5}$ nucleotide substitutions/site/year. The virus therefore circulates in serum as a population of very closely related genetic variants, referred to as a quasispecies. Although a lot of these variants would have mutations that would be deleterious to the virus, as a result of constraints imposed by the overlapping ORFs, some would be advantageous, either offering a replication advantage or facilitating immune escape. These are discussed below in the clinical settings in which they have been described.

Markers of Infection

Serological diagnosis of HBV infection relies on the detection of HBsAg in serum, and its persistence for longer than 6 months indicates progression to chronic infection. Appearance of anti-HBs (antibody to HBsAg) indicates recovery from infection, or acquired immunity after preventive vaccination. Detection of HBeAg denotes active viral replication, as does the detection of serum HBV-DNA by qualitative or quantitative PCR tests. Seroconversion to anti-HBe occurs after recovery from acute infection, and less often during the chronic phase, either spontaneously or after therapeutic intervention. In the latter case, this leads to a quiescent phase of disease that can be long term, but does not necessarily mean that virus replication ceases completely (see below). Detection of antibody to core antigen (anti-HBc) of IgM class at high level is a marker of acute infection, whereas total anti-HBc (primarily IgG) is detectable during both acute and chronic infection.

Natural History of the Disease

Exposure to HBV may result in asymptomatic, acute icteric, or, in some instances, fulminant hepatitis (0.1–0.5%). Approximately 5% of adults and 95% of perinatally infected young children become persistently infected. The outcome depends on the age of the patient and genetic factors determining the efficiency of the host immune response. Genetic factors influencing outcome (in more than one study) include polymorphisms of the MHC class II glycoproteins, which influence presentation of viral peptides during induction of the cellular immune response, and mannin-binding lectins, which bind to mannose-terminated carbohydrate residues such as those present on the C-terminus of the Pre-S2 region of the middle envelope protein facilitating phagocytosis. The risk of chronicity in children decreases with increasing age. A small proportion of carriers each year may become HBsAg negative (0.05–2%, depending on age of infection), thus leading to resolution of the hepatitis.

Acute HBV Infection

The incubation period following exposure is 3–6 months. In the week before icterus appears, some patients develop a serum sickness-like syndrome including arthralgia, fever, and urticaria. The clinical picture varies from asymptomatic anicteric infection to protracted icterus and, in some patients (<1%), liver failure (fulminant hepatitis). The acute infection is self-limiting and most patients recover within 1–2 months after the onset of icterus.

Chronic HBV Infection

This is defined as persistent viremia of more than 6 months duration and accompanied by hepatic inflammation. The latter is based on histological examination of liver biopsy material that is followed by assigning of scores for necroinflammatory activity (out of 18) and stage of fibrosis (out of 6), which are used to decide whether a patient needs therapy.

Course of Chronic Infection

Chronic HBV infection is quite variable and is typically characterized by four phases. These phases are the immune tolerant, the immune clearance, the nonreplicative (immune-controlled low-level infection), and the reactivation phase that may be seen in some patients, particularly in Southern Europe and the Far East (**Figure 6**). During the immune-tolerant phase, the patient is HBsAg- and HBeAg-positive with high levels of HBV-DNA, but with near-normal or minimally elevated alanine aminotransferase (ALT) levels. Children infected at birth or soon after are more likely to go through this phase, which may last for 2–3 decades. During the immune clearance phase more commonly seen in those infected in adult life, HBeAg and HBV-DNA levels decrease, ALT levels increase, and necroinflammatory changes are seen in liver biopsies. Loss of HBeAg may be accompanied by an ALT flare, culminating in seroconversion to anti-HBe and entry to the nonreplicative phase when the infection is under

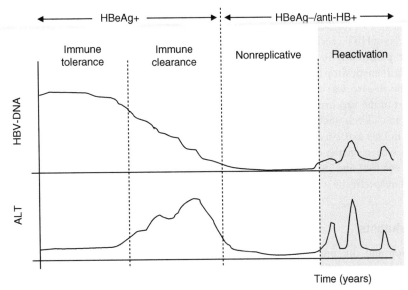

Figure 6 Diagram of the natural history of chronic HBV infection showing the immune tolerant, immune clearance, nonreplicative, and reactivation phases. Reproduced from Karayiannis P, Carman WF, and Thomas HC (2005) Molecular variations in the core promoter, precore and core regions of hepatitis B virus, and their clinical significance. In: Thomas HC, Lemon S, and Zuckerman AJ (eds.) *Viral Hepatitis* 3rd edn., pp. 242–262. London: Blackwell, with permission from Blackwell Publishing.

immune control. Viral DNA integration into the host genome may take place during chronic infection and persist during the nonreplicative (low replicative) phase. During this phase, plasma HBV-DNA may or may not be detectable, while ALT levels return to normal. This serological profile characterizes the 'inactive carrier state', which is maintained thereafter. Some patients, however, for reasons that still remain unknown, show disease reactivation accompanied by ALT rises and return of viremia. Such patients may exhibit fluctuations in ALT levels with occasional severe exacerbations. Continued necroinflammatory activity may lead to fibrosis, and faster development of cirrhosis and HCC.

Mutant Viruses and Chronic Infection

Anti-HBe-positive patients in the reactivated phase of the disease are also referred to as the HBeAg-negative viremic group. Genomic analyses has revealed that such patients carry natural mutants of the virus that have either reduced levels (core promoter variants) or complete abrogation of HBeAg (precore variants) production. These variants are selected at the time of, or soon after, seroconversion, and become dominant during the reactivation phase. The most common precore mutation is the G1896A substitution, which creates a premature stop codon in the precursor protein from which HBeAg is elaborated. This mutation affects the stem of the ε encapsidation signal, but leads to stronger base pairing with the A1896 change in genotypes with a T at position 1858 of the precore region, such as B, C, D, and E. The double

mutation affecting the core promoter region (A1762T, G1764A) is thought to result in decreased transcription of the precore mRNA, with a knockon effect on HBeAg production, while pgRNA production remains the same or is even upregulated. It is now apparent that additional mutations in this region may contribute to this phenotype.

Vaccination

Prophylactic vaccination offers the only means of interrupting the transmission of the virus. Vaccines currently used consist of recombinantly expressed HBsAg in yeast such as *Saccharomyces cerevisiae*. In adults, the vaccine is administered intramuscularly into the deltoid at 0, 1, and 6 months. In countries of high and medium seroprevalence, universal vaccination programmes have been instituted, and HBV vaccination is recommended for infants born to carrier mothers within 12 h of birth, given together with hepatitis B immune globulin (HBIg). The response to the vaccine is determined by measuring anti-HB levels 1–4 months after the last dose of the vaccine, and the minimum protection level is set at 10 mIU ml^{-1}.

Development of anti-HBs following vaccination has been recorded in 90–95% of healthy individuals, with lower response rates in hemodialysis and hemophiliac patients (70%). Recent studies on the duration of antibodies have shown maintenance of levels above the 10 mIU ml^{-1} cutoff for 12 years, in up to 80% of individuals immunized at a young age. Booster immunizations therefore may not be required for at least 10 years after vaccination, and some countries are reconsidering the necessity for this.

The beneficial effects of HBV vaccination are becoming increasingly apparent, particularly in reducing new infections. There has been a dramatic drop in HBV prevalence in populations where the disease was endemic. In Taiwan, 15 years after the start of the vaccination programme, the prevalence of HBsAg in children under 15 years of age has decreased from 9.8% in 1984 to 0.9% in 1999. Similarly, the incidence of HCC has been on the decline from 0.7 per 100 000 children between 1981 and 1986, to 0.57 and 0.36 in 1986–90 and 1990–94, respectively.

Vaccine Escape Mutants

In spite of vaccination and the presence of a satisfactory antibody level, it has been observed that in some instances breakthrough infections occur, the commonest of which involves a mutant with a G145R substitution in the '*a*' determinant region of HBsAg. This and additional mutations in this region have been shown to result in altered antigenicity, accompanied by failure of HBsAg recognition by neutralizing antibody. Such mutant viruses have also been described in the liver transplantation setting, where use of HBIg or monoclonal anti-HBs is recommended in an attempt to prevent infection of the new liver graft.

Treatment

The agents currently available for the treatment of chronic HBV infection are divided into two main groups: the immunomodulators, which include interferon-alpha (IFN-α), and nucleos(t)ide analogs such as lamivudine (3TC), adefovir dipivoxil (Hepsera), entecavir (Baraclude), and telbivudine (Tyzeka or Sebivo), which are currently approved for this purpose. The immunomodulators act by promoting cytotoxic T-cell activity for lysis of infected hepatocytes and by stimulating cytokine production for control of viral replication. Nucleos(t)ide analogs on the other hand are chain terminators acting at the stage of DNA synthesis.

HBeAg-Positive Patients

Treatment with pegylated IFN-α-2, the current standard treatment administered once a week for up to 1 year, achieves seroconversion to anti-HBe in 32% of patients, compared to 18%, 12%, 21%, and 23% with lamivudine, adefovir, entecavir, and telbivudine, respectively. The latter drugs are taken orally daily, in contrast to the weekly intramuscular injections of pegylated interferon. These responses are sustainable in over 95% of patients.

HBeAg-Negative Patients

Treatment of these patients with pegylated interferon for a year results in virologic remission (HBV-DNA <20 000 IU ml^{-1}; equivalent to 105 copies ml^{-1}) in about 44% of them, followed by ALT normalization. This response appears durable in around 20%. Similarly, treatment with nucleos(t)ide analogs for a year leads to HBV-DNA becoming undetectable in between 65% and 90% of treated patients. However, on stopping therapy, only a small minority have a sustained response at the end of 24 weeks of follow up.

Protracted Treatment

To manage such relapses following initial interferon treatment, nucleos(t)ide therapy should be started and continued long term in both HBeAg-positive and -negative patients not achieving a sustained response after a trial of pegylated interferon for 6–12 months. In HBeAg-positive patients, prolonged treatment with lamivudine, for example, leads to increased seroconversion rates from 17% in year 1 to 27% and 40% for years 2 and 3, respectively. Besides, prolonged treatment leads to normalization of ALT levels and an obvious improvement in the histological findings of liver biopsy material. Unfortunately, in many cases, there are breakthrough infections which are attributed to the development of resistance as described below. In such cases, virological breakthrough is soon accompanied by biochemical (ALT rise) and histological relapse. The latter can be avoided by switching to a different nucleos(t)ide analogue that has no cross-resistance with the previous one. Monitoring at three monthly intervals for viral resistance, using molecular assays, is essential.

Resistance

Lamivudine resistance develops in about 24% of patients at year 1 rising to >70% by year 5. Adefovir resistance on the other hand is delayed, being 0% at year 1, 3% at year 2, and rising to 28% by year 4. Entecavir resistance has only been seen so far in patients with lamivudine resistant strains. Longer term follow-up with this nucleoside analogue is ongoing. Nevertheless, it appears that this analog has a high genetic resistance barrier while lamivudine has a low one. Resistance to telbivudine is already a problem after a year of treatment but it appears initially to be more potent than lamivudine.

Molecular Basis of Drug Resistance

The rt domain of the HBV polymerase contains six subdomains (A–F) that are spatially separated, but closely associated with, the normal function of the protein. The characteristic YMDD (tyrosine-methionine-aspartate-aspartate) motif of the catalytic site is located within subdomain C. Subdomains A, C, and D are most likely involved with dNTP binding and catalysis, whereas subdomains B and E interact with the pgRNA template and primer. Amino acid substitutions that confer resistance to lamivudine predominantly affect the YMDD motif, so that the methionine (M) at position 204 is changed either to valine (YVDD, rtM204V) or isoleucine (YIDD, rtM204I). The former mutation is almost always associated with a second one in subdomain B, involving a substitution of leucine with methionine at position 180 (rtL180M). Adefovir resistance is conferred by mutations rtN236T in subdomain D and rtA181V in subdomain B. In the small number of entecavir-resistant cases detected so far, in addition to the lamivudine-resistant substitutions additional ones that include rtI169T, rtT184G, rtS202I, and rtM250V have been identified.

See also: Hepatitis A Virus; Hepadnaviruses: General Features.

Further Reading

Carman WF, Jazayeri M, Basune A, Thomas HC, and Karayiannis P (2005) Hepatitis B surface antigen (HBsAg) variants. In: Thomas HC, Lemon S,, and Zuckerman AJ (eds.) *Viral Hepatitis,* 3rd edn., pp. 225–241. London: Blackwell.

Ganem D and Prince AM (2004) Hepatitis B virus infection – Natural history and clinical consequences. *New England Journal of Medicine* 350: 1118–1129.

Hadziyannis SJ and Papatheodoridis GV (2006) Hepatitis B e antigen-negative chronic hepatitis B: Natural history and treatment. *Seminars in Liver Disease* 26: 130–141.

Hunt CM, Mc Gill JM, Allen MI, *et al.* (2000) Clinical relevance of hepatitis B viral mutations. *Hepatology* 31: 1037–1044.

Karayiannis P (2003) Hepatitis B virus: Old, new and future approaches to antiviral treatment. *Journal of Antimicrobial Chemotherapy* 51: 761–785.

Karayiannis P, Carman WF, and Thomas HC (2005) Molecular variations in the core promoter, precore and core regions of hepatitis B virus, and their clinical significance. In: Thomas HC, Lemon S,, and Zuckerman AJ (eds.) *Viral Hepatitis,* 3rd edn., pp. 242–262. London: Blackwell.

Thomas HC (2006) Hepatitis B and D. *Medicine* 35: 39–42.

Zoulim F (2006) Antiviral therapy of chronic hepatitis B. *Antiviral Research* 71: 206–215.

Hepatitis C Virus

R Bartenschlager and S Bühler, University of Heidelberg, Heidelberg, Germany

Glossary

Pseudotypes Retroviral vector particles bearing heterologous glycoproteins on their surfaces.

Replicon DNA or RNA molecule capable of self-replication in a cell or in an adequate *in vitro* system (e.g., cell lysate).

Sustained virological response (SVR) Continuous absence of HCV RNA from the serum starting 6 months after cessation of antiviral therapy.

Introduction

In the 1970s, when blood tests for the detection of hepatitis A virus (HAV) and hepatitis B virus (HBV) became available, many blood samples responsible for post-transfusion hepatitis were negative when tested for these two viruses. Therefore, this third form of transfusion-associated hepatitis was named non-A, non-B hepatitis. However, in 1989, Choo and co-workers discovered hepatitis C virus (HCV) as the causative agent of parenterally transmitted non-A, non-B hepatitis. Initially, they isolated a viral complementary DNA clone from the serum of a chimpanzee experimentally infected with non-A, non-B hepatitis and used it to establish a screening test for antibodies in patients infected with this agent. By using this initial cDNA clone as a hybridization probe, Choo and colleagues then isolated a near full-length viral genome that was readily classified as a close relative of the animal pathogenic pestiviruses based on similarities of genome organization and virion properties.

Taxonomy and Geographical Distribution

HCV has been classified as the only member of the genus *Hepacivirus* and grouped together with the genera *Pestivirus, Flavivirus,* and tentatively the GB-viruses, in the family *Flaviviridae.* According to phylogenetic analyses, HCV is more closely related to the pestiviruses than to the flaviviruses.

Based on genomic heterogeneity, six major genotypes, having more than 30% nucleotide sequence divergence, and more than 70 subtypes differing from each other by 10–30% at the nucleotide sequence level, have been defined. Subtypes are designated by lowercase letters following the number of the genotype (e.g., genotype 1 subtype b = 1b). While genotype 1 and 2 viruses are prevalent almost worldwide, HCV genotypes 3–6 are to a large extent restricted to distinct geographical regions, including the Indian subcontinent and Southeast Asia (genotype 3), Africa and Middle East (genotype 4), South Africa (genotype 5), and Southeast Asia (genotype 6). Individual genotypes have not been ascribed to particular disease manifestations, except for a higher prevalence of steatosis with patients infected with genotype 3 viruses, but genotypes are important predictors of therapy outcome (see below).

Transmission

HCV is mainly transmitted by parenteral exposure to blood and blood products. The development of effective screening tests for blood and blood products and the implementation of viral disinfection procedures have almost excluded this route of transmission in countries where these measures are in place. Thus, the major remaining risk factor for acquiring HCV infection in developed countries is the use of contaminated needles in injection drug use. In some countries, HCV infection has been spread primarily by the use of inadequately sterilized medical instruments. In contrast to HBV infection, sexual transmission and maternal–infant spread of HCV are much less frequent.

Clinical Manifestation

Acute HCV infections are usually asymptomatic or, in about 30% of cases, associated with nonspecific symptoms such as abdominal pain, fatigue, weakness, poor appetite, and nausea. During an incubation period of 15–75 days, HCV RNA becomes detectable in serum by

reverse transcription-polymerase chain reaction (RT-PCR), and virus titers usually peak at 10^5–10^7 genomes/ml between weeks 6 and 10, irrespective of disease outcome (**Figure 1(a)**). Two to four weeks after onset of viremia serum alanine aminotransferase (ALT) levels begin to rise, indicative of hepatocellular injury. Due to these nonspecific signs and symptoms, acute infection often remains unrecognized. The duration of viremia in acute hepatitis C is unpredictable and can vary from 2 to more than 4 months. Some patients even become HCV RNA negative during early convalescence but later on viremia rebounds. Overall 50–80% of HCV infections lead to a chronic carrier state (**Figure 1(b)**). About 30% of these chronically infected persons progress to liver cirrhosis 10–30 years after primary infection and hepatocellular carcinoma occurs in up to 2.5% of these patients. In contrast to chronic hepatitis B, in case of persistent HCV infection a hepatocellular carcinoma only develops on the basis of prior cirrhosis.

Pathology and Histopathology

Hepatocytes are the primary target of HCV. Therefore, the histological alterations of chronic hepatitis C are hepatocellular injury, portal and parenchymal inflammation, and necrosis. The injury of the hepatocyte is thought to be induced primarily by the immune reaction rather than by viral cytopathogenicity. Liver damage is typically spotty and focal with accompanying chronic inflammatory cells, macrophages, and, eventually, variable degrees of fibrosis. The progression rate of hepatic fibrosis is the major determinant for the outcome of chronic hepatitis C in terms of developing cirrhosis and hepatocellular carcinoma. Unfortunately, there are only a few histological markers that are more often associated with hepatitis C than with other causes of hepatitis, such as steatosis.

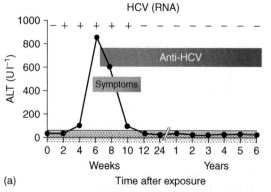
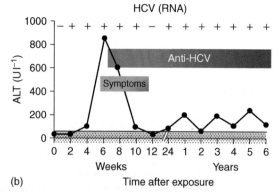

Figure 1 Course of acute and chronic HCV infection. (a) In acute HCV infection, viral RNA is typically detectable between weeks 2 and 10 after virus exposure. ALT levels rise between weeks 4 and 10 peaking around week 6. This is also the time when the first symptoms manifest. HCV-specific antibodies arise late in infection. In self-limiting infection HCV is cleared as measured by RNA levels and ALT returns to normal levels. (b) In chronic hepatitis C the early phase is similar to acute infection but later on the virus persists. In the chronic phase, ALT levels fluctuate as does viremia.

Although the liver is the primary target, persistent HCV infection is often associated with extrahepatic symptoms, such as renal complications, lymphoma, and diabetes. A high proportion of patients with chronic hepatitis C develop cryoglobulinemia, which may account for some of these extrahepatic manifestations.

Genome Organization

The genome of HCV is a 9.6 kb single-stranded RNA molecule of positive polarity (**Figure 2(a)**). It is flanked by two highly structured nontranslated regions (NTRs). The 5′ NTR contains an internal ribosome entry site (IRES) (**Figure 2(b)**), mediating cap-independent translation of a polyprotein of *c.* 3000 amino acids in length. The 3′ NTR is composed of a 40-nt-long variable region,

a polypyrimidine tract (heterogeneous length), and the 98-nt-long highly conserved 3′ terminal X-tail (**Figure 2(b)**). Both the 5′ and the 3′ NTRs contain *cis*-acting RNA elements (CREs) that are required for viral replication. Within the 3′ terminal part of the NS5B gene, three additional CREs are localized (5BSL3.1–5BSL3.3), wherein 5BSL3.2 is absolutely required for viral RNA replication by forming a long-distance RNA–RNA interaction with the middle loop in the X-tail.

The organization of the HCV polyprotein and the functions of the individual gene products are depicted in **Figure 2(a)**. The structural proteins, core and the envelope proteins 1 (E1) and 2 (E2), are located within the N-terminal part of the polyprotein preceding the p7 protein which appears to be an ion channel and therefore was grouped into the viroporin protein family. The nonstructural (NS) proteins NS2, NS3, NS4A, NS4B, NS5A, and NS5B are

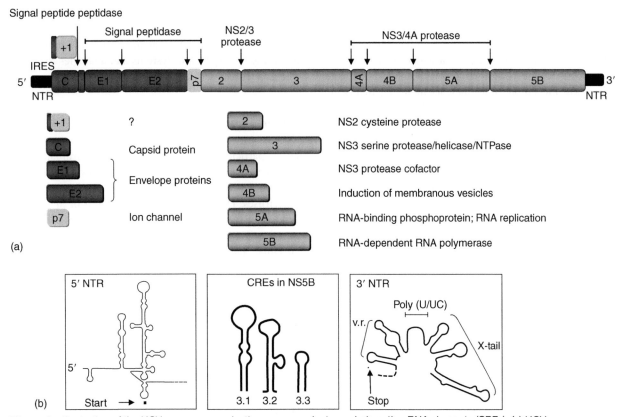

Figure 2 Illustration of the HCV genome organization, gene products, and *cis*-acting RNA elements (CREs). (a) HCV genome organization, gene products, and their functions in the replication cycle. The HCV coding region is shown as bar with arrows above indicating the positions of polyprotein cleavage and involved proteases. The structural region in the N-terminal third of the polyprotein is drawn in orange, and the region encoding the nonstructural proteins is drawn in green. The core+1 protein(s) and the p7 protein are drawn in gray. The HCV coding region is flanked by two nontranslated regions (5′ and 3′ NTR), indicated in dark gray. The 5′ NTR contains an internal ribosome entry site (IRES). Functions of the individual gene products are given in the lower panel. (b) Schematic representation of CREs. The 5′ NTR (left panel) contains the IRES as well as structures important for viral RNA replication. Three CREs are located in the 3′ terminal part of the NS5B coding region (middle panel). The loop region of stem–loop 5BSL3.2 forms a long-distance RNA–RNA interaction essential for RNA replication with the loop region of the middle stem–loop in the X-tail. The right panel displays the organization of the 3′ NTR with variable region (v.r.), poly(U/UC) tract, and X-tail. Positions of start and stop codons are indicated with dots.

encoded in the remainder. The NS2 protein together with the N-terminal protease domain of NS3 is responsible for the autocatalytic cleavage of the NS2–NS3 junction (**Figure 2(a)**). It is a dimeric cysteine protease with a composite active site. The same NS3 protein domain carries a serine-type protease that after association with its cofactor NS4A cleaves the residual junctions between the NS proteins. Moreover, the same protease also cleaves two cellular signaling molecules involved in the induction of the innate immune response (see below). Two additional enzymatic activities (RNA helicase and nucleoside triphosphatase) reside in the C-terminal two-thirds of NS3. Alterations of intracellular membranes, in particular membranous vesicles, are mainly induced by the 27 kDa integral membrane protein NS4B. These vesicles accumulate in the perinuclear region, are called the membranous web, and are the site of viral RNA replication. So far, the role of the phosphorylated zinc metalloprotein NS5A in the viral replication cycle is unclear. NS5A is composed of an N-terminal amphipathic α-helix serving as a membrane anchor and three largely cytosolic domains. The X-ray crystal structure of RNA-binding domain I was resolved and shown to form homodimers resulting in a basic groove. NS5A phosphorylation is mediated by cellular kinases, in particular the α isoform of the protein kinase CKI. The NS5A phosphorylation state appears to affect replication efficiency indicating that NS5A is an important replication factor. Furthermore, NS5A may also contribute to interferon-alpha (IFN-α) resistance that is often observed with genotype 1 and 4 viruses. The 68 kDa protein NS5B is the RNA-dependent RNA polymerase (RdRp). It is a membrane-associated enzyme with a structural organization similar to that of other polymerases with palm, finger, and thumb subdomains. However, it differs from most other RdRps by having a fully encircled active site, which is due to tight interactions between the finger and thumb subdomains.

In addition to the polyprotein, a heterogeneous group of HCV proteins is expressed either by ribosomal frameshifting into the +1 ORF or by internal translation initiation. The resulting proteins, collectively designated core +1, are not essential for replication and virus production in cell culture, and their role *in vivo*, if any, remains to be elucidated.

HCV Replication Cycle

HCV infection starts by binding the envelope glycoprotein E1/E2 complex on the surface of the virus particle to its cognate receptor(s) presumably leading to clathrin-mediated endocytosis and a subsequent fusion step from within an acidic endosomal compartment (**Figure 3**). Cellular factors implicated in virus binding and entry are glycosaminoglycans, scavenger receptor class B type 1 (SR-B1), CD81, and low-density lipoprotein (LDL) receptor. However, for most of these factors, the

precise role is not well understood and one or several additional factors may be required for productive entry. Upon release of the RNA genome, the polyprotein is expressed by IRES-dependent translation occurring at the rough endoplasmic reticulum (rER) where host cell signal peptidases, signal peptide peptidases, and viral proteases catalyze polyprotein cleavage.

During or after cleavage, the membrane-associated replication complex, which catalyzes the RNA amplification via negative-strand RNA intermediates, is formed (**Figure 3**). These membrane-associated complexes are composed of viral RNA, viral proteins, and most likely host cell factors. Newly synthesized positive-strand RNAs either are used for translation or serve as templates for further RNA synthesis or interact with the core protein to form the viral nucleocapsid. The E-proteins are retained at rER membranes indicating that viral envelopes are generated by budding into the lumen of this organelle. Progeny particles are thought to be exported by the secretory pathway and after fusion of the transport vesicle with the plasma membrane, virions are released. However, most of these steps are poorly understood and several assumptions were made that are based on studies with heterologous expression systems and analogies to closely related viruses.

Virion Properties

HCV particles are enveloped and spherical and have a diameter of 55–60 nm as determined by filtration and electron microscopy (**Figure 4**). By analogy to other flaviviruses, HCV particles are composed of at least the genomic RNA, the core protein, and the two envelope proteins E1 and E2 which are embedded into the lipid envelope. The core protein forms the internal viral capsid (presumably 30–35 nm in diameter) that shelters the single-stranded RNA genome (**Figure 4**). The S_{20W} is approximately 200S and infectious HCV virions isolated from the plasma sample of infected patients and chimpanzees have low buoyant densities in the range of $1.05–1.10 \, \text{g ml}^{-1}$.

Tissue Tropism and Host Range

Hepatocytes are considered to be the natural target cells for HCV. Viral RNA was also detected in peripheral blood mononuclear cells (PBMCs) and bone marrow cells but it is unclear whether productive infection occurs in these cells. In cell culture, HCV RNA replication was demonstrated in non-liver cells like human T- and B-cell lines or embryonic kidney cells (293). Furthermore, certain mouse cell lines can support replication of HCV replicons demonstrating that the viral replication machinery is also functional in a murine host cell environment.

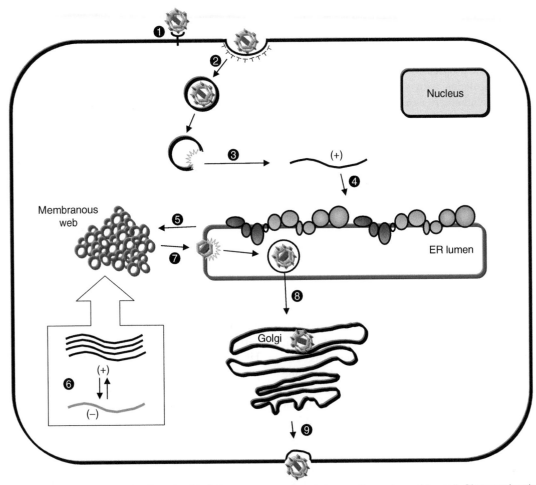

Figure 3   HCV replication cycle. (1) HCV virion binds to one or several receptors on the surface of the cell. Glycosaminoglycans, SR-B1, CD 81, and eventually LDL receptor are required for or contribute to virus binding and entry. (2) The virus particle supposedly enters the cell via clathrin-mediated endocytosis. (3) After a low-pH-mediated fusion step from within an acidic endosome and uncoating, the HCV genome is liberated into the cytoplasm of the host cell. (4) The viral RNA genome is translated at the rough endoplasmic reticulum (rER). (5) The membranous web presumably originating from ER membranes is formed. (6) It is the site of viral RNA amplification which occurs via negative-strand RNA intermediates. Newly synthesized positive-strand RNA is either used for translation or replication or the RNA is packaged into nascent capsids (7). This may occur at the ER where the E-proteins are retained. It is assumed that virions are generated by budding into the ER lumen. (8) Progeny virions are thought to be exported by the secretory pathway and, after fusion of the transport vesicle with the plasma membrane, virions are released (9).

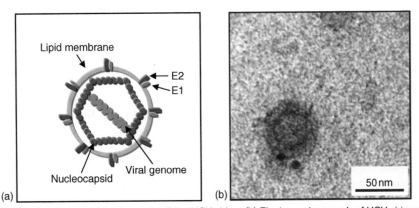

Figure 4   Composition of HCV particles. (a) Schematic of the HCV virion. (b) Electron micrograph of HCV virion produced in cell culture. The spherical particle has an outer diameter of about 60 nm and an inner core of about 30 nm. E2 was detected by immunoelectron microscopy using an E2-specific antibody and a secondary antibody conjugated to 10 nm gold particles.

Experimental Systems

Animal Models

Possibilities to propagate HCV *in vivo* are rare. For many years HCV could be propagated only in chimpanzees after experimental inoculation with virus containing samples from patients or synthetic *in vitro* transcripts derived from cloned infectious genomes. More recently, transgenic mice xenografted with primary human hepatocytes were found to be susceptible to HCV infection. Virus replication occurs in the transplanted human tissue but, given the technical challenge, this mouse model is not widely available. Alternative models to study HCV *in vivo* are the closely related GB-viruses, especially GBV-B that replicates in tamarins (*Sanguis* sp.), causing an acute self-limiting infection of the liver or, under certain experimental conditions, a persistent infection.

Cell Culture Systems

Development of efficient cell culture systems for HCV propagation was difficult and was not successful until more than 10 years after the discovery of the virus. The first breakthrough was the development of subgenomic replicons composed of the NTRs, a selectable marker (*neo*), and a heterologous IRES directing translation of the HCV replicase (NS3–NS5B) (**Figure 5(a)**). When transfected into a human hepatocarcinoma cell line (Huh-7) and subjected to selection (e.g., with G418 in case of replicons containing the *neo* gene), stable cell lines were established that carry autonomously replicating HCV replicons. These viral RNAs replicate to very

high levels and are maintained persistently when the cells are passaged under conditions of continuous selective pressure (e.g., G418). Owing to its high efficiency, this replicon system was of enormous value for studying HCV replication and HCV–host interaction, and for the development of antivirals targeting any of the viral replicase components (e.g., NS5B RdRp or the NS3 protease).

Since the first description of this system in 1999 numerous improvements have been made. These include the identification of replication-enhancing mutations (so-called adaptive mutations), different replicon formats allowing short-term replication analyses, and high-throughput screening assays. Thus far, replicons from different HCV isolates and two genotypes (1 and 2) are available, as are various cell lines, including two of murine origin.

Studies of the early steps of the HCV replication cycle are often performed using HCV pseudoparticles (HCVpp) (**Figure 5(b)**). These are retroviral capsids harboring a retroviral vector RNA into which a reporter gene has been inserted and which are surrounded by a lipid envelope carrying mature HCV E1/E2 glycoprotein complexes. This HCVpp system is an important tool to analyze the infection process and to measure HCV neutralization.

Robust production of infectious HCV particles in cell culture finally became possible in 2005 (**Figure 5(c)**). Key to this achievement is a particular HCV isolate designated JFH-1 (abbreviation for Japanese fulminant hepatitis) that was cloned from the serum of a patient with fulminant hepatitis C. When the JFH-1 genome is introduced into Huh-7 cells, virus particles are released that are infectious for naive Huh-7 cells, chimpanzees, and mice with human

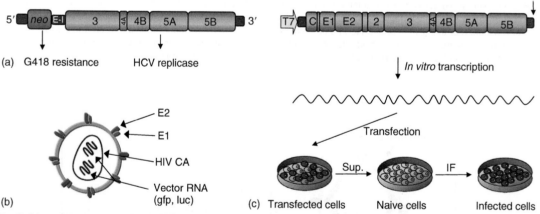

Figure 5   Cell-based systems for HCV. (a) Schematic illustration of the structure of a subgenomic HCV replicon carrying the selectable marker *neo* that confers G418 resistance. Translation of *neo* is directed by the 5′ NTR of HCV whereas translation of the replicase (NS3 to NS5B) is directed by the encephalomyocarditis virus (EMCV)-IRES. (b) Schematic of an HCV pseudoparticle (HCVpp). The retroviral vector RNA carries a reporter gene encoding, for example, for the green fluorescent protein (gfp) or the luciferase (luc). Two copies of vector RNA are packaged into the viral capsids surrounded by a lipid envelope carrying functional E1/E2 complexes. (c) Principle of the HCV infection system. Viral genomes are synthesized by *in vitro* transcription using a plasmid encoding a DNA copy of the viral genome. The T7 promoter at the 5′ end and a ribozyme or a restriction site (arrow) at the 3′ end are used to obtain run off transcripts with authentic termini. *In vitro* transcripts are transfected into Huh-7 cells and virus containing supernatant is transferred onto naive Huh-7 cells. Infection of these cells is detected, for example, by immunofluorescence (IF).

liver xenografts. Efficiency of this virus system has been increased by the construction of chimeric JFH-1 genomes, cell-culture-adapted virus variants, and by using highly permissive Huh-7 cell clones for HCV replication and entry. Very recently, a highly cell-culture-adapted variant of a genotype 1a HCV isolate has been constructed that also supports virus production in Huh-7 cells, but virus titers are extremely low.

HCV–Host Interaction

Replication Factors

Several cellular proteins appear to contribute to HCV replication. For example, the ubiquitously expressed human vesicle-associated membrane protein-associated protein A (VAP-A) and its isoform VAP-B were identified as interaction partners of NS5A and NS5B. NS5A hyperphosphorylation seems to disrupt the VAP-A association and thereby negatively regulates HCV RNA replication. It is thought that VAP-A directs HCV nonstructural proteins to cholesterol-rich, detergent-resistant membranes, which are the presumed sites of HCV RNA replication.

Another host cell factor interacting with NS5A is FBL-2 belonging to the family of proteins that contain an F box and multiple leucine-rich repeats. FBL-2 is modified by geranylgeranylation which is important for NS5A interaction. FBL-2 appears to be required for HCV RNA replication. Likewise, Cyclophilin B (CyPB), a cellular protein interacting with the NS5B RdRp, seems to contribute to replication of genotype 1 isolates by promoting RNA-binding capacity of NS5B. CyPs are a family of peptidyl-prolyl *cis–trans*-isomerases which catalyze the *cis–trans*-interconversion of peptide bonds N-terminal of proline residues, facilitating changes in protein conformation. Cyclosporine or derivatives thereof potently block HCV RNA replication and it is assumed that this is due in part to sequestration of CyPB, which binds to cyclosporine with high affinity.

Also the host cell lipid metabolism plays a fundamental role in the HCV replication cycle. Treatment of replicon cells with lovastatin, an inhibitor of 3-hydroxy-3-methylglutaryl CoA reductase, or with an inhibitor of protein geranylgeranyl transferase I induced the disintegration of the HCV replication complex. Fatty acids can either stimulate or inhibit HCV replication, depending on their degree of saturation. Saturated and monounsaturated fatty acids stimulate viral replication, whereas polyunsaturated fatty acids impair replication.

Innate Immunity

Both in cell culture and in the majority of patients treated with IFN-α, a rapid and efficient block of HCV replication occurs. This result is somewhat surprising given the high rate of persistence of HCV infections (50–80%) and the finding that, in infected liver, type 1 IFN-induced genes are activated. In several studies it was concluded that HCV proteins, such as core, interfere with the various steps of the IFN-α/β-induced signaling and that some HCV proteins appear to block individual IFN-α/β-induced effectors. One prominent example is NS5A, assumed to block activity of the double-strand RNA-activated protein kinase PKR by binding to PKR via a particular NS5A region. This region overlaps with the so-called interferon-sensitivity-determining region in NS5A, assumed to correlate with outcome of antiviral therapy. However, this original assumption is still contradictory and it is still unclear whether HCV indeed interferes with one or several type 1 IFN-induced effector molecule(s). It also remains to be clarified by which mechanism interferons block HCV RNA replication.

Much less controversial are the mechanisms by which HCV interferes with the induction of innate antiviral defense. Several studies have shown that the NS3 protease proteolytically cleaves two signal-transducing molecules: TRIF, linking the activation of Toll-like receptor 3 to kinase complexes responsible for the phosphorylation of interferon response factor-3 (IRF-3) and CARDIF (also called MAVS, ips-1, VISA) relaying the activation of retinoic-acid-inducible gene 1 (RIG-1) also to IRF-3 phosphorylation. As a result, IRF-3-dependent genes are not expressed including IFN-β and IRF-7 and cells remain sensitive to virus infection. Although linking the block of IFN-β expression to persistence is attractive, it is unclear if and to what extent that is the case. On one hand blocking IRF-3 activation would not affect the antiviral program induced by type 1 IFN (e.g., produced by activated dendritic cells or administered during therapy), whereas on the other hand this block may affect the secretion of cytokines required for the development of a vigorous adaptive immune response and its attenuation may facilitate persistence.

Adaptive Immunity

The role of HCV-specific antibodies in controlling viral infection is not clear. They appear to be dispensable for viral clearance and do not protect from reinfection, neither in experimentally infected chimpanzees nor in humans after multiple exposure to HCV. However, there is evidence that the presence of HCV-specific antibodies at least partially attenuates infection. For instance, antibodies neutralizing HCV virions of different genotypes have been detected in sera of chronic hepatitis C patients but the frequency of these antibodies appears to be low. Control of acute HCV infection is primarily achieved by a rigorous and multispecific T-cell response. Thus, successful antiviral response generally encompasses multiple major histocompatibility complex (MHC) class-I and class-II restricted T-cell epitopes and a profound expansion of $CD8^+$ and $CD4^+$ T cells. In contrast, persistent infections are characterized by oligoclonal T-cell responses and a low frequency of HCV-specific T cells. The underlying reasons for the weak response in the majority of patients are not clear but several possibilities have been suggested: (1) an impaired antigen presentation that might be due to interference of HCV with dendritic cell function; (2) $CD4^+$ T-cell failure due to deletion or anergy; (3) mutational escape in important T- (and B-)cell epitopes; and (4) functional impairment of HCV-specific $CD8^+$ T cells. How T-cell impairment is brought about is unclear but one attractive possibility is that the defect induced in innate immunity results in a defect in $CD4^+$ T-cell help. In fact, HCV-induced loss of T-cell help appears to be the key event of immune evasion.

Diagnosis

Routine screening tests for detecting HCV infections are based on serological assays measuring HCV-specific antibodies (most often by enzyme-linked immunosorbent assay (ELISA)) and nucleic acid-based tests to determine viral RNA. Current ELISA assays have a specificity of >99% and they are positive in 99% or more of immunocompetent patients in whom viral RNA is detectable. Given the higher sensitivity, the diagnostic window can be reduced by using nucleic acid-based tests. Qualitative RNA detection assays have been implemented in many blood banks in European Union countries and in the US. The risk to acquire transfusion-associated hepatitis C in such countries has been reduced to <1/million blood donations. Determination of HCV genotypes, which is an important parameter for current antiviral therapy, is based on analyzing viral RNA either by hybridization or direct sequence analysis or by using genotype-specific primers for PCR.

Treatment

Current antiviral therapy is based on the combination of a polyethylene glycol conjugated form of IFN-α with ribavirin resulting in an overall sustained virological response (SVR) of about 60%. However, the success rate depends very much on the genotype of the infecting virus. While up to 85% of genotype 2- and 3-infected patients develop SVR, only about 45% of patients infected with genotype 1 viruses do so. In addition, this therapy has numerous side effects, such as flu-like symptoms, including increased body temperature, headache and muscle pain; neuropsychiatric alterations and hemolytic anemia are also severe side effects of this combination therapy. Thus, therapy often has to be discontinued and many patients are not eligible for this treatment. Numerous efforts are therefore undertaken to develop selective drugs targeting viral functions without causing side effects. The first promising candidates are currently in clinical trials and have shown potent antiviral efficacy. Most advanced are inhibitors of the NS3 protease and the NS5B RdRp. However, monotherapy with these compounds leads to rapid selection for therapy-resistant HCV variants. Future therapy of HCV infection most likely will be based on a combination therapy, which may include a selective drug and IFN.

See also: Hepatitis A Virus; Hepatitis B Virus: General Features.

Further Reading

Appel N, Schaller T, Penin F, et al. (2006) From structure to function: New insights into hepatitis C virus RNA replication. *Journal of Biological Chemistry* 281: 9833–9836.

Bartenschlager R (2006) Hepatitis C virus molecular clones: From cDNA to infectious virus particles in cell culture. *Current Opinion in Microbiology* 9: 416–422.

Bartenschlager R, Frese M, and Pietschmann T (2004) Novel insights into hepatitis C virus replication and persistence. *Advances in Virus Research* 63: 71–180.

Bartosch B and Cosset FL (2006) Cell entry of hepatitis C virus. *Virology* 348: 1–12.

Blight KJ, Kolykhalov AA, and Rice CM (2000) Efficient initiation of HCV RNA replication in cell culture. *Science* 290: 1972–1974.

Bowen DG and Walker CM (2005) Adaptive immune responses in acute and chronic hepatitis C virus infection. *Nature* 436: 946–952.

Choo QL, Kuo G, Weiner AJ, et al. (1989) Isolation of a cDNA clone derived from a blood-borne non-A, non-B viral hepatitis genome. *Science* 244: 359–362.

Foy E, Li C, Sumpter R, et al. (2003) Regulation of interferon regulatory factor-3 by the hepatitis C virus serine protease. *Science* 300: 1145–1148.

Gale M Jr. and Foy M (2005) Evasion of intracellular host defence by hepatitis C virus. *Nature* 436: 939–945.

Lindenbach BD and Rice CM (2005) Unravelling hepatitis C virus replication from genome to function. *Nature* 436: 933–938.

Lindenbach BD, Evans MJ, Syder AJ, et al. (2005) Complete replication of hepatitis C virus in cell culture. *Science* 309: 623–626.

Lohmann V, Körner F, Koch J, et al. (1999) Replication of subgenomic hepatitis C virus RNAs in a hepatoma cell line. *Science* 285: 110–113.

Manns MP, Wedemeyer M, and Cornberg M (2006) Treating viral hepatitis C: Efficacy, side effects, and complications. *Gut* 55: 1350–1359.

Wakita T, Pietschmann T, Kato T, et al. (2005) Production of infectious hepatitis C virus in tissue culture from a cloned viral genome. *Nature Medicine* 11: 791–796.

Zhong J, Gastaminza P, Cheng G, et al. (2005) Robust hepatitis C virus infection *in vitro*. *Proceedings of the National Academy of Sciences, USA* 102: 9294–9299.

Hepatitis Delta Virus

J M Taylor, Fox Chase Cancer Center, Philadelphia, PA, USA

Glossary

Antigenome For hepatitis delta virus (HDV), the antigenome refers to an exact complement of the genome. It also is a single-stranded circular RNA.

Editing In recent years it has become clear that many RNAs undergo nucleotide sequence changes relative to the nucleic acid templates from which they are derived. There are many different forms of this process, collectively known as editing. It can occur during or after the process of RNA transcription. HDV RNA undergoes a specific form of post-transcriptional editing in which certain adenosines are deaminated to inosine.

Genome For a virus the genome is that nucleic acid species present within virus particles. For HDV, the genome is a single-stranded circular RNA.

Ribozyme When it was realized that certain RNA molecules could have enzymatic activities similar to certain proteins, such RNAs were defined as ribozymes. Both the genomic and antigenomic RNAs of HDV contain regions that undergo specific self-cleavage, and are thus defined as ribozymes.

Rolling-circle replication For agents that have a circular genome, whether it be of DNA or RNA, there is the possibility that replication can initiate at one or more locations, leading to the synthesis of species longer than the original circle. Such multimers may then undergo processing (e.g., by cleavage and ligation) to form new unit-length products. Such a mechanism, which is referred to as rolling-circle replication, applies to certain agents and has been implicated for the replication of HDV.

Viroid Among the infectious agents of plants there are small circular single-stranded RNAs that seem to replicate without the aid of a helper virus or the synthesis of any encoded protein. These agents do not fulfill the definition of a virus and so have been named viroids.

Classification

Hepatitis delta virus or hepatitis D virus (HDV) was discovered in patients with a more severe form of human hepatitis B virus (HBV) infection. HDV is a subviral satellite of HBV. HDV is often called a virus but strictly speaking it does not satisfy the definition of a virus and should be called subviral; HDV infection and assembly of new virus particles depends upon the envelope protein provided by the natural helper virus, HBV. HDV is also called a satellite of HBV because there is no nucleotide homology between the genomes of HBV and HDV.

No other infectious agents of animals resemble HDV. There are agents in plants that share several important characteristics of RNA genome structure and replication. These plant agents include the viroids and certain satellite RNAs and satellite viruses. Nevertheless, there are also enough major differences between HDV and these plant agents that the International Committee on Taxonomy of Viruses has agreed to assign HDV as a separate genus, *Deltavirus*, with only itself as a member.

Structure

HBV, the natural helper virus of HDV, encodes three envelope proteins. These are also used for the assembly of HDV, but in a different way.

Infectious HBV particles are roughly spherical with a diameter of about 42 nm. Inside these is an icosahedral nucleocapsid of about 27 nm diameter. HBV assembly is inefficient in that infectious particles are found in serum in the presence of a 1000–1 000 000-fold excess of empty particles. These empty particles consist of 25 nm spheres and filaments with a 22 nm diameter and a heterogenous length.

Infectious HDV particles contain a ribonucleoprotein composed of the HDV RNA genome in a complex with more than 70 copies of the delta antigen, the only protein encoded by HDV. It is considered from electron microscopy and filtration studies that infectious HDV particles are spherical and at least 38 nm in diameter. However, such studies are not as clear-cut as for HBV. First, they do not show which particles actually contain RNA. Second, they do distinguish which of the RNA-containing particles are infectious. What seems clear is that the same HBV envelope protein domains are needed for HDV and HBV infectivity. That is, it is likely that for infection HDV uses the same as yet unidentified receptor as HBV.

The internal ribonucleoprotein complex of the HDV RNA genome and delta proteins has been demonstrated but the actual structure has not been clarified yet.

Replication

The RNA genome (**Figure 1**) is a single-stranded RNA of about 1700 nt in length. It is unique for many reasons

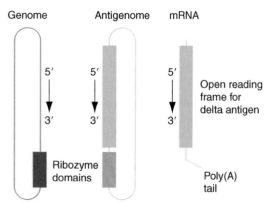

Figure 1 A representation of the three RNAs detected during the replication of HDV. The first is the 1679 nt single-stranded circular RNA found within virions, and thus defined as the genome. The second is an exact complement of the genome, defined as the antigenome, and it along with the genome is found in infected cells. A third RNA, the least abundant, is cytoplasmic, 5'-capped and 3'-polyadenylated, and is the mRNA for the translation of the delta protein. The genome and antigenomic circles are drawn as elongated in order to represent their ability to form extensive intramolecular base pairing and fold into an unbranched rod-like structure. Note that both the genome and the antigenome each contain a domain that will act as a self-cleaving ribozyme.

including its very small size and its circular conformation. The replication takes place by a mechanism that is fundamentally different from the reverse transcription pathway used by the helper virus HBV. HDV replicates with RNA rather than DNA intermediates. Inside infected cells we find not only the circular RNA genome but also an exact complement, the antigenome, which is also circular (**Figure 1**). A third RNA is also complementary to the genome. It is about 800 nt in length, 5'-capped and 3'-polyadenylated, and acts as the mRNA for the translation of the delta protein (**Figure 1**).

HDV genome replication seems to take place in the nucleus and involves redirection of the host RNA polymerase II. Because the genomic RNA is circular, it is possible for transcription to make multimeric RNAs from this template, in what is called a rolling-circle mechanism. Both the genomic and antigenomic RNAs contain a ribozyme that cleaves the RNA at a unique location. A detailed structure for one of these ribozymes has been reported. Ribozyme cleavage allows the processing of the multimeric RNAs into unit-length species, that are then somehow ligated to makes circles. The RNases of animal cells are mainly exonucleases and so circular RNAs are much more stable than the corresponding linear species. In infected liver tissue, the circular genomic RNAs accumulate to around 300 000 copies per average cell.

The mRNA of an infectious HDV needs to be translated into what is known as the small delta protein. This 195 amino acid protein is highly basic. It can dimerize using a region near the N-terminus, through what is

known as an antiparallel coiled-coil domain. It can also bind with specificity to HDV RNAs, and localize to the nucleus. For a combination of these and maybe additional reasons, the small delta protein is essential for genome replication. However, during this replication, some of the antigenomic RNAs are post-transcriptionally modified at a specific location, by a form of RNA-editing. The editing involves a double-stranded RNA-specific adenosine deaminase, now known as ADAR. The editing occurs in the middle of the amber termination codon for the open reading frame of the small delta protein. This leads to the translation of a protein that is 19 amino acids longer. This 214-amino-acid long delta protein is a dominant negative inhibitor of genome replication. However, it also has a positive role. Most of it becomes farnesylated at a cysteine located four amino acids from the new C-terminus. This modified protein is essential for the late phase of HDV replication, the assembly of new virus particles, using the envelope proteins of the helper virus, HBV.

Epidemiology

HDV infections are transmitted via infected blood or blood products. There are two main classifications of HDV infection. A co-infection is one in which the individual receives both HBV and HDV at the same time. A superinfection is one in which the individual has a prior infection with HBV, usually a chronic infection, and is then infected with HDV. Such superinfections have a much greater chance of being more extensive and also a greater chance of going on to chronicity.

It was not realized until 1980 that HDV was an infectious agent. Convenient tests for HDV were soon developed and epidemiological information gathered. The initial test was for antibody directed against the delta antigen and then tests were developed for the antigen itself. Now we have much more sensitive tests for the RNA, but such tests are not routinely used.

HDV was first studied among populations in southern Italy. Of course it is only found in situations where HBV is also present, but the converse is not always true. There are geographic populations in which HBV infections are more likely to be associated with HDV. Data indicate that the fraction of HBV infections that are also HDV-associated can range from <1% to >10%. The high levels have been reported for areas such as the Amazon basin in South America and southern regions of the former Soviet Union. Also, within a geographic population there may be individuals, such as intravenous drug users who share needles, where the fraction is very high, >70%.

Levels of HDV infection have been greatly reduced in recent years. This is in part due to changes in the behavior of susceptible individuals, especially the intravenous drug users, and also due to screening of blood supplies.

In addition, the introduction of widespread immunization against HBV, which simultaneously protects against HDV, will ultimately reduce both the number of chronic HBV carriers and HDV infections.

Clinical Features

The replication of HBV is not directly cytopathic. The liver damage arises because of the involvement of the host immune response to these infections. The same is probably also true for HDV. In addition, there are experimental situations where HDV infections can be directly cytopathic.

In certain geographic areas, such as the Amazon basin, HDV infections can have a very high risk of producing a fulminant hepatitis, sometimes with death in less than 1 week.

Control

Immunization against the natural helper virus, HBV, confers protection against HDV. However, for nonimmunized individuals and especially for those already chronically infected with HBV, the risks remain high.

For an individual infected with HDV, there is no good therapy that directly targets the HDV infection. In one study, treatment with high doses of interferon was associated with some cures. Of course the interferon therapy also attacks the HBV infection.

Recently, antiviral therapies based upon inhibitors of the HBV reverse transcriptase are being directed against HBV infections. One might expect that these therapies would indirectly inhibit cycles of HDV replication, but such has not been the case.

See also: Hepatitis B Virus: General Features.

Further Reading

Casey JL (ed.) (2006) *Current Topics in Microbiology and Immunology, Vol. 307: Hepatitis Delta Virus.* Berlin: Springer.
Farci P, Roskams T, Chessa L, *et al.* (2004) Long-term benefit of interferon alpha therapy on chronic hepatitis D: Regression of advanced hepatic fibrosis. *Gastroenterology* 126: 1740–1749.
Handa H and Yamaguchi Y (eds.) (2006) *Hepatitis Delta Virus.* Georgetown, TX: Landes Bioscience.
Taylor JM (2006) Hepatitis delta virus. *Virology* 344: 71–76.

Hepatitis E Virus

X J Meng, Virginia Polytechnic Institute and State University, Blacksburg, VA, USA

Glossary

Animal reservoir A large animal population serving as a source of virus supply for the transmission of virus(es) to other animals including humans.
Enzootic An epidemiology term describing multiple continuous disease presence in an animal population in a defined geographic region and time period.
Zoonosis Infectious diseases transmissible under natural conditions from vertebrate animals to humans.

Introduction

The initial evidence for the existence of a new form of enterically transmitted viral hepatitis came from serological studies of waterborne epidemics of hepatitis in India in 1980, as cases thought to be hepatitis A were tested negative for antibodies to the hepatitis A virus (HAV). To conform to the standard nomenclature of viral hepatitis, this new form of viral hepatitis was named hepatitis E. In 1983, viral hepatitis E was successfully transmitted to a human volunteer via fecal–oral route with a stool sample collected from a non-A, non-B hepatitis patient, and virus-like particles were visualized by electron microscope in the stool of the infected volunteer. Subsequently, the agent was also successfully transmitted to nonhuman primates. However, the identity of the virus was not known until 1990 when the genomic sequence of the new virus, named hepatitis E virus (HEV), was determined. The recent identification and characterization of animal strains of HEV, swine hepatitis E virus (swine HEV) from pigs in 1997 and avian hepatitis E virus (avian HEV) from chickens in 2001, have broadened the host ranges and diversity of the virus, and also provided two unique homologous animal model systems to study HEV replication and pathogenesis.

Convincing evidence indicates that hepatitis E is a zoonotic disease, and pigs and perhaps other animal species are reservoirs for HEV.

Properties and Structure of Virions

HEV is a symmetrical, icosahedral, spherical virus particle of approximately 32–34 nm in diameter without an envelope (**Figure 1**). The capsid protein encoded by the open reading frame (ORF) 2 gene of HEV is the only known structural protein on the virion. The N-terminal truncated capsid protein, which contains amino acid residues 112–660, can self-assemble into empty virus-like particles when expressed in baculovirus. The buoyant density of HEV virions is reportedly 1.35–1.40 g cm^{-3} in CsCl, and 1.29 g cm^{-3} in potassium tartrate and glycerol. The virion sedimentation coefficient is 183 S. HEV virion is sensitive to low-temperature storage and iodinated disinfectants but is reportedly stable when exposed to trifluorotrichloroethane. HEV virion is more heat labile than is HAV, another enterically transmitted hepatitis virus. HAV was only 50% inactivated at 60 °C for 1 h but was almost totally inactivated at 66 °C. In contrast, HEV was about 50% inactivated at 56 °C and almost totally inactivated (96%) at 60 °C. The fecal–oral route of transmission indicates that HEV is resistant to inactivation by acidic and mild alkaline conditions in the intestinal tract.

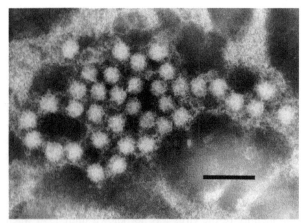

Figure 1 Electron micrograph of 30–35 nm diameter particles of an avian strain of the HEV. The virus particles were detected from a bile sample of a chicken with hepatitis–splenomegaly syndrome. Scale = 100 nm. Reproduced from Haqshenas G, Shivaprasad HL, Woolcock PR, Read DH, and Meng XJ (2001) Genetic identification and characterization of a novel virus related to human hepatitis E virus from chickens with hepatitis–splenomegaly syndrome in the United States. *Journal of General Virology* 82: 2449–2462, with permission from Society for General Microbiology.

Taxonomy and Classification

HEV was initially classified in the family *Caliciviridae* on the basis of its superficial similarity in morphology and genomic organization to caliciviruses. However, subsequent studies revealed that the HEV genome does not share significant sequence homology with caliciviruses, and that the codon usage and genomic organization of HEV are also different from that of caliciviruses. Therefore, in the *Eighth Report of the International Committee on Taxonomy of Viruses* (ICTV), HEV was declassified from the family *Caliciviridae*, and was placed in the sole genus *Hepevirus*. The proposed family name *Hepeviridae* has yet to be officially approved by ICTV.

The species in the genus *Hepevirus* includes the four recognized major genotypes of HEV (**Figure 2**): genotype 1 (primarily Burmese-like Asian strains), genotype 2 (a single Mexican strain), genotype 3 (strains from rare endemic cases in the United States, Japan, and Europe, and swine strains from pigs in industrialized countries), and genotype 4 (variant strains from sporadic cases in Asia, and swine strains from pigs in both developing and industrialized countries). A tentative new species in the genus *Hepevirus* is the recently discovered avian HEV from chickens (**Figure 1**). The nucleotide sequence identity differs by 20–30% between genotypes, and by *c*. 40–50% between avian HEV and mammalian HEVs. Despite the extensive nucleotide sequence variations, however, it appears that there exists a single serotype of HEV.

Genome Organization and Gene Expression

The genome of HEV, which possesses a cap structure at its 5′ end, is a single-stranded, positive-sense RNA molecule of approximately 7.2 kb in length. The viral genome consists of a short 5′ noncoding region (NCR) of approximately 26 bp, three open reading frames (ORFs 1–3), and a 3′ NCR. ORF3 overlaps ORF2, but neither ORF2 nor ORF3 overlaps with ORF1 (**Figure 3**). The ORF1 at the 5′ end encodes viral nonstructural proteins that are involved in viral replication and protein processing.

Functional motifs, characteristic of methyltransferases, papain-like cystein proteases, helicases, and RNA-dependent RNA polymerases (**Figure 3**), were identified in ORF1 based upon sequence analyses and analogy with other single-strand positive-sense RNA viruses. ORF2, located at the 3′ end, encodes the major capsid protein that contains a typical signal peptide sequence, and three potential glycosylation sites. The capsid protein contains the most immunogenic epitope, induces neutralizing antibodies against HEV, and is the target for HEV vaccine development. ORF3 encodes a small

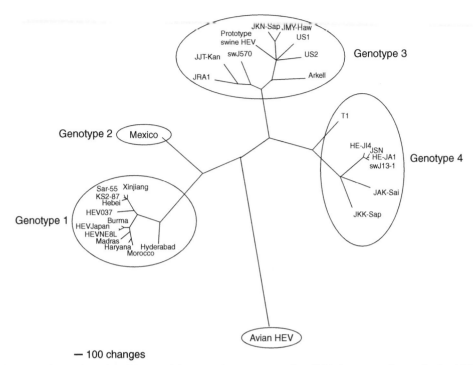

— 100 changes

Figure 2   A phylogenetic tree based on the complete genomic sequences of available human, swine, and avian HEV strains. The tree was constructed with the aid of the PAUP program by using heuristic search with 1000 replicates. A scale bar, indicating the number of character state changes, is proportional to the genetic distance. The four recognized major genotypes of HEV are indicated. The avian HEV in a branch distinct from mammalian HEV is tentatively classified as a separate species. Reproduced from Huang FF, Sun ZF, Emerson SU, et al. (2004) Determination and analysis of the complete genomic sequence of avian hepatitis E virus (avian HEV) and attempts to infect rhesus monkeys with avian HEV. *Journal of General Virology* 85: 1609–1618, with permission from Society for General Microbiology.

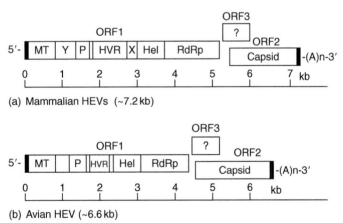

Figure 3   Schematic diagram of the genomic organization of HEV: a short 5′ (solid box at the 5′ end), a 3′ NCR (solid box at the 3′ end), and three ORFs. ORF2 and ORF3 overlap each other but neither overlaps ORF1. ORF1 encodes nonstructural proteins including putative functional domains, ORF2 encodes putative capsid protein, and ORF3 encodes a small protein with unknown function. MT, methytransferase; X, 'X' domain; Y, 'Y' domain; P, a proline-rich domain that may provide flexibility; HVR, a hypervariable region; Hel, helicase; RdRp, RNA-dependent RNA polymerase.

cytoskeleton-associated phosphoprotein. The N-terminus of ORF3 has a cysteine-rich region, binds to HEV RNA, and enters into a complex with the capsid protein. The C-terminal region of the ORF3 protein is a multifunctional domain, and may be involved in HEV virion morphogenesis and viral pathogenesis. Antibodies to ORF3 protein have been detected in some animals (rhesus monkeys and chickens) experimentally infected with HEV; however, it remains unknown if ORF3 is a structural protein in the virion.

The transcription and translation mechanisms of HEV genes are still poorly understood, largely due to the lack of an efficient cell culture system for the propagation of HEV. By using an *in vitro* HEV replicon system, a bicistronic subgenomic mRNA was identified and found to encode both ORF2 and ORF3 proteins. Subgenomic mRNAs were also detected in infected liver tissues. The ORF3 gene contains a *cis*-reactive element and encodes a protein that is essential for virus infectivity *in vivo*. However, recent studies showed that the expression of ORF3 protein is not required for virus replication, virion assembly, or infection of hepatoma cells *in vitro*. The translation and post-translational processes of the ORF1 polyprotein remain largely unknown. When expressed in baculovirus, the nonstructural ORF1 polyprotein was found to process into smaller proteins that correlate with predicted functional domains in ORF1. However, no processing of the ORF1 polyprotein was detected when it was expressed in bacterial or mammalian expression systems.

Epidemiology

HEV is transmitted primarily through the fecal–oral route, and contaminated water or water supplies are the main sources of infection. Hepatitis E, generally affecting young adults, is an important public health disease in many developing countries of the world where sanitation conditions are poor. Rare epidemics are associated with fecal contamination of water, and are generally restricted in developing countries of Asia and Africa, and in Mexico. Most cases of acute hepatitis E occurred as endemic or sporadic forms worldwide in both industrialized and developing countries. The genotypes 1 and 2 HEV strains are associated with epidemics, whereas genotypes 3 and 4 strains cause sporadic cases of hepatitis E. A unique feature of HEV infections is the high mortality rate, up to 25%, in infected pregnant women, although the mechanism of fulminant hepatitis during pregnancy is still not known.

Seroprevalence of HEV antibodies is age dependent, with the highest rate occurring in young adults of 15–40 years of age. In endemic countries, the seroprevalence rate, generally ranging from 3% to 27%, is much lower than expected, although higher seroprevalence rates have been reported in some endemic countries such as Egypt. Surprisingly, a significant proportion of normal blood donors in the United States (4–36%) and other industrialized countries were tested seropositive for immunoglobulin G (IgG) anti-HEV antibodies, suggesting prior infections with HEV (or an antigenically related agent). The source of seropositivity in individuals from industrialized countries is not clear but a zoonotic origin via direct contact with infected animals or consumption of raw or undercooked animal meats has been suggested.

Swine HEV

The identification and characterization of swine HEV from pigs in the United States lend credence to the zoonosis concept for HEV. Since the initial report in 1997, swine HEV has now been identified from pigs in more than a dozen countries. Thus far, the viruses identified from pigs worldwide belong to either genotype 3 or 4, which both cause sporadic cases of acute hepatitis E. Recently, a genotype-1-like swine HEV was reportedly identified from a pig in Cambodia but independent confirmation of this finding is still lacking. Genetic and phylogenetic analyses of the complete genomic sequences of swine HEV revealed that swine HEV is very closely related, or identical in some cases, to the genotype 3 and 4 strains of human HEV (**Figure 2**). Seroepidemiological studies demonstrated that swine HEV is ubiquitous in pigs in the Midwestern United States, and that about 80–100% of the pigs in commercial farms in the United States were infected. Similar findings were also reported in more than a dozen other developing and industrialized countries, indicating that swine HEV infection in pigs is common worldwide. The ubiquitous nature of swine HEV infection in pigs provides a source of virus supply for zoonotic infection. Swine HEV infection generally occurs in pigs of 2–4 months of age. The infected pigs remain clinically normal, although microscopic evidence of hepatitis has been observed.

Avian HEV

Avian HEV was first isolated and characterized in 2001 from bile samples of chickens with hepatitis–splenomegaly (HS) syndrome in the United States, although a big liver and spleen disease virus (BLSV) with 62% nucleotide sequence identity to HEV (based on a 523 bp genomic region) was reported in 1999 from chickens in Australia. HS syndrome is an emerging disease of layer and broiler breeder chickens in North America characterized by increased mortality and decreased egg production. Dead birds have red fluid or clotted blood in their abdomens, and enlarged livers and spleens. Avian HEV shared *c.* 80% nucleotide sequence identity with the Australian BLSV, suggesting that big liver and spleen disease (BLS) in Australia and HS syndrome in North America are caused by variant strains of the same virus.

Avian HEV is morphologically, genetically, and antigenically related to human HEV. The complete genomic sequence of avian HEV is about 6.6 kb in length (**Figure 3**), which is about 600 bp shorter than that of human and swine HEVs. Although avian HEV shares only *c.* 50–60% nucleotide sequence identity to mammalian HEVs, the genomic organization, functional motifs, and common antigenic epitopes are conserved between avian and mammalian HEVs (**Figure 3**). Phylogenetic analyses indicated that avian HEV is distinct from mammalian HEV (**Figure 2**) and may represent either a fifth genotype of HEV or a separate species within the genus *Hepevirus*. Like swine HEV, avian HEV infection in chickens is widespread in the United States: *c.* 71% of chicken flocks and 30% of chickens are positive for IgG antibodies to avian HEV. Like human and swine HEVs, avian HEV antibody prevalence is also age dependent: *c.* 17% of chickens younger than 18 weeks are seropositive, as compared to *c.* 36% of adult chickens. Avian HEV isolates recovered from chickens with HS syndrome in the United States displayed 78–100% nucleotide sequence identities to each other, and 56–61% identities to known strains of human and swine HEVs.

Host Range and Cross-Species Infection

Swine HEV has been shown to cross species barriers and infect both rhesus monkey and chimpanzee. Infection of nonhuman primates, the surrogates of man, with swine HEV demonstrated the possibility of human infection with swine HEV. Conversely, genotype 3 human HEV has been shown to infect pigs under experimental conditions. However, attempts to experimentally infect pigs with genotypes 1 and 2 strains of human HEV were unsuccessful. Cross-species infection of HEV has also been reported in other animal species. Lambs were reportedly infected with human HEV isolates. Similarly, Wistar rats were reportedly infected with a human stool suspension containing infectious HEV, although others failed to confirm the rat transmission results. Cross-species infection by avian HEV has also been demonstrated, as avian HEV recovered from a chicken with HS syndrome was able to successfully infect turkeys. However, an attempt to experimentally infect two rhesus monkeys with avian HEV was unsuccessful. Thus, it appears that, unlike swine HEV, avian HEV may not readily infect humans.

There is potentially a wide host range of HEV infection. In addition to swine and chickens, antibodies to HEV have been reportedly detected in several other animal species including rodents, dogs, cats, sheep, goats, cattle, and nonhuman primates, suggesting that these animals have been exposed to HEV (or a related agent) and thus might serve as reservoirs. However, the source of seropositivity in these animal species, with the exception of pigs and chickens, could not be definitively identified since virus was either not recovered from these species or the recovered virus could not be sequenced to confirm its identity. A significant proportion of wild rats caught in different geographic regions of the United States (ranging from 44% to 90%) and other countries tested positive for IgG anti-HEV antibodies. Rodents are frequently found in both urban and rural environments and, thus, could potentially play an important role in HEV transmission. The existence of a wide host range of animal species positive for HEV antibodies further supports the zoonosis concept for HEV.

Pathogenesis and Tissue Tropism

The pathogenesis of HEV is largely unknown. It is believed that HEV enters the host through the fecal–oral route. However, the primary site of HEV replication is not known. In primates and pigs experimentally infected with human and swine HEVs, virus replication in the liver has been demonstrated. It is believed that, after replication in liver, HEV is released to the gallbladder from hepatocytes and then is excreted in feces. In pigs experimentally infected with human and swine HEVs, in addition to the liver, HEV replication was also identified in extrahepatic tissues including small intestine, colon, hepatic, and mesenteric lymph nodes. Although the clinical and pathological significance of these extrahepatic sites of virus replication is not known, it is believed that HEV may first replicate in the gastrointestinal tract after oral ingestion of the virus, and subsequently spreads to the target organ liver via viremia. It has been well documented that pregnancy increases the severity and mortality of the disease. The overall mortality rate caused by HEV in infected pregnant women can reach up to 25%, although, under experimental conditions, fulminant hepatitis E could not be reproduced in infected pregnant rhesus monkeys or infected pregnant sows. Therefore, the mechanism of fulminant hepatitis E in infected pregnant women remains unknown.

Zoonotic Risk

Hepatitis E is now considered a zoonotic disease, and pigs (and possibly other animal species) act as reservoirs. It has been demonstrated that pig handlers such as pig farmers and swine veterinarians in both developing and industrialized countries are at increased risk of HEV infection. For example, swine veterinarians in the United States are 1.51 times (swine HEV antigen, $p = 0.03$) more likely to be positive for HEV antibodies than age- and geography-matched normal blood donors. Also, it has been reported that HEV antibody prevalence in field workers from the Iowa Department of Natural Resources is significantly higher than that in blood donors, suggesting that human populations with occupational exposure to wild animals also have a higher risk of HEV infection. Transmissions of hepatitis E from a pet cat and a pet pig to human owners were also reported.

As a fecal–orally transmitted disease, waterborne epidemics are the characteristic of hepatitis E outbreaks in humans. Large amounts of viruses are excreted in feces of infected pigs and other animals. Therefore, swine and other animal manure and feces could be a source of contamination of irrigation water or coastal waters with concomitant contamination of produce or shellfish. Strains of HEV of both human and swine origin have been detected in sewage water. Consumption of contaminated shellfish has been implicated in sporadic cases of acute hepatitis E. Sporadic and cluster cases of acute hepatitis E have also been epidemiologically and genetically linked to the consumption of raw or undercooked pig livers. Approximately 2% of the pig livers sold in local grocery stores in Japan and 11% in the United States were tested positive for swine HEV RNA. The contaminating virus in commercial pig livers sold in the grocery stores of the United States remains fully infectious. Most importantly, the virus sequences recovered from pig livers in grocery stores are closely related, or identical in a few cases, to the viruses recovered from human hepatitis E patients in Japan. Recently, a cluster of four cases of acute hepatitis E were definitively linked to the consumption of raw deer meat in two families in Japan. The viral sequence recovered from the leftover frozen deer meat was 99.7–100% identical to the nucleotide sequence of viruses recovered from the four human patients. Family members who ate none or little deer meats were not infected. Taken together, these data provide convincing evidence of zoonotic HEV transmission either via direct contact with animals or animal wastes or via consumption of infected animal meats. Recently, numerous novel strains of HEV genetically closely related to swine HEV have been identified from patients with acute hepatitis E in many countries, suggesting that these novel strains of human HEV may be of swine origin.

Transmission and Natural History

The primary transmission route for HEV is fecal–oral. Feces from infected humans and other animals contain large amounts of viruses and are likely the main source of virus for transmission. However, under experimental conditions, reproduction of HEV infection in nonhuman primates and pigs via the oral route of inoculation has proven to be difficult, even though the animals can be readily infected by HEV via the intravenous route of inoculation. Chickens were successfully infected via the oral route of inoculation with avian HEV. Other route(s) of transmission cannot be ruled out.

The natural history of HEV is not known. The identification of HEV strains from swine and chickens and their demonstrated ability of cross-species infection and the existence of a wide host range of seropositive animals has

further complicated the understanding of HEV natural history. Since human-to-human transmission is uncommon for HEV, therefore a speculative scenario is that HEV is constantly circulating among different animal species, and that each species is infected by a unique strain that is enzootic in respective animal species. Some species, but not all, carry HEV strains that are genetically very similar to human HEV and are transmissible to humans. Therefore, HEV can infect humans through direct contact with infected domestic or farm animals or with feces-contaminated water or via consumption of infected raw or undercooked animal meats. If this happens in a developing country, it may result in an endemic or epidemic due to the poor sanitation conditions. However, if this happens in an industrialized country with good sanitation measures, it will occur only as a sporadic case. It will now be important to determine whether there are basic differences in host range or pathogenicity between epidemic or endemic strains in humans and enzootic strains that are mainly circulating in animal species.

Immunity

The immune response to HEV infection, characterized by a transient appearance of immunoglobulin M (IgM) HEV antibodies followed by long-lasting IgG antibodies, appears late during the period of viremia and virus shedding in stool. The HEV capsid protein is immunogenic and induces protective immunity. The capsid proteins between mammalian and avian HEV strains share common antigenic epitopes, and all HEV strains identified thus far appear to belong to a single serotype. Cross-challenge experiments in primates have demonstrated cross-protection following infection with different genotypes of human HEV strains. The cell-mediated immune response against HEV infection is largely unknown.

Prevention and Control

A vaccine against HEV is not yet available. The experimental recombinant HEV vaccines appear to be very promising; however, their efficacies against the emerging strains of HEV including animal strains with zoonotic potential need to be thoroughly evaluated. In the absence of a vaccine, important preventive measures include the practice of good hygiene, and avoiding drinking water of unknown purity or consuming raw or undercooked pig livers. The demonstrated ability of cross-species infection by swine HEV raises a public health concern, especially for high-risk groups such as pig handlers. An effective measure to prevent potential zoonotic transmission for pig and other animal handlers is to wash hands thoroughly after handling infected animals.

See also: Hepatitis A Virus.

Further Reading

Emerson SU, Anderson D, Arankalle A, *et al.* (2004) Hepevirus. In: Fauquet CM, Mayo MA, Maniloff J, Desselberger U,, and Ball LA (eds.) *Virus Taxonomy, Eighth Report of the International Committee on Taxonomy of Viruses*, pp. 851–855. San Diego, CA: Elsevier Academic Press.

Emerson SU and Purcell RH (2003) Hepatitis E virus. *Reviews in Medical Virology* 13: 145–154.

Haqshenas G, Shivaprasad HL, Woolcock PR, Read DH, and Meng XJ (2001) Genetic identification and characterization of a novel virus related to human hepatitis E virus from chickens with hepatitis–splenomegaly syndrome in the United States. *Journal of General Virology* 82: 2449–2462.

Huang FF, Sun ZF, Emerson SU, *et al.* (2004) Determination and analysis of the complete genomic sequence of avian hepatitis E virus (avian HEV) and attempts to infect rhesus monkeys with avian HEV. *Journal of General Virology* 85: 1609–1618.

Meng XJ (2000) Novel strains of hepatitis E virus identified from humans and other animal species. Is hepatitis E a zoonosis? *Journal of Hepatology* 33: 842–845 (editorial).

Meng XJ (2003) Swine hepatitis E virus: Cross-species infection and risk in xenotransplantation. *Current Topics in Microbiology and Immunology* 278: 185–216.

Meng XJ (2005) Hepatitis E as a zoonosis. In: Thomas H, Zuckermann A,, and Lemon S (eds.) *Viral Hepatitis*, 3rd edn., pp. 611–623. Oxford: Blackwell.

Meng XJ and Halbur PG (2005) Swine hepatitis E virus. In: Straw BE, Zimmerman J, D' Allaire S,, and Taylor DJ (eds.) *Diseases of Swine*, 9th edn., pp. 537–545. Ames, IA: Blackwell/Iowa State University Press.

Meng XJ, Purcell RH, Halbur PG, *et al.* (1997) A novel virus in swine is closely related to the human hepatitis E virus. *Proceedings of the National Academy of Science, USA* 94: 9860–9865.

Meng XJ, Shivaprasad HL, and Payne C (in press) Hepatitis E virus infections. In: Saif M (ed.) *Diseases of Poultry*, 12th edn., ch. 14. Ames, IA: Blackwell/Iowa State University Press.

Purcell RH and Emerson SU (2001) Hepatitis E virus. In: Knipe D, Howley P, Griffin D, *et al.* (eds.) *Fields Virology*, 4th edn., pp. 3051–3061. Philadelphia: Lippincott Williams and Wilkins.

Herpesviruses: General Features

A J Davison, MRC Virology Unit, Glasgow, UK

Introduction

The family *Herpesviridae* consists of a substantial number of animal viruses that have large, double-stranded DNA genomes and share a defining virion structure. Herpesviruses have been discovered in vertebrates from fish to humans, and one has been found in invertebrates (bivalves). They exhibit a wide range of pathogenic properties, ranging from inapparent in many instances to life-threatening (including cancer) in some, and have the ability to establish lifelong latent infections that can reactivate periodically. This chapter introduces the fundamental molecular properties of the herpesviruses: structure, replication, classification, genome, genes, and evolution.

Virion Structure

Herpesvirus particles (virions) are spherical and have an approximate diameter of 200 nm. They have a unique morphology consisting of four basic components (**Figure 1**).

Core

The core is occupied by the virus genome, which is a large, linear, double-stranded DNA molecule packaged at high density.

Capsid

The capsid is an icosahedron of diameter 125–130 nm. It is fashioned from 161 protein capsomeres, which are contributed by 150 hexons and 11 pentons, plus the portal in the 12th pentonal position. The hexons and pentons contain six and five copies each, respectively, of the major capsid protein, each copy of which in the hexons is decorated by a small, external protein. The portal consists of 12 copies of the portal protein and forms the vertex through which DNA enters and leaves the capsid. The capsomeres in the capsid shell are joined together via complexes known

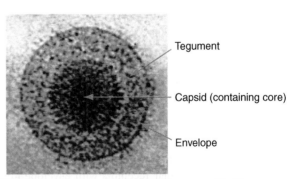

Figure 1 Structure of the herpesvirion exemplified by a cryoelectron microscope image of HSV-1. Adapted from Rixon FJ (1993) Structure and assembly of herpesviruses. *Seminars in Virology* 4: 135–144, with permission from Elsevier.

as triplexes, which contain two copies of one protein and one copy of another.

The immature capsid shell is constructed in the cell nucleus around a scaffold that consists of approximately 1200 copies of the scaffold protein plus approximately 150 copies of an N-terminally extended form of this protein that contains a protease domain in the additional region. The scaffold is replaced by the virus genome during DNA packaging in a process that involves proteolytic cleavage and loss of all the scaffold protein fragments except for the protease domain.

Tegument

The capsid is embedded in the tegument, and is often not located centrally therein. The tegument contains many virus protein species and is poorly defined structurally except for the region close to the capsid, where a degree of icosahedral symmetry exists.

Envelope

The tegument is wrapped in the lipid envelope, which contains several virus membrane glycoproteins as well as some cellular proteins.

Replication Cycle

The lytic replication cycle has been studied in detail for relatively few herpesviruses, most information having come from herpes simplex virus type 1 (HSV-1). As a consequence, there is a substantial degree of generalization – and even controversy – about applying conclusions from one virus across the whole family. This is especially pertinent to aspects of virus growth involving functions that are not genetically conserved. The mechanisms involved in establishment of, and reactivation from, latency are in this class, with different groups of herpesviruses having evolved different ways of ensuring that the virus stays with the host for life. Herpesviruses possess elaborate means of modulating the host responses to infection, and the genetic functions involved are largely not conserved across the family.

In broad outline, the phases of the lytic replication cycle are as follows. Details on the lytic and latent replication cycles (and pathogenic properties) of specific viruses are available in the relevant articles.

Entry

The virion envelope fuses to the cell membrane via the interactions of cellular receptors with envelope glycoproteins, and the capsid and tegument enter the cytoplasm. Some – perhaps many – of the incoming tegument proteins have specific roles in modulating the replication

cycle, for example, in inhibiting host macromolecular synthesis and initiating virus transcription. Some tegument proteins also reach the nucleus, perhaps independently of the capsid.

Expression

Capsids are transferred via microtubules to nuclear pores, through which the virus genome enters the nucleus. The genome is transcribed into mRNA by host RNA polymerase II in three major, regulated phases of transcription. Transcription of immediate early genes, unlike that of later phases, is not dependent on protein synthesis. Some of the immediate early proteins regulate the expression of early and late genes. Functions involved in DNA replication or nucleotide metabolism, and a subset of structural proteins, are in the former class, and many virion proteins are in the latter class.

Some polyadenylated RNAs, or introns derived therefrom, appear to function via pathways not requiring translation into proteins. In some herpesviruses, small, noncoding RNAs are transcribed by RNA polymerase III. The functions of these RNAs are largely unknown.

Replication

In the nucleus, DNA replication initiates at one or more specific sequences (origins of replication) to generate head-to-tail concatemeric genomes, probably by a rolling circle mechanism. Unit-length genomes are cleaved from the concatemers and packaged into preformed capsids.

Maturation

Capsids acquire some tegument proteins in the nucleus and gain a temporary envelope by budding through the inner nuclear membrane. This envelope is lost upon transit across the outer nuclear membrane into the cytoplasm. Further tegument proteins are added in the cytoplasm, and the tegumented capsids gain their final envelope by budding into a post-Golgi compartment.

Exit

Mature virions are released from the cell by reverse endocytosis.

Classification

The task of classifying viruses, including herpesviruses, commenced in 1966 and is undertaken by the International Committee on Taxonomy of Viruses (ICTV). Various criteria have been utilized, as enabled by developments in knowledge and technology. The current taxonomy of

Table 1 Present and proposed herpesvirus classification schemes. Species other than the type species of each genus are not included

Taxon level	Current taxon	Proposed taxon	Common name of virus
Order		Herpesvirales	
Family	Herpesviridae	Herpesviridae	
Subfamily	Alphaherpesvirinae	Alphaherpesvirinae	
Genus	Simplexvirus	Simplexvirus	
Type species	Human herpesvirus 1	Human herpesvirus 1	Herpes simplex virus type 1
Genus	Varicellovirus	Varicellovirus	
Type species	Human herpesvirus 3	Human herpesvirus 3	Varicella-zoster virus
Genus	Mardivirus	Mardivirus	
Type species	Gallid herpesvirus 2	Gallid herpesvirus 2	Marek's disease virus type 1
Genus	Iltovirus	Iltovirus	
Type species	Gallid herpesvirus 1	Gallid herpesvirus 1	Infectious laryngotracheitis virus
Subfamily	Betaherpesvirinae	Betaherpesvirinae	
Genus	Cytomegalovirus	Cytomegalovirus	
Type species	Human herpesvirus 5	Human herpesvirus 5	Human cytomegalovirus
Genus	Muromegalovirus	Muromegalovirus	
Type species	Murid herpesvirus 1	Murid herpesvirus 1	Murine cytomegalovirus
Genus	Roseolovirus	Roseolovirus	
Type species	Human herpesvirus 6	Human herpesvirus 6	Human herpesvirus 6
Genus		Proboscivirus	
Type species		Elephantid herpesvirus 1	Endotheliotropic elephant herpesvirus
Subfamily	Gammaherpesvirinae	Gammaherpesvirinae	
Genus	Lymphocryptovirus	Lymphocryptovirus	
Type species	Human herpesvirus 4	Human herpesvirus 4	Epstein–Barr virus
Genus	Rhadinovirus	Rhadinovirus	
Type species	Saimiriine herpesvirus 2	Saimiriine herpesvirus 2	Herpesvirus saimiri
Genus		Macavirus	
Type species		Alcelaphine herpesvirus 1	Wildebeest-associated malignant catarrhal fever virus
Genus		Percavirus	
Type species		Equid herpesvirus 2	Equine herpesvirus 2
Family		Alloherpesviridae	
Genus	Ictalurivirus	Ictalurivirus	
Type species	Ictalurid herpesvirus 1	Ictalurid herpesvirus 1	Channel catfish virus
Family		Malacoherpesviridae	
Genus		Ostreavirus	
Type species		Ostreid herpesvirus 1	Oyster herpesvirus

herpesviruses, as laid out in the *Eighth Report of the ICTV* (2005), is summarized in **Table 1**. The family *Herpesviridae* is divided into three subfamilies populated by herpesviruses of higher vertebrates (mammals and birds): *Alphaherpesvirinae* (containing four genera: *Simplexvirus, Varicellovirus, Mardivirus,* and *Iltovirus*), *Betaherpesvirinae* (containing three genera: *Cytomegalovirus, Muromegalovirus,* and *Roseolovirus*), and *Gammaherpesvirinae* (containing two genera: *Lymphocryptovirus* and *Rhadinovirus*). The family also contains a genus (*Ictalurivirus*) that is not linked to any subfamily and has a single fish herpesvirus as a member.

In proposals under consideration by the ICTV (**Table 1**), an order (*Herpesvirales*) is introduced as the highest taxon. The family *Herpesviridae* is redefined as restricted to viruses of higher vertebrates (which in this context will eventually include reptiles as well as mammals and birds). Within this redefined family, an additional genus (*Proboscivirus*) is added to the *Betaherpesvirinae*, and two new genera (*Macavirus* and *Percavirus*) are split from the

Rhadinovirus genus in the *Gammaherpesvirinae*. Two new families are also created: *Alloherpesviridae* to accommodate viruses of lower vertebrates (amphibians and fish), and *Malacoherpesviridae* for the single herpesvirus of invertebrates (bivalves).

The formal names of herpesvirus species follow a taxonomic designation derived from the natural host followed by the word 'herpesvirus' and a number (e.g., *Human herpesvirus 4* – the fourth of the eight species whose members infect humans). However, many herpesviruses are better known by common names (e.g., Epstein–Barr virus rather than human herpesvirus 4), and in this respect are characterized by a dual nomenclature. In addition, vernacular terms are often used to imply members of the family (e.g., herpesvirus), subfamily (e.g., gammaherpesvirus), or genus (e.g., rhadinovirus).

Herpesviruses are defined as separate species if their nucleotide sequences differ in a readily assayable and distinctive manner across the entire genome and if they occupy different ecological niches by virtue of their distinct epidemiology and pathogenesis or their distinct natural hosts. This definition implies that several criteria are employed in identifying a new species, and their application is to some extent arbitrary. The criteria are outlined below.

Morphological Criteria

Assignment of a virus to the family *Herpesviridae* depends primarily upon virion morphology, as described above.

Biological Criteria

The three subfamilies *Alphaherpesvirinae*, *Betaherpesvirinae*, and *Gammaherpesvirinae* were defined initially on the basis of biological criteria, in the application of which a degree of generality is implicit: host range in cell culture, length of replication cycle, cytopathology, and characteristics of latency. Alphaherpesviruses exhibit a variable host range, have a short replication cycle, spread quickly with efficient destruction of infected cells, and establish latent infections primarily in sensory ganglia. Betaherpesviruses have a narrow host range and a long replication cycle with slow spread and cell enlargement. Viruses may become latent in secretory glands and lymphoreticular cells. Gammaherpesviruses are associated with lymphoproliferative diseases, and latent virus is present in lymphoid tissue. They infect B- or T-lymphocyte cells *in vitro*, in which infection is frequently arrested so that infectious progeny are not produced. However, some gammaherpesviruses are able to cause lytic infections in fibroblastoid or epithelial cell lines.

Serological Criteria

Closely related viruses may be detected using antisera or specific antibodies.

Genomic Criteria

The general layout of a genome in terms of unique and repeat regions (see below) is limited as a criterion since, although particular structures are found more commonly in certain subfamilies or genera, similar structures have evidently evolved more than once. The DNA sequences of herpesviruses are sufficiently diverged to limit extensive nucleic acid similarity (detectable by hybridization) to closely related viruses.

Sequence Criteria

Phylogenetic analysis based on sequence comparisons between conserved genes has become the predominant criterion in classification of herpesviruses at all taxonomic levels. **Figure 2** shows one example of a phylogenetic tree supporting the current classification scheme. In recent

years, many herpesviruses have been detected in animal tissues solely by polymerase chain reaction (PCR) of short sequences. Given the multifactorial nature of the herpesvirus species definition (see above), the absence of other information renders formal classification problematic in these cases.

Genome Organization

The herpesvirus genomes studied to date range in size from approximately 124 kbp (simian varicella virus) to 295 kbp (koi herpesvirus) and in nucleotide composition from 32% to 74% G+C. Alphaherpesviruses are not deficient in the $5'$ CG dinucleotide, betaherpesviruses are deficient in very limited regions, and gammaherpesviruses are deficient throughout their genomes. $5'$ CG deficiency is thought to be a consequence of spontaneous deamination of methylated cytosine residues in DNA over evolutionary time to produce $5'$ TG. There is evidence that methylation of certain regions of the Epstein–Barr virus genome resident in peripheral blood lymphocyte cells may be involved in perpetuating infection. Extensive methylation of the $5'$ CG dinucleotide has been found in the virion DNA of two frog herpesviruses, both of which encode the enzyme DNA (cytosine-5-)-methyltransferase.

Herpesvirus genomes differ in the arrangements of direct and inverted repeat regions with respect to unique (nonrepetitive) regions. **Figure 3** illustrates the five types of structure that have been confirmed adequately. The type A structure (e.g., human herpesvirus 6) consists of a unique region (U) flanked by a direct terminal repeat (TR) at the genome ends. Type B genomes (e.g., human herpesvirus 8, also known as Kaposi's sarcoma-associated herpesvirus) contain variable numbers of a TR at each end of the genome. The type C structure (e.g., Epstein–Barr virus) has in addition a variable number of copies of an internal direct repeat (IR), which is unrelated to TR, and the presence of IR splits U into two unique regions (U_L and U_S). The type D structure (e.g., pseudorabies virus) also has two unique regions (U_L and U_S), with U_S flanked by an inverted repeat (TR_S/IR_S). In some type D genomes (e.g., varicella-zoster virus), U_L is flanked by a very small, unrelated inverted repeat (TR_L/IR_L). By virtue of recombination between inverted repeats, the two orientations of U_S are present in equimolar amounts in virion DNA populations, and U_L is present completely or predominantly in a single orientation. In the type E structure (e.g., HSV-1), TR_L/IR_L is larger and the two orientations of U_L and U_S are each present in equimolar amounts in virion DNA populations, giving rise to four genome isomers. A direct repeat (the *a* sequence) is also present at the termini, and an inverted copy (*d*) is present internally.

In addition to large-scale repeats, regions consisting of tandem repeats of short sequences are found at various

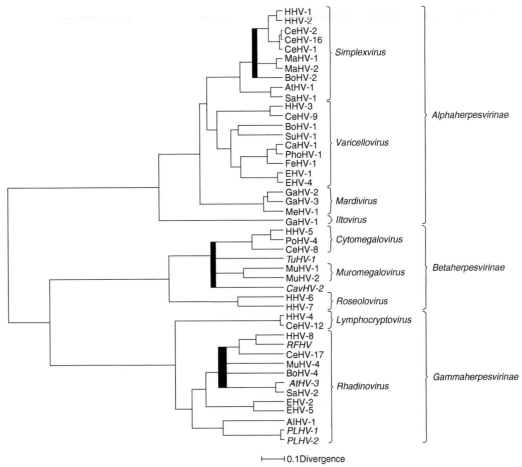

Figure 2 Phylogenetic tree for herpesviruses. The scope is limited to the three subfamilies that comprise the revised family *Herpesviridae*; see **Table 1**. The tree is a composite derived from sequence alignments of up to eight sets of core proteins, analyzed using the maximum-likelihood method with a molecular clock imposed. Thick lines denote regions of uncertain branching. Prefixes denote host species: H, human; Ce, cercopithecine; Ma, macropodid; Bo, bovine; At, ateline; Sa, saimiriine; Su, suid; Ca, canid; Pho, phocid; Fe, felid; E, equid; Ga, gallid; Me, meleagrid; Po, pongine; Tu, tupaiid; Mu, murid; Cav, caviid; and Al, alcelaphine. Other virus name abbreviations are: RFHV, retroperitoneal fibromatosis herpesvirus of macaques; and PLHV-1 and PLHV-2, porcine lymphotropic herpesviruses 1 and 2. Viruses that are not yet incorporated into genera are in italics. Genera and subfamilies are on the right. Adapted from McGeoch DJ, Dolan A, and Ralph AC (2000) Toward a comprehensive phylogeny for mammalian and avian herpesviruses. *Journal of Virology* 74: 10401–10406, with permission from American Society for Microbiology.

locations in many herpesvirus genomes. The elements that make these up may be identical to each other or merely similar, giving rise to simple or complex repeats, and their presence in variable numbers causes genome size heterogeneity.

Gene Content

To date, the genome sequences of herpesviruses belonging to 42 species have been published, with more than one strain determined for several of these species. Details are available via the genomic biology Web pages at the National Center for Biotechnology Information. In addition, a large amount of data is available for portions of other herpesvirus genomes. Analyses of these sequences provide detailed views of genetic content and phylogeny.

Herpesvirus genomes consist mostly of protein-coding sequences. Gene complements range from about 70 to 170 and are arranged about equally between the two DNA strands. They are not generally located in functionally related groups. Overlap between protein-coding regions in different reading frames on the same or opposing strands is infrequent and, where it does occur, is not extensive. In instances where extensive or complete overlap of two protein-coding regions has been mooted, evidence that both encode functional proteins is invariably unconvincing.

Most herpesvirus genes are transcribed from their own promoters and thus specify mRNAs with unique 5′ ends. Groups of genes are frequently arranged tandemly on the same DNA strand and share a common polyadenylation site, with mRNAs sharing the same 3′ end. Most genes are not spliced, particularly among the alphaherpesviruses.

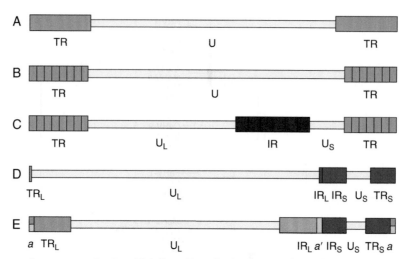

Figure 3   Types of herpesvirus genome structure. The disposition of unique regions (yellow), direct repeats (blue), and inverted repeats (red) are shown (not to scale). Within a structure, unique regions are unrelated to each other, and only the repeats depicted in the same color and shade are identical. Among the structures, repeats represented in the same color and shade are not necessarily related to each other. In the type E structure, an inverted copy of a direct repeat (*a*) at the genome termini is present internally (*a'*).

RNA polymerase II transcripts that do not encode proteins but may have other functions, and micro-RNAs, have been identified in representatives of all three subfamilies, and RNA polymerase III transcripts in certain gammaherpesviruses. The functions of such transcripts are largely unknown. Herpesvirus genomes also contain *cis*-acting signals in addition to those involved in transcriptional control, such as origins of DNA replication.

Sequence comparisons among members of the revised family *Herpesviridae* indicate that a set of 43 core genes has been inherited from the ancestor of the three subfamilies. This number of core genes is an approximation, since its derivation assumes that the *Alphaherpesvirinae* was the first subfamily to diverge (as indicated by molecular phylogeny; see **Figure 2**). Moreover, it is based not simply on primary sequence conservation but, in some cases, on positional and functional similarities. Three of the core genes derived from the ancestor have been lost subsequently from certain lineages. The core genes are generally arranged collinearly among members of the same subfamily, but in members of different subfamilies blocks of genes have been rearranged and sometimes inverted.

The most strongly represented functional categories among the core genes are involved in central aspects of lytic replication. Particularly prominent are genes encoding capsid proteins (six genes) or proteins involved in replication (seven genes) or processing and packaging of DNA (eight genes). Also featured are genes with roles in nucleotide metabolism or DNA repair (five genes), and, to a lesser extent, genes encoding tegument (seven genes) or envelope proteins (five genes). Genes with roles in niche-specific aspects of the life cycle, such as modulation of the host response and regulation of latency, do not generally belong to the core set. This feature illustrates the high degree of evolutionary flexibility that herpesviruses have

exhibited in colonizing particular ecological niches. The fact that over half (in some cases well over half) of the genes in a herpesvirus genome may be removed individually without eliminating viral growth in cell culture, when all presumably have a role *in vivo*, testifies to the extensive interactions that the virus has with its host during natural growth and transmission.

The comments above refer to the revised family *Herpesviridae*, where most information is available. Similar points may be made about the proposed family *Alloherpesviridae*, though the number of core genes is considerably fewer (probably not more than 20), presumably due to the greater antiquity of the common ancestor.

Herpesvirus Evolution

The processes that have occurred during evolution of the three subfamilies of the *Herpesviridae* from their common ancestor are the same as in other organisms, and include the gradual effects of nucleotide substitution, deletion, and insertion to modify existing genes or produce genes *de novo*, and the recombinational effects of gene capture, duplication, and rearrangement. These processes are also evident in the proposed family *Alloherpesviridae*.

Herpesviruses are usually restricted to a single species in the natural setting, and severe symptoms of infection are often limited in the natural host to young or immunosuppressed individuals. This indicates that a substantial degree of co-adaptation and co-evolution have taken place over the long term between herpesviruses and their hosts. Although some exceptions suggesting ancient interspecies transfer have been registered, phylogenetic studies provide strong support for co-evolution as a general historic characteristic, in some instances supporting the idea that the viruses have speciated along with their hosts. This correspondence has allowed a timescale for herpesvirus evolution to be proposed on the basis of accepted dates for host evolution. For example, the most recent analyses suggest divergence dates of 400 million years (before present) for the three subfamilies, 120 million years for the genera *Simplexvirus* and *Varicellovirus* of the *Alphaherpesvirinae*, and 8 million years for HSV-1 and HSV-2. These dates are approximate, especially the further back they go, and vulnerable to the vicissitudes of estimated host dates and developments in analytical approaches.

The three lineages populated by the revised family *Herpesviridae* and the two proposed families *Alloherpesviridae* and *Malacoherpesviridae* share similarities in capsid structure and replication that indicate evolution from a common ancestor, the forerunner of all herpesviruses. However, in comparison with the situation within the families, detectable amino acid sequence similarity among proposed families is very limited, with evidence for a common ancestor focused on a single gene (encoding a subunit of the terminase complex responsible for DNA packaging). These features imply that the divergence events that gave rise to the three lineages are very ancient. Moreover, structural considerations focused on the capsid continue to stimulate the notion that herpesviruses might share an even earlier ancestor with T4-like bacteriophages.

Note: The proposals for new taxa mentioned in this article have been accepted by the ICTV.

Further Reading

Davison AJ (2002) Evolution of the herpesviruses. *Veterinary Microbiology* 86: 69–88.

Davison AJ, Eberle R, Hayward GS, *et al.* (2005) Family *Herpesviridae*. In: Fauquet CM, Mayo MA, Maniloff J, Desselberger U,, and Ball LA (eds.) *Virus Taxonomy: Eighth Report of the International Committee on Taxonomy of Viruses*, pp. 193–212. San Diego, CA: Elsevier Academic Press.

Grunewald K, Desai P, Winkler DC, *et al.* (2003) Three-dimensional structure of herpes simplex virus from cryo-electron tomography. *Science* 302: 1396–1398.

Kieff E and Rickinson AB (2001) Epstein–Barr virus and its replication. In: Knipe DM and Howley PM (eds.) *Fields Virology*, 4th edn., pp. 2511–2573. Philadelphia, PA: Lippincott Williams and Wilkins.

McGeoch DJ, Dolan A, and Ralph AC (2000) Toward a comprehensive phylogeny for mammalian and avian herpesviruses. *Journal of Virology* 74: 10401–10406.

McGeoch DJ and Gatherer D (2005) Integrating reptilian herpesviruses into the family *Herpesviridae*. *Journal of Virology* 79: 725–731.

McGeoch DJ, Rixon FJ, and Davison AJ (2006) Topics in herpesvirus genomics and evolution. *Virus Research* 117: 90–104.

Mocarski ES and Tan Courcelle C (2001) Cytomegaloviruses and their replication. In: Knipe DM and Howley PM (eds.) *Fields Virology*, 4th edn., pp. 2629–2673. Philadelphia, PA: Lippincott Williams and Wilkins.

Moore PS and Chang Y (2001) Kaposi's sarcoma-associated herpesvirus. In: Knipe DM and Howley PM (eds.) *Fields Virology*, 4th edn., pp. 2803–2833. Philadelphia: Lippincott Williams and Wilkins.

Rixon FJ (1993) Structure and assembly of herpesviruses. *Seminars in Virology* 4: 135–144.

Roizman B and Pellett PE (2001) Herpes simplex viruses and their replication. In: Knipe DM and Howley PM (eds.) *Fields Virology*, 4th edn., pp. 2399–2459. Philadelphia, PA: Lippincott Williams and Wilkins.

Zhou ZH, Dougherty M, Jakana J, *et al.* (2000) Seeing the herpesvirus capsid at 8.5 Å. *Science* 288: 877–880.

Human Cytomegalovirus: General Features

E S Mocarski Jr., Emory University School of Medicine, Emory, GA, USA
R F Pass, University of Alabama School of Medicine, Birmingham, AL, USA

Introduction

Cytomegaloviruses, also known as salivary gland viruses, are widely distributed, species-specific herpesviruses, with an evolutionarily related representative identified in most mammalian hosts when cells of the same species have been used for isolation. Human cytomegalovirus (HCMV), formally called human herpesvirus 5 (HHV-5), infects a majority of the world population by adulthood, but causes acute disease in only a small proportion of immunocompetent individuals. Developing areas of the world typically exhibit widespread transmission early in life, whereas more developed areas show a broader range of patterns. Individuals may escape infection early in life and remain susceptible during the childbearing years. Once rubella was controlled by vaccination, transplacental transmission of HCMV emerged as the major infectious cause of congenital hearing loss preventable by vaccination. HCMV is an opportunistic pathogen associated with disease in immunocompromised hosts, predominating in the settings of genetic or acquired immunodeficiency, allograft tissue and organ transplantation, and pregnancy. Disease pathogenesis requires active viral replication and focuses on different target tissues and organs in different clinical settings, particularly in circumstances where the ability to mount a cellular immune response has been compromised. Transmission of this virus in the general population depends on direct contact with infected bodily secretions.

History and Classification

HCMV is designated formally in the species *Human herpesvirus 5* and belongs to genus *Cytomegalovirus* in subfamily *Betaherpesvirinae* of the family *Herpesviridae*. Human herpesvirus 6 (HHV-6; often considered as two variants, HHV-6A and HHV-6B) and human herpesvirus 7 (HHV-7) belong to the species *Human herpesvirus 6* and *Human herpesvirus 7*, respectively, and represent genus *Roseolovirus* in the same subfamily. All betaherpesviruses replicate slowly in cell culture, remain cell-associated, and exhibit species specificity.

Starting in the early 1930s, the most severe form of HCMV-associated congenital disease, cytomegalic inclusion disease (CID), was recognized by an 'owl's eye' cytopathology in salivary gland, liver, lung, kidney, pancreas, and thyroid autopsy materials from infants. By the early 1950s, CID diagnosis was based on the presence of inclusion-bearing cells in urine, and viral etiology was established by isolation on cultured human fibroblasts. By the early 1970s, the host species specificity of viral replication, widespread distribution of HCMV-like agents in mammals, and tissue and cell type distribution in the diseased host were well recognized. Most importantly, the relationship between transplacental transmission and neurological damage in newborns was established and the social cost of the major sequela, progressive sensorineural hearing loss, placed a high priority on control of this infection through vaccination, which has not been realized to this day. Although primary infection results in the most severe disease with congenital infection, less frequent transmission following recurrent maternal infection nevertheless remains important in the overall epidemiology of disease. Placental infection appears to be considerably more frequent than transplacental transmission, which overall is on the order of 0.5–1% of live births in the USA or Europe. Transplacental transmission is less frequent during recurrent infection (<1% of newborns) than during primary infection (~30–40% of newborns). Young children are a major reservoir of this virus, often responsible for transmitting primary infection in pregnant women.

The second prominent setting of HCMV disease is in the immunocompromised host, and this has driven initiatives for therapeutic intervention. HCMV is associated with various diseases in which T-lymphocyte immune surveillance is compromised. Infection of immunocompetent individuals, ranging from immediately postpartum through adulthood, does not generally lead to significant illness other than occasional (heterophile negative) mononucleosis. A remarkably strong and broad T-cell response, particularly the cytotoxic T-cell response, contributes to lifelong suppression of active virus replication. Immunosuppressive therapy necessary to prevent T-cell-mediated allograft rejection reduces HCMV immunosurveillance, allowing the virus to replicate to levels that lead to various diseases. The incidence of HCMV pneumonia in allogeneic hematopoietic cell transplantation (HCT) and the widespread incidence of HCMV retinitis in acquired immune deficiency syndrome (AIDS) contributed to the development of the antiviral drugs ganciclovir, foscarnet, and cidofovir, and to the later development of the orally administered drug, valganciclovir, as well as ongoing investigation of maribavir. HCMV plays a suspected role in chronic vascular diseases, and this is best illustrated by cardiac allograft vascular disease incidence in heart transplantation and the contribution of this virus to incidence of bacterial and fungal infections in allogeneic HCT settings.

Geographic and Seasonal Distribution

As a ubiquitous virus, HCMV does not show a particular seasonal distribution, although initial acquisition varies with living circumstances. In general, prevalence is more widespread in younger individuals in developing countries than in developed countries, and, within developed countries, it is more widespread in urban than in suburban groups, and low-socioeconomic groups than in high-socioeconomic groups. In a US-based survey, overall HCMV prevalence was approximately 60%, with a higher prevalence in females (64%) than males (54%) and in non-Hispanic blacks (76%) and Mexican Americans (82%) than in non-Hispanic whites (51%). There is a doubling in the prevalence of HCMV infection between childhood and old age, which rises to include 75–85% of the population regardless of demographic considerations. In addition to age and socioeconomic level, early acquisition of HCMV is observed in immigrants and is associated with fewer years of education, large family size, and residence in the southern states.

Host Range and Virus Propagation

Cytomegaloviruses are most readily propagated in fibroblasts cultured from the origin host species, although efficient replication of HCMV in human fibroblasts is facilitated by mutations in the viral genome that reduce the ability to replicate in other host-cell types. Studies on autopsy materials from immunocompromised individuals with acute HCMV disease have shown evidence of virus replication in epithelial, endothelial, macrophage, and dendritic cells. HCMV antigens are also readily detected in nonpermissive peripheral blood (PB) neutrophils of diseased individuals, probably as a result of phagocytosis, and this has become the basis of an important diagnostic assay (antigenemia) specific for a major viral structural antigen (pp65). Fresh clinical isolates replicate efficiently on primary or secondary cultures of epithelial, endothelial, macrophage, and dendritic cells, but this tropism is lost when virus is propagated in fibroblasts due to mutations that accumulate in the viral genome. Extensively passaged laboratory strains acquire a variety of large and small deletions that remove or disrupt tropism genes as well as other genes that are dispensable for replication in cultured fibroblasts. Variants of common laboratory strains, all used under a single name (e.g., AD169, Towne), have arisen via independent propagation since their isolation in different laboratories around the world. Although cellular receptors for HCMV are important determinants of entry into host cells, species specificity and human cell tropism is not determined solely by the distribution of receptors for this virus; nonpermissive fibroblasts from other species generally allow viral attachment and penetration, but are blocked at an early postentry step. An exception appears to be HCMV isolated and adapted to fibroblasts, during which variants arise that lack the ability to enter primary human endothelial cells, epithelial cells, and myeloid cells due to acquisition of mutations.

Genetics and Replication

Betaherpesviruses have linear DNA genomes with direct terminal repeats that contain the *cis*-acting signals for cleavage and packaging of progeny viral DNA during replication. Based on a subset of protein-coding genes conserved across mammalian members of the *Herpesviridae* (the core genes), all herpesviruses likely follow common pathways of DNA replication, DNA encapsidation, and virion maturation. Otherwise, betaherpesvirus genomes exhibit some divergent characteristics. Primate cytomegaloviruses undergo genome rearrangement similar to some alphaherpesviruses. HCMV packages any one of four isomers and has a genome organization that includes a unique long (U_L) component surrounded by a set of inverted repeats (*ab–b'a'*, or TRL–IRL) and a unique short component (U_S) also surrounded by a second set of inverted repeats (*a'c'–ca*, or TRS–IRS) (**Figure 1**). HHV-6 and HHV-7 do not rearrange, and have genomes with a large terminal repeat. Murine or rat CMV genomes also do not rearrange and have terminal repeats that are the smallest (<50 bp) of any characterized herpesvirus.

Genome sequence analysis has revealed evolutionary relationships and codified the classification of herpesviruses. Betaherpesvirus genomes are collinear and exhibit more extensive genetic similarity with each other than with other herpesviruses, where the 40 core genes are arranged in different clusters. Betaherpesviruses encode approximately 170 protein-coding gene homologs, 40 of which are common to alphaherpesviruses and 46 of which are common to gammaherpesviruses. **Figure 1** depicts these gene sets along with an estimate of the overall genomic coding capacity.

The HCMV virion has typical herpesvirus structure, although somewhat larger than alphaherpesviruses or gammaherpesviruses, at 200–300 nm diameter. The 125 nm icosahedral nucleocapsid is composed of five herpesvirus core proteins: the major capsid protein (MCP) comprising the hexons and pentons, the minor capsid protein (mCP or TRI2) together with the minor capsid protein-binding protein (mCP-BP or TRI1) comprising the intercapsomeric triplexes, the small capsid protein (SCP) that decorates the hexon tips, and the portal protein (PORT) that comprises one penton position and is used for encapsidation of viral DNA. The nucleocapsid encloses a single linear molecule of DNA as well as origin of lytic DNA replication (*ori*Lyt)-associated RNA. The nucleocapsid is embedded in a tegument (or matrix) containing at least 27 relatively abundant virus-encoded phosphoproteins as well as many more proteins and RNAs that are present in small amounts. About a dozen herpesvirus core as well as a dozen betaherpesvirus-specific structural proteins are considered tegument components. These appear to be involved in the earliest steps of infection and uncoating and release of the viral genome into the nucleus, as well as at late stages of replication for encapsidation of progeny viral DNA, capsid egress from nuclei, and, importantly, final envelopment and egress from the cytoplasm. Tegument proteins also modulate events in the host cell to block intrinsic resistance mechanisms that impede viral replication. The tegument is surrounded by a lipid bilayer envelope derived from cellular endoplasmic reticulum (ER)–Golgi intermediate compartment (ERGIC) membranes and into which some 20 or more virus-encoded glycoproteins are inserted. Unlike other herpesviruses that encode subgroup-specific envelope glycoproteins central to entry, the most prominent HCMV envelope glycoproteins are herpesvirus core gene products. These are known by common nomenclature as glycoprotein (g)B, gH:gL, and gM:gN, and all play essential replication functions. None of the numerous additional glycoproteins encoded by HCMV are essential for replication in cultured fibroblasts. Overall, HCMV is the most structurally complex herpesvirus, reflecting the large number of gene products encoded by this virus. During infection in cell culture, HCMV produces an abundance of noninfectious particles, including dense bodies that lack a nucleocapsid as well as other defective, capsid-containing particles. These particles constitute at least 99% of virion preparations, producing particle-to-PFU ratios of 100 or greater.

Complete or largely complete genome sequences have been determined for a number of laboratory and low-passage HCMV strains. All HCMV strains exhibit an average of >95% DNA sequence identity, although large deletion mutations are present in many highly propagated strains. Wild-type HCMV is estimated to carry a minimum of 166 protein-coding genes, the great majority of which are conserved in the closest relative of HCMV, chimpanzee CMV. A liberal upper estimate of 252 ORFs has been suggested. In addition to protein-coding genes

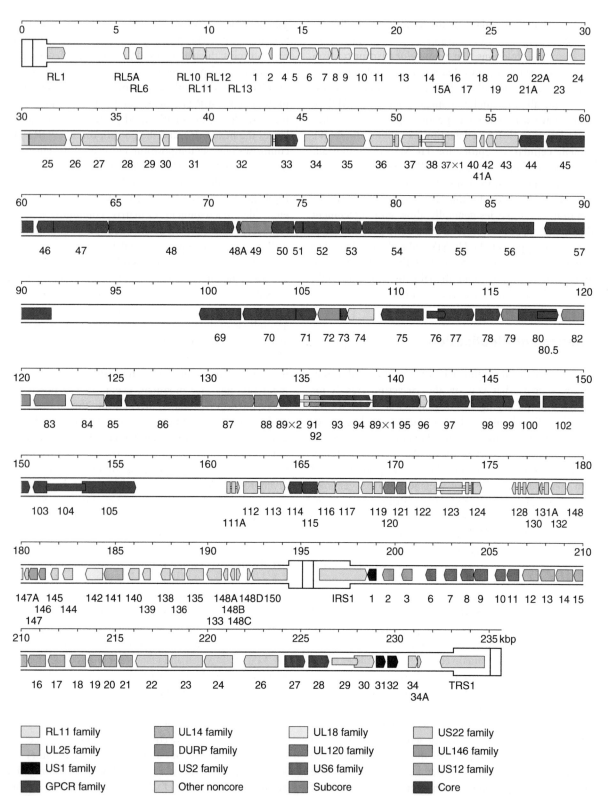

Figure 1   Genetic organization and content of wild-type human HCMV, based on low passage strain Merlin. The inverted repeats TRL/IRL (*ab–b′a′*) and TRS/IRS (*a′c′–ca*) are shown in a thicker format than U$_L$ and U$_S$. Protein-coding regions are indicated by arrows and gene names are listed below. Introns are shown as narrow bars. Genes corresponding to those in TR$_L$/IR$_L$ and TR$_S$/IR$_S$ of strain AD169 are given their full nomenclature, but the UL and US prefixes have been omitted from UL1–UL150 and US1–US34A. Herpesvirus core genes (inherited from the ancestor of the alpha-, beta-, and gammaherpesviruses), subcore genes (inherited from the ancestor of beta- and gammaherpesviruses), other unique genes (homologs present only in betaherpesviruses), and members of families of related genes are color-coded as depicted in the key. Adapted from Dolan A, Cunningham C, Hector RD, *et al.* (2004) Genetic content of wild type human cytomegalovirus. *Journal of General Virology* 85: 1301–1312, with permission from Society for General Microbiology.

and potential miRNA-like elements, the HCMV genome has three types of resident signals that act to control gene expression, DNA replication, and DNA packaging during replication. The genes on the viral genome are controlled by promoter-regulatory signals that are recognized by host-cell RNA polymerase II and influenced by viral regulatory proteins, and are expressed in a temporal cascade that initiates following penetration of the host cell.

Entry into cells depends upon envelope glycoproteins and release of virion DNA into the nucleus depends upon

tegument proteins. Entry initiates with a series of distinct steps involving (1) binding to specific cell surface receptors, (2) fusion of the virion envelope with the cellular membrane to release nucleocapsids into the cytoplasm, (3) nucleocapsid association with cytoskeletal elements and translocation toward the nucleus, (4) nucleocapsid interaction with nuclear pores, and (5) release of the viral genome into the nucleus (**Figure 2**). Expression of the immediate early (IE) class of viral genes follows entry and is influenced by virion tegument proteins (virion

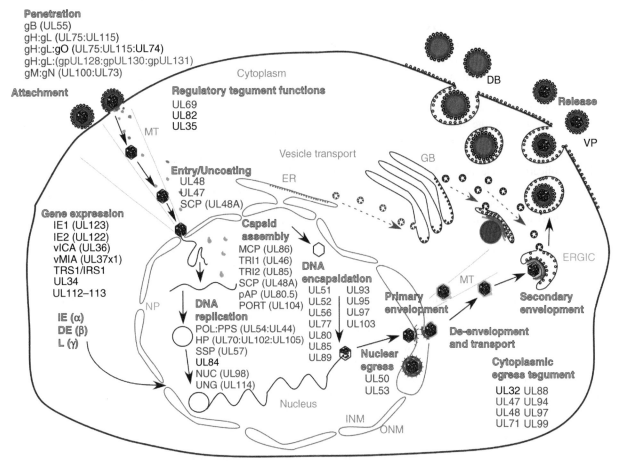

Figure 2 Summary of the HCMV replication pathway with focus on herpesvirus core (red) and betaherpesvirus-conserved (black) gene products playing known or predicted roles in replication. Major steps in productive replication are indicated in large gray outlined font, and black arrows indicate the procession of steps with individual functions identified by abbreviated names. The entry pathway shown employs direct fusion at the plasma membrane (attachment and penetration) although an endocytic pathway may also be important in certain cell types. Entry requires gB, gH:gL, possibly with gO, or gpUL128-gpUL130-gpUL131, and gM:gN. Virion tegument functions (UL69, UL82, UL35) are involved in regulation. UL47, UL48, and SCP are predicted to mediate transport on microtubules, docking at nuclear pores, and release of virion DNA from the capsid into the nucleus. Transcriptional regulation of viral and host-cell gene expression is mediated by IE genes (IE1, IE2) or DE genes (UL34, UL35, UL112-UL113). Cell death suppression is mediated by IE gene products vICA and vMIA. DNA replication depends on several core proteins (POL:PPS, HP, SSB, NUC, and UNG) as well as one betaherpesvirus-specific function (UL84). Capsid assembly uses core functions MCP, TRI1:TRI2, SCP, PORT, and pAP. Preformed capsids likely translocate to sites of DNA replication where several core proteins (UL51, UL56, UL77, UL80.5, UL85, UL89, UL93, UL95, UL97, UL103 gene products) are likely to be involved in encapsidation of viral DNA. Nuclear egress is likely to be controlled by UL50 and UL53 gene products, which are core proteins. Cytoplasmic egress (black arrows) and secondary (final) envelopment are controlled by core functions (UL47, UL48, UL71, UL88, UL94, UL97, UL99 gene products) as well as one betaherpesvirus-specific protein (UL32 gene product). Nucleocapsids are likely transported on microtubules and virion envelope glycoproteins follow vesicle transport to sites of final envelopment in the cytoplasm. Golgi body (GB), microtubules (MTs), and ER and ERGIC, as well as both virus particle (VP) and dense body (DB) final release steps are identified in the cytoplasm. Nuclear pores (NPs), inner nuclear membrane (INM), and outer nuclear membrane (ONM) are identified in the nucleus. The cellular vesicle transport pathway from the ER to GB is also designated (dashed gray arrow).

transactivators). IE genes include viral functions that regulate gene expression by activating transcription and suppressing host repression systems, cell death, and major histocompatibility complex class I gene expression. As in all herpesviruses, different temporal classes of genes are interspersed across the HCMV genome. The IE genes are not clustered and map to diverse locations in the U_L, U_S, and IR_S/TR_S regions of the viral genome. Expression of the next set of genes, the delayed early (DE) genes, depends on the expression of regulatory IE gene products. DE genes control the initiation of viral DNA replication and a wide range of host-cell modulatory functions. Viral DNA synthesis initiates on the viral genome at oriLyt and relies on six core virus-encoded DNA synthesis proteins well as additional functions that facilitate this process. Expression of late (L) genes occurs last and includes a majority of virion structural proteins, a great many of which are herpesvirus core functions. DE and L gene classes also include as many as 100 immunomodulatory functions that impact the host cell and the immune response of the host, only a fraction of which have been studied (**Table 1**).

The replication cycle of HCMV is slow, requiring 48–72 h to begin the release of progeny, with a switch from E to L phase being delayed until 24–36 h post infection (hpi) and maximum levels of virus release starting at 72 –96 hpi. The basic features of HCMV capsid formation and maturation are likely to be common to all herpesviruses. Encapsidation of viral DNA is under the control of a set of viral proteins that package and cleave viral DNA molecules into preformed capsids. Seven herpesvirus core encapsidation proteins likely act as a complex to process a concatemeric DNA template via cleavage/packaging (*pac*) sites located within the terminal *a* sequences, and following the insertion of genome-length viral DNA, cleave to produce a filled nucleocapsid. The nucleocapsid follows a complex two-stage envelopment and egress process that starts in the nucleus and leads to virion release by exocytosis at the plasma membrane. This process depends upon many core herpesvirus functions and starts with primary envelopment at the inner nuclear membrane followed by a de-envelopment event at the outer nuclear membrane, a process that releases the nucleocapsid into the cytoplasm (**Figure 2**). Secondary envelopment occurs in the cytoplasm at ERGIC membranes with the resulting vesicles transporting mature virions to the cell surface using the cellular exocytic pathway. Dense bodies form in the cytoplasm, following only the cytoplasmic steps (**Figure 2**). Once maturation starts, infected fibroblasts continue to produce virus at peak levels for several days, depending on the viral strain and constellation of cell-death suppressors encoded by the strain. Based on systematic mutagenesis, about 80 viral genes play important roles in replication, with roughly 45 being essential for replication in fibroblasts.

Evolution

HCMV has a 236 kbp genome and the capacity to encode in excess of 166 gene products, including several gene families (**Figure 1**). This is considerably more than HHV-6 and HHV-7, whose smaller genomes (145–162 kbp) encode an estimated 84 or 85 gene products. Cytomegaloviruses from a wide variety of host species conserve the same 70 betaherpesvirus-common genes, as do HHV-6 and HHV-7. Betaherpesviruses exhibit the greatest divergence observed in the herpesviruses, with even the most closely related primate cytomegaloviruses exhibiting differences in gene content and different CMV strains containing a subset of strikingly variable genes. Human roseoloviruses and HCMVs lack detectable DNA sequence homology. The deduced protein-coding capacity of cytomegaloviruses is also highly diverged, although a set of betaherpesvirus-conserved proteins emerges from bioinformatic analysis of potential protein-coding regions and greater levels of conservation are observed in cytomegaloviruses of closely related host species. The diversity of genes observed in biologically related viruses may be a product of immune clearance pressure through co-evolution with particular hosts. Each betaherpesvirus appears to have co-evolved with its host species and exhibits little genetic evidence of cross-species transmission.

Pathogenesis and Latency

HCMV transmission is via contact with virus-positive body fluids and requires direct contact with infectious material, as is the case with most human herpesviruses. HCMV is shed for prolonged periods of time in urine, saliva, tears, semen, and cervical secretions, as well as in breast milk. HCMV transmission rates are highest where contact with body fluids occurs, such that HCMV is an important sexually transmitted disease as well as an infection that is transmitted among children in day-care centers and from young children to parents and other care providers. Thus, two distinct types of exposure are associated with horizontal transmission of HCMV: sexual activity among adults and direct contact with urine or saliva from young children. Children in day-care centers, who frequently transmit virus to each other through casual contact, continue to shed virus in saliva and urine for years without symptoms. Day-care workers have markedly increased rates of HCMV infection as do parents of young children who attend day-care centers, where transmission rates of 10% or greater per year have been reported. Hygiene is thought to play a role in transmission, and regular hand washing has been recommended to reduce transmission. Although shedding of HCMV is common among hospitalized individuals, medical-care professionals who are known to use good

Table 1 HCMV gene characteristics and functions.

HCMV[a,b]	HCMV gene family/gene name[c]	Function/comments/abbreviation[d]
RL1		
RL5A	RL11 fam	
RL6	RL11 fam	
RL10	Virion env-gp	
RL11	RL11 fam; IgG Fc-binding glycoprotein	Modulation of antibody activity
RL12	RL11 fam; put mem-gp	
RL13	RL11 fam; put mem-gp	
UL1	RL11 fam	
UL2	Put mem	
UL4	RL11 fam; env-gp	
UL5	RL11 fam; virion envelope protein?	
UL6	RL11 fam; put mem-gp	
UL7	RL11 fam; put mem-gp	
UL8	RL11 fam; put mem-gp	
UL9	RL11 fam; put mem-gp	Temperance
UL10	RL11 fam; put mem-gp	Temperance
UL11	RL11 fam; mem-gp	
UL13	Put sec	
UL14	UL14 fam; put mem-gp	
UL15A	Put mem	
UL16	Mem-gp	Inhibits NK cell cytotoxicity via NKG2D ligands MICA and ULBPs; temperance
UL17		
UL18	UL18 fam; put mem-gp; MHC class I homolog	LIR-1 ligand
UL19		
UL20	T-cell receptor γ chain homolog	
UL21A[¥]		
UL22A	Virion env, sec-gp	CC chemokine-binding protein (also called UL21.5); possibly temperance
UL23	US22 fam; teg	Temperance
UL24	US22 fam; teg	
UL25	UL25 fam: teg	Temperance
UL26[¥]	US22 fam; teg	Activator of major IE promoter; regulates teg phosphorylation
UL27		Maribavir resistance
UL28[¥]	US22 fam	
UL29[¶]	US22 fam	Temperance
UL30[¥]		
UL31[¶]	dUTPase-related protein (DURP) fam	
UL32[†]	Major teg-pp (pp150); highly immunogenic	Binds to capsids, cytoplasmic envelopment of virions
UL33x1/ UL33x2	GPCR fam, virion env	Constitutive signaling
UL34[†]		Represses US3 transcription
UL35[¶]	UL25 fam; teg-pp	Interacts with UL82 protein; regulates virion transactivation and assembly
UL36x1/ UL36x2	US22 fam; IE, teg; inhibitor of caspase-8-induced apoptosis	Cell death suppression (vICA)
UL37x1[¶]	IE; mitochondrial inhibitor of apoptosis	Cell death suppression (vMIA)
UL37	IE glycoprotein	Gene regulation, vMIA domain at amino terminus
UL38[¶]	Mem-gp	Cell death suppression
UL40	Mem-gp	Signal peptide binds HLA-E to inhibit NK cell cytotoxicity via CD94:NKG2A
UL41A	Virion env-gp	Also called UL41.5
UL42	Put mem	
UL43	US22 fam; teg	
UL44[†]	(core) DNA polymerase processivity subunit	Increases DNA pol product length (PPS)
UL45	(core) Teg	Large subunit ribonucleotide reductase homolog (enzymatically inactive); virion protein (RR1)
UL46[†]	(core) Capsid	Component of capsid triplexes (minor capsid binding protein; TRI1)
UL47[¶]	(core) Teg	Intracellular capsid transport; binds to UL48 protein? (LTPbp)

Continued

Table 1   Continued

HCMV[a,b]	HCMV gene family/gene name[c]	Function/comments/abbreviation[d]
UL48[†]	(core) Largest teg	Intracellular capsid transport? (LTP)
UL48A[†]	(core) Smallest capsid	Located on tips of hexons in capsids; capsid transport? (SCP) (also called UL48.5)
UL49[†]		
UL50[†]	(core) Inner nuclear mem	Nuclear egress of capsids; virion protein? (NEMP)
UL51[†]	(core) Terminase component	DNA packaging (TER3)
UL52[†]	(core)	Capsid transport in nucleus
UL53[†]	(core) Teg	Nuclear matrix protein; capsid egress; nuclear egress lamina protein
UL54[†]	(core) DNA polymerase	DNA polymerase catalytic subunit (POL)
UL55[†]	(core) Virion env-gp B (gB)	Homomultimers; heparan-binding; role in entry and signaling
UL56[†]	(core) Terminase component	Binds to DNA packaging motif, exhibits nuclease activity (TER2)
UL57[†]	(core)	Single-stranded DNA-binding protein (SSB)
ori Lyt[†]		DNA replication origin for productive infection (cis-acting); positional conservation, sequence divergence in betaherpesviruses.
UL69[✠]	(core) Multiple regulatory protein; teg	Tegument protein; contributes to cell cycle block; exhibits nucleocytoplasmic shuttling; promotes nuclear export of unspliced mRNA (MRP)
UL70[†]	(core) DNA helicase primase subunit	Unwinding DNA, primase homology (HP2)
UL71[†]	(core) Teg	Cytoplasmic egress
UL72	(core) DURP fam	Deoxyuridine triphosphatase homolog (enzymatically inactive) (dUTPase)
UL73[†]	(core) Virion env-gp N (gN)	Complexes with gM; entry
UL74[¶]	Virion env-gp O (gO)	Complexes with gH:gL
UL75[†]	(core) Virion env-gp H (gH)	Associates with gL; complexes with gO or UL128-UL130-UL131; entry role
UL76[†]	(core) Virion-associated regulatory	
UL77[†]	(core) Portal capping	DNA packaging (PCP)
UL78	GPCR fam; put chemokine receptor, env-gp	
UL79[†]		
UL80[†]	(core)	Precursor of maturational protease (PR; N terminus) and capsid assembly (scaffold) protein (AP; C terminus)
UL80.5[†]	(core)	Precursor of capsid assembly (scaffold) protein (pAP)
UL82[✠]	DURP fam; teg-pp (pp71; upper matrix)	Virion transactivator; ND10 localized; degrades Daxx
UL83	DURP fam; major teg-pp (pp65; lower matrix)	Suppresses interferon response
UL84[†]	DURP fam	Role in organizing DNA replication; exhibits nucleocytoplasmic shuttling; binds IE2
UL85[†]	(core) Capsid	Component of capsid triplexes (minor capsid protein; TRI2)
UL86[†]	(core) Major capsid	Component of hexons and pentons (MCP)
UL87[†]		
UL88[¶]	(core) Teg	Cytoplasmic egress
UL89x1[†]/ UL89x2	(core) Terminase component	ATPase subunit (TER1)
UL91[†]		
UL92[†]		
UL93[†]	(core) Teg	Capsid transport
UL94[†]	(core) Teg	Binds single-stranded DNA; cytoplasmic egress
UL95[†]	(core)	Encapsidation chaperone protein
UL96[†]	Teg	
UL97[¶]	(core) Viral serine-threonine protein kinase; teg	Phosphorylates ganciclovir; inhibited by maribavir; roles in DNA synthesis, DNA packaging and nuclear egress; mimics cdc2/CDK1 (VPK)
UL98[†]	(core) Deoxyribonuclease	(NUC)
UL99[†]	(core) Myristylated teg-pp pp28	Cytoplasmic egress tegument protein
UL100[†]	(core) Virion env-gp M (gM)	Complexes with gN
UL102[†]	(core) DNA helicase primase subunit	Unwinding DNA (HP3)
UL103[¶]	(core) Teg	Nuclear egress
UL104[†]	(core)	Portal protein; DNA encapsidation (PORT)
UL105[†]	(core) DNA helicase primase subunit	Unwinding DNA; helicase homology (HP1)
UL111A	CMV interleukin 10	(cmvIL-10) and latency-associated (LA) vIL-10

Continued

Table 1   Continued

HCMV[a,b]	HCMV gene family/gene name[c]	Function/comments/abbreviation[d]
UL112[¥]/ *UL113[¥]*		*Transcriptional activation, orchestration of DNA replication*
UL114[¶]	*(core) Uracil-DNA glycosylase*	*Roles in excision of uracil from DNA and temporal regulation of DNA replication (UNG)*
UL115[†]	*(core) Virion env-gp L (gL)*	*Associates with gH; complexes with gO or UL128-UL130-UL131; entry*
UL116	Put mem-gp	
UL117[¥]		
UL119	IgG Fc-binding glycoprotein; virion env-gp	Mem related to OX-2; modulation of antibody activity
UL120	UL120 fam; put mem-gp	
UL121	UL120 fam; put mem-gp	
UL122[†]	*IE2 transactivator*	*Interacts with transcriptional machinery; repression via specific DNA-binding activity; cell cycle modulation (IE2)*
UL123[¥]	*Major immediate early 1 co-transactivator*	*Enhances activation by IE2; indirect effect on transcription machinery; binds HDACs; disrupts ND10 (IE1)*
UL124	*Mem-gp, latent protein*	
UL128	Put sec	Endothelial and epithelial cell tropism, env-gp complexes with gH:gL
UL130	Put sec	Endothelial and epithelial cell tropism, envelope gp complexes with gH:gL
UL131A	Put sec	Endothelial and epithelial cell tropism; envelope gp complexes with gH:gL
UL132[¶]	Virion env-gp	Temperance
UL148	Put mem-gp	
UL147A	Put mem	
UL147	UL146 fam; put sec-gp;	Put CXC chemokine
UL146	UL146 fam; sec-gp	hCXCR2-specific CXC chemokine
UL145		
UL144	Mem-gp; TNF receptor homolog	Regulates lymphocyte activation via BTLA
UL142	UL18 fam; put mem-gp; MHC class I homolog	Inhibits NK cytotoxicity
UL141	UL14 fam; mem-gp	Inhibits NK cell cytotoxicity by downregulating CD155 (CD226 ligand)
UL140	Put mem	Inhibits NK cytotoxicity
UL139	Put mem-gp	
UL138	Put mem	
UL136	Put mem	
UL135	Put sec	
UL133	Put mem	
UL148A	Put mem	
UL148B	Put mem	
UL148C	Put mem	
UL148D	Put mem	
UL150	Put sec	
IRS1	*US22 fam; IE protein; teg*	*Transcriptional activator, blocks PKR-mediated shutoff of translation*
US1	US1 fam	
US2	US2 fam; mem-gp	Degradation of MHC class I and possibly MHC class II
US3	US2 fam; IE gene; mem-gp	Inhibits processing and transport of MHC class I and possibly MHC class II
US6	US6 fam; put mem-gp	Inhibits TAP-mediated ER peptide transport
US7	US6 fam; mem-gp	
US8	US6 fam; mem-gp	Binds to MHC class I
US9	US6 fam; mem-gp	Cell-to-cell spread
US10	US6 fam; mem-gp	Delays trafficking of MHC class I
US11	US6 fam; mem-gp	Selective degradation of MHC class I
US12	US12 fam; put 7TM, GPCR?	
US13[¶]	US12 fam; put 7TM, GPCR?	
US14	US12 fam; put 7TM, GPCR?	
US15	US12 fam; put 7TM, GPCR?	
US16	US12 fam; put 7TM, GPCR?	Temperance
US17	US12 fam; put 7TM, GPCR?	Nuclear, fragmented
US18	US12 fam; put 7TM, GPCR?	
US19	US12 fam; put 7TM, GPCR?	Temperance
US20	US12 fam; put 7TM, GPCR?	
US21	US12 fam; put 7TM, GPCR?	

Continued

Table 1   Continued

HCMV[a,b]	HCMV gene family/gene name[c]	Function/comments/abbreviation[d]
US22	*US22 fam; teg*	*Released from cells*
US23[¶]	US22 fam; teg	
US24	US22 fam; teg	
US26[ˠ]	US22 fam	
US27	GPCR fam; virion env-gp	
US28	GPCR fam; env-gp	CC and CX3C chemokine receptor
US29	Put mem-gp, necessary in RPE cells	
US30	Put mem-gp	Temperance
US31	US1 fam	
US32	US1 fam	
US34	Put sec	
US34A	Put mem-gp	
TRS1[¶]	US22 fam; IE protein; teg pp	*Transcriptional activator; blocks PKR-mediated shutoff of translation*

[a]Commonly annotated ORFs of HCMV (see **Figure 1**). Based on the replication properties of HCMV mutant viruses, most genes are dispensable in cell culture (normal type). Viruses with mutations that influence replication efficiency exhibit one of three broad growth deficient phenotypes: failure to replicate ([¶]), very poor replication ([ˠ]), or slight replication defect ([¶]) when assayed in human fibroblasts. Mutations of putative HCMV ORFs UL60 and UL61 are interpreted as disrupting *ori*Lyt rather than any protein-coding ORF. Certain mutant virus phenotypes vary depending on viral strain and strain variant tested.
[b]Betaherpesvirus-common genes are in italics, and include 40 herpesvirus core functions, labeled as 'core'. Gene family, characteristics, and functional information are provided for HCMV and a blank indicates the lack of information.
[c]Abbreviations: fam, family; pp, phosphoprotein; teg, tegument; gp, glycoprotein; mem-gp, membrane gp; env-gp, envelope gp, TM-gp, transmembrane gp; sec, secreted; put, putative; GPCR, G-protein-coupled receptor; 7TM, seven transmembrane-spanning; IE, immediate early.
[d]Functional information is speculative in some cases.

hygiene practices do not exhibit any increased risk of HCMV infection. Horizontal transmission may also occur through blood transfusion, blood and marrow (hematopoietic cell) allograft transplantation, and in the clinically important setting of solid organ transplantation from HCMV seropositive donors to naive recipients.

HCMV is transmitted vertically during pregnancy, as well as during the birthing process or from mother's milk. Transplacental transmission is a characteristic of HCMV and possibly roseoloviruses, and is not observed with alphaherpesviruses or gammaherpesviruses. Primary infection has been reported to occur in 1–4% of pregnant women, and is associated with a significant risk for transplacental transmission. Between 20% and 40% of newborns delivered by women with primary infection are HCMV infected, compared to between 1% and 2% of newborns delivered by women with past infection. Primary infection is associated with more severe forms of congenital disease, although disease occurrence has been well documented in both settings. Transmission at birth as well as through mother's milk helps maintain HCMV infection in the population, with 25–50% of infants nursed by seropositive mothers acquiring HCMV by 1 year of age. Importantly, there are no known disease sequelae associated with intrapartum or postpartum acquisition of HCMV in healthy term newborns.

Although serotypes of HCMV have not been useful for epidemiology, various molecular genetic approaches that assess viral genome sequence variation have been used to differentiate viral strains in circulation. Comparison of polymerase chain reaction (PCR)-amplified segments of specific, highly variable genomic regions and protein-coding genes has been most useful, notably the noncoding genomic L–S junction (*a* sequence) as well as genes UL144, UL146, UL73, and UL74. To date, no particular viral strain has been unambiguously linked to any clinical disease.

HCMV appears to reside latent in progenitor cells of the myeloid lineage and to reactivate when these progenitors are stimulated by pro-inflammatory cytokines. HCMV is persistently detected in saliva approximately 3–5% of the time. Based on the distribution and levels of viral DNA, natural latency occurs in bone marrow-derived myelomonocytic cells that give rise to macrophages and dendritic cells, with approximately 0.01–0.001% of cells infected and each cell carrying two to ten genome copies of HCMV DNA. Little is known about sporadic reactivation in immunocompetent individuals, which leads to shedding in saliva and other bodily fluids. However, reactivation in allogeneic transplant settings appears to follow the elaboration of pro-inflammatory cytokines that are a component of tissue rejection. Patients with compromised immunity to HCMV amplify virus to levels that become a clinical threat. HCMV reactivation also occurs in settings without allogeneic stimulation. Pregnancy appears to allow reactivation at levels that are not a threat to women but may be a threat to a developing fetus. Severely immunocompromised patients, such as terminal AIDS patients, appear to support sufficiently high levels of HCMV replication for disease to occur.

Clinical Features and Pathology

HCMV infection in the immunocompetent host is typically clinically silent. A small percentage of mononucleosis is due to HCMV, which is typically less severe than that caused by Epstein–Barr virus. Severe or systemic HCMV disease affecting one or more organs only occurs in immunocompromised hosts and has been known to unveil underlying immunodeficiency in individuals with a previously unrecognized immune deficit.

Congenital disease is the hallmark of HCMV pathogenesis and follows transplacental transmission to the fetus any time during pregnancy, and is a particular risk for woman with primary infection. Congenital disease remains the most important medical and public health concern for HCMV, and is difficult to identify because primary infection is typically asymptomatic. A significantly lower rate of congenital disease follows recurrent compared to primary maternal infection during pregnancy, providing the key evidence that universal vaccination would benefit the population. In addition, primary infection at an earlier gestational age is most likely to manifest as disease in the newborn. HCMV disease recognized at birth often reflects neuronal damage (hearing loss, retinitis, optic neuritis, microcephaly, or encephalopathy) as well as damage to the reticuloendothelial system (hepatomegaly, splenomegaly, petechiae, or jaundice). Prematurity and poor intrauterine growth are common among newborns with symptomatic congenital HCMV infection. Although the majority of infected newborns are asymptomatic at birth, some still develop sequelae, notably sensorineural hearing loss, over the first few years of life. Most newborns with congenital HCMV infection, even those severely affected at birth, survive; congenital HCMV infection takes its toll by affecting hearing, eyesight, and mental capacity.

Very low birth weight premature infants who acquire HCMV infection during birth or postpartum (from human milk or transfusion) may develop systemic disease that is distinct from conventional congenital disease. Risk factors include very low birth weight, exposure to multiple units of blood and birth to a seronegative mother (lack of passive immunity). Transfusion-associated HCMV disease in newborns has been controlled by the use of seronegative (or leukocyte-depleted) blood products. Whether or not transmission of HCMV from a mother's milk to a very low birth weight premature newborn should be prevented remains an area of controversy.

HCMV has become one of the most common opportunistic pathogens as allograft transplantation has grown and as the AIDS epidemic has unfolded. Solid organ and hematopoietic cell allograft recipients all receive strong post-transplant immunosuppressive therapy and AIDS patients progress to a T-lymphocyte deficit that provides an opportunity for HCMV to replicate to high levels and cause disease. Active infection arises from primary infection of naive individuals, reinfection with additional strains of virus, and reactivation of latent virus. This aspect of disease pathogenesis is complicated because HCMV shedding and viremia are common in the face of impaired cellular immunity even when HCMV disease is absent. Clinically silent HCMV infection may predominate even in the face of antiviral prophylaxis, and may only progress to disease as T-cell-mediated immune surveillance becomes severely compromised, such as occurs in AIDS patients with very low CD4 T-cell counts.

Clinical manifestations of disease in solid organ transplant patients include systemic, febrile illness (CMV syndrome, with malaise, arthralgia and rash; neutropenia, thrombocytopenia, and elevated liver enzymes), as well as a direct or indirect impact on specific organs. This disease risk has been reduced but not eliminated by preemptive therapy or prophylaxis with antiviral drugs. Clinical detection of infection using assays for viral antigens or nucleic acids without the need for virus culture successfully reduced the incidence of acute HCMV disease in the first few weeks following transplantation. Preemptive therapy has been beneficial in other high-risk patients such as allogeneic blood and marrow (hematopoietic cell) transplantation where late-onset disease and indirect effects have become more prominent. The detection of HCMV antigens (usually pp65 antigenemia) or nucleic acids (usually PCR detection of viral DNA in plasma or leukocytes) in blood is used to implicate this virus in disease. Solid organ transplant recipients may acquire HCMV pneumonitis, or gastrointestinal lesions, hepatitis, retinitis, pancreatitis, myocarditis, and, in rare circumstances, encephalitis or peripheral neuropathy, whereas hematopoietic cell transplant recipients suffer HCMV pneumonitis or gastrointestinal disease. Establishing an etiologic role for HCMV requires detection of virus in affected tissue or bronchoalveolar lavage or quantitation of HCMV in blood or plasma. The principal indirect effects of HCMV, particularly during solid organ transplantation, include allograft rejection, vascular disease complications, and increased risk of opportunistic fungal and bacterial infections. Primary infection is most likely to lead to disease when a naive recipient receives an organ from an HCMV seropositive donor, although the particular organ and immunosuppression regimen also influence outcome.

Although antiviral prophylaxis has proved to be very effective in preventing HCMV disease in solid organ transplant recipients, late-onset HCMV disease may follow prophylaxis in as many as 5% of patients. Prophylactic or preemptive antiviral treatment in hematopoietic cell transplant recipients reduces the incidence of HCMV disease during the first 3–4 months to around 5%; however, late-onset disease, usually more than 100 days after transplant, remains a problem. In all clinical transplant settings, HCMV has been associated with chronic disease consequences that prophylaxis and preemptive therapy have not completely alleviated. In the nontransplanted individual, HCMV has been a suspected cofactor in atherosclerotic vascular disease and in autoimmune vasculitis.

Highly active antiretroviral therapy (HAART) reduces incidence of HCMV retinitis and gastrointestinal disease in AIDS patients due to reconstitution or preservation of cellular immune function, although HCMV remains a significant risk to human immunodeficiency virus (HIV)-positive individuals when CD4 T-cell counts drop to low levels.

Four antiviral agents are currently approved in the USA for treatment of HCMV disease, ganciclovir, valganciclovir, cidofovir, and foscarnet, with intravenous ganciclovir and orally administered prodrug valganciclovir being first choices in most settings. These two are also common choices for prophylaxis and preemptive therapy. All of the anti-HCMV drugs have potentially significant toxicity and are limited to use in patients with disabling or life-threatening disease risk. Thus, additional drugs are under development. Prolonged use of any investigational or licensed drug may select for resistant virus, but drug-resistant mutants have not been observed to circulate in the population.

Immune Response, Prevention, and Control

Prevention of HCMV infections during pregnancy to reduce congenital disease risk is an important public health goal, and universal vaccination during childhood is believed to be the appropriate route to achieve this control. Attempts to develop live, attenuated, killed, and subunit vaccines over the past 30 years have not yet resulted in success. The Centers for Disease Control and Prevention (CDC) currently recommends that parents and caregivers of young children be informed of how HCMV is transmitted and of hygienic measures that reduce transmission, particularly to women who care for young children and may become pregnant.

Natural HCMV infection is highly immunogenic, resulting in broad humoral antibody and cellular T-lymphocyte responses that persist for life. The parameters of CD4 and CD8 T-lymphocyte responses vary with age and other characteristics, but the continued high levels of response in a majority of infected individuals

suggests that virus antigen provides a continuous immunogenic stimulus throughout life. In addition to the adaptive immune response, innate cellular clearance by natural killer (NK) cells appears to be important in the initial stages of infection.

HCMV encodes a very large array of gene products that deflect intrinsic host-cell antiviral responses mediated at the transcriptional level through activation of the interferon pathways or cell death. In addition, this virus encodes a wide range of functions aimed at disarming the innate NK cell response as well as the effectiveness of adaptive humoral and T-cell responses. These functions provide an impression that this virus survives in tight balance with host immune clearance mechanisms, and are summarized in **Table 1**. In addition, accumulating evidence from animal models of HCMV pathogenesis implicates pro-inflammatory viral gene products in creating the appropriate environment to allow efficient growth and dissemination to important tissue sites to assure transmission to new hosts.

Future Perspectives

Although there have been tremendous gains in knowledge of HCMV molecular biology and pathogenesis, this virus continues to be a very important cause of disease especially for immunocompromised hosts and for the fetus. To date, antiviral chemotherapy has been only partially successful in controlling HCMV infection in transplant and other immunocompromised patients and there remains a need for vaccination to reduce the incidence of congenital HCMV infection. An important goal for future research will be to translate the large and growing body of basic knowledge of HCMV biology into improved treatments and effective vaccines.

See also: Herpesviruses: General Features; Human Herpesviruses 6 and 7.

Further Reading

Davison AJ and Bhella D (2007) Comparative betaherpesvirus genome and virion structure. In: Arvin AM, Mocarski ES, Moore P, *et al.* (eds.) *Human Herpesviruses: Biology, Therapy and Immunoprophylaxis*, pp 177–203. Cambridge: Cambridge University Press.

Dolan A, Cunningham C, Hector RD, *et al.* (2004) Genetic content of wild type human cytomegalovirus. *Journal of General Virology* 85: 1301–1312.

Mocarski ES, Jr. (2007) Betaherpesvirus-common genes and their functions. In: Arvin AM, Mocarski ES, Moore P, *et al.* (eds.) *Human Herpesviruses: Biology, Therapy and Immunoprophylaxis*, pp 202–228. Cambridge: Cambridge University Press.

Mocarski ES Jr., Shenk T, and Pass RF (2006) Cytomegalovirus. In: Knipe DM, Howley PW, Griffin DE, *et al.* (eds.) *Fields Virology*, 5th edn., pp. 2701–2772. Philadelphia, PA: Lippincott Williams and Wilkins.

Human Herpesviruses 6 and 7

U A Gompels, University of London, London, UK

Introduction

The roseoloviruses human herpesviruses 6 and 7 (HHV-6 and HHV-7) infect almost all babies to give an 'infant fever', sometimes with rash (then termed 'exanthema subitum' or 'roseola infantum'), and persist throughout the host's lifetime. Infections with these viruses are generally regarded as benign and self-limiting, although severe complications have been recorded, with occasional associated fatalities, during some primary as well as secondary, reactivated infections in immunosuppressed (human immunodeficiency virus/acquired immune deficiency syndrome (HIV/AIDS) or transplantation) patients. These viruses infect and can remain latent in leukocyte stem cells and neuronal cell types, with lytic replication in CD4+ T-lymphocytes. Immunomodulatory gene products can aid persistence and contribute to pathogenesis. There are two sides to this. On the one hand, studies on such a widespread, well-adapted virus allow a greater understanding of human immunity to infection and the possible development of new immunotherapies. On the other hand, recent associations of HHV-6 (in particular) with neurological disease, including 'status epilepticus', encephalitis, and multiple sclerosis (MS), have led to reevaluations of the pathogenic potential of the roseoloviruses. To date, there are no licensed vaccines or antiviral treatments available.

History and Classification

The first isolates of HHV-6 were characterized in 1986–88 in the USA (strains GS and Z29) and the UK (strain U1102), followed by Japan (strain HST). Using reagents derived from these laboratory strains, it was found that there are two strain groups, termed variants, HHV-6A (strains GS and U1102) and HHV-6B (strains Z29 and HST). Subsequently, HHV-6B was shown to be more prevalent in these countries, and most of the available data concern this variant. In comparison, HHV-6A appears to be an emergent infection. Complete genome sequences were derived from plasmid clones for HHV-6A (strain U1102; 159 kbp; accession X83413) and HHV-6B (strain Z29; 162 kbp; accession AF157706) in 1995 and 1999, respectively. These laboratory strains have subsequently been denoted as the prototype reference strains. They were isolated from viruses reactivated from adult immunosuppressed HIV/AIDS patients from African countries: HHV-6A strain U1102 from Uganda and HHV-6B strain Z29 from the Democratic Republic of Congo. Other laboratory strains include HHV-6A strain GS, the first report of HHV-6 infection, which was isolated from an adult HIV/AIDS patient in the USA; HHV-6A strain AJ, from an adult HIV/AIDS patient in the UK; and HHV-6B strain HST, from a pediatric patient with 'exanthema subitum' in Japan. HHV-6B strain HST is the only isolate from primary childhood infection to have been sequenced completely (accession AB021506), and partial genome sequences are available for HHV-6A strains GS and AJ.

HHV-7 was isolated in 1990 from an immunocompetent blood donor. Infections with this virus appear less severe, although the virus is as widespread as HHV-6 and persists at higher levels in the blood (possibly lacking 'true latency'), with frequent secretions in saliva as with HHV-6. HHV-7 can reactivate latent HHV-6 infections. Both viruses appear to give rise to 'exanthema subitum', although HHV-6 infection is earlier and predominates. The genomes of two strains of HHV-7 have also been sequenced: JI (145 kbp; U43400) and RK (153 kbp; AF037218).

The species *Human herpesvirus 6* and *Human herpesvirus 7* are classified in genus *Roseolovirus*, subfamily *Betaherpesvirinae*, family *Herpesviridae*, and are related to genus *Cytomegalovirus* in the same subfamily. The human virus that is most closely related to HHV-6 and HHV-7 is therefore human cytomegalovirus (HCMV). The DNA sequences of the HHV-6A and HHV-6B variants are very closely related overall (>95%), with most variation located in repetitive sequences at the ends of the genomes. Hypervariable loci are also present in other regions of the genome mostly near the ends, and include genes encoding the viral chemokine vCCL (U83), immediate early transcriptional regulators (U86 and U90), glycoprotein gQ (U100), and, at the center of the genome, glycoprotein gO (U47). These regions of substantial variation presumably contribute to the different biological properties of the variants. Comparisons of the genomes of HHV-6B strains Z29 and HST show less variation (1–2%).

Geographical Distribution

Serological studies show that HHV-6 and HHV-7 are widespread throughout the world, with over 95% of adults infected. However, the geographical distribution of HHV-6A and HHV-6B is difficult to establish. There is currently no serological assay that can distinguish between the variants, since the genes encoding immunodominant proteins belong largely to the well-conserved group. The variable genes, which are diagnostically attractive, do not encode consistently immunogenic proteins. Thus, current estimates of the distribution of HHV-6A and HHV-6B have been derived using conventional polymerase chain reaction (PCR) of virus DNA or reverse transcription-polymerase chain reaction (RT-PCR) of virus RNA from tissue, blood, saliva, or cerebrospinal fluid (CSF) samples, with the use of additional techniques such as quantitative PCR, restriction endonuclease digestion, and sequencing of variable genes. In analyses of specific patient groups in North America (USA), Europe (UK), and East Asia (Japan), HHV-6B causes most (>97%) of the primary pediatric infections that give rise to HHV-6-associated infant fever with or without the 'exanthema subitum' rash. HHV-6A is detected, but as a minor component in mother–child pairs. In studies of adult bone marrow transplantation (BMT) and solid organ transplantation patients in the USA and the UK, the distribution of the variants seems similar to that in childhood infections, with primarily HHV-6B identified. In contrast, HHV-6A and HHV-6B were shown to be equally prevalent in hospitalized febrile infants in southern Africa (Zambia). Thus, there appear to be geographical differences in the distribution of HHV-6A and HHV-6B.

Biological differences may also be driven by certain variable genes, thus compounding any differences in geographic distribution. For example, in comparison to HHV-6B, HHV-6A infections are more neurotropic and more prevalent in CSF samples and congenital infections, as well as in early infections of infants less than 3 months old. In analyses of adult lung samples in the USA, both HHV-6A and HHV-6B were detected with equal prevalence. Some analyses have detected HHV-6A DNA in sera but not in peripheral blood mononuclear cells (PBMCs). Thus, the biological compartmentalization of the variants *in vivo* may differ, contributing an additional dimension to the geographical distribution of the variants.

Cellular Tropism, Laboratory Culture, and Latency

HHV-6 and HHV-7 are T-lymphotropic and neurotropic viruses. They have both been adapted to grow in CD4+ T-leukemic cell lines: for example, J-JHAN (Jurkat), HSB2, and Molt-3 cells for HHV-6; and SupT-1 cells for HHV-6 and HHV-7. However, higher titers of both HHV-6 and HHV-7 are obtained in activated cord blood lymphocytes or mononuclear cells (CBLs or CBMCs) or in peripheral blood lymphocytes (PBLs) or PBMCs. Screening of these cells is required prior to use, as infection with laboratory strains can result in reactivation of resident latent virus from adult blood and occasionally from cord blood.

CD4+ T-lymphocytes are permissive for replication and virus production, as shown *in vitro* and *in vivo* during viremia from acute infection. Infection results in cell death by necrotic lysis, with associated apoptosis in bystander cells. Lytic replication results in a characteristic cytopathic effect of ballooning cells (cytomegalia) and fused, multinucleated cells (syncytia). Studies *in vitro* show that CD4+, CD8+, and γδ T-lymphocytes can be infected, particularly by HHV-6A, which may have a wider tropism. HHV-7 binds to CD4 on T-lymphocytes, contributing to cellular tropism. HHV-6 binds to CD46, a ubiquitous receptor, and there may also be a specific co-receptor.

Similar to HCMV, and a feature of the betaherpesviruses in general, latency occurs within myeloid subsets or bone marrow progenitor cells. There is also evidence, particularly for HHV-6A, for replication in glial cells, including oligodendrocytes, astrocytes and a microglial cell type with similarities to monocytic/macrophage cells, which may also be a site of persistence in the central nervous system (CNS). HHV-7 circulates at higher levels than HHV-6, and can reactivate HHV-6. Both HHV-6 and HHV-7 can be shed asymptomatically in saliva, and salivary glands may be a site of persistence.

Recent studies indicate that 0.2% or 0.8% of blood donors in Japan or the UK, respectively, exhibit germline integration of HHV-6 genomes (either HHV-6A or HHV-6B). How this relates to latency or pathogenesis is being evaluated, but it can lead to high levels of virus DNA being detected in the blood (in cells and in sera due to cell breakage) in the absence of virus production, although a limited number of genes may be expressed. Germline integration can confound diagnoses by quantitative PCR, since in these individuals high levels of DNA do not correlate with viremia or symptoms. However, gene expression from the integrated genomes may contribute to chronic disease or immunity to HHV-6 infection.

Genome Organization

The roseolovirus genomes consist of a large unique region (U) flanked by a terminal direct repeat (DR).

The variation in size among the genomes is primarily due to differences in the size of DR. DR is itself bounded by smaller repeats (t) that are related to human telomeric repeats, and there is some suggestion that this arrangement may mediate a latent chromosome-like state or facilitate the rare integrations into the human genome that are observed (see above). At the ends of DR are 'pac' sequences for cleavage and packaging of unit-length genomes from replicative head-to-tail concatamers. Other repetitive sequences with known functions include the origin of lytic DNA replication (ORI) in the center of the genome. This combines features of ORIs in betaherpesviruses (e.g., HCMV) and alphaherpesviruses (e.g., herpes simplex virus (HSV)). HHV-6 ORI is relatively large, as in HCMV, and contains binding sites for an origin-binding protein (OBP), as in HSV. HHV-6 and HSV each encode an OBP, whereas HCMV lacks a homolog to this gene.

The protein-coding regions predicted from the genome sequences (see **Figure 1**) are available in the sequence database accessions. The prototypic HHV-6 genome layout from HHV-6A strain U1102 is shown in **Figure 1**, with main differences between HHV-6 and HHV-7 as marked and cited below. Approximately 30% of the genome is

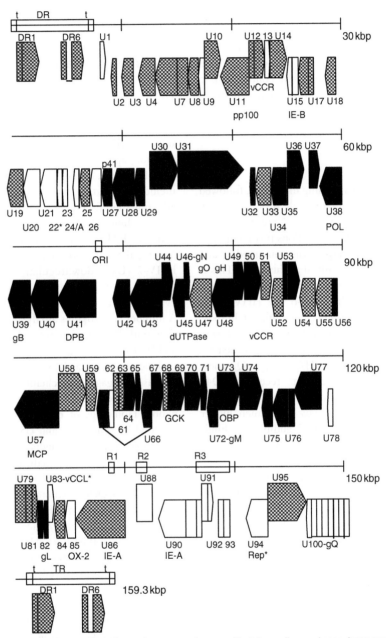

Figure 1 HHV-6 genome organization and locations of conserved genes. Protein-coding regions whose amino acid sequences are conserved among herpesviruses are indicated in black, those conserved only among betaherpesviruses are indicated as patterned, and those conserved in the roseoloviruses are indicated in white. HHV-6-specific genes are U22, U83, and U94 as asterisked, with additional possibly specific genes being U1, U9, U61, and U78. The U prefix is omitted from some gene names to enhance clarity. Repetitive sequences are marked: DR, terminal direct repeat; t, telomeric repeat; ORI, origin of lytic DNA replication; and R1, R2, and R3, locally repetitive sequences. Ancillary information is provided for certain genes mentioned in the text: p101, the major immunodominant tegument phosphoprotein; U94 Rep, the parvovirus Rep homolog and gene/replication regulatory latency gene; IE-A and IE-B, immediate early regulatory genes; POL, DNA polymerase; gB, gH, gL, gO, gM, gN, and gQ, envelope glycoproteins; vCCR, viral chemokine receptors; GCK, ganciclovir kinase; and chemokine vCCL.

taken up with genes encoding proteins that are conserved among mammalian and avian herpesviruses. These proteins dictate common features of replication, and include glycoproteins mediating virus entry by cell fusion, enzymes and accessory factors in the DNA replicase complex, and proteins for making the characteristic herpesvirus icosahedral nucleocapsid and packaging the genome into it. Proteins that are specific to betaherpesviruses are generally transcription factors controlling the gene expression cascade, functions for modulating the specificity of glycoproteins mediating virus entry by cell fusion, or proteins for modifying DNA virus replication. Functions specific to roseoloviruses that affect gene control and, in particular, immunomodulation presumably mediates latency and persistence.

Replication Cycle

Infection is initiated by virus binding to the cell, followed by penetration via virus-mediated cell fusion. As with other herpesviruses, HHV-6 and HHV-7 are first loaded onto the cell via proteoglycan interactions involving heparin or heparan sulfate. The herpesvirus-conserved gB and roseolovirus-specific gQ are involved at this stage. This is followed by membrane fusion mediated by the herpesvirus-conserved gH/gL complex. In HHV-6 and HHV-7, the gH/gL dimer also forms multimers, one with betaherpesvirus-specific gO, and the other with gQ (in two forms, gQ1 and gQ2). So far, no receptor has been identified for the gH/gL/gO complex, but the gH/gL/gQ1/gQ2 complex binds to the ubiquitous cellular receptor CD46 (which is also the measles virus co-receptor). The HHV-6A gH/gL/gQ1/gQ2 complex binds with much higher affinity than that of HHV-6B. HHV-7 additionally binds to the CD4 molecule (like HIV), but the virus attachment protein has not been identified.

Following transport of the nucleocapsid to the nucleus and release of the genome, expression of immediate early genes initiates the transcription cascade. The two spliced IE-A genes (U90 and U86) are positional counterparts of the well-characterized HCMV transcription factors, IE1 and IE2. U90 is particularly variable in sequence between HHV-6A, HHV-6B, and HHV-7. Like the corresponding region in HCMV, this major immediate early gene region is subject to CpG suppression, which is indicative of gene control by DNA methylation. This appears to be a common strategy for betaherpesviruses, which are latent in myeloid cells.

DNA replication is initiated at ORI utilizing a conserved replicase complex modified by the U55 protein, which corresponds to HCMV replication protein UL84, and also by the HHV-6-specific replication modulator, the U94 Rep protein. U94 Rep appears to be a latency-specific factor, and its absence from HHV-7 possibly contributes to the 'leaky latency' observed for this virus. The pac sites at the ends of the genome mediate cleavage of concatamers into unit-length genomes, which are then packaged into preformed nucleocapsids composed of herpesvirus-conserved capsid proteins. The virus buds through the nuclear membrane utilizing herpesvirus-conserved functions, and probably exits via the de-envelopment–re-envelopment pathway involving the *trans*-Golgi network (TGN), as has been shown for alphaherpesviruses.

Immunomodulation

HHV-6 and HHV-7 can have both direct and indirect modulatory effects on the immune system to favor persistence in immune cells. Direct effects include lysis of infected CD4+ lymphocytes during virus replication. In addition, apoptosis of bystander cells has been shown for both HHV-6- and HHV-7-infected cells. Indirect effects include modulation of the receptors on immune cells, thus affecting their function or specificity in immune activation or signaling. HHV-6 downregulates CD3 expression. Whereas HHV-7 downregulates CD4 expression, HHV-6 upregulates it. A protein encoded by both HHV-6 and HHV-7 (U21) downregulates major histocompatibility complex class I expression, which can lead to immune evasion of the antiviral TH1 cytotoxic T-cell response. A number of cytokines are dysregulated by HHV-6 infection, with IL-2 downregulated and IL-10, IL-12, TNFα, and IL-1 upregulated.

Like other primarily blood-borne herpesviruses, roseoloviruses engage the chemokine inflammatory system either to effect immune evasion or enhance virus dissemination. Homologs of chemokine receptors (vCCRs) are encoded by genes U12 and U51, and mimic properties of the human receptors in mediating immune cell traffic either constitutively, in homing to the lymph node, or inducibly, in the inflammatory response to infection. The HHV-6 vCCRs are betachemokine receptors that bind novel combinations of betachemokine ligands, including those with specificity for monocytic/macrophage cell types. Signaling by the U51 vCCR is affected by binding of different ligands and by G-protein levels in the cell. Early in infection when the U51 vCCR is produced, signaling leads to downregulation of the human CCR1-, CCR3-, and CCR5-specific chemokine Rantes/CCL5. In contrast, the HHV-7 vCCRs appear to mimic the constitutive homing chemokine receptors. HHV-6 infection can also mimic the constitutive receptor CCR7, which could allow homing of infected cells to sites of ligand secretion in the lymph node.

The HHV-6 U83 gene encodes a chemokine, vCCL. This gene is hypervariable between HHV-6A and HHV-6B but absent from HHV-7, and thus is a candidate for contributing to differences in virulence. HHV-6A vCCL has a high potency for human CCR1, CCR4,

CCR5, CCR6, and CCR8, which are present on mature monocytic/macrophage and T-cell subsets (TH2, skin homing) and immature dendritic cells. HHV-6B vCCL has a low potency for human CCR2 present on monocytes. These activities could aid immune evasion and virus dissemination, thus contributing to differences in tropism between the variants. They may also aid persistence via the chemoattraction of cell types for efficient antigen presentation and immune control.

In vivo reactivation of HHV-6 in BMT patients can lead to inhibition of outgrowth of cellular lineages. This is supported by *in vitro* data. HHV-6 infection is associated with monocyte dysfunction and suppression of macrophage maturation from bone marrow cultures. Similarly, HHV-6 infection can result in suppression of differentiation and colony formation from hematopoietic progenitor cells. For HHV-7, infection results in inhibition of megakaryocyte survival or differentiation.

Pathogenesis and Disease Associations

Infant Fever with or without Rash

HHV-6 and HHV-7 infect up to 95% of infants. Both HHV-6A and HHV-6B cause primary infant fever, and most infections occur following a drop in maternal immunity after 6 months of age. In the USA, HHV-6B accounts for 97% and HHV-6A for 3% of these infant infections. However, further studies in the USA and the UK show that in less common, earlier infections acquired either congenitally, during delivery, or heritably from germline integration, HHV-6A infections are more frequent, with a prevalence similar to that of HHV-6B. In southern Africa, infant febrile infections detected by PCR analysis of whole blood also indicate equal prevalence. Studies on acquisition of HHV-6B show that infection is symptomatic, with a fever of longer duration than other infections being the most common symptom (3–4 days, 39.4–39.7 °C in various studies). This is a frequent cause of referrals to physicians or hospital. HHV-7 is acquired later, in early childhood, with similar symptoms. As HHV-7 can reactivate HHV-6, the infections can be difficult to distinguish.

The main route of transmission appears to be spread by secretion of reactivated or persistent virus in the saliva from parents or siblings. Congenital infections with HHV-6, but not HHV-7, occur in 1% of births, a prevalence similar to that of HCMV, although HHV-7 has been detected in the placenta. Infections appear as asymptomatic compared to HCMV, although there is one report of neonatal HHV-6B infection associated with neurological disease, seizures, and mental retardation.

A minority of infants have other symptoms or complications, which may be mild or severe. Up to 10% have a skin rash similar to that of measles or rubella, which can confound diagnoses of those infections. This macular or papular rash spreads on face or trunk or both, and has previously been called 'exanthema subitum', 'roseola infantum', or sixth disease. The mean age for acquiring HHV-6 with rash is 7 months. Although this is primarily a benign, self-limiting disease, severe and occasionally life-threatening complications can develop, including lymphadenopathy, diarrhea, myocarditis, myelosuppression, and neurological disease. Indeed, HHV-6 has been reported to account for a third of childhood febrile seizures and direct or indirect mechanisms (via fever) are being evaluated. In the USA, where childhood infections by HHV-6B predominate, links with 'status epilepticus' have been suggested, HHV-6-associated childhood encephalitis cases can occasionally be fatal. The complications previously associated solely with HHV-6 rash are also found in HHV-6 infant fever without rash, and thus up to 90% of symptomatic HHV-6 infections may be undiagnosed or unrecognized.

Immunocompromised People

Solid organ transplantation

Owing to efficient and widespread early childhood transmission of HHV-6 and HHV-7, infections in the adult are primarily reactivations of latent virus, particularly in immunocompromised people such as transplantation patients. Where monitored, co-infections with HCMV present with more severe pathology ('CMV disease'), with a subgroup of delayed graft rejections in liver or kidney transplantation patients. HHV-6-linked encephalitis has occasionally been recorded in these patients, and also in cardiac and heart/lung transplantation patients. Immune suppression using monoclonal antibody to CD3 enhances HHV-6 reactivation and CMV disease; this treatment can also enhance HHV-6 replication *in vitro*. Where symptomatic correlates have been made, HCMV has a greater influence than HHV-6, and HHV-6 has a greater effect than HHV-7. Anecdotal correlates of HHV-6 infection in this context include fever, rash, pneumonitis, encephalitis, hepatitis, and bone marrow suppression. However, it is rare that HCMV reactivates in an HHV-6- or HHV-7-negative patient, as HHV-6 usually reactivates first, then HHV-7 concurrent with HCMV. Thus CMV disease is usually contingent on roseolovirus reactivation. An immunomodulatory role has been presented for HHV-6 reactivations that correlate with increased opportunistic infections, including those associated with HCMV and fungi. Occasional primary infections in the adult have been observed in rare HHV-6- or HHV-7-naive patients who become infected via the donor organ and experience more severe symptoms.

Bone marrow and hematopoietic stem cell transplantation

HHV-6 reactivation is associated with disease in BMT and hematopoietic or cord blood stem cell transplantation (SCT). HHV-6B predominates in Europe and the USA, where typing has been done, reflecting the prevalence of this variant in primary infections of children there. Half of the patients have HHV-6 reactivations 2–4 weeks post-transplantation, with both direct and indirect immunomodulatory effects. Direct effects of reactivation can lead to HHV-6-associated encephalitis and reduced outgrowth of progenitor lineages, called 'bone marrow suppression' or stem cell inhibition. Indirect immunomodulatory effects leading to HCMV reactivation have also been recorded. The presence of virus DNA in the blood has been demonstrated by quantitative PCR, prior to encephalitis or CNS disease developing by 2–3 weeks post-transplantation. The highest levels were shown for cord blood SCT. Retrospective studies have shown that both HHV-6 reactivation and the use of monoclonal antibody to CD3 are independent risk factors for the development of encephalitis. Amnesia, delirium, or 'confusion' following HHV-6 reactivation have been reported, with estimates of 40% mortality for HHV-6-linked encephalitis in SCT patients. Further investigations are required, and should include possible complications in future stem cell therapy; prospective studies are underway to assess neurological involvement in BMT and SCT.

HIV/AIDS

Like HIV, both HHV-6 and HHV-7 can infect and kill or remain latent in CD4+ T-lymphocytes as well as monocytic/macrophage cells. In addition to direct effects via reactivation of HHV-6 and HHV-7, there may also be indirect interactions between these viruses. As the CD4 count in blood decreases with AIDS progression, so does detection of HHV-6 and HHV-7. However, in studies of disseminated reactivated infections, increased levels of HHV-6 DNA in various organs correlate with higher levels of HIV, suggesting interactions during AIDS progression. HHV-6 reactivations have been identified with HIV in lymph nodes, and have been associated with the early phases of lymphadenopathy syndrome. Individual case studies have recorded HHV-6A-associated fatalities in HIV/AIDS patients from pneumonitis and encephalitis. Furthermore, HHV-6-associated retinitis (on its own or in association with HCMV) has been identified in HIV/AIDS patients. However, the use of antiretroviral therapy in some countries has restored immune control of opportunistic infections such as HCMV, and probably HHV-6 and HHV-7.

Studies *in vitro* and in animal models point to possible mechanisms of interaction between HIV and HHV-6. HHV-6A has been shown to reactivate HIV from latency in monocytes *in vitro*. Ongoing studies of HHV-6A coinfection with simian immunodeficiency virus (SIV) in monkey models show enhanced disease. HHV-7 binds to CD4 and can compete with HIV *in vitro* for interaction with this receptor, and so inhibit infection. HHV-6A can induce CD4, thus enhancing infection with HIV in

different cell types *in vitro*, whereas HHV-6A chemokine U83A can bind to CCR5, the HIV co-receptor, and inhibit infection. However, the HHV-6A U51 vCCR can bind, sequester, and downregulate the CCR5 ligand and the HIV-1 inhibitor, Rantes/CCL5, and thus enhance HIV-1 infection. Expression of the other HIV-1 co-receptor, CXCR4, is downregulated by HHV-6 infection and may inhibit progression. Thus, complex interactions between HIV-1 and HHV-6 may either inhibit or enhance HIV-1, depending on virus strain, specific gene expression, cell type, and stage of the lytic/latent life cycle.

Neuroinflammatory Disease and Persistence in the Brain

HHV-6 and HHV-7 have been identified as commensals in the brain, with latent or persistent infection in the CNS, and it is a major challenge to distinguish these silent infections from any locally activated ones associated with neurological disease. This problem is further complicated by the rare occurrence of germline integration of HHV-6A or HHV-6B as noted above. In studies of postmortem brain samples, HHV-6 has been identified more frequently than HHV-7 (*c.* 40% compared to 5%). Where genotyped, 75% of the HHV-6 was HHV-6B, reflecting the greater prevalence of this variant in childhood infections in the populations studied (China and the UK).

In the case of encephalitis, most data concern HHV-6, where active infections have been detected by a combination of identifying virus DNA in the CSF and sera and, where biopsies are available, by *in situ* hybridization in order to detect expression of lytic genes in various temporal classes. RT-PCR of virus RNA in blood may also identify specific viremia, but may often miss relevant localized reactivations in the CNS. Encephalitis associated with HHV-6A and HHV-6B has been identified as a rare complication during primary infection in childhood, and in adults. As described above, SCT and BMT patients are at most risk, since frequent HHV-6 infection/reactivation is linked with life-threatening HHV-6-associated encephalitis; further prospective studies are required.

Links with other neurological conditions have been described, including that of HHV-6B with 'status epilepticus' noted above, and prospective studies are underway. Evidence for active lesions associated with mesial temporal lobe specific regions of the brain, particularly the hippocampus, has been presented and evaluated for links with mesial temporal lobe epilepsy. Interestingly, this region of the brain is also associated with memory, and virus reactivation here may correlate with observations of amnestic periods linked with HHV-6 reactivations in some SCT and BMT patients. Neurological symptoms associated particularly with HHV-6A reactivations have also been linked with subsets of chronic fatigue syndrome patients (and in some cases termed HHV-6A encephalopathy), but the data are conflicting and prompt further studies.

Multiple sclerosis

Roseoloviruses have also been linked with a subset of MS patients, in particular the active HHV-6A infections in a subset of the relapsing remitting form of the disease, and in some studies they have been correlated with exacerbations. These HHV-6A infections occur in countries where the most prevalent childhood infections would be HHV-6B, although there are also some data for multiple reactivations along with HHV-6B or HHV-7. Thus, HHV-6A infections linked with MS could represent rare primary infections occurring during adulthood with this more neurotropic variant. Alternatively, an underlying condition may permit infection with multiple strains.

There is some evidence supporting mechanisms that link HHV-6 with MS. In one study, T-cells from MS patients had lower frequencies of activity against the immunodominant HHV-6 p101 (or pp100) protein (U11), suggesting defects in virus clearance. Furthermore, in situ hybridization and immunostaining of biopsy material from MS lesions showed the presence of HHV-6 DNA in oligodendrocytes, lymphocytes, and microglia, plus antigen expression in astrocytes and microglia. Studies on an oligodendrocyte cell line showed some productive infection with HHV-6A but abortive infection with HHV-6B; similar results were found using progenitor-derived astrocytes. In vitro studies on glial precursor cell infection by HHV-6 suggest that early virus proteins act in cell cycle arrest, thus inhibiting differentiation to the myelin-producing oligodendrocytes essential for repair of demyelination. In a study conducted in the USA, β-interferon treatment of MS patients resulted in lower amounts of detectable HHV-6 in sera. β-interferon also inhibited growth of HHV-6 cell culture. It has been suggested that tests with antiviral agents such as ganciclovir (GCV) will be required to examine the role of HHV-6 in MS. This will require careful selection of patients and use of appropriate controls, particularly if HHV-6 contributes only to a subsection of this disease.

Immune Response, Diagnosis, and Control

Protective Immunity

In immunocompetent people, HHV-6 and HHV-7 infections give rise to lifelong protective immunity. However, subsequent infections with multiple strains, either HHV-6A or HHV-6B, have been recorded even during early primary infection, with milder or no symptoms. Prior infection with HHV-6 does not prevent infection with HHV-7, but it may provide some cross-protective immunity.

Neutralizing antibodies can be generated after primary infection. Targets include gB as well as the gH/gL/gQ complex. As with other infections, not all antibodies are neutralizing, and thus high serological titers do not always correspond to protection against infection.

Cellular immunity also develops in response to these infections. It is usually HHV-6- or HHV-7-specific, but sometimes cross-reactive. HHV-6- or HHV-7-specific CD4+ T- and NK-cell clones have been isolated, as well HHV-6 antigen-specific clones to p101. Thus, efficient cellular immunity develops after infection, and immunomodulation of lymphoid and myeloid cells may contribute to a possible strategy for effective persistence.

Control

Compounds with activity specifically against HHV-6 are not available and require development. However, HHV-6 and HHV-7 share with HCMV genes encoding proteins involved in replication, and these serve as targets for certain antiviral compounds. Thus, many drugs that are active against HCMV and other herpesviruses also show some activity against HHV-6 and HHV-7. These include GCV, foscarnet, and cidofovir. Acyclovir, which is used to treat alphaherpesvirus, and sometimes gammaherpesvirus, infections, is not effective in vitro against HHV-6 or HHV-7, as these viruses do not have the thymidine kinase gene required for activity. The oral prodrug form of GCV (valganciclovir, vGCV) has some anecdotal efficacy during virus reactivations in BMT patients, but is not as efficacious as it is with HCMV, and some HHV-6 or HHV-7 antigenemia can still be observed after vGCV prophylaxis. However, as for HCMV, HHV-6 GCV-escape mutants have been observed in vivo in transplantation patients, indicating that there is some efficacy against virus replication. Mutations occur in gene U69, which encodes the homolog of the HCMV GCV kinase (GCK), or in gene U38, which encodes the DNA polymerase (POL). In vitro, the HHV-6 GCK is tenfold less active than that of HCMV, which perhaps explains the differences in response between these two betaherpesviruses. Prospective clinical trials are required to demonstrate clinical efficacy in vivo, and are underway with vGCV for herpesvirus-associated CNS disease.

Acknowledgments

The author is grateful for support from the Biotechnology and Biological Sciences Research Council (BBSRC, UK) and the Bill and Melinda Gates Foundation.

See also: Herpesviruses: General Features; Human Cytomegalovirus: General Features; Human Eye Infections.

Further Reading

DeBolle L, Michel D, Mertens T, *et al.* (2002) Role of the human herpesvirus 6 U69-encoded kinase in the phosphorylation of ganciclovir. *Molecular Pharmacology* 62: 714–721.

Dewin DR, Catusse J, and Gompels UA (2006) Identification and characterization of U83A viral chemokine, a broad and potent beta-chemokine agonist for human CCRs with unique selectivity and inhibition by spliced isoform. *Journal of Immunology* 176: 544–556.

Dietrich J, Blumberg BM, Roshal M, *et al.* (2004) Infection with an endemic human herpesvirus disrupts critical glial precursor cell properties. *Journal of Neuroscience* 24: 4875–4883.

Dominguez G, Dambaugh TR, Stamey FR, Dewhurst S, Inoue N, and Pellett PE (1999) Human herpesvirus 6B genome sequence: Coding content and comparison with human herpesvirus 6A. *Journal of Virology* 73: 8040–8052.

Fotheringham J, Akhyani N, Vortmeyer A, *et al.* (2007) Detection of active human herpesvirus-6 infection in the brain: Correlation with polymerase chain reaction detection in cerebrospinal fluid. *Journal of Infectious Diseases* 195: 450–454.

Gompels UA (2004) Roseoloviruses: Human herpesviruses 6 and 7. In: Zuckerman AJ, Banatvala JE, Pattison JR, Griffiths PD, and Schoub BD (eds.) *Principles and Practice of Clinical Virology,* 5th edn., pp. 147–168. Chichester, UK: Wiley.

Gompels UA and Kasolo FC (2006) HHV-6 genome: Similar and different. In: Krueger G and Ablashi D (eds.) *Perspectives in Medical Virology, Vol. 12: Human Herpesvirus-6,* 2nd edn., pp. 23–46. Elsevier: New York.

Gompels UA, Nicholas J, Lawrence G, *et al.* (1995) The DNA sequence of human herpesvirus-6: Structure, coding content, and genome evolution. *Virology* 209: 29–51.

Goodman AD, Mock DJ, Powers JM, Baker JV, and Blumberg BM (2003) Human herpesvirus 6 genome and antigen in acute multiple sclerosis lesions. *Journal of Infectious Diseases* 187: 1365–1376.

Hall CB, Caserta MT, Schnabel KC, *et al.* (2006) Characteristics and acquisition of human herpesvirus (HHV)-7 infections in relation to infection with HHV-6. *Journal of Infectious Diseases* 193: 1063–1069.

Hall CB, Long CE, Schnabel KC, *et al.* (1994) Human herpesvirus-6 infection in children: A prospective study of complications and reactivation. *New England Journal of Medicine* 331: 432–438.

Isegawa Y, Mukai T, Nakano K, *et al.* (1999) Comparison of the complete DNA sequences of human herpesvirus 6 variants A and B. *Journal of Virology* 73: 8053–8063.

Ward KN, Leong HN, Thiruchelvam AD, Atkinson CE, and Clark DA (2007) Human herpesvirus 6 DNA levels in cerebrospinal fluid due to primary infection differ from those due to chromosomal viral integration and have implications for diagnosis of encephalitis. *Journal of Clinical Microbiology* 45: 1298–1304.

Zerr DM, Corey L, Kim HW, Huang ML, Nguy L, and Boeckh M (2005) Clinical outcomes of human herpesvirus 6 reactivation after hematopoietic stem cell transplantation. *Clinical Infectious Diseases* 40: 932–940.

Zerr DM, Meier AS, Selke SS, *et al.* (2005) A population-based study of primary human herpesvirus 6 infection. *New England Journal of Medicine* 352: 768–776.

Human Respiratory Syncytial Virus

P L Collins, National Institute of Allergy and Infectious Diseases, Bethesda, MD, USA

Published by Elsevier Ltd.

Glossary

Fractalkine The sole known CX3C cytokine. It is present as a membrane-bound form that is upregulated by inflammation and promotes adhesion of monocytes and lymphocytes and as a secreted form that promotes chemotaxis of monocytes and lymphyocytes.

Furin A subtilisin-like cellular endoprotease present in the exocytic pathway with the consensus cleavage sequence Arg-X-Arg/Lys-Arg↓.

Glycosaminoglycan Long, unbranched, highly negatively charged polysaccharides that consist of repeating disaccharide subunits and are located on the cell surface or in the extracellular matrix.

Humanized antibody Substitution, by recombinant DNA techniques, of the antigen binding sequences of a nonhuman antibody molecule into the backbone of a human antibody molecule.

Mucin A family of large, heavily glycosylated, secreted or transmembrane proteins that form a protective barrier on the respiratory, gastrointestinal, and reproductive tracts.

Polylactosaminoglycan Carbohydrate of unknown function formed in the Golgi apparatus by the addition of a variable number of repeating units of lactosamine (galactose-β-1,4-N-acetylglucosamine-β-1,3) to an N-linked core oligosaccharide.

Rhinorrhea Runny nose.

Ribavirin A nucleoside analog (1-β-D-ribofuranosyl-1,2,4-triazole-3-carboxamide) that has antiviral activity against a number of RNA viruses.

Syncytium A multinucleated cell, formed in the case of human respiratory syncytial virus by fusion of the plasma membrane of an infected cell with those of its neighbors.

Tachykinin A family of biologically active peptides (prototype, substance P) that can be potent vasodilators and can induce smooth muscle contraction directly or indirectly.

History

Human respiratory syncytial virus (HRSV) was first isolated in 1956 from a laboratory chimpanzee with upper respiratory tract disease. Shortly thereafter, an apparently identical virus was recovered from two children ill with pneumonia or croup and was identified as a human virus. HRSV quickly became recognized as the leading viral agent of pediatric respiratory tract disease worldwide. It has also gained recognition as a significant cause of morbidity and mortality in the elderly and severely immunocompromised individuals. Its inefficient growth in cell culture and propensity to easily lose infectivity due to physical instability impede research. HRSV lacks an approved vaccine or clinically effective antiviral therapy, although, as described below, passive immunoprophylaxis is available for infants at high risk for serious HRSV disease.

Classification

HRSV is a member of family *Paramyxoviridae* of order *Mononegavirales*, the nonsegmented negative-strand RNA viruses. *Paramyxoviridae* has two subfamilies: (1) subfamily *Paramyxovirinae* contains five genera whose members include Sendai virus, the human parainfluenza viruses (HPIVs), and mumps and measles viruses among others; and (2) subfamily *Pneumovirinae* contains genus *Metapneumovirus*, which includes avian and human metapneumoviruses, and genus *Pneumovirus*, which includes HRSV, bovine respiratory syncytial virus (BRSV), ovine respiratory syncytial virus (RSV), and pneumonia virus of mice (PVM). **Figure 1(a)** compares gene maps of the two genera of *Pneumovirinae* with those of a representative genus (*Respirovirus*) of *Paramyxovirinae*. **Figure 1(b)** illustrates the relatedness among members of the two genera of *Pneumovirinae* based on the nucleotide sequence of the N gene. HRSV is most closely related to BRSV. One might speculate that HRSV originally emerged in the past from infection of humans with BRSV-like virus.

Virion Structure and Viral Proteins

HRSV virions consist of spherical particles of 80–350 nm in diameter and filamentous particles that are 60–200 nm in diameter and up to 10 μm in length (**Figure 2**).

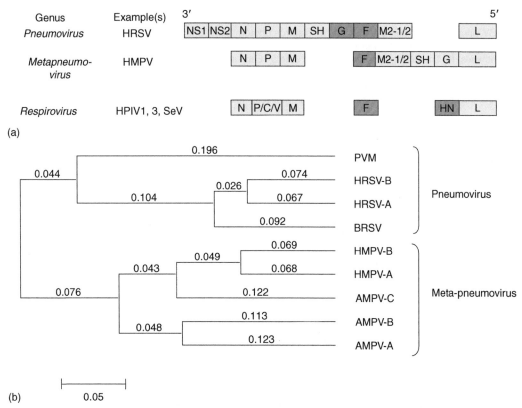

Figure 1 Comparison of human respiratory syncytial virus (HRSV) with other selected members of family *Paramyxoviridae*. (a) Alignment of the gene maps of HRSV, human metapneumovirus (HMPV), human parainfluenza virus (HPIV) types 1 and 3, and Sendai virus (SeV). (b) Relationships among the members of the two genera of subfamily *Pneumovirinae* based on the nucleotide sequence of the N gene. The scale bar represents approximately 5% nucleotide difference between pairs.

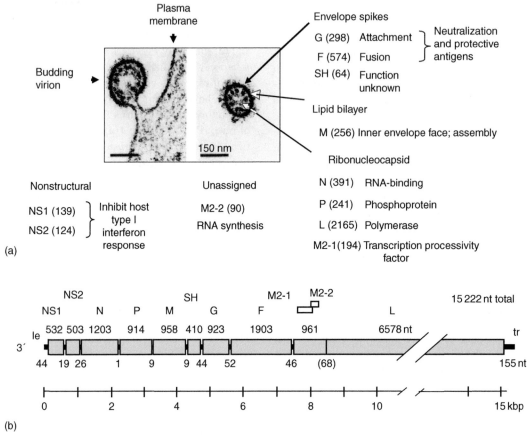

Figure 2 HRSV virion, proteins, and genome. (a) The electron photomicrographs illustrate an RSV virion budding from the plasma membrane of an infected cell (left) and a free virion (right). The viral proteins are indicated, with the amino acid length of the unmodified protein in parentheses. (b) The RNA genome is illustrated 3′ to 5′. Each large rectangle indicates a gene that is transcribed into a separate mRNA, with the gene nucleotide length shown above. The overlapping open reading frames of the M2 gene are indicated. The nucleotide lengths of the extragenic leader (le), intergenic, and trailer (tr) regions are shown underneath. The overlap between the M2 and L genes is indicated by its nucleotide length in parentheses. Nucleotide and amino acid lengths are for strain A2.

Filaments appear to be the predominant form produced in cell culture. The virion contains a helical nucleocapsid (diameter 12–15 nm compared to 18 nm for *Paramyxovirinae*) packaged in a lipoprotein envelope acquired from the host cell plasma membrane during budding. The outer surface of the envelope contains a fringe of surface projections or spikes of 11–12 nm. HRSV lacks a hemagglutinin or neuraminidase.

HRSV encodes 11 proteins. Four are associated with the nucleocapsid: the major nucleocapsid protein N (56 kDa), the nucleocapsid phosphoprotein P (33 kDa), the transcription processivity factor M2-1 (22 kDa), and the large L protein (250 kDa). The N protein binds tightly along the entire length of genomic RNA as well as its positive-sense replicative intermediate that is called the antigenome. L is the major polymerase subunit containing the catalytic domains. P is thought to associate with free N and L to maintain them in soluble form for association with the nucleocapsid and probably also participates as a cofactor in RNA synthesis. N, P, and L are the viral proteins that are necessary and sufficient to direct RNA replication. They also direct transcription, but this is poorly processive unless the M2-1 protein is also present.

There are three transmembrane viral glycoproteins that are expressed on the surface of infected cells and are packaged in the virion: the large G glycoprotein (90 kDa), the fusion F glycoprotein (70 kDa), and the small hydrophobic SH protein (7.5–60 kDa, depending on the amount of added carbohydrate). These assemble separately into homo-oligomers that constitute the surface spikes: F assembles into trimers, G assembles into trimers or tetramers, and SH has been detected as a pentamer.

The G glycoprotein mediates viral attachment. It is a type II glycoprotein: there is a signal/anchor sequence near the N-terminus, with the C-terminal two-thirds of the molecule oriented extracellularly. G is heavily glycosylated, with several N-linked carbohydrate side chains and an estimated 24–25 O-linked side chains. The unglycosylated protein has an M_r of 32 500 compared to 90 000 for the mature protein. Most of the ectodomain is thought to have an extended, heavily glycosylated, mucin-like structure. In the middle of the ectodomain there is a predicted disulfide-linked tight turn (cystine noose) in the secondary structure. The cystine noose is overlapped on its N-terminal end by a 13-amino-acid conserved sequence of unknown significance and on its C-terminal end by a C–X3–C motif that it is embedded in a region of limited sequence relatedness with the CX3C chemokine fractalkine. A synthetic peptide containing this sequence has fractalkine-like chemotactic activity *in vitro*. The role of this apparent chemokine mimicry in the biology of HRSV is unclear. The tight turn, the conserved domain, and the fractalkine domain can be deleted from recombinant HRSV without significantly reducing its replication efficiency in cell culture or in the respiratory tract of mice. Thus, the region of G that is necessary for attachment has not been identified.

The F glycoprotein mediates cell-surface membrane fusion, which is responsible for delivering the viral nucleocapsid to the cytoplasm. In addition, F expressed at the cell surface mediates fusion of infected cells with their neighbors, resulting in the formation of syncytia. F is a type I glycoprotein, with an N-terminal cleaved signal anchor and a C-proximal membrane anchor. It has four or five N-linked carbohydrate side chains. F is synthesized as a precursor, F_0, which is cleaved intracellularly at two sites (amino acids 109/110 and 136/137) by a furin-like cellular protease. This yields the following fragments, in N- to C-terminal order: F_2 (109 amino acids), p27 (27 amino acids), and F_1 (438 amino acids). F_2 and F_1 remain linked by a disulfide bond and represent the active form of F. In BRSV, the p27 fragment has tachykinin activity and may play a role in promoting inflammation, but p27 of HRSV does not resemble a tachykinin.

The function of the SH glycoprotein is not known. Molecular modeling suggests that it might be an ion-channel-forming protein, although the significance of this to HRSV biology is unclear. SH is anchored in the membrane by a centrally located signal/anchor sequence, with the N-terminus oriented intracellularly and the C-terminus extracellularly. A portion of SH present intracellularly and in virions is unglycosylated (M_r 7500), a portion has a single N-linked side chain (M_r 13 000–15 000), and a portion has the further modification of polylactosaminoglycan added to the N-linked sugar (M_r 21 000–60 000 or more). This multiplicity of forms is conserved in *Pneumovirinae* but its significance is unknown.

Remarkably, the G and SH genes can be deleted individually or in combination from viable HRSV. Deletion of SH does not reduce the efficiency of replication in cell culture and has only a modest attenuating effect on replication in mice, chimpanzees, or humans (the last observation is based on trials of experimental live vaccines). Deletion of G was attenuating in HEp-2 cells but not Vero cells, and was highly attenuating in mice and humans. Since SH and G are dispensable, at least in cell

culture, it is thought that F can function as an alternative attachment protein in that setting.

The nonglycosylated M protein is thought to be located on the inner surface of the envelope and to have a central role in organizing the envelope and directing packaging of the nucleocapsid.

The M2-2 protein is expressed at a low level and its status as structural or nonstructural is unknown. Recombinant HRSV from which the M2-2 coding sequence was deleted replicates more slowly than wild-type HRSV in cell culture and is attenuated *in vivo*. This deletion virus exhibits an increase in transcription and a decrease in RNA replication, suggesting that M2-2 normally is involved in downregulating transcription and upregulating RNA replication.

NS1 and NS2 are small proteins and do not appear to be packaged significantly in the virion. Both proteins inhibit the host interferon response. NS1, and to a lesser extent NS2, inhibit the induction of interferon α/β by blocking activation of interferon regulatory factor 3. In addition, NS2, and to a lesser extent NS1, inhibit interferon α/β-induced signaling through the Janus kinases/ signal transducers and activators of transcription (JAK/STAT) pathway, thus inhibiting the amplification of the interferon response, the upregulation of interferon-stimulated genes, and the development of the antiviral state. This appears to involve enhanced degradation of STAT2. Deletion of NS1 and NS2 individually or in combination yields viable viruses that replicate almost as efficiently as wild-type HRSV in cells that do not make interferon, but which are attenuated in interferon-competent cultured cells and *in vivo*.

Genome Organization, Transcription, and Replication

The HRSV genome is a single negative-sense strand of RNA that ranges in length from 15 191 to 15 226 nt for the strains that have been sequenced to date (**Figure 2(b)**). Its organization, expression, and replication follow the general pattern of *Mononegavirales*. The genome is neither capped nor polyadenylated. It is tightly encapsidated with N protein both in the virion and intracellularly. Based on the prototype A2 strain, the genomic RNA has a 44 nt 3'-extragenic leader at the 3' end. This is followed in order by the NS1, NS2, N, P, M, SH, G, F, M2, and L genes. The L gene is followed by a 155 nt extragenic trailer region that comprises the 5' end. The first nine genes are separated by intergenic regions of 1–52 nt. The last gene, L, initiates within the downstream nontranslated region of the M2 gene, and thus these two genes overlap by 68 nt.

In transcription, the viral polymerase initiates at a single promoter at the 3' end of the genome and copies the genes by a sequential stop–start mechanism that yields subgenomic mRNAs. The upstream and downstream boundaries of each gene contain transcription signals: the upstream end consists of a conserved 10 nt gene-start motif that directs transcriptional initiation, and the downstream end consists of a moderately conserved 12–13 nt gene-end motif that directs termination and polyadenylation. The intergenic regions appear to lack any conserved motifs and seem to be nonspecific spacers. Between genes, the majority of polymerase remains template-bound and scans for the next gene. However, some polymerase dissociates from the template during transcription, yielding a polar gradient such that upstream genes are expressed more efficiently than downstream ones.

The HRSV mRNAs contain a virally synthesized $5'$ cap [$m^7G(5')ppp(5')Gp$] and a $3'$ polyadenylate tail. The latter is produced by reiterative copying by the viral polymerase on a tract of 4–7 U residues at the downstream end of each gene-end signal. Each mRNA encodes a single major viral protein except for the M2 mRNA, which contains two open reading frames (ORFs) that overlap by approximately 32 nt and encode two distinct proteins, M2-1 and M2-2 (**Figure 2(b)**). Expression of the downstream M2-2 ORF appears to be coupled to translation of the upstream M2-1 ORF and presumably involves a ribosomal stop–restart mechanism.

In RNA replication, the viral polymerase initiates in the same promoter region and ignores the gene-start and gene-end signals to make a full-length positive-sense copy called the antigenome. The antigenome is neither capped nor polyadenylated. It is tightly encapsidated with N protein and serves as the template for the synthesis of progeny genomes.

The first 11 nt at the $3'$ end of the viral genome are essential for both transcription and RNA replication. The two processes involve overlapping sets of residues. For replication, nucleotides 16–32 are required in addition for encapsidation and the synthesis of complete antigenome. For transcription, nucleotides 36–43 are required in addition for full activity. The first 24 nt at the $3'$ end of the antigenome have 81% sequence identity with the $3'$ end of the genome, indicative of a conserved promoter element.

Viral Infection in Cell Culture and Experimental Animals

HRSV can infect and produce virus, with varying degrees of efficiency, in a surprisingly wide array of cell lines from various tissues and hosts. Replication is most efficient in epithelial cells, in particular the human HEp-2 line. HRSV that has been propagated *in vitro* generally retains its virulence.

Efficient infection by HRSV of established cell lines *in vitro* involves binding to cellular glycosaminoglycans, in particular heparan sulfate and chondroitin sulfate. Both G and F can mediate this binding. It is not known whether this represents attachment in total or whether it is an initial interaction that is followed by a second, higher-affinity step that remains to be identified. It is also not known how closely this mirrors the attachment process *in vivo*.

All events in HRSV infection occur in the cytoplasm. Viral mRNAs and proteins can be detected intracellularly by 4–6 h post infection. The accumulation of mRNAs has been reported to plateau by 14–18 h. This apparent shut-off of transcription might be due to accumulation of the M2-2 regulatory factor, since it does not appear to occur when the M2-2 coding sequence has been deleted. Apart from this, there is no apparent temporal regulation of gene expression. The release of progeny virus begins by 10–12 h, reaches a peak after 24 h, and continues until the cells deteriorate by 30–48 h. Although most of the infected cells in the culture are killed, persistent infections *in vitro* can readily be established.

In an *in vitro* model of human airway epithelium, HRSV infection was strictly limited to ciliated cells of the apical surface. Remarkably, HRSV infection caused little gross cytopathic effect despite ongoing infection over several weeks. In particular, infection did not result in the formation of syncytia. The expression of the F protein was polarized to the apical surface, which might have prevented contact with neighboring cells and might explain the lack of syncytia. Thus, HRSV is not inherently a highly cytopathic virus in the absence of syncytia formation, and much of the damage to infected cells that occurs *in vivo* might be a consequence of immune attack rather than direct viral effects. HRSV infection causes a modest reduction in cellular DNA, RNA, and protein synthesis. Apoptosis does not occur until late in infection. The virus buds at the plasma membrane. In polarized cells, this occurs at the apical surface.

HRSV does not replicate to high titer *in vitro*. Most of the virus remains cell associated and is released by freeze–thawing or sonication. HRSV can rapidly lose infectivity during unfrozen storage or freeze–thawing. Stability can be improved by adjusting the harvested culture supernatants to pH 7.5 and 0.1 M magnesium sulfate, or by including 15% w/v sucrose. The yield of virus is relatively low: 10 PFU per cell is typical. Most of the infectious particles produced *in vitro* were trapped by a 0.45 μm filter, suggesting that the infectious unit is in the form of large filaments or aggregates. The instability and size heterogeneity of the virus produced *in vitro* makes purification and concentration difficult.

The most permissive hosts for HRSV are the human and the chimpanzee, and these are the only hosts in which respiratory tract disease can reliably be observed. HRSV can also replicate in the respiratory tract of several species of monkey as well as in hamsters, guinea pigs, infant ferrets, cotton rats, and mice. However, infection in these animals is only semipermissive, particularly in the case of rodents. In the BALB/c mouse, the most commonly used experimental model, intranasal infection with 10^6 PFU yields only 10^6 PFU in lungs harvested at the peak of virus replication 4 days post infection.

Genetics

Like RNA viruses in general, HRSV has a high misincorporation rate (approximately one substitution in 10^4 nt), providing the potential for diversity. RNA recombination involving exchange between viruses appears to be exceedingly rare. Defective interfering particles presumably occur but have not been described molecularly.

Negative-sense RNA is not directly infectious alone. However, as for *Mononegavirales* in general, complete infectious recombinant virus can be produced entirely from cloned cDNAs (reverse genetics). This involves transfecting cells with plasmids that express a complete antigenomic RNA and the proteins of the nucleocapsid, which in the case of HRSV are the N, P, M2-1, and L proteins. These components assemble (inefficiently) into a nucleocapsid that initiates a productive infection. This method can be used to introduce desired changes into infectious virus via the cDNA intermediate.

Another system that has been very useful for basic studies involves helper-dependent mini-replicons. These are short, internally truncated versions of genomic or antigenomic RNA in which the viral genes have been replaced by one or more reporter genes under the control of HRSV transcription signals. When complemented by the appropriate mix of plasmid-encoded HRSV proteins, a mini-replicon can be encapsidated, transcribed, replicated, and packaged into virus-like particles. The small size and simplicity of a mini-replicon makes it ideal for detailed structure–function studies.

Antigens and Antigenic Subgroups

The F and G proteins are the only known HRSV neutralization antigens. They have markedly different antigenic properties. Many of the available F-specific monoclonal antibodies (MAb's) efficiently neutralize HRSV *in vitro*, whereas most of those for G neutralize weakly or not at all. However, polyclonal antibodies specific to G neutralize infectivity efficiently. The high content of O-linked carbohydrate in the G protein may be a factor in its unusual antigenic properties, and indeed the sugars have been shown to be important, directly or indirectly, in the binding of many, but not all, MAb's. The sugar side chains might mask the viral polypeptide. In addition, microheterogeneity might exist in the placement and composition of the side chains, which might alter or mask epitopes. In seropositive humans, most of the HRSV proteins have been shown to stimulate HRSV-specific memory CD8+ T lymphocytes.

HRSV has a single serotype. However, isolates can be segregated into two antigenic subgroups A and B. These exhibit a fourfold difference in cross-neutralization *in vitro* by postinfection sera. Epitopes in F tend to be conserved whereas those for G are not, such that antigenic relatedness between the two subgroups is greater than 50% for the F protein compared to only 5% or less for G. At the amino acid level, F is 89% identical between subgroups while G is the most divergent of the proteins and is only 53% identical, with most of the diversity occurring in the ectodomain. Other proteins range from 76% (SH) to 96% identical (N). Thus, the two antigenic subgroups have substantial differences throughout the genome and represent two divergent lines of evolution, as opposed to differing at only a few antigenic sites.

In a 2 year window following infection, there was a 64% reduction in the incidence of infection by the same subgroup versus a 16% reduction against the heterologous subgroup. In epidemics, typically, there is an alternating pattern with a 1–2 year interval with regard to the predominant subgroup. These observations indicate that antigenic dimorphism contributes to the ability of HRSV to reinfect, although its effect is modest rather than absolute.

Viral isolates obtained over successive years or decades exhibit some evidence of progressive amino acid changes and some changes in reactivity detectable with MAb's. However, all isolates retained a high level of antigenic relatedness and thus HRSV did not exhibit significant antigenic drift during this time frame.

Epidemiology and Clinical Factors

HRSV is the most important cause of serious viral respiratory tract disease in the pediatric population worldwide. In many areas it outranks all other microbial pathogens as a cause of bronchiolitis and pneumonia in infants less than 1 year of age. HRSV is conservatively estimated to cause 64 million infections and 160 000 deaths annually in the pediatric population. In the United States, HRSV is estimated to account for 73 400–126 300 hospitalizations annually for bronchiolitis and pneumonia in children of under 1 year of age, and is responsible for 90–1900 pediatric deaths annually. Hospitalization rates in developed countries are approximately one in 100–200 infections.

In a 13 year study of infants and children in the United States, HRSV was detected in 43%, 25%, 11%, and 10% of those hospitalized for bronchiolitis, pneumonia, bronchitis, and croup, respectively, and in aggregate accounted for 23% of pediatric hospitalizations for respiratory tract disease as a conservative estimate. Middle ear infection is a common complication. As another complication, approximately 40–50% of infants hospitalized with HRSV bronchiolitis have subsequent episodes of wheezing during childhood. HRSV infection also can exacerbate asthma.

Infection and reinfection with HRSV are frequent during the first years of life. Sixty to seventy percent of infants and children are infected by HRSV during the first year of life. The peak of serious disease is approximately 1–2 months of age (**Figure 3**). By age 2, 90% of children have been infected once with HRSV and 50% have been infected twice. The greatest incidence of serious disease occurs between 6 weeks and 6 months of age. Maternal antibodies account for the relative sparing of newborns. The major risk factors for serious HRSV disease in the pediatric population include chronic lung disease, congenital heart disease, prematurity, and young age (<6 months). While underlying disease is an important risk factor, the majority of infants hospitalized for HRSV disease were previously healthy.

Reinfection of older children and adults is common. For example, hospital staff members on pediatric wards have an infection rate of 25–50% during HRSV epidemics. Healthy individuals usually suffer only a common cold syndrome. However, HRSV is also an important cause of morbidity and mortality in the elderly, with an impact that is estimated to approach that of nonpandemic influenza virus. HRSV has been estimated to cause 17 000 deaths annually in the elderly in the United States. HRSV infection is also associated with a high mortality rate in children and adults with immunodeficiency or immunosuppression, particularly hematopoietic cell transplant recipients.

HRSV is highly contagious and is readily spread in day-care settings, to family members, in nursing homes, and in the hospital. Spread involves close contact and inoculation of conjunctival or mucosal surfaces by large droplets or by contaminated hands or objects. In experimental infections, HRSV had an incubation period of 4–5 days. Virus typically is shed for 7–12 days coincident with clinical disease, although sometimes shedding is longer and can continue after recovery.

Most primary infections are symptomatic, with upper respiratory tract disease and sometimes a fever. Twenty-five to forty percent of primary infections progress to the lower respiratory tract with the primary manifestations of serious disease being bronchiolitis or pneumonia. There is profuse rhinorrhea, coughing, intermittent fever, expiratory wheezes, and, frequently, middle-ear disease. Seriously ill infants have increased coughing and wheezing, rapid respiration, and hypoxemia, requiring the administration of humidified oxygen.

HRSV causes yearly epidemics that are centered in the winter months in temperate climates (**Figure 4**) or in the rainy season in the tropics, although there can also be local variations to this pattern.

The most definitive diagnosis is by virus isolation in cell culture. Rapid diagnosis can be made by (1) detection of viral antigen using an antigen-capture enzyme-linked immunosorbent assay (ELISA) or by an immunofluorescence analysis of exfoliated cells with HRSV-specific antibody or (2) detection of nucleic acid by reverse transcriptase polymerase chain reaction (RT-PCR). The sensitivity of detection can be over 90%.

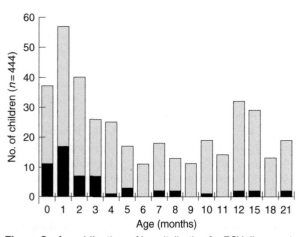

Figure 3 Age at the time of hospitalization for RSV disease at the Johns Hopkins Hospital during 1993–96. The filled bars indicate more severe disease. Adapted from Karron RA, Singleton RJ, Bulkow L, *et al.* (1999). Severe respiratory syncytial virus disease in Alaska native children. *Journal of Infectious Diseases* 180: 41–49.

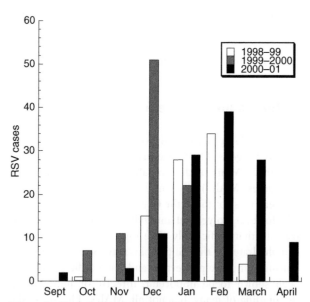

Figure 4 Variation in the timing of the RSV epidemic during three successive years at the Johns Hopkins Hospital. Unpublished data kindly provided by Karron RA, Johns Hopkins School of Hygiene and Public Health and School of Medicine.

Pathogenesis and Immunity

HRSV replicates primarily in the epithelial cells that line the lumen of the respiratory tract. It can also infect macrophages and dendritic cells and modify their functioning. Immunohistochemistry of airway tissues from infected individuals suggests a patchy distribution of infection, with only superficial cells expressing viral antigen. There is destruction of the epithelium and an influx of mononuclear cells, lymphocytes, plasma cells, and macrophages. Tissues become edematous and the secretion of mucus is excessive. Mucus, inflammatory cells, and debris from dead infected cells accumulate in the airways and can cause obstruction, which is a particular problem in infants due to the small diameter of their airways. With pneumonia, the alveolar spaces may fill with fluid and the interalveolar walls may thicken due to mononuclear cell infiltration.

HRSV is an acute infection that typically is completely cleared by host immunity, although sometimes shedding can persist for weeks. Studies in experimental animals and in the clinic indicate that virus-neutralizing secretory IgA antibodies, virus-neutralizing serum antibodies, and cytotoxic CD8+ T lymphocytes participate in resolving infection. These same effectors also confer protection against reinfection. Protection conferred by cytotoxic T lymphocytes appears to diminish within several weeks or months and thus is more important in the short term. Virus-neutralizing secretory IgA antibodies are particularly effective in restricting infection; this response is short-lived following primary infection but can increase in duration following reinfection. Virus-neutralizing serum antibodies provide long-lasting protection. However, they gain access to the respiratory lumen by the inefficient process of transudation, and thus protection is not efficient, particularly in the upper respiratory tract.

Perhaps the most important determinant of HRSV pathogenesis is its ability to infect young infants early in life despite the presence of maternal serum antibodies (**Figure 3**). Why HRSV seems more able than most other respiratory pathogens to evade maternal antibodies and infect very early in life is not understood. The fact that the virus can infect in early infancy when disease is less easily supported and airways are small and more easily obstructed probably accounts for much of its impact.

The immune response during the first months of life is reduced due to immunologic immaturity as well as the immunosuppressive effects of maternal antibodies on humoral responses. This probably contributes to difficulty in controlling the virus and facilitates reinfection early in life. The Th2-biased nature of immune responses in early infancy has also been speculated to contribute to HRSV disease and reduced immune responses. In addition, the tropism of HRSV to the superficial epithelium might reduce its exposure to immune effectors and might also provide reduced immune stimulation.

There is some evidence that HRSV might have suppressive effects on cell-mediated immunity, although the significance and magnitude of these effects are unclear. The cystine noose of the G protein has been shown to inhibit innate immune responses in human monocytes. The inefficiency of virus-neutralizing serum antibodies in controlling HRSV presumably is also a factor in its ability to reinfect throughout life.

Treatment and Immunoprophylaxis

Treatment of severe disease is largely supportive, including mechanical ventilation in the most severe cases. Ribavirin has potent antiviral activity in cell culture and experimental animals, but it has not been clearly beneficial clinically and is not routinely used in most hospitals. Anti-inflammatory therapies have not been beneficial to date but are still being investigated. Animal studies suggest a benefit of combining antiviral and anti-inflammatory therapies. Bronchodilators are commonly used but have, at most, modest benefits.

Passive immunoprophylaxis is available for infants who are at high risk for serious HRSV disease. This involves monthly intramuscular injections during the HRSV season of an HRSV-neutralizing MAb called palivizumab (Synagis), developed by MedImmune, Inc. This is a humanized version of a mouse MAb specific to the F protein.

A vaccine is not available. A major obstacle to developing a pediatric vaccine is that immunization ideally should start during the first weeks of life. As already noted, immune responses during the first few months of life are reduced due to immunologic immaturity and the immunosuppressive effects of maternal antibodies.

A vaccine consisting of formalin-inactivated, concentrated HRSV (FI-RSV) was evaluated in the 1960s. FI-RSV was found to be poorly protective and, unexpectedly, primed for immune-mediated enhanced HRSV disease that occurred on subsequent natural infection. In subsequent studies, FI-RSV was shown to induce antibodies that bound efficiently to viral antigen but did not efficiently neutralize infectivity. Antigen–antibody complexes might contribute to enhanced disease. In addition, compared to natural infection, FI-RSV caused a disproportionate stimulation of the Th2 subset of CD4+ T lymphocytes, whose role in enhanced disease was confirmed by depletion studies in experimental animals. Disease enhancement appears to be specific to killed or protein subunit HRSV vaccines and might occur because these nonreplicating vaccines do not efficiently stimulate natural killer cells and CD8+ T lymphocytes, which in turn play an important role in regulating the

T-helper-cell response via secreted interferon γ. Disease enhancement appears to be an issue only for immunization early in life, and thus protein subunit vaccines appear to be safe in HRSV-experienced individuals.

Because of the phenomenon of vaccine-related disease enhancement, pediatric vaccine development is focused on the development of live-attenuated HRSV strains for intranasal administration. A number of candidate live vaccines developed by reverse genetics are presently in clinical trials. There is also a need for an HRSV vaccine for the elderly. Subunit vaccines are presently being developed for that age group.

See also: Human Respiratory Viruses.

Further Reading

Collins PL and Crowe JE, Jr. (2006) Respiratory syncytial virus and metapneumovirus. In: Knipe DM and Howley PM (eds.) *Fields Virology,* 5th edn., pp. 1601–1646. Philadelphia, PA: Lippincott Williams and Wilkins.

Collins PL and Murphy BR (2005) New generation live vaccines against human respiratory syncytial virus designed by reverse genetics. *Proceedings of the American Thoracic Society* 2: 166–173.

Crowe JE, Jr. and Williams JV (2003) Immunology of viral respiratory tract infection in infancy. *Paediatric Respiratory Reviews* 4: 112–119.

Hall CB (2001) Respiratory syncytial virus and parainfluenza virus. *New England Journal of Medicine* 344: 1917–1928.

Hussel T, Baldwin CJ, O'Garra A, and Oppenshaw PJ (1997) T cells control Th2-driven pathology during pulmonary respiratory syncytial virus infection. *European Journal of Immunology* 27: 3341–3349.

Karron RA, Singleton RJ, Bulkow L, et al. (1999). Severe respiratory syncytial virus disease in Alaska native children. *Journal of Infectious Diseases* 180: 41–49.

McGivern DR, Collins PL, and Fearns R (2005) Identification of internal sequences in the 3 leader region of human respiratory syncytial virus that enhance transcription and confer replication processivity. *Journal of Virology* 79: 2449–2460.

Melero JA, Garcia-Barreno B, Martinez I, Pringle CR, and Cane PA (1997) Antigenic structure, evolution, and immunobiology of human respiratory syncytial virus attachment (G) protein. *Journal of General Virology* 78: 2411–2418.

Murphy BR, Sotnikov AV, Lawrence LA, Banks SM, and Prince GA (1990) Enhanced pulmonary histopathology is observed in cotton rats immunized with formalin-inactivated respiratory syncytial virus (RSV) or purified F glycoprotein and challenged with RSV 3–6 months after immunization. *Vaccine* 8: 497–502.

Polack FP, Irusta PM, Hoffman SJ, et al. (2005) The cysteine-rich region of the respiratory syncytial virus attachment protein inhibits the innate immune response elicited by the virus and endotoxin. *Proceedings of the National Academy of Sciences, USA* 102: 8996–9001.

Singleton RJ, Bulkow L, et al. (1999). Severe respiratory syncytial virus disease in Alaska native children. *Journal of Infectious Diseases* 180: 41–49.

Spann KM, Collins PL, and Teng MN (2003) Genetic recombination during co-infection of two mutants of human respiratory syncytial virus. *Journal of Virology* 77: 11201–11211.

Teng MN and Collins PL (2002) The central conserved cystine noose of the attachment G protein of human respiratory syncytial virus is not required for efficient viral infection *in vitro* or *in vivo. Journal of Virology* 76: 6164–6171.

Tripp RA, Jones LP, Haynes LM, et al. (2001) Cytokine mimicry by respiratory syncytial virus G glycoprotein. *Nature Immunology* 2: 732–738.

Wright PF, Karron RA, Madi SA, et al. (2006) The interferon antagonist NS2 protein of respiratory syncytial virus is an important virulence determinant in humans. *Journal of Infectious Diseases* 193: 573–581.

Young J (2002) Development of a potent respiratory syncytial virus-specific monoclonal antibody for the prevention of serious lower respiratory tract disease in infants. *Respiratory Medicine* 96 (supplement B): S31–S35.

Zhang L, Peeples ME, Boucher RC, et al. (2002) Respiratory syncytial virus infection of human airway epithelial cells is polarized, specific to ciliated cells, and without obvious cytopathology. *Journal of Virology* 76: 5654–5666.

Human Respiratory Viruses

J E Crowe Jr., Vanderbilt University Medical Center, Nashville, TN, USA

Glossary

Bronchiolitis A disease condition characterized by trapping of air in the lungs with difficulty expiring (i.e., wheezing), caused by inflammation or infection of the bronchioles, the smallest and highest-resistance airways.

Croup A disease condition characterized by a difficulty in inspiration, associated with a barky cough, caused by inflammation or infection of the larynx, trachea, and bronchi.

Lower respiratory tract The anatomical region below the vocal cords, including the trachea, bronchi, bronchioles, and lung.

Pneumonia Infection of the alveolar space of the lungs.

Introduction

Respiratory virus infections of humans are the most common and frequent infections of man. Hundreds of different viruses can be considered respiratory viruses. Viruses that enter through the respiratory tract include viruses that replicate and cause disease that is restricted to the respiratory epithelium, and other viruses that enter through the mucosa but also spread by viremia causing systemic disease. An example of the latter is measles virus. SARS coronavirus is another. In general, viruses that do not cause viremia are capable of reinfecting the same host multiple times throughout life. In contrast, infections with systemic viruses induce lifelong immunity. Probably, the high rate of reinfection of mucosally restricted viruses reflects the difficulty and metabolic cost of maintaining a high level of immunity at the vast surface area of the mucosa. Virus-specific IgA levels are maintained at high levels generally only for several weeks or months after infection.

The Human Respiratory Tract

The anatomy and the cell types of the respiratory tract dictate to a large degree the type of disease observed during respiratory virus infection. The demarcation between the upper and lower respiratory tracts is the vocal cords. The structures of the upper respiratory tract, which are all interconnected, include the nasopharynx, the larynx, the Eustachian tube and middle ear space, and the sinuses. Significant collections of lymphoid tissue reside in the upper respiratory tract, the tonsils and the adenoids. The lower respiratory tract structures include the trachea, bronchi, bronchioles, alveoli, and lung tissue. The cell types that line the respiratory tract are complex, and exhibit different susceptibilities to virus infection. The predominant cell types are ciliated and nonciliated epithelial cells, goblet cells, and Clara cells. Smooth muscle cells are prominent features of the airways down to the level of the bronchioles, and the lung possesses type I and II pneumocytes.

Disease Syndromes

The disease syndromes that are associated with respiratory viruses generally follow the anatomy of the respiratory tract. Different viruses appear to have tropisms for different cells or regions of the respiratory tract; therefore, there are particular associations of viruses with clinical syndromes. The clinical diagnoses for infections with disease manifestations in the respiratory tract are rhinitis and the common cold, sinusitis, otitis media, conjunctivitis, pharyngitis, laryngitis, tracheitis, acute bronchitis, bronchiolitis, pneumonia, and exacerbations of reactive airway disease or asthma. Clinical syndromes with more systemic illness due to respiratory viruses include the influenza syndrome, measles, severe acute respiratory syndrome (SARS), and hantavirus pulmonary syndrome (HPS).

Viruses That Cause Respiratory Illness in Immunocompetent Humans

The principal causes of acute viral respiratory infections in children became apparent through large epidemiologic studies conducted soon after cell culture techniques became available. The landmark studies of association of viruses with clinical syndromes were performed in the 1960s and 1970s. Recent studies have increased our understanding of the causes of viral respiratory infection in infants, especially because of the advent of molecular tests such as the polymerase chain reaction (PCR), which is more sensitive than cell culture. Respiratory syncytial virus (RSV), parainfluenza viruses (PIVs), adenoviruses, and influenza viruses were identified initially as the most common causes of serious lower respiratory tract disease in infants and children. More recently, human metapneumovirus (hMPV) was identified as a major cause of serious illness. In the last 10 years, a number of additional viruses have been associated with respiratory illness, as discussed below. However, still, infectious agents are not identified in 30–50% of clinical illnesses in large surveillance studies, even using sensitive diagnostic techniques such as viral culture on multiple cell lines, antigen detection assays, and RT-PCR based methods. It is not known if these illnesses are due to identified pathogens that are simply not detected due to low titers of virus in patient samples or if there are novel agents that are yet to be identified.

Immunocompromised Hosts

Reactivation of latent viruses, such as the herpesviruses HSV and CMV, and adenoviruses occurs in immunocompromised humans, particularly subjects with late-stage HIV infection, those with organ transplantation, and patients with leukopenia and neutropenia caused by chemotherapy. CMV is the most frequently recovered virus from diagnostic procedures such as bronchoalveolar lavage in immunosuppressed patients with pneumonia. These patients also suffer more frequent and more severe disease including mortality with common respiratory viruses, including RSV, hMPV, PIV, influenza viruses, rhinoviruses, and adenoviruses. Nosocomial transmission including large unit outbreaks is not uncommon, and can result in high frequency of transmission.

Specific Viral Causes of Respiratory Disease

Picornaviridae

A wide variety of picornaviruses cause respiratory disease, including rhinoviruses, the enteroviruses A to D including coxsackieviruses A/B, echoviruses, non-polio enteroviruses, and parechoviruses 1–3. Enterovirus infections occur most commonly in the summer months in temperate areas, which differs from the season of many of the other most common respiratory viruses such as paramyxoviruses and influenza virus. Rhinovirus infections occur year-round.

Rhinoviruses

Rhinovirus is a genus of the family *Picornaviridae* of viruses. Rhinoviruses are the most common viral infective agents in humans, and a causative agent of the common cold. There are over 105 serologic virus types that cause cold symptoms, and rhinoviruses are responsible for approximately half of all cases of the common cold. Rhinoviruses have single-stranded positive-sense RNA genomes. The viral particles are icosahedral in structure, and they are nonenveloped. Rhinovirus-induced common colds may be complicated in children by otitis media and in adults by sinusitis. Most adults, in fact, have radiographic evidence of sinusitis during the common cold, which resolves without therapy. Therefore the primary disease is probably best termed rhinosinusitis. Rhinovirus infection is associated with exacerbations of reactive airway disease in children and asthma in adults. It is not clear whether rhinovirus is restricted to the upper respiratory tract and induces inflammatory responses that affect the lower respiratory tract indirectly, or whether the viruses spread to the lower respiratory tract. In the past, it was thought that these viruses did not often replicate or cause disease in the lower respiratory tract. However, recent studies discern strong epidemiological associations of RVs with wheezing and asthma exacerbations, including episodes severe enough to require hospitalization. Likely, rhinoviruses can infect the lower airways to some degree, inducing a local inflammatory response. Another possibility is that significant local infection of the upper respiratory tract might induce regional elaboration of mediators that causes lower airways disease. Association of rhinovirus infection with lower respiratory tract illness is difficult to study because cell diagnosis by cell culture is not sensitive. RT-PCR diagnostic tests are difficult to interpret because they are often positive for prolonged periods of time and even asymptomatic individuals may have a positive test. Comprehensive serologies to confirm infection are difficult because of the large number of serotypes. Nevertheless, most experts believe rhinoviruses are a common cause of lower respiratory tract illness.

Coxsackieviruses

These viruses cause oral lesions and often are associated in children with a disease syndrome termed 'hand-foot-and-mouth disease'. The pharyngitis associated with this infection often is marked by the very characteristic findings of herpangina, a clinical syndrome of ulcers or small vesicles on the palate and often involving the tonsillar fossa associated with the symptoms of fever, difficulty swallowing, and throat pain. Outbreaks commonly occur in young children, in the summer.

Enteroviruses

Non-polio enteroviruses are common and distributed worldwide. Although infection often is asymptomatic, these viruses cause outbreaks of clinical respiratory disease, sometimes with fatal consequences. Studies have associated particular types with clinical syndromes, as enterovirus 68 with wheezing and enterovirus 71 with pneumonia.

Echoviruses

The term 'echo' in the name of the virus is an acronym for enteric cytopathic human orphan, although this may be an archaic notion since most echoviruses are associated with human diseases, most commonly in children. There are at least 33 echovirus serotypes. Echoviruses can be isolated from many children with upper respiratory tract infections during the summer months. Echovirus 11 has been associated with laryngotracheitis or croup. Epidemiology studies also have associated echoviruses with epidemic pleurodynia, an acute illness characterized by sharp chest pain and fever.

Parechoviruses

These viruses have been assigned a new genus of the family *Picornaviridae* because of distinctive laboratory-based molecular properties. The most common member of the genus *Parechovirus*, human parechovirus 1 (formerly echovirus 22) is a frequent human pathogen. The genus also includes the closely related virus, human parechovirus 2 (formerly echovirus 23). Human parechoviruses usually cause mild respiratory or gastrointestinal illness. Most infections occur in young children. There is a high seroprevalence for parechoviruses 1 and 2 in adults, and a few clear descriptions of neonatal cases of severe disease.

Paramyxoviridae

Respiratory syncytial virus

RSV is a single-stranded negative-sense nonsegmented RNA genome virus of the family *Paramyxoviridae*, genus *Pneumovirus*. It is one of the most infectious viruses of humans and infects infants at a very young age, often in the first weeks or months of life. It is the most common viral cause of severe lower respiratory tract illness in children and one of the most important causes of hospitalization in infants and children throughout the world. There is one serotype, but circulating viruses exhibit an antigenic dimorphism such that there are two antigenic subgroups designated A and B. Reciprocal cross-neutralization studies using human sera showed that the antigenic groups are about 25% related. Reinfection is common and can be caused by viruses of the same subgroup. Yearly, epidemics of disease often peak between January and March in temperate regions. RSV infection causes mild upper respiratory tract infection in most infants and young children, but results in hospitalization in 0.5–1% of infants. Most children have been infected by the age of 2 years. There is an association of RSV infection early in life and subsequent asthma, although a causal relationship is controversial. Most hospitalized infants are otherwise healthy, but some groups are considered high risk for severe disease such as premature infants especially those with chronic lung disease and infants born with congenital heart disease. Immunocompromised patients of any age are at risk of severe disease.

Human parainfluenza viruses

These viruses constitute a group of four distinct serotypes (types 1–4) of single-stranded RNA viruses belonging to the family *Paramyxoviridae*. When considered as a group, they are the second most common cause of lower respiratory tract infection in young children. PIV3 is the most common cause of severe disease. Repeated infection throughout life is common. First infections are more commonly associated with lower respiratory tract disease, especially croup, while subsequent infections typically are limited to the upper respiratory tract. PIVs are detected using cell culture with hemadsorption or immunofluorescent microscopy, and RT-PCR.

Human metapneumovirus

In 2001, investigators in the Netherlands described a new human respiratory virus, hMPV. Evidence of near universal seroconversion was found in the general population by 5 years of age, suggesting ubiquitous infection in early childhood. This virus, a member of the genus *Pneumovirus* with RSV, differs from RSV in that it lacks the NS1 and NS2 nonstructural genes that counteract host interferons and it possesses a slightly different gene order. Studies of the role of hMPV in pediatric lower respiratory tracts infection (LRI) in otherwise healthy children in the United States, using a prospectively collected 25-year database and sample archive representing about 2000 children, revealed that nearly 12% of LRI in children was associated with a positive hMPV test. This and similar studies suggested that the virus is one of the major respiratory pathogens of early childhood. The clinical features of hMPV LRI were similar to those of other paramyxoviruses, most often resulting in cough, coryza, and a syndrome of bronchiolitis or croup. Interestingly, hMPV seemed to be clinically intermediate between RSV and PIV in that it tended to cause bronchiolitis with similar frequency to RSV but more frequently than PIV, while causing croup less often than the latter. Studies in subjects with conditions predisposing to increased risk of respiratory illness suggest that hMPV plays a significant role in exacerbations of asthma in children and adults, LRI in immunocompromised subjects, and in the frail and elderly.

Measles virus

Measles virus, a paramyxovirus of the genus *Morbillivirus* causes infection with systemic disease, also known as rubeola. The virus is spread both by direct contact/fomite transmission and by aerosol transmission, and therefore is one of the most highly contagious infections of man. The classical symptoms of measles include 3 or more days of fever that is often quite high and a clinical constellation of symptoms termed 'the three Cs': cough, coryza, and conjunctivitis. A characteristic disseminated maculopapular rash appears soon after onset of fever. Transient mucosal lesions in the mouth of a characteristic appearance (Koplik's spots) are considered diagnostic when identified by an experienced clinician. The virus causes a number of systemic effects and can be complicated by severe pneumonia, especially when primary infection occurs in an unvaccinated adult or immunocompromised person of any age. Mortality in developing countries is high, especially when infection occurs in the setting of malnutrition.

Hendra and Nipah viruses

These emerging pathogens that are grouped in their own new genus *Henipaviruses* may not be respiratory pathogens in a conventional sense, but they are paramyxoviruses that probably infect humans by the respiratory route. Nipah virus is a newly recognized zoonotic virus, named after the location in Malaysia where it was first identified in 1999. It has caused disease in humans with contact with infectious animals. Hendra virus (formerly called equine morbillivirus) is another closely related zoonotic paramyxovirus that was first isolated in Australia in 1994. The viruses have caused only a few localized outbreaks, but their wide host range and ability to cause high mortality raise concerns for the future. The natural host of these viruses is thought to be a certain species of fruit bats present in Australia and the Pacific. Pigs may be an intermediate host for transmission to humans in Nipah infection, and horses in the case of Hendra. Although the mode of transmission from animals to humans is not defined, it is likely that inoculation of infected materials onto the respiratory tract plays a role. The clinical presentation usually appears to be an influenza-like syndrome, progressing to encephalitis, may include respiratory illness, and causes death in about half of identified cases.

Orthomyxoviridae

Influenza viruses

Influenza is a single-stranded segmented negative-sense RNA genome virus of the family *Orthomyxoviridae*. There are three types of influenza viruses: influenza virus A, influenza virus B, and influenza virus C. Influenza A and C infect multiple species, while influenza B infects humans almost exclusively. The type A viruses are the most virulent human pathogens among the three influenza types, and cause the most severe disease. The influenza A virus can be subdivided into different subtypes based on the antibody response to these viruses. The subtypes that have been confirmed in humans in seasonal influenza, ordered by the number of known human pandemic deaths, are: H1N1 which caused the 1918 pandemic, and H2N2 which caused the 1957 pandemic of avian influenza that originated in China, H3N2 which caused the pandemic of 1968. Currently, H3N2, H1N1, and B viruses cause annual seasonal epidemics. In addition, H5N1 virus infection of humans occurred during an epizootic of H5N1 influenza in Hong Kong's poultry population in 1997. The disease affected animals of many species and exhibited a high rate of mortality in humans. The virus is spreading throughout Asia, carried by wild birds. Human-to-human transmission does not occur efficiently at this time; however, there is widespread current concern about the potential for an H5N1 pandemic if the virus acquired transmissibility among humans. The H7N7 avian virus also has unusual zoonotic potential. In 2003 this virus caused an outbreak in humans in the Netherlands associated with an outbreak in commercial poultry on several farms. One death occurred and 89 people were confirmed to have H7N7 influenza virus infection. H1N2 virus appears to endemic in pigs and humans. H9N2, H7N2, H7N3, and H10N7 human infections have been reported. Influenza B virus is almost exclusively a human pathogen, and is less common than influenza A. It mutates less rapidly than influenza A, and there is only one influenza B subtype. In humans, common symptoms of influenza infection and syndrome are fever, sore throat, myalgias, headache, cough, and fatigue. In more serious cases, influenza causes pneumonia, which can be fatal, particularly in young children and the elderly. Influenza pneumonia has an unusually high rate of complication by bacterial superinfection with staphylococcal and streptococcal bacterial pneumonia occurring in as many as 10% of cases in some clinical series.

Adenoviridae

Viruses of the family *Adenoviridae* infect both humans and animals. Adenoviruses were first isolated in human lymphoid tissues from surgically removed adenoids, hence the name of the virus. In fact, some serotypes establish persistent asymptomatic infections in tonsil and adenoid tissues, and virus shedding can occur for months or years. These double-stranded DNA viruses are less than 100 nm in size, and have nonenveloped icosahedral morphology. The large dsDNA genome is linear and nonsegmented. There are six major human adenovirus species (designated A through F) that can be placed into 51 immunologically distinct serotypes. Human respiratory tract infections are mainly caused by the B and C species. Adenovirus infections can occur throughout the year. Sporadic outbreaks occur with many of the serotypes, while others appear to be endemic in particular locations. Respiratory illnesses include mild disease such as the common cold and lower respiratory tract illness, including croup, bronchiolitis, and pneumonia. Conjunctivitis is associated with infection by species B and D. There is a particular constellation of symptoms called 'pharyngo-conjunctival fever' which is very frequently associated with acute adenovirus infection. In contrast, gastroenteritis has been associated most frequently with the serotype 40 and 41 virus of species F. Immunocompromised subjects are highly susceptible to severe disease during infection with respiratory adenoviruses. The syndrome of acute respiratory disease (ARD), especially common during stressful or crowded living conditions, was first recognized among military recruits during World War II and continues to be a problem for the military following suspension of vaccination. ARD is most often associated with adenovirus types 4 and 7.

Coronaviridae

Members of the genus *Coronavirus* also contribute to respiratory illness including severe disease. There are dozens of coronaviruses that affect animals. Until recently, only two representative strains of human coronaviruses were known to cause disease, human coronavirus 229E (HCoV-229E) and HCoV-OC43. A recent outbreak of SARS-associated coronavirus (SARS-CoV) showed that animal coronaviruses have the potential to cross species to humans with devastating effects. There has been one major epidemic to date, between November 2002 and July 2003, with over 8000 cases of the disease, and mortality rates approaching 10%. SARS-CoV causes a systemic illness with a respiratory route of entry. SARS is a unique form of viral pneumonia. In contrast to most other viral pneumonias, upper respiratory symptoms are usually absent in SARS, although cough and dyspnea occur in most patients. Typically, patients present with a nonspecific illness manifesting fever, myalgia, malaise, and chills or rigors; watery diarrhea may occur as well. Recently, investigators reported the identification of a fourth human coronavirus, HCoV-NL63, a new group 1 coronavirus. Evidence is emerging that HCoV NL63 is a common respiratory pathogen of humans, causing both upper and lower respiratory tract illness. Human coronavirus (HCoV) HKU1 was first described in January 2005 following detection in a patient with pneumonia. Several cases of respiratory illness have been associated with the virus, but the infrequent identification suggests to date that this putative group 2 coronavirus causes a low incidence of illness.

Herpesviridae

Several herpes viruses cause upper respiratory infections, especially infection of the oral cavity. Herpes simplex pharyngitis is associated with characteristic clinical findings, such as acute ulcerative stomatitis and ulcerative pharyngitis. Herpes simplex virus 1 (HSV-1) and herpes simplex virus 2 (HSV-2), also called human herpesvirus 1 (HHV-1) and human herpesvirus 2 (HHV-2), respectively, cause oral lesions, although over 90% of oral infections are caused by HSV-1. Primary oral disease can be severe, especially in young children, who sometimes are admitted for rehydration therapy due to poor oral intake. A significant proportion of individuals suffer recurrences of symptomatic disease consisting of vesicles on the lips. Epstein–Barr virus (EBV) mononucleosis syndrome is often marked by acute or subacute exudative pharyngitis; in some cases, the swelling of the tonsils in EBV pharyngitis is so severe that airway occlusion appears imminent. Most of the viruses of the family *Herpesviridae* can cause severe disease in immunocompromised patients (especially hematopoietic stem cell transplant patients), including cytomegalovirus (CMV), EBV, varicella-zoster virus, herpesvirus 6, herpesvirus 7, and herpesvirus 8.

Parvoviridae

Human bocavirus

A new virus was identified recently in respiratory samples from children with lower respiratory tract disease in Sweden. Sequence analysis of the viral genome revealed that the virus is highly related to canine minute virus and bovine parvovirus and is a member of the genus *Bocavirus*, subfamily *Parvovirinae*, family *Parvoviridae*. This virus was tentatively named human bocavirus (HBoV). HBoV has been identified as the sole agent in a limited number of respiratory samples from children hospitalized with respiratory tract disease. It remains to be seen whether the virus is causative of or merely associated with disease in these preliminary studies.

Bunyaviridae

Hantavirus

Over 400 cases of HPS have been reported in the United States. The disease was first recognized during an outbreak in 1993. About a third of recognized cases end in death. The Four Corners area outbreak is well known; however, cases now have been reported in 30 states. Patients with HPS usually present with a febrile illness beginning with symptoms of a flu-like illness. Physical examination is not specific, often only with findings of fever, and increased heart and respiratory rates. In addition to the respiratory symptoms, abdominal pain and fever are common. Diagnosis is often delayed until a severe illness occurs requiring mechanical ventilation.

Reoviridae

Rotavirus

Rotaviruses are dsRNA enteric viruses that are the most common cause of severe viral infectious gastroenteritis in children. Clinical series suggest that some children with gastroenteritis suffer upper respiratory symptoms during the prodrome of disease manifestation, and virus can be recovered from respiratory secretions. Some reports suggest that rotavirus infection is associated with lower respiratory tract illness, although this association is unclear.

Reovirus

These dsRNA viruses (named using an acronym for respiratory enteric orphan virus) are not clearly associated with respiratory disease, but seroconversion rate is high in the first few years of life, and they probably cause minor or subclinical illness.

Retroviridae

Human immunodeficiency virus

Pharyngitis occurs with primary HIV infection and may be associated with mucosal erosions and lymphadenopathy.

Papovaviridae

Polyomaviruses

Polyomaviruses are small dsDNA genome nonenveloped icosahedral viruses that may be oncogenic. There are two polyomaviruses known to infect humans, JC and BK viruses. Eighty percent or more of adult US subjects are seropositive for these viruses. JC virus can infect the respiratory system, kidneys, or brain. BK virus infection causes a mild respiratory infection or pneumonia and can involve the kidneys of immunosuppressed transplant patients.

Co-Infections

Given the overlap in the winter season of these viruses in temperate areas, it is not surprising that co-infections with two or more viruses occur. In general, when careful studies using cell culture techniques were used for virus isolation, more than one virus was isolated from respiratory secretions of otherwise healthy subjects with acute respiratory illness in about 5–10% of cases in adults and 10–15% in children. There is little evidence that more severe disease occurs during co-infections, although there is insufficient evidence on this point to be definitive. The incidence of two molecular diagnostic tests being positive (generally RT-PCR, for these RNA viruses) is expected to be higher than that of culture, because molecular tests can remain positive for an extended period of time after virus shedding has ended.

Transmission

Respiratory viruses generally have two main modes of transmission, large particle aerosols of respiratory droplets transmitted directly from person-to-person by coughing or sneezing, or by fomites. Fomite transmission occurs indirectly when infected respiratory droplets are deposited on hands or on inanimate objects and surfaces with subsequent transfer of secretions to a susceptible subject's nose or conjunctiva. Most respiratory viruses, unlike measles virus or varicella zoster virus, do not spread by small particle aerosols across rooms or down halls. Therefore, contact and droplet precautions are sufficient to prevent transmission in most settings; handwashing is critical in healthcare settings during the winter season.

Antiviral Drugs for Respiratory Viruses

Ribavirin is a nucleoside antimetabolite pro-drug that is activated by kinases in the cell, resulting in a 5′ triphosphate nucleotide form that inhibits RNA replication. The drug was licensed in an aerosol form in the US in 1986 for treatment of children with severe RSV lower respiratory tract infection. The efficacy of aerosolized ribavirin therapy remains uncertain despite a number of clinical trials. Most centers use it infrequently, if ever, in otherwise healthy infants with severe RSV disease. Intravenous ribavirin has been used for adenovirus, hantavirus, measles virus, PIV, and influenza virus infections, although a good risk/benefit profile has not been established clearly for any of these uses.

A humanized mouse monoclonal antibody directed to the F protein of RSV, 'palivizumab', is licensed for prevention of RSV hospitalization in high-risk infants. It is efficacious in half or more of high-risk subjects. A more potent second-generation antibody is being studied in clinical trials. Experimental treatment of both immunocompetent and immunocompromised RSV-infected subjects has been reported but the efficacy of this approach is not established.

There are four licensed drugs in the US for treatment or prophylaxis of influenza. 'Amantadine' and 'rimantadine' are two of the drugs that interfere with the ion channel activity caused by the viral M2 protein of influenza A viruses, which is needed for viral particle uncoating following endocytosis. The other two drugs, 'oseltamivir' and 'zanamivir', are neuraminidase inhibitors that act on both influenza A and B viruses by serving as transition state analogs of the viral neuraminidase that is needed to release newly budded virion progeny from the surface of infected cells. The cell surface normally is coated heavily with the viral receptor sialic acid. Resistance to the ion channel inhibitors arises rapidly during prophylaxis or treatment, and in 2006 resistance levels became so common in circulating viruses that the CDC no longer recommends use of these drugs.

'Interferon-α' has been shown to protect against rhinovirus infections when used intranasally. This biological drug causes some side effects, such as nasal bleeding, and resistance to the drug developed during experimental use, so the molecule is no longer being developed for this purpose. 'Pleconaril' has been tested for treatment of rhinovirus infection, as it is an oral drug with good bioavailability for treating infections caused by picornaviruses. This drug acts by binding to a hydrophobic pocket in the VP1 protein and stabilizing the protein capsid, preventing release of viral RNA into the cell. The drug reduced mucus secretions and other symptoms and is being further examined.

'Acyclovir' and related compounds are guanine analog antiviral drugs used in treatment of herpes virus infections. HSV stomatitis in immunocompromised patients is treated with 'famciclovir', or 'valacyclovir', and immunocompetent subjects with severe oral disease compromising oral intake are sometimes treated. These compounds have also been used prophylactically to prevent recurrences of outbreaks, with mixed results. Intravenous acyclovir is effective in HSV or varicella zoster virus pneumonia in immunocompromised subjects. 'Ganciclovir' with human immunoglobulin may reduce the mortality associated with CMV pneumonia in hematopoietic stem cell transplant recipients and has been used as monotherapy in other patient groups.

'Cidofivir' is a nucleotide analog with activity against a large number of viruses, including adenoviruses. Intravenous cidofovir has been effective in the management of severe adenoviral infection in immunocompromised patients but may cause serious nephrotoxicity.

Vaccines

There are licensed vaccines for influenza viruses. In the US, both a trivalent (H3N2, H1N1, and B) inactivated intramuscular vaccine and a live attenuated trivalent vaccine for intranasal administration is available. The efficacy of these vaccines is good when the vaccine strains chosen are highly related antigenically to the epidemic strain. Antigenic drift caused by point mutations in the HA and NA molecules leads to antigenic divergence, requiring new vaccines to be made each year. The influenza genome is segmented, which allows reassortment of two viruses to occur during co-infection, which sometimes leads to a major antigenic shift resulting in a pandemic. Pandemics occur every 20–30 years on average. There is current concern about the potential for an H5N1 pandemic, and experimental vaccines are being tested for this virus. To date, H5N1 vaccines have been poorly immunogenic compared to comparable seasonal influenza vaccines. Vaccines were developed for adenovirus serotypes 4 and 7, and these were approved for preventing epidemic respiratory illness among military recruits. Essentially, these were unmodified viruses given by the enteric route in capsules, instead of the respiratory route, which is the natural route of infection leading to disease. Inoculation by the altered route resulted in an immunizing asymptomatic infection. All US military recruits were vaccinated against adenovirus from 1971 to 1999 with near complete prevention of the disease in this population, but the sole manufacturer of the vaccine halted production in 1996 and supplies ran out 3 years later. Since 1999, adenovirus infection has reemerged as a significant problem in the military with approximately 10% of all recruits suffering illness due to adenovirus infection during basic training; some deaths have occurred. Live attenuated vaccine candidates are under development and being tested in phase I and II clinical trials for RSV and the PIVs. Mutant strains with reduced pathogenicity were isolated in the laboratory, tested, and sequenced. Now, vaccine candidates are being optimized by combining mutations from separate biologically derived viruses into single strains using recombinant techniques for generating RNA viruses from cDNA copies, a process called reverse genetics. Subunit vaccines have been developed for RSV, but there are safety concerns about their use in young infants because formalin inactivated vaccine induced a more severe disease response to infection in the 1960s. There are no vaccines against rhinoviruses as there is little or no cross-protection between serotypes, and it is not feasible to develop a vaccine for over 100 serotypes. Efforts to develop coronavirus vaccines are in the preclinical stage.

Summary

Viruses are the leading causes of acute lower respiratory tract infection in infancy. RSV is the most common pathogen, with hMPV, PIV-3, influenza viruses, and rhinoviruses accounting for the majority of the remainder of acute viral respiratory infections. Humans generally do not develop lifelong immunity to reinfection with these viruses; rather, specific immunity protects against severe and lower respiratory tract disease.

See also: Human Respiratory Syncytial Virus.

Further Reading

Booth CM, Matukas LM, Tomlinson GA, et al. (2003) Clinical features and short-term outcomes of 144 patients with SARS in the greater Toronto area. *JAMA* 289: 2801–2809.

Booth CM, Matukas LM, Tomlinson GA, et al. (2003) Clinical features and short-term outcomes of 144 patients with SARS in the greater Toronto area – Erratum. *JAMA* 290: 334.

Collins PL and Crowe JE Jr. (2006) Respiratory syncytial virus and metapneumovirus. In: Knipe DM and Howley PM (eds.) *Fields Virology*, 5th edn., pp. 1601–1646. Philadelphia: Lippincott, Williams and Wilkins.

Fisher RG, Gruber WC, Edwards KM, et al. (1997) Twenty years of outpatient respiratory syncytial virus infection: A framework for vaccine efficacy trials. *Pediatrics* 99: E7.

Glezen WP, Frank AL, Taber LH, and Kasel JA (1984) Parainfluenza virus type 3: Seasonality and risk of infection and reinfection in young children. *Journal Infectious Diseases* 150: 851–857.

Glezen WP, Paredes A, Allison JE, Taber LH, and Frank AL (1981) Risk of respiratory syncytial virus infection for infants from low-income families in relationship to age, sex, ethnic group, and maternal antibody level. *Journal of Pediatrics* 98: 708–715.

Heymann PW, Carper HT, Murphy DD, et al. (2004) Viral infections in relation to age, atrophy, and season of admission among children hospitalized for wheezing. *Journal of Allergy and Clinical Immunology* 114: 239–247.

Karron RA and Collins PL (2006) Parainfluenza viruses. In: Knipe DM and Howley PM (eds.) *Fields Virology*, 5th edn., pp. 1497–1526. Philadelphia, PA: Lippincott Williams and Wilkins.

Martinez FD (2002) What have we learned from the Tucson Children's Respiratory Study? *Paediatric Respiratory Reviews* 3: 193–197.

Parrott RH, Kim HW, Arrobio JO, et al. (1973) Epidemiology of respiratory syncytial virus infection in Washington, DC. Part II. Infection and disease with respect to age, immunologic status, race, and sex. *American Journal of Epidemiology* 98: 289–300.

Subbarao K, Klimov A, Katz J, et al. (1998) Characterization of an avian influenza A (H5N1) virus isolated from a child with a fatal respiratory illness. *Science* 279: 393–396.

Williams JV, Harris PA, Tollefson SJ, et al. (2004) Human metapneumovirus and lower respiratory tract disease in otherwise healthy infants and children. *New England Journal of Medicine* 350: 443–450.

Winther B, Hayden FG, and Hendley JO (2006) Picornavirus infections in children diagnosed by RT-PCR during longitudinal surveillance with weekly sampling: Association with symptomatic illness and effect of season. *Journal of Medical Virology* 78: 644–650.

Wright PF, Neumann G, and Kawaoka Y (2006) Orthomyxoviruses. In: Knipe DM and Howley PM (eds.) *Fields Virology*, 5th edn., pp. 1691–1740. Philadelphia, PA: Lippincott Williams and Wilkins.

Influenza

R A Lamb, Howard Hughes Medical Institute at Northwestern University, Evanston, IL, USA

Glossary

Antigenic drift The gradual accumulation of amino acid changes in the surface glycoproteins of influenza viruses.

Antigenic shift The sudden appearance of antigenically novel surface glycoproteins in influenza A viruses.

Pandemic The rapid spread of an infection involving many countries.

Reassortment The exchange of genome RNA segments among influenza A viruses.

Recombinant virus A virus generated through reverse genetics techniques.

Reverse genetics Techniques which allow the introduction of specific mutations into the genome of an RNA virus.

Subtype Classification of influenza A virus strains according to the antigenicity of their HA and NA proteins.

Introduction: The Disease

The disease influenza is caused by influenza virus (family *Orthomyxoviridae*). Symptoms include fever, headache, cough, nasal congestion, sneezing, and whole-body aches. Influenza virus remains an important viral pathogen of significant medical importance causing mortality statistics comparable to human immunodeficiency virus (HIV) and producing considerable morbidity in the population. There were about 22 000 deaths from acquired immune deficiency syndrome (AIDS) in the US in 1993 compared with an estimated 20 000 influenza-associated deaths in the US in each of the epidemic years between 1972–73 and 2005–06. Influenza epidemics continue to infect large numbers of people worldwide, despite the availability of inactivated vaccines derived from the current circulating strains, because of frequent natural variation of the hemagglutinin (HA) and neuraminidase (NA) envelope proteins of the virus. This variation allows the virus to escape neutralization by preexisting circulating antibody in the blood stream, present as a result of either previous natural infection or immunization.

Taxonomy and Nomenclature

The *Orthomyxoviridae* comprises five genera: *influenzavirus A*; *influenzavirus B*; *influenzavirus C*; *thogotovirus* which are tick-borne viruses; and *isavirus* which includes infectious salmon anemia virus. Influenza A viruses are further classified into subtypes based on the antigenic properties of their surface spike glycoproteins, the HA, and NA. There are 16 known HA subtypes (H1–H16) and nine NA subtypes (N1–N9). Both influenza A and B virus strains cause disease, but influenza A virus strains, in most epidemic years, are usually more widespread. All human pandemics have been caused by influenza A virus strains. Retrospective seroepidemiology indicates that the 1889–91 pandemic was caused by an H3-like virus. The 1918–19 pandemic was caused by an H1N1 virus, the 1957 pandemic by an H2N2 virus, and the 1967–68 pandemic by an H3N2 virus. In 1977, there was a reintroduction in the human population of a co-circulating H1N1 virus, and since 2001 the reassortant virus H1N2 has been isolated. Since 1997 a highly pathogenic avian virus (H5N1) has infected millions of domestic fowl, and as of 12 March 2007 is known to have infected 278 humans resulting in 168 deaths.

Transmission and Tissue Tropism

Influenza viruses of humans and other mammals are spread by aerosols, including sneezing. The virus replicates in the cells of the upper and lower respiratory tract, reaching a peak at 2–3 days after infection, and the virus is usually cleared in 7 days. Children experiencing their first infection can shed virus up to 13 days.

Influenza viruses of birds are usually spread by fecal contamination of water but can also be spread by aerosols (e.g., high pathogenicity H5N1). Avian influenza viruses replicate in both the respiratory tract and the lower intestinal tract, hence the shedding of high concentrations of virus into feces.

Virus Isolation and Propagation

The first influenza virus was isolated from pigs in 1930 and the first human virus in 1933 (influenza A virus). Influenza B virus was isolated in 1940 and influenza C virus in 1946. Influenza viruses can either be propagated in tissue culture cells (particularly Madin–Darby canine kidney cells) or in the allantoic cavity of embryonated chicken eggs.

The Virus – Structure, Genome, and Proteins

The *Orthomyxoviridae* are enveloped viruses of 150–200 nm diameter. In the electron microscope, the shape of the viruses ranges from roughly spherical to pleomorphic, and filamentous viruses over a micron in length are observed from some hosts (**Figure 1**). The lipid envelope of influenza viruses is derived from the plasma membrane of the host cell in which the virus is grown. Influenza A and B virions are morphologically indistinguishable, whereas influenza C virions can be distinguished from the other genus as the glycoprotein spike is organized into orderly hexagonal arrays.

The influenza A, B, and C viruses can be distinguished on the basis of antigenic differences between their nucleocapsid (NP) and matrix (M) proteins. Influenza A viruses are further divided into subtypes based on the antigenic nature of their HA and NA glycoproteins. Other important characteristics that distinguish influenza A, B, and C viruses are given as follows.

1. Influenza A viruses infect naturally a wide variety of avian species, humans, and several other mammalian species including swine and horses. Influenza B virus appears to naturally infect only humans, but influenza C virus has been isolated mainly from humans and also from swine in China.
2. The HA and NA of influenza A viruses exhibit much greater amino-acid-sequence variability than their counterparts in the influenza B viruses. Influenza

C virus has only a single multifunctional glycoprotein, HA-esterase-fusion protein (HEF).
3. Although influenza A, B, and C viruses possess similar proteins, each virus type has distinct mechanisms for encoding proteins.
4. Influenza A and B viruses each contain eight distinct RNA segments whereas influenza C viruses contain seven RNA segments.

The most striking feature of the influenza A virion is a layer of about 500 spikes radiating outward (10–14 nm) from the lipid envelope. These spikes are of two types: rod-shaped spikes of HA and mushroom-shaped spikes of NA. The ratio of HA to NA varies but is usually 4–5 to 1. Influenza A, B, and C viruses also encode other integral membrane proteins, the M2 (influenza A virus), NB and BM2 (influenza B virus), and CM2 (influenza C virus) proteins, respectively. Biochemical evidence indicates that these proteins are only present in a few copies in virions. The viral matrix protein (M1) is thought to underlie the lipid bilayer and to associate with the cytoplasmic tails of the glycoproteins and the ribonucleoprotein (RNP) core of the virus.

Inside the virus, observable by thin sectioning of virus or by disrupting particles, are the RNP structures which can be separated into different size classes and contain eight different segments of single-stranded RNA. The RNPs have the appearance of flexible rods. The RNP strands often exhibit loops on one end and a periodicity of alternating major and minor grooves, suggesting that the structure is formed by a strand that is folded back on

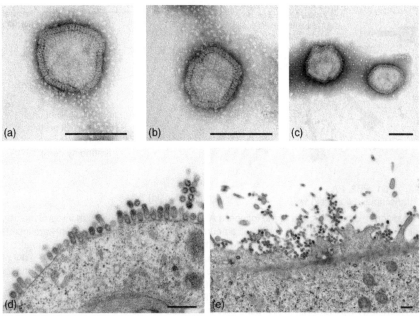

Figure 1 Electron micrographs of purified influenza virus virions (A/Udorn/72) (a–c) and A/WSN/33 virions budding from the surface of infected MDCK cells (d, e). Scale = 100 nm (a–c), 500 nm (d, e). Data provided by Dr. George Leser, Northwestern University, Evanston, IL, USA.

itself and then coiled on itself to form a type of twin-stranded helix. The RNPs consist of four protein species and RNA. NP is the predominant protein subunit of the nucleocapsid and coats the RNA, approximately 20 nucleotides per NP subunit. Associated with the RNPs is the RNA-dependent RNA polymerase complex consisting of the three P (polymerase) proteins – PB1, PB2, and PA – which are only present at 30–60 copies per virion. The NS2/NEP protein is present at 130–200 molecules per virion (**Figure 2**).

Influenza A and B viruses each contain eight segments of single-stranded RNA (for influenza A virus 2341 nucleotides to 890 nucleotides chain length), and influenza C viruses contain seven segments of single-stranded RNA (influenza C viruses lack an NA gene). The gene assignment for influenza A virus is as follows: RNA segment 1 codes for PB2, 2 for PB1 and in some strains also PB1-F2, 3 for PA, 4 for HA, 5 for NP, 6 for NA, 7 for M1 and M2, and 8 for NS1 and NS2/NEP. PB1, PB2, and PA form the RNA-dependent RNA polymerase and together with the NP protein form the RNPs. HA has receptor (cell surface expressed sialic acid (SA)) binding activity and HA through multivalent interactions attaches the virus to the surface of a cell. HA also mediates the entry of the virus into cells by causing virus–cell membrane fusion. NA has neuraminidase activity that cleaves SA from complex carbohydrate molecules. Although seemingly an opposing activity to HA-binding SA, HA binding and NA activity work at different pHs and at different times in the virus life cycle. Thus, NA activity is the receptor-destroying activity necessary for virus release from cells. The viral matrix protein (M1) is thought to underlie the lipid bilayer and to associate with the cytoplasmic tails of the glycoprotein and the RNP core of the virus. The NS2 protein forms an association with the M1 protein, which is thought to be an essential interaction in the virus life cycle for export of the RNP complex from the nucleus. The NS1 protein is a multifunctional protein. It mediates the block of transport of host cell mRNAs from the nucleus, it interacts with phosphatidylinositol-3-kinase blocking phosphorylation of the downstream effector molecule Akt, and NS1 has major roles in defeating the innate immune system and limiting the production of interferons. PB1-F2 is thought to be involved in promoting apoptosis of host cells. The influenza A virus

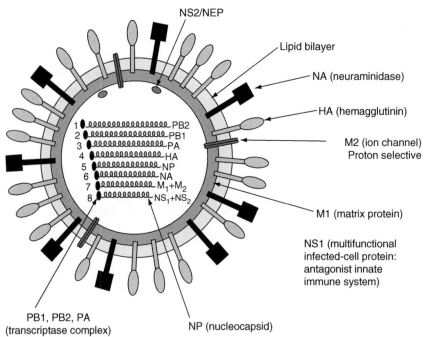

Figure 2 A schematic diagram of the structure of the influenza A virus particle. Three types of integral membrane protein – hemagglutinin (HA), neuraminidase (NA), and small amounts of the M2 ion channel protein – are inserted through the lipid bilayer of the viral membrane. The virion matrix protein M1 is thought to underlie the lipid bilayer and also to interact with the helical RNPs. The NS2/NEP protein associates with the M1 protein and is required for export of the RNPs out of the nucleus. Within the envelope are eight segments of single-stranded genome RNA (ranging from 2341 to 890 nucleotides) contained in the RNP. Associated with the RNPs are small amounts of the transcriptase complex, consisting of the proteins PB1, PB2, and PA. The coding assignment of the eight RNA segments are also illustrated. RNA segments 7 and 8 each code for more than one protein (M1 and M2, and NS1 and NS2/NEP, respectively). NS1 is found only in infected cells and is not thought to be a structural component of the virus. NS1 is a multifunctional protein and its functions include being an antagonist of the innate immune system. Adapted from Lamb RA and Krug RM (2001) *Orthomyxoviridae*: The viruses and their replication. In: Knipe DM and Howley PM (eds.) *Fields Virology*, 4th edn., pp. 1487–1531. Philadelphia, PA: Lippincott Williams and Wilkins.

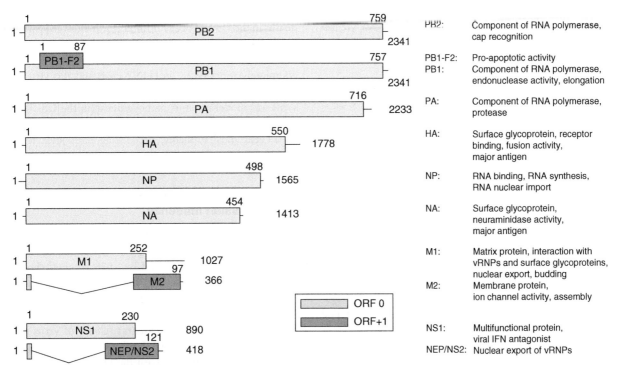

Figure 3 Genome structure of influenza A/Puerto Rico/8/34 virus. RNA segments (in nucleotides) shown in positive sense and their encoded proteins (in amino acids). The lines at the 5′ and 3′ termini represent the noncoding regions. The PB1 segment contains a second ORF in the +1 frame resulting in the PB1-F2 protein. The M2 and NEP/NS2 proteins are encoded by spliced mRNAs (the introns are indicated by the V-shaped lines). Adapted from Palese P and Shaw ML (2006) *Orthomyxoviridae: The viruses and their replication.* In: Knipe DM and Howley PM (eds.) *Fields Virology*, 5th edn., pp. 1647–1689. Philadelphia, PA: Lippincott Williams and Wilkins.

M2 protein and the influenza B virus BM2 protein are proton-selective ion channels that cause acidification of the interior of the virus particle during uncoating of the virion in endosomes. M2 protein is the target of the antiviral drug amantadine. The function of the influenza B virus NB protein is not known. NB is not essential for replication of the virus in tissue culture cells but it appears to confer a growth advantage in infections of mice. The influenza C virus CM2 protein has been suggested to be the counterpart of M2 and BM2 and to have ion channel activity, but this has not been shown rigorously (**Figure 3**).

Evolution of Influenza Virus

The finding that all known HA and NA subtypes are maintained in avian species together with phylogenic analysis of genome nucleotide sequences led to the hypothesis that all mammalian influenza A viruses are derived from the avian influenza virus pool. The evolutionary rates for avian virus both at the nucleotide and amino acid level are significantly lower than for human viruses, a finding which suggests that the influenza viruses of aquatic birds are in evolutionary stasis and thus are optimally adapted to their hosts. Thus, although mutations occur, they do not lead to amino acid changes. In contrast, mammalian and domestic poultry viruses

continue to accumulate amino acid changes. Among human influenza viruses, the genes accumulate mutations at different rates despite the RNA polymerase having a constant mutation rate, for example, HA is evolving faster than the genes for the internal proteins, probably because of selection pressure. The H3 HA gene has evolved in a single lineage since 1968 when it was first introduced into humans with a mutation rte of 4×10^{-3} substitutions per nucleotide per year and 5×10^{-3} substitutions per residues per year in HA1. Most of these amino acid changes occur in the antigenic epitopes (sites) and it is for this reason that the influenza virus vaccine has to be reformulated each year. In contrast to influenza A virus, type B and C viruses appear to be at or near an evolutionary equilibrium in humans.

Influenza Virus Genetics

Reassortment

Reassortment is the switching of viral RNA (gene) segments in cells infected with two different influenza viruses. The term recombination is often used incorrectly for the process of reassortment. Although reassortment occurs for influenza A, B, and C viruses, it does not occur among the different types. The 1957 and 1968 pandemic viruses have been determined to be reassortments between HA and NA

(1957) and HA and PB1 (1967) of avian virus origin into a human virus genetic background, and the H5N1 viruses circulating between 1997 and 2007 arose from multiple reassortment events among avian influenza viruses.

Recombination

Recombination is a rare event caused by the virion-associated RNA polymerase switching templates. Recombination has led to the insertion of nonviral nucleotide sequences into the HA gene and to the generation of defective-interfering (DI) RNAs.

Reverse Genetics

Several systems are available for the generation of influenza viruses from cloned DNA. The process is highly efficient and novel viruses, including reconstruction of 1918 influenza virus, have been generated. The reverse genetic systems for influenza virus have permitted a detailed structure–function analysis of the viral proteins and their role in the virus life cycle, pathogenesis, and host range.

Influenza Pandemics

Pandemics are outbreaks that occur in very large geographic areas, usually involving more than one continent, and affecting large percentages of the population in a short period of time.

The Pandemic of 1918–19 – Spanish Influenza

The 1918–19 pandemic killed more than 25 million people worldwide and reduced life expectancy in the US by 10 years. Approximately one-third of the US population became sick and the mortality rate is estimated to be greater than 2.5%. The mortality pattern was different from that observed for other influenza virus pandemics. Usually the highest death rates are found in very young children and in the elderly. However, for 1918, a large number of deaths occurred in young adults (15–35 years old). Analysis of the reconstructed 1918 virus indicates that this virus is highly pathogenic for mice and nonhuman primates and the available data suggest that the 1918 virus causes a 'cytokine storm' leading to inflammatory cell infiltration and hemorrhage.

The Pandemics of 1957 (Asian Influenza) and 1968 (Hong Kong Influenza)

In 1957, a newly identified H2N2 influenza virus that is a reassortment between avian and human genes (see the section titled 'Reassortment') was identified as the causative agent of influenza. Although the ensuing pandemic was not extraordinarily pathogenic, the increased mortality (70 000 deaths in the US and over 1 million worldwide) is attributed to the lack of preexisting immunity for HA and NA among humans. In 1968 the H2N2 Asian influenza virus was completely replaced by an H3N2 virus and this virus was also a reassortment between avian and human viruses. This virus was moderate in its pathogenicity (in the US, 33 800 excess mortality) but the attack rate (40%) was highest in 10–14 year olds. Probably, preexisting antibodies to the N2NA moderated the disease in older humans.

The Re-Emergence of H1N1 Viruses in 1977 – Russian Influenza

In May 1977, an outbreak of influenza occurred on the Russian–Chinese border that spread rapidly in the former Soviet Union and China, and by 1978 reached the US. The virus was identified as an H1N1 virus that was very closely related to H1N1 viruses that circulated in the 1950s. It was suggested at the time, and it is still the prevailing view, that an accidental release of virus from a laboratory started the pandemic. In 2007, this H1N1 virus is still co-circulating with the H3N2 virus.

The H5N1 'Bird Flu' Outbreak

In Hong Kong, in May 1997 a 3-year-old boy died of influenza that was identified as being caused by an H5N1 virus that was entirely of avian origin. This was the first known occurrence of transmission of an avian virus to humans with a fatal outcome. In the fall of 1997, 17 additional cases were reported with five fatal outcomes. However, importantly, there was no evidence of human-to-human transmission. Culling of all poultry in Hong Kong's live bird markets is attributed to preventing further human infections. Nonetheless, the potential for avian influenza viruses transmitting to humans was not fully realized until these cases occurred. The observed mortality rate of 33% is atypical for influenza virus infections and this formed the basis for the worldwide concern that there may be a looming pandemic of grave consequences.

In July 2003 a new outbreak of H5N1 virus started in Thailand, Vietnam, and Indonesia. Since then the virus has spread over much of Asia, reached southeast Europe, and Africa, particularly Nigeria. The virus had led to the depopulation or death through disease of over 100 million poultry. These more recent H5N1 viruses have caused severe disease in limited numbers of humans. As of 12 March 2007, there have been 278 known human infections resulting in 168 deaths. These more recent H5N1 viruses cause systemic infections in humans, with virus being recovered from the stool and cerebrospinal fluid in addition to respiratory organs. Again, to date, there is no conclusive evidence for extensive human-to-human spread of disease.

Influenza Virus in Humans

Antigenic Drift

Antigenic drift is caused by point mutations and is defined as the minor gradual antigenic changes in the HA or NA protein. Influenza A virus drift variants result from the positive selection of spontaneously arising mutants by neutralizing antibodies, that is, antibody escape mutants. Mutations on the human virus HA or NA amino acid sequence occur at a frequency of less than 1% per year. Nonetheless, antigenic drift variants can cause epidemics and often prevail for 2–5 years before being replaced by a different variant.

HA is the major antigenic spike glycoprotein and from the atomic structure of prefusion HA and mapping of both natural virus HA variants and laboratory-derived monoclonal antibody escape mutants, it was possible to determine that HA possessed five antigenic sites (epitopes). These antigenic sites are all located in HA1 at or near the top of the molecule and mostly are found in protein loops. Similarly, antigenic drift has been found for NA and the sites of antigenic drift mapped to specifc regions of the NA atomic structure.

Antigenic Shift

Antigenic shift involves major antigenic changes and it occurs through the introduction, in a new human virus, of immunologically distinct HA and/or NA molecules. Antigenic shift leads to high infection rates in an immunologically naïve population and is the cause of influenza pandemics. As discussed above (reassortment) antigenic shift occurs through mixing of human and avian genes.

Influenza Virus in Animals

The natural host (reservoir) for influenza A viruses are aquatic birds, but influenza A viruses infect a wide variety of animals in addition to humans. These include land birds and poultry, swine, horses, dogs, cats, whales, and seals. In the hosts, apart from humans and poultry, influenza viruses usually cause asymptomatic infections and the viruses are in evolutionary stasis. Even H5N1 viruses are in evolutionary stasis in aquatic birds (with notable exceptions). However, on introduction into land-based poultry or mammalian species, they evolve rapidly.

In aquatic birds, influenza viruses replicate in the epithelial cells of the intestinal tract and these birds shed influenza viruses in high concentration in feces. Influenza viruses have been isolated routinely from lakes or ponds where migratory birds have congregated. In contrast, human influenza viruses replicate in the upper respiratory tract of ducks, but not in their intestinal tract. In part, this is thought to be due to the difference in linkage of receptor molecules used by avian and human viruses (SA linked to galactose via α2,3 vs. α2,6 linkages) and corresponding amino acids located in the receptor-binding sites on the tip of the HA molecule.

Avian influenza viruses are classified as highly pathogenic (HPAI) or low pathogenicity (LPAI) viruses. LPAI viruses cause mild respiratory disease, whereas HPAI viruses cause extensive mortality. Although multiple genes are involved in virulence, high pathogenicity is always associated with the HA molecule containing a series of basic residues at the cleavage site such that the HA molecules are cleaved to the two chains HA1 and HA2 intracellularly in the *trans*-Golgi network by the endogenous enzyme furin. In contrast, low pathogenicity viruses contain an HA molecule that contains a single basic residue in the HA cleavage site and HA is cleaved/activated by extracellular trypsin-like enzymes.

There have been many outbreaks of HPAI since 1955 and these have always involved the H5 or H7 subtypes. Although LPAI viruses had been thought to be innocuous, it is now clear that HPAI arises from LPAI of the same H5 and H7 subtypes.

Several studies have indicated a role for pigs in the emergence of pandemic influenza. This includes the finding that pigs can be naturally or experimentally infected with avian influenza viruses and that the pig trachea contains both avian (α2,3-linked SA) and human-type receptors (α2,6-linked SA). Replication of avian viruses in pigs leads to variants that prefer human-type receptors. Taken together, these finding suggest that pigs can host genetically diverse viruses and lead to the notion that pigs may be the 'mixing vessel', that is, pigs can be infected simultaneously with avian and human viruses which permits the generation of reassortant viruses that could cause pandemic influenza.

H7N7 and H3N8 viruses have historically been associated with equine influenza. The horse-racing industry has promoted the use of both killed and live-attenuated vaccines for these equine-tropic viruses.

In the laboratory, although not a natural host, mice are used extensively as an animal model. Except for mouse adapted strains (e.g., A/WSN/33 and A/PR/8/34) that have been passaged multiple times through mouse brains, most human viruses do not cause mouse lethality, but they do replicate in mice and cause transient weight loss. Interestingly, recently isolated H5N1 viruses are lethal for mice without prior adaptation. Most inbred strains of mice lack the interferon-induced Mx gene and thus although mice may be a convenient small animal model it is not a perfect model.

Ferrets are readily infected by influenza A or B viruses and they develop a febrile rhinitis. The long trachae of the ferret is thought to resemble the human trachea and pathological changes of bronchitis and pneumonia resemble those seen in humans. The drawback of ferrets is that they are much more difficult to handle than mice.

Both Old and New World primates can be infected with influenza viruses. Recently, cynomolgus macaques have been used as a model system for H5N1 viruses and found to develop acute respiratory distress syndrome with fever, analogous to the disease observed in H5N1-infected humans.

Molecular Determinants of Host Range Restriction and Pathogenesis

Three proteins, HA, PB2, and NS1, have been identified as major determinants in host range restriction and pathogenicity of influenza viruses.

The HA Protein

Cleavage of HA

HA is synthesized as a precursor polypeptide chain that for HA to be active in mediating virus-cell fusion, the precursor HA0 has to be cleaved at a specific site – the cleavage site – in two chains HA1 and HA2. The atomic structure of HA shows that HA1 contains the receptor-binding site and the sites of the antigenic epitopes and HA2 is the domain of the protein-mediating membrane fusion. The cleavage site of HPAI H5 and H7 viruses contains mutiple basic residues and are recognized by proteases resident in the *trans*-Golgi network such as furin or PC6 and thus can be cleaved in multiple different organs. In contrast, HA of LPAI and human viruses contain a single arginine residue in the cleavage site that has to be cleaved by extracellullar trypsin-like proteases and is cleaved in only a few organs.

Receptor specificity

The HA of human viruses bind preferentially to SA that is linked to the penultimate galactose (Gal) residue by an $\alpha2,6$-linkage, whereas most avian and equine viruses have a higher binding affinity for SA linked to galactose via an $\alpha2,3$-linkage. Nonciliated epithelial cells express $SA\alpha2,6$ Gal oligosaccharides and are predominantly infected by human influenza virus. It has also been found that whereas $SA\alpha2,6Gal$ oligosaccharides are dominant on epithelial cells in nasal mucosa, trachea, and bronchi, $SA\alpha2,3Gal$ oligosaccharides are found on nonciliated bronchiolar cells at the junction between the respiratory bronchiole and alveolus and also on type cells lining the alveolar wall.

Receptor specificity is determined by the nature of the amino acids that form the receptor-binding pocket. The residues at positions 226 and 228 play an important role in receptor specificity for the H2 and H3 HAs and receptor specificity can be switched by mutations of these amino acid residues. For H1 HAs receptor specificity is determined in large part by the nature of the residues found at position 190 (H3 residue numbering).

The NS1 Protein

In addition to affecting the transport of host mRNAs out of the nucleus, NS1 functions as an interferon (INF) antagonist. Probably, all viruses need a system to defeat INF action in INF-competent hosts. The NS1 protein targets both IFN β production and the activation of INF-induced genes that are required for establishing the antiviral state. Although there are 200–300 IFN-stimulated genes, the biological properties of the encoded proteins are known only for a few, for example, dsRNA-activated protein kinase (PKR), Mx proteins, $2',5'$ oligo-adenylate synthetase and RNAase L. NS1 interferes with PKR and RNase L.

NS1 protein from different influenza viruses appears to have different abilities to counteract the IFN system and thus this affects pathogenicity of the virus. Viruses that defeat the IFN system well are more pathogenic than those that only cause partial inactivation of the IFN system. Several findings suggest that the NS1 protein of highly pathogenic viruses may cause the cytokine imbalance and that has been observed in patients infected with H5N1 virus or macaques infected with 1918 H1N1 virus.

The PB2 Protein

The PB2 protein is part of the RNA-dependent RNA polymerase complex. PB2 binds to ^{7}MeGpppG cap structures on host mRNAs; the cap structure and 10–13 nucleotides of the host mRNA are cannibalized by the influenza virus RNA polymerase to act as primers for mRNA transcription. The PB2 protein and the residue found at position 627 (glutamic acid in LPAI and lysine in HPAI) have emerged as important determinants of virulence. How the mechanism by which these residue changes affect the polymerase activity is not fully elucidated. However, it appears that viruses with lysine at position 627 grow faster than those with glutamic acid at this position.

The NA Protein

HA of the A/WSN/33 human influenza virus contains a single arginine residue at the HA cleavage site; yet, for plaque formation in tissue culture unlike other human influenza virus strains, WSN does not require trypsin for multiple rounds of virus replication and plaque formation. However, the ability of A/WSN/33 to form plaques without trypsin requires the A/WSN/NA gene. It was determined that the WSN NA protein has lost a carbohydrate chain as compared to other N1NA proteins and that the lack of the carbohydrate chain permits the WSN NA to bind plasminogen, the precursor to the protease plasmin. It is envisaged that the tethered plasmin cleaves HA.

Antivirals

Amantadine and Rimantadine: M2 Ion Channel Blockers

Amantadine, and its methyl derivative rimantadine, were discovered as anti-influenza viral drugs in the 1960s by workers at DuPont. Rimantadine is licensed in the US for both the treatment and prophylaxis of influenza and at one time was being used extensively for prophylaxis in nursing homes. The drugs target the pore (transmembrane domain) of the M2 proton-selective ion channel. A drawback to the use of rimantadine is that drug-resistant variant viruses arise in humans within 4 days of drug treatment. Quite remarkably in 2005–06, the circulating H3N2 viruses were almost all rimantadine resistant despite little use of rimantadine. It has been postulated that the rimantadine-resistance mutation in M2 piggy-backed with another change in HA which conferred viral fitness.

NA Inhibitors

Two neuraminidase inhibitors are licensed in the US for the treatment and prophylaxis of influenza. Zanamivir is a derivative of the transition state intermediate 2-deoxy-2,3-dihydro-N-acetylneuraminic acid and the drug binds in the NA active site and has a K_i of 2×10^{-10}. The drug has to be administered intranasally or inhaled. Oseltamivir is another derivative of the transition state intermediate 2-deoxy-2,3-dihydro-N-acetylneuraminic acid and it contains a lipophilic group, which improves its bioavailability, and the drug can be taken orally. Although when used for treatment of influenza these drugs only reduce the duration of illness by a day or two, this may be highly significant (beneficial) in infections of high pathogenicity viruses.

Resistant variants to the NA inhibitors have been selected both *in vitro* and *in vivo* but at a much lower frequency than for amantadine-resistant variants. In part, this is because the drugs interact with several residues in the active site and each of these residues is important for enzyme activity. Thus, mutation of a residue in the active site leads to a lowered K_i and a lowered enzyme activity. Interestingly, emergence of resistance is first detected by finding mutations in the SA-binding site of HA, which compensates for reduced NA activity; the affinity of HA for its receptor is lowered. Later mutations occur in NA in the framework residues that surround the active site and stabilize its structure.

Vaccines

Inactivated Vaccines

Inactivated influenza A and B virus vaccines are licensed for administration in humans. The vaccine is reformulated each year to include the strains thought most likely to be prevailing. The choice of seed virus is made by the World Health Organization (WHO) and the US Centers for Disease Control (CDC). The vaccine virus is currently grown in embryonated eggs but because many human influenza virus isolates do not grow to high yield in eggs, a reassortment virus is made using the high egg-yielding PR/8/34 genetic backbone and the HA and NA genes of the candidate virus. Reverse genetics procedures speed up the time needed to produce a high-yielding reassortment over the former method of mixed infection and selecting the virus from random plaques. Vaccine is manufactured by harvesting allantoic fluid and concentrating the virus by zonal centrifugation and inactivation of infectivity with formalin or beta-propiolactone. One egg yields one to three doses of vaccine. The vaccine is administered intramuscularly. Vaccination with inactivated virus has been shown to consistently confer resistance to illness (reduced frequency and severity of disease), and to a somewhat lesser extent infection with influenza A and B viruses.

Live Virus Vaccines

A live attenuated vaccine (Flumist) has been licensed. The vaccine virus is based on the genetic backbone of a cold-adapted virus (A/Ann Arbor/6/60) and a reassortment made to incorporate the current HA and NA genes. The cold-adapted virus replicates efficiently in the nasopharynx to induce protective immunity. However, replication is restricted at higher temperatures, including those present in the lower airways and lungs. In clinical studies with matched strains, the live virus vaccine demonstrated 87% efficacy in children and 85% in adults. There is continued interest in the use of a live influenza virus vaccine because infection of the respiratory tract stimulates both systemic and local immunity, and in principle should stimulate cell-mediated immunity. Thus, all components of the human immune response are brought into action. Furthermore, there is the added advantage of acceptance of a nasal spray rather than a needle injection in young children.

See also: Emerging and Reemerging Virus Diseases of Vertebrates; Zoonoses.

Further Reading

Fouchier RA, Schneeberger PM, Rozendaal FM, *et al.* (2004) Avian influenza A virus (H7N7) associated with human conjunctivitis and a fatal case of acute respiratory distress syndrome. *Proceedings of the National Academy of Sciences, USA* 101: 1356–1361.
Gamblin SJ, Haire LF, Russell RJ, *et al.* (2004) The structure and receptor binding properties of the 1918 influenza hemagglutinin. *Science* 303: 1838–1842.

Garcia-Sastre A (2004) Indentification and characterization of viral antagonists of type 1 interferon in negative-strand RNA viruses. *Current Topics in Microbiology and Immunology* 283: 249–280.

Goto H and Kawaoka Y (1998) A novel mechanism for the acquisition of virulence by a human influenza A virus. *Proceedings of the National Academy of Sciences, USA* 95: 10224–10228.

Guan Y, Poon LL, Cheung CY, et al. (2004) H5N1 influenza: A protean pandemic threat. *Proceedings of the National Academy of Sciences, USA* 101: 8156–8161.

Gubareva LV, Kaisr L, and Hayden FG (2000) Influenza virus neuraminidase inhibitors. *Lancet* 355: 827–836.

Kawaoka Y and Webster RG (1988) Sequence requirements for cleavage activation of influenza virus hemagglutinin expressed in mammalian cells. *Proceedings of the National Academy of Sciences, USA* 85: 324–328.

Lamb RA, Holsinger LJ, and Pinto LH (1994) The influenza A virus M_2 ion channel protein and its role in the influenza virus life cycle. In: Wimmer E (ed.) *Receptor-Mediated Virus Entry into Cells*, pp. 303–321. Cold Spring Harbor, NY: Cold Spring Harbor Press.

Lamb RA and Krug RM (2001) Orthomyxoviridae: The viruses and their replication. In: Knipe DM and Howley PM (eds) *Fields Virology*, 4th edn., pp. 1487–1531. Philadelphia, PA: Lippincott Williams and Wilkins.

Mastrosovich MN, Mastrosovich TY, Gray T, et al. (2004) Human and avian influenza viruses target different cell types in cultures of human airway epithelium. *Proceedings of the National Academy of Sciences, USA* 101: 4620–4624.

Neumann G, Watanabe T, Ito H, et al. (1999) Generation of influenza A viruses entirely from cloned cDNAs. *Proceedings of the National Academy of Sciences, USA* 96: 9345–9350.

Palese P and Shaw ML (2006) *Orthomyxoviridae*: The viruses and their replication. In: Knipe DM and Howley PM (eds.) *Fields Virology*, 5th edn, pp. 1647–1689. Philadelphia, PA: Lippincott Williams and Wilkins.

Skehel JJ and Wiley DC (2000) Receptor binding and membrane fusion in virus entry: The influenza hemagglutinin. *Annual Review of Biochemistry* 69: 531–569.

Tumpey TM, Basler CF, Aguilar PV, et al. (2005) Characterization of the reconstructed 1918 Spanish influenza pandemic virus. *Science* 310: 77–80.

Varghese JN, Laver WG, and Colman PM (1983) Structure of the influenza virus glycoprotein antigen neuramindase at 2.9 A resolution. *Nature* 303: 35–40.

Wright PF, Neumann G, and Kawaoka Y (2006) Orthomyxoviruses. In: Knipe DM and Howley PM (eds.) *Fields Virology*, 5th edn, pp. 1691–1740. Philadelphia, PA: Lippincott Williams and Wilkins.

Kaposi's Sarcoma-Associated Herpesvirus: General Features

Y Chang and P S Moore, University of Pittsburgh Cancer Institute, Pittsburgh, PA, USA

History

Kaposi's sarcoma (KS) was first described by Moritz Kaposi in 1872 as a rapidly fatal, 'idiopathic, pigmented sarcoma' of the skin. Although initially associated with men of Eastern European, Ashkenazi Jewish and Mediterranean ancestry, by the 1950s KS was recognized to be the third most common malignancy in sub-Saharan Africa. The unusual geographic distribution of this cancer led to speculation about a viral cause, speculation that intensified with the onset of the acquired immune deficiency syndrome (AIDS) epidemic in the early 1980s. AIDS patients were 100 000-fold more likely to develop KS than the general population and the tumor took on a more aggressive and frequently lethal form in AIDS patients.

Two epidemiologists, Harold Jaffe and Valerie Beral, examined patterns among AIDS surveillance data and concluded that KS is caused by a viral agent other than human immunodeficiency virus (HIV) and that the agent is uncommon in the general population but sexually transmitted efficiently among gay men. These predictions were later found to be strikingly accurate. Over 20 possible culprits were described as 'the KS agent'. As early as 1972, Giraldo and colleagues suggested that human cytomegalovirus might cause KS. These findings were discounted after further study,

but in 1984 Walter and colleagues succeeded in directly observing herpesvirus particles in KS tumor specimens, thus reviving the possibility that KS is a herpesvirus disease.

In 1993, Chang and Moore used representational difference analysis to isolate two small DNA fragments from a KS lesion similar to, but distinct from, known herpesvirus sequences. Collaborating with Ethel Cesarman, they were then able to show that this putative new virus was present in virtually all KS tumors, was more likely to be found at the tumor site than distal tissues, and was not present in control tissues from patients without AIDS. The virus was given the common name Kaposi's sarcoma-associated herpesvirus (KSHV) and recognized to be the eighth human herpesvirus (HHV-8).

A B-cell lymphoma, called primary effusion lymphoma (PEL), was quickly identified as harboring KSHV. These lymphomas were known to be common secondary malignancies among KS patients, and isolation of PEL cells allowed the first *in vitro* culture of KSHV. These early cell lines were coinfected with both Epstein–Barr virus (EBV) and KSHV, but nonetheless accurate first generation serologic assays were developed using them. A second neoplastic disorder called multicentric Castleman's disease (MCD) was also recognized to be frequently infected with KSHV by Soulier and colleagues.

Once the virus was identified, its characterization proceeded rapidly. Studies demonstrated that all forms of KS, both HIV-positive and HIV-negative, are uniformly infected with KSHV. Extensive HIV/AIDS cohort databanks were used for serologic test development and showed that KSHV infection preceded onset of disease. These early studies also revealed that KSHV infection is uncommon in the general population of the USA and Europe – despite technical confusion resulting from highly cross-reactive assays – and patterns of infection mirror KS tumor rates among high risk populations, following closely the Beral-Jaffe predictions for the KS agent. Parravincini and colleagues showed that KS arising among transplant patients could either be due to reactivation of preexisting infection or to *de novo* infection from the organ allograft, helping to explain the association of this tumor with transplantation.

Virologic characterization was equally rapid. In 1996, Ganem's group isolated a KSHV-infected PEL cell line free of EBV infection, and performed the first studies on viral replication. While KSHV had been previously cultured *in vitro* in EBV-coinfected cell lines, this was a major breakthrough allowing unambiguous characterization of the virus. That same year, Chang and Moore finished sequencing the 165 kbp viral genome, almost exactly 2 years after reports of its initial discovery. These studies revealed that the virus makes extensive use of molecular piracy, encoding homologs to multiple known cellular oncogenes. Shortly thereafter, research groups identified KSHV inhibitory proteins targeting p53 and retinoblastoma protein, interferon regulatory proteins, and KSHV paracrine-signaling molecules regulating cell growth control, providing key molecular clues on how this virus might initiate tumorigenesis.

Shortly after its initial description, KSHV was widely recognized to be the infectious cofactor causing KS and related diseases. With the onset of the AIDS epidemic, KS is now the most common tumor reported in sub-Saharan Africa, resulting in an enormous, unappreciated morbidity and mortality. In contrast, the introduction of highly effective retroviral therapy into developed countries in the mid-1990s has reduced KS incidence among AIDS patients by nearly 90% – a remarkable public health success story.

Taxonomy, Classification and Evolution

KSHV is a gammaherpesvirus (subfamily *Gammaherpesvirinae*) belonging to the genus *Rhadinovirus*, which is distinct from the genus *Lymphocryptovirus* containing EBV (**Figure 1**). While rhadinoviruses are distributed among both primates and nonprimates (e.g., mice, cattle, and horses), EBV-like viruses are found exclusively among primates.

The genus *Rhadinovirus* contains three evolutionarily distinct lineages of primate viruses. One lineage is found

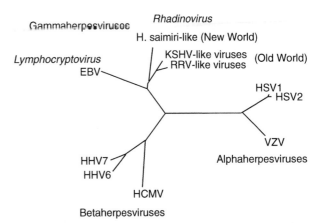

Figure 1 Relationship of KSHV to other herpesviruses. KSHV belongs to a lineage of rhadinoviruses infecting Old World primates. A second rhadinovirus lineage, exemplified by rhesus rhadinovirus (RRV), has been discovered infecting Old World primates. No human infections with an RRV-like virus have been described.

among New World monkeys and two parallel but distinct lineages (including KSHV) infect Old World primates including humans. KSHV was first recognized to be closely related to the New World squirrel monkey virus, herpesvirus saimiri. In the search for KSHV-like viruses among nonhuman primates, similar viruses were found among rhesus macaques as well as baboons, gorillas, and chimps, suggesting an evolutionary codivergence for these viruses with their hosts.

A second rhadinovirus lineage found in rhesus macaques (and hence commonly called rhesus rhadinovirus, RRV) was quickly extended to other Old World primate hosts. The importance of this finding is that no human RRV-like virus has been described. If it exists, and evolutionary evidence strongly suggests that it might, then it would become HHV-9.

Molecular epidemiology studies based on variation of the K1 gene and the right-hand end of the genome reveal at least four unique viral clades called A–D that largely match patterns of human migration from Africa. There are several conserved alleles of the right-hand end of the genome (called M, N, O, and P) found across clades suggesting that these viruses are chimeric and have arisen by recombination.

Geographic Distribution

Unlike most human herpesviruses, KSHV is not a ubiquitous human infection. KSHV infection is hyperendemic throughout sub-Saharan Africa with estimated adult infection rates of 30–60%. Other isolated populations, including indigenous Amazonian tribes, may also have infection rates at this level or higher. The prevalence of infection declines among Mediterranean basin countries such that general adult infection rates in Sicily average about 10% and continue to decline at more northern latitudes in Italy. In the USA and Northern Europe, approximately 2% of blood donors are KSHV infected. While general infection rates are low in the USA and Europe, gay men are recognized to have a rate of infection 10–20 times higher than heterosexuals.

Transmission

In the absence of underlying immunosuppression, KSHV infection appears to be asymptomatic, or perhaps associated with transient fever and rash. KSHV is recognized to have several patterns of transmission, and modes of transmission differ dramatically between developed and developing countries. It is secreted from the oral mucosa through salivary secretions. In developed countries, there is a strong sexual component to transmission among gay and bisexual men but the precise sexual behavior responsible for transmission is unknown. Two possibilities include deep kissing and use of saliva as a sexual lubricant. In contrast, heterosexual transmission is apparently rare.

In developing countries, and possibly endemic regions of Europe and the Middle East, casual transmission is common. Again precise mechanisms of transmission are unknown, but KSHV transmission is much more efficient in sub-Saharan Africa where, unlike Northern Europe and the USA, significant rates of infection occur among children and adolescents. While intrauterine transmission and transmission through breast milk is uncommon, maternal-child transmission does occur during infancy and early childhood.

Of increasing concern, KSHV is also transmitted both through organ allografts and through blood transfusion. KS arising during transplantation is an important clinical problem with rates among all transplant patients between 0.2% and 6% depending on the geographic locale and background endemicity for viral infection. KS in this setting has a high mortality and morbidity since primary treatment involves removing immunosuppression. The bulk of KS among transplant recipients derives from reactivation of preexisting, quiescent infection which subsequently flares during immunosuppression, but transmission from donor allografts has been documented. Interestingly, one study has demonstrated that KS tumor cells rather than virus itself can be transmitted during transplantation.

Blood transfusion has in the past been considered a minor component of KSHV transmission. Several studies have shown a relationship between non-AIDS KS and past transfusion history, but this relationship has been obscured by the overwhelming risk of sexual transmission among HIV/AIDS patients. Transfusion transmission has recently been documented to occur among a fraction of infected blood samples. Whether a public health response to this is needed remains unknown.

Host Range and Virus Propagation

KSHV is grown in the laboratory using PEL-derived cell lines and can be activated into lytic virus production by treatment with chemicals such as protein kinase C activators or histone deacetylase inhibitors. The virus cannot be maintained in cultured cells from KS tumor explants and is rapidly lost within a few passages.

KSHV can, however, be readily transmitted to a range of human and nonhuman cell lines in culture, although it is lost unless it is kept under some form of selection. The virus is commonly transmitted in culture to endothelial cell lines, which undergo transformation into a spindle growth pattern resembling KS. Receptors for virus binding and entry include extracellular heparan, integrin $\alpha 3\beta 1$, the cystine transporter xCT, and DC-SIGN. It is not yet clear which of these receptors act in concert or independently of each other to allow different steps of binding, internalization, and entry. Transmission to nonobese diabetic/severe combined immunodeficiency (NOD/SCID) mice has been documented, although the consequences of infection have not been fully examined.

Although whole virus transmission to animal models is limited, single gene expression studies have proved valuable. The K1 protein, for example, has been placed into a herpesvirus saimiri backbone and caused lymphatic tumors in rhesus macaques. Many KSHV genes, including those encoding viral interleukin 6 (vIL6), viral interferon regulatory factor 1 (vIRF1), and kaposin, transform rodent cell lines and cause tumors in mice. In addition, expression of the viral G protein-coupled receptor (vGPCR) in transgenic mice results in paracrine development of endothelial cell tumors that closely resemble human KS tumors.

Virus Genetics and Molecular Biology

KSHV is a ∼165 kbp double-stranded DNA virus with a long unique region (LUR) containing all protein-coding sequences that is flanked by high G + C content direct terminal repeats (TRs) on both ends. The TRs are 801 bp in length each, with 20 or more units in a typical virus, and are the site for circularization (latency) or linearization (lytic replication). One KSHV protein, latency-associated nuclear antigen 1 (LANA1), acts similarly to a corresponding EBV protein, EBNA1, to bridge between the viral episome and host cell chromosomes during latency, allowing equal segregation of virus to daughter cells. During latent replication, in which the virus is in a circular state, the origin of DNA replication is located within the TR region.

The LUR encodes over 90 independent protein-coding open reading frames (ORFs), and alternative splicing may markedly increase the expressed number of viral proteins. During latency, the KSHV genome is largely quiescent with only a few genes constitutively expressed, primarily from the right-hand latency locus and including LANA1, viral cyclin (vCYC), viral FLICE-inhibitory protein (vFLIP), and approximately 12 micro-RNAs.

KSHV, like other herpesviruses, has a highly choreographed cascade of gene expression during lytic replication. Lytic replication is initiated by a single transactivator protein, RTA, expressed from ORF50. This leads to sequential early, delayed-early, and late gene expression. Ultimately, the viral polymerase is expressed and linear KSHV chromosomes are replicated through a rolling circle mechanism.

KSHV genes are commonly divided into 'latent' and 'lytic' classes based on whether or not they are activated during the lytic replication cycle. This is clearly too simplistic a categorization to be meaningful. A large group of nonstructural protein genes have long been known to be expressed at low levels during viral latency but are upregulated during lytic replication (so called type II genes). Notch signaling, which activates the transcription factor RBP-Jk that acts in concert with RTA to initiate lytic replication, has recently been found to activate expression of these genes without late gene expression or virion production. Increased notch signaling is present in PEL cells and appears to be responsible for low level expression of type II genes during viral latency.

Molecular Piracy by KSHV

Rhadinoviruses show the most extensive piracy of host genes among the herpesviruses. KSHV genes that have been directly acquired from the host genome include those encoding proteins involved in DNA synthesis (thymidine kinase, dihydrofolate reductase, thymidylate synthase, ribonucleotide reductase subunits, and formyglycinamide ribotide amidotransferase (FGARAT)), deoxyuridine metabolism (dUTPase), paracrine signaling (viral complement control protein, vIL6, viral chemokine ligands 1, 2 and 3 (vCCL1, vCCL2, and vCCL3)) and vGPCR, interferon signaling (vIRF1, vIRF2, and LANA2), major histocompatibility class (MHC) regulation (modulator of immune recognition 1 and 2 (MIR1 and MIR2)), and cell cycle (vCYC) and apoptosis control (vBCL-2, vFLIP, and viral inhibitor of apoptosis (vIAP)). These proteins frequently fall into the type II expression pattern described above.

All of these proteins have recognizable sequence similarity to their human counterparts and appear to act in the same regulatory pathways. The primary difference between the viral and human homologs is at the level of protein regulation, in which the viral protein generally escapes from normal regulatory controls imposed on the human protein. vCYC, for example, targets the retinoblastoma protein for phosphorylation by recruiting cellular cyclin-dependent kinases. This allows the viral protein to initiate unscheduled S-phase entry of the cell cycle. vCYC resembles cellular D-type cyclins but differs in a key characteristic in that it is resistant to cyclin-dependent kinase inhibitors that control cellular cyclin function. Expression of these proteins, together with viral proteins that have no cellular counterparts, such as LANA1, is thought to be responsible for the tumorigenic capacity of this virus.

While the range of these homologous nonstructural proteins is unique to KSHV among the human herpesviruses, careful inspection reveals that the functions of these proteins are similar to those found in other viruses. There is a close functional correspondence between latent EBV proteins and latent KSHV proteins despite the fact that there is little or no sequence similarity. In general, EBV nonstructural proteins act as signaling molecules to activate specific cellular pathways, whereas KSHV has pirated members of these pathways to act in a similar fashion.

Immune Response

Infection with KSHV generates a strong antibody response that can be measured by indirect immunofluorescence assays (IFA), ELISA, and western blotting. In the absence of lytic stimulation, the nuclear antigen LANA1 commonly elicits antibody titers exceeding 1:50 000. This protein migrates aberrantly as a 223–234 kDa doublet band on western blotting. While LANA1 immunoreactivity is highly specific for KSHV infection, approximately 20% of AIDS-KS patients do not have immunoreactivity. For this reason, attempts to increase test sensitivity using lytic genes have been made. Whole cell lytic immunoassays can be highly sensitive but have demonstrated cross-reactivity that can be measured using adsorption with formalin-fixed KSHV-negative cell line antigen. Use of lytic cell assays led to considerable confusion in early studies about the prevalence of KSHV infection in various low-risk populations.

Two recombinant structural antigens, the ORF65 and K8.1 proteins, have been valuable in maintaining high sensitivity with low levels of cross-reactivity. Assays based on these antigens have been further refined using peptide epitopes in ELISA assays. Together with a recombinant LANA1, ELISA sensitivity and specificity of greater than 90% for KSHV detection can be routinely achieved. Complicating the serologic detection of KSHV is the fact that much of this work is based on patients with end-stage AIDS-KS. These patients routinely lose antibody reactivity due to loss of CD4+ helper activity.

The surge in KS among AIDS patients revealed the importance of cellular immunity, particularly CD4+ based immunity, to KS tumor control. Cell-mediated immunity assays have measured cellular immune responses against a number of KSHV protein epitopes, including those found on both structural and latent antigens. Among AIDS patients, these responses closely follow regression of KS tumors during highly active antiretroviral therapy (HAART).

Surprisingly, cellular immunity to the constitutively expressed LANA1 protein is generally low. The corresponding EBV protein, EBNA1, escapes immune surveillance by inhibiting its own proteosomal degradation and retarding its own translational synthesis. The latter effect appears to inhibit the formation of misfolded EBNA1 defective ribosomal products that are rapidly processed into MHC class I (MHC I) presented peptides. A similar mechanism seems to be at work for KSHV LANA1. Although the two proteins are not homologous, the nucleotide sequence of a central repeat region of both viral proteins is similar but is frameshifted between the two viruses. It remains to be seen whether the nucleotide sequence or the individual protein sequences are responsible for this immunoevasion effect.

KSHV also evades MHC I immune processing by expressing two proteins, MIR1 and MIR2, that ubiquitinate MHC I and other immune accessory proteins, causing them to be internalized and degraded. Although MIR1 and MIR2 are generally expressed during lytic replication, MIR1 is expressed at low levels during latency and can be upregulated by notch signaling.

In addition to cell-mediated immune response evasion, KSHV encodes a number of proteins that act to overcome innate immune signaling pathways. vIRF1 and the ORF45 protein act to sequester interferon-regulated transcription factors, effectively shutting off interferon signaling during infection. vIL6 signals in a similar manner to human IL-6 but it can bind directly to the signal transducer molecule gp130 to initiate signaling. One consequence of this effect is to abrogate signaling from interferon receptors to downstream signaling machinery.

KSHV-Associated Diseases

Kaposi's Sarcoma

KS is an endothelial tumor having molecular markers suggesting that it originates from lymphatic endothelium (**Figure 2**). Microscopically, the tumor is characterized by tumor spindle cells forming disorganized vascular clefts that fill with blood cells, giving the tumor a bruised like appearance. KSHV is detected in virtually all spindle cells, but tumors also show active neoangiogenesis in which more organized vessels lace the tumor mass. KSHV is generally absent from these cells and the intrusion of neovascular and immune cell components give the

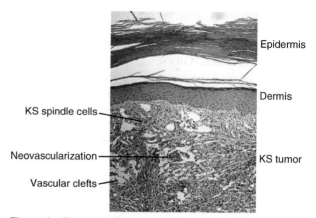

Figure 2   Photomicrograph of a KS tumor showing spindle tumor cells forming irregular vascular clefts that fill with blood. While near-universal KSHV infection of spindle cells is generally seen, the virus is generally absent from the neovascularization that can also be present in tumors. Frequently an inflammatory infiltrate is also seen in KS tumors.

tumors a mixed cellular origin. Thus, the pathology of KS strongly suggests that the tumor has both neoplastic and hyperplastic components. Conflicting data exist as to whether or not KS tumors are cellularly monoclonal, and studies of viral TRs suggest that KS tumors may originate from both polyclonal and monoclonal infection. It is likely that tumor cells evolve from polyclonal populations and gradually evolve into monoclonal or oligoclonal entities over time, helping to explain conflicting studies on the origin of the tumor.

Similarly, there is mixed evidence for the virus contributing to KS tumor growth through virus-transforming and paracrine activities. In tumors, virtually all tumor spindle cells are infected with KSHV, suggesting that the virus drives cell multiplication through intracellular expression of specific oncoproteins while the overwhelming majority of tumor cells are in a tight latency expression pattern. In line with this, antiherpesvirus drugs, such as ganciclovir, are effective in preventing KS but, once tumors are established, have little impact on disease. In contrast, KS tumors show marked hyperplasia and cellular cytokine overexpression. Since the virus is rapidly lost from tumor cells once the tumor is disaggregated and put into culture, there is strong evidence that the tumor environment maintains KSHV infection through paracrine signaling mechanisms. The best animal model for KS involves transgenic expression of vGPCR, which is known to induce factors such as VEGF in T cells, resulting in disorganized proliferation of endothelial cells. Taken together, these data suggest that the virus contributes to tumorigenesis through both neoplastic and hyperplastic mechanisms.

KS tumors from all sites and geographic settings are nearly universally infected with KSHV. While KS in the past has been split into categories depending on the epidemiologic setting, such as endemic KS, classical KS, iatrogenic KS, and epidemic KS, all forms of the tumor are pathologically indistinguishable. Cellular immune status appears to be key to the clinical expression of the tumor among infected persons. In the absence of HIV, KS primarily occurs in those with immune compromise such as the extreme elderly and patients on immunosuppressive therapy. The incubation period from infection to KS has been reported to average 3 years among HIV/AIDS patients, but this appears to be determined by degree of underlying immunosuppression at time of infection. In one case, transient KS was detected in an AIDS patient weeks after initial infection. While KSHV is largely asymptomatic in immunologically intact individuals, it has a very high degree of tumor expression among those who are immunosuppressed. Up to half of early AIDS patients develop KS and among transplant patients infected with KSHV, and 20–60% have been reported to develop clinical disease.

Primary Effusion Lymphoma

PEL is a rare, postgerminal center B-cell tumor accounting for less than 3% of B-cell lymphomas from various clinical series in developed countries. The tumor can form malignant effusions in body cavities, and among AIDS patients it generally has an aggressive course. Unlike KS, PELs are monoclonal. Tumor cells lack most B-cell markers, although V(D)J rearrangement studies confirm their B-cell origin and they express syndecan-1. PEL tumor cells have been reported to be autocrine-dependent on human IL10 and viral IL6. The latter cytokine is peculiar since it appears to form a 'xenocrine' loop in which vIL6 signaling abrogates cellular interferon responses resulting from virus infection that would otherwise stop growth of the tumor cell. PEL cells are uniformly infected with KSHV and can be grown stably in culture with each cell maintaining 40–150 copies of the viral episome. Cell lines derived from PEL tumors, particularly from AIDS patients, frequently have EBV coinfection, but EBV-negative, KSHV-positive tumors are also found.

Multicentric Castleman's Disease

Unlike PEL, MCD is considered a hyperproliferative lymphoid disorder, with affected individuals displaying a high rate for subsequent development of other lymphoid malignancies. Among HIV-negative persons, only about 50% of MCD tumors show evidence of KSHV infection whereas >90% of HIV-positive MCD patients have KSHV present.

The primary characteristic of MCD is the formation of adventitious germinal centers with marked hyperplasia in lymphoid organs. Examination of these KSHV-positive tumors reveals scattered KSHV infected cells in the marginal zone of the germinal centers, with the bulk of the cells being uninfected. Aberrant IL6 signaling has been demonstrated to be central to the pathogenesis of MCD, and KSHV-positive tumors have marked

expression of vIL6, with little human IL6 expression, while KSHV-negative tumors show extensive overexpression of the human cytokine.

Unlike KS and PEL, KSHV-infected tumor cells in MCD show a broad range of viral gene expression and perhaps full lytic viral replication. While standard treatment of KSHV-positive tumors has a high mortality, recent studies have reported marked success in treatment using anti-CD20 antibodies together with ganciclovir.

Other KSHV-Related Disorders

Transplant patients have been reported to develop bone marrow failure after graft infection with KSHV. The extent and consequences of this nonmalignant complication are unknown. In addition, a plasmacytic post-transplant lymphoproliferative disorder from KSHV has been reported to occur among transplant patients.

KSHV has been reported to be associated with a number of other malignant and autoimmune diseases, including multiple myeloma, sarcoidosis, post-transplant skin tumors, and idiopathic pulmonary hypertension. Despite initial enthusiasm, subsequent studies have largely failed to demonstrate any association between the virus and these diseases. It remains formally possible that KSHV causes a subset of one or more of these conditions with the majority of disease cases caused by other agents or conditions.

Diagnosis, Treatment, and Prevention

At present, there are no clinically certified tests to detect KSHV infection, although individual research laboratories have the capacity to test samples under special conditions. This presents a major public health problem, particularly in the setting of transplantation and in blood transfusions in highly endemic areas of the world. Treatment of KSHV-related diseases also generally does not directly target underlying viral infection, instead relying on traditional surgical and chemotherapy. An exception to this are ongoing clinical studies of MCD in which the lytic form of the virus is controlled with ganciclovir. Similarly, blinded clinical trials among high-risk AIDS patients show that antiherpesviral treatment can be highly effective in preventing KS. The introduction of HAART therapy has dramatically reduced the risk of KS among these patients, and thus attempts to extend these results have been limited. Since HAART does not target KSHV, it is expected that a resurgence of KS may occur with aging of the AIDS population.

There is currently no development of vaccines that might be useful to developing country populations. The exquisite sensitivity of KSHV-associated tumors to immune reconstitution and the loss of KSHV from developed populations throughout the world provides evidence that an appropriate vaccine might be extremely effective in controlling this virus infection.

In summary, the public health importance of this virus is clear: KS is the most common malignancy in sub-Saharan Africa and remains an important cause of cancer death among transplant and immunocompromised patients. It remains distressing that the wealth of basic science data available for this virus has yet to be used in a significant fashion to prevent or treat diseases caused by KSHV.

See also: Epstein–Barr Virus: General Features; Herpesviruses: General Features.

Further Reading

Beral V, Peterman TA, Berkelman RL, and Jaffe HW (1990) Kaposi's sarcoma among persons with AIDS: A sexually transmitted infection? *Lancet* 335: 123–128.

Chang Y, Cesarman E, Pessin MS, *et al.* (1994) Identification of herpesvirus-like DNA sequences in AIDS-associated Kaposi's sarcoma. *Science* 265: 1865–1869.

Ganem D (2006) KSHV-induced oncogenesis. In: Arvin A, Campadelli-Fiume G, Moore PS, Mocarski E, Roizman B, Whitley R, and Yamanishi K (eds.) *The Human Herpesviruses: Biology, Therapy and Immunoprophylaxis*, ch. 56, pp. 1007–1030. Cambridge, UK: Cambridge University Press.

Jarviluoma A and Ojala PM (2006) Cell signaling pathways engaged by KSHV. *Biochimica Biophysica Acta* 1766: 140–158.

Kaposi M (1872) Idiopathic multiple pigmented sarcoma of the skin. *Archives of Dermatology and Syphilology* 4: 265–273.

Martin J (2006) Epidemiology of KSHV. In: Arvin A, Campadelli-Fiume G, Moore PS, Mocarski E, Roizman B, Whitley R, and Yamanishi K (eds.) *The Human Herpesviruses: Biology, Therapy and Immunoprophylaxis*, ch. 5, pp. 960–985. Cambridge, UK: Cambridge University Press.

Mendez JC and Paya CV (2000) Kaposi's sarcoma and transplantation. *Herpes* 7: 18–23.

Russo JJ, Bohenzky RA, Chien MC, *et al.* (1996) Nucleotide sequence of the Kaposi sarcoma-associated herpesvirus (HHV8). *Proceedings of the National Academy of Sciences, USA* 93: 14862–14867.

Measles Virus

R Cattaneo, Mayo Clinic College of Medicine, Rochester, MN, USA
M McChesney, University of California, Davis, Davis, CA, USA

Glossary

Oncolytic virotherapy The experimental treatment of cancer patients based on the administration of replication-competent viruses that selectively destroy tumor cells but leave healthy tissue unaffected.

RNA editing The introduction into a RNA molecule of nucleotides that are not specified by the gene; the measles virus polymerase introduces a single G nucleotide in the middle of the phosphoprotein messenger RNA by reading twice over a C template (polymerase stuttering).

Subacute sclerosing panencephalitis (SSPE) A rare but always lethal brain disease caused by measles virus.

Syncytia Fused cells with multiple nuclei characteristic of measles virus infection.

Introduction and Classification

Measles virus (MV) is an enveloped nonsegmented negative-strand RNA virus of the family *Paramyxoviridae*, genus *Morbillivirus*. The *Paramyxoviridae* are important agents of disease, causing age-old diseases of human and animals (measles, mumps, respiratory syncytial virus (RSV), the parainfluenza viruses), and newly recognized emerging diseases (Nipah, Hendra, morbilliviruses of aquatic mammals).

Among negative-strand RNA viruses, the *Paramyxoviridae* are defined by having a protein (F) that causes fusion of viral and cell membranes at neutral pH. The organization and expression strategy of the nonsegmented genome of *Paramyxoviridae* including MV is similar to that of the *Rhabdoviridae*.

The defining characteristics of the genus *Morbilliviruses* are the lack of neuraminidase activity, and cell entry through the primary receptor signaling lymphocyte activation molecule (SLAM, CD150): MV, canine distemper virus, and rinderpest virus all enter cells through SLAM (human, canine, or bovine, respectively). The cellular distribution of SLAM overlaps with the sensitivity of different cell types to wild type MV infection, and explains immunosuppression.

Viral Particle Structure and Components

MV particles are enveloped by a lipid bilayer derived from the plasma membrane of the cell in which the virus was grown. They have been visualized as pleomorphic or spherical, depending on the methods used for their purification. Their diameter ranges from 120 to 300–1000 nm, implying that their cargo volume may differ by a factor 30 and that the large particles are polyploid. Inserted into the envelope are glycoprotein spikes that extend about 10 nm from the surface of the membrane and can be visualized by electron microscopy (**Figure 1**). A schematic diagram of an MV particle is shown in **Figure 2(a)**.

Inside the viral membrane is the nucleocapsid core, typically including several genomes. Each genome has 15 894 nucleotides tightly encapsidated by a helically arranged nucleocapsid (N) protein (**Figure 2(a)**). Two

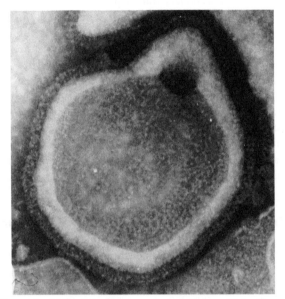

Figure 1 MV particle. Electron micrograph from Claire Moore and Shmuel Rozenblatt, Tel-Aviv University, Israel.

other proteins, a polymerase (L for large) and a polymerase cofactor (P for phosphoprotein), are associated with the RNA and the N protein to form a replicationally active ribonucleoprotein (RNP) complex. The MV RNP is condensed by the matrix (M) protein and then selectively covered by the two envelope spikes, consisting of oligomers of the F and H proteins.

The F protein spike is trimeric, whereas the H protein forms covalently linked dimers that may form noncovalently linked tetramers. The H protein contacts the cellular receptors, whereas F executes fusion. This protein is cleaved and activated by the ubiquitous intracellular protease furin. In the assembly process viral proteins are preferentially incorporated into nascent viral particles, whereas the majority of host proteins are excluded.

Genome, Replication Complex, and Replication Strategy

The MV negative-strand genome begins with a 56 nt 3′ extracistronic region known as leader, and ends with a 40 nt extracistronic region known as trailer. These control regions are essential for transcription and replication and flank the six genes. The term gene refers here to contiguous, nonoverlapping transcription units separated by three untranscribed nucleotides. There are six genes coding for eight viral proteins, in the order (positive strand): 5′-N-P/V/C-M-F-H-L-3′ (**Figure 2(b)**). The P gene uses overlapping reading frames to code for three proteins, P, V, and C. Complete sequences of several MV wild type and vaccine strains have been obtained.

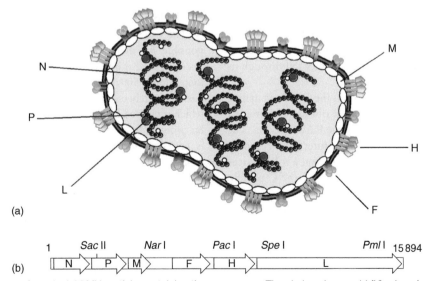

Figure 2 (a) Diagram of a polyploid MV particle containing three genomes. The viral nucleocapsid (N), phosphoprotein (P), polymerase (large, L), matrix (M), fusion (F), and hemagglutinin (H) proteins are indicated with different symbols. (b) Schematic representation of the MV antigenome (plus strand). The open reading frames of the six largest proteins are indicated with open arrows. The P gene codes for three proteins, P, V, and C. Unique restriction enzyme sites used for reverse genetics are indicated above the genome.

The first gene codes for the N protein. Each N protein covers 6 nt, and about 13 N proteins may constitute a turn in the RNP helix. RNPs are formed when N is expressed in the absence of other viral components, suggesting that N–N interactions drive RNP assembly. Two domains have been identified in the N protein: a conserved N-terminal N core (about 400 amino acids) and a variable C-terminal N tail (about 100 amino acids). N core is essential for self-assembly, RNA binding, and replication activity, whereas N tail interacts with a C-terminal domain of the P protein. N protein exists in at least two forms in infected cells: one associated with RNA in a RNP structure and a second unassembled soluble form named N^0 that may encapsidate the nascent RNA strand during genome and antigenome replication.

The second gene codes for three proteins implicated in transcription or innate immunity control: P, V, and C. Two of these proteins have a modular structure: the 231 N-terminal residues of V are identical with those of P, but its 68 C-terminal residues are translated from a reading frame accessed by insertion of a nontemplated G residue through co-transcriptional editing (polymerase stuttering). This V domain is highly conserved in paramyxoviruses, with cysteine and histidine residues binding two zinc molecules per protein. The main function of the V protein is to counteract the innate immune response; V interferes with intracellular signaling pathways supporting the interferon response and sustains virus spread in the host immune system.

The main function of the P protein is to support viral replication and transcription; it is an essential component of the polymerase, and of the protein complex mediating RNA encapsidation by N^0 protein. The P protein N-terminal segment, identical with the V protein N-terminus, is phosphorylated on serines and threonines and contains regions of high intrinsic disorder, possibly facilitating interactions with multiple viral and cellular proteins. P self-assembles as a tetramer through a central region in its unique domain, and interacts with N tail through its C-terminus.

The third protein expressed from the P gene is named C. Its reading frame is accessed by ribosomes initiating translation 22 bases downstream of the P AUG codon. The MV C protein not only inhibits the interferon response but also has infectivity factor function, and a role in virus particle release has been demonstrated for the C protein of the related Sendai virus.

The third, fourth, and fifth genes code for envelope-associated proteins that are discussed below in the context of receptor recognition and membrane fusion. The large (L) sixth and last codes for the RNA-dependent RNA polymerase, believed to possess all enzymatic activities necessary to synthesize mRNA: nucleotide polymerization, capping and methylation, and polyadenylation. L adds poly-A tails to nascent viral mRNAs cotranscriptionally, by stuttering on a stretch of U residues occurring at the end of each viral gene. Sequence comparison identified six highly conserved domains in the L protein that were tentatively assigned different catalytic functions, whereas interaction of this 200 kDa protein with the P and other viral proteins was mapped to nonconserved regions.

The N, P, and L proteins are associated with the RNA to form the replicationally active RNP complex that starts primary transcription after cell entry. The negative-strand genome is then used to synthesize positive-strand 'antigenomes' that produce more genomes, completing one amplification cycle. Amplification produces the genomic templates for secondary transcription.

The polymerase transcribes the viral genome with a sequential 'stop–start' mechanism. It accesses it through an entry site located near its 3′ end, transcribes the first gene (N) with high processivity, polyadenylates the N mRNA, and reinitiates P mRNA synthesis. The frequency of reinitiation is less than 100%, resulting in a gradient of transcript levels; N is transcribed at the highest levels, the most promoter-distal L gene (coding for a catalytic enzyme) at the lowest. The gene order and transcription strategy are fundamental characteristics that MV shares with all other paramyxoviruses.

Envelope Proteins and Cellular Receptors

The M protein, coded by the third gene, is a somewhat hydrophobic protein visualized as an electron-dense layer underlying the lipid bilayer. M is not an intrinsic membrane protein but can associate with membranes. It also binds RNPs, associates with the F and H protein cytoplasmic tails and modulates cell fusion. Thus, it is considered the assembly organizer and may also drive virus release/budding.

The two spike glycoproteins F and H are primarily responsible for membrane fusion and receptor attachment, respectively. An interesting peculiarity of the F gene is the long (almost 500 nt) 5′ untranslated region, whose function has not yet been characterized. The trimeric F protein, which is cleaved and activated by the ubiquitous intracellular protease furin, executes membrane fusion. This process is necessary for MV not only to enter cells, but also to spread through cell–cell fusion forming giant cells (syncytia). Membrane fusion activity depends not only on F protein proteolytic activation, but also on receptor recognition by the cognate H protein, which transmits a signal to F eliciting a conformational change and membrane fusion.

Since the MV H protein can hemagglutinate certain nonhuman primate red cells but lacks neuraminidase activity, it is named H and not HN. Other *Paramyxoviridae* use sialic acid as receptor and need neuraminidase to destroy receptor activity while budding from a host cell. Morbilliviruses do not use sialic acid as a receptor and do not need neuraminidase.

Two MV receptors have been characterized: Wild-type and vaccine MV target SLAM, whose expression is limited to immune cells. This protein was originally identified on activated B and T lymphocytes, but it is also expressed constitutively on immature thymocytes, memory T cells, and certain B cells. Other cell types including monocytes and dendritic cells (DCs) express SLAM only following activation. This cellular distribution overlaps with the sensitivity of different cell types to wild-type MV infection. Another strong argument for the central role of SLAM in MV tropism is the fact that three morbilliviruses (MV, canine distemper virus, and rinderpest virus) enter cells through SLAM (human, canine, or bovine, respectively).

The live attenuated MV vaccine strain Edmonston can also use the regulator of complement activation membrane cofactor protein (MCP; CD46) as a receptor. CD46's primary function is to bind and promote inactivation of the C3b and C4b complement products, a process protecting human cells from lysis by autologous complement, a function that requires ubiquitous expression. The question of the relevance of an ubiquitous receptor for the pathogenesis of a lymphotropic virus was raised when it was shown that the H protein of the attenuated Edmonston strain interacts much more efficiently with CD46 than the proteins of certain wild-type MV strains, and then again when the MV receptor function of human SLAM was discovered. The relevance of CD46 has been discussed in the context of both MV virulence and attenuation.

Clinical Features

Measles, one of the most contagious infectious diseases of man, was recognized clinically by the rash and other signs from early historical times and it was differentiated from small pox by Rhazes in the tenth century, who noted that it could be more fatal than small pox. Transmitted by aerosol droplets, the infection has an incubation period of 7–10 days, with onset of fever, cough, and coryza, followed in about 4 days by the skin rash which begins on the face and spreads to the whole body. The skin rash fades after about 5 days and clinical resolution is usually uneventful. Measles is typically an infection of childhood and protective immunity is lifelong, such that a second case of measles in a child or adult would be highly unusual. Prior to widespread vaccination against measles in the 1960s, the infection had a case–fatality rate of less than 5% in children, higher in infants and in children in developing countries, where fatality rates of up to 20% can still occur. Complications include pneumonia,. encephalitis, otitis media, blindness, and secondary infections by common bacteria and viruses. In developing countries, common complications are diarrheal illness and wasting. 'Atypical measles', a severe MV infection that occurred following the use of whole, inactivated virus vaccine from 1963 to 1967, is characterized by high and persistent fever, a different body rash that resembles Rocky Mountain spotted fever, and lobar pneumonia with effusions. This unusual clinical manifestation is discussed in the section titled 'Pathology and histopathology'.

Compared to infections by other viruses of the *Paramyxoviridae*, measles has more serious clinical potential than infection by RSV or the parainfluenza viruses, possibly because the latter infections are usually confined to the respiratory tract and not systemic; but measles in man causes less disease and death than infections due to the most closely related morbilliviruses, rinderpest in cattle, or canine distemper in dogs.

Latent tuberculosis may be reactivated following a case of measles. A regular complication of measles virus-induced immunosuppression was initially studied by von Pirquet, who observed, in 1908, that the tuberculin skin test response is suppressed during measles. MV-induced immunosuppression has an onset near to the peak of viremia, such that the primary immune responses to MV are not impaired, but the immunosuppression is global and lasts for several months. Several distinct mechanisms of virus–cell interaction have been elucidated to account for impaired functions of lymphocytes and antigen presenting cells by MV *in vitro*, but the global and sustained nature of immunosuppression *in vivo* is not understood. Infections by other morbilliviruses are also associated with immunosuppression and this complication was a hallmark of epidemic disease in harbor seals that resulted in the discovery of a new morbillivirus, the phocine distemper virus. In the extreme case, immunosuppression with massive lymphocyte depletion is fatal in canine distemper virus-infected ferrets.

Immune Response and Complications

The primary immune responses to MV, initially IgM antibody, type 1 CD4 and CD8+ T-cell responses, followed by neutralizing IgG antibody, are completely effective in controlling viral replication and resolution of the infectious process. Both primary and secondary immunodeficiencies that impair T-cell responses, for example, the DiGeorge syndrome or advanced HIV infection, are a significant risk for failure of the host to control MV infection, resulting in persistent infection and death or serious disease in the lower respiratory tract and central nervous system. In contrast, deficiency of the antibody response does not impair the immune control of MV replication.

These fundamental insights about antiviral immunity, based upon the tragic consequences of immunodeficiency diseases or childhood leukemia, were confirmed by the experimental infection of rhesus monkeys with MV. CD8+ T-cell depletion of monkeys at the time of viral inoculation resulted in prolonged viremia until the T cells repopulated, but depletion of B cells had no significant effect on MV infection. Persistent and/or fatal MV infection has occurred in HIV-infected children who contracted measles and this happened in a young, HIV-infected man who was vaccinated with live, attenuated MV. However, the risk of serious disease with measles in the immunocompromised host (50% or greater case fatality) outweighs the risk of vaccination, and measles vaccination is recommended for HIV-infected infants and children unless they have severe immunodeficiency with low, age-adjusted CD4+ T-cell counts in blood.

Persistent MV infection can result in giant cell pneumonia or two neurological diseases: measles inclusion body encephalitis and subacute sclerosing panencephalitis (SSPE). Another rare neurologic complication, acute demyelinating encephalomyelitis, not due to continuing viral replication in the brain, is associated with autoimmunity to myelin. Several other diseases, including multiple sclerosis, inflammatory bowel disease, and autism, have been linked to MV infection, either anecdotally or by inference or deduction, but causal connections to MV infection or vaccination have never been established.

Pathology and Histopathology

The histopathological hallmark of MV infection is the formation of syncytia, or multinucleated giant cells. Mediated by the viral fusion protein, syncytial cells are not unique to MV infection but they are characteristic. MV infects cells of ectodermal, endodermal, and mesenchymal origin and synctial cells have been observed in all of these cell types. Multinucleated giant cells are readily observed in the organized lymphoid organs and in mononuclear cell aggregates in many tissues, including the inflamed lung, where they are referred to as Warthin–Finkeldy giant cells. These syncytia are of lymphocyte, macrophage, dendritic, or reticular cell origin. Syncytial cells are also readily observed in many epithelia, including the columnar epithelieum of the trachea and bronchi, the stratified squamous epithelium of the skin and buccal mucosa, and the transitional epithelium of the urinary bladder and urethra. Endothelial syncytial cells were observed in small pulmonary arteries of monkeys infected with MV. Eosinophilic cytoplasmic and nuclear inclusion bodies can be seen in measles giant cells. The syncytial cells of measles are not long lived and they disappear with resolution of the infection.

The major pathologic changes of measles are due to inflammation and necrosis followed by tissue repair without fibrosis. Secondary infections by bacterial or other viral agents are common and they alter the pathologic process

accordingly, especially in the respiratory and gastrointestinal tracts. Pathology in the lower respiratory tract is mainly peribronchiolar inflammation and necrosis with a mild exudate, but interstitial pneumonitis with mononuclear cell infiltrates may occur. In the brain and central nervous system, perivascular mononuclear infiltrates can occur with a few necrotic endothelial cells, microglia, and neurons. In lymph nodes, spleen, and thymus, the major changes are mild to moderate lymphocyte depletion and multinucleated giant cells. Lymph node and splenic follicular hyperplasia are not seen in primary measles but are present if the host was previously infected or vaccinated against measles.

The unexpected occurrence of atypical measles following vaccination with whole-inactivated virus and subsequent infection with live, attenuated vaccine virus or wild-type virus was thought to be due to an aberrant, anamnestic host immune response resulting in an Arthus reaction or delayed hypersensitivity. Similar immunopathology was seen in children exposed to RSV following vaccination with whole-inactivated RSV. Atypical measles was experimentally induced in monkeys vaccinated with whole-inactivated MV and then challenged with wild type virus. Compared to monkeys vaccinated with live, attenuated MV, the aberrant immune responses associated with atypical measles resulted in immune complex deposition and eosinophilia. A marked skewing of T-cell cytokine responses toward type 2, with abnormal interleukin 4 production was also observed.

Diagnosis, Prevention and Control

As measles becomes a rare illness in regions with high vaccine coverage where the virus has been eliminated or controlled, the diagnosis of MV infection will be a challenge. The typical punctate, maculopapular skin rash, and the prodromal signs and symptoms are not specific for this viral infection and measles diagnosis requires differentiation from other pathogens causing exanthems of children, including infectious mononucleosis (Epstein–Barr virus) and cytomegalovirus infections, rubella, scarlet fever, typhus, toxoplasmosis, meningococcus, and staphylococcus. An enanthem with small white lesions on the buccal, labial, or gingival mucosal (Koplik's spots) is considered specific for MV infection and it typically occurs a few days before the skin rash. A buccal swab smeared on a glass slide, fixed and stained (e.g., Wright–Giemsa), may show multinucleated syncytia of epithelial cells. Secondary infections due to MV-induced immunosuppression are caused by the common pathogens in a geographic region. Detection of the early IgM response in blood by antibody-capture ELISA is diagnostic. MV can be cultured from peripheral blood mononuclear cells and from oral or nasal aspirates. Rescue of wild-type MV is readily done using B95a cells or Vero cells transfected with human SLAM. The virus can be detected by reverse transcription polymerase chain reaction (RT-PCR) from these samples and from urine. Filter paper spot assays of blood, buccal, or nasopharyngeal swabs have recently been developed for the detection of viral antibodies or viral RNA. The World Health Organization (WHO) hosts a website with descriptions of measles diagnostic samples and assays.

Measles remains the leading cause of vaccine-preventable illness and death in the world. The WHO and other international bodies have proposed the global eradication of MV in the twenty-first century, following the current campaign to eradicate poliovirus. This is an achievable goal as humans are the only known host species for this virus, although nonhuman primates are susceptible hosts. Regional elimination of MV has been achieved. Endogenous, circulating MV has been eliminated from the Americas in the last 20 years by the vaccination of children with the live, attenuated vaccines in current usage.

Many countries are planning to increase vaccination coverage as they progress toward targeted reductions in measles mortality or elimination of transmission. Recent experience in both developed and developing countries has shown that the maintenance of effective herd immunity against MV requires a two-dose vaccination strategy. Because of the highly contagious nature of this infection, about 95% of susceptibles will require vaccination to prevent the circulation of MV in a population of more than several hundred thousand. Greater than 90% measles vaccine coverage has been achieved in most countries but more than 25% of countries have not achieved this level of vaccination (**Figure 3**). The HIV pandemic presents a potential obstacle to MV eradication globally, especially in Africa and Asia, but HIV-infected children that are not immunocompromised can be safely vaccinated with live, attenuated MV (see above). The importation of MV into countries where elimination has been achieved is a very real challenge for diagnosis and control which has been successfully met by molecular genetic methods of rapid viral genomic sequencing and taxonomy.

The New Frontiers: MV-Based Multivalent Vaccines and Oncolysis

The live attenuated measles vaccine, which has an outstanding efficacy and safety record, is being developed as pediatric vaccine eliciting immunity against additional pathogens. An infectious cDNA with the identical coding capacity of a vaccine strain but with regularly spaced restriction sites has been engineered, and vectored MV expressing the hepatitis B surface antigen (HBsAg) generated by reverse genetics. One of these vectored MV vaccines induced protective

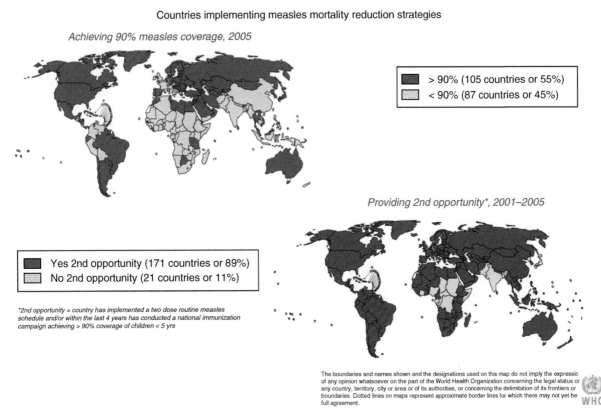

Figure 3 Global MV vaccine coverage, 2005. Reproduced from World Health Organization (2005) *Progress Towards Global Immunization Goals – 2005: Summary presentation of key indicators*, with permission.

levels of HBsAg antibodies while protecting Rhesus macaques against measles challenge. Another vectored MV expressing the West Nile virus envelope protein protected mice from West Nile virus encephalitis. A distinctive advantage of immunization with a di- or multivalent MV-based vaccine is delivery of an additional immunization safely without additional cost.

The knowledge gained from basic research has also been applied to the development of vectors for targeting and eliminating cancer cells. Oncolytic virotherapy is the experimental treatment of cancer patients based on the administration of replication-competent viruses that selectively destroy tumor cells but leave healthy tissue unaffected. MV is one of several human vaccine strains, or apathogenic animal viruses, currently being genetically modified to improve oncolytic specificity and efficacy. These modifications include targeting cell entry through designated receptors expressed on cancer cells like CD20 (lymphoma), CD38 (myeloma), or carcinoembryonic antigen (colon cancer).

Moreover, cancer cell specificity can be enhanced by silencing the expression of proteins that counteract the interferon system, often inactivated in cancer cells. Finally, proteolytic activation of the F protein has been engineered for exclusive cleavage through matrix metalloproteinases, enzymes degrading the extracellular matrix and promoting cancer invasiveness. Clinical trials of MV-based oncolysis for ovarian cancer, myeloma, and glioma are ongoing. These trials will soon profit from second generation targeted oncolytic MV with enhanced cancer specificity.

See also: Parainfluenza Viruses of Humans; Mumps Virus.

Further Reading

Cathomen T, Mrkic B, Spehner D, et al. (1998) A matrix-less measles virus is infectious and elicits extensive cell fusion: consequences for propagation in the brain. EMBO Journal 17: 3899–3908.
Cattaneo R (2004) Four viruses, two bacteria, and one receptor: Membrane cofactor protein (CD46) as pathogens' magnet. Journal of Virology 78: 4385–4388.
Griffin DE (2007) Measles virus. In: Knipe DM, Howley PM, Griffin DE, et al. (eds.) Fields Virology, 5th edn., vol. 2, pp. 1551–1586. Philadelphia, PA: Lippincott Williams and Wilkins.
Katz SL (2004) Measles (rubeola). In: Gershon AA, Hotez PJ,, and Katz SL (eds.) Krugman's Infectious Diseases of Children, 11th edn., pp. 353–372. Philadelphia: Mosby.
Lamb RA and Parks GD (2007) Paramyxoviridae: The viruses and their replication. In: Knipe DM, Howley PM, Griffin DE, et al. (eds.) Fields Virology, 5th edn., vol. 1, pp. 1449–1496. Philadelphia, PA: Lippincott Williams and Wilkins.
McChesney MB, Miller CJ, Rota PA, et al. (1997) Experimental measles. Part I. Pathogenesis in the normal and the immunized host. Virology 233: 74–84.
Moss WJ and Griffin DE (2006) Global measles elimination. Nature Reviews Microbiology 4: 900–908.
Panum P (1939) Observations made during the epidemic of measles on the Faroe Islands in the year 1846. Medical Classics 3: 829–886.
Rager M, Vongpunsawad S, Duprex WP, and Cattaneo R (2002) Polyploid measles virus with hexameric genome length. EMBO Journal 21: 2364–2372.
Rima BK and Duprex WP (2006) Morbilliviruses and human disease. Journal of Pathology 208: 199–214.
Springfeld C and Cattaneo R (in press) Oncolytic virotherapy. In: Schwab M (ed.) Encyclopedia of Cancer, 2nd edn. Heidelberg: Springer.
von Messling V and Cattaneo R (2004) Toward novel vaccines and therapies based on negative-strand RNA viruses. Current Topics in Microbiology and Immunology 283: 281–312.
von Messling V, Svitek N, and Cattaneo R (2006) Receptor (SLAM [CD150]) recognition and the V protein sustain swift lymphocyte-based invasion of mucosal tissue and lymphatic organs by a morbillivirus. Journal of Virology 80: 6084–6092.
von Pirquet C (1908) Das Verhalten der kutanen Tuberkulinreaktion während der Masern. Deutsche medizinische Wochenschrift 34: 1297–1300.
World Health Organization (2005) Progress Towards Global Immunization Goals – 2005: Summary Presentation of Key Indicators. http://www.who.int/immunization_monitoring/data/SlidesGlobalImmunization.pdf.
World Health Organization (2007) Manual for the Laboratory diagnosis of Measles and Rubella virus Infections, 2nd edn., http://www.who.int/immunization_monitoring/LabManualFinal.pdf (accessed December 2007).
Yanagi Y, Takeda M, and Ohno S (2006) Measles virus: Cellular receptors, tropism and pathogenesis. Journal of General Virology 87: 2767–2779.

Relevant Website

http://www.ncbi.nlm.nih.gov – National Center for Biotechnological Information.

Molluscum Contagiosum Virus

J J Bugert, Wales College of Medicine, Heath Park, Cardiff, UK

Glossary

Acanthoma A tumor composed of epidermal or squamous cells.

Anamnesis The complete history recalled and recounted by a patient.

Epicrisis A series of events described in discriminating detail and interpreted in retrospect.

History and Classification

The typical molluscum lesion, a smooth, dome-shaped, flesh-colored protrusion of the skin with a typical central indentation, was first described by Edward Jenner (1749–1823) as a 'tubercle of the skin' common in children. Thomas Bateman (1778–1821) first used the term 'molluscum contagiosum' (MC). In 1841, 'molluscum bodies', intracytoplasmic inclusions in the epidermal tissues of MC lesions, were independently observed by Henderson and Paterson. Similarities of molluscum bodies to the 'Borrel' bodies in fowlpox-infected tissues were noted later by Goodpasture, King, and Woodruff. At the beginning of the last century, Juliusberg demonstrated that the etiological agent of MC cannot be removed by filtration through Chamberland filters. Filtrates were used to infect human volunteers, who developed MC between 25 and 50 days after inoculation. Short of fulfilling all the Koch postulates, an animal model for MC has not been established to this day. Smaller elementary bodies inside the molluscum bodies were observed by Lipschütz in 1911. Electron microscopy revealed these elementary bodies to be poxvirus particles with dimensions of 360 nm × 210 nm.

Virion, Genome, and Evolution

Molluscum contagiosum virus (MCV) particles have a typical poxviral morphology (**Figure 1**). The virions are enveloped, pleomorphic, but generally ovoid to brick-shaped, with a dumbbell-shaped central core and lateral bodies similar to those in orthopoxvirus virions. MCV cores show complex structural patterns. Virions are often found to have membrane fragments loosely attached to them, indicating a noncontinuous lipid envelope wrapping the core.

The genome of MCV is a double-stranded DNA molecule of 190 289 bp (GenBank accession U60315: MCV type 1/80) with covalently closed termini (hairpins) and about 4.2 kbp of terminally inverted repeats (**Figure 2**). This excludes 50–100 bp of terminal hairpin sequences that could not be cloned or sequenced because replicative intermediates are not apparent in DNA from MCV biopsy specimens. The genomes of MCV (genus *Molluscipoxvirus*, subfamily *Chordopoxvirinae*), crocodilepox virus, and parapoxviruses stand out in the family *Poxviridae* because they have G+C contents of over 60%.

The MCV genome encodes 182 nonoverlapping open reading frames of more than 45 codons (**Figure 2**), almost half of which have no similarities to known proteins. Hypothetical MCV structural proteins and proteins encoding enzymes of the replication and transcription apparatus share obvious homologies to other poxvirus proteins. Less-obvious homologies exist between MCV and avipoxviruses (MC130, MC133, and MC131 A-type inclusion body-like proteins) and notably between MCV, parapoxviruses, and crocodilepox virus (MC026 modified RING protein and a number of proteins shared between only two of the above poxviruses). Unique MCV nonstructural proteins that are not involved in replication or transcription can be divided into two functional classes: (1) proteins dealing with the host immune system (host-response-evasion factors), such as the MCV chemokine antagonist (MC148) and the interleukin-18 (IL18)-binding protein (MC054), and (2) proteins supporting MCV replication in the host cell or the host tissue (host cell/tissue-modulating factors), such as the antiapoptotic selenoprotein MC066 and the Hrs-binding protein MC162.

An epidermal growth factor (EGF) homolog similar to the ones expressed by other poxviruses was not found in the genome of MCV. The only other poxvirus that

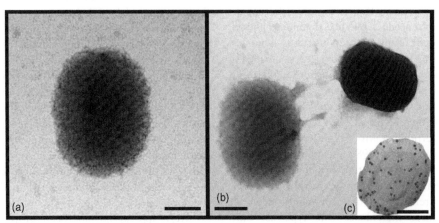

Figure 1 Electron microscope images of MCV particles negatively stained using the ammonium molybdate technique. (a) MCV particle showing the typical core protein pattern. (b) MCV particles: one that has lost the envelope appears larger and shows the typical core protein pattern, while the other is still wrapped in membrane and appears smaller. (c) Five nanometer gold particles bound to mouse antihuman antibodies, detecting human polyclonal patient antibodies binding to the surface of an MCV particle. Scale = 100 nm (a–c). Electron microscopy: Bugert and Hobot, Cardiff University School of Medicine, 2005.

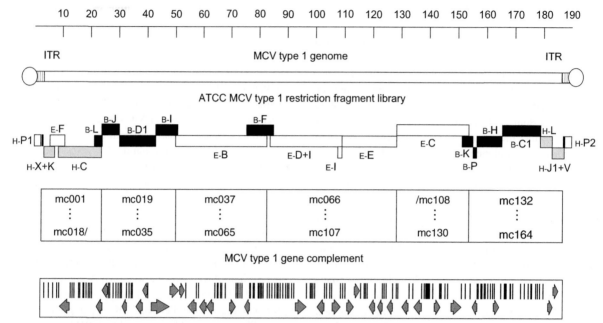

Figure 2 The MCV genome. The scale at the top is in kbp. The inverted terminal repeats (ITRs) are shown as vertical stripes flanking the genome, pointing inward from both covalently closed ends. The ITRs do not contain any complete coding sequences. The area covered by the ATCC MCV genome fragment library is shown as white (EcoRI restriction fragments), gray (HindIII restriction fragments), and black (BamHI restriction fragments) boxes representing the respective size of the viral sequence insert of each clone. The terminal HindIII restriction fragments P1 and P2 do not contain protein-coding regions and were not cloned. MCV genes are given the lowercase prefix 'mc', whereas (in the text) MCV proteins are given the uppercase prefix 'MC'. The MCV genes encoded in different parts of the genome, as defined by the boundaries of defined restriction fragments, are indicated in white boxes. The slashes signify ORFs that straddle a restriction site used for cloning and that are therefore not completely contained in any one plasmid on either side of the restriction site. Two MCV genes (mc036 and mc131) are split between two cloned restriction fragments, and therefore not listed. The numbering of MCV genes ends at mc164, the original number of genes larger than 90 codons. An additional 18 genes have been identified as being larger than 45 codons and are numbered as appendices of preceding genes (e.g., mc004.1). Protein-coding regions of the MCV type 1 gene complement are shown at the bottom as arrows (larger than 1.5 kbp) or small rectangles.

does not encode this factor is swinepox virus. However, MCV-infected basal keratinocytes seem to increase EGF receptor and transferrin receptor expression, in comparison to uninfected epidermis. Inducing EGF receptor expression may be an indirect mechanism causing epidermal hyperproliferation. MCV is the only chordopoxvirus that does not encode a J2R-like thymidine kinase.

In a phylogenetic analysis of 26 poxvirus genomes, MCV (representing the molluscipoxviruses) formed a group by itself among the subfamily of chordopoxviruses, separate from avipoxviruses (fowlpox virus), orthopoxviruses (vaccinia and variola viruses), and all other genera.

Four main genetic subtypes of MCV have been identified by DNA fingerprinting. MCV type 1 prototype (p) is the most common genetic type (98%) in immune-competent hosts in Western Europe. MCV type 1 (including variants) is the most common genetic type worldwide. MCV types 2–4 are relatively more commonly seen in immunocompromised individuals. One type has only been described in Japan. MCV genotypes discernible by DNA fingerprinting do not change when the viruses are transmitted between family members or in larger contact groups, indicating a low overall mutation rate.

Host Range and Virus Propagation

MCV, like smallpox virus, is considered to be an exclusive pathogen of man. Reports of MCV in a number of animals, including horses, chimpanzees, and kangaroos, have not been supported by DNA sequence confirmation. Many pox-like infections of vertebrates, most of them caused by orthopoxviruses, can be confused with MCV by their clinical appearance. Conventional immune-competent laboratory animals, including mice, rats, guinea pigs, and tree shrews, do not support MCV replication in their skin. MCV-infected human keratinocytes have been transplanted into mice with severe combined immune deficiency (SCID) and typical MCV lesions have subsequently developed in these non-natural hosts. Attempts to passage the virus in SCID mice were unsuccessful. However, despite the absence of molecular evidence, an animal reservoir of MCV cannot be excluded.

MCV has so far not been grown in conventional human cell lines, including immortalized tumorigenic/virus-transformed and nontumorigenic skin keratinocytes (HaCaT, NIKS). Experiments with *ex vivo* cultures of human skin cells (raft cultures) are ongoing. MCV may use a vegetative mechanism for replicating in differentiating keratinocytes.

In the absence of culturable virus, classical virological research on MCV is severely restricted. All progress so far has been made by studying MCV genes in isolation, based on the complete MCV genome sequence gained from an overlapping redundant MCV genome fragment library. This reagent has been made available to the ATCC. The entire MCV gene complement is covered by 18 recombinant bacterial plasmid clones harboring viral sequences from the EcoRI, BamHI, and HindIII restriction fragment libraries of MCV type 1/80 (**Figure 2**).

Further research is being carried out using abortive cell culture systems. MCV induces a remarkable cytopathogenic effect (CPE) in human fibroblasts, both in primary cells (MRC5) and in telomerase-transduced immortal cell lines (hTERT-BJ-1). The CPE starts 4 h post infection (p.i.) and reaches a maximum at 24 h p.i., with the cells looking as if they have been trypsinized, partially detaching from the monolayer, rounding, and clumping. Cells settle down at 48–72 h p.i., but show a morphological transformation from an oblong fibroblast to a more square epithelial-looking cell type. MCV transcribes early mRNA in these cells. The CPE is not induced by UV-inactivated virions or in the presence of cycloheximide, indicating that expression of viral proteins is required. mRNA transcription can be detected by reverse transcriptase-polymerase chain reaction (RT-PCR) for months in serially passaged infected cells. A productive MCV infection cannot be rescued nongenetically by co-infection with other chordopoxviruses in these cells. MCV can infect human HaCaT keratinocytes and transcribes mRNA in these cells, but does not induce a CPE. MCV cannot infect nonhuman cells. It induces type 1 interferons in mouse and human embryo fibroblasts and IL8 in human lung epithelial cells, which it cannot infect, suggesting involvement of surface pathogen-associated molecular pattern (PAMP) receptors like TLR2 or TLR4. Removal of interferon pathways from cell lines susceptible for MCV infection would be worth investigating, in order to exclude interference causing abortive MCV infections. MCV is currently isolated from human-infected skin biopsies. MCV purified from biopsy material can be used for infection studies, electron microscopy, viral DNA extraction, and analyses of early mRNA synthesized by *in vitro* transcription of permeabilized virions.

Clinical Features and Pathology

The mean incidence of MC in the general population is 0.1–5%. Seroepidemiological studies have shown that antibody prevalence in persons over 50 years of age is 39%. This indicates that MC is a very common viral skin infection, which is supported by its common occurrence in dermatological practice. MCV outbreaks occur in crowded populations with reduced hygienic standards. Outbreaks with more than 100 cases have been described in kindergartens, military barracks, and public swimming pools. MC was found to be very common in the Fiji Islands.

MC is most often seen as a benign wart-like condition (German: *dellwarze*) with light pruritus in preadolescent children, but can occur in immuncompetent adults. MC is more severe in immunocompromised people or individuals with atopic dermatitis, where it can lead to giant molluscum and eczema molluscum. The lesions generally occur on all body surfaces, but not on the palm of the hand or on mucous membranes. They may be associated with hair follicles. MC lesions can grow close to mucous membranes on the lips and eyelids. When situated near the eye, they can lead to conjunctivitis. MC is transmitted by smear-infection with the infectious fluids discharged from lesions and by direct contact with contaminated objects. MC is not very contagious and therefore infection depends on a high inoculating dose. It is a sexually transmitted disease when lesions are located on or in the vicinity of sexual organs.

MC lesions are generally globular, sometimes ovate, 2–5 mm in diameter and sit on a contracted base. Cellular semiliquid debris can be expressed from the central indentation at the top of the lesion. The infection spreads via contact with this fluid. Histologically, the tumors are strictly limited to the epidermal layer of the skin and have a resemblance to hair follicles. They are therefore classified as acanthomas.

If not mechanically disturbed, MC lesions will persist for months and even years in immune-competent hosts, but can disappear spontaneously, probably when virus-infected tissue is exposed to the immune system. To expose the infection by limited (sterile) trauma is a way of treatment.

Scratching or disturbing the lesions leads to a quicker resolution but can complicate the condition through bacterial superinfection. This must be avoided in severely immunocompromised hosts, who develop widespread MC with hundreds of lesions of larger size and can succumb to sepsis following bacterial superinfection. MCV is a marker of late-stage disease in human immunodeficiency virus (HIV)-infected individuals, and in HIV-infected populations the incidence of MC was 30% before the onset of human cytomegalovirus (HCMV) prophylaxis with cidofovir.

MCV probably enters the epidermis through microlesions. The typical MCV lesion contains conglomerates of hyperplastic epithelial cells organized in follicles and lobes, which all develop into a central indentation toward the surface of the skin in a process similar to holocrine secretion. The whole lesion has the appearance of a hair follicle where the hair is replaced by the virus-containing plug. The central indentation is filled with cellular debris and is rich in elementary viral particles in a waxy plug-like structure. This plug becomes mobilized and spreads the infection to other areas of surrounding skin or contaminates objects. The periphery of the MCV lesion is characterized by basaloid epithelial cells with prominent nuclei, large amounts of heterochromatin, slightly basophilic cytoplasm, and increased visibility of membranous structures. These cells are larger than normal basal keratinocytes, they divide faster than normal basal cells, their cytoplasm contains a large number of vacuoles, and they are sitting on top of an intact basal membrane. The lesion is a strictly intraepidermal hyperplastic process (acanthoma). Distinct poxviral factories (molluscum bodies or Henderson– Patterson bodies) appear about four cell layers away from the basal membrane in the stratum spinosum. The inclusion bodies grow and obliterate cellular organelles. Cells with inclusion bodies do not divide further. The cytoplasm of MCV-producing cells shows keratinization, which is not expected at that stage of keratinocyte differentiation and indicates dyskeratinization in the sense of abnormal differentiation.

Immune Response

In undisturbed MC lesions, histological studies have shown a conspicuous absence of effectors of the cellular immune system, in particular skin-specific tissue macrophages (Langerhans cells). This is in contrast to papillomata, where a vigorous cellular immune response, including cytotoxic T lymphocytes (CTLs), is mounted immediately. The absence of macrophages has been attributed to the activity of various MCV genes that are suspected to make the MC lesion immunologically 'invisible'. This includes a biologically inactive IL8 receptor-binding beta-chemokine homolog (MC148), which may suppress the immigration of neutrophils; a major histocompatibility complex (MHC) class I homolog that may upset MHC class I antigen presentation on the surface of infected cells, or natural killer cell recognition; and an IL18-binding protein, which underlines the importance of this cytokine for the local immune response in human skin. As for the humoral response, MCV-specific antibodies have been detected in several studies, showing a seroprevalence of MCV of up to 40% in the general population, much higher than previously expected. However, these antibodies do not seem to confer a neutralizing immunity. MCV genes were expressed in a cowpox virus expression system and two antigenetically prominent MCV proteins identified: mc133L (70 kDa protein: MC133) and mc084L (34 kDa protein: MC084). These proteins are presumably glycosylated and present on the surface of MCV virions, where they allow binding of antibodies and detection by immune electron microscopy (**Figure 1(c)**).

Diagnosis, Treatment, and Prevention

MCV is readily diagnosed by its clinical appearance and by the typical histopathology found in sections of lesion biopsies. After the eradication of smallpox, MCV is the most commonly diagnosed poxviral infection. Ortho- and parapoxviral zoonoses are rare. In the differential diagnosis of MC, smallpox must be considered along with other ortho- and parapoxviruses. The anamnesis must cover contacts with pets, especially gerbils and chipmonks of African origin (monkeypox) as well as local rodents and cats (cowpox). Always looming in the background is the possibility of a smallpox bioterrorist attack. An actual example for the management of such a contingency is the epicrisis of a

Table 1   Suggested MC treatments, side effects, and success rates

Symptom	Therapy	Side effects	Success rates
Pruritus	Antihistamine ointments	Tiredness	High
Acanthoma	Curettage (surgical) with sharp spoon. Local anesthetics required for children	Scar, pain impractical for large lesion numbers	High
	Lancing of lesion with needle	Pain, infection	High
	Cryosurgery with topical anesthesia	Pain, no scars	Medium
	Topical salicylic acid colloid, for example, occlusal (26% salicylic acid in polyacrylic vehicle)		High
	Immune modulators	Predisposition for bacterial and fungal skin infections	Low
	Tacrolimus 0.1% ointment		
	Pimecrolimus 0.5% ointment		
	Imiquimod 0.5% ointment		
	Podophyllotoxin 0.5% ointment		
	Antivirals (high cost)	Allergy	High
	DNA polymerase inhibitors		
	Acyclic nucleoside phosphonates (e.g., topical cidofovir)		
	Topoisomerase inhibitors		
	Lamellarin		
	Coumermycin		
	Cyclic depsipeptide sansalvamide A		

monkeypox outbreak in Wisconsin, USA, in 2003 published by the Centers for Disease Control and Prevention (CDC). The most likely nonpoxviral differential diagnosis is varicella-zoster virus. Other viral agents can be excluded by - electron microscopy and PCR. Further differential diagnoses include syphilis, papilloma, and skin malignancies such as melanoma.

MC lesions are generally self-limiting, with an average of 6 months to 5 years for lesions to disappear. Patients with immune dysfunction or atopic skin conditions have difficulty clearing lesions. Therapy is recommended for genital MC to avoid sexual transmission, and should include antipruritics to prevent scratching and bacterial superinfection.

Treatment options cover a wide range of invasive and topical treatment strategies (**Table 1**). Topical application of salicylic acid or removal by curettage emerge as the two most successful strategies for large and small numbers of lesions, respectively. Needling of lesions has been reported to work and may expose MCV to immune effectors. In immune-suppressed individuals with widespread MC, topical immune modulators like imiquimod have been tried with limited success. Topical antivirals work but are not cost-effective.

MC is best prevented by exposure prophylaxis. The vaccine against smallpox (vaccinia virus) does not protect against MCV, underlining the fundamental antigenic differences between ortho- and molluscipoxviruses.

See also: Cowpox Virus; Poxviruses; Smallpox and Monkeypox Viruses.

Further Reading

Brown T, Butler P, and Postlethwaite R (1973) Non-genetic reactivation studies with the virus of molluscum contagiosum. *Journal of General Virology* 19: 417–421.

Bugert JJ (2006) Molluscipoxviruses. In: Mercer A, Schmidt A,, and Webber O (eds.) *Advances in Infectious Diseases*, pp. 89–112. Basel: Birkhauser.

Bugert JJ and Darai G (1991) Stability of molluscum contagiosum virus DNA among 184 patient isolates: Evidence for variability of sequences in the terminal inverted repeats. *Journal of Medical Virology* 33: 211–217.

Bugert JJ and Darai G (2000) Poxvirus homologues of cellular genes. *Virus Genes* 21: 111–133.

Buller RM, Burnett J, Chen W, and Kreider J (1995) Replication of molluscum contagiosum virus. *Virology* 213: 655–659.

Konya J and Thompson CH (1999) Molluscum contagiosum virus: Antibody responses in persons with clinical lesions and seroepidemiology in a representative Australian population. *Journal of Infectious Diseases* 179: 701–704.

McFadden G, Pace WE, Purres J, and Dales S (1979) Biogenesis of poxviruses: Transitory expression of molluscum contagiosum early functions. *Virology* 94: 297–313.

Melquiot NV and Bugert JJ (2004) Preparation and use of molluscum contagiosum virus from human tissue biopsy specimens. *Methods in Molecular Biology* 269: 371–384.

Porter CD and Archard LC (1992) Characterisation by restriction mapping of three subtypes of molluscum contagiosum virus. *Journal of Medical Virology* 38: 1–6.

Postlethwaite R and Lee YS (1970) Sedimentable and non-sedimentable interfering components in mouse embryo cultures treated with molluscum contagiosum virus. *Journal of General Virology* 6: 117–125.

Reed RJ and Parkinson RP (1977) The histogenesis of molluscum contagiosum. *American Journal of Surgical Pathology* 1: 161–166.

Scholz J, Rosen-Wolff A, Bugert J, et al. (1998) Molecular epidemiology of molluscum contagiosum. *Journal of Infectious Diseases* 158: 898–900.

Senkevich TG, Bugert JJ, Sisler JR, Koonin EV, Darai G, and Moss B (1996) Genome sequence of a human tumorigenic poxvirus: Prediction of specific host response-evasion genes. *Science* 273: 813–816.

Thompson CH, Yager JA, and Van Rensburg IB (1998) Close relationship between equine and human molluscum contagiosum virus demonstrated by *in situ* hybridisation. *Research in Veterinary Science* 64: 157–161.

Viac J and Chardonnet Y (1990) Immunocompetent cells and epithelial cell modifications in molluscum contagiosum. *Journal of Cutaneous Pathology* 17: 202–205.

Vreeswijk J, Leene W, and Kalsbeek GL (1976) Early interactions of the virus molluscum contagiosum with its host cell. Virus-induced alterations in the basal and suprabasal layers of the epidermis. *Journal of Ultrastructural Research* 54: 37–52.

Mumps Virus

B K Rima and W P Duprex, The Queen's University of Belfast, Belfast, UK

Glossary

Editing Process by which mRNAs are altered during or after transcription of the gene.

Mononegavirales Order of viruses consisting of four families with nonsegmented negative-stranded RNA genomes.

Nucleocapsid The ribonucleoprotein of mumps virus consisting of the RNA genome, the nucleocapsid protein, and associated proteins.

Pleomorphic From the Greek 'having many forms'.

Polyploid Having more than one genome copy per virion.

R₀ Index used in epidemiology, indicating the number of secondary cases that could originate from a single index case of viral infection.
Viremia Presence of virus in blood.
Virion The virus particle.

History

The primary clinical manifestation in mumps is swelling of the salivary glands because of parotitis. This symptom is so characteristic that the disease was recognized very early as different from other childhood illnesses which give rise to skin rashes. Hippocrates described mumps as a separate entity in the fifth century BC. He also noted swelling of the testes (orchitis) as a common complication of mumps. Infection in the central nervous system (CNS) and meninges in some cases of mumps was first noted by Hamilton in 1790. In 1934, Johnson and Goodpasture demonstrated the filterable nature of the causative agent and Koch's postulates were fulfilled by infection of human volunteers with virus propagated in the salivary glands of monkeys.

Taxonomy and Classification

Mumps virus (MuV) is sensitive to ether and other membrane-destroying reagents and has hemagglutinating and neuraminidase (HN) activity. It contains a nonsegmented negative-stranded RNA genome. MuV is thus classified in the family *Paramyxoviridae* and placed in the genus *Rubulavirus*. MuV is the prototype species, and two other human rubulaviruses, human (h) parainfluenza virus 2 (hPIV2)

and hPIV4, have been identified. Other rubulaviruses infect a range of vertebrates – for example, Mapuera virus infects bats. Simian virus 5 (SV5) was originally isolated from rhesus and cynomolgus monkey kidney-cell cultures and thus designated as a primate virus. Sometimes SV5 is referred to as canine parainfluenza virus although it has a more extended host range and it has been suggested the virus be renamed PIV5. Porcine rubulavirus (PoRv) caused a fatal encephalomyelitis in neonatal pigs. Newcastle disease virus and a number of avian paramyxoviruses were included in the genus although these have recently been assigned to the genus *Avulavirus*.

Properties of the Virion

Paramyxoviruses consist of an inner ribonucleoprotein (RNP) core surrounded by a lipid bilayer membrane from which spikes protrude (**Figure 1**). The MuV virion appears to be roughly spherical and normally diameters range from 100 to 300 nm when the virus is grown in cell culture or embryonated eggs. Sometimes bizarre rod-shaped and other pleomorphic particles have been observed. Electron microscopy (**Figure 1(a)**) shows that MuV has the typical paramyxovirus structure with a lipid bilayer membrane surrounding an internal RNP complex, the nucleocapsid. The nucleocapsid displays the herring-bone structure characteristic of *Paramyxoviridae* (arrow, **Figure 1(a)**) and is approximately 1 μm in length with a diameter of 17 nm and an internal central core of 5 nm. Some of the pleomorphic particles have been reported to contain more than one RNP structure. The biological significance of such polyploid particles has not been investigated.

The RNP contains the RNA genome covered with nucleocapsid (N) protein as well as a phosphoprotein (P)

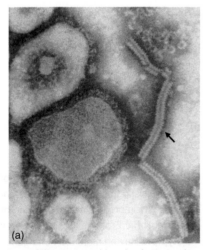

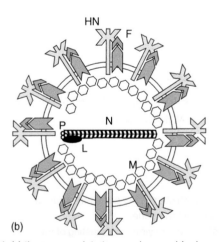

(a)   (b)

Figure 1   The structure of the mumps virion. In electron micrograph (a) the arrow points to a nucleocapsid released from a virus particle showing the characteristic herringbone structure. Schematic representation (b) indicates the location of the major viral structural proteins (see **Figure 2** for an explanation of the shapes and abbreviations).

and the large protein (L). The RNP is surrounded by a lipid bilayer membrane derived from the host cell in which the matrix protein (M) of the virus is embedded (**Figure 1(b)**). This protein interacts with the internal core N protein and the viral glycoproteins. Spikes (10–15 nm in length) protrude from the membrane and these contain the viral glycoproteins, the hemagglutinin–neuraminidase protein (HN) and the fusion (F) protein. The HN protein is probably a homo-tetramer, the fusion protein a homo-trimer. The ratio of HN and F protein molecules in the spike complex has not been elucidated yet. The spikes are also involved in the hemolysis of erythrocytes of different origins. The hemolysis reflects the ability of the virus to fuse with infected cells. Fusion is required for the entry of the RNP cores into cells.

Properties of the Genome

MuV has a single nonsegmented negative-stranded RNA genome (**Figure 2(a)**). The nucleotide sequence of the entire genome of several strains is known and all of these are 15 384 nt in length. The order of the genes of MuV and transcription of the genome is similar to that of other paramyxoviruses, especially to that of PIV5. There are seven transcription units which are separated by intergenic (Ig) sequences. The basic unit of infectivity is the negative-stranded, encapsidated RNP (**Figure 2(d)**).

Properties of the Proteins

The properties of the MuV proteins are summarized in **Table 1** and the number of amino acid residues in each viral protein is given in **Figure 2(c)**. It should be emphasized that this assignment is largely based on analogy of the MuV proteins with those of other paramyxoviruses, as gene identifications have not been carried out directly. However, the similarities to other paramyxoviruses are so striking that this assignment is beyond dispute. The presence of six structural proteins, namely, the N, P, M, and L proteins, as well as two glycosylated membrane-spanning proteins, the HN and F proteins, has been demonstrated in MuV virions. Furthermore, the virus induces the synthesis of at least two nonstructural proteins (V and W) from transcripts of the V/W/P gene. The presence of a small hydrophobic (SH) protein has been demonstrated in MuV-infected cells using antisera to peptides derived from the deduced amino acid sequence. It is not clear whether the protein is incorporated into virions. At least one strain (Enders) expresses the SH gene as a tandem readthrough transcript with the F gene in tissue culture. It is unlikely that the SH protein is translated from such an F–SH bicistronic mRNA and growth of this strain in tissue culture may not require the expression of this protein. A recombinant virus lacking the SH protein has been shown to be unaffected in growth in several cell types, formally proving the nonessential nature of the protein.

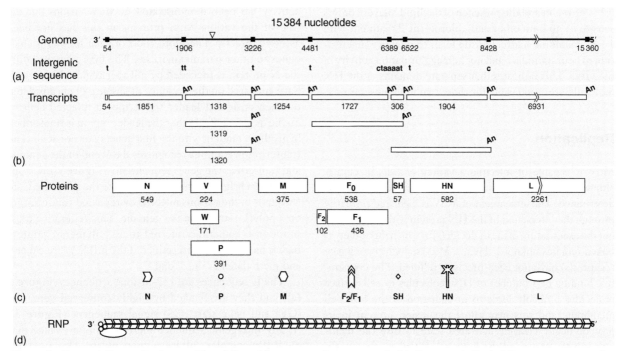

Figure 2 Transcription, replication, and translation of the mumps virus genome. In this figure are indicated: the mumps gene order and size and the position, sequence (positive strand) of the intergenic sequences (a); the major transcripts derived from the MuV genome and their sizes (b); the proteins and their sizes in numbers of amino acid residues and their schematic representations (c), and the replicative intermediates (d).

Table 1   Properties of the proteins of MuV

Protein	Size in SDS-PAGE (kDa)	Function
Nucleocapsid (N)	68–73	Phosphorylated structural protein of RNP; protects genome from RNases, possible role in regulation of transcription and replication (S antigen)
Phosphoprotein (P)	45–47	Phosphorylated protein associated with the RNP; possible role in solubilization of the N protein, role in RNA synthesis
Large (L)	>200	Protein with RdRp polymerase activity associated with the RNP; role in capping, methylation, and polyadenylation
Matrix (M)	39–42	Hydrophobic protein associated with inner side of membrane; role in budding by interactions with the N, HN, and F proteins
Fusion (F)	65–74	Acylated, glycosylated protein F_2–F_1 heterodimer activated by proteolytic cleavage; fusion of virion membrane with the plasma membrane which also involves HN (hemolysis antigen)
Hemagglutinin–neuraminidase (HN)	74–80	Acylated and glycosylated protein with hemagglutinin and neuraminidase activity; accessory role in fusion of virion membrane with the plasma membrane (major V antigen)
Small hydrophobic (SH)	6	Membrane protein with unknown function; present in infected cells but not detected in virions to date
Nonstructural V (earlier NS1)	23–28	Phosphorylated protein with a cysteine-rich domain which may be involved in metal binding; leads to the proteasomal degradation of STAT1 and targets STAT3 for ubiquitination
Nonstructural W (earlier NS2)	17–19	Phosphorylated protein with unknown role, possibly an artifact of misediting

SDS-PAGE, sodium dodecyl sulfate-polyacrylamide gel electrophoresis; kDa, mass of the protein in kilodaltons.

Physical Properties

The MuV virion is very susceptible to heat and treatment with ultraviolet (UV) light. The UV target size is one genome equivalent of RNA. The virus is inactivated by 0.2% formalin and the presence of the lipid bilayer confers sensitivity to both ether and chloroform. Treatment with 1.5 M guanidine hydrochloride leads to selective inactivation of neuraminidase and not hemagglutination activity of the virus. This indicates that separate domains of the HN molecule are responsible for these two functions.

Replication

MuV is capable of infecting a variety of cells in culture although whether this is the case *in vivo* remains to be determined. The attachment of MuV is mediated primarily through the interaction of the HN protein with a sialic acid, but the exact nature of the molecule(s) to which this moiety is linked remains unknown. Hence, MuV sialoglycoconjugate receptor(s) have not been precisely defined. The cooperative binding of a number of HN molecules to cell surface molecules probably leads to invagination of the host cell membrane and this may allow the fusion protein in its proteolytically cleaved, activated state to fuse the membrane of the virus and the host cell. Whether viropexis is another mechanism of entry of MuV is not known.

After introduction of the RNP into the cell, primary transcription of the negative-stranded genome occurs.

This is probably mediated by the viral L and P proteins of the virion and leads primarily to the synthesis of positive-strand, monocistronic mRNAs (**Figure 2(b)**). In addition, a number of polycistronic mRNAs have been identified. RNA-dependent RNA polymerase (RdRp) activity has been demonstrated in MuV virions but the role of the various viral proteins in this has not been assessed directly. Therefore, most of what follows is analogous to other paramyxoviruses. The first gene encoding the N protein is preceded by a leader region. No reports have appeared on the presence or absence of encapsidated or unencapsidated leader transcripts in infected cells or on the question of whether the leader region is transcribed by itself, in tandem with the first gene(s), or not at all. The transcription complex recognizes the 3′ end of the genome and transcribes the genes sequentially (**Figure 2(c)**), stopping at each Ig sequence to synthesize the polyadenylate (An) tails of the various mRNAs by repeated transcription on a poly(U) stretch in the genome. This reiterative transcription is sometime referred to as 'polymerase stuttering'. It has not been determined if the mRNAs are capped and methylated at the 5′ end.

The Ig sequences are 1–7-nt-long sequences (**Figure 2(a)**) and they are flanked by highly conserved gene end (GE) and gene start (GS) signal sequences (**Figure 3**). At any intergenic sequence there is a finite chance that the RdRp complex will leave the template. This gives rise to a transcription gradient so that the 3′ proximal N gene is most frequently transcribed and the 5′ proximal L gene is transcribed very infrequently. The gradient has not

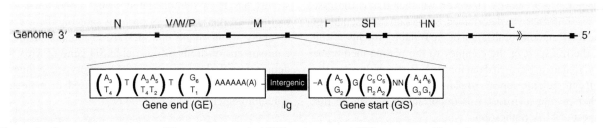

Figure 3 Consensus sequences of the seven gene start (GS) and gene end (GE) sequences. The various consensus sequences are shown as positive strand sequences. The specific intergenic sequences and their positions in the genome are shown in **Figure 2(a)**.

been quantified in MuV-infected cells. Occasionally, the GE and GS sequences are ignored and tandem read-through transcripts of two or more genes are generated. Recognition of transcription signals appears to be dependent on host as well as viral factors. Thus, strains which have been adapted to growth in eggs only give rise to monocistronic mRNAs in chicken embryo fibroblasts, whereas only large tandem readthrough transcripts are generated if mammalian cells in culture are infected with these strains.

Co-transcriptional editing is responsible for the generation of mRNAs encoding the P and W proteins of MuV. Insertion of one or up to five extra G residues at a site in the V/W/P gene with a sequence similar to the polyadenylation signal leads to the formation of mRNAs that encode the W and P protein or V, W, or P proteins with an extra glycine residue (**Figures 2(b)** and **2(c)**).

The mRNAs are translated by cellular ribosomes and there is no indication for shutoff of host mRNA translation or preferential translation of viral mRNAs in MuV-infected cells. Early reports of temporal translational control and control of transcription and translation of host mRNAs by the presence of viral glycoproteins in the cell membrane have not been confirmed. Some of the viral proteins are modified post-translationally (**Table 1**). The processing pathway for the HN protein differs from that for the F protein. The HN protein forms oligomers during transport through the Golgi apparatus, and carbohydrate side chains are modified slowly in the *trans*-Golgi cisternae, whereas the F protein rapidly matures with respect to its glycosylation. The proteolytic cleavage and consequent activation of the F_0 precursor into the F_1 and F_2 complex occurs in the *trans*-Golgi cisternae. Both the F and the HN proteins appear to play a role in fusion of virus-infected cells and syncytium formation. This is indicated by the observations that first, fusing as well as nonfusing strains contain cleaved activated F protein (i.e., the F_1 and F_2 complex); second, levels of neuraminidase are higher in nonfusing strains; and third, proteolytic cleavage of the HN protein can activate fusion. Co-expression of F and HN from eukaryotic expression vectors leads to the formation of multinucleated syncytia in transiently transfected cells which are indistinguishable

from those generated in an MuV infection. These fusion assays have been useful in assessing the effect of site-directed mutagenesis on the biological function of the proteins and in determining where oligomerization takes place in the cell. Co-transfection of an equivalent construct containing the M gene has shown that this does not alter syncytium size.

Replication of the genome starts at the 3′ end of the (−) RNP. In replication mode the RdRp ignores the GE, Ig, and GS signals to generate one single positive-stranded RNA molecule. This RNA is concomitantly encapsidated by N protein immediately after the start of its synthesis leading to the formation of a (+)RNP. It is not known for MuV if the transcriptase complex and the replicase complex are identical or whether they involve different host factors, as is the case for vesicular stomatitis virus, another virus in the order *Mononegavirales*. The intracellular concentration of N protein may regulate the balance between transcription and replication. The positive-stranded RNAs in the newly formed RNPs then form the template for further negative-strand synthesis, again with concomitant encapsidation by N protein. The resulting (−)RNPs reach the cell surface by an unknown mechanism where they are incorporated into progeny virions. The budding process itself and its regulation have not been studied in great detail for MuV. Virion budding probably takes place as a consequence of the interaction of the M protein with the RNP (most probably the C-terminal part of the N protein) and the cytoplasmic tails of the viral glycoproteins which accumulate in patches on the plasma membrane. Both (+)RNPs, containing the genome, and (−)RNPs, containing the antigenome, can be incorporated into MuV virions. However, whether the budding process is selective in favoring inclusion of (−)RNPs into virions is not yet clear.

There are a number of outstanding issues with respect to the life cycle of MuV which are not yet clear, some of which are specific to the virus. The role(s) of the V and W (earlier called NS1 and NS2, respectively) nonstructural proteins in the processes of replication, transcription, translation, and assembly has yet to be elucidated. Neither is it clear what role the SH protein plays. A functional role, preventing apoptosis in infected *in vitro* cells, has been suggested (see above). However, whether this is the case *in vivo* remains to be determined. Studies on the assembly of the RNP and the localization of the P and L proteins as well as the transport of the complex to the plasma membrane also remain to be carried out for MuV. Particularly, since the cell cytoskeleton appears to play a role in the replication of other paramyxoviruses, it is important to investigate this aspect of MuV replication.

Geographic and Seasonal Distribution

The virus has a worldwide distribution and requires a minimum population for it to continue to be able to circulate by continuous infection. The minimum population size is assumed to be of a similar order of magnitude to that for measles virus (*c.* 250 000) although no systematic study has been undertaken to ascertain this for MuV. Before successful control of mumps by vaccination had been achieved, outbreaks of mumps were more often observed in the winter and spring than in the summer, at least in the temperate Northern Hemisphere. Such a seasonal pattern was not observed in the tropics.

Host Range and Viral Propagation

Man is the only known host for the virus. Dogs can be naturally infected and show parotid swelling, although they do not pass on the virus. MuV can be used to infect a variety of animals experimentally, including monkeys, cats, dogs, ferrets, and a number of rodent species such as rabbits, suckling rats and mice, hamsters, and guinea pigs. Its adaptation to growth in 8-day-old embryonated eggs allowed the biological activities of the virus to be studied before the advent of tissue culture. The virus infects a wide range of cells in culture and causes a distinct cytopathic effect in most cell cultures with either rounding off or detachment of the cells from the substratum or widespread syncytium formation. Cytopathic effect varies from strain to strain and fusing and nonfusing variants have been described. The virus also readily establishes persistent infection in tissue culture systems, a property shared with many of the other viruses in the family *Paramyxoviridae*. Only low titers of virus are produced in such infections. However, the clinical significance of these observations is questionable as they do not reflect any known pathological outcome of the acute infection.

Serologic Relationships and Variability

MuV is a monotypic virus, and tests with human sera indicate the existence of only a single serotype. Polyclonal sera from infected individuals show a low level of cross-reactivity with hPIV2 and PIV5. Variability between strains has been demonstrated using monoclonal antibodies with the HN and N proteins showing the greatest diversity when single epitopes are examined. Sequence comparisons of the highly variable SH gene of MuV has demonstrated the existence of 12 genotypes. Sequence analysis of the SH gene is routinely used in molecular epidemiological studies (see below).

Evolution and Genetics

Human populations only became dense enough to sustain MuV from about 4000 years ago and, therefore, it has been suggested that the virus must have evolved from an animal pathogen. However, no closely related primate or other animal pathogen has yet been identified. Neither temperature-sensitive nor any other conditional lethal mutants of MuV have been reported nor has recombination been described in any nonsegmented negative-strand RNA virus. Although host range mutants have not been isolated, adaptation of the virus to growth in eggs or in chicken embryo fibroblasts requires a number of blind passages. Strains adapted in this way do not readily grow and fail to generate syncytia when they are used to infect mammalian cells in culture. As MuV is a neuropathogenic virus some clinical isolates have been adapted to grow in the CNS of experimental animals to study this biological property. These viruses are currently being used in reverse genetics approaches to attempt to identify the molecular determinant of neuropathogenesis. At present neutralizing monoclonal antibody escape mutants of the HN protein are the only type of MuV mutants which have been described.

Epidemiology

Outbreaks of mumps show annual periodicities although the length of the cycle may vary from 2 to 7 years as a result of factors that are poorly understood. Historically, the virus caused severe problems when troops were assembled for war and it was observed that male recruits from rural populations were affected in greater numbers. It is, therefore, assumed that children in isolated rural or island populations are exposed to the virus later in life than those in densely populated conurbations. The infection gives rise to lifelong immunity from disease, but it is not clear whether a single dose of live-attenuated vaccine achieves the same. Based on an ongoing outbreak involving a number of vaccinated individuals some have suggested that vaccinees may indeed be susceptible. However, at present this idea should be treated with caution until a systematic retrospective analysis has been performed and the data are considered alongside the known rates of seroconversion after vaccination. The existence of a number of different genotypes has allowed the development of molecular epidemiology for mumps. Specific genotypes appear to dominate in Japan and China, respectively. In some European outbreaks, co-circulation of two genotypes has been described. Changes in the nucleotide sequences of viruses isolated during an epidemic have not been studied although differences between isolates obtained over several years from a given geographical area indicate that the virus gradually accumulates nonexpressed and, to a lesser extent, expressed mutations. However, strains isolated more than 40 years apart can still easily be recognized as belonging to a specific genotype.

Transmission and Tissue Tropism

The virus replicates in the upper respiratory tract and the salivary glands and is transmitted in salivary droplets. Patients are infectious from 3 days before until approximately 4 days after the onset of clinical symptoms. Mumps can also cause viruria but this is not considered important in transmission. Transmission occurs only in the acute phase and from the level of infection observed in naive populations, it can be concluded that the virus is highly contagious ($R_0 = 5$–12) but not as contagious as, for example, measles virus ($R_0 = 16$–450) or chickenpox viruses. The infection is systemic and the virus multiplies in a wide variety of tissues in the human host. The tropism for the pancreas, particularly the β-cells, has been suggested as an explanation for the temporal link between MuV infection and juvenile onset diabetes mellitus. However, direct evidence for such a link is missing (**Table 2**).

Clinical Features of the Infection

In humans the normal MuV incubation period ranges from 14 to 21 days although occasionally this period has been estimated to extend for over 50 days. In infected individuals as many as one-third of MuV infections are subclinical. When symptoms ensue the most common clinical manifestation is parotitis. Other complications, such as orchitis, are not infrequent (**Table 2**). Contrary to popular belief, orchitis has not been linked to an increase in male sterility. Mastitis occurs in females with the same frequency and the incidence of both these clinical features increases with the age at which MuV infection is contracted. Before the development of the currently used live-attenuated vaccine, MuV was the most common cause of viral meningitis and encephalitis in the USA. The encephalitis is usually benign although minor neurological changes, learning, and concentration impairments and sudden deafness are well-documented sequelae in a

Table 2 Clinical features, complications and prognosis of mumps virus infection in various organs

Organ	Clinical features	Frequency	Pathology	Prognosis
Salivary gland	Parotitis (bilateral or unilateral)	95% of symptomatic cases	Blockage of duct of Stensen	Swelling disappears usually in 3–4 days
Submaxillary and sublingual salivary glands	Swelling	Rare		Swelling subsides in 3–4 days
Testes	Orchitis (mostly unilateral; some bilateral)	25% of males (especially adult males)		Good; mostly only transient depression of sperm production
Breast	Mastitis	15% of females		Good; cause of virus in breast milk
Ovaries	Oophoritis	Rare		
Meninges	Meningitis fever/ vomiting	Mononuclear pleocytosis in CSF in 40–60% of cases	Ependymal epithelium destroyed by virus	Benign and self-limiting: ataxia (some permanent damage possible)
Brain	Encephalitis	2% of cases (<1% = fatal)	Virus spreads by neuronal pathways	Poor
Kidney				Good/cause of viruria
Pancreas	Pancreatis with nausea and vomiting	50% of cases	Could be due to interferon responses rather than specific tissue infection	Good/no established link to IDDM
Middle ear	Deafness	Very rare (<3%)	Cochlear infection	Permanent deafness is very rare
Heart	Myocarditis	Very rare	Fibroelastosis	Altered ECG; can cause myocardial infection
Blood	Immunosuppression	All cases	Infection in macrophages and lymphocytes	Viremia resolves
Fetus	Abortion in first trimester	Frequent	Virus is widespread in tissues of aborted fetus	In live births CMI response in the absence of humoral response

number of patients. More rare complications are oophoritis, thyroiditis, pancreatitis, otitis, retinitis, conjunctivitis, and keratitis (**Table 2**).

Pathology and Histopathology

Upon infection, the virus replicates primarily in the nasal mucosa and the epithelial layer of the upper respiratory tract. After penetrating the draining lymph nodes, a transient viremia occurs and thereafter various target organs such as the salivary glands, the kidney, pancreas, and the CNS are infected. Infection in the salivary glands produces parotitis which is the most predominant clinical feature of the virus. Viral replication leads to tissue damage and the subsequent immune response leads to inflammation and swelling of the gland. Dissemination into the kidneys can lead to prolonged infection of this organ and viruria. Virus can be isolated from throat swabs, blood, saliva, and urine. Involvement of the CNS may be as high as 50% of cases and parotitis is not required for this to take place. MuV can be readily isolated from the cerebrospinal fluid (CSF) in cases of meningoencephalitis.

Pathogenicity

A number of MuV strains give rise to varying degrees of pathogenicity in experimental animal infections, for example, mice and hamsters. However, this does not seem to extend to natural human infections above and beyond some variation in the level of meningitis which tends to be associated with particular MuV strains (see below). The neurovirulence of MuV strains and vaccine batches is assessed using a monkey neurovirulence test (MNVT), but recently an alternative approach was devised based on the level of viral replication and hydrocephalus in neonatal rats. This rat neurovirulence test (RNVT) has apparently better predictive power than the MNVT. Some neutralizing monoclonal antibody escape mutants show alterations in neuropathogenicity in a hamster model.

Immune Response

It is not known whether the humoral or cell-mediated immune (CMI) response is the most important in clearing MuV from an infected host. Both play a role although neither seems to be required exclusively for successful control of the infection. Eleven days after infection, the humoral immune response is well established and the presence of neutralizing viral antibodies probably terminates viremia. Similarly, the appearance of IgA in the salivary fluid stops excretion of infectious MuV in the saliva. The precise time at which MuV reactive cytotoxic T lymphocytes first appear is unclear and these have been demonstrated in both the blood from patients with the natural disease and in vaccinees. The magnitude and effectiveness of this response may be related to the genetic human leukocyte antigen (HLA) background of the host. A complication in the development of the CMI response is the tropism of the virus for T and B cells. Reduction in CMI responses to antigens previously recognized has been observed, although the mechanism is unclear. It is less severe and of shorter duration than the immunosuppression associated with measles virus infection. The virus grows well in activated but not in resting T lymphocytes and infection of the CNS during MuV infection is thought to occur via transfer of infected monocytes into the choroid plexus. Perinatal exposure of the fetus to MuV via the placenta does not appear to lead to infection of fetal tissues. However, this can give rise to anomalous immune responses to MuV in the newborn child. In these children, CMI but no humoral responses are detectable. Neutralizing B-cell epitopes have been defined in the HN gene of MuV but no other B- or T-cell epitopes have been delineated, as yet.

Prevention and Control

Adaptation of MuV to growth in embryonated eggs and chicken embryo fibroblasts allowed the early development of live-attenuated vaccines for mumps. In 1946, Enders observed that adaptation of MuV to chicken cells was associated with the loss of virulence for monkeys. In the past, killed virus preparations were used for human vaccination although these did not lead to lifelong protective immunity and their use has been discontinued. In general, the appearance of atypical cases of measles and respiratory syncytial virus infection after vaccination with killed virus has led to the exclusive use of live-attenuated vaccines for the control of paramyxoviruses. Mumps vaccination has substantially reduced the incidence of the disease worldwide. After successful licensing of the vaccine in 1967 in the USA, the incidence of mumps dropped from 76 to 2 cases per 100 000 population. There are now a number of live-attenuated vaccine strains, for example, the Jeryl Lynn (JL) strain, which are usually administered in a trivalent vaccine containing live-attenuated strains of measles and rubella viruses as well as MuV (MMR). At present most developed countries have chosen to adopt a two-dose schedule for MMR vaccination and the vaccine is administered at 15 months and *c.* 4 years of age. The JL strain of MuV is most frequently used in the MMR vaccine and interestingly it has been shown to be comprised of two strains, the major (JL5) and the minor (JL2) components. The Urabe strain has been removed from MMR vaccines since reports in several countries indicated a higher incidence of meningitis associated with the use of this strain of MuV.

MuV and Inclusion Body Myositis

In the past MuV has been implicated in inclusion body myositis. However, neither *in situ* hybridization nor the polymerase chain reaction or immunocytochemistry has been able to link MuV to the paramyxovirus-nucleocapsid-like structures observed in muscle cells of patients with this disease. In contrast, myocarditis in patients with fibro-elastosis has been associated with the presence of mumps viral RNA with reverse transcription-polymerase chain reaction (RT-PCR). The link to arthritis is also unclear (**Table 2**).

Future Perspectives

Over the last ten years, the development of reverse genetics systems for all members of the *Mononegavirales* has had a significant impact on our understanding of these viruses. Such systems have been generated for PIV5, hPIV2, and MuV, and to date they have been used to begin to define the structural and functional relationships and the roles that various proteins play in attenuating these viruses. The opportunity to examine the contribution of individual proteins from neurovirulent strains, such as Urabe, to neuropathogenesis in animal models should help to identify virulence determinants, something which is important if it proves necessary to develop new MuV vaccines. Expression of individual proteins may also allow a dissection of the humoral and cellular immune response and this should help improve our understanding of the role that these have in virus clearance.

One of the key challenges for the next number of years is to systematically monitor the immune status of vaccines and assess their susceptibility to reinfection by currently circulating MuV genotypes. Furthermore, documenting the occurrence of sequelae after the introduction of large-scale vaccination is vital. This should be underpinned by comprehensive molecular epidemiological approaches to ensure that the currently circulating genotypes are rapidly detected. Such approaches are particularly important given the recent large number of vaccinated individuals who have been reportedly infected in recent and ongoing outbreaks in both the UK and the USA. Linking MuV genotypes to particular phenotypes, such as neurovirulence, is crucial for our understanding of this ubiquitous human pathogen and the key goal in the medium term is to move from unproven association to formal proof. It is in this arena that reverse genetics approaches for MuV should prove most useful.

See also: Measles Virus; Parainfluenza Viruses of Humans.

Further Reading

Carbone KM and Rubin S (2006) Mumps virus. In: Knipe DM, Howley PM, Griffin DE, *et al.* (eds.) *Fields Virology,*, 5th edn, pp. 1527–1550. Philadelphia: Lippincott Williams and Wilkins.

Feldmann HA (1989) Mumps. In: Evans AS (ed.) *Viral Infections of Humans,* ch. 17, p471. New York: Plenum.

Gupta RK, Best J, and MacMahon E (2005) Mumps and the UK epidemic 2005. *British Medical Journal* 330: 1132–1135.

Noroviruses and Sapoviruses

K Y Green, National Institutes of Health, Bethesda, MD, USA

Glossary

Fomites An object that in itself is not harmful, but that can harbor a pathogenic organism and therefore serve as an agent of its transmission.

Gastroenteritis An inflammation of the stomach and intestines, often characterized by symptoms of vomiting and diarrhea.

Introduction

Diarrheal illnesses have a major impact on public health. The association of bacteria with such illness was recognized over a century ago with the discovery of bacterial pathogens such as *Vibrio cholerae* and *Shigella dysenteriae*. The role of viruses in diarrheal illness was established much later. Volunteer studies in the 1940s showed that bacteria-free filtrates of feces obtained from individuals

Table 1 Taxonomy of the *Caliciviridae*

Genus	Species	Type strain
Norovirus (NoV)	*Norwalk virus* (NV)	Hu/NoV/GI.1/Norwalk/1968/US
Sapovirus (SaV)	*Sapporo virus* (SV)	Hu/SaV/GI.1/Sapporo/1982/JP
Lagovirus (LaV)	*Rabbit hemorrhagic disease virus* (RHDV)	Ra/LaV/RHDV/GH/1988/DE
	European brown hare syndrome virus (EBHSV)	Ha/LaV/EBHSV/GD/1989/FR
Vesivirus (VeV)	*Vesicular exanthema of swine virus* (VESV)	Sw/VeV/VESV/VESV-A48/1948/US
	Feline calicivirus (FCV)	Fe/VeV/FCV/F9/1958/US

Calicivirus strains are written in a cryptogram format that is organized as follows: Host species from which the virus was obtained/genus/species (or genogroup)/strain name/year of occurrence/country of origin. Abbreviations for the host species are: Fe, feline; Ha, Hare; Hu, Human; Sw, Swine; Ra, Rabbit. Country abbreviations are: DE, Germany; FR, France; JP, Japan; US, United States. GenBank Accession numbers of representative viruses: Norwalk virus, M87661; Sapporo virus, U65427; RHDV, M67473; VESV, AF181082; FCV, M86379

with diarrheal disease could induce a similar illness in volunteers who were challenged orally with the inoculum. In 1972, the Norwalk virus was identified in human feces and shown to be the etiologic agent of an outbreak of gastroenteritis that occurred in an elementary school in Norwalk, Ohio in 1968. The Norwalk virus became the prototype strain for a large group of related caliciviruses known now as the noroviruses. A second group of distantly related caliciviruses, the sapoviruses, was discovered soon afterwards.

The family *Caliciviridae* includes several important human and animal pathogens, including the noroviruses and sapoviruses associated with acute gastroenteritis (**Table 1**). The human noroviruses, named for the prototype strain *Norwalk virus*, are now recognized as a major cause of gastroenteritis in all age groups. Norovirus outbreaks often occur in settings such as communities, nursing homes, schools, hospitals, cruise ships, camps, social gatherings, families, and military personnel. Norovirus illnesses can also occur sporadically in the community. A common name for norovirus gastroenteritis is 'stomach flu', but this is a misnomer because the noroviruses are not related to influenza virus. The acute, symptomatic phase of the illness, which often includes either vomiting or diarrhea, or both, generally lasts from 24 to 48 h. In most cases, norovirus gastroenteritis is mild and self-limiting, but it can be incapacitating during the symptomatic phase. The illness can sometimes be severe and prolonged in certain individuals such as either the very old or young, or those compromised by pre-existing illness or immunosuppressive therapy.

The sapoviruses, named for the prototype strain, *Sapporo virus*, are characteristically associated with pediatric gastroenteritis, but outbreaks and illness in older individuals can occur. Although illness is characteristically mild, severe disease has been reported. The sapoviruses do not appear to be a major cause of epidemic gastroenteritis, in contrast to the noroviruses. It should also be noted that although sapoviruses and noroviruses have both been associated with pediatric gastroenteritis, and the noroviruses are considered to be the second most important cause of such illnesses,

Table 2 Natural host range and disease syndromes associated with caliciviruses

Calicivirus Genus	Host	Disease syndrome
Norovirus	Human	Gastroenteritis
	Porcine	Gastroenteritis
	Bovine	Gastroenteritis
	Murine	Asymptomatic enteric infection in wild type mice severe systemic disease in mice lacking STAT1
Sapovirus	Human	Gastroenteritis
	Porcine	Gastroenteritis
	Mink	Gastroenteritis
Vesivirus[a]	Porcine	Vesicular exanthema, abortion
	Sea lion	Vesicular lesions
	Chimpanzee	Vesicular lesions
	Canine	Gastroenteritis
	Walrus	None described
	Mink	None described
	Bovine	None described
	Reptilian	None described
	Skunk	None described
	Amphibian	None described
	Cetacean	None described
	Feline	Upper respiratory, pneumonia, oral ulceration
Lagovirus	Rabbit	Hepatitis, disseminated intravascular coagulation
	Hare	Hepatitis, disseminated intravascular coagulation

[a]There is a report documenting human infection with a vesivirus isolated from a sea lion.

the major cause by far of severe nonbacterial diarrhea in infants and young children is the rotavirus, which belongs to a different virus family, the *Reoviridae*.

Caliciviruses have been detected in a large number of animal species and are associated with a diverse range of clinical syndromes (**Table 2**). Veterinary pathogens of note in the *Caliciviridae* include feline calicivirus (FCV), an important cause of respiratory illness in cats, and rabbit hemorrhagic disease virus (RHDV), an often-fatal acute infection in rabbits.

Taxonomy and Classification

The taxonomy of the noroviruses and sapoviruses is based primarily on the phylogenetic relationships among strains (**Figure 1**). Members of the family *Caliciviridae* apparently share a common ancestor, and the four major phylogenetic groups define the four genera: *Norovirus*, *Sapovirus*, *Lagovirus*, and *Vesivirus* (**Table 1**). Members within each genus share common features in their genomic organization, but host range and disease manifestations may vary among members of each genus. Each genus is further divided into one or more species, with each species represented by a 'type' strain (**Table 1**). The genus *Lagovirus* is comprised of two species, *Rabbit hemorrhagic disease virus* and *European brown hare syndrome virus*, and the genus *Vesivirus* is subdivided into two species, *Vesicular exanthema of swine virus* and *Feline calicivirus*. Presently, the genera *Norovirus* and *Sapovirus* have only one species each, designated as *Norwalk virus* and *Sapporo virus*, respectively.

The official classification system of viruses by the International Committee on Taxonomy of Viruses (ICTV) does not address classification below the species level. However, several genetic typing systems have been developed to facilitate communication among researchers in tracking the spread of epidemic strains. These genetic typing systems are based on sequence relatedness in a selected region of the viral genome. One such approach is based on comparisons of the major capsid protein-encoding gene as illustrated for the noroviruses and sapoviruses in **Table 3**. In these genetic typing systems, the noroviruses and sapoviruses are first divided by sequence relatedness into

major branches within the genus termed 'genogroups'. For example, noroviruses are presently divided into five distinct genogroups designated I, II, III, IV, and V. Each genogroup is further divided into genetic clusters that are designated as 'genotypes'. For example, genogroup I of the noroviruses is divided into eight genotypes, and genogroup II is divided into 19 genotypes (**Table 3**). The role of genetic diversity in the natural history of the noroviruses and sapoviruses, and the correlation of genotypes with antigenicity is not yet known. However, the classification and genetic typing systems allow the utilization of a cryptogram to describe strains. The cryptogram is organized as follows: Host species from which the virus was obtained/genus/species or genetic type/strain name/year of occurrence/country of origin. For example, Norwalk virus would be designated as: Hu/NoV/GI.1/Norwalk/1968/US.

Virion Structure and Composition

Virus particles are isometric, ranging from 27 to 35 nm in diameter, with icosahedral symmetry. Human caliciviruses such as Norwalk virus (representing the noroviruses) and Parkville virus (representing the sapoviruses) can be observed in stool specimens by negative-stain-electron microscopy (EM) as shown in **Figure 2**. Cryo-EM and computer-generated reconstructions of recombinant virus-like particles produced by expression of the major capsid protein (VP1) of the Norwalk or Parkville virus illustrates the presence of the cup-shaped depressions on the surface, a common feature of caliciviruses that inspired the family *Caliciviridae* (*calix* means 'cup' in Latin) (**Figure 2**). The mature virion contains two structural proteins, VP1 and VP2. VP1 (approximately 60 kDa in most strains) is the predominant capsid protein and is present in 180 copies per virion. The VP1 contains the major antigenic and receptor binding sites of the virus. The VP2 (ranging in size from approximately 8 to 29 kDa) is present in an estimated one or two copies per virion, and may play a role in particle assembly and stability. A third protein found in virions is the VPg, an approximately 15 kDa protein that is covalently linked to the viral RNA genome. The presence of the VPg protein on the viral RNA is required for the efficient initiation of an infection following entry of the viral RNA into cells, most likely because of the proposed role of VPg in mediating interactions between the viral RNA and the host cell translation machinery.

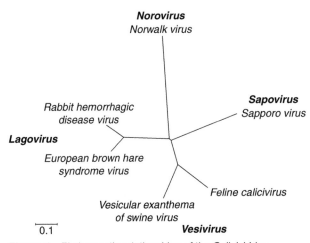

Figure 1 Phylogenetic relationships of the *Caliciviridae*. Caliciviruses in the four genera (*Norovirus*, *Sapovirus*, *Lagovirus*, and *Vesivirus*) cluster into four major groups when the nucleotide sequences of full-length genomes are compared in a phylogenetic analysis (Neighbor-joining, Jukes-Cantor distance parameter). Each genus can be further divided into groups that represent distinct species.

Genome Organization and Expression

The genome of the caliciviruses is a positive-sense RNA molecule ranging in length from approximately 7.4 to 8.3 kbp. The 5'-end of the genome is covalently linked to a

Table 3   Norovirus and sapovirus genetic typing systems

Reference virus	Genogroup	Genotype	GenBank accession number
Noroviruses			
Hu/NoV/GI.1/Norwalk/1968/US	I	1	M87661
Hu/NoV/GI.2/Southampton/1991/UK	I	2	L07418
Hu/NoV/GI.3/Desert Shield 395/1990/SA	I	3	U04469
Hu/NoV/GI.4/Chiba 407/1987/JP	I	4	AB042808
Hu/NoV/GI.5/Musgrove/1989/UK	I	5	AJ277614
Hu/NoV/GI.6Hesse 3/1997/DE	I	6	AF093797
Hu/NoV/GI.7/Winchester/1994/UK	I	7	AJ277609
Hu/NoV/GI.8/Boxer/2001/US	I	8	AF538679
Hu/NoV/GII.1/Hawaii/1971/US	II	1	U07611
Hu/NoV/GII.2/Melksham/1994/UK	II	2	X81879
Hu/NoV/GII.3/Toronto 24/1991/CA	II	3	U02030
Hu/NoV/GII.4/Bristol/1993/UK	II	4	X76716
Hu/NoV/GII.5/Hillingdon/1990/UK	II	5	AJ277607
Hu/NoV/GII.6/Seacroft/1990/UK	II	6	AJ277620
Hu/NoV/GII.7/Leeds/1990/UK	II	7	AJ277608
Hu/NoV/GII.8/Amsterdam/1998/NL	II	8	AF195848
Hu/NoV/GII.9/VA97207/1997	II	9	AY038599
Hu/NoV/GII.10/Erfurt546/2000/DE	II	10	AF427118
Sw/NoV/GII.11/Sw918/1997/JP	II	11	AB074893
Hu/NoV/GII.12/Wortley/1990/UK	II	12	AJ277618
Hu/NoV/GII.13/Fayetteville/1998/US	II	13	AY113106
Hu/NoV/GII.14/M7/1999/US	II	14	AY130761
Hu/NoV/GII.15/J23/1999/US	II	15	AY130762
Hu/NoV/GII.16/Tiffin/1999/US	II	16	AY502010
Hu/NoV/GII.17/CS-E1/2002/US	II	17	AY502009
Sw/NoV/GII.18/OH-QW101/2003/US	II	18	AY823304
Sw/NoV/GII.19/OH-QW170/2003/US	II	19	AY823306
Bo/NoV/GIII.1/Jena/1980/DE	III	1	AJ011099
Bo/NoV/CH126/1998/NL	III	2	AF320625
Hu/NoV/GIV.1/Alphatron 98–2/1998/NL	IV	1	AF195847
Mu/NoV/GV.1/MNV-1/2003	V	1	AY228235
Sapoviruses			
Hu/SaV/GI.1/Sapporo/1982/JP	I	1	U65427
Hu/SaV/GI.2/Parkville/1994/US	I	2	U73124
Hu/SaV/GI.3/Stockholm/1997/SE	I	3	AF194782
Hu/SaV/GII.1/London/1992/UK	II	1	U95645
Hu/SaV/GII.2/Mex340/1990/MX	II	2	AF435812
Hu/SaV/GII.3/Cruise ship/2000/US	II	3	AY289804
Sw/SaV/GIII/PEC-Cowden/1980/US	III	1	AF182760
Hu/SaV/GIV/Hou7–1181/1990/US	IV	1	AF435814
Hu/SaV/GV/Argentina39/AR	V	1	AY289803

Note: Norovirus and sapovirus typing systems from Zheng *et al.*, and Farkas *et al.*, respectively.

protein, VPg, and the 3′-end of the genome contains a poly (A) tract. There is a relatively short nontranslated region (NTR) at both the 5′- and 3′-ends of the genome that flank the open reading frames (ORFs). Genomes of the caliciviruses are organized into either two or three major ORFs, depending on the genus (**Figure 3**). The first ORF (beginning near the 5′-end) of all caliciviruses encodes the nonstructural (NS) proteins of the virus, whereas the terminal ORF encodes the minor structural protein, VP2. The major difference in reading frame usage among the caliciviruses relates to the coding sequence of the major

capsid protein, VP1. In the noroviruses and vesiviruses, the VP1 is encoded in a separate reading frame (ORF2), whereas in the sapoviruses and lagoviruses, the VP1 is encoded in the same ORF (ORF1) as the NS proteins. Thus, the norovirus genome is organized into three major ORFs, and the sapovirus genome is organized into two major ORFs.

Caliciviruses encode six to seven mature NS proteins, depending again on the genus. This variation is due to differences among the proteolytic processing strategies used by viruses to cleave the ORF1 polyprotein. In the lagoviruses, the virus-encoded cysteine proteinase cleaves

Genus: *Norovirus*

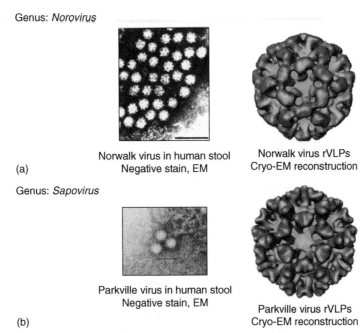

(a)

Norwalk virus in human stool
Negative stain, EM

Norwalk virus rVLPs
Cryo-EM reconstruction

Genus: *Sapovirus*

Parkville virus in human stool
Negative stain, EM

(b)

Parkville virus rVLPs
Cryo-EM reconstruction

Figure 2 Structural features of noroviruses and sapoviruses. (a) Genus: *Norovirus*. (Left panel) Norwalk virus, a norovirus, as seen in human stool material by negative-staining and immune EM (IEM). The size of Norwalk virus in stool material has been described as 27–32 nm in diameter. Scale = 100 nm. (Right panel) Norwalk virus recombinant virus-like particles (rVLPs) were expressed in the baculovirus system, purified, and analyzed with the technique of cryo-EM. (b) Genus: *Sapovirus*. (Left panel) Parkville virus, a sapovirus, as seen in human stool material by negative staining and EM. Scale = 50 nm. (Right panel) Parkville virus rVLPs were analyzed by cryo-EM. The cryo-EM computer-generated images of both Norwalk virus and Parkville virus rVLPs show that the surfaces of the particles have cup-shaped depressions, a structural hallmark of the caliciviruses. (a, left panel) Image provided by A. Z. Kapikian, National Institutes of Health. (a, b, right panel) Image provided by B. V. Prasad, Baylor College of Medicine. (b, left panel) Image provided by C. D. Humphrey, Centers for Disease Control and Prevention.

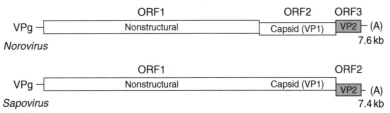

Figure 3 Genome organization of noroviruses and sapoviruses. The positive sense RNA genome of Norwalk virus (representing the noroviruses) is organized into three major ORFs. The genome of Manchester virus (representing the sapoviruses) is organized into two major ORFs, with the VP1capsid coding sequence in frame with that of the NS proteins. (The Norwalk virus and Manchester virus genome sequences correspond to GenBank accession numbers M87661 and X86560, respectively.)

the ORF1 polyprotein at six cleavage sites to release seven mature NS proteins, designated as NS1 through NS7 (**Table 4**). In some genera, cleavage between certain NS proteins has not been detected during virus replication. This includes the NS1 and NS2 precursor of the noroviruses (designated as NS1–2 in this nomenclature system, and known also as the N-terminal protein or p48) and the NS6 and NS7 precursor of the vesiviruses (NS6–7, also known as ProPol). The calicivirus NS proteins and their functions, if known, are summarized in **Table 4**. Key enzymes include an NTPase (NS3), a cysteine proteinase (NS6), and an RNA-dependent RNA polymerase (NS7).

Table 4 Calicivirus proteins

Virion proteins (VP)

VP1	Major structural protein of virion (~60 kDa)
VP2	Minor structural protein, function unknown
VPg	Covalently linked to genomic RNA

Nonstructural proteins (NS)

NS1	N-terminal protein of ORF1, function unknown
NS2	Function unknown
NS3	NTPase
NS4	Function unknown
NS5	Becomes linked to RNA as VPg, role in translation and replication
NS6	Proteinase (Pro)
NS7	RNA-dependent RNA Polymerase (Pol)

Replication

Cell culture systems are not available for all caliciviruses, but those that grow in cell culture, such as FCV and murine norovirus characteristically grow efficiently and form plaques (**Figure 4**). Like other positive-strand RNA viruses, caliciviruses replicate in the cytoplasm of infected cells. The positive-strand RNA genome functions as a messenger RNA that is translated following entry of the virus particle into the cell. This initial translation event produces NS proteins that are used in the replication of the viral RNA genome and the production of new progeny. Replication of the RNA occurs on intracellular membranes and extensive membrane rearrangements are observed in infected cells (**Figure 4**). The viral capsids can sometimes be seen in infected cells as paracrystalline

Plaque morphology

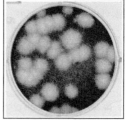 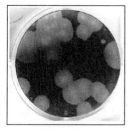

Feline calicivirus   Murine norovirus

Intracellular membrane rearrangements

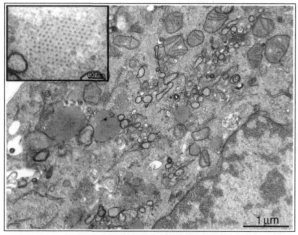

FCV-infected feline kidney cells

Figure 4 (Upper panel) Plaque morphology and membrane rearrangements in an infected cell. Feline calicivirus and murine norovirus induce a rapid cytopathic effect in permissive cell culture. Plaques can be detected in a cell monolayer by 24 h post infection. (Lower panel) Caliciviruses, like other positive strand RNA viruses, induce membrane rearrangements and vesicles in infected cells. The inset shows a paracrystalline array of capsid proteins produced in an FCV-infected cell. Images provided by A. Weisberg.

arrays (**Figure 4**). There are two major positive-strand RNA species detected in infected cells – one corresponds to the full-length genome, and the other corresponds to an abundant subgenomic RNA co-terminal with the 3'-end region of the genome. The NS proteins are translated from the full-length RNA. The subgenomic RNA serves as a messenger RNA for translation of the VP1 and VP2, the two structural proteins.

Evolution

Comparative sequence analysis suggests that members of the *Caliciviridae* have a common ancestor. A distant evolutionary relationship has been proposed between the *Caliciviridae* and members of the family *Picornaviridae*. A striking feature among the caliciviruses is their extensive genetic variation. This variation is due, in part, to the high error rate inherent in positive-strand RNA virus replication, which employs an RNA-dependent RNA polymerase without a known editing function for correcting mistakes. There is compelling evidence also that recombination occurs between related strains, which would then allow the emergence of new viruses. Potential recombination sites have been identified in norovirus genomes at several positions, including the junction between the ORF1 and ORF2, which would allow a virus to emerge with a new subgenomic region that would encode a different VP1 capsid protein.

Transmission and Host Range

Transmission of the noroviruses and sapoviruses occurs by several modes, including direct person-to-person contact, ingestion of contaminated food or water, or exposure to contaminated fomites. Noroviruses are a major cause of foodborne gastroenteritis. The route of transmission is predominantly fecal–oral, and viruses can be shed in feces for days to weeks following infection. The virus has been detected in vomitus, and transmission may occur also via exposure to aerosolized droplets of vomitus. Good personal hygiene and frequent hand washing is important in controlling the spread of these highly infectious viruses.

Noroviruses have been found in several mammalian species, including humans, pigs, cattle, and mice, and it is likely that additional hosts will be identified. Sapoviruses have also been found in several hosts thus far, including humans, pigs, and mink. There is little evidence that zoonotic transmission of animal caliciviruses to humans (or humans to animals) plays a role in the natural history of these viruses, but such transmission might be possible considering that certain human norovirus strains can infect chimpanzees and pigs in experimental challenge studies.

Pathogenicity

Noroviruses and sapoviruses replicate in the enteric tract, and viral antigen-expressing cells (for both groups of viruses) have been identified in the small intestinal epithelial cells of swine. The cell types supporting the replication of the human noroviruses and sapoviruses have not been verified *in vivo*, but intestinal biopsies have shown blunting of the intestinal villi following infection of adult volunteers with Norwalk virus. The mechanisms responsible for diarrhea are not known, but the lesion caused by blunting of the intestinal villi may affect absorption and the osmotic balance. Murine norovirus is shed in feces and can be found in multiple organs of asymptomatic normal mice, including the intestine, liver, spleen, and mesenteric lymph nodes. However, certain strains of murine norovirus can cause a highly lethal infection in immunodeficient mice lacking key components of the innate immune system. In these mice, a lethal, disseminated infection occurs leading to encephalitis, meningitis, vasculitis, hepatitis, and pneumonia.

Clinical Features of Infection

Norovirus gastroenteritis is characterized by a short incubation period and an acute onset of illness. Symptoms include one or more of the following: diarrhea, vomiting, fever, malaise, and abdominal cramps. The illness is generally considered mild and self-limiting, but severe illness can occur. Treatment is aimed toward the prevention of dehydration, and includes either oral rehydration or intravenous administration of fluids. Noroviruses have been identified in several studies as the second most important viral agent (but considerably less than rotaviruses) associated with severe gastroenteritis in infants and young children.

The sapoviruses have been associated predominantly with diarrhea that can range from mild to severe. The illness is usually self-limiting, but the prevention of dehydration is important.

Noroviruses, sapoviruses, and other caliciviruses have been associated with asymptomatic infection, and persistent infection has been documented. Shedding of the virus can occur for prolonged periods (weeks to months) following resolution of symptoms in some patients.

Immune Response

Immunity to the noroviruses is poorly understood, because it has been difficult to study the role of neutralizing antibodies in the absence of a cell culture system. Adult volunteer challenge studies have been the only available approach for the study of resistance to illness in humans. It was noted early in these volunteer studies that the presence of pre-existing serum or local intestinal antibodies to the virus did not correlate with resistance to illness, but rather was associated with susceptibility to infection and illness. In contrast, later studies suggested that local immunity in the intestine played an important role in mediating protection, but immunity to Norwalk virus was short term. Susceptibility to infection may also be associated with host genetic factors relating to the presence or absence of receptors for the virus on intestinal epithelial cells. There is evidence that noroviruses bind to histo-blood group antigens on intestinal epithelial cells, and these antigens might serve as receptors or binding ligands for the virus. Because histo-blood group antigens vary among individuals, and variation among norovirus strains has been detected in the recognition of these antigens, it has been postulated that this might, in part, provide an explanation for varying host susceptibility. The understanding of immunity to the noroviruses is complicated by the marked antigenic diversity among circulating strains. Limited cross-challenge studies have found evidence for at least two distinct serotypes, represented by the Norwalk and Hawaii norovirus strains, but the number of serotypes is presently unknown.

The predominant association of sapovirus gastroenteritis with individuals in younger age groups suggests that immunity to sapoviruses may be acquired early in life.

Prevention and Control

There are presently no vaccines or antiviral therapies for the control of norovirus and sapovirus gastroenteritis. Prevention and control strategies currently consist of standard infection control procedures, such as frequent hand washing, avoidance of exposure, and disinfection of contaminated areas.

Diagnosis

Norovirus outbreaks characteristically have the following epidemiological features, known as the 'Kaplan criteria': (1) a mean (or median) illness duration of 12–60 h, (2) a mean (or median) incubation period of 24–48 h, (3) more than 50% of people with vomiting, and (4) no bacterial agent previously found. Although these features are generally highly specific for the provisional diagnosis of a norovirus outbreak, laboratory tests are recommended for ruling out bacteria and confirming a viral etiology. The most widely used method for detection of noroviruses and sapoviruses is reverse transcriptase-polymerase chain reaction (RT-PCR) analysis of viral RNA in stool specimens. The extensive genetic variation among the noroviruses has been problematic in the design of broadly reactive primer pairs, and many laboratories use more than one primer pair for detection.

Noroviruses and sapoviruses can be observed in stool specimens by EM, but this technique often requires the use of antibodies to facilitate detection (immune EM). Commercial immunoassays are becoming available for clinical use in which broadly reactive antibodies are used to detect norovirus antigen in stool specimens.

Vaccination

Vaccines are not available for the noroviruses, but studies are in progress to identify and evaluate potential vaccine candidates. Most vaccine candidates are based on the production of recombinant norovirus VP1, the major capsid protein. The VP1 will spontaneously self-assemble into virus-like particles (VLPs) that are antigenically similar to native virions and can be produced in high yields in expression systems such as baculovirus. The VLPs are immunogenic when administered orally to humans.

Vaccines have been developed and are in use for caliciviruses such as FCV (for use in cats) and RHDV (for use in rabbits). Because FCV grows efficiently in cell culture, a live attenuated vaccine has been developed, as well as an inactivated vaccine.

Future Perspectives

Noroviruses are the major cause of nonbacterial gastroenteritis outbreaks, and large numbers of illnesses occur each year. The sapoviruses play a lesser role in epidemic gastroenteritis, but further studies are needed. Efforts will continue to focus on the development of improved diagnostic tests and in the establishment of a cell culture system for the human noroviruses and sapoviruses. It will also be important to determine whether vaccines or antiviral drugs will be effective in controlling norovirus disease. A norovirus vaccine candidate based on the expression of recombinant virus-like particles is under investigation in early clinical trials. Promising new tools for study of the noroviruses include the first efficient cell culture system (murine norovirus), a human norovirus infectivity assay using a three-dimensional cell culture system, a cell-based human norovirus replicon system (Norwalk virus), a reverse genetics system for the murine noroviruses, and an animal disease model (pigs) for the human noroviruses. In addition, advances in the elucidation of the structure and function of individual viral proteins may lead to a better understanding of replication in this important group of viruses.

See also: Enteric Viruses.

Further Reading

Asanaka M, Atmar RL, Ruvolo V, Crawford SE, Neill FH, and Estes MK (2005) Replication and packaging of Norwalk virus RNA in cultured mammalian cells. *Proceedings of the National Academy of Sciences, USA* 102: 10327–10332.

Atmar RL and Estes MK (2006) The epidemiologic and clinical importance of norovirus infection. *Gastroenterology Clinics of North America* 35: 275–290.

Chang KO, Sosnovtsev SV, Belliot G, King AD, and Green KY (2006) Stable expression of a Norwalk virus RNA replicon in a human hepatoma cell line. *Virology* 353: 463–473.

Cheetham S, Souza M, Meulia T, Grimes S, Han MG, and Saif LJ (2006) Pathogenesis of a genogroup II human norovirus in gnotobiotic pigs. *Journal of Virology* 80: 10372–10381.

Chen R, Neill JD, Noel JS, et al. (2004) Inter- and intragenus structural variations in caliciviruses and their functional implications. *Journal of Virology* 78: 6469–6479.

Estes MK, Prasad BV, and Atmar RL (2006) Noroviruses everywhere: Has something changed? *Current Opinion in Infectious Diseases* 19: 467–474.

Farkas T, Zhong WM, Jing Y, et al. (2004) Genetic diversity among sapoviruses. *Archives of Virology* 149: 1309–1323.

Green KY, Ando T, Balayan MS, et al. (2000) Taxonomy of the caliciviruses. *Journal of Infectious Diseases* 181: S322–S330.

Hansman GS, Natori K, Shirato-Horikoshi H, et al. (2006) Genetic and antigenic diversity among noroviruses. *Journal of General Virology* 87: 909–919.

Hardy ME (2005) Norovirus protein structure and function. *FEMS Microbiology Letters* 253: 1–8.

Jiang X, Graham DY, Wang K, and Estes MK (1990) Norwalk virus genome cloning and characterization. *Science* 250: 1580–1583.

Kapikian AZ (2000) The discovery of the 27-nm Norwalk virus: An historic perspective. *Journal of Infectious Diseases* 181: S295–S302.

Kapikian AZ, Wyatt RG, Dolin R, Thornhill TS, Kalica AR, and Chanock RM (1972) Visualization by immune electron microscopy of a 27-nm particle associated with acute infectious nonbacterial gastroenteritis. *Journal of Virology* 10: 1075–1081.

Le Pendu J, Ruvoen-Clouet N, Kindberg E, and Svensson L (2006) Mendelian resistance to human norovirus infections. *Semin Immunology* 18: 375–386.

Noel JS, Liu BL, Humphrey CD, et al. (1997) Parkville virus: A novel genetic variant of human calicivirus in the Sapporo virus clade, associated with an outbreak of gastroenteritis in adults. *Journal of Medical Virology* 52: 173–178.

Sosnovtsev SV, Belliot G, Chang KO, et al. (2006) Cleavage map and proteolytic processing of the murine norovirus nonstructural polyprotein in infected cells. *Journal of Virology* 80: 7816–7831.

Straub TM, Höner zu Bentrup K, Orosz-Coghlan P, et al. (2007) In vitro cell culture infectivity assay for human noroviruses. *Emerging Infectious Diseases* 13(3): 396–403.

Tacket CO, Sztein MB, Losonsky GA, Wasserman SS, and Estes MK (2003) Humoral, mucosal, and cellular immune responses to oral Norwalk virus-like particles in volunteers. *Clinical Immunology* 108: 241–247.

Ward VK, McCormick CJ, Clarke IN, et al. (2007) Recovery of infectious murine norovirus using pol II-driven expression of full-length cDNA. *Proceedings of the National Academy of Sciences, USA* 104: 11050–11055.

Wobus CE, Thackray LB, and Virgin HW (2006) Murine norovirus: A model system to study norovirus biology and pathogenesis. *Journal of Virology* 80: 5104–5112.

Zheng DP, Ando T, Fankhauser RL, Beard RS, Glass RI, and Monroe SS (2006) Norovirus classification and proposed strain nomenclature. *Virology* 346: 312–323.

Parainfluenza Viruses of Humans

E Adderson and A Portner, St. Jude Children's Research Hospital, Memphis, TN, USA

Introduction

The human parainfluenza viruses (hPIVs) are an important cause of respiratory disease in infants and children. Four types were discovered between 1956 and 1960. hPIV-1, hPIV-2, and hPIV-3 were first isolated from infants and children with lower respiratory tract (LRT) disease and subsequently shown to be a major cause of croup (type 1) and pneumonia and bronchiolitis (type 3). hPIV-4 was initially isolated from young adults and has been associated with mild upper respiratory tract disease of children and adults. Other viruses antigenically and structurally related to the human paramyxoviruses have been isolated from animals. Sendai virus, a natural pathogen of mice and not of humans, was the first PIV isolated and is antigenically related to human PIV-1. Simian virus (SV5) now PIV-5, recovered from primary monkey kidney cells, causes croup in dogs and is related to human type 2, and bovine shipping fever virus is a subtype of type 3.

Taxonomy and Classification

The PIVs belong to two genera, human parainfluenza virus types 1 and 3 to *Respirovirus* and human parainfluenza virus types 2, 4a, and 4b to *Rubulavirus*, of the subfamily *Paramyxovirinae* in the family *Paramyxoviridae*. Some other species found in the *Rubulavirus* are mumps virus, which causes disease in humans and in the genus *Respirovirus* Sendai virus in mice and Bovine parainfluenza type 3. The family *Paramyxoviridae* belongs to the order *Mononegavirales*, the distinctive feature of which is a negative-stranded RNA genome and a similar strategy of replication, suggesting that all negative-stranded viruses may have evolved from an archetypal virus.

Virion Structure, Genome Organization, and Protein Composition

The hPIVs are roughly spherical, lipoprotein enveloped particles 150–250 nm in diameter with an internal helical nucleocapsid containing the negative-sense single-stranded RNA genome. Projecting from the surface of the virion are the hemagglutinin–neuraminidase (HN) and fusion (F) glycoproteins. These glycoproteins are anchored to the plasma membrane of the infected cell or the virion envelope by a hydrophobic transmembrane region. In paramyxoviruses the transmembrane domain of HN is located near the N-terminus of the molecule and F near the C-terminus.

Extending into the cytoplasm of the infected cell or inside the virion membrane is a short hydrophilic tail region, which plays a role in viral assembly through its interaction with the matrix (M) protein which lines the inner surface of the plasma membrane and itself interacts with the nucleocapsid. Inside the lipid bilayer of the viral particle is the RNA nucleocapsid which houses the nonsegmented negative-stranded RNA genome. The genomes of hPIV-1, hPIV-2, and hPIV-3 are approximately 15 000 nt and all genes except L have been sequenced for hPIV-4a and -4b and are certain to fall in this range once the sequencing is complete. The RNA genome serves as a template for transcription of mRNAs specifying six virion structural proteins linked in tandem in the order of 3′-nucleoprotein (NP)–polymerase-associated protein (P/V)–matrix protein (M)–fusion protein (F)–hemagglutinin-neuraminidase (HN)–large protein (L)-5′. The P gene alone is unique in its capacity to express, in addition to the P protein, various other proteins by utilizing internal initiation codons in the same or different reading frames or by RNA editing of the P gene mRNA through insertion of nontemplated G residues. Besides P, these other proteins have been designated V, C, and D, depending on the PIV. The helical nucleocapsid is 18 nm in diameter, contains approximately 2000 molecules of NP bound to the RNA genome, about 200 P and 20 L molecules. The P protein, which forms a polymerase complex with L, is essential for the enzymatic processes of viral RNA transcription and replication including the 3′ addition of poly(A), modification of the 5′ end, and nucleotide polymerization of viral transcripts. The approximate molecular weights in daltons of the PIV proteins as exemplified by PIV-3 are: NP, 58 000; P, 68 000; M, 40 000; F, 63 000; HN, 72 000; and L, 256 000. A cartoon and an electron micrograph of a naturally occurring PIV are shown in **Figure 1**.

Attachment Protein

The process of infection is initiated by the action of the HN glycoprotein, which binds the virion to sialic acid-containing glycoprotein or glycolipid receptors on the host cell surface. The same process is responsible for the hemagglutination of avian and mammalian erythrocytes. HN also causes the enzymatic (neuraminidase) cleavage of sialic acid residues from the carbohydrate moiety of glycoproteins and glycolipids, which functionally serves to prevent the self-aggregation of virus during release and likely aids in the spread of virus from infected cells. Besides attachment, HN provides an unknown

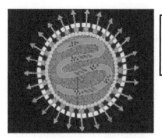

Membrane proteins
- HN: receptor-binding, neuraminidase, fusion promotion
- F: membrane fusion
- M: assembly

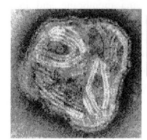

Nucleocapsid
- NP: encapsidate viral RNA
- P: forms polymerase complex with L
- L: RNA synthesis, capping, polyadenylation

Figure 1   Parainfluenza virus structure.

function that is either essential or enhances the fusion activity of the F protein. It is proposed that HN directly interacts with F, possibly altering its conformation, thereby stimulating the fusion activity of F.

The morphology of HN based on studies of PIVs such as Sendai virus is envisioned as an N-terminal stalk region of approximately 130 amino acids anchoring a large glycosylated hydrophilic globular head region to the viral envelope. A small uncharged hydrophobic peptide located near the N-terminus spans the viral envelope, and a small hydrophilic domain is internal to the membrane. The globular head contains the active site for virus attachment, neuraminidase activity, and antigenic determinants that induce neutralizing antibodies for hPIVs, as well as the other members of the *Respirovirus* and *Rubulavirus* such as Sendai virus. HN exits on the surface of the virion as disulfide-linked homodimers or tetramers.

Solution of the three-dimensional structure of the HN protein of NDV and more recently of hPIV-3 and SV5 has resolved many of the previous issues concerning the structure and functions of HN. A significant advance was the determination that the HN sialic acid-binding site and the neuraminidase active site were the same and for NDV that conformational change of the site switches HN activity from sialic acid binding (attachment) to sialic acid hydrolysis (neuraminidase activity). However, similar conformational changes may not occur for hPIV-3 and SV5 HN.

Fusion Protein

Following virus attachment, F, the other surface glycoprotein, mediates the fusion of the virion and host cell-surface membranes, which allows the nucleocapsid to be deposited in the cell cytoplasm where gene expression begins. F expressed on the surface of infected cells also mediates fusion, allowing the extension of infection to uninfected cells.

All F proteins are synthesized as inactive precursors (FO) which are post-translationally cleaved by a host cell trypsin-like protease to form the biologically active molecule. For the paramyxoviruses in general, the cleavage site is located about 100 amino acids from the N-terminus of FO. The cleavage site is characterized by a short span of basic amino acids on the amino side of the site and a longer stretch of about 30 hydrophobic residues on the carboxyl side. The number and location of basic amino acids on the amino side of the cleavage site varies with individual PIVs. hPIV-1 and Sendai virus have one basic amino acid immediately adjacent to the cleavage site (Arg), whereas PIV-2 and PIV-3 have two (Arg–Lys) and PIV-5 has five (all Arg). The motif of paired basic amino acids at the cleavage site increases the efficiency of cleavage, host and tissue tropism, and pathogenicity, as the dibasic motif is recognized by a ubiquitous protease, whereas the enzymes that cleave at a monobasic site are found in a limited number of tissues. Cleavage of FO results in two disulfide-linked fragments; the larger one, Fl, forms the new hydrophobic N-terminus, which causes membrane fusion. The smaller product, F2, is the original approximately 100 N-terminal residues of FO.

Recent solutions of the crystal structure of the F in its prefusion and postfusion conformations reveals dramatic alterations in the F protein structure during membrane fusion and offers insight into the mechanism of F activation.

M Protein

The M protein lines the inner surface of the viral envelope and is thought to play a role in virus maturation by interacting with the envelope glycoproteins and the nucleocapsid. During infection M associates with the inner leaflet of the plasma membrane where it orchestrates the release (budding) of progeny virus by interacting with specific sites on the cytoplasmic tail of the viral glycoproteins and the nucleocapsid and in transport of viral components to the budding site.

Transcription, Translation, and Replication

The negative-strand strategy of viral replication involves the synthesis of unique mRNA species of each paramyxovirus gene during infection. After introduction of the infecting nucleocapsid into the host cell, transcription is the first step in gene expression. Transcriptional regulation of mRNA abundance is determined by the gene order; the closer the gene is to the 3′ end of the genome, the more efficient is the transcription. Thus, the abundance of paramyxovirus proteins is determined mainly by the polarity of the genome. Once protein synthesis is underway, replication of the genome begins, which provides additional templates for transcription and replication.

Development of 'reverse genetics' systems for SV and hPIV-3 as well as other members of the paramyxovirus family, in which the RNA genomes of these viruses are expressed from a DNA template, has provided tools and facilitated our understanding of PIV protein structures and function, virus assembly, regulation of RNA transcription and replication, and viral pathogenesis.

Geographic and Seasonal Distribution

All of the hPIV types 1–4 have a wide geographic distribution. PIV-1–PIV-3 have been identified in most areas where facilities are available for the study of childhood respiratory tract diseases. PIV-4 has been isolated in fewer areas but this is likely to be due to the difficulty of isolation and it is probably widely distributed.

Host Range and Viral Propagation

The four hPIV types were originally isolated from humans: they cause disease in humans and humans are the primary host. Other laboratory animals can serve as experimental hosts; hamsters, guinea pigs, and ferrets can be infected with hPIV-1, hPIV-2, and hPIV-3 but these infections are usually asymptomatic. hPIV-3 can

also infect cotton rats, rhesus, and patas monkeys and chimpanzees, but these animals are not good model systems for studying disease caused by PIVs.

Embryonated hen's eggs can support the growth of some strains of hPIV-1, hPIV-2, and hPIV-3, but are much less sensitive than monkey kidney cells for primary isolation. Sendai virus, a murine subtype of PIV-1, is an exception in that it grows exceedingly well in eggs.

All four hPIV types grow well in primary monkey or human kidney cells, which are also used in the isolation of virus from clinical samples. LLC-MK2, a rhesus monkey kidney cell line, offers an efficient system for the isolation of PIVs and an experimental tissue culture system. PIV-2 and PIV-1 require trypsin in the medium to cleave the F glycoprotein for cell growth, but not PIV-3 strains. Viral infection of tissue culture can be detected by hemadsorption with chicken and guinea pig erythrocytes and the cytopathic effects produced by the viruses.

Genetics and Evolution

The entire genomic sequences of hPIV-1, hPIV-2, and hPIV-3 have been completed. The genomes of other members of the genera *Respirovirus* and *Rubulavirus* (Sendai virus, bPIV-3, and PIV-5) have been sequenced as well. In general, the genome organization is remarkably similar, but differences exist in sequence, intergenic regions, and nonstructural proteins expressed from the P gene. Sequence and immunological analyses suggest that human hPIV-1 and Sendai virus are closely related type 1 PIVs, as is PIV-3 of human and bovine origin. hPIV-1 and -3 are more closely related to each other than to hPIV-2, PIV-5, mumps virus and NDV, which in turn show a closer evolutionary relationship to each other. Evolutionary divergence of hPIV-3 and hPIV-1 is greatest for the P protein (a phenomenon of paramyxovirus P proteins in general), less for the HN and F glycoproteins, and least for M, NP, and L. Similarly, hPIV-1 and Sendai virus, and human and bovine PIV-3, show the greatest divergence in the P protein and least for NP.

Serologic Relationships and Variability

The human paramyxoviruses can be divided into two antigenic groups, comprised of PIV-1/PIV-3 and PIV-2/PIV-4/mumps virus. Human PIVs share certain antigenic determinants, but structural and antigenic variation occurs between serotypes and, to a lesser degree, within strains belonging to the same type. Antigenic diversity is not generally progressive, but may contribute to PIVs' propensity to cause recurrent infection. Antibody to F and HN correlates with neutralizing antibody and protective immunity.

Table 1   Proportion of viral respiratory tract infections caused by PIV

	Proportion (%)	Most common type
Rhinitis (common cold)	20	
Pharyngitis	20	
Laryngotracheitis (croup)	50–70	PIV-1
Bronchiolitis	20	PIV-3
Pneumonia	10	PIV-1, PIV-3
Otitis media (middle ear)	10	

Epidemiology and Transmission

The hPIVs are an important cause of respiratory tract infections (**Table 1**). hPIV-3 infections are endemic, whereas infections caused by other PIVs occur in outbreaks. Infections are common before 2 years, especially with hPIV-3, and almost universal by 5 years. hPIVs are highly communicable by respiratory droplets and by contact with surfaces contaminated by respiratory secretions. The incubation period is 2–6 days. Virus is typically shed for 4–21 days.

Pathogenicity

hPIVs bind to specific receptors on upper respiratory tract epithelial cells and may subsequently spread to the LRT. Optimal fusion efficiency requires the coordinated action of both F and HN. The virus and host factors contributing to disease pathogenesis are not completely understood. Both viral (F and HN structure) and host features (genetic susceptibility, host cell proteases, immunocompetence) are likely to influence the severity of infection.

Clinical Features

hPIVs cause between 15% and 65% of viral respiratory infections, most notably laryngotracheitis (croup) and bronchiolitis (**Table 1**). Although infections are generally mild, PIVs are responsible for over 10% of pediatric hospitalizations for respiratory infection. Life-threatening LRT infection occurs in patients with cellular immunodeficiencies, particularly those with severe combined immunodeficiency and hematopoietic stem cell and solid organ transplants. Rare cases of parotiditis, myocarditis, aseptic meningitis, and encephalitis have been reported.

The gold standard for diagnosis of hPIV infections is culture on primary monkey kidney, human embryonic kidney, or human lung carcinoma cells, which typically requires incubation for 4–7 days. Detection of epithelial cell-associated viral antigens in nasopharyngeal or bronchoalveolar washings is rapid and has a sensitivity and specificity of >80% compared to culture. Polymerase chain reaction (PCR) is rapid and more sensitive, but is not widely available. Detection of specific IgM and IgG in paired acute and convalescent sera has limited utility in the diagnosis of acute infections.

Pathology

hPIV has direct cytopathic effects, causing ciliary damage, epithelial necrosis, and recruitment of a mononuclear inflammatory response. Recent studies suggest that host inflammatory responses, rather than the direct effects of viral replication, are most accountable for the signs and symptoms of PIV infection. Alterations in HN receptor-binding or -activity influence host inflammatory responses independent of viral replication or the ability to infect epithelial cells. PIV infection may trigger long-term bronchial hyperreactivity in genetically susceptible persons.

Immune Response

Viral shedding is more prolonged and disease severity increased in persons with T-cell immunodeficiencies, implying cellular immunity is important in the control of acute hPIV infection. Protection from reinfection is associated with the development of serum and secretory antibody against F and HN. The duration of protection after acute illness is relatively short however, especially in infants, and protection from infection by heterotypic stains is incomplete.

Prevention and Control

Most hPIV infections require supportive care only. Children with moderate-to-severe croup benefit from inhaled vasoconstrictors or inhaled or systemic corticosteroids, which reduce airway edema. Anecdotal reports describe the successful use of ribavirin in immunocompromised patients. There are currently no licensed vaccines to prevent hPIV. Early formalin-inactivated vaccines were poorly immunogenic and had the potential to enhance pulmonary inflammatory responses to infection with wild-type virus.

Future Perspectives

Novel antiviral therapies being developed for PIV infections include selective inhibitors of HN, fusion, and IMP dehydrogenase, and siRNA against phosphoprotein mRNA. Vaccines currently in early clinical trials include live attenuated human PIV-3, bovine PIV-3, human-bovine chimeras, and bovine PIV or Sendai virus expressing heterologous human PIV F and HN proteins. Besides vaccines, antiviral drugs may be designed that curtail viral replication or prevent viral spread. Knowledge of the three-dimensional structure of HN and F, especially those regions involved in viral attachment, penetration, and release, will be important in drug design.

See also: Human Respiratory Viruses.

Further Reading

Karron RA and Collins PL (2006) Parainfluenza viruses. In: Knipe DM, Howley PM, Griffin DE, *et al.* (eds.) *Fields Virology,* 5th edn., pp. 1497–1526. Philadelphia, PA: Lippincott Williams and Wilkins.

Lamb RA and Parks GD (2006) *Paramyxoviridae:* The viruses and their replication. In: Knipe DM, Howley PM, Griffin DE, *et al.* (eds.) *Fields Virology,* 5th edn., pp. 1449–1496. Philadelphia, PA: Lippincott Williams and Wilkins.

Lamb RA, Paterson RG, and Jardetzky TS (2006) Paramyxovirus membrane fusion: Lessons from the F and HN atomic structures. *Virology* 344(1): 30–37.

Morrison T and Portner A (1991) Structure, function and intracellular processing of the glycoproteins of the *Paramyxoviridae.* In: Kingsbury DW (ed.) *The Paramyxoviruses,* pp. 347–382. New York: Plenum.

Subbarao K (2003) Parainfluenza viruses. In: Long SS, Pickering LK, and Prober CG (eds.) *Principles and Practice of Pediatric Infectious Diseases,* 2nd edn., p. 1131. Philadelphia, PA: Churchill Livingstone.

Takimoto T and Portner A (2004) Molecular mechanism of paramyxovirus budding. *Virus Research* 106: 133–145.

Parvoviruses: General Features

P Tattersall, Yale University Medical School, New Haven, CT, USA

The Family *Parvoviridae*: An Overview

The family *Parvoviridae* comprises small, isometric, nonenveloped viruses that contain single-stranded DNA genomes that are linear, a set of properties unique in the known biosphere. The parvovirus virion contains a single genomic molecule 4–6 kbp long, which terminates in short palindromic sequences that can fold back on themselves to create duplex hairpin telomeres. These terminal hairpins are different from one another, both in sequence and predicted structure, in heterotelomeric genomes, while in homotelomeric genomes they form part of a terminal repeat (TR) that can be inverted or direct. These terminal hairpins are essential for the unique rolling-hairpin strategy of parvovirus DNA replication, and are therefore an invariant hallmark of the family.

The bulk of the parvovirus genome lies between these hairpins, and comprises two gene cassettes, with transcripts from one half of the genome, by convention the left-hand side, programming synthesis of the DNA replication initiator protein(s), while the right-hand encodes an overlapping set of capsid polypeptides. All parvovirus initiator proteins incorporate two separate enzymatic cores. The N-terminal of these is a site-specific single-strand nuclease domain, comprising active-site motifs common to all rolling-circle initiator proteins, which recognize and nick the replication origin(s). Carboxy-terminal to this nickase lies a helicase domain, which belongs to the superfamily III (SF3) group of viral 3'-to-5' helicases. Parvovirus genomes replicated using a unidirectional, strand-displacement mechanism called rolling-hairpin replication (RHR),

which appears to be an evolutionary adaptation of the ancient rolling-circle replication mechanism used by bacteriophages with circular single-stranded DNA genomes. The parvovirus genome contains two viral origins of DNA replication, one embedded in each hairpin telomere. During RHR, these hairpins can unfold to be copied, then refold to allow continuous amplification of the linear template. Viral replication exhibits two distinct phases, the first of which is an amplification phase, during which high-molecular-weight duplex replicative form (RF) DNA intermediates are generated and subsequently processed back down to monomeric duplexes by the action of the viral nickase. Later in the infectious process, a genome displacement phase predominates, in which individual progeny single strands are displaced from duplex forms and encapsidated.

To initiate the first phase of RHR, the 3' nucleotide of incoming virion DNA pairs with an internal base to create a DNA primer, which allows a host polymerase to initiate synthesis of a complementary DNA strand. This generates a monomer-length, duplex intermediate in which the two strands, designated plus or minus with respect to transcription, are covalently linked, or hairpinned, by a single copy of the original viral telomere. For homotelomeric parvoviruses, these hairpinned structures create replication origins that can be acted upon by NS1 or Rep proteins, in a process called terminal resolution, which converts them into duplex palindromic telomeres. For heterotelomeric viruses, however, the left-end telomere in its hairpin form can be refractory to nicking by NS1, and replication proceeds through an obligatory dimer RF.

For both types of parvovirus, further DNA amplification proceeds by unidirectional strand displacement, where the initiator protein also serves as the 3′-to-5′ replicative helicase, while all other replication proteins are commandeered from the host cell. Replication continues to the end of the genome where the hairpin is displaced and copied to create a palindromic, or extended form, telomere. These terminal palindromes can be melted and rearranged in hairpins such that the 3′ end can act as a primer for further replication, using the newly synthesized product as a template. Where the template ends in a hairpinned telomere, this is copied by the replication fork, switching the direction of synthesis back toward the initiating telomere, creating a dimer. Thus the RHR process creates a series of palindromic duplex dimeric and tetrameric concatemers, in which the unit-length genomes are fused in left-end:left-end and right-end:right-end combinations.

Site-specific single-strand nicks are subsequently introduced, by the viral initiator protein, into the duplex telomeric origins embedded in these concatemers, allowing successive rounds of replication to be initiated, or progeny single strands to be excised and ultimately displaced. Nicking involves a trans-esterification reaction that generates a base-paired 3′ nucleotide and leaves the initiator nuclease covalently attached, by a phosphotyrosine bond, to the 5′ nucleotide at the nick. Displaced progeny single strands re-enter the replication pool unless sequestered by the packaging machinery and encapsidated into empty particles. Thus packaging appears to be driven by ongoing viral DNA synthesis, and is entirely dependent upon the availability of preformed capsids. The efficiency of excision, displacement, and packaging of each strand sense depends upon the efficiency of the replication origin producing it. Thus it follows that all homotelomeric parvoviruses generate equal numbers of each strand as packaging precursors, and therefore produce virion populations containing equal numbers of plus and minus strands, each packaged in a separate particle. The ratio of plus to minus strands packaged by the heterotelomeric parvoviruses depends upon the relative efficiencies of the two different DNA replication origins embedded in their disparate telomeres. In all cases where this has been determined, the origin at the 5′ end of the transcription template strand, by convention the right-hand end of the minus strand, is the predominant origin, and drives the displacement and packaging of the minus strand at ratios between 10:1 and 100:1 over that of the plus strand. Thus, all of the heterotelomeric parvoviruses examined to date are effectively negative-strand DNA viruses.

Independent of the sense of strand they contain, parvovirus particles are physically very stable and are antigenically and structurally quite simple. A combination of protein chemistry, X-ray crystallography and cryo-electron microscopy, has established that the virion is an icosahedral structure exhibiting $T = 1$ symmetry, constructed from two to four species of structural protein. These polypeptides are encoded as a nested sequence set in the right half of the genome, and the capsid shell comprises 60 copies of the common, usually C-terminal, 60–70 kDa region of the polypeptide set. Each polypeptide contains an eight-membered β-barrel, or jelly-roll, fold, found in most viral capsid proteins. The surface of the particle is formed by several of the loops between these β-strands, such that differences in length and primary amino acid sequence of these loops gives rise to the marked differences in topology observed between members of separate genera, as shown in **Figure 1**. Virions are resistant to inactivation by organic solvents, thus lack essential lipids, and there is no evidence that any of the capsid polypeptides are glycosylated, although they may be modified post-translationally by phosphorylation. The N-terminal region of the largest structural polypeptide, VP1, is an extension of the common structural region, and, in most parvoviruses, contains a functional phospholipase A_2 (PLA_2) enzymatic core whose activity is essential for escape from endosomal compartment into the cytosol, early in viral entry.

Only two antigenic sites have been identified on the virion surface, as defined by mutations that allow escape from neutralization by monoclonal antibodies. Since this relatively simple antigenic structure is very stable, serotype has been a useful adjunct to sequence-based phylogenetic analysis for taxonomic classification, particularly for the parvoviruses of vertebrates. Parvoviruses encode several well-recognized functional protein domains that might serve as linearly descended evolutionary 'tags'. Foremost among these is the relatively contiguous set of well-defined functional subdomains, called Walker boxes, within the SF3 helicase domain of the replication initiator protein of all known parvoviruses. Interestingly, SF3 helicases have also been identified within genes encoded by DNA viruses as diverse as members of the families *Poxviridae, Baculoviridae, Papillomaviridae, Polyomaviridae,* and *Circoviridae,* as well as in the genomes of small RNA viruses such as members of the families *Picornaviridae* and *Comoviridae.* However, this class of helicase has not been found encoded in cellular genomes, and their phylogenetic branch within the AAA + ATPase superfamily diverged from the rest of the tree of life before the separation of the archaea, bacteria, and eukarya. This suggests that the SF3 class of helicases might have originally evolved in primitive replicons that are only represented by viruses in the present biosphere, and that the SF3 helicase domain evident in present-day parvoviruses might represent an uninterrupted vertical link to the first common ancestor of the entire family *Parvoviridae.*

The family *Parvoviridae* is divided into two subfamilies, the subfamily *Parvovirinae,* whose members infect vertebrate hosts, and the subfamily *Densovirinae,* whose members infect arthropods. Using DNA sequence-based phylogenetic analysis, members of the subfamily *Parvovir-*

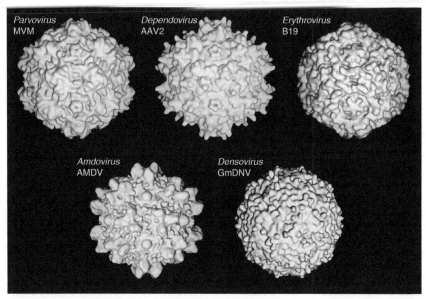

Figure 1 Molecular topography of representative virions from the family *Parvoviridae*. Low-resolution surface maps of minute virus of mice (MVM), adeno-associated virus-2 (AAV2), B19, mature aleutian mink disease virus (AMDV), and galleria mellonella densovirus (GmDNV), at 13 Å resolution. The surface map image of AMDV was generated from a pseudoatomic model built into cryo-EM density, while the others were generated directly from atomic coordinates, as described by Agbandje-McKenna and Chapman in 2006, and were graciously provided by Lakshmanan Govindasamy and Mavis Agbandje-McKenna.

Table 1   The taxonomic structure of the family *Parvoviridae*

Subfamily	Genus
Parvovirinae	Parvovirus
	Dependovirus
	Erythrovirus
	Amdovirus
	Bocavirus
Densovirinae	Densovirus
	Pefudensovirus
	Iteravirus
	Brevidensovirus

inae have been divided into five genera, and those of the subfamily *Densovirinae* into four genera, as listed in **Table 1**. As listed in **Tables 2** and **3**, these nine genera contain 34 species accepted as such by the International Committee for the Taxonomy of Viruses, with 25 species tentatively assigned to individual genera and a further nine virus isolates currently unassigned within the subfamily *Densovirinae*.

Genera in the Subfamily *Parvovirinae*

Genus *Parvovirus*

Viruses belonging to species within the genus *Parvovirus* have heterotelomeric genomes ~5 kbp in length. The packaged strands are predominantly negative-sense with respect to their monosense transcription strategy, although parvovirus LuIII virus packages both strands, in separate particles, in an approximately equimolar ratio. The terminal hairpin at the 3'-end of the negative strand, by convention the left-hand end of the genetic map, is 115–121 nucleotides (nt) long, whereas their right-hand hairpins vary between 200 and 248 nt in length. As shown in **Figure 2**, there are two transcriptional promoters, at map units ~4 and ~40, from the left-hand end, and transcripts co-terminate at a single polyadenylation site near the right-hand end of the genome. Many viruses belonging to this genus encode a second, smaller, nonstructural protein, NS2, in addition to the major DNA replication initiator protein NS1. NS2 is involved in several aspects of viral replication and capsid assembly, but is dispensable in some cell types. Infecting virions lack accessory proteins, chromatin or even a duplex transcription template, and therefore remain silent within their host cell nucleus until the cellular synthetic machinery manufactures a complementary DNA strand, creating the first transcription template. Typically, this occurs when the host cell enters S-phase, of its own volition, and it is followed rapidly by expression of viral transcripts driven from the left-hand promoter. These viruses can persist both in nondividing cells in culture and within the intact host animal, and, in the latter case, frequently re-emerge following immunosuppression. Despite convincing serologic and PCR evidence for long-term persistence by many parvoviruses, at present essentially nothing is known of the mechanisms underlying this type of latency. Members of many species within this

Table 2   Subfamily *Parvovirinae*

Genus *Parvovirus*
Species

Minute virus of mice – type species	(MVM)
Feline panleukopenia virus	(FPV)
H-1 parvovirus	(H-1PV)
Kilham rat virus	(KRV)
LuIII virus	(LuIIIV)
Mouse parvovirus 1	(MPV-1)
Porcine parvovirus	(PPV)
HB parvovirus[a]	(HBPV)
Lapine parvovirus[a]	(LPV)
RT parvovirus[a]	(RTPV)
Tumor X virus[a]	(TXV)

Tentative species[b]

Hamster parvovirus	(HaPV)
Rat minute virus 1	(RMV-1)
Rat parvovirus 1	(RPV-1)

Genus *Dependovirus*
Species

Adeno-associated virus-1	(AAV1)
Adeno-associated virus-2 – type species	(AAV2)
Adeno-associated virus-3	(AAV3)
Adeno-associated virus-4	(AAV4)
Adeno-associated virus-5	(AAV5)
Avian adeno-associated virus	(AAAV)
Bovine adeno-associated virus	(BAAV)
Duck parvovirus	(BDPV)
Goose parvovirus	(GPV)
Canine adeno-associated virus[a]	(CAAV)
Equine adeno-associated virus[a]	(EAAV)
Ovine adeno-associated virus[a]	(OAAV)

Tentative species[b]

Adeno-associated virus-7	(AAV7)
Adeno-associated virus-8	(AAV8)
Adeno-associated virus-9	(AAV9)
Adeno-associated virus-10	(AAV10)
Adeno-associated virus-11	(AAV11)
Adeno-associated virus-12	(AAV12)
Serpentine adeno-associated virus	(SAAV)
Caprine adeno-associated virus	(Go.1 AAV)
Bovine parvovirus type 2[c]	(BPV2)

Genus *Erythrovirus*
Species

Human parvovirus B19 – type species[d]	(B19V-Au)

Tentative species[b]

Chipmunk parvovirus	(ChpPV)
Pig-tailed macaque parvovirus	(PmPV)
Rhesus macaque parvovirus	(RmPV)
Simian parvovirus	(SPV)
Bovine parvovirus type 3[c]	(BPV3)

Genus *Amdovirus*
Species

Aleutian mink disease virus – type species	(ADV-G)

Genus *Bocavirus*
Species

Bovine parvovirus 1 – type species	(BPV1)
Canine minute virus	(CnMV)

Tentative species[b]

Human bocavirus[c]	(HBoV)

[a]Formally accepted by ICTV, but no representative genomes have been sequenced.
[b]Representative genome sequenced, but not formally accepted as a species by ICTV.

genus, particularly those whose natural host are rodents, have been found to be markedly oncolytic in transformed human cells, both in culture and in xenotransplanted tumor models.

Genus *Dependovirus*

The genus *Dependovirus*, as the name implies, originally comprised only the helper-dependent adeno-associated viruses. However, phylogenetic analysis now places the autonomously replicating viruses from the *Goose parvovirus* and *Duck parvovirus* species solidly within this genus. Except for members of these two avian parvovirus species, all other viruses belonging to this genus that have been isolated to date are dependent upon helper adenoviruses or herpes viruses for efficient replication. Most primate adeno-associated virus (AAV) serotypes isolated to date appear to be simian viruses. On the other hand, sero-epidemiologic evidence clearly indicates that AAV2 and AAV3 are human viruses, while AAV5, which is most closely related to caprine AAV, has been isolated from humans only once.

So far, all members of this genus have been found to be homotelomeric, and their virions contain equivalent numbers of positive or negative DNA strands, between 4.7 and 5.1 kbp in size. Typically, the AAV genome has TRs of ~145 nt, the first ~125 nt of which form a palindromic hairpin sequence, while members of the autonomously replicating avian parvovirus species have ITRs that are much larger, between 444 and 457 nt. As shown in **Figure 2**, three distinct transcriptional strategies have been elucidated for members of this genus. Two subtypes, represented by AAV2 and AAV5, have three transcriptional promoters (P5, P19, and P40), but differ in the positions of their functional polyadenylation sites. For both of these subtypes there is one polyadenylation site at the right-hand end of the genome, but for the AAV5-like viruses another site, located in the middle of the genome, is also used. The GPV-like viruses have a polyadenylation site arrangement like that of AAV5, but differ from the other two subtypes by not having a functional middle, P19, promoter.

Under certain conditions, such as the treatment of host cells with mutagens or hydroxyurea, AAV DNA replication can be detected in the absence of helper viruses. However, infections without helper virus generally result in a persistent latent infection. Three modes of persistence have been demonstrated for AAV. First, AAV2

[c]Genome sequenced or partially sequenced by PCR-based virus discovery techniques, but virus not yet isolated physically or biologically.
[d]Three major genotypes, represented by B19V-Au, B19-LaLi, and B19-V9. Species names are italicized, abbreviations for individual viruses are given in parentheses.

Table 3 Subfamily *Densovirinae*

Genus *Densovirus*
Species
    Junonia coenia densovirus – type species
        Junonia coenia densovirus   (JcDNV)
    Galleria mellonella densovirus
        Galleria mellonella densovirus   (GmDNV)

Tentative species[a]
    Diatraea saccharalis densovirus   (DsDNV)
    Mythimna loreyi densovirus   (MlDNV)
    Toxorhynchites splendens densovirus   (TsDNV)
    Pseudoplusia includens densovirus   (PiDNV)

Genus *Pefudensovirus*
Species
    Periplaneta fuliginosa densovirus – type species
        Periplaneta fuliginosa densovirus   (PfDNV)

Genus *Iteravirus*
Species
    Bombyx mori densovirus – type species
        Bombyx mori densovirus   (BmDNV)

Tentative species[a]
    Casphalia extranea densovirus   (CeDNV)
    Sibine fusca densovirus   (SfDNV)

Genus *Brevidensovirus*
Species
    Aedes aegypti densovirus – type species
        Aedes aegypti densovirus   (AaeDNV)
    Aedes albopictus densovirus
        Aedes albopictus densovirus   (AalDNV)

Tentative species[a]
    Penaeus stylirostris densovirus[b]   (PstDNV)
    Aedes pseudoscutellaris densovirus   (ApDNV)
    Simulium vittatum densovirus   (SvDNV)

[a]Representative genome sequenced, but not formally accepted as a species by ICTV.
[b]This is also called infectious hypodermal and hematopoietic necrosis virus (IHHNV) of penaeid shrimps.
Species names are italicized, acronyms for individual viruses are given in parentheses.

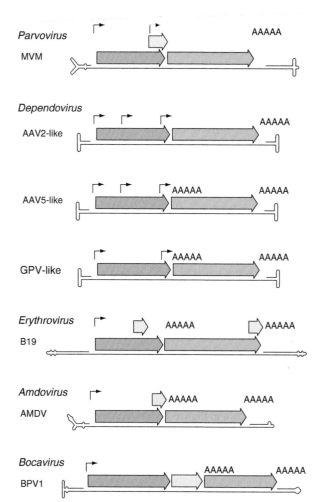

Figure 2 Genetic strategies of representative viruses from genera in the subfamily *Parvovirinae*. Genomes from viruses belonging to the type species of each genus, and an additional two subtypes from the genus *Dependovirus*, are denoted as a single line terminating in hairpin structures. The hairpins are drawn to represent their predicted structures, and are scaled about 20× with respect to the rest of the genome. Open reading frames are represented by arrowed boxes, colored green for the major SF3 domain-containing replication initiator protein, blue for the structural proteins of the capsid, and yellow for the ancillary nonstructural proteins. Transcriptional promoters are indicated by solid arrows and polyadenylation sites by the AAAAA sequence block.

and some other serotypes can integrate their genomes site-specifically into a 4 kbp locus on human chromosome 19q13-qter, designated AAVS1. This occurs by a replication-dependent mechanism, requiring low-level expression of Rep, and depends upon sequences in AAVS1 that can function as an AAV DNA replication origin. The second mode, which is independent of Rep gene expression, is primarily seen with recombinant AAV (rAAV) genomes used in gene transduction scenarios, and proceeds through nonspecific integration. Typically, a transgene, flanked by AAV ITRs and packaged in an AAV capsid, is used to infect target tissues in a host animal. Integration of rAAVs occurs at multiple positions throughout the host genome, with a bias toward actively transcribed loci, and is enhanced by the presence of double-strand breaks in host DNA. A third form of persistence, again exploited in rAAV-based gene transduction

strategies, results from the establishment of monomeric, and later concatemeric, circular duplex episomes, following vector delivery at high copy number to postmitotic tissues, such as liver or skeletal muscle. Similar episomes have also been detected *in vivo* in latently infected human tissues, although it is not known whether they are created by cellular repair mechanisms or by annealing of complementary strands. Recent studies have shown that the tissue most efficiently targeted by rAAV vectors depends upon the serotype of AAV providing the capsid gene, although a consensus hierarchy of target preference across all of the serotypes continues to evolve.

Genus *Erythrovirus*

Until recently, the only known human pathogenic member of the family *Parvoviridae* was human parvovirus B19 (B19V). This virus is responsible for transient aplastic crisis in patients with a variety of hemolytic anemias, and is the causative agent of *Erythema Infectiosum*, a widespread childhood rash-like disease also referred to as 'fifth disease'. Intrauterine transmission of B19V from an infected mother to her fetus can result in *hydrops fetalis*, particularly in the second trimester of pregnancy. Recently it has become apparent that there are at least three distinct genotypes of B19V, circulating in different human subpopulations. While these are all serotypically equivalent, and thus are considered members of the same species, retrospective PCR analysis of archival tissues has shown that they have predominated in the human population during different periods in the recent past. Additional erythroviruses have been identified in other primate species, which share B19V's specificity for erythroid progenitor cells and cause a similar disease in their hosts.

The erythrovirus genome is homotelomeric, with inverted terminal repeats (ITRs) of 383 nt, and populations of mature B19V virions contain equivalent numbers of positive- and negative-sense DNA strands, each ~5.5 kbp in size. As shown in **Figure 2**, viral transcription is driven by a single promoter at map unit 6 and terminates at alternative polyadenylation sites, one near the middle of the genome, the other at the right-hand end, which generates transcripts encoding NS1 and VP1, respectively. The B19V genomes contain two additional small open reading frames (ORFs), which are accessed by alternatively splicing and translation initiation. One of these encodes an 11 kDa protein containing three proline-rich regions containing consensus Src homology 3 domains, while the other encodes a 7.5 kDa polypeptide of unknown function.

Genus *Amdovirus*

The genus *Amdovirus* contains a single species, *Aleutian mink disease virus*. Mature Aleutian mink disease virus (AMDV) virions contain a predominantly negative-strand, heterotelomeric genome of 4748 nt whose sequence is markedly divergent from other members of the subfamily *Parvovirinae*. As shown in **Figure 2**, the ADMV transcription strategy resembles that of the erythroviruses, in having a single promoter and two alternative polyadenylation sites. The major distinguishing feature of AMDV is its VP1 N-terminus, which is quite short and completely lacks a phospholipase 2A enzymatic core. As seen in **Figure 1**, AMDV virion structure is also somewhat distinctive. Permissive replication has only been achieved in cell culture for the ADV-G isolate, which replicates in Crandell feline kidney cells and is relatively apathogenic in mink. Several highly pathogenic strains of AMDV exist and differ in

their disease potential depending upon the age and genetic background of the infected host. Thus infected mink kits develop interstitial pneumonia involving direct attack on type II pneumocytes, while adult mink develop an autoimmune disease characterized by massive hypergammaglobulinemia and fatal glomerulonephritis. As the virus' name suggests, the latter condition is exacerbated in mink carrying the Aleutian coat color allele, which is tightly linked to an antigen presentation disorder in this genetic background. While mostly studied in mink, serologic evidence suggests that this virus also circulates naturally in several other species within the superfamily *Musteloidea*.

Genus *Bocavirus*

The bocaviruses package heterotelomeric genomes ~5.5 kbp in length, and the bovine virus, bovine parvovirus 1 (BPV1), has been shown to package negative-sense and positive-sense DNA strands at a 10:1 ratio. The bocavirus transcription strategy resembles that of the erythroviruses and AMDV in having a single promoter at the left-hand end, and two alternative polyadenylation sites. The bocaviruses differ, however, from all other members of the subfamily *Parvovirinae* in encoding a 22.5 kDa nuclear phosphoprotein, NP1, that is distinct from any other parvovirus-encoded polypeptide. As shown in **Figure 2**, the ORF encoding NP1 sits immediately downstream of that encoding NS1, and immediately upstream of the middle polyadenylation site. NP1, whose function is currently unknown, is abundantly expressed from transcripts that have been spliced to remove the NS1 ORF, and can be polyadenylated at either site. Human bocavirus (HBoV) was discovered in 2005 and subsequent PCR-based surveys have indicated that it is a common human respiratory pathogen, mostly of infants and young children. Although sero-epidemiologic assays remain to be developed, studies so far indicate that HBoV is likely the cause of a substantial proportion of undiagnosed respiratory tract disease, and appears to be distributed worldwide.

Genera in the Subfamily *Densovirinae*

Genus *Densovirus*

The homotelomeric densovirus genome is typically about 6 kbp in length, with long ITRs. The genome contains a >500 nt long ITR, the first ~100 nt of which are predicted to be able to fold as a T-shaped structure. These viruses, along with the pefudensoviruses described below, represent a paradigm shift for the members of the family *Parvoviridae*, since they exhibit ambisense organization. Although they appear to maintain the division of the genome into separate nonstructural and structural gene cassettes typical of all other family members, these

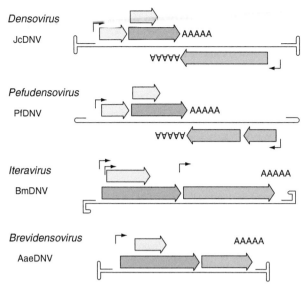

Figure 3 Genetic strategies of a representative of the type species from genera in the subfamily *Densovirinae*. Genomes from viruses belonging to the type species of each genus are diagrammed as in the legend to **Figure 2**.

cassettes are inverted with respect to one another, as shown in **Figure 3**. Populations of virions encapsidate equal numbers of positive and negative strands. The positive strand, by convention the strand encoding the nonstructural proteins, contains three ORFs, which are predicted to encode three NS proteins, and which are accessed by alternative splicing of mRNAs transcribed rightward from a promoter just within the ITR at the left-hand end. The negative, or complementary, strand expresses four structural proteins by alternative translation initiation, from an mRNA transcribed leftward from the homologous promoter just inside the right-hand ITR.

Genus *Pefudensovirus*

Like the members of the genus *Densovirus*, viruses belonging to the genus *Pefudensovirus* exhibit an ambisense organization. The homotelomeric genome is ~5.5 kbp in length, with a rightward promoter at 3 map units and a leftward promoter at 97 map units, located within the opposing 201 nt ITRs. As can be seen in **Figure 3**, the VP gene is located in the 5′ half of the complementary strand, and is split into a small upstream ORF and a large downstream ORF, which appear to be spliced in order to code for the largest VP, expression of which also appears to require frameshifting after splicing. Unlike other members of the family *Parvoviridae*, in which the PLA2 domain is expressed in the N-terminus of the largest structural protein, in pefudensoviruses this motif is centered 60–70 amino acids from the C-terminus of the ORF predicted to encode the small VP protein. The ORFs predicted to encode the three pefudensovirus nonstructural proteins

are organized in the same way as for those of the genus *Densovirus*, and are of similar sizes.

Genus *Iteravirus*

The homotelomeric iteravirus genome is ~5 kbp in length, and populations of virions encapsidate equal numbers of plus and minus strands, in separate particles. The monosense genome, diagrammed in **Figure 3**, has an ITR of 230 nt, the first 159 of which are predicted to fold in a 'J-shaped' hairpin structure. There are two ORFs for nonstructural proteins and one ORF encoding the structural proteins, located on the same strand. A predicted transcriptional promoter resides upstream of each nonstructural ORF, such that each is expressed from its own transcript. A further putative promoter, lying downstream of the nonstructural genes, is predicted to drive production of the structural gene transcript, from which the synthesis of four or five overlapping structural proteins is proposed to occur by a leaky scanning translational initiation process.

Genus *Brevidensovirus*

The monosense genomes of members of the genus *Brevidensovirus* are the smallest within the family, being about 4 kbp in length. This is the only genus within the subfamily *Densovirinae* that have heterotelomeric genomes, and their virions encapsidate predominantly (85%) negative-sense strands. The left-hand end of a representative of the type species, *Aedes aegypti densovirus*, comprises a palindromic sequence of 146 nt while the right-hand end is a palindromic sequence of 164 nt. While different in sequence, both terminal sequences are predicted to fold into a T-shaped structure. As shown in **Figure 3**, the genome contains two transcriptional promoters, at map units 7 and 60. Two overlapping ORFs encoding the nonstructural proteins occupy more than half of the genome, the balance being occupied by a single ORF encoding the structural polypeptides. The genome does not contain any translated sequence recognizable as a PLA2 domain. Viruses belonging to this genus are evolutionarily extremely remote from all other members of the family *Parvoviridae*, and infect arthropod species as diverse as mosquito and shrimp. The latter include viruses that cause hypodermal and hematopoietic necrosis, infecting all multiple organs of ectodermal and mesodermal origin of the shrimp, but not the midgut. These viruses quite closely resemble the mosquito viruses in both genome size and organization. Recently, however, a number of parvoviruses have been isolated from shrimp that infect hepatopancreatic epithelial cells. While these cluster phylogenetically with the brevidensoviruses when their common sequences are compared, they are more than 50% larger, and differ from them substantially in genome organization. Namely, their two nonstructural ORFs are arranged in tandem, and their structural protein genes are also substantially longer, although they are still devoid of a recognizable PLA2 domain. Thus, in contrast to the founding members of this genus, these shrimp viruses have the largest genomes in the family *Parvoviridae*, and it is not yet clear whether they represent a new genus separate from the genus *Brevidensovirus*.

Acknowledgments

The author would like to thank Susan Cotmore, David Pintel, and Peter Tijssen for much helpful discussion, and Lakshmanan Govindasamy and Mavis Agbandje-McKenna for providing the images for **Figure 1**. The author was supported by PHS grants AI26109 and CA29303 from the National Institutes of Health.

Further Reading

Agbandje-McKenna M and Chapman M (2006) Correlating structure with function in the viral capsid. In: Kerr J, Cotmore SF, Bloom ME, Linden RM,, and Parrish CR (eds.) *The Parvoviruses*, ch. 10, pp. 125–139. London: Hodder Arnold.

Carter BJ, Burstein H, and Peluso RW (2004) Adeno-associated virus and AAV vectors for gene delivery. In: Templeton NS (ed.) *Gene and Cell Therapy: Therapeutic Mechanisms and Strategies*, ch. 5, pp. 71–102. New York: Dekker.

Cotmore SF and Tattersall P (2006) Genome structure and organization. In: Kerr JR, Cotmore SF, Bloom ME, Linden RM,, and Parrish CR (eds.) *The Parvoviruses*, ch. 7, pp. 73–94. London: Hodder Arnold.

Cotmore SF and Tattersall P (2006) Parvoviruses. In: DePamphilis M (ed.) *DNA Replication and Human Disease*, ch. 29, pp. 593–608. Cold Spring Harbor, NY: Cold Spring Harbor Laboratory Press.

Qiu J, Yoto Y, Tullis G, and Pintel DJ (2006) Parvovirus RNA processing strategies. In: Kerr J, Cotmore SF, Bloom ME, Linden RM,, and Parrish CR (eds.) *The Parvoviruses*, ch. 18, pp. 253–273. London: Hodder Arnold.

Tattersall P (2006) The evolution of parvoviral taxonomy. In: Kerr J, Cotmore SF, Bloom ME, Linden RM,, and Parrish CR (eds.) *The Parvoviruses*, ch. 1, pp. 5–14. London: Hodder Arnold.

Tattersall P, Bergoin M, Bloom ME, *et al.* (2005) *Parvoviridae*. In: Fauquet CM, Mayo MA, Maniloff J, Desselberger U,, and Ball LA (eds.) *Virus Taxonomy: Eighth Report of the International Committee on Taxonomy of Viruses*, pp. 353–369. San Diego, CA: Elsevier Academic Press.

Tijssen P, Bando H, Li Y, *et al.* (2006) Evolution of densoviruses. In: Kerr J, Cotmore SF, Bloom ME, Linden RM,, and Parrish CR (eds.) *The Parvoviruses*, ch. 5, pp. 55–68. London: Hodder Arnold.

Wu Z, Asokan A, and Samulski RJ (2006) Adeno-associated virus serotypes: Vector toolkit for human gene therapy. *Molecular Therapy* 14: 316–327.

Young NS and Brown KE (2004) Parvovirus B19. *New England Journal of Medicine* 350: 586–597.

Poliomyelitis

P D Minor, NIBSC, Potters Bar, UK

Introduction

A funerary stele from about 1300 BC currently in the Carlsberg museum at Copenhagen shows the priest Rom with the withered single limb and down-flexed foot typical of motor neuron destruction caused by poliovirus. It is considered to be the first documentary evidence for an infectious disease of humans. Two highly effective vaccines were developed in the 1950s, and a major program of the World Health Organization (WHO) is underway which may make poliomyelitis the second human disease to be eradicated globally after smallpox.

Pathogenesis and Disease

Poliomyelitis gets its name from the specificity of the virus for the motor neurons that form the gray matter (*polios* and *myelos*, Greek for gray and matter, respectively) of the anterior horn. Despite the obvious physical signs of muscle atrophy and motor neuron degeneration, few cases of poliomyelitis are identifiable in the literature before the end of the nineteenth century, and it is believed that it was extremely rare. However, at this time, the disease began to occur in large epidemics, initially in Scandinavia (particularly Sweden), and then in the USA, most commonly affecting young children (hence the alternative name of infantile paralysis). The legs are more commonly affected than the arms, and paralysis tends to occur in one limb rather than symmetrically.

Poliovirus occurs in three antigenically distinct serotypes designated 1, 2, and 3, such that infection with one serotype confers solid protection only against other viruses of that serotype. Infections primarily occupy the gut, and most are entirely silent, but in a small number of cases they lead to a systemic infection (the minor disease) 3–7 days post exposure, characterized by fever, rash, or sore throat. Depending on the strain or type of virus, usually less than 1% of all infections lead to the major disease or poliomyelitis which develops on average 7–30 days after infection. Spinal poliomyelitis resulting in lower limb paralysis or bulbar poliomyelitis in which the breathing centers are affected occurs when the lower or upper regions, respectively, of the spinal cord are affected. In the mid-twentieth century, about 10% of cases recovered without sequelae, 80% had permanent residual paralysis, and the remainder died. Encephalitis occurs but is rather rare. Meningitis, also known as abortive or nonparalytic poliomyelitis, occurs at a rate of about 5% of poliomyelitis cases.

Infection is mainly fecal–oral, although the virus can also be transmitted by the respiratory route from the throats of infected individuals. The primary site of infection in the gut is not known but may be the lymphoid tissues, specifically the Peyer's patches and tonsils or the mucosal surfaces in the gut or throat; infectious virus can be found in the local lymph nodes and in more distal mesenteric lymph nodes but it is not clear that the virus necessarily replicates there. The Peyer's patch-associated M-cells are believed by many to be the major infected cells in the gut.

Viremia may occur about 7 days after infection, corresponding roughly to the appearance of the minor disease. It is believed to seed sites including the peripheral and central nervous systems resulting in the major disease. Thus humoral antibodies should prevent poliomyelitis by blocking viremia; the protective effect of passively administered humoral antibodies was shown in the 1950s. This explains the change in the epidemiology of the disease at the start of the twentieth century as hygiene improved, and children were exposed to infection later in life when maternal antibody levels had declined to levels no longer able to confine the infection to the gut.

The Virus Genome

The virus contains a single strand of messenger sense RNA of about 7500 nt. A long highly structured 5′ noncoding region of about 740 nt which serves as an internal ribosomal entry site (IRES) is followed by a single open reading frame and terminates in a 3′ noncoding region of c. 70 nt followed by a polyadenylate tract. The 5′ end of the genome is covalently linked to a virus-encoded protein termed VPg. The single open reading frame encodes the structural proteins which make up the capsid (collectively termed the P1 region) followed by the regions encoding the non-structural proteins P2 and P3. P1 is divided into VP1, VP3, and VP0 (VP2 plus VP4). P2 is cleaved into $2A^{pro}$, 2B, and 2C, and P3 into 3A, 3B (or VPg), $3C^{pro}$, and $3D^{pol}$ by virus-encoded proteases. $3D^{pol}$ is the viral polymerase, but all proteins in the nonstructural part of the genome play a role in RNA replication, which also depends on RNA structural elements and host cell membranes which are extensively rearranged in the course of infection.

The Virus Particle

The infectious virus particle consists of 60 copies each of VP1, VP2, VP3, and the smaller protein VP4; VP2 and VP4 are generated by autocatalytic cleavage of VP0, in the last stage of the maturation of the particle. The proteins are arranged with icosahedral symmetry such that VP1 is found at the pentameric apex of the icosahedron and VP2 and VP3 alternate around the pseudo-sixfold axes of symmetry of the triangular faces of the icosahedron. VP4 is located internally about the pentameric apex and is myristylated. The pentameric apex of the particle is surrounded by a dip or canyon into which the cellular receptor for poliovirus fits. The atomic structure of the virus was solved in 1985.

The Poliovirus Receptor

Although some strains of type 2 poliovirus are able to infect normal mice, only the higher primates and Old World monkeys are susceptible to infection by all serotypes as they possess the specific receptor site required, and this species restriction is one of the factors that makes eradication theoretically possible. The receptor site was identified in 1986 and is a three-domain membrane protein of the immunoglobulin superfamily termed CD155. It is necessary and sufficient for the infection of cells *in vitro*, and transgenic mice carrying the gene for the polio receptor can be infected by all poliovirus types, developing paralysis when infected with wild-type virus. Such mice have been developed as alternatives to monkeys in the safety testing of live polio vaccines.

The tissue distribution of the receptor site does not explain the targets of infection of the virus and it is possible that innate immunity plays a significant role in its highly specific tropism in normal individuals.

Classification

The members of the family *Picornaviridae* to which poliovirus belongs are small nonenveloped viruses of about 30 nm in diameter when hydrated, essentially featureless when examined by electron microscopy and containing a single strand of an RNA molecule of messenger sense. The family is currently split into nine genera on the basis of sequence similarities, as shown in **Table 1**.

The genus *Enterovirus*, of which poliovirus is the archetypal species, is further subdivided into eight species of which *A* to *D* and the *Poliovirus* infect humans. The classification is summarized in **Table 2**, with examples of the viruses within the species.

The sequences of the capsid region of the viruses within a species define a virus type while sequences of

Table 1   Genera within the family *Picornaviridae*

Genus
  Enterovirus
  Rhinovirus
  Cardiovirus
  Aphthovirus
  Hepatovirus
  Parechovirus
  Erbovirus
  Kobuvirus
  Teschovirus

Table 2   Species within the genus *Enterovirus*

Species	Serotype
Poliovirus	1, 2, 3
Human enterovirus A	Coxsackievirus A2, 3, 5, 7, 8, 10, 12, 14, 16
	Enterovirus 71
Human enterovirus B	Coxsackievirus B 1–6, coxsackievirus A 9
	Human echovirus 1–7, 9, 11–21, 24–27, 29–33
	Human enterovirus 69
Human enterovirus C	Coxsackie virus A 1, 11, 13, 15, 17–22, 24
Human enterovirus C	Human enterovirus 68, 70
Bovine enterovirus	Bovine enterovirus 1, 2
Porcine enterovirus A	Porcine enterovirus 8
Porcine enterovirus B	Porcine enterovirus 9, 10

other regions of the genome do not. This suggests that viruses within a particular species can exchange genome segments more or less freely. On this basis, polioviruses should be assigned to the species *C enterovirus* but at the time of writing they remain a separate species because of the unique human disease they cause.

The comparison of the sequence of field isolates has proved a very valuable tool in the WHO program to eradicate polio. Viruses from the same geographical region tend to cluster in terms of their sequence largely independent of the year of isolation. Thus it is possible to identify a virus from a case as indigenous to the region where it was isolated or an importation. Similarly, as virus circulation is obstructed by effective vaccination programs, the variety of sequences found declines, indicating progress long before the disease is eradicated. Finally, it is possible to identify strains as wild type or vaccine derived. It has become clear that the rate at which the sequence of a vaccine or wild-type virus lineage drifts in an epidemic or during chronic infection of immunodeficient individuals unable to clear the virus is amazingly constant at about 2–3% silent substitutions

per year, or 1% for all substitutions. Thus the comparison of viral sequences can date the common ancestor of two polioviruses accurately and therefore how long they have been circulating.

Vaccines

Inactivated polio vaccine (IPV) was developed by Salk. It consists of wild-type virus that has been treated with low concentrations of formalin sufficient to inactivate the virus without affecting its antigenic properties to any great extent. The vaccine was first licensed in 1955 in the USA and reduced the number of cases by over 99%. It has been shown to be capable of eradicating the disease in certain countries, notably Scandinavia and the Netherlands. However, there remained controversy over whether a nonreplicating vaccine could eradicate disease and the virus altogether in less-developed countries where exposure is more intense, and it was possible that live-attenuated vaccines imitating natural infection might give better protection against infection by wild-type viruses. The live-attenuated vaccines given by mouth (oral polio vaccine, OPV) that form the basis of the current eradication campaign were developed by Sabin and introduced in the early 1960s. The Sabin vaccines have been shown to be able to interrupt epidemics and to break transmission if used correctly, resulting in the eradication of the virus in entire regions and possibly eventually the world.

It was also known that the Sabin vaccines altered in the vaccine recipients, becoming more neurovirulent particularly in the case of the type 3 component, and that in rare instances, now estimated at about 1 case per 750 000 first-time vaccinees, the vaccine could cause poliomyelitis in recipients and their immediate contacts. Both IPV and OPV contain a single representative of each of the three serotypes.

Attenuation of the Sabin Vaccine Strains

The genome of poliovirus is of positive (messenger) RNA sense and therefore infectious. Complete genomes of the virulent precursors of the Sabin vaccine strains or isolates from vaccine-associated cases were cloned, sequenced, and mutations introduced or segments exchanged. Virus recovered from RNA transcribed from the modified plasmids was tested in monkeys or in transgenic mice carrying the poliovirus receptor. It was possible to identify two differences between Leon, the virulent precursor of the Sabin type 3 vaccine strain which would attenuate Leon or would de-attenuate the Sabin strain, one in the 5′ noncoding region, the other in capsid protein VP3.

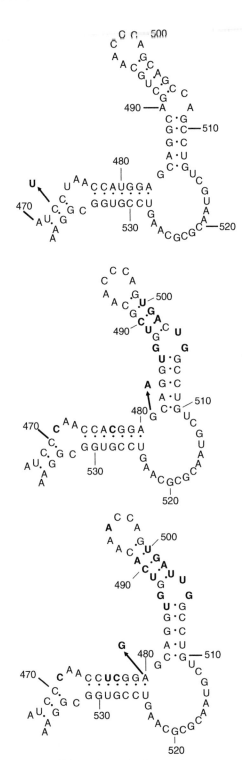

Figure 1 Structure of RNA domain in the 5′ noncoding region of polio involved in attenuating the neurovirulence of the Sabin live-attenuated vaccine strains. Top: type 3; center: type 2; bottom: type 1. Differences from the type 3 sequence are shown in bold, illustrating the general conservation of the base-paired structures. Base changes involved in attenuation are shown by arrows for the three types. Note that for types 1 and 3, the changes result in weaker but allowed base pairing compared to the wild-type sequence.

Similarly, there were two major attenuating mutations in the type 2 strain, one in the 5′ noncoding region, the other in capsid protein VP1. The story with type 1 was more complicated. Again there was one mutation in the 5′ noncoding region but several throughout the capsid region. All three of the 5′ noncoding mutations affect the highly structured region shown in **Figure 1**.

All 5′ noncoding mutations have been shown to affect initiation of protein synthesis, all involve allowed but altered base pairing, and all revert or are suppressed in vaccine recipients when sequential isolates are made. Excretion of virus following vaccination with OPV continues on average for 4 or 5 weeks and the reversions observed occur early in the excretion period, usually within 1 or 2 days for the type 3 strain and within a week for the other two types. Other changes also take place, including the reversion or more usually direct or indirect suppression of the VP3 mutation in the type 3 strain.

In addition, the viruses recombine with each other at high frequency. The type 3 strain in particular is usually excreted as a recombinant from about 11 days post immunization with the part of the genome encoding the nonstructural genes from the type 1 or type 2 strains. Complex recombinants with portions from different serotypes are also common, although their selective advantage is not known. The adaptation of the virus to the gut is therefore rapid and subtle and by a variety of mechanisms including reversion, second site suppression, and suppression of the phenotype of poor growth by enhancing fitness by an entirely unrelated route, and may involve mutation or recombination. Once adapted, virus excretion persists typically for several weeks. The drift in the viral sequence over prolonged periods of time referred to above occurs in addition to these selected changes, and appears to be a consequence of a purely stochastic process.

The Global Polio Eradication Program

For many years, it was thought that OPV could not be effective in tropical countries, and despite large-scale use its impact was in fact minimal. The reasons put forward included interference by other enteric infections, and many other factors, including breast-feeding. The most plausible explanations are that the vaccine used in routine vaccination programs was probably poorly looked after and therefore inactive, and the epidemiology of the disease was different in tropical and temperate climates. In countries of Northern Europe, poliomyelitis is highly seasonal, occurring essentially only in summer. Thus a routine vaccination campaign in which children are immunized at a set age is able to reduce the number of susceptibles during the winter when the virus is not freely circulating, so that circulation of the wild-type virus in the summer is impaired. Eventually, the wild-type virus dies out. In tropical climates, however, exposure is less seasonal, so that there is no respite during which immune populations can be built up by immunization; it remains a matter of chance whether a child is exposed first to vaccine or wild-type virus, and the impact on disease is correspondingly less. The strategy required is to immunize large proportions of the population at once. This approach was successfully followed in the 1960s in the USA in the southern states, where the climate is more tropical and routine immunization was less effective. However, it was not until the 1980s that the strategy was used in developing countries in South America when vaccine was given in mass campaigns termed National Immunization Days (NIDs). The success of the program led to a resolution in 1988 by WHO to eradicate polio from the world by the year 2000. While this has still not been achieved at the time of writing, there are only four countries from which poliovirus has never been eradicated: India, Pakistan, Afghanistan, and Nigeria. Northern India has proven extremely difficult and some children have contracted poliomyelitis after 10 or more immunizations with OPV. One approach that has been adopted is to use monovalent vaccine instead of the trivalent form containing all three serotypes. The rationale is that in the trivalent vaccine the different serotypes compete so that the most relevant serotype may not infect and immunize, whereas a monovalent type 1 vaccine used in an area where this is the problem serotype will be effective. There is evidence that this gives faster immune responses, and it was first used in Egypt where it eradicated the final type 1 strains. Monovalent vaccines are becoming the major tool in the current stages of eradication.

While there are few countries in which poliomyelitis has not been eradicated, many countries have suffered reintroductions. This is shown in **Figure 2**, which shows cases of the regions where polio has not been completely eliminated.

The first examples of this phenomenon were in central Africa. A decision was taken because of shortage of funds to concentrate immunization efforts on Nigeria which had many cases (**Figure 2(a)**). Thus immunization in the surrounding countries suffered, and at the same time resistance to immunization grew in northern Nigeria because of local concerns about supposed contaminants in the vaccine. During the period when immunization ceased, there was a resurgence in polio in Nigeria, which spread to adjacent countries where the immunization activities had been reduced (**Figure 2(b)**). As a result, polio spread from Nigeria across much of central Africa, being brought under control eventually by coordinated NIDs across most of the continent, an operation of un-

precedented scale. Shortly after this, with polio still endemic in Nigeria, the annual pilgrimage to Mecca resulted in the introduction of polio from northern Nigeria into Yemen and Indonesia (**Figure 2(c)**). In 2006, polio got introduced into several African countries from northern India (**Figure 2(d)**).

The difficulties of eradication are hard to overestimate, and are compounded by the fact that most infections are entirely silent. It is clear that so long as one country remains a source of the virus the world remains at risk. This complicates the strategies to be followed once there is some confidence that the virus has in fact been eradicated in the wild, which are further complicated by the fact that OPV is a live vaccine derived from wild-type virus that is able to change in the infected vaccinee, from whom virus may be isolated for significant periods.

Vaccine-Derived Poliovirus

Vaccine-associated paralytic poliomyelitis (VAPP) cases were recognized from the first use of the Sabin vaccine strains, although their unambiguous identification required the molecular methods applied in the 1980s. They occur in primary vaccinees at a rate of about 1 per 750 000 but can also occur in contacts and those previously vaccinated. The occurrence of such cases, while rare, indicates that the vaccine strains can revert to virulence in recipients and that it is possible for the vaccine strains to spread from person to person.

In 2001, it was recognized for the first time that the Sabin vaccine strains could be the cause of outbreaks of poliomyelitis when about 22 cases were identified in Hispaniola, comprising Haiti and the Dominican Republic. Sequencing of the strains showed that they were very closely related to the type 1 Sabin vaccine strains and not to the previous endemic strains of which the last had been isolated 20 years earlier. Moreover, the sequence diversity indicated that the outbreak strains had been circulating unnoticed for c. 2 years, as they differed from the vaccine strain by about 2% overall. In addition, they were shown to be recombinant strains with a major portion of the nonstructural regions of the genome from viruses identified as species C enteroviruses unrelated to the vaccine strains. At least three different genomic structures were identified. Subsequently, it was reported that between 1988 and 1993 all supposed wild type 2 strains isolated from poliomyelitis cases in Egypt were in fact heavily drifted vaccine-related strains. Outbreaks in the Phillipines in 2001, two in Madagascar in 2002 and 2005, one in China in 2004, and one in Indonesia in 2005 have since been recorded. The most likely explanation is that vaccination programs become less vigorous once polio is eliminated from a country and other health issues take priority, so that while administration of OPV continues, coverage is less than 100% giving perfect conditions for the selection of transmissible strains. For reasons that are not understood, all such strains to date have been recombinants with unidentified species C enteroviruses. So far the outbreaks have been limited and easy to control; this was particularly shown in Indonesia where a type 1 outbreak from a virus introduced from Nigeria occurred at the same time as an outbreak of circulating vaccine-derived poliovirus (CVDPV). The wild-type outbreak persisted longer.

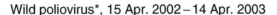

Wild poliovirus*, 15 Apr. 2002 – 14 Apr. 2003

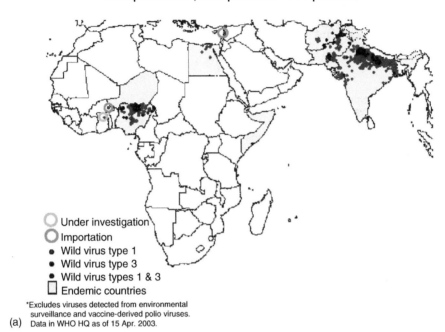

○ Under investigation
○ Importation
● Wild virus type 1
● Wild virus type 3
● Wild virus types 1 & 3
☐ Endemic countries

*Excludes viruses detected from environmental surveillance and vaccine-derived polio viruses.
(a)   Data in WHO HQ as of 15 Apr. 2003.

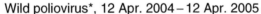

Wild poliovirus*, 12 Apr. 2004 – 12 Apr. 2005

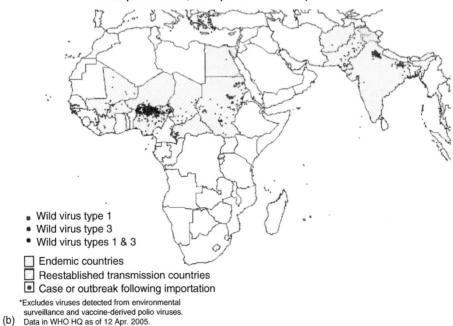

● Wild virus type 1
● Wild virus type 3
● Wild virus types 1 & 3

☐ Endemic countries
☐ Reestablished transmission countries
☐ Case or outbreak following importation

*Excludes viruses detected from environmental surveillance and vaccine-derived polio viruses.
(b)   Data in WHO HQ as of 12 Apr. 2005.

Figure 2   Continued

Wild poliovirus*, 25 Jan. 2005–24 Jan. 2006

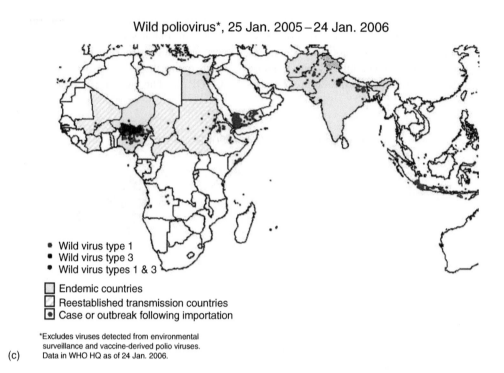

- Wild virus type 1
- Wild virus type 3
- Wild virus types 1 & 3

☐ Endemic countries
☐ Reestablished transmission countries
☑ Case or outbreak following importation

*Excludes viruses detected from environmental
surveillance and vaccine-derived polio viruses.
(c)   Data in WHO HQ as of 24 Jan. 2006.

Wild poliovirus*, 30 Aug. 2005–29 Aug. 2006

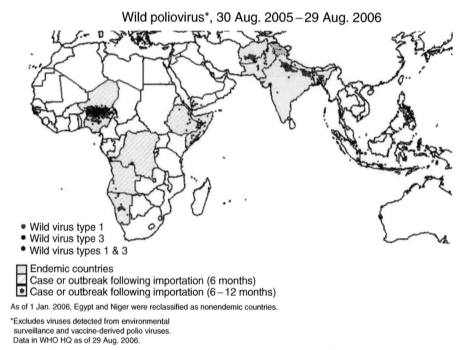

- Wild virus type 1
- Wild virus type 3
- Wild virus types 1 & 3

☐ Endemic countries
☐ Case or outbreak following importation (6 months)
☑ Case or outbreak following importation (6–12 months)

As of 1 Jan. 2006, Egypt and Niger were reclassified as nonendemic countries.

*Excludes viruses detected from environmental
surveillance and vaccine-derived polio viruses.
(d)   Data in WHO HQ as of 29 Aug. 2006.

Figure 2   Occurrence of cases of poliomyelitis in remaining areas of infection from 2002 to 2006. Source: World Health Organization (WHO).

Virologically, there is no real reason why vaccine-derived viruses should not become as aggressive as wild-type viruses from which they derived, although this does not seem to have happened at the time of writing. The occurrence of such viruses is clearly a problem when cessation of vaccination is considered.

A second issue is the occasional case of long-term excretion of polioviruses by individuals deficient in humoral immunity. The viruses are termed immunodeficient vaccine-derived polioviruses (IVDPVs). Probably only a few percent of these hypogammaglobulinemic individuals will become long-term excreters of virus even if given OPV, and most stop shedding virus spontaneously after a period, which may be 2 or 3 years. Occasionally virus excretion may continue for much longer; in one instance isolates, were available for 12 years, and the sequence data and medical history of the patient suggest that virus has been shed for well over 20 years. The patient remains entirely healthy, although the virus is highly virulent in animal models. No treatment has been successfully applied to such individuals, although there are claims for success with an antiviral compound in one case. It is of interest that the mechanism by which virus is cleared is still not known. An infected individual can be expected to excrete virus for over 4 weeks and will continue to do so after an immune response is detectable. Immune-deficient patients can stop excreting virus spontaneously with no evidence of an immune response and while termination of excretion correlates in general with a rise in fecal IgA levels, this is neither necessary nor sufficient.

Cessation of Vaccination

OPV is the major tool of the eradication efforts that have been so successful in most of the world. While the remaining pockets of infection seem to be particularly intransigent, it is likely that polio can be eradicated possibly serotype by serotype by the increasing usage of monovalent OPV. In fact, the last known wild type 2 virus was isolated in October 1999, proving that eradication is possible in principle. This leads to the need to stop vaccinating while ensuring that the disease does not re-emerge. So far as CVDPVs are concerned the safest strategy might be to stop vaccinating abruptly after one last mass immunization, so that OPV is not continuously dripped into a population with overall declining immunity. The assumption would be that the virus dies out before susceptibles build up to a sufficient extent to maintain circulation. The strategy would require careful monitoring to ensure that the virus was not returning. IVDPVs are more difficult in that there is no known treatment and the only strategy currently may be to ensure that the populations around the cases have a high level of immunity, which clearly cannot involve the administration of OPV as this would risk starting the cycle all over again.

It is therefore likely that IPV will play a bigger role as time goes by, and many developed countries have already switched to its use, including the USA, Canada, and most of western Europe. IPV is both more expensive and difficult to administer than OPV and currently cannot be easily given in mass campaigns. It tends to be used in countries with higher incomes. However, it is possible that IPV could be combined with other vaccines such as diphtheria and tetanus for use in developing countries.

A remaining problem is that the production of IPV at present involves the growth of very large amounts of wild-type poliovirus. There have been at least two instances of virus escaping from such production facilities, although this may be less likely now that the issue has been recognized and containment at the major production sites greatly improved as a result. IPV production still poses a risk and if IPV were to be the only vaccine against polio production would probably have to increase in scale. Possibilities such as the use of the Sabin vaccine strains to make IPV are being examined as a possibly safer option, but raise complex issues of immunogenicity and yield as well as logistic concerns to do with the clinical trials of novel vaccine formulations which may be necessary.

The most likely current scenario for stopping vaccination seems to be that well-off countries and the better-off in developing countries will continue be immunized, but with IPV rather than OPV, while vaccination for the remainder will simply cease after a major last mass campaign.

See also: Smallpox and Monkeypox Viruses.

Further Reading

Bodian D (1955) Emerging concept of poliomyelitis infection. *Science* 122: 105–108.

Fine PE and Carneiro IA (1999) Transmissibility and persistence of oral polio vaccine viruses: Implications for the global poliomyelitis eradication initiative. *American Journal of Epidemiology* 150: 1001–1021.

Hammon WD, Coriell LL, Wehrle PF, *et al.* (1953) Evaluation of Red Cross gammaglobulin as a prophylactic agent for poliomyelitis. Part 4: Final report of results based on clinical diagnosis. *JAMA* 151: 1272–1285.

Kew O, Morris-Glasgow V, Landarverde M, *et al.* (2002) Outbreak of poliomyelitis in Hispaniola associated with circulating type 1 vaccine-derived poliovirus. *Science* 296: 356–359.

Minor PD (1992) The molecular biology of poliovaccines. *Journal of General Virology* 73: 3065–3077.

Minor PD (1997) Poliovirus. In: Nathanson N, Ahmed R, Gonzalez-Scarano F, *et al.* (eds.) *Viral Pathogenesis*, pp, 555–574. Philadelphia: Lippincott-Raven Publishers.

Minor PD, John A, Ferguson M, and Icenogle JP (1986) Antigenic and molecular evolution of the vaccine strain of type 3 poliovirus during the period of excretion by a primary vaccinee. *Journal of General Virology* 67: 693–706.

Nkowane BU, Wassilak SG, and Orenstein WA (1987) Vaccine associated paralytic poliomyelitis in the United States: 1973 through 1984. *JAMA* 257: 1335–1340.

Paul JR (1971) *A History of Poliomyelitis.* New Haven, CT: Yale University Press.

Sabin AB (1956) Pathogenesis of poliomyelitis: Reappraisal in the light of new data. *Science* 123: 1151–1157.

Sabin AB, Ramos-Alvarez M, Alvarez-Amesquita J, *et al.* (1960) Live orally given poliovirus vaccine: Effects of rapid mass immunization on population under conditions of massive enteric infection with other viruses. *JAMA* 173: 1521–1526.

Relevant Website

http://www.polioeradication.org – The Global Polio Eradication Initiative.

Polyomaviruses

M Gravell and E O Major, National Institutes of Health, Bethesda, MD, USA

Classification

Prior to the Seventh Report of the International Committee on Taxonomy of Viruses, polyomaviruses and papillomaviruses were classified in the family *Papovaviridae*. Commensurate with the release of this report, the genus *Polyomavirus* was removed from this family and elevated to independent status as the family *Polyomaviridae*. Capsid and genome size differences between polyomaviruses and papovaviruses were instrumental in prompting this change. Polyomavirus capsids are 40–45 nm in diameter and their genomes contain about 5000 bp, whereas papillomavirus capsids are 50–55 nm in diameter and their genomes contain 6800–8400 bp. Major differences in the replication cycles of polyomaviruses and papillomaviruses have also been described. The family *Polyomaviridae* currently comprises 13 members: four from monkeys, three from humans, two from mice, and one each from bird, hamster, rabbit, and cow. One virus, athymic rat polyomavirus, has been tentatively assigned to the family.

Morphological, Physicochemical, and Physical Properties

Members of the family *Polyomaviridae* have similar virion structures and the same general genome organization. Virions of polyomaviruses are nonenveloped, icosahedral particles composed of 360 copies of the major structural protein, VP1, and 30–60 copies of the minor structural proteins, VP2 and VP3. These molecules form 72 pentameric capsomers arranged in a skewed ($T = 7$d) lattice. Each capsomer is composed of five copies of VP1 and one copy of VP2 or VP3, each added to the internal cavity formed by association of the 5 VP1 molecules. The C-terminal ends of VP1 molecules extend to anchor neighboring capsomeres together. The VP2 and VP3 molecules are present within, but are not covalently linked to, the virion. In the course of virion assembly, occasional mistakes sometimes occur and aberrant capsid structures (such as empty particles, microcapsids, and tubular structures) are made.

Being nonenveloped, polyomaviruses are ether and acid resistant and relatively heat stable (50 °C, 1 h). However, they are unstable in 1 M $MgCl_2$. Virions have a sedimentation coefficient ($S20_w$) of 240S and an M_r of 2.5×10^7 Da. The buoyant densities of polyomaviruses are 1.2 and 1.34–1.35 g ml^{-1} in sucrose and CsCl gradients, respectively.

When the VP1 DNA sequence of the human polyomaviruses JC virus (JCV) or BK virus (BKV) is inserted into a baculovirus plasmid vector and expressed in insect cells as a recombinant gene, pentamers form resembling virion capsomeres. When these pentameric capsomere-like structures are purified and placed in a solution of physiological pH and ionic strength containing Ca^{2+} ions, directed self-assembly of pentamers into genome-free virions occurs. The capsids formed, which are called virion-like particles (VLPs), have the size, icosahedral symmetry and antigenicity of native virions. Practical use has been made of VLP production. JCV or BKV VLPs have been used in enzyme immunoassays (EIA) to measure titers of JCV- or BKV-specific antibodies elicited by infection with these viruses. Because of the greater sensitivity, specificity, and safety of these genome-free VLPs, their use in EIAs has now largely replaced hemagglutination assays as the preferred method to measure levels of JCV- or BKV-specific antibodies.

Genome

The genome in each polyomavirion contains a single, supercoiled molecule of closed circular, double-stranded DNA of about 5000 bp. It makes up about 10–13% by weight of the virion, the remainder being protein. The genome is composed of three functional regions: the genetically conserved early and late coding regions separated by the hypervariable regulatory region that contains the origin of DNA replication (ORI). Host cell histone proteins H2a, H2b, H3, and H4 associate with the supercoiled genome to form a mini-chromosome-like structure. Polyomavirus DNA synthesis occurs exclusively within the S-phase of the cell cycle. However, although cellular DNA replicates only once during each cellular S-phase, multiple cycles of viral genome replication can occur.

Proteins

Proteins produced during the course of polyomavirus replication are divided into those produced during the early and late stages of infection. The early proteins are nonstructural, and are called the large T and small t proteins (or antigens) based on their sizes; T (in either case) is derived from the word tumor. These T proteins are considered the master regulators because they stimulate cells to produce the enzymes and other factors required for cellular DNA replication, thereby setting up the conditions required for late events during viral DNA replication and virion assembly. The T proteins interfere with aspects of cell cycle regulation and cause cell transformation and sometimes tumorigenesis. They are translated from 2 to 5 mRNAs generated by alternative splicing from a common pre-mRNA.

The T protein genes are transcribed from one of the genomic DNA strands in the counterclockwise direction, and the late genes are transcribed in a clockwise direction from the other genomic strand from the opposite side of ORI. Polyomavirus replication occurs exclusively within the cellular S-phase. Binding of T protein to the hypophosphorylated retinoblastoma susceptibility protein (pRb) permits premature release of the E2F transcription factor, thus stimulating cell entry into S-phase. After recruitment of the host cell DNA polymerase complex to ORI, bidirectional replication is initiated. Activation of the late viral promoter by T protein and association with specific cellular transcription factors results in expression of late virus genes. These include the genes for the virion structural proteins, VP1, VP2, and VP3 and the nonstructural regulatory agnoprotein.

The three structural capsid proteins (VP1, VP2, and VP3) originate from a common precursor mRNA by alternative splicing. The VP2 precursor mRNA contains the coding sequence for the complete VP3 protein, and each protein is translated by virtue of different start codons in the same mRNA. More than 70% of the polyomavirus capsid protein is composed of VP1, the major structural protein. For the polyomaviruses simian virus 40 (SV40), mouse polyomavirus (mPyV), and JCV, the minor capsid proteins (VP2 and VP3) have been reported to be required for proper import of virion proteins to specific nuclear localization sites for assembly. VP2 and VP3 share an identical C-terminal sequence that contains the DNA-binding domain and the VP1-interacting domain. Disulfide bonds and calcium ions are required for maintenance of structural stability of virion capsids. Virion assembly occurs exclusively in the nucleus and has been linked to the presence of a higher calcium ion concentration in the nucleus than in the cytoplasm.

The nonstructural agnoprotein functions in the life cycle of polyomaviruses in several ways. In JCV replication, it has been implicated in regulating transcription and maturation. It has also been shown to interact functionally with YB-1, a cellular transcription factor, and to regulate JCV gene transcription negatively. More recently, it was reported to participate in JCV cell transformation by interfering with the ability of a DNA-dependent protein kinase repair complex, composed of a 470 kDa catalytic subunit and a K70/K80 heterodimer regulatory subunit, to repair breaks in double-stranded cellular DNA, thus inhibiting its role in cellular DNA repair.

Replication Cycle

Nuclear Entry

Major advances have been made in recent years in understanding mechanisms that polyomaviruses use to attach and penetrate cells in order to gain entry into the cytoplasm. All events, both early and late, required for polyomavirus replication occur in the nucleus. Although many steps in this process are now understood, the question of how, where, and in what state the virus minichromosome traverses the nuclear membrane is not fully understood. Intact polyomavirions have been seen inside the nucleus by electron microscopy prior to expression of T proteins, suggesting that the virions that initiate infection enter the nucleus in an undegraded state and are uncoated therein. However, partially uncoated virions have also been seen in the cytoplasm. Whether these partially uncoated intermediates are the entities that initiate virus DNA replication and virion assembly in the nucleus is uncertain. The site of entry and mechanism of virion entry into the nucleus is also not clearly defined. Virions in cytoplasmic vesicles and their fusion with the nuclear membrane have been observed, but whether this is the mechanism of virus genome entry into the nucleus is not clear. Two sites that have been implicated in virion entry into the nucleus are the endoplasmic reticulum and the nuclear pore complex.

Evidence that BKV enters the nucleus via passage through the endoplasmic reticulum follows. To enter the cytoplasm, BKV employs a caveolae-mediated endocytic pathway, which is generally slower than clathrin-mediated endocytosis. It is generally thought that cellular microtubules are involved in the shuttling of newly formed endocytic vesicles to various intracellular locations. Treatment of Vero cells with nocodazole does not prevent the endocytic uptake of BKV into the cytoplasm, but it does cause disassembly of the cellular microtubule network and inhibits movement of endocytic vesicles. BKV replication is inhibited if added to nocodazole-treated cells during the first 8 h of infection, which is the time period generally required for BKV to traverse the cytoplasm to the nucleus where replication begins. Microtubule disassembly prevents directional movement of endocytic vesicles, stopping them from passing through the endoplasmic reticulum to reach the Golgi. Treatment of LNCaP cells with brefeldin A, which blocks transport from the endoplasmic reticulum to the Golgi apparatus, prevents BKV infection of these cells. These results were interpreted to suggest that the route BKV uses for nuclear entry is via the endoplasmic reticulum.

Receptors and Modes of Cytoplasmic Entry

Polyomavirus entry into the cytoplasm has been studied in the greatest detail for mPyV, SV40, JCV, and BKV.

The mechanisms of attachment and penetration are described below.

mPyV

This virus was the first polyomavirus for which sialic acids were implicated as an attachment receptor. The receptor studies were initiated in response to finding plaque size variants that produced small or large plaques. Upon sequencing the genomes of these size variants, it was found that the size differences in plaques resulted from a single amino acid change at VP1 position 92, in which glutamic acid was changed to glycine. Studies yielded evidence that the differences between small and large plaques originated from the capability of virus to bind to sialic acids. The small plaque isolates bound well to the straight chain α(2–3)-linked sialic acids and the branched moieties containing both α(2–3)- and α(2–6)-linked sialic acids. In contrast, the large plaque variant bound well to only the straight chain α(2–3)-linked structure and poorly to the branched structure. The single amino acid change from glutamic acid to glycine was shown to occur in a site responsible for mPyV hemagglutination of erythrocytes and receptor-binding to permissive cells. Because of this single amino acid change, the small plaque variant gained a receptor attachment advantage over the large plaque variant that translated to production of higher titers of infectious virus and virus having a higher cell transformation efficiency. These results illustrated that even a single amino acid change in a receptor site could produce major changes in virus yield and virulence.

Subsequent to implicating sialic acids as an attachment receptor for mPyV, the protein component of the receptor was found to be α4β1 integrin. Endocytosis of mPyV has been shown to occur by either of two mechanisms: (1) by caveolae-mediated endocytosis, or (2) by an alternative clathrin, caveolin-1, dynamin-1 pathway. The target cell influences the pathway chosen. Recent evidence also has implicated gangliosides as a receptor for mPyV infection. Treatment with ganglioside GD1 of mouse cells lacking a functional receptor for permissive mPyV infection imparted susceptibility to infection to these cells.

SV40

Of the four polyomaviruses described herein, all except SV40 utilize a sialic acid component as receptor. By comparing the crystal structure of the SV40 capsid with that of mPyV, it was shown that the inability of SV40 to bind to sialic acid resided in truncation of an eight amino acid residue segment of an external loop on the capsid essential for binding to sialic acid.

The receptor by which SV40 initiates infection was found to be major histocompatability complex (MHC) class I molecules. Although these molecules mediate binding to cells, they neither envelop virions nor enter cells during the infectious process. Evidence suggests that after SV40 binds to MHC class I molecules, it sends an intracellular signal that facilitates its entry into cells by caveolae-mediated endocytosis. As with mPyV, gangliosides have been implicated as a receptor for SV40 attachment and cellular entry. GM1 gangliosides are important in initiating SV40 infection.

JCV

Evidence that sialic acid is a receptor for JCV attachment came from initial studies showing that treatment of red blood cells (RBCs) and permissive glial cells with crude neurominodase abrogated hemagglutination of RBCs and infection of permissive glial cells. However, treatment of these cell types with an α(2–3)-specific neuraminidase did not cause inhibition, providing evidence that sialic acid might be a receptor, but not the α(2–3)-linked sialic acid moiety. Results defining the specific sialic acid receptor came from several additional experiments. Binding of high concentrations of JCV to permissive glial cells was shown to block binding of the α(2–6)-linked straight chain specific lectin, *Sambucus nigra* lectin (SNA). Use of specific O-linked and N-linked glycosylation inhibitors further showed that the JCV-specific receptor was an N-linked glycoprotein with a terminal α(2–6)-linked sialic acid.

Chlorpromazine and the related compound clozapine both block clathrin-dependent endocytosis, and also JCV infection. These drugs belong to a class known as serotonin-dopamine inhibitors. Glial cells susceptible to JCV infection coexpress receptors for both serotonin and dopamine. To identify whether serotonin or dopamine is the receptor component required for JCV infection, glial cells permissive to JCV infection were treated with the dopamine antagonists bromocriptine and miniprine, and a dopamine agonist, pergolide. These agents did not block JCV infection and had only minimal influence on serotonin receptors. In contrast, treatment of glial cells with metoclopramide, chlorpromazine, or clozapine, all of which are antagonists of the $5HT_{2A}$ serotoninergic receptor, significantly inhibited JCV infection. Furthermore, monoclonal antibodies specific to $5HT_{2A}$ and $5HT_{2C}$ receptors inhibited JCV infection of glial cells, but monoclonal antibodies to the dopamine receptor did not. The specificity of these antibodies to JCV infection was further illustrated by their failure to inhibit SV40 replication in treated glial cells. This is as expected, since SV40 and JCV utilize different receptors for cell attachment and enter cells by different endocytic pathways.

HeLa cells are mostly refactory to JCV infection, but because they contain the N-terminal α(2–6)-linked sialic acid receptor component on their surface, they bind JCV as well as permissive cells. When transfected with JCV genomic DNA, HeLa cells acquire the capacity to support JCV early gene expression. However, stable or transient transfection of HeLa cells with a $5HT_{2A}$ receptor-containing construct reversed their susceptibility to JCV infection. This illustrates the necessity of having both receptor components, N-terminal α(2–6)-linked sialic acid and a 5HT$_{2A}$ protein serotonergic component present on cells for susceptibility to JCV infection. Other than establishing the requirement for both cellular receptors, the mechanism by which 5HT$_{2A}$ transfection into HeLa cell alters their susceptibility to JCV infection has not been explained.

After entry into the cell interior, polyomaviruses must enter the nucleus for replication and assembly. For nuclear entry, components of the cellular cytoskeleton have been shown to be important in intracellular movement of virus through the cell cytoplasm, as described above. After virion entry into the cell interior, an intact microtubule network has been reported to be important in the early phase of JCV infection. Furthermore, SVG cells (an astroglial cell line highly susceptible to JCV infection) was shown to require an intact actin cytoskeleton to maintain its susceptibility to JCV infection. It has been suggested that the actin cytoskeleton system does not participate directly in viral movement through the cytoplasm, but may be important in assembling the clathrin machinery necessary for JCV endocytosis. Participation of intermediate filaments is also required for permissive JCV infection of cells.

The etiological link between JCV and progressive multifocal leukoencephalopathy (PML) and the high concentrations of gangliosides in the human brain make them attractive candidates as JCV receptors. The sialic acids of glycoproteins and glycol lipids have been shown to bind to JCV VLPs at their VP1-binding sites. Pretreatment of JCV virions with the ganglioside GT1b also inhibited their ability to infect susceptible glial cells. This evidence was used to infer that GT1b ganglioside bound to JCV VP1 receptor sites, thereby blocking the ability of the virus to initiate infection of the highly JCV susceptible cell lines IMR-32 and SVG and suggesting that both glycoproteins and glycolipids may function as JCV receptors. JCV has been reported to have specificity for N-terminal α(2–6) sialic acids of glycoproteins in order to initiate infection, and has also been reported to bind JCV VLPs at various α(2–3) and α(2–6) structures. These results suggest that both glycoproteins and glycolipids may function as JCV receptors. The question of whether glycolipids are involved in JCV infection of the brain has not been resolved.

BKV

The role of sialic acids as a receptor for BKV entry was reported recently. The cellular receptor that BKV uses to initiate infection is a glycoprotein with an N-linked α(2–3) sialic acid. This was demonstrated by treatment of Vero cells with sialidase S, an enzyme that specifically removes α(2–3)-linked sialic acid from glycoproteins and complex carbohydrates. Reconstitution of the asialo Vero cells by α(2–3)-specific sialyltransferase restored susceptibility of these cells to infection by BKV, but restoration by an α(2–6)-specific sialyltransferase did not. Evidence that the sialic acid was N-linked was obtained by showing that treatment with tunicamycin, an inhibitor of N-linked glycosylation, reduced BKV infection, whereas treatment with the O-linked glycosylation inhibitor benzylGalNac did not.

The protein component of the BKV receptor has not been determined. However, gangliosides have been implicated in binding to BKV and altering cell susceptiblity to BKV infection. BKV binding to erythrocyte membranes has been investigated by use of sucrose flotation assays. It was shown that binding was to a neuraminidase-sensitive, proteinase K-resistant molecule. It was suggested that the terminal α(2–8)-linked disialic acid motif, present on both GT1b and GD1b gangliosides, was responsible for inhibiting BKV binding to erythrocyte membranes. Furthermore, it was shown that LNCaP cells, which are normally resistant to BKV infection, became susceptible to BKV infection after treatment with gangliosides GT1b and GD1b. Also, it has been reported that recoating cells stripped of sialic acid and galactose with a mixture of all gangliosides derived from Vero cells restored their capacity to be infected by BKV. These results suggest that gangliosides have a role as receptors in BKV attachment and infection. The mechanisms that gangliosides employ in reversing cell susceptibility to BKV infection have not been determined.

In addition to glycolipids, the phospholipid bilayer has also been implicated in BKV hemagglutination and infection. Pre-incubating BKV with phospholipids decreases its ability to infect Vero cells, presumably because BKV binds to the exogenously added lipid, thus blocking its receptor sites from interacting with the host cell. Treating cells with either phospholipase A2 or D cleaves fatty acids, and reduces their permisssiveness to BKV infection and their ability to hemagglutinate RBCs. These parameters can be restored to the native state by adding back various preparations of phospholipids, such as L-α phosphatidylcholine and phospholipids derived from Vero cells. Hemagglutination titers of RBCs treated with phospholipase C are elevated compared to those of untreated controls, although the reason for these results is not completely understood. They point out that gangliosides are important to BKV hemagglutination and infection. Adding various gangliosides to cells has been shown to alter their susceptibility to BKV infection. Currently, four subtypes of BKV have been identified, although no clear-cut link has been established between any of these subtypes and increased BKV virulence. The receptor for BKV attachment has been linked to a region of VP1 between amino acid residues 61 and 83. This sequence aligns with a hydrophilic region that aligns with the the BC loop of the SV40 capsid. It has not been determined whether all of the BKV subtypes share the same amino acid receptor sequence for cellular attachment. As previously explained for mPyV, a single amino acid change in its receptor sequence translated to altered plaque size, hemagglutination activity, virus output, and virulence.

Host Cell Susceptibility

Although the human polyomaviruses JCV and BKV share about 75% DNA sequence homology, they differ widely in many biological properties, including host cell range, cellular receptors, cell entry mechanisms, tissue tropisms, and disease manifestations. A defining feature of these polyomaviruses is the hypervariability of their non-coding regulatory regions. The makeup of these regions affects levels of transcription and influences host cell range and tissue tropism. For an in-depth discussion of JCV variants, based on the nucleotide sequences of their noncoding region, refer to the work by Jensen and Major listed in the 'Further reading' section. The notion that polyomavirus replication is controlled at the intracellular, molecular level came from the similarity in results obtained for host cell susceptibility and virus output when native virions or transfected genomic DNA were used to infect various cell types. Results supporting this conclusion are presented below.

A family of DNA-binding proteins called NF-1, composed of four subtypes called A, B, C, and D (or X) has been linked with site-coding specific transcription of viral genes and JCV replication. Elevated levels of NF-1 class X (NF-1X) mRNA were expressed by brain glial cells that are highly susceptible to JCV infection, but not by nonsusceptible HeLa cells. $CD34^+$ precursor cells of the KG-1 line, when treated with phorbol ester 12-myristate 13-acetate (PMA), differentiated to cells with macrophage-like characteristics and lost susceptibility to JCV infection. To determine whether loss of JCV susceptibility in these cells was linked to reduced levels of NF-1X expression, reverse transcription-polymerase chain reaction (RT-PCR) was used to evaluate levels of mRNA of each of the four NF-1 subtypes found in PMA-treated KG-1 cells. Different levels of specific subtypes of mRNA were observed in the PMA-treated macrophage-like cultures compared with controls. Northern blot hybridization confirmed that the levels of NF-1X expressed by PMA-treated KG-1 cells were lower than those produced by untreated KG-1 cells. Use of gel mobility shift assays later confirmed this finding by showing the induction of specific NF-1-DNA complexes in KG-1 cells undergoing PMA treatment. These results suggested that the binding pattern of NF-1 class members may change in hematopoietic precursor cells, such as KG-1, as they undergo differentiation to macrophage-like cells. Transfection of PMA-treated KG-1 cells with an NF-1X expression vector restored their susceptibility to JCV infection. Transfection of PMA-treated KG-1 cells with NF-1 subtypes A, B, and C vectors failed to restore JCV susceptibility. These data collectively show the importance of NF-1X expression for JCV replication.

The importance of NF-1X expression for JCV replication has also been shown in multipotential human nervous system progenitor cells. By use of selective growth conditions, these progenitor cells were cultured from fetal brain tissue as undifferentiated, attached cell layers. Selective culture techniques yielded highly purified population of neurons or astrocytes. Infection with JCV virions or with a plasmid encoding the JCV genome demonstrated the susceptibility of astrocytes and, to a lesser degree, their undifferentiated progenitors. However, neurons remained nonpermissive for JCV replication. Expression of the NF-1X transcription factor was much higher in astrocytes than in neurons. Transfection of an NF-1X expression vector into progenitor-derived neuronal cells, prior to JCV infection, yielded JCV protein production. These results indicate that susceptibility to JC infection is regulated at the molecular level. Furthermore, they suggest that differential recognition of viral promoter sequences can predict lineage pathways of multipotential progenitor cells in the human nervous system.

Perspectives

Phylogenetic evidence indicates that polyomaviruses have evolved from a common ancestor. Despite their very similar morphological, physical, and chemical characteristics, events in the life cycle of closely related species can vary considerably. This article contains information of recent vintage on the variety of mechanisms involved in polyomavirus attachment, penetration and movement within the cell to reach the cell nucleus, where replication occurs. Our understanding of the role of sialic acid receptors in polyomavirus replication has been greatly expanded, especially those associated with glycoproteins. Recent work has also implicated various gangliosides as receptor molecules, and much new information should be available shortly on how they contribute to the infectious process.

Information is also presented on how levels of specific cellular transcription factors, such as NF-1X, can influence the infectability of specific cell types by JCV. Much new information has also been published on how the noncoding regulatory region of JCV changes from the archetype arrangement found in most urine isolates to those found in other tissues, such as lymphocytes, tonsils, and in brains of individuals with PML. Modifications to this promoter/enhancer structure can alter cellular host range and may be responsible for switching infection from the latent to lytic states. The importance of immunosuppression in JCV- or BKV-caused disease, and the predominant role of cellular immunity in their prevention, have been firmly established.

The tumorigenicity of JCV and BKV for animals has been widely known for many years. Their nucleic acids have been detected in tumor and surrounding tissue by sensitive PCR techniques. Also, polyomavirus T proteins that impair the cell-cycle regulatory functions of p53 and pRb have been detected by sensitive immunochemical techniques in human colon, gastric, brain, and pancreatic tumors. JCV and BKV persistently infect a high percentage of the human population worldwide. The range of cell types infectable by JCV or BKV has also increased in recent years, establishing the possibility that tumor cells could become infected after tumorigenesis begins.

See also: Polyomaviruses of Humans; Simian Virus 40.

Further Reading

Cole CN and Conzen SD (2001) *Polyomaviridae*: The viruses and their replication. In: Fields BN, Knipe DM, Howley PM, *et al.* (eds.) *Fields Virology*, 4th edn., vol. 2, pp. 2141–2174. Philadelphia, PA: Lippincott Williams and Wilkins.

Eash S, Manley K, Gasparovic M, Querbes W, and Atwood WJ (2006) The human polyomaviruses. *Cellular and Molecular Life Sciences* 63: 865–876.

Gee GV, Dugan AS, Tsomaia N, Mierke DF, and Atwood WJ (2006) The role of sialic acid in human polyomavirus infections. *Glycoconjugate Journal* 23: 19–26.

Imperiale MJ and Major EO (2007) Polyomaviruses. In: Knipe DM, Howley PM, *et al.* (eds.) *Fields Virology*, 5th edn., vol. 2, pp. 2263–2298. Philadelphia, PA: Lippincott Williams and Wilkins.

Jensen PN and Major EO (2001) A classification scheme for human polyomavirus JCV variants based on the nucleotide sequence of the noncoding regulatory region. *Journal of Neurovirology* 7: 280–287.

Poxviruses

G L Smith, P Beard, and M A Skinner, Imperial College London, London, UK

Introduction

Poxviruses have been isolated from birds, insects, reptiles, marsupials, and mammals. The best known is variola virus (VARV), the cause of smallpox, an extinct disease that claimed millions of victims and influenced human history. All poxviruses have complex, enveloped virions that are large enough to be visible by the light microscope and contain double-stranded DNA (dsDNA) genomes with terminal hairpins linking the two DNA strands into a single polynucleotide chain. Poxvirus genes are transcribed by the virus-encoded RNA polymerase and associated transcriptional enzymes, which are packaged into the virion. Virus morphogenesis and entry have unique features, such as the possession of a thiol-oxidoreductase system to enable disulfide bond formation and morphogenesis in the cytoplasm, and a complex of several proteins for the fusion of infecting virions with the cell membrane. The large genome enables poxviruses to encode many virulence factors that are nonessential for virus replication in cell culture but which influence the outcome of infection *in vivo*. Diseases caused by poxviruses range from mild infections to devastating plagues, such as smallpox in man, mousepox in the laboratory mouse, and myxomatosis in the European rabbit.

Classification

The family *Poxviridae* comprises two subfamilies, the *Entomopoxvirinae* (**Table 1**) and *Chordopoxvirinae* (**Table 2**), whose members infect insects and chordates, respectively. The subfamily *Entomopoxvirinae* is divided into three genera: *Alphaentomopoxvirus*, *Betaentomopoxvirus*, and *Gammaentomopoxvirus*, which are typified by the species *Melolontha melolontha entomopoxvirus* (the virus name is abbreviated to MMEV), *Amsacta moorei entomopoxvirus 'L'* (AMEV), and *Chironomus luridus entomopoxvirus* (CLEV), respectively (**Table 1**). Alphaentomopoxviruses infect beetles (Coleoptera), betaentomopoxviruses infect butterflies and moths (Lepidoptera), and gammaentomopoxviruses infect mosquitoes and flies (Diptera). Compared to the *Chordopoxvirinae*, relatively few data are available for entomoxpoviruses and only two genomes have been sequenced. Nonetheless, these sequences revealed considerable divergence such that, although both sequenced viruses had originally been assigned to the same genus, *Melanoplus sanguinipes entomopoxvirus* (MSEV) was subsequently removed from this genus and the virus is now an unassigned member of the subfamily. Many features of the replication of entomopoxviruses are likely to be similar to those of chordopoxviruses, as exemplified by the orthopoxvirus *Vaccinia virus* (VACV). However, the morphology of entomopoxviruses differs from that of chordopoxviruses and there are also differences between the three entomopoxvirus genera (see below).

The subfamily *Chordopoxvirinae* is divided into eight genera: *Avipoxvirus*, *Capripoxvirus*, *Leporipoxvirus*, *Orthopoxvirus*, *Parapoxvirus*, *Suipoxvirus*, *Tanapoxvirus*, and *Yatapoxvirus* (**Table 2**). There are also several unassigned poxviruses that might form additional genera once their phylogenetic relationships have been established. For instance, the genome sequences of viruses isolated from Nile crocodiles (*Crocodylus niloticus*) and mule deer (*Odocoileus hemionus*) in North America indicate that these will form additional genera. Within each genus there are distinct

Table 1   Family *Poxviridae*, subfamily *Entomopoxvirinae*

Genus	Species[a] (abbreviation of virus name)	Genome accession no.	Genome size (bp)
Alphaentomopoxvirus	*Anomala cuprea entomopoxvirus* (ACEV)		
	Aphodius tasmaniae entomopoxvirus (ATEV)		
	Demodema boranensis entomopoxvirus (DBEV)		
	Dermolepida albohirtum entomopoxvirus (DAEV)		
	Figulus subleavis entomopoxvirus (FSEV)		
	Geotrupes sylvaticus entomopoxvirus (GSEV)		
	Melolontha melolontha entomopoxvirus (MMEV)		
Betaentomopoxvirus	*Acrobasis zelleri entomopoxvirus 'L'* (AZEV)	AF250284	232392
	Amsacta moorei entomopoxvirus 'L' (AMEV)		
	Arphia conspersa entomopoxvirus 'O' (ACOEV)		
	Choristoneura biennis entomopoxvirus 'L' (CBEV)		
	Choristoneura conflicta entomopoxvirus 'L' (CCEV)		
	Choristoneura diversuma entomopoxvirus 'L' (CDEV)		
	Choristoneura fumiferana entomopoxvirus 'L' (CFEV)		
	Chorizagrotis auxiliars entomopoxvirus 'L' (CXEV)		
	Heliothis armigera entomopoxvirus 'L' (HAVE)		
	Locusta migratoria entomopoxvirus 'O' (LMEV)		
	Oedaleus senigalensis entomopoxvirus 'O' (OSEV)		
	Operophtera brumata entomopoxvirus 'L' (OBEV)		
	Schistocera gregaria entomopoxvirus 'O' (SGEV)		
Gammaentomopoxvirus	*Aedes aegypti entomopoxvirus* (AAEV)		
	Camptochironomus tentans entomopoxvirus (CTEV)		
	Chironomus attenuatus entomopoxvirus (CAEV)		
	Chironomus luridus entomopoxvirus (CLEV)		
	Chironomus plumosus entomopoxvirus (CPEV)		
	Goeldichironomus haloprasimus entomopoxvirus (GHEV)		
Unassigned species in the subfamily	*Diachasmimorpha entomopoxvirus* (DIEV)		
Unassigned virus in the subfamily	*Melanoplus sanguinipes entomopoxvirus* (MSEV)	AF063866	236120

[a]Type species shown in bold.
Data from the International Committe on Taxonomy of Viruses (ICTV) (http://www.ncbi.nlm.nih.gov/ICTVdb/Ictv/index.htm) and the Poxvirus Bioinformatics Resource Center (http://www.poxvirus.org).

species and strains thereof. At least one genome sequence is available from each genus and in some cases large numbers of viruses have been sequenced. The orthopoxviruses have been studied most extensively and the poxvirus website lists genome sequences of 48 strains of VARV, 14 strains of VACV, and 9 strains of monkeypox virus (MPXV).

Virion Structure

Poxviruses have large virions with an oval or brick-shaped morphology. The best-studied poxvirus is VACV, which has dimensions of approximately 250 nm × 350 nm. Each infected cell produces two different forms of infectious virion called intracellular mature virus (IMV) and extra-cellular enveloped virus (EEV). These two forms differ in that EEV is surrounded by an additional membrane containing several virus proteins that are absent from IMV. The EEV form can be produced either by IMV budding through the plasma membrane or by exocytosis

of a triple enveloped virus (see 'Morphogenesis', under 'Replication cycle').

The surface of the IMV particle contains surface tubules that have either an irregular appearance (in ortho-poxviruses and avipoxviruses) or a basket-weave symmetry (in orf virus (ORFV), a parapoxvirus). The structure of the VACV IMV has been studied most intensively and there are differing views. Some investigators reported that the virus is surrounded by a double lipid membrane, whereas others propose that the outer layer comprises a single membrane surrounded by a protein coat. The evidence now strongly favors the one membrane model. The virus core has a dumbbell shape and there are lateral bodies of unknown function located in the core concavities. The virus core is surrounded by a palisade of protein spikes of 18 nm and the core wall contains pores through which virus mRNAs might extrude during early transcription. The virus genome is packaged in the core together with transcriptional enzymes and capsid proteins.

Table 2   Family *Poxviridae*, subfamily *Chordopoxvirinae*

Genus	Species[a] (abbreviation of virus name)	Genome accession no.	Genome size (bp)
Avipoxvirus	Canarypox virus (CNPV)	AY318871	359853
	Fowlpox virus (FWPV)	AF198100, AJ581527	288539, 266145
	Juncopox virus (JNPV)		
	Mynahpox virus (MYPV)		
	Pigeonpox virus (PGPV)		
	Psittacinepox virus (PSPV)		
	Quailpox virus (QUPV)		
	Sparrowpox virus (SRPV)		
	Starlingpox virus (SLPV)		
	Turkeypox virus (TKPV)		
	Crowpox virus (CRPV)		
	Peacockpox virus (PKPV)		
	Penguinpox virus (PEPV)		
Capripoxvirus	Goatpox virus (GTPV)	AY077836, AY077835	149723, 149599
	Lumpy skin disease virus (LSDV)	AF325528, AF409137	150773, 150793
	Sheeppox virus (SPPV)	AY077833, AY077834, NC_004002	150057, 149662, 149955
Leporipoxvirus	Hare fibroma virus (FIBV)		
	Myxoma virus (MYXV)	AF170726	161773
	Rabbit fibroma virus (RFV)	AF170722	159857
	Squirrel fibroma virus (SQFV)		
Molluscipoxvirus	**Molluscum contagiosum virus** (MOCV)	U60315	190289
Orthopoxvirus	Camelpox virus (CMLV)	AY009089, AF438165	202205, 205719
	Cowpox virus (CPXV)	AF482758, X94355, DQ437593	224499, 223666, 228250
	Ectromelia virus (ECTV)	AF012825,	209771, 207620
	Monkeypox virus (MPXV)	AF380138, DQ011156, AY753185, DQ011157	196858, 200256, 199469, 198,780
	Raccoonpox virus (RCNV)		
	Taterapox virus (TATV)	DQ437594	198050
	Vaccinia virus (VACV)	U94848, M35027, AF095689, AY243312	177923, 191737, 189274, 194711
	Variola virus (VARV)	L22579, X69198, Y16780, DQ441447	186103, 185578, 186986, 188251
	Volepox virus (VPXV)		
	Horsepox virus (HSPV)	DQ792504	212633
	Skunkpox virus (SKPV)		
	Uasin Gishu disease virus (UGDV)		
Parapoxvirus	Bovine papular stomatitis virus (BPSV)	AY386265	134431
	Orf virus (ORFV)	AY386264, DQ184476	139962, 137,820
	Parapoxvirus of red deer in New Zealand (PVNZ)		
	Pseudocowpox virus (PCPV)		
	Squirrel parapoxvirus		
	Auzduk disease virus		
	Camel contagious ecthyma virus		
	Chamois contagious ecthyma virus		
	Sealpox virus		
Suipoxvirus	**Swinepox virus** (SWPV)	AF410153	146454
Yatapoxvirus	Tanapox virus (TANV)		
	Yaba-like disease virus (YLDV)	AJ293568	144575
	Yaba monkey tumor virus (YMTV)	AY386371	134721
Unassigned viruses in the family	Nile crocodile poxvirus (CRV)	NC_008030	190054
	Mule deer poxvirus (DPV)	AY689436, AY689437	166259, 170560
	California harbor seal poxvirus (SPV)		
	Cotia virus (CPV)		
	Dolphin poxvirus (DOPV)		

Continued

Table 2   Continued

Genus	Species[a] (abbreviation of virus name)	Genome accession no.	Genome size (bp)
	Embu virus (ERV)		
	Grey kangaroo poxvirus (KXV)		
	Marmosetpox virus (MPV)		
	Molluscum-like poxvirus (MOV)		
	Quokka poxvirus (QPV)		
	Red kangaroo poxvirus (KPV)		
	Salanga poxvirus (SGV)		
	Spectacled caiman poxvirus (SPV)		
	Yoka poxvirus (YKV)		

[a]Type species shown in bold. Virus names in normal type (not italic) are tentative or unassigned.
Data from the International Committe on Taxonomy of Viruses (ICTV) (http://www.ncbi.nlm.nih.gov/ICTVdb/Ictv/index.htm) and the Poxvirus Bioinformatics Resource Center (http://www.poxvirus.org).

The structures of entomopoxvirus virions differ from those of chordopoxviruses. Virions of alphaentomopoxviruses have dimensions of approximately 350 nm × 450 nm and have a concave core with a single lateral body. The betaentomopoxvirus virions are a little smaller at about 250 nm × 350 nm with a cylindrical core and a lateral body that has a sleeve-like appearance. The gammaentomopoxvirus virions are 320 nm × 230 nm and are more like chordopoxviruses in having a biconcave core and two lateral bodies.

The general lack of symmetry of poxvirus virions contrasts with the icosahedral capsid of another family of large dsDNA viruses, the herpesviruses. Consequently, the structure of poxviruses is presently refractory to determination by current methods such as cryoelectron microscopy reconstruction and X-ray crystallography.

Genome Structure

Poxvirus genomes are dsDNA molecules that are linked at each terminus by a hairpin loop. The genome length varies from 134.4 kbp for bovine papular stomatitis virus, a parapoxvirus, to 359.9 kbp for canarypox virus, an avipoxvirus. When deproteinized, poxvirus genomes lack infectivity because the virus DNA-dependent RNA polymerase is required for transcription of poxvirus genes. The genomes of chordopoxviruses all show the same basic arrangement. Adjacent to each terminus there is an inverted terminal repeat (ITR) so that the sequence at one end of the genome is repeated at the other end in the opposite orientation. The length of the ITR varies considerably and may be less than 1 kbp and lacking protein coding sequences (e.g., VARV) or >50 kbp and containing numerous genes that are consequently diploid (e.g., some cowpox virus (CPXV) strains). Adjacent to each hairpin there is a short conserved sequence called the concatemer resolution sequence that is required for DNA replication.

The central region (approximately 100 kbp) of chordopoxvirus genomes encodes proteins that are conserved between chordopoxviruses and (mostly) essential for virus replication. Approximately equal numbers of genes from this region are transcribed leftward and rightward. In contrast, genes within the left and right terminal regions of the genome are transcribed predominantly toward the genome termini. These genes are more variable between viruses in both their type and number, and for the most part are nonessential for virus replication. Instead, these genes encode proteins that affect virus virulence, tropism, and interactions with the host immune system. Within chordopoxviruses the gene order in the central genome region is fairly well conserved, with two exceptions. First, in the avian viruses there are inversions and transpositions of blocks of genes. Second, in both avipoxviruses and crocodilepox virus (CRV) there are groups of inserted genes that are absent from other poxvirus genomes.

The entomopoxvirus genomes contain some of the genes conserved throughout the chordopoxviruses, but differ in that these genes are scattered throughout the genome and are not arranged centrally and in the specific order found in chordopoxviruses.

The nucleotide composition of poxvirus genomes varies considerably. The two sequenced entomopoxviruses are very rich in A + T (82.2% and 81.7%). Several chordopoxviruses are also (A + T)-rich, but less so than the insect viruses. For instance, sheeppox virus (SPPV) and VACV are 75% and 67% A + T, respectively. At the other end of the spectrum, the genome of molluscum contagiosum virus (MOCV) is 36% A + T. Despite these wide variations in base composition, the encoded proteins display considerable similarity.

Gene Content

Comparisons of sequenced chordopoxviruses have identified c. 90 genes that are present in every virus. These genes encode proteins that are essential for virus replication, such as capsid proteins and enzymes for transcription and DNA replication. All of these genes are located in the central region of the genome, and are likely to represent the core genome of an ancestral virus from which modern poxviruses have evolved. As poxviruses evolved and adapted to particular hosts, they seem to have acquired additional genes that are located predominantly in the terminal regions of the genome and give each virus its particular host range and virulence. For instance, many of the immunomodulatory proteins expressed by orthopoxviruses are absent from viruses of avian and reptile hosts and also from MOCV, which has a different set of immunomodulators.

If the entomopoxviruses are included in the above comparison, the number of conserved genes falls to fewer than 50. As more poxvirus genomes are sequenced the number of genes conserved in all poxviruses (the minimal gene complement) is likely to be reduced.

Phylogeny

Phylogenetic comparisons of poxviruses indicate that the entomopoxviruses are quite divergent from chordopoxviruses, but the exact relationships of most entomopoxviruses remain unknown owing to lack of sequence data. However, for the chordopoxviruses the situation is clearer. Genome sequences are available for at least one member of each genus, and a phlyogenetic tree (**Figure 1**) shows that the genera *Yatapoxvirus, Suipoxvirus, Leporipoxvirus,* and *Capripoxvirus* and deerpox virus (DPV) cluster together. The orthopoxviruses are the nearest genus to this cluster, but have slightly larger genomes and other distinguishing features. The remaining genera, *Molluscipoxvirus, Parapoxvirus,* and *Avipoxvirus,* as well as the recently sequenced CRV are more divergent from the genera mentioned above. The avian poxviruses and CRV are most divergent and their genomes are distinguished by a lower degree of amino acid similarity, greater numbers of genes that are unique to that genus, and divergent gene order. The next most divergent genus is *Molluscipoxvirus,* which like VARV infects only humans but has very different immunomodulatory proteins compared to orthopoxviruses. Interestingly, there are some genes shared by only MOCV and CRV. Lastly, the parapoxviruses form a quite distinct genus.

Although only eight chordopoxvirus genera have been recognized so far by the International Committee for the Taxonomy of Viruses, the genomes of DPV and CRV are distinct from all other genera and so are likely to represent new genera.

Replication Cycle

Details of the poxvirus replication cycle have been obtained primarily by study of VACV and for greater

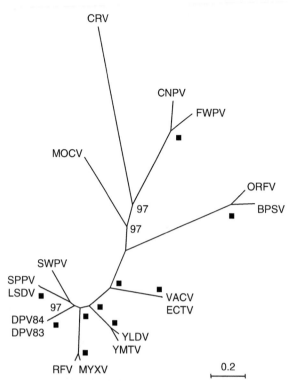

Figure 1 Phylogenetic relationships between chordopoxviruses based on a concatenated amino acid sequence alignment of 83 conserved proteins. Abbreviations: CRV, crocodilepox virus; CNPV, canarypox virus; FWPV, fowlpox virus; ORFV, orf virus; BSPV, bovine papular stomatitis virus; VACV, vaccinia virus; ECTV, ectromelia virus; YLDV, Yaba-like disease virus; YMTV, Yaba monkey tumor virus; MYXV, myxoma virus; RFV, rabbit fibroma virus; DPV, deerpox virus; LSDV, lumpy skin disease virus; SPPV, sheeppox virus; SWPV, swinepox virus; MOCV, molluscum contagiosum virus. Bootstrap values of greater than 70 are indicated at the appropriate nodes and black squares indicate values of 100. Reproduced from Afonso CL, Tulman ER, Delhon G, *et al.* (2006) Genome of crocodilepox virus. *Journal* of *Virology* 80: 4978–4991, with permission from the American Society for Microbiology.

detail the reader is referred to the article on that virus. Here only an overview is given.

Entry

VACV forms two distinct virion types (IMV and EEV), which are surrounded by different numbers of membranes. These different virions are also produced by viruses from several chordopoxvirus genera, and may be universal for poxviruses. IMV enters by fusion of its membrane with either the plasma membrane or the membrane of an intracellular vesicle following endocytosis. EEV entry is complicated by the second membrane that is shed on contact with the cell by a ligand-dependent nonfusogenic process. This places the IMV from within the EEV envelope against the plasma membrane and thereafter entry takes place as for free IMV. A remarkable feature of VACV fusion is the presence of a complex of nine proteins that are all required for fusion but not binding to the cell. In contrast, the fusion machinery of other enveloped viruses is often only a single protein. The fusion proteins of VACV are conserved in many other poxviruses, suggesting a common mechanism of entry. After a virus core has entered the cell, it is transported on microtubules deeper into the cell (see **Figure 2(d)** for an image of a virus core).

Gene Expression

Within minutes of infection the early virus genes are transcribed by the virus-associated DNA-dependent RNA polymerase within the core. The mRNAs are capped and polyadenylated, and are not spliced. They are extruded from the core and translated on host ribosomes. Early genes encode proteins that initiate DNA replication or combat the host response to infection (see 'Immune evasion' under 'Pathogenesis'). Once DNA replication has started, the intermediate class of genes is transcribed and, after expression of intermediate proteins, late transcription starts. Generally, late proteins encode structural proteins, which are expressed at higher levels than the early proteins involved in replication. Unusual features of late mRNAs are that they have a polyA tract just after the 5′ cap structure as well as at the 3′ end, and are heterogeneous in length due to a failure to terminate transcription at specific sites.

DNA Replication

DNA replication occurs in virus factories in the cytoplasm, and is catalyzed by the virus DNA polymerase and

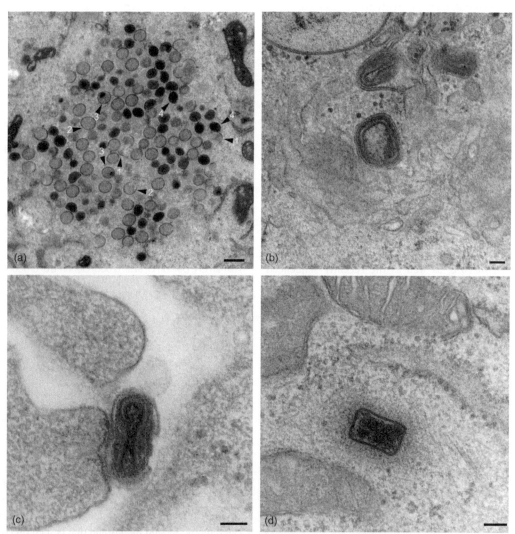

Figure 2 Electron micrographs of VACV. (a) Virus factory showing the different stages of VACV morphogenesis: (1) virus crescent; (2) immature virus, (3) immature virus showing stages of condensation and eccentric nucleoid formation, (4) IMV. (b) Wrapping of IMV to form IEV. The virion at top is partly wrapped while the virion in the center is completely wrapped. (c) CEV on the surface of an actin tail protruding from the cell surface. (d) Virus core within the cytosol shortly after infection. Scale = 500 nm (a), 100 nm (b–d). Reproduced by permission of Michael Hollinshead, Imperial College London.

associated factors. The terminal hairpins and the adjacent concatemeric resolution sequence are essential for this process. Replication starts with the introduction of a nick near a terminal hairpin, followed by unfolding of the hairpin to enable self-priming from the free 3'-hydroxyl group. After extension to the genome terminus, separation of the parental and daughter strands, and refolding, DNA replication proceeds by strand displacement to form concatemeric molecules in either head-to-head or tail-to-tail configuration. Resolution of the concatemers occurs at the concatemer resolution sequence using the activity of a resolvase. Unit-length monomers are then packaged into virions. For additional details, see the article on VACV.

Morphogenesis

Virus assembly takes place in modified areas of the cytoplasm called factories or virosomes (**Figure 2**). The first structure seen by electron microscopy is crescent shaped, and is composed of host lipid and virus protein. This grows into immature virus (IV) in which the virus genome is packaged together with transcriptional enzymes. Once the virus membrane is sealed, the core condenses, some capsid proteins are cleaved proteolytically, and an IMV is formed. IMV may be released from cells following cell lysis either as free virions or within proteinaceous bodies. The latter are produced by some orthopoxviruses (including ectromelia virus (ECTV), raccoonpox virus, and some strains of CPXV), some avipoxviruses, and entomopoxviruses. These proteinaceous bodies are thought to give the virions extra stability outside the host until taken up by a new susceptible host. Interestingly, the proteinaceous body of entomopoxviruses is disassembled by high pH (as found in the insect gut) whereas the inclusion bodies of CPXV are disaggregated by low pH.

Not all IMVs remain in the cell until cell lysis, as some are exported from the cell by two distinct pathways that each results in formation of EEV. The first pathway, exemplified by VACV, starts with transport of IMV away from factories on microtubules and the wrapping by a double layer of host membrane derived from the *trans*-Golgi network or early endosomes that has been modified by the insertion of virus proteins (**Figure 2(b)**). The wrapping process produces an intracellular enveloped virus (IEV), which contains three membranes, and this particle is transported to the cell surface on microtubules. At the cell surface, the outer membrane fuses with the plasma membrane to release a virion by exocytosis. The virion is called cell-associated enveloped virus (CEV) if it remains on the cell surface (**Figure 2 (c)**) and EEV if it is released. The majority of EEVs made by VACV are produced in this way. The second pathway, illustrated by fowlpox virus (FWPV), is the budding of an IMV through the plasma membrane to release EEV.

In addition to being released as EEV, CEV can also induce formation of long cellular projections, which are driven by polymerization of actin (**Figure 2(c)**). These are important for efficient cell-to-cell dissemination of virus, because virus mutants that are unable to induce formation of actin tails form small plaques.

Pathogenesis

Diseases caused by poxviruses vary greatly and may be associated with high mortality or cause minor, local, or asymptomatic infections. Examples of systemic diseases caused by chordopoxviruses include smallpox, monkeypox, mousepox, camelpox, sheeppox, and myxomatosis.

Smallpox was the most serious human disease caused by a poxvirus and produced a systemic infection in which VARV spread sequentially through the body, culminating in the formation of skin lesions through which the virus was released to infect new hosts. A feature of smallpox that distinguished it from chickenpox (caused by varicella-zoster virus, a herpesvirus) was the centrifugal distribution of lesions (abundant on the face and limbs but less so on the trunk). The mortality rate associated with infection of immunologically naive subjects with variola major virus was 30–40%, whereas infection with variola minor virus caused only 1–2% mortality. That VARV was such a dangerous human pathogen may never be fully understood, but VARV contains many immunomodulatory proteins that subvert the host response to infection, especially the innate immune response (see below). Comparisons of the sequences of variola major and variola minor viruses revealed many differences, such that it was not possible to deduce which change(s) was (were) responsible for the large difference in virulence.

Human monkeypox is a systemic infection that is similar to smallpox but, unlike smallpox, the infection spreads very poorly from human to human. The virulence of MPXV depends on the virus strain. Viruses isolated from central Africa (e.g., Zaire) caused up to 10% mortality, whereas those from West Africa are less virulent. For instance, the zoonotic introduction of a West African strain into the USA in 2003 infected at least 37 people but no mortalities were recorded. The genomes of MPXV and VARV are significantly different, such that it is unlikely that MPXV would mutate into a VARV-like virus with efficient human-to-human transmission.

SPPV and goatpox virus (GTPV) are two very closely related members of the genus *Capripoxvirus*, and are of considerable veterinary importance because they are responsible for severe, systemic disease in sheep and goats. The viruses are endemic in parts of Africa, Asia, and the Middle East with a propensity of spreading to neighboring areas, as revealed by recent outbreaks in Vietnam, Mongolia, and Greece. The viruses are transmitted by direct contact, environmental contamination, or biting insects, and cause the most severe disease in young animals where the mortality can reach 100%. The affected animals exhibit typical poxviral disease with discrete, circumscribed cutaneous lesions most numerous in sparsely haired areas. Lesions are also found in the lung, gasterointestinal tract, and mucous membranes.

ECTV causes mousepox in inbred mouse colonies and can have very high mortality rates. For instance, in susceptible mouse strains the lethal dose 50 (LD50) of ECTV is less than one plaque-forming unit. Some features of mousepox have similarity with smallpox and consequently it is being used by some investigators as a model for smallpox. The natural host of ECTV is uncertain but is likely to be wild rodents.

Camelpox virus (CMLV) causes a severe systemic disease in camels that also has some features resembling smallpox. Sequencing of the CMLV genome showed that VARV and CMLV are closely related, although there remain many differences, especially within the terminal regions of the virus genome, so mutation of CMLV into a VARV-like virus is unlikely.

Myxomatosis is a disease caused by myxoma virus (MYXV) in the European rabbit (*Oryctolagus cuniculus*). However, the natural host for MYXV is the jungle rabbit (*Sylviagus brasiliensis*) or brush rabbit (*S. bachmani*), in which the outcome of MYXV infection is mild. MYXV infection in the European rabbit has been used as a model for poxvirus pathogenesis. MYXV virus is also famous as the virus used in Australia in the 1950s to control the European rabbit population, which increased from 13 in 1859 to more than 500 million early in the twentieth century. The spread of MYXV in Australian rabbits is an excellent example of host–pathogen evolution: very soon after release of the highly virulent virus into the rabbit population, the virus strains isolated from infected rabbits were of more modest virulence such that they did not kill all available hosts. Likewise, surviving rabbit populations were more resistant to the effects of virus infection.

Immune Evasion

Poxviruses encode many proteins that block or subvert the host response to infection. The genes encoding these proteins are mostly located within the terminal regions of the genomes and are nonessential for virus replication in cell culture. The proteins are directed predominantly against the innate response to infection, but target a wide range of host molecules both inside and outside the cell. Poxvirus intracellular proteins may block signaling pathways resulting from engagement of Toll-like receptors or receptors for cytokines or interferons. Additionally, intracellular proteins may inhibit the antiviral activity of interferon (IFN)-induced proteins or the pathways leading to induction of apoptosis. Extracellular proteins may inhibit the action of complement, cytokines, chemokines, or IFNs by binding these proteins in solution and preventing them from reaching their natural receptors on cells. Some poxviruses also subvert the cytokine or chemokine systems by encoding cytokines (e.g., interleukin-10, transforming growth factor beta) or chemokine mimics, or by the expression of chemokine receptors on the surface of infected cells. In general, the removal of individual immunomodulatory proteins has caused modest attenuation of virulence in one model or another, but the outcome is uncertain and in some cases an increase in virulence was reported. Very often, the attenuation deriving from loss of an immunomodulatory protein is modest compared to that caused by deletion of a gene involved in virus intracellular transport or release, but there are exceptional cases where loss of an immunomodulator has caused a several log increase in the virus LD50. The wide variety of immunomodulators expressed by poxviruses makes these viruses excellent models for studying virus–host interactions and provides a logical means by which the immunogenicity of recombinant poxviruses being considered as vaccine vectors can be improved.

Acknowledgments

G. L. Smith is a Wellcome Principal Research Fellow and P. M. Beard holds a Wellcome Trust Intermediate Clinical Fellowship.

See also: Cowpox Virus; Molluscum Contagiosum Virus; Smallpox and Monkeypox Viruses.

Further Reading

Afonso CL, Tulman ER, Delhon G, *et al.* (2006) Genome of crocodilepox virus. *Journal of Virology* 80: 4978–4991.

Buller RM, Arif BM, Black DN, *et al.* (2005) *Poxviridae.* In: Fauquet CM, Mayo MA, Maniloff J, Desselberger U,, and Ball LA (eds.) *Virus Taxonomy: Eighth Report of the International Committee on Taxonomy of Viruses*, pp. 117–133. San Diego, CA: Elsevier Academic Press.

Fenner F, Henderson DA, Arita I, Jezek Z, and Ladnyi ID (1988) *Smallpox and Its Eradication.* Geneva: World Health Organization.

Fenner F, Wittek R, and Dumbell KR (1989) *The Orthopoxviruses.* London: Academic Press.

Mercer AA, Schmidt A, and Weber O (2007) *Poxviruses.* Berlin: Birkhäuser Verlag.

Moss B (2007) *Poxviridae*: The viruses and their replication. In: Knipe DM, Howley PM, Griffin DE, *et al.* (eds.) *Fields Virology,* 5th edn., pp. 2905–2946. Philadelphia, PA: Lippincott Williams and Wilkins.

Relevant Website

http://www.poxvirus.org – Poxvirus Bioinformatics Resource Center.

Rabies Virus

I V Kuzmin and C E Rupprecht, Centers for Disease Control and Prevention, Atlanta, GA, USA

Glossary

Apoptosis One of the main types of programmed cell death which involves a series of biochemical events leading to morphological changes and death.

Chiropteran Pertaining to members of the order of flying mammals commonly called 'bats'.

Gliosis Proliferation of astrocytes in damaged areas of the central nervous system.

Hematophagous The habit of certain animals of feeding on blood.

Herpestidae A vertebrate family which includes mongooses.

Meninges The system of membranes which envelope the central nervous system. The meninges consist of three layers: the dura mater, the arachnoid mater, and the pia mater.

Neuronophagia Phagocytic destruction of nerve cells.

Paraesthesia A sensation of tingling, pricking, or numbness of a person's skin with no apparent physical effect.

Introduction

Rabies is fatal encephalitis caused by rabies virus and other lyssaviruses. This important zoonosis has been known for over 4000 years, but still causes more than 50 000 human deaths annually besides enormous economic losses, primarily developing countries of Asia and Africa where dog rabies is enzootic. Once symptoms appear, the disease is almost invariably fatal. Since the first successful use of rabies vaccine by Louis Pasteur in 1885, pre-exposure and post-exposure prophylaxis have been improved significantly, and canine rabies has been eliminated from Western Europe and large parts of North America. Nevertheless, the continuing burden of the disease in other parts of the world poses requirements for further development of affordable protective biologicals and treatment regimens for rabies.

Disclaimer: The findings and conclusions in this report are those of the authors and do not necessarily represent the views of the funding agency.

Genome and Morphology

Rabies virus is classified as the type species of the genus *Lyssavirus*, family *Rhabdoviridae*, order *Mononegavirales*. The negative-sense single-stranded RNA (ssRNA) genome is *c.* 12 kbp in length (**Figure 1**) and encodes a short leader sequence (*c.* 50 nt), followed by five structural protein genes, separated by nontranscribed intergenic regions. The N gene consists of 1350–1353 nt and codes for the nucleoprotein. Due to its abundance and ease of the detection by fluorescent antibody and RNA-based methods, the nucleoprotein and the N gene are the most common targets of diagnostic tests, and antigenic and phylogenetic typing. The P gene consists of 891–915 nt and codes for the phosphoprotein. This protein is composed of two domains: the NH_2-terminal portion contains an L protein binding site, as well as a weak N protein binding site; the COOH-terminal portion contains a strong N protein binding site. The M gene consists of 606 nt and codes for the matrix protein. This protein is involved in later steps of virion formation, such as tightening of the ribonucleoprotein complex (RNP) into a compressed helical structure and the budding of nucleocapsids at cell membranes to obtain the viral envelope. The G gene consists of 1566–1599 nt and codes for the transmembrane glycoprotein. The glycoprotein interacts with receptors on the cell surface and is responsible for neutralizing antibody production. It is composed of four distinct domains: a signal peptide, ectodomain, transmembrane peptide, and cytoplasmic domain. The glycoprotein, and particularly the ectodomain, play a crucial role in rabies virus (RABV) pathogenicity. For example, one arginine residue at position 333 of the ectodomain is important for peripheral infectivity of RABV. Replacement of this amino acid in vaccine strains significantly attenuates pathogenicity. The L gene is 6381–6426 nt length and codes for the RNA-dependent RNA polymerase. This is a highly conserved polypeptide responsible for replication and transcription of the viral genome.

The RABV virion is bullet-shaped (**Figure 2**), 50–100 nm × 100–430 nm in dimensions, and composed of two structural units: an internal helical RNP, about 50 nm in diameter, and a lipid envelope which is derived from the host cytoplasmic membrane during budding. The RNP is comprised of the RNA genome and N nucleoprotein in tight association. The heavily phosphorylated phosphoprotein and polymerase are also bound to the RNP. The exact position of the matrix protein remains controversial, and may be either contained in the

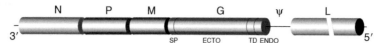

Figure 1 Structure of the rabies virus genome. N, nucleoprotein gene; P, phosphoprotein gene; M, matrix protein gene; G, glycoprotein gene (including SP, signal peptide; ECTO, ectodomain; TD, transmembrane domain; ENDO, endodomain); Ψ, large G-L intergenic region, sometimes referred to as a pseudogene; L, RNA-dependent RNA polymerase gene.

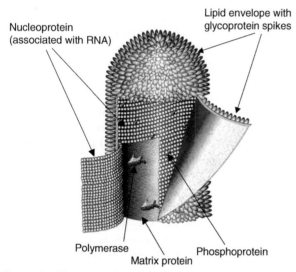

Figure 2 Structure of the rabies virus virion.

central channel of RNP or embedded into the inner layer of the virion membrane. Knobbed glycoprotein spikes, consisting of three glycosylated ectodomains and serving for binding of the virions to host cell receptors, protrude through the virion membrane.

Phylogeny and Evolution

RABV is the most broadly distributed member of the genus *Lyssavirus*, circulating in both carnivorous and chiropteran hosts. Phylogenetic lineages of RABV reflect the geographic distribution and association with a particular host species (**Figure 3**). In general, the RABV lineage is split into two large clusters. One includes viruses circulating worldwide among terrestrial carnivores (predominantly canids and mongoose). The second cluster is indigenous to the New World, and includes viruses circulating among raccoons, skunks, and a variety of bats. The first cluster includes the major 'cosmopolitan' canid RABV lineage, believed to have originated in Europe and widely disseminated as a consequence of global colonization during the sixteenth to nineteenth centuries. Presently, these viruses circulate in moderate latitudes of Eurasia, the Middle East, Africa, and the Americas. The majority of RABV vaccine strains, such as PV, ERA (SAD), PM, and HEP, belong to the 'cosmopolitan' RABV lineage. The lineage of Arctic and Arctic-like rabies viruses is monophyletic but, ancestrally, it is linked to the 'cosmopolitan' group. Viruses comprising the Arctic

portion of this lineage are distributed in circumpolar regions of Eurasia and North America, whereas distinct groups of Arctic-like rabies viruses circulate in some regions of the Middle East, and southern and eastern Asia. Representatives of some African virus lineages of Canidae and Herpestidae origin are more distantly related. The most divergent representatives of the Old World RABVs circulate in dogs in South Asia. Among the indigenous New World RABV lineages, the majority are tightly associated with particular bat species.

RABV is one of the most slowly evolving negative-stranded RNA viruses, with substitution rates of approximately 2×10^{-4} to 5×10^{-4} per site per year. No recombination has been reported in RABV genomes. Mutations occur due to the lack of proofreading and post-replication error correction by RNA polymerase. However, there is clear evidence of negative selection, as RABV and other lyssaviruses are subjected to strong constraints against amino acid substitutions, probably related to their unique pathobiology. There is some limited evidence that positive selection may have occurred at a few sites in the G gene, such as codons 156, 160, 183, and 370, but the role of these residues is not currently known. Although descriptions of a disease similar to rabies are known from 4000-year-old manuscripts, the origin of current RABV diversity has been estimated at 800–1500 years for separation of the major bat and terrestrial virus lineages, 1200–1800 years for the closest ancestor of current American bat rabies viruses, and 280–500 years for the 'cosmopolitan' group.

Pathogenesis

After delivery into a wound, RABV can infect several types of cells and replicate at the inoculation site, as has been shown for skeletal muscle cells and fibroblasts. Attachment to cell membrane receptors is mediated by the glycoprotein spikes protruding from the virion membrane. Several types of putative receptors for RABV attachment have been suggested: nicotinic acetylcholine receptor, carbohydrate moieties, phospholipids, and gangliosides. Once bound, the virus enters the cell by endocytosis. Following a decrease in pH in the endosomal vesicle, the viral membrane fuses with the endosomal membrane, and the RNP is released into the cytoplasm. Because RABV RNA has negative polarity, it must be transcribed to produce the complementary positive-sense mRNA.

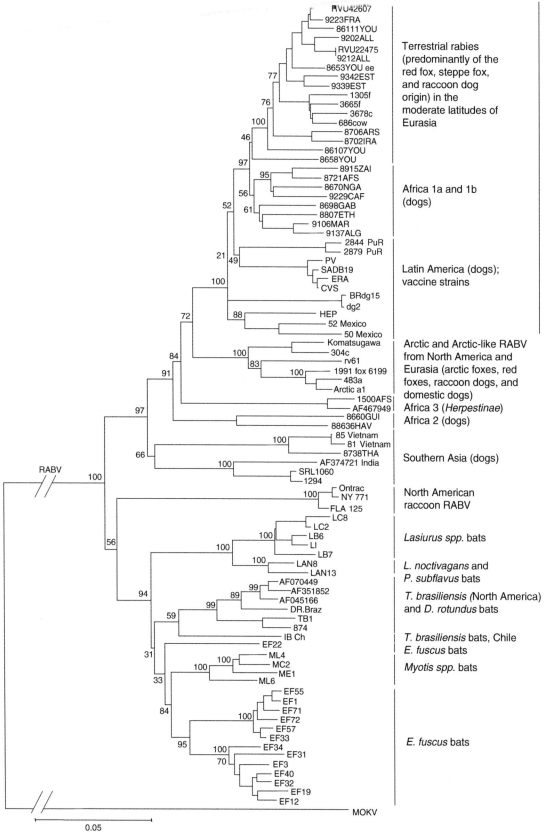

Figure 3 Phylogenetic tree of the major rabies virus lineages based on the sequences of the entire nucleoprotein gene. Bootstrap support values are presented for key nodes, and branch lengths are drawn to scale.

This process is mediated by the viral RNA-dependent RNA polymerase. The RNP serves as a template for transcription and replication, and protects the RNA from nuclease activity. Translation of the viral mRNAs is ensured by the cellular protein synthesis machinery. All processes of transcription, translation, and replication take place in the cytoplasm. The glycoprotein is synthesized at the rough endoplasmic reticulum and delivered to the cytoplasmic membrane. The other viral proteins are expressed in the cytosol by free polyribosomes. At the final stage, transcription and replication are inhibited, the RNP becomes intensively condensed and assembled into mature nucleocapsids, which are subsequently delivered to the cell membrane for the budding of complete virions. During the budding process, virions acquire the lipid envelope and the glycoprotein which is embedded in the cell membrane.

After several replication cycles at the inoculation site, RABV penetrates peripheral nerves and spreads to the central nervous system (CNS) by retrograde axonal transport. Neuronal pathways shield the virus from host immune surveillance, resulting in the absence of an early antibody response. Once delivered to the CNS, the virus disseminates rapidly in the spinal cord, medulla, thalamus, pons, hippocampus, striatum, cerebellum, and cortex. The spread of infection within the CNS occurs from one neuron to another by both axonal and trans-synaptic transport. Neuropathological changes observed in the infected brain are relatively mild histologically and include gliosis, slight neuronophagia, and perivascular infiltration with inflammatory cells, with rare involvement of meninges. Occasionally, more severe brain damage occurs, such as spongiform lesions, extensive neuronal degeneration, and widespread inflammation. Functional alteration of the CNS is much more significant than morphological changes. Apoptosis as a response to RABV infection is an additional prominent factor of neuron damage. Generalized CNS dysfunction leads to a lethal outcome.

Reverse dissemination of virus from the CNS during the clinical period of rabies occurs along peripheral nerves. The RABV RNA may be detected in a variety of organs and tissues at the end of clinical period. However, infectious virus can be isolated from extraneural tissues only occasionally and in low titers. The exception is the salivary glands, where virus passes additional replication cycles and is released into the saliva to enable transmission.

Although a bite is the main method of transmission, non-bite exposures also may occur under unusual circumstances. For instance, two human rabies cases have been attributed to airborne exposure in laboratories, and another two cases have been attributed to airborne exposures in a bat-infested cave in Texas. Aerosol transmission has been demonstrated experimentally, only in very specific conditions with a highly concentrated viral aerosol. Several cases of human-to-human RABV transmission have occurred due to transplantation of cornea, liver, kidneys,

and associated tissues obtained from donors who died of rabies. Exposure may occur by direct contact of saliva, nervous or other infected tissues from a rabid animal with mucous membranes, or from scratches. For example, several cases have occurred in trappers who skinned rabid animals without suitable protection.

Various mammalian species exhibit different susceptibilities to the variety of RABV variants, including mutual adaptation of virus and principal host. For example, canids are highly sensitive to homologous RABV variants, and develop the furious form of rabies with high titers of virus in salivary glands. These peculiarities ensure transmission of the infection to a critical number of susceptible individuals, before the death of the rabid animal. A very low level of seroprevalence has been detected in natural populations of foxes, indicating that most RABV contact events lead to a fatal infection. In contrast, a high level of seroprevalence has been detected among bats. These gregarious mammals demonstrate moderate to low susceptibility to RABV. In many cases, bats develop antibody rather than disease when they encounter RABV. In general, RABV evades immunological responses after entering into the nervous system. Development of antibodies could be attributed to peripheral virus activity rather than to CNS infection. There is contradictory evidence as to whether bats or other mammals can survive rabies. Initial observations made at the beginning of the twentieth century on vampire bats suggested that they can be 'asymptomatic carriers' of RABV. More recent reports from Spain have described some cases in which viral RNA was detected in extraneural tissues and oral swabs of naturally infected bats that were negative for rabies infection in brain tissue. Experimental studies of vampire bats have demonstrated intermittent shedding of RABV in saliva. However, a number of other experiments and field surveillance performed in Europe and the USA provided no evidence in support of a 'carrier' state: bats that developed rabies always died, and virus was detected only in those animals but not in healthy survivors. Some survivors do develop virus-neutralizing antibodies, suggesting a form of abortive infection. Most likely, this abortive infection occurs at the inoculation site. The susceptibility of other mammalian species, that do not serve as principal RABV hosts, is variable. Susceptibility of primates, including humans, is low to moderate, depending on the virus variant.

Indeed, rare cases of survival after the manifestation of clinical signs of rabies are occasionally registered in different animal species. However, these sporadic events cannot be taken in support for a theory of RABV persistence *in vivo*. At least six cases of human recovery after clinical rabies have been published. Five of the patients were vaccinated before clinical onset, and in one case no vaccination was performed. Rabies diagnosis in each case was based on a history of exposure, compatible symptoms, and increasing titers of anti-RABV antibodies in the serum and cerebrospinal fluid (CSF). However, no virus isolates were obtained from these patients.

Clinical Spectrum

The incubation period of rabies can vary from less than 10 days to more than 6 years. The reason for this variability is not yet clear. Some reports attribute long incubation periods to virus replication in the skeletal myocytes before entering the nerves, whereas short incubation periods may be associated with immediate penetration of the nerves and transfer to CNS. Most typical incubation periods after peripheral inoculation of natural hosts and humans vary from 3 to 14 weeks.

Prodromal symptoms are nonspecific: general malaise, fever, chills, sore throat, headache, nausea and vomiting, and sometimes diarrhea, anxiety, and irritability. Humans often suffer from a paresthesia or pain in the inoculation site, and the wound may become slightly inflamed. The prodromal period usually continues for 1–3 days before development of encephalitic symptoms.

Historically, two main clinical forms of rabies have been recognized, based on predominating symptoms: furious (encephalitic) or dumb (paralytic). However, mixed forms occur as well. When the disease is furious, animals or humans become agitated and aggressive. Insomnia, irritability, and anxiety are commonly observed. Other signs, such as pupillary dilation, altered phonation, aimless wandering, drooling of saliva, and muscle tremors and seizures may be noted. Humans often develop hallucinations and delirium. Some symptoms, which have been considered as 'classic' but are observed in 50% or less of patients, are hydrophobia (painful throat seizures at attempts to drink or even due to seeing or hearing running water), aerophobia, photophobia, and phonophobia (seizures in response to airflow, bright lights, and loud sounds, respectively). Subsequently, progressive pareses and paralysis appear. Sick animals or humans become comatose and die, usually due to respiratory failure.

Paralytic rabies is characterized by a greater prevalence of pareses and paralysis from the beginning of disease manifestations, whereas agitation and anxiety are moderate or absent. In part, the form of the disease may depend on the virus variant and animal species. For instance, vampire bat RABVs commonly cause paralytic rabies in cattle and bats. Canine RABV variants from both North America and Eurasia often cause furious rabies. Once symptoms appear, death occurs usually within 1–10 days. Ventilatory support may prolong survival to 3–4 weeks, but no effective treatment exists to date. On occasion, no rabies-specific symptoms can be observed, especially when the paralytic form of disease occurs. Rabies should be considered a possible cause in each case of encephalitis when the etiologic agent is unclear and the probability of lyssavirus exposure cannot be rejected.

Diagnosis

The direct fluorescent antibody test, performed on impressions of infected brain on glass slides, is the gold standard for rabies diagnosis. The brainstem and cerebellum are tissues of choice. Commercially available fluorescein-labeled anti-rabies antibodies, either polyclonal or monoclonal, react with the nucleocapsid of the whole spectrum of RABV variants described to date. The RNP in the infected neurons is condensed into 'inclusions' which are easily observed under the ultraviolet (UV) microscope. The indirect fluorescent antibody test, employing nonlabeled anti-nucleocapsid monoclonal antibodies (N-MAbs), is used commonly for typing of lyssaviruses. Among other methods for RABV antigen capture, some modifications of the enzyme-linked immunosorbent assay (ELISA), including an immuohistochemistry test, have been described and used in research laboratories worldwide.

RABV isolation can be attempted if replication-competent virus is needed for further investigations, or to confirm a negative result obtained by antigen-capturing methods. Isolation can be performed in laboratory mice, aged from suckling to 4 weeks old. Intracerebral inoculation is preferred because the susceptibility of mice to peripheral inoculation is usually 100–10 000 times less than susceptibility to intracerebral inoculation. Incubation periods in mice inoculated intracerebrally usually vary from 3 to 14 days, depending on the dose and particular properties of the isolate, but may be prolonged up to 6 weeks. Development of typical rabies signs, particularly paralysis and death, is characteristic. The inoculation result must be verified by detection of lyssavirus antigen in the brain of moribund mice. Among available cell cultures, those which derive from mammalian neurons are preferred (e.g., use of mouse neuroblastoma cell culture (MNA) is common in diagnostic laboratories). Susceptibility of MNA cells to RABV is similar to the susceptibility of suckling mice. The result can be detected after 48–72 h of incubation. The disadvantage of cell culture compared to mouse inoculation is related to the quality of the inoculum. Field specimens are often cytotoxic and so can be tested *in vitro* only after filtration or high dilution, reducing sensitivity of the test.

The reverse transcription-polymerase chain reaction (RT-PCR) test is a powerful adjunct diagnostic tool, particularly for antemortem diagnosis of rabies in humans. It is also useful for amplifying small quantities of RNA from infected tissues for use in genetic sequencing and phylogenetic analyses. PCR primer selection depends on the survey aim. For diagnostic purposes, when the virus variant is not known, the choice of primer and PCR regimen is a compromise between specificity and sensitivity. The N gene is targeted most commonly for diagnostic purposes because of its conservation, relative abundance in infected cells, and because it is well studied and represented in the public domain (GenBank).

For phylogenetic comparisons, it is useful to amplify a variable region of a gene, but the primers should target flanking conserved regions to ensure specific annealing. For the N gene, the first 400 and the last 320 nucleotides are variable, whereas the space between them (*c.* 600 nt) is conserved. Nested and hemi-nested PCR methods have been developed for RABV. Although they are more sensitive than conventional RT-PCR, nonspecific amplification may still occur, and the result must be verified by molecular hybridization or sequencing of the PCR products. If used properly, and the result is verified, nested PCR is the most sensitive test among PCR-based methods available to date. A real-time PCR test for RABV has also been described. As for other real-time PCR applications, exceptional specificity has been demonstrated for RABV RNA detection. The real-time PCR test can detect highly degraded RNA because very short nucleotide chains (<100 nt) are amplified, and allows quantification of the load of viral RNA. A disadvantage of the specificity of the real-time method is the possibility that it could fail to detect genetically divergent viruses. Therefore, real-time PCR is especially suitable for experimental studies when the genetic sequence of the virus is known.

In some cases, particularly for human antemortem diagnosis, the detection of increasing titers of anti-RABV antibodies in serum, and particularly in the CSF, provides a suitable confirmatory diagnosis of rabies.

Epidemiology

RABV is global in distribution with the exception of Australia, Antarctica, and some isolated insular territories that are inaccessible to many viral hosts. Mammals and birds are susceptible to experimental infection, but only the former are relevant in the epidemiology of the disease. In the Old World, RABV circulates among terrestrial mammals (predominantly of the order Carnivora, families Canidae, and Herpestinae). Tropical Asia and Africa are endemic for dog rabies. These territories also encounter the greatest number of human rabies cases (40 000–60 000 annually). Nearly all occur after exposure to dogs. Dogs in Asia and Africa maintain circulation of different RABV lineages but the 'cosmopolitan' variant is distributed most broadly. Dog populations within moderate latitudes of Eurasia are more limited, and implementation of comprehensive vaccination programs has eliminated dog rabies, at least in developed countries. However, RABV still circulates in these countries among wild canids (e.g., red foxes, steppe foxes, raccoon dogs). Developed countries of western Europe are nearing eradication of terrestrial rabies in wildlife because of the implementation of oral rabies vaccination (ORV), but in other territories of the Palearctic, rabies is broadly distributed in wild canids. Some regions, such as conifer forests (taiga), are apparently free of the infection because of extremely low host population densities which are apparently incapable of maintaining RABV. The Arctic variant of RABV, harbored predominantly by Arctic foxes with involvement of other species, such as red foxes, wolves, and dogs, is distributed circumpolarly in the Arctic and subarctic zones.

In the New World, besides the Arctic and 'cosmopolitan' RABV variants introduced from Eurasia and circulating among canids, a number of indigenous RABV lineages are represented. Raccoon rabies emerged in the southeastern US during the 1950s and, to date, has occupied a broad territory along the eastern coast of North America. Skunks maintain circulation of distinct RABV lineages, such as 'south-central skunk', 'north-central skunk', and 'California skunk', and are involved often in the circulation of other lineages, originating from dogs, raccoons, and even bats. For example, a population of striped skunks in Arizona has maintained circulation of an RABV variant which is regularly isolated from big brown bats, indicative of a host shift. At least seven distinct RABV variants have been described to date among hematophagous and insectivorous bats in both North and South America. Migratory species, such as *Lasiurus* spp., *Tadarida brasiliensis*, etc., facilitate virus spread within broad territories along their migration pathways. The number of identified bat-associated RABV lineages will definitely increase with the improvement of surveillance systems, particularly in South America. Bat RABV variants (predominantly associated with the silver-haired bat, *Lasionycteris noctivagans*, and the eastern pipistrelle bat, *Pipistrellus subflavus*) have been responsible for nearly 90% of domestic human rabies cases reported in the USA during the last 10 years. Many of the bat exposure cases are 'cryptic' in that the circumstances of human exposure to bats frequently are peculiar and little attention is paid to rather small lesions caused by bat bites.

Mongooses also acquire and maintain circulation of distinct RABV variants in some regions. In some instances, they maintain circulation of viruses indistinguishable from those that circulate among dogs (the 'cosmopolitan' variant in the Caribbean and Indian dog variant in southern Asia). In Africa, mongooses harbor a specific RABV variant that circulates exclusively among herpestides of several species.

Prevention and Control

Rabies can be successfully prevented by immunization, not only prior to an exposure, but also after exposure. However, post-exposure prophylaxis (PEP) should commence soon as possible, before virus entry into magistral nerves and CNS, where it becomes largely inaccessible to the immune system due to the blood–brain barrier.

Two primary kinds treatment are used for PEP: vaccines, which lead to the development of active immunity;

and anti-rabies immune globulins (RIGs), which provide passive immunity at early stages of immunization when immune response to the vaccine is limited.

Modern commercial human vaccines are pure, potent, safe, and efficacious against all RABV variants described to date. Most human vaccines are derived from the Pasteur virus strain, and are inactivated. Vaccines are manufactured using cell lines or primary cell cultures (such as human diploid cell, avian embryos, Vero, and BHK cells) from which virions are concentrated and partly purified to avoid allergic and adverse reactions. Older generations of nervous-tissue-derived vaccines (sheep or suckling mouse brain) are still used in some developing countries. Due to low potency, they must be administered in significantly higher doses and for longer courses of application. Adverse reactions are more common during vaccination.

Domestic animals are vaccinated against rabies to prevent virus circulation in the population, to eliminate important sources of human exposure, and to avoid economic losses. Most modern veterinary vaccines are inactivated, and potent in the ability to induce appropriate protection for 12–48 months after one dose. Vaccination of dogs and cats is recommended in all territories where contact with RABV is possible. Immunization regulations for other species of domestic and agricultural animals differ depending on the specific epizootic surroundings, geographic and economic circumstances, etc. Quarantine for animals imported from rabies-endemic territories is another measure implemented in some states or districts free of terrestrial rabies.

Outstanding progress in rabies prophylaxis in wildlife has been achieved by implementation of oral vaccination. Oral vaccines contain live-attenuated RABV or recombinant viruses (such as vaccinia virus) expressing the RABV glycoprotein. Wildlife oral vaccination campaigns have been conducted in North America and Europe. As a result, rabies epizootics in wild canids have been significantly reduced or eliminated in most West European countries,

Canada, and in parts of the USA. The oral vaccination of raccoon populations, performed in the eastern USA, has prevented further westward spread. Due to very high population density of raccoons, oral vaccination is challenging in this species. To date, oral vaccination programs have not been applied to bats.

Further Reading

Baer GM (ed.) (1991) *The Natural History of Rabies,* 2nd edn. Boca Raton, FL: CRC Press.

Centers for Disease Control and Prevention (CDC) (1999) Human rabies prevention – United States, 1999. Recommendations of the Advisory Committee on Immunization Practices (ACIP). Morbidity and Mortality Weekly Report, vol. 48(no. RR-1), pp. 1–21. Atlanta, GA: CDC.

Jackson AC and Wunner WH (eds.) (2007) *Rabies,* 2nd edn. New York: Academic Press.

Krebs JW, Wilson ML, and Childs JE (1995) Rabies – Epidemiology, prevention, and future research. *Journal of Mammalogy* 76: 681–694.

Meltzer MI and Rupprecht CE (1998) A review of the economics of the prevention and control of rabies. Part 1: Global impact and rabies in humans. *Pharmacoeconomics* 14: 365–383.

Meltzer MI and Rupprecht CE (1998) A review of the economics of the prevention and control of rabies. Part 2: Rabies in dogs, livestock and wildlife. *Pharmacoeconomics* 14: 481–498.

Meslin F-X, Kaplan MM,, and Koprowski H (eds.) (1996) *Laboratory Techniques in Rabies,* 4th edn. Geneva: World Health Organization.

Rupprecht CE, Dietzschold B,, and Koprowski H (eds.) (1994) *Lyssaviruses.* Berlin: Springer.

Smith JS (1995) Rabies virus. In: Murray PR, Baron EJ, Pfaller MA, Tenover FC,, and Yolken PH (eds.) *Manual of Clinical Microbiology,* pp. 997–1003. Washington, DC: ASM Press.

Tordo N, Charlton K, and Wandeler A (1998) Rhabdoviruses: Rabies. In: Collier LH (ed.) *Topley and Wilson's Microbiology and Microbial Infections,* pp. 666–692. London: Arnold.

Tsiang H (1993) Pathophysiology of rabies virus infection of the central nervous system. *Advances in Virus Research* 42: 375–412.

World Health Organization (1996) WHO recommendations on rabies post-exposure treatment and the correct technique of intradermal immunization against rabies. *WHO/EMC/ZOO/96.6.* Geneva: World Health Organization.

World Health Organization (2005) WHO expert consultation on rabies. First report. *WHO Technical Report Series*, vol. 931. WHO: Geneva.

Reoviruses: General Features

P Clarke and K L Tyler, University of Colorado Health Sciences, Denver, CO, USA

Glossary

Caspase 3−/− mice Mice that do not express caspase 3.

CTL (cytotoxic T lymphocyte) A lymphocyte capable of inducing the death of infected somatic or tumor cells. CTLs express T-cell receptors

(TcRs) that can recognize a specific antigenic peptide bound to class I MHC molecules, present on all nucleated cells, and a glycoprotein called CD8.

EHBA (extrahepatic biliary atresia) A progressive congenital disorder that destroys the external bile duct structure of the liver, impairing normal bile flow (cholestasis).

SCID mice Mice with severe combined immunodeficiency, that is, cannot make T or B lymphocytes.

History

In 1959, AB Sabin proposed the designation reovirus (respiratory enteric orphan) for a subgroup of respiratory and enteric viruses not known to be associated with human disease. These viruses had particular distinguishing characteristics including: (1) their size, which at ≤ 75 nm was larger than other known enteric viruses; (2) their capacity to produce cytoplasmic inclusions in monkey kidney cells in tissue culture; (3) their pathogenicity for newborn but not adult mice; and (4) their capacity to hemagglutinate human type O erythrocytes. The first reovirus, isolated from an aboriginal child in 1951 by NF Stanley and colleagues, was named hepatoencephalomyelitis virus. Later, in 1953, M Ramos-Alvarez and AB Sabin isolated the prototype virus for reovirus serotype 1 (reovirus serotype 1 strain Lang, T1L) from the stool of a baby named Lang. In 1955, Ramos-Alverez and Sabin also isolated the prototypes for reovirus serotype 2 from the stool of a child named Jones who had a summer diarrheal illness (reovirus serotype 2 strain Jones, T2J) and for reovirus serotype 3 from the stool of a child named Dearing (reovirus serotype 3 strain Dearing, T3D). A second prototype for reovirus serotype 3 was isolated from an anal swab from a baby named Abney (reovirus serotype 3 strain Abney, T3A) by L Rosen in 1957.

With the isolation and characterization of additional viruses, the acronym 'reo' was retained for the encompassing family of viruses, the *Reoviridae*, all members of which could be called reoviruses. The prefix ortho was added to the names of the initial isolates (orthoreoviruses) and their genus (*Orthoreovirus*) to distinguish them from other members of the family (see below). Despite these formal changes in nomenclature, the orthoreoviruses are still commonly referred to as reoviruses.

Taxonomy and Classification

Currently, the *Reoviridae* is the largest of all the six double-stranded (ds) RNA virus families and its members are also the most diverse in terms of host range (**Table 1**). The genomes of these viruses comprise 10, 11, or 12 segments of dsRNA, each encoding one to three proteins (usually one) on only one of the complementary strands. Their mature virions have characteristic sizes (60–85 nm excluding the extended fiber proteins that project from the surface of some members), no lipid envelope, and proteins arranged in two or three concentric layers that generally reflect icosahedral symmetry. A distinguishing feature of their replication cycles, also found in dsRNA viruses in other families, is the synthesis of viral mRNAs by virally encoded enzymes within the icosahedral particles.

Viruses in the 12 recognized genera of the family *Reoviridae* can be distinguished by differences in relative size, capsid number and structure, genome segment number, nature and number of structural proteins and patterns of reactivity with antisera (**Table 1**). Regions of significant sequence similarity across genus lines are few and of limited length; hence, exchanges of genetic material between genera are unlikely. Viruses in a subset of the genera have a turret-like projection from the innermost capsid layer (**Table 1**). This article focuses on the genus *Orthoreovirus*. The characteristics of other genera of the *Reoviridae* are discussed elsewhere in this encyclopedia.

The genus *Orthoreovirus* currently contains five species including *Mammalian orthoreovirus* (MRV) as species I, *Avian orthoreovirus* (ARV) as species II, *Nelson Bay orthoreovirus* (NBV) as species III, *Baboon orthoreovirus* (BRV) as species IV, and *Reptilian orthoreovirus* (RRV) as species V. All orthoreoviruses, except MRV, are fusogenic and induce syncytia.

Members of the genus *Orthoreovirus* have 10 segments of dsRNA contained in two concentric protein capsids of approximately 85 nm diameter (**Table 1**). Orthoreovirus genomes comprise three large (L1–L3), three medium (M1–M3), and four small (S1–S4) segments (**Table 2**). Most of the genome segments are mono-cistronic, except for S1 which is bi-cistronic in MRV, BRV, and RRV and tri-cistronic in ARV and NBV. Further details on the molecular biology of orthoreoviruses is described elsewhere in this encyclopedia.

Fusogenic Orthoreoviruses

The fusogenic orthoreoviruses include the species ARV, NBV, BRV, and RRV. Avian orthoreoviruses can be isolated from both domestic and wild birds and cause a variety of diseases including tenosynovitis (arthritis), a gastrointestinal maladsorption syndrome, and runting. Although some avian reoviruses can be adapted for growth in mammalian cells, or will grow in mammalian cells under certain conditions, there is little or no evidence for natural infection of mammals. Nelson Bay virus, isolated from an Australian flying fox, has traits intermediate between classical mammalian and avian orthoreoviruses. Although NBV was isolated from a mammal and replicates in mammalian cell cultures, it induces syncytia formation in those cultures and is thus fusogenic. Baboon reovirus, isolated from a colony in Texas, has similar properties to NBV, including replication and syncytia formation in

Table 1 The family *Reoviridae*

Genera	No. of genome segments	No. of capsid layers	Hosts
Turreted[a]			
Orthoreovirus	10	2	Mammals, birds, reptiles
Aquareovirus	11	2	Fish, mollusks
Cypovirus	10	1[b]	Insects
Fijivirus	10	2	Plants, insects[c]
Oryzavirus	10	2	Plants, insects[c]
Myocoreovirus	11/12	2	Fungi
Idnoreovirus	10	2	Insects
Nonturreted			
Rotavirus	11	3	Mammals, birds
Orbivirus	10	3	Mammals, birds, arthropods[c]
Coltivirus	12	3	Mammals, arthropods[c]
Phytoreovirus	12	3	Plants, insects[c]
Seadornavirus	12	3	Mosquitoes[c], mammals, humans

[a]Two groups of genera are designated based on the presence or absence of turrets or spikes situated at the 12 icosahedral vertices of either the virus or core particle.
[b]Most cypovirus particles are characteristically occluded within a matrix of proteinaceous crystals called polyhedra.
[c]Serve as vectors for transmission to other hosts.
Modified from Nibert ML and Schiff LA (2001). Reoviruses and their replication. In: Knipe DM and Howley PM (eds.) *Fields Virology*, 4th edn., pp. 1679–1728. Philadelphia, PA: Lippincott Williams and Wilkins, with permission from Lippincott Williams and Wilkins.

Table 2 List of the dsRNA segments of mammalian orthoreovirus-3De (MRV-3De), their encoded proteins, and selected functions

Gene segment	Protein	Location	Function
L1	λ3 (Pol)	Core	RNA polymerase (Pol)
L2	λ2 (Cap)	Core Spike	Guanylyl transferase, methyl transferase (capping enzyme). 'Turret' protein
L3	λ1 (Hel)	Core	Inner capsid structural protein, binds dsRNA and zinc, helicase (Hel)
M1	μ2	Core	NTPase
M2	μ1	Outer capsid	Multimerizes with σ3. Cleaved to form μ1C and μ1N which assume $T = 13$ symmetry in the outer capsid. μ1C is further cleaved to δ and ϕ during entry
M3	μNS μNSC	Nonstructural (NS)	Binds ssRNA and cytoskeleton. μNSC results from an alternate translational start site and has unknown function.
S1	σ1 σ1s	Outer capsid NS	Viral attachment protein Nonstructural, blocks cell-cycle progression
S2	σ2	Core	Inner capsid structural protein
S3	σNS	NS	ssRNA binding, genome packaging?
S4	σ3	Outer capsid	dsRNA binding, multimerizes with σ1, nuclear and cytoplasmic localization, translational control

Reproduced from Chappell JD, Duncan R, Mertens PPC, and Dermody TS (2005) *Othoreovirus*. In : Fauquet CM, Mayo MA, Maniloff J, Desselberger U, and Ball LA (eds.) *Virus Taxonomy: Eighth Report of the International Commitee on Taxonomy of Viruses*, pp. 455–465. San Diego, CA: Elsevier Academic Press, with permission from Elsevier.

mammalian cultures, but is distinguishable in other respects. Nucleotide sequence analysis indicates that NBV and BRV represent additional phylogenetic groups within the genus *Orthoreovirus*. Fusogenic isolates from snakes represent yet another distinct phylogenetic group within the genus.

Fusogenic reoviruses encode a unique group of small (95–140 amino acids) fusion-associated, small transmembrane (FAST) proteins. Three distinct members of the FAST protein family have been described; the homologous p10 proteins of ARV and NBV, and the unrelated p14 and p15 proteins of RRV and BRV, respectively. Unlike the well-characterized fusion proteins of enveloped viruses, the FAST proteins

are nonstructural viral proteins and are not involved in viral entry into the cell. They appear to mediate cell to cell, rather than virus to cell, membrane fusion.

The fusogenic orthoreoviruses are less well characterized, by far, than the non-fusogenic mammalian reoviruses. The rest of this article focuses on mammalian reovirues.

Mammalian Reoviruses

Serotypes and Strains

The three major MRV serotypes (MRV-1, MRV-2, and MRV-3) represent numerous isolates including the early

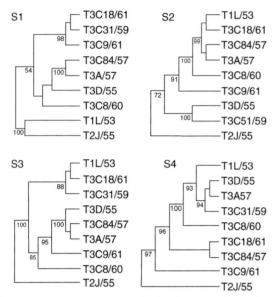

Figure 1 Phylogenetic trees indicating the potential evolutionary relationship and degree of diversity or relatedness between reovirus strains based on the nucleotide sequences of the reovirus S1, S2, S3, and S4 dsRNA segments. Each tree is rooted at the midpoint of its longest branch. Reproduced from Virgin HW, IVth, Tyler KL, and Dermody TS (1997) Reovirus. In: Nathanson N (ed.) *Viral Pathogenesis*, p. 669. Philadelphia, PA: Lippincott-Raven, with permission from Lippincott Williams and Wilkins.

human reovirus prototype isolates T1L (now MRV-1La), T2J (now MRV-2Jo), and T3D (now MRV-3De). A fourth MRV serotype, Ndelle (MRV-4Nd) contains only one isolate. MRV serotype is determined by the cell attachment protein, σ1 (**Table 2**). The S1 genome segment, which encodes σ1, shows the greatest sequence diversity of all the genome segments (**Figure 1**), with only 26–49% identity between viruses belonging to different serotypes. In contrast, S1 sequence identity between viruses of the same serotype is 86–99%, which is similar to the sequence identity of other genome segments between viruses belonging to different serotypes (**Figure 1**). This suggests that three versions of the S1 genome segment, corresponding to the three major MRV serotypes, arose from progenitors at different times and have subsequently diverged at a rate similar to that of other segments. Detailed phylogenetic analyses of the evolutionary relationship between a number of MRV strains from different serotypes based on the nucleotide sequence of their S1, S2, S3, and S4 gene segments are shown in **Figure 1**. Interestingly, the phylogenetic trees of individual MRV strains differ depending on the dsRNA segment chosen for comparison, indicating that reassortment of MRV gene segments occurs under natural circumstances.

MRV reassortants can easily be generated by co-infection of susceptible cells or mice with two distinct MRV serotypes. This capacity to exchange genetic material by genome reassortment during mixed infections to produce viable progeny virus strains can be used to identify individual species within the genus *Orthoreovirus*. In contrast

to the evidence supporting reassortment of dsRNA segments between reovirus strains within a species, there is an absence of evidence of genetic recombination between either homologous or heterologous dsRNA segments.

Distribution and Host Range

Mammalian orthoreoviruses are ubiquitous in their geographic distribution. Studies of variation in the seasonal pattern of human infection are limited but an increased incidence of childhood illnesses associated with MRV-2 infection in the Northern Hemisphere summer (June–September) has been reported. In addition, many of the initial human reovirus isolates were from infants and children with summer diarrheal illnesses. Evidence of MRV infection has been found in animals of an enormous variety of species including humans, a wide variety of nonhuman primates, swine, horses, cattle, sheep, goats, dogs, cats, rabbits, rats, mice, guinea pigs, voles, bats, and a large number of marsupials.

Epidemiology

The majority of humans develop detectable serum antibodies against all three of the major MRV serotypes by late childhood. In a recent study of 272 serum specimens from young children, rapid loss of maternal antibody was detected between 0 and 6 months of age, seroprevalence was 0% in children 6–12 months of age, and then increased steadily throughout early childhood reaching 50% in children 5–6 years of age. The majority of cases of MRV infection in humans appear to be sporadic in nature, although outbreaks of infection caused by MRV-1 have been described. Age-related susceptibility to MRV infection has also been observed in both natural and experimental infection of animals. Calves, foals, piglets, and neonatal mice thus all appear more susceptible to MRV infection than their adult counterparts. Experimental studies in mice indicate that host immune status is another important factor in determining the nature and outcome of MRV infection. Immunocompetent adult mice develop an immune response but do not generally show clinical or pathological evidence of disease following reovirus infection. By contrast, after MRV infection, SCID mice develop prominent and often lethal hepatic disease. SCID mice and mice with targeted disruptions of the transmembrane exon of IgM (i.e., antibody and B-cell-deficient mice) also show altered patterns of viral clearance following peroral inoculation with MRV.

Transmission

Mammalian orthoreovirus transmission (horizontal spread) under natural circumstances involves respiratory aerosols and secretions, and fecal–oral transmission. In mice, there is an excellent correlation between the capacity of MRVs to grow in the intestine, the amount of virus subsequently shed in the stool, and the efficiency with which an infected animal transmits disease to its uninfected litter mates. The viral L2 gene, which encodes the core spike protein λ2, is the primary determinant of the efficiency of viral transmission following peroral inoculation. Both the L2 (see above) and the S1 gene (which encodes the virus cell attachment protein, σ1, and the small nonstructural protein, σ1s) influence growth and survival of reovirus in intestinal tissue (**Figure 2**).

Transmission is also influenced by the capacity of the virus to survive the environment after being shed from an infected host. Most MRVs are generally stable below room temperature although, at higher temperatures, strain-specific differences in thermostability become apparent. For example, MRV-1La has a half-life of 19 h at 37 °C, compared to 2.6 h for MRV-3De. MRVs are also stable in aerosols especially in the presence of high relative humidity. Viral outer capsid proteins appear to be the major determinants of virion stability.

Pathogenesis

The basic steps in the pathogenesis of mammalian orthoreovirus infection have been studied extensively in experimental animals, including mice and rats. After peroral or intratracheal inoculation, virions adhere to the surface of epithelial M (microfold) cells, which overlie collections of lymphoid tissue in the small intestine and bronchi that form part of the systems of gut-associated lymphoid tissue (GALT) and bronchus-associated lymphoid tissue (BALT). In the intestinal lumen, virions are partially digested by proteases to generate intermediate subviral particles (ISVPs). It appears that, at least in the intestine,

ISVPs are the form of virus particles that bind to M cells. After binding, ISVPs and/or virions are transported across these cells to the underlying intestinal lymphoid tissue. Studies of intestinal infection suggest that replication may occur in macrophages within mucosal lymphoid tissue.

Spread of virus from the site of primary infection to distant tissues and organs, by means of the lymphatic system, blood stream, or by axoplasmic transport within neurons, results in systemic disease. MRV serotypes differ both in their capacity to generate and sustain viremia and the efficiency with which they utilize neuronal transport. Following footpad or intramuscular infection in neonatal mice, reovirus MRV-1La spreads to the central nervous system (CNS) primarily through the blood stream, whereas MRV-3De spreads predominantly through neural pathways. In this model the viral S1 gene determines both the pathway of spread in the infected host and the extent of extra-intestinal spread (**Figure 2**).

Depending on the viral strain, the route of inoculation and host factors such as age and immune status, MRVs can produce injury in a variety of target tissues. Among the most extensively studied targets of viral infection in murine model systems are the CNS, the lung, the heart, the hepatobiliary system, and the gastrointestinal tract (**Figure 2**). The specific pathology induced in these various organ systems is discussed extensively in the references included at the end of this article.

MRV strains often show striking differences in their pattern of organ and tissue tropism. For example, MRV-3De infects neurons and retinal ganglion cells, whereas MRV-1La infects ependymal cells and cells in the anterior lobe of the pituitary gland. Differences in tropism within the brain, the pituitary gland, and the retina are all determined by the viral S1 gene. Studies

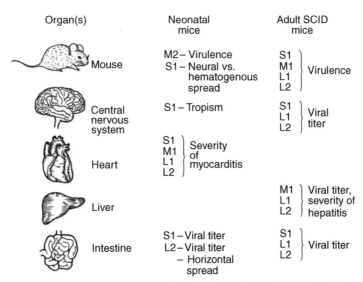

Figure 2 Reovirus dsRNA segments shown to have a role in determining organ-specific virulence in mice. Reproduced from Virgin HW, IVth, Tyler KL, and Dermody TS (1997) *Reovirus*. In: Nathanson N (ed.) *Viral Pathogenesis*, p. 669. Philadelphia, PA: Lippincott-Raven.

with monoclonal antibody resistant σ1 variants of MRV-3De indicate that a single amino acid substitution in this gene is sufficient to alter neurovirulence, CNS growth, and pattern of CNS tropism.

Attachment and Penetration

The cell attachment protein, σ1, consists of an elongated fibrous tail that inserts into the virion, and a virion-distal globular head. Four distinct and tandemly arranged morphologic regions within the σ1 tail have been designated (T(i)–T(iv)) based on proximity to the virion surface. A conserved surface at the base of the σ1 head domain of all three of the major MRV serotypes appears to determine virus binding to a serotype-independent receptor junction adhesion molecule-A (JAM-A). The σ1 protein of MRV-3De also contains a receptor binding domain in the T(iii) region of the tail that binds α-linked sialic acid. The relative importance of the JAM-A and sialic acid receptor binding domains of MRV-3De σ1 for efficient attachment and infection of host cells varies between different target cells. MRV-1La also binds a carbohydrate moiety but the nature of the glycosyl ligand remains uncertain. In contrast to MRV-3De σ1, the carbohydrate binding domain of MRV-1La σ1 has been mapped to tail region T(iv). Whereas there seems to be some flexibility on the binding of sialic acid and JAM-A for reovirus growth, both these receptors are required for the ability of reovirus to induce apoptosis in infected cells (see below).

In addition to receptor binding, β-1 integrin has recently been shown to facilitate reovirus internalization suggesting that viral entry occurs by interactions of reovirus virions with independent attachment and entry receptors on the cell surface.

Virus–Cell Interactions

Members of the MRV species induce apoptosis in cultured cells. MRV serotypes differ in this capacity with MRV-1La producing less apoptosis than MRV-3 strains. Serotype-specific differences in the capacity to induce apoptosis are determined by the S1 and M2 genome segments.

As noted above, the S1 genome segment encodes two proteins, the cell attachment protein (σ1) and a nonstructural protein (σ1s), which promotes G_2/M cell-cycle arrest. Several lines of evidence indicate that, at least in some cells in tissue culture, σ1 is the S1-encoded determinant of virus-induced apoptosis. First, apoptosis can be induced by UV-inactivated replication-incompetent virions, which lack σ1s. Second, apoptosis can be induced at nonpermissive temperatures by a variety of reovirus temperature-sensitive (ts)-mutants, which fail to synthesize σ1s in infected cells. Finally, the σ1s null-mutant MA, which fails to induce G2/M arrest in virus

infected cells in tissue culture, retains the capacity to induce apoptosis, indicating that σ1s is not required for this process. Recent studies have, however, demonstrated that σ1s is a determinant of the magnitude and extent of reovirus-induced apoptosis *in vivo*, in both the heart and CNS.

The M2 gene encodes the major viral outer capsid protein μ1/μ1c. Apoptosis is inhibited following incubation of infected cells with MAbs directed against μ1 proteins and in cells infected with a temperature-sensitive (ts) membrane-penetration-defective M2 mutant. The μ1 protein is also sufficient to induce apoptosis in transfected cells. These observations support the role of the M2 genome segment in virus-induced apoptosis. In addition, recent studies suggest that binding of σ1 to JAM-A and sialic acid may be dispensable for virus-induced apoptosis and that the M2 gene segment is the only viral determinant of apoptosis when infection is initiated via Fc receptors.

As the M2 gene is a determinant of apoptosis, and as both anti-μ1 and anti-σ3 MAbs (which inhibit the virion-uncoating but not virus-cell attachment) can inhibit apoptosis, early events during virus entry, but subsequent to engagement with cellular receptors, appear to be required for apoptosis. This interpretation has subsequently been supported by experiments indicating that virus-uncoating but not replication is required for apoptosis.

MRV-induced apoptosis is associated with regulation of cellular MAPK signaling pathways, including c-Jun N terminal kinase (JNK) signaling, and transcription factors, including c-Jun and nuclear factor-kappa B (NF-κB). MRV-induced apoptosis also involves both the intrinsic and extrinsic apoptotic signaling pathways. Further details of reovirus-induced apoptotic signaling are provided in the references at the end of the article.

MRVs also induce apoptosis *in vivo* in the CNS and heart where virus infected and apoptotic cells co-localize to regions of viral injury. Virus-induced activation of caspase 3, injury, and viral load are diminished in the presence of chemical inhibitors of apoptosis or in caspase 3−/− mice (**Figure 3**). In addition, MRV-infected caspase 3−/− mice show increased survival compared to wild-type controls (**Figure 3**). These studies indicate that apoptosis is an important mechanism of virus-induced injury in the host and suggest that apoptosis inhibitors may provide useful antiviral therapies.

MRV infection is also associated with other cellular responses that influence virus growth and pathogenesis including: (1) increased expression of inducible NADPH-dependent nitric oxide (NO) synthase (iNOS) in the brains of MRV-infected mice, suggesting that NO may play an antiviral role during reovirus infection; and (2) increased phosphorylation of the eukaryotic initiation factor 2α which facilitates reovirus replication. Global expression analysis using microarrays indicates that, by 24 h following reovirus infection, the expression of 309 cellular genes (2.6% of the total number of genes present

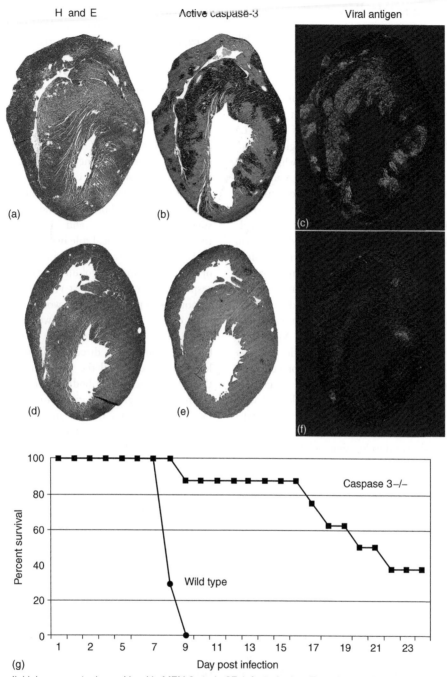

Figure 3 Myocardial injury, apoptosis, and load in MRV-3 strain 8B-infected mice. Two-day-old Swiss-Webster mice were infected with MRV-3 strain 8B followed by intraperitoneal administration of the pharmacologic caspase inhibitor Q-VD-OPH (50 mg kg^{-1} day^{-1}) or its diluent control on days 3–6 post infection. The animals were sacrificed on day 7. Consecutive sections were analyzed for histologic injury (H and E staining), active caspase 3 (brown diaminobenzadine staining), and virus antigen (fluorescent green staining). (a–c) Sections from Q-VD-OPH treated mice or (d–f) controls are shown. (g) Survival curves for MRV-3 strain 8B-infected caspase 3−/− animals and wild-type controls are also shown. Reproduced from DeBiasi RL, Robinson BA, Sherry B, *et al.* (2004) Caspase inhibition protects against reovirus-induced myocardial injury *in vitro* and *in vivo*. *Journal of Virology* 78: 11040–11050, with permission from American Society for Microbiology.

on the array) is altered in infected cells. Many of these genes are involved in cell-cycle regulation, apoptosis, and DNA repair. Further analysis of the 5′ upstream sequences of the most differentially expressed genes has revealed highly preserved sequence regions (modules) and higher-order patterns of modules (supermodules) containing binding sites for multiple transcription factors. This suggests a coordinated mechanism for virus-induced control of the expression of genes involved in similar biological processes.

Clinical Features and Infection

Human orthoreoviruses remain as much human orphan viruses as when they were first described. Human infection occurs during early childhood (see above) and is either asymptomatic or produces mild symptoms of upper respiratory or intestinal infections or, in some cases, exanthema with fever. The predominant symptoms observed in children during an outbreak of MRV-1La infection included rhinorrhea (81%), pharyngitis (56%), and diarrhea (19%), although the extent to which these were attributable exclusively to the MRV-1La infection itself is unclear. Over half the children shed virus in the stool for at least 1 week and 21% shed virus for at least 2 weeks. The longest reported duration of stool shedding was 5 weeks. Deliberate inoculation of adult human volunteers with MRVs produces similar patterns of infection to those that appear to occur under natural circumstances. Nasal inoculation of seronegative volunteers with MRV-1La, MRV-2Jo, or MRV-3De is associated with seroconversion and shedding of virus in the stool but is typically asymptomatic. Approximately one-third of MRV-1La-inoculated individuals do develop symptomatic infection (fever, headache, coughing, sneezing, rhinorrhea, and generalized malaise) lasting 4–7 days and beginning 24–48 h after viral challenge. Individuals challenged with MRV-3De sometimes develop mild rhinitis. In general, individuals with pre-existing antireovirus antibody prior to challenge with reovirus do not develop signs of clinical disease and do not shed significant amounts of reovirus in stools.

MRV-3De infection of mice produces a disease with clinical and pathological features that resemble human extrahepatoic biliary atresia (EHBA). However, attempts to link reovirus infection to human EHBA have produced conflicting results. Some studies show a higher frequency or higher titers of anti-reovirus antibodies in children with EHBA as compared to controls, whereas other studies do not. Similarly, some studies show that reovirus dsRNA can be amplified from patient tissues with increased frequency compared to controls, whereas other studies do not. Reovirus has not been directly isolated from pathological specimens obtained at biopsy, surgery, or autopsy from patients with EHBA; nor has reovirus been detected in the liver or biliary tissues of patients by immunocytochemistry.

One of the hallmarks of MRV infection in rodents is CNS disease. It is therefore not surprising that several case reports associating reovirus with CNS disease have appeared. Among the most convincing is a case of aseptic meningitis in a previously healthy 3-month-old. The child seroconverted and a serotype 1 MRV was isolated from cerebral spinal fluid (CSF) after inoculation onto green monkey kidney cells. In addition, a serotype 3 MRV strain was isolated from the CSF of a 6.5-week-old child with meningitis. This virus was capable of systemic spread in newborn mice after peroral inoculation and produced lethal encephalitis. Other rare reports of an association between MRV infection and human diseases including encephalitis, keratoconjunctivitis, and pneumonia exist. However, it is important to recognize that reoviruses are responsible for a vanishingly small percentage of the total number of cases of these various illnesses.

Immune Response

As noted above, both SCID mice and antibody and B cell deficient mice show increased susceptibility to MRV infection and diminished capacity to clear the virus. Similar results have been found with immunocompetent neonatal mice depleted of CD4+ and/or CD8+ T cells. This suggests that both B and T cell-mediated immune responses play a critical role in controlling MRV infection.

Following natural or experimental infection, the bulk of both the immunogobulin (Ig)A and IgG antibody response is directed against viral structural proteins and is not serotype-specific, as would be expected by the high degree of homology between proteins of viruses belonging to different serotypes. Serotype-specific antibody responses are directed against $\sigma 1$ which is the least conserved of all the MRV proteins. The nature of the MRV-specific antibody response is influenced by the route of viral inoculation. Following peroral inoculation with MRV-1La, there is an increase in the number of reovirus-specific IgA-producing cells in intestinal Peyers patches and in the spleen. Enteric infection is also associated with the induction of IgG antibody, predominantly of the IgG2a and IgG2b subclasses. Variations in the dominant IgG antibody subclass are influenced both by the route of virus inoculation and the strain of mouse.

T cell responses are also induced during reovirus infection. Following peroral inoculation, MRV-1La-specific MHC-restricted cytotoxic T lymphocytes can be found in Peyer's patches and among the intraepithelial intestinal lymphocyte population. These cells are CD8+, bear the alpha/beta T cell receptor (TCR), are capable of MHC-restricted lysis of virus-infected target cells and increase dramatically after intestinal infection. Perforin, Fas-FasL, and TRAIL pathways are involved in intestinal lymphocyte cytoxicity against MRV-1La. Studies of Vβ TCR usage indicate that MRV infection is associated with oligoclonal expansion of specific TCR subpopulations. Serotype-specific MRV CTL responses are again directed against products of the S1 gene, whereas nonserotype-specific CTL responses are presumably directed against epitopes on other proteins or conserved epitopes within the S1-encoded proteins.

Both antibody and MRV-specific lymphocytes can protect mice against challenge with a variety of MRV strains and from infection by a variety of different routes. Passively transferred MRV-specific immune cells seem more effective than antibody in controlling viral replication at primary sites, whereas antibody may be more effective in controlling growth and spread of virus within certain tissues or organs, including the CNS.

Passive protection can be conferred by monoclonal antibodies specific for each of the viral outer capsid proteins (σ1, μ1C, σ3) and is associated with inhibited replication at primary sites, reduced viral spread to critical target tissues, and diminished growth and spread of virus within these tissues. Both CD4+ and CD8+ T cells are required for optimal protection following passive transfer of MRV-specific T cells. There is currently no evidence that intestinal intraepithelial γ/δ TCR+ T cells, as opposed to α/β TCR+ T cells, play a significant role in immunity to MRV infection.

In addition to humoral and cellular immune responses, cytokines and other mediators may play a role in modulating MRV infection. MRV-induction of interferon (IFN) depends on both the viral strain and the host cell and differs between mice of different strains. MRV-3De, for example, is a better inducer of IFN in mouse L-cell fibroblasts than MRV-1La. MRV-3De also induces higher levels of chemokine mRNA expression for TNFα and MIP-2 than MRV-1la in pulmonary cells *in vitro* and within the lung following *in vivo* infection.

MRVs are also susceptible to β-IFN, although strains differ strikingly in sensitivity, with MRV-3De being much more sensitive than MRV-1La. Differences in the levels of IFN-induced dsRNA-dependent protein kinase (PKR) may play a role in mediating effects of β-IFN on MRV replication. The σ3 protein inhibits the activation of PKR, by preventing its interaction with dsRNA. Differences in IFN sensitivity of reovirus strains may thus depend, in part, on their σ3 proteins. In cardiac myocyte cultures, reovirus induction of β-IFN is determined by viral core proteins and inversely correlates with the capacity of viruses to induce cytopathic effect *in vitro* and myocarditis *in vivo*. Depletion of β-IFN enhances the myocarditic potential of nonmyocarditic viral strains, suggesting a

protective effect for β-IFN. These results contrast with studies of experimental reovirus serotype 2-induced murine diabetes, in which the severity of insulitis in mice correlates with increased expression of γ-IFN, and is ameliorated by administration of anti-γ-IFN antibody. This suggests that IFN induction may play a pathogenetic rather than a protective role in this setting.

See also: Orbiviruses; Rotaviruses.

Further Reading

Barton ES, Chappell JD, Connolly JL, Forrest JC, and Dermody TS (2001) Reovirus receptors and apoptosis. *Virology* 290: 173–180.

Chappell JD, Duncan R, Mertens PPC, and Dermody TS (2005) *Orthoreovirus*. In: Fauquet CM, Mayo MA, Maniloff J, Desselberger U,, and Ball LA (eds.) *Virus Taxonomy: Eighth Report of the International Committee on Taxonomy of Viruses*, pp. 455–465. San Diego, CA: Elsevier Academic Press.

Clarke P, Richardson-Burns SM, DeBiasi RL, and Tyler KL (2005) Mechanisms of apoptosis during reovirus infection. In: Griffin DE (ed.) *Role of Apoptosis in Infection. Current Topics in Microbiology and Immunology*, 289: pp. 1–24. Heidelberg: Springer.

Clarke P and Tyler KL (2003) Reovirus-induced apoptosis. *Apoptosis* 8: 141–150.

DeBiasi RL, Robinson BA, Sherry B, *et al.* (2004) Caspase inhibition protects against reovirus-induced myocardial injury *in vitro* and *in vivo*. *Journal of Virology* 78: 11040–11050.

Mertens PPC, Attoui H, Duncan R, and Dermody TS (2004) *Reoviridae*. In: Fauquet CM, Mayo MA, Maniloff J, Desselberger U,, and Ball LA (eds.) *Virus Taxonomy: Eighth Report of the International Committee on Taxonomy of Viruses*, pp. 447–454. San Diego, CA: Elsevier Academic Press.

Nibert ML and Schiff LA (2001) Reoviruses and their replication. In: Knipe DM and Howley PM (eds.) *Fields Virology*, 4th edn., pp. 1679–1728. Philadelphia, PA: Lippincott Williams and Wilkins.

Tyler KL (2001) Mammalian reoviruses. In: Knipe DM and Howley PM (eds.) *Fields Virology*, 4th edn., pp. 1729–1746. Philadelphia, PA: Lippincott Williams and Wilkins.

Tyler KL and Oldstone MBA (eds.) (1998) *Reoviruses. Current Topics in Microbiology and Immunology*, 223 and 224. Heidelberg: Springer.

Virgin HW, IVth, Tyler KL, and Dermody TS (1997) *Reovirus*. In: Nathanson N (ed.) *Viral Pathogenesis*, p. 669. Philadelphia, PA: Lippincott-Raven.

Retroviruses: General Features

E Hunter, Emory University Vaccine Center, Atlanta, GA, USA

Glossary

Lenti From Latin *lentus*, 'slow'; refers to the slow development of pathology associated with lentivirus infections.

Retro From Latin *retro*, 'backward'; refers to the activity of reverse transcriptase and the transfer of genetic information from RNA to DNA.

Spuma From Latin *spuma*, 'foam'; refers to the vacuolated morphology of spumavirus infected cells.

Introduction

The family *Retroviridae* contains a large and diverse group of viruses that infect vertebrates. They are enveloped viruses that undergo a unique replication cycle, which clearly distinguishes them from other viruses. Virions generally contain a single-stranded RNA genome that upon introduction into the target cell is converted to a double-stranded DNA (dsDNA) copy by a process termed reverse transcription. This DNA version of the viral genome is then integrated into the chromosomal DNA of the cell, allowing the virus to persist and produce progeny for as long as the cell lives and providing a mechanism for lifelong infection in the vertebrate host.

The retrovirus family includes two human pathogens, human immunodeficiency virus (HIV), the causative agent of acquired immune deficiency syndrome (AIDS), and human T-lymphotropic virus 1 (HTLV-1), which induces T-cell lymphomas and degenerative nervous system disease in man. The family also includes important pathogens of horses, cows, sheep, cats, and rodents, where members induce cancers, anemias, arthritis, immunodeficiencies, and degenerative disease.

Retroviruses are an ancient group of viruses with archival evidence in the form of endogenous genomes pointing to infections that date back tens of millions of years. They have provided new tools and insights into molecular biology, have yielded clues to the basis of cancer, and continue to impact mankind through their pathogenic potential.

History

Although in 1904 equine infectious anemia was the first retroviral disease to be described, it was not recognized until much later that this was the result of viral infection. Four years later, however, Ellerman and Bang showed that chicken leukosis, a form of leukemia, was caused by a virus, and 3 years after that (1911) Peyton Rous reported cell-free transmission of sarcomas in the chicken. This virus, Rous sarcoma virus (RSV), named after its discoverer, together with the avian leukosis viruses (ALVs), is representative of the genus *Alpharetrovirus*. In part because these observations were made in birds, the scientific community did not immediately appreciate the importance of these oncogenic virus discoveries and it was 25 years before John Bittner identified the first mammalian retrovirus. He demonstrated that mouse mammary tumors were caused by a milk-transmitted, filterable agent. Then in 1957, Ludwik Gross described the development and serial cell-free passage of a highly potent strain of mouse leukemia virus. This was followed over the next two decades by the discovery and isolation of many oncogenic retroviruses from mice, cats, cows, and nonhuman primates.

It was also in the 1950s (1954) that Sigurdsson described visna, a neurological disease in sheep that slowly and progressively induced paralytic symptoms in its host. This led the authors to put forward the concept of slow viral infections and to the nomenclature that now describes members of the genus *Lentivirus* (derived from Latin: *lentus*, slow).

Spumaviruses are unusual in that they were not isolated from a specific disease state but rather from cell cultures derived from a healthy monkey contaminated by a simian member of this genus in 1954. In cell culture, the viruses induce a characteristic foamy appearance in the cytoplasm of the cell and this led to the nomenclature of the genus (derived from Latin: *spuma*, foam).

The first human retrovirus to be described in 1980 was HTLV-1, a member of the genus *Deltaretrovirus*, which induces a cutaneous T-cell lymphoma in a small number of individuals infected years earlier with the virus. It was only 3 years later that human immunodeficiency virus type-1 (HIV-1 – initially called lymphadenopathy-associated virus (LAV)) was isolated from patients with early manifestations of AIDS by Montagnier and his co-workers, and in 1984 that the link between this lentivirus (initially termed HTLV-III) and AIDS was conclusively established by Gallo and his colleagues. Since then numerous nonhuman primate, feline, and bovine members of the genus *Lentivirus* have been described, and they provide powerful animal models for the study of HIV/AIDS.

The archival evidence of previous retroviral infections in the form of endogenous proviruses that are found in high copy number in the genome of several mammalian species, including human, argues for multiple instances of widespread retroviral infections in mammals. Endogenous proviruses can vary from intact genomes capable of producing complete virus (modern endogenous viruses) to highly mutated variants that have evolved with the host and date back tens of millions of years (ancient endogenous retroviruses).

Taxonomy and Classification

The family *Retroviridae* contains two subfamilies: the *Orthoretrovirinae* and the *Spumaretrovirinae*. Differentiation between subfamilies is based on morphological characterization, replication differences, and variation in the expression and function of viral proteins. Six genera are present in the *Orthoretrovirinae*: *Alpharetrovirus*, which includes the avian leukosis and sarcoma viruses; *Betaretrovirus*, which includes mouse mammary tumor virus (MMTV) and Mason–Pfizer monkey virus (M-PMV); *Gammaretrovirus*,

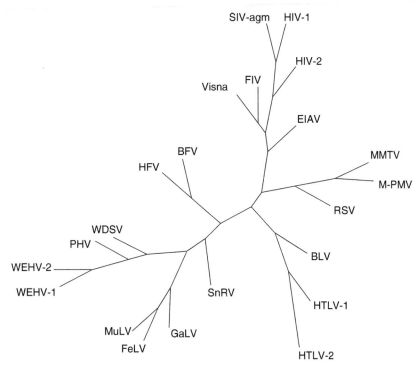

Figure 1 Phylogenetic relationships: phylogenetic analysis of conserved regions of the pol genes of retroviruses. An unrooted neighbor-joining phylogenetic tree was constructed based on an alignment of the amino acid residues of reverse transcriptase genes of several retroviruses. Courtesy of Quackenbush S and Casey J. Reproduced from *Virus Taxonomy: Seventh Report of the International Committee on Taxonomy of Viruses*, Elsevier/Academic Press, with permission.

which contains the mammalian 'C-type' retroviruses, including rodent and primate leukemia and sarcoma viruses and the avian reticuloendotheliosis virus (REV); *Deltaretrovirus*, which includes bovine leukemia virus (BLV) an HTLV-1; *Epsilonretrovirus*, comprising the fish retroviruses, including the walleye dermal sarcoma virus (WDSV); and *Lentivirus*, which include HIV-1 and HIV-2, as well as viruses from ungulates such as visna-maedi and equine infectious anemia virus (EIAV). The subfamily *Spumaretrovirinae* is comprised of a single genus, *Spumavirus*, which contains the prototype foamy virus (PFV; originally named human foamy virus but more recently shown to be of chimpanzee origin). Members of this genus have been isolated from cats, cows, horses, and a variety of nonhuman primates but not from humans. Spumaviruses have replication characteristics intermediate between the orthoretroviruses and members of the *Hepadnaviridae*. Their genomic organization is similar to other retroviruses and reverse transcription of the viral genome is a prerequisite for infection, assembly and budding occur on intracellular membranes, DNA transcription from the RNA genome occurs prior to virus release from the cell, and the viral (reverse) transcriptase is translated independently from a spliced mRNA and requires the viral genome for incorporation (**Figure 1**).

Genome Structure and Organization

The viral genome is genetically diploid, consisting of two linear, positive-sense, single-stranded RNAs that range in size from 7 to 11 kbp depending on the species in question. The RNA monomers are held together in a (70S) dimer through hydrogen bonds in a 5′-located dimer linkage structure. Each monomer of RNA is polyadenylated at the 3′ end and has a cap structure (type 1) at the 5′ end. The purified virion RNA is not infectious and must be converted into a dsDNA provirus via a process of reverse transcription in order for the virus life cycle to proceed. Each RNA monomer has a specific tRNA molecule base-paired to a region (termed the primer binding site) near the 5′ end of the genomic RNA. This tRNA acts as the primer for DNA synthesis on the RNA template.

Infectious viruses have a minimum of four genes that encode the virion structural and replication proteins in the order: 5′-*gag–pro–pol–env*-3′. The *gag* gene encodes the viral structural proteins that are translated initially as a gag polyprotein precursor; *pro* encodes the viral aspartyl proteinase (PR), which mediates polyprotein cleavage during virus maturation; *pol* codes for the reverse transcriptase enzyme (RT) and the viral integrase (IN). RT is responsible for converting the viral RNA genome into a dsDNA provirus, which must then be integrated into the chromosomal DNA of the target cell by the IN protein (**Figure 2**).

Members of the genera *Deltaretrovirus*, *Epsilonretrovirus*, *Lentivirus*, and *Spumavirus* encode additional genes encoding nonstructural proteins important for the regulation of gene expression and for virus replication. The primate lentiviruses appear to have the most complex set of six accessory genes that include *tat*, which encodes a 'transactivator of transcription', and '*rev*', which codes for a protein (Rev) that transports unspliced and partially spliced viral RNA transcripts out of the nucleus. Genes encoding proteins with similar transcription enhancing and RNA transport functions are found in the deltaretroviruses (*tax* and *rex*) and spumaviruses (*tas*).

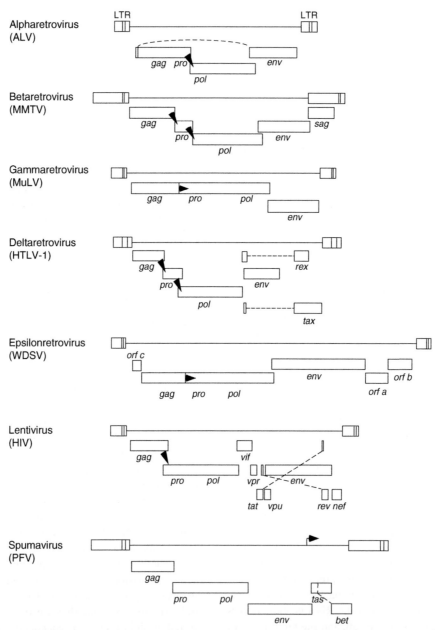

Figure 2 Genomic organization of retroviruses: the different prototypical provirus genomes for each genus are shown indicating the positions of the LTRs and encoded structural genes (*gag, pro, pol, env*) and certain other nonstructural genes (e.g., *tax* and *rex* in the deltaretroviruses) as well as their reading frames (ribosomal frameshift or ribosomal readthrough sites: arrowheads). LTR, long terminal repeat.

Some members of the alpharetroviruses and the gammaretroviruses carry cell-derived sequences that are important in pathogenesis. These cellular sequences are either inserted in a complete retrovirus genome (e.g., some strains of RSV), or in the form of substitutions for deleted viral sequences (e.g., murine sarcoma virus). Such deletions render the virus replication defective and dependent on replication-competent helper viruses for production of infectious progeny. In many cases, the cell-derived sequences form a fused gene with a viral structural gene that is then translated into one chimeric protein (e.g., gag-onc protein).

Virus Morphology

The virions are spherical, enveloped particles 80–100 nm in diameter, that for the most part derive their lipid bilayer from the plasma membrane of an infected cell. Inserted into the viral envelope are glycoprotein surface projections, which are about 8 nm in length and have the appearance of knobbed spikes. An internal core encapsidates the viral ribonucleoprotein and associated replicative enzymes. This structure has a spherical appearance in members of the genera *Alpharetrovirus*, *Gammaretrovirus*, and *Deltaretrovirus* of the subfamily *Orthoretrovirinae* and in members of the subfamily *Spumaretrovirinae*. It is spherical or rod shaped for members of the genus *Betaretrovirus*, and has a truncated cone shape in virions from the genus *Lentivirus*. Retroviruses have a characteristic buoyant density of 1.16–1.18 g cm^{-3} and a sedimentation coefficient (S_{20w}) of approximately 600S in sucrose (**Figure 3**).

Two distinct morphogenic pathways exist. Members of the genera *Alpharetrovirus* and *Gammaretrovirus*, which assemble their immature capsids at the plasma membrane, were historically classified as C-type viruses based on electron microscopy, and members of the genus *Lentivirus* are also assembled via this pathway. In contrast, members of the genus *Betaretrovirus* assemble immature capsids (previously termed A-type particles) in the cytoplasm, which are then enveloped at the plasma membrane with either a B-type (MMTV) or D-type (M-PMV) morphology. Members of the subfamily *Spumaretrovirinae* also assemble immature capsids in the cytoplasm, but these are enveloped primarily at intracellular membranes.

Viral Proteins

The surface of the virion is studded by envelope glycoprotein (Env) spikes comprised of three copies each of two envelope proteins: SU (surface) and TM (transmembrane). These individual components are synthesized as part of a single Env precursor, which is encoded by the viral env gene and is proteolytically cleaved during intracellular transport and prior to assembly into the virus. The number of Env trimers/virion can vary from an estimated low of 7–14 for HIV to a high of more than 150 for primate foamy viruses. SU acts as the receptor-binding component and TM as a membrane-spanning anchor that mediates virus and cell membrane fusion during virus entry.

For members of the *Orthoretrovirinae*, virions contain 3–6 internal, nonglycosylated structural proteins (encoded by the *gag* gene). These are, in order from the N-terminus, (1) MA (matrix protein), (2) a protein, frequently phosphorylated, that in some viruses plays a role in viral budding (3) CA (capsid protein), (4) NC (nucleocapsid protein), and (5) a small C-terminal protein, found in some viruses, that can play a role in assembly and/or budding. These proteins are translated as a single gag polyprotein precursor, which is cleaved by a virus-encoded aspartyl proteinase to the mature products. The MA is often modified with a myristic acid moiety that is covalently linked to the N-terminal glycine. This modification combined with basic residues in the MA domain form a bipartite signal that facilitates intracellular transport of the gag precursor and its association with the plasma membrane. Viruses of the genera *Alpha-*, *Beta-*, and *Gammaretrovirus* encode a protein between MA and CA, which contains one or two motifs that recruit host factors (ESCRT proteins) necessary for successful release of the budding virus from the cell. In primate lentiviruses, these motifs are encoded in a protein at the C-terminus of gag. The CA domain of the Gag precursor plays a key role in immature capsid assembly as well as in the formation of the mature viral core, which encapsidates the viral genome and replicative enzymes. Coating of the viral RNAs by NC appears to facilitate the compact packing of the viral genome into the core.

For members of the subfamily *Spumaretrovirinae*, the Gag protein is only cleaved once near the C-terminus and there are no mature cleavage products analogous to MA or NC of the *Orthoretrovirinae*. Gag also lacks features of other retroviral Gag proteins such as the addition of myristic acid at the N-terminus, the Cys-His boxes of NC, and the major homology region (MHR) of CA. Instead there are three glycine–arginine-rich (GR) boxes near the C-terminus, which are likely involved in assembly and/or RNA binding.

In all retroviruses three nonstructural, enzymatic proteins are incorporated into virions. These are the aspartyl protease (PR, encoded by the *pro* gene), the reverse transcriptase (RT, encoded by the *pol* gene), and integrase (IN, encoded by the *pol* gene). PR is required for cleavage of the Gag precursor, an obligate step in maturation and for

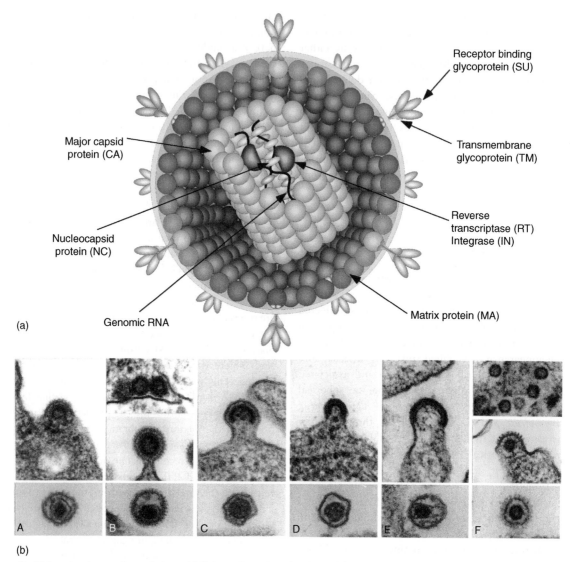

(a)

(b)

Figure 3 Virion structure and morphology. (a) Schematic cartoon (not to scale) shows the inferred locations of the various structures and proteins. (b) A, *Alpharetrovirus*: avian leukosis virus (ALV), type 'C' morphology; B, *Betaretrovirus*: mouse mammary tumor virus (MMTV), type 'B' morphology; C, *Gammaretrovirus*: murine leukemia virus (MLV); D, *Deltaretrovirus*: bovine leukemia virus (BLV); E, *Lentivirus*: human immunodeficiency virus 1 (HIV-1); F, *Spumavirus*: human foamy virus (HFV). The bar represents 100 nm. Reproduced from *Virus Taxonomy: Seventh Report of the International Committee on Taxonomy of Viruses*, Elsevier/Academic Press, with permission.

virus infectivity. In some viruses a dUTPase (DU, role unknown) is also present. Proteins constitute about 60% of the virion dry weight.

Retrovirus Replication Cycle

Attachment and Penetration

Entry into the host cell is mediated by an interaction between the virion glycoproteins and specific protein receptors at the surface of the host cell. This interaction, sometimes aided by low pH in endosomal vesicles,

induces a conformational change in the Env trimer that allows the fusion peptides of the TM proteins to be inserted into the target cell membrane and additional rearrangements of TM, which bring the viral and cell membranes together. Fusion of the viral envelope with the plasma membrane then occurs. Retroviral receptors are cell-surface proteins. For HIV, both the CD4 protein, which is an immunoglobulin-like molecule with a single transmembrane region, and a chemokine receptor (CCR5 or CXCR4), which span the membrane seven times, are required for membrane fusion. The receptors for ecotropic murine leukemia virus (MLV), amphotropic

MLV, and gibbon ape leukemia virus (GALV) as well as M-PMV are involved in the transport of small molecules. These transporters have a complex structure with multiple transmembrane domains. For the ALVs two receptors have been identified: that for subgroup A viruses is a small molecule with a single transmembrane domain, distantly related to a cell receptor for low-density lipoprotein while that for subgroup B viruses is related to the TNF-receptor family of proteins.

Once the viral membrane has fused with that of the target cell, the viral core is exposed to the intracellular environment of the cytoplasm. It is not clear whether a specific uncoating event occurs or whether initiation of nucleic acid transcription is sufficient to partially disassemble the viral core. Subsequent early reverse transcription events are carried out in the cytoplasm in the context of a nucleoprotein complex derived from the mature capsid.

Reverse Transcription

Replication of the viral genome starts with reverse transcription by RT of virion genomic RNA into cDNA. This process was so termed because at the time of its discovery, it reversed the accepted flow of genetic information in the cell. The 3′ end of the genome-associated tRNA acts as a primer for synthesis of a negative-sense cDNA transcript (**Figure 4(b)**). Because the primer binding site is located near the 5′ end of the genome, the initial short product (minus-strand strong stop) must transfer to the 3′ end of the genome through duplicated sequences (R) that are present at each end of the viral RNA. The transferred transcript can now prime continued cDNA synthesis (**Figure 4(c)**).

The RT enzyme is structured such that the DNA synthetic active site is located in close proximity to an RNase H active site that specifically digests the RNA template strand present in the newly formed RNA–DNA

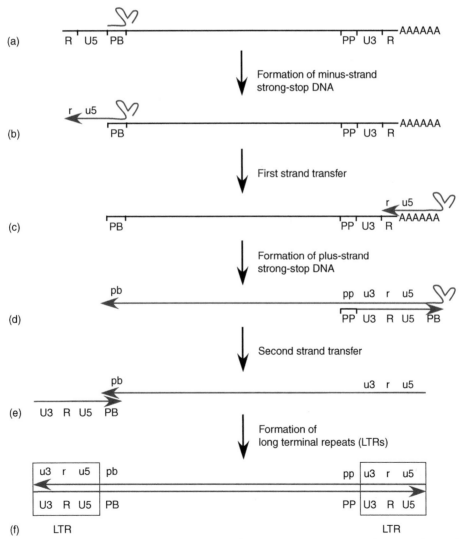

Figure 4 Reverse transcription: process of reverse transcription of the retroviral genome. RNA (black lines), DNA (red lines).

hybrid. Reverse transcription thus involves the concomitant synthesis of DNA and digestion of the viral RNA. Short undigested (purine-rich) RNA products of this process act to prime virus-sense cDNA synthesis on the negative-sense DNA transcripts (**Figure 4(d)**). One of these polypurine primers (PP) located near the 3′ end of the genome initiates a second (plus-strand strong stop) strand transfer, this time using homologies in the tRNA primer-binding site (PB, **Figure 4(e)**). Both strand transfers result in duplication of 5′ and 3′ genomic RNA sequences respectively, so that in its final form the single linear dsDNA transcript derived from the diploid viral genome contains long terminal repeats (LTRs) composed of sequences from the 3′ (U3) and 5′ (U5) ends of the viral RNA that now flank the R sequence (**Figure 4(f)**). A high frequency of recombination is observed during the process of reverse transcription when, following co-infection of a cell, two genetically distinct RNAs are packaged into a retrovirus. This appears to reflect the frequent transfer of the elongating RT from one template RNA to the other, and implies that the RNAs are packaged in the core in a fashion that facilitates this.

Integration

The linear, double-stranded, greater-than-genome-length DNA product of reverse transcription complexed with the viral integrase is called the pre-integration complex (PIC). It must be transported into the nucleus in order for the viral DNA to be integrated into the chromosomal DNA of the host to form an integrated provirus. For most retroviruses, nuclear membrane breakdown during cell division is required for entry of the PIC, but the lentivirus PIC can be transported into the nucleus via nuclear pores, allowing proviral integration in nondividing cells. Integration is mediated by the viral IN protein. The ends of the virus DNA are joined to cell DNA, following the removal of two nucleotides from the ends of the linear viral DNA. Integration generates a short duplication of cell sequences at the integration site, the length of which is virus specific. Proviral DNA can integrate randomly at many sites in the cellular genome with no specific sequence being targeted, although there does appear to be a preference for integration in or near actively transcribed genes. Once integrated, a sequence is generally incapable of further transposition within the same cell. The map of the integrated provirus is collinear with that of unintegrated viral DNA. Integration appears to be a prerequisite for virus replication.

Genomic and mRNA Transcription

The integrated provirus is transcribed by cellular RNA polymerase II into virion RNA and mRNA species in response to transcriptional signals in the U3 region of the viral LTRs. In some genera, virus-encoded transactivating proteins also regulate transcription. Transcription starts at the beginning of the 5′ R region and proceeds to the end of the 3′ R′ sequence. Signals in the U5 region of the 3′ LTR promote cleavage and polyadenylation of the RNA at this site. There are several classes of mRNA depending on the virus and the genetic organization of the retrovirus. With the exception of the spumaviruses, an mRNA comprising the whole retroviral genome serves for the translation of the *gag, pro*, and *pol* genes. This results in the formation of polyprotein precursors, which are the source of the structural proteins, protease, RT, and IN, respectively. A smaller mRNA consisting of the 5′ end of the genome spliced to sequences from the 3′ end of the genome that include the *env* gene and the U3 and R regions, is translated into the precursor of the envelope proteins. In viruses that contain additional genes, various additional forms of spliced mRNA are also made; however, all these spliced mRNAs share a common sequence at their 5′ ends. Spumaviruses are unique in that they make use of an internal promoter (IP) located in the *env* gene upstream of the accessory protein reading frames. Most primary translational products in retrovirus infections are polyproteins, which require proteolytic cleavage before becoming functional. The *gag, pro*, and *pol* products are generally produced from a nested set of primary translation products. For *pro* and *pol*, translation involves bypassing translational termination signals by ribosomal frameshifting or by readthrough at the *gag-pro* and/or the *pro-pol* boundaries (**Figure 1**).

Assembly and Release of Virions

Immature capsids assemble either at the plasma membrane (a majority of the genera) or at intracytoplasmic particles (*Betaretrovirus* and *Spumavirus*). Little is known about the intracellular targeting of Gag precursor proteins within the cell, although the myristic acid modification at the N-terminus of Gag and positively charged amino acids in the MA domain appear to provide a bipartite signal to initiate budding at the plasma membrane. For the betaretroviruses, a short (cytoplasmic targeting/retention) signal (CTRS) in the MA domain of Gag interacts with components of the dynein motor so that translating polysomes are transported to the pericentriolar region (microtubule organizing center) of the cell, where immature capsid assembly occurs. Mutations in the CTRS result in plasma membrane assembly of immature capsids. A similar mechanism for intracellular targeting and assembly of Gag appears to be utilized by the spumaviruses.

Most retroviruses are released from the cell by a process of budding from a region of the plasma membrane where viral glycoproteins must also be targeted. There is evidence in several genera that interaction of Gag and Env components occurs at an intracellular location prior to co-localization at the budding site. This process of budding, however, does not appear to require the Env proteins since expression of Gag alone is sufficient for release of virus particles. The final pinching-off and release of virus requires the complex cellular machinery (ESCRT) normally involved in multivesicular body formation, which is recruited to the site of budding by sequence motifs in Gag. Polyprotein processing of the internal proteins occurs concomitant with or just subsequent to release of virus from the cell and is accompanied by maturation of the virion. This includes morphological changes that include condensation of the viral RNA into an electron-dense ribonucleoprotein core and the acquisition of infectivity.

Pathogenesis

Members of the family *Retroviridae* establish persistent lifelong infections in their hosts – a reflection of their replication cycle and their ability to insert a copy of the proviral genome into the chromosome of a target cell. Because retroviruses are in general noncytopathic to their host cells and function as effective parasites that siphon off only a small percentage of the macromolecular machinery, continued production of progeny viruses over the lifespan of the cell is thus the norm. Moreover, in the context of the vertebrate host, this means that curing infection is effectively impossible, since a single retrovirus-infected cell can be the source of systemic infection.

Viruses from several retroviral genera are capable of inducing tumor formation in their natural hosts. It was the 'acute transforming' retroviruses, exemplified by RSV, that provided the key to our initial understanding of how retroviruses induce cancer in their hosts. These viruses, members of the genera *Alpha-* and *Gammaretrovirus*, have transduced cellular genes (now known as proto-oncogenes) that function in the signal transduction pathways involved in growth factor upregulation of cell proliferation. With the exception of certain RSV isolates, these acutely ransforming retroviruses are generally replication defective, since the inserted oncogene replaces replicative genes, and require a helper virus to provide the missing replicative functions. Nevertheless, they are capable of rapidly inducing a variety of cancers in their hosts. The replication-competent WDSV, a member of the genus *Epsilonretrovirus*, also induces cell transformation through expression of a cell-derived gene, although in this case it is related to the cyclin family of regulators.

For the so-called 'chronic transforming' members of the genera *Alpha-*, *Beta-*, and *Gammaretrovirus*, persistent infection with the high numbers of associated viral integration events eventually results in the insertional activation of cellular oncogenes. This was first defined for ALV where, in birds with this form of leukemia, frequent integrations just upstream of the *c-myc* oncogene

in malignantly transformed cells were found to result in its unregulated expression. Related mechanisms that deregulate cellular oncogene expression have been described for MMTV, MuLV, and other vertebrate 'leukemia' viruses. The human pathogen HTLV-1 induces T-cell-derived tumors in a fraction of infected individuals but this appears in part to be the result of *trans*-activation of cellular genes such as Il-2 and Il-2 receptors as well as inactivation of cell-cycle regulators such as p53 by Tax, which leads to unregulated proliferation of T-cells.

Members of the genus *Lentivirus*, including visna-maedi virus, EIAV, caprine arthritis encephalitis virus (CAEV), and HIV-1, generally establish persistent infections that progressively impose a defined pathology on their host. It was the progressive central nervous system degeneration in sheep induced by visna virus that led to the term 'slow infections' and to the nomenclature for this genus. The human pathogen HIV-1 is typical of members of the genus; although it is cytopathic in CD4+ T-lymphocytes, it establishes a persistent disease through constant cycles of infection of lymphocytes and macrophages in lymphoid tissues. Generally, it takes several years for depletion of the immune system to progress to a level where opportunistic infections and cancers, which are the hallmark of AIDS, develop. Interestingly, the simian immunodeficiency viruses (SIVs) do not appear to cause disease in their natural hosts, where presumably there has been co-evolution of virus and host to reach a nonpathogenic equilibrium.

See also: AIDS: Disease Manifestation; AIDS: Global Epidemiology; Retroviral Oncogenes.

Further Reading

Desrosiers R (2007) Nonhuman lentiviruses. In: Knipe DM, Howley PM, Griffin DE, *et al.* (eds.) *Fields Virology*, 5th edn., pp. 2215–2241. Philadelphia, PA: Lippincott Williams and Wilkins.

Freed EO and Martin MA (2007) HIVs and their replication. In: Knipe DM, Howley PM, Griffin DE, *et al.* (eds.) *Fields Virology*, 5th edn., pp. 2107–2185. Philadelphia, PA: Lippincott Williams and Wilkins.

Goff SP (2007) *Retroviridae*: The retroviruses and their replication. In: Knipe DM, Howley PM, Griffin DE, *et al.* (eds.) *Fields Virology*, 5th edn., pp. 1999–2069. Philadelphia, PA: Lippincott Williams and Wilkins.

Kuritzkes DR and Walker B (2007) HIV-1: Pathogenesis, clinical manifestations, and treatment. In: Knipe DM, Howley PM, Griffin DE, *et al.* (eds.) *Fields Virology*, 5th edn., pp. 2187–2214. Philadelphia, PA: Lippincott Williams and Wilkins.

Lairmore MD and Franchini G (2007) Human T-cell leukemia viruses types 1 and 2. In: Knipe DM, Howley PM, Griffin DE, *et al.* (eds.) *Fields Virology*, 5th edn., pp. 2070–2105. Philadelphia, PA: Lippincott Williams and Wilkins.

Linial M (2007) Foamy viruses. In: Knipe DM, Howley PM, Griffin DE, *et al.* (eds.) *Fields Virology*, 5th edn., pp. 2245–2262. Philadelphia, PA: Lippincott Williams and Wilkins.

Linial ML, Fan H, Hahn B, *et al.* (2004) *Retroviridae*. In: Fauquet CM, Mayo MA, Maniloff J, Desselberger U, and Ball LA (eds.) *Virus Taxonomy: Eighth Report of the International Committee on Taxonomy of Viruses*, pp. 421–440. San Diego, CA: Elsevier Academic Press.

Rhinoviruses

N W Bartlett and S L Johnston, Imperial College London, London, UK

Glossary

Afebrile Without a fever.

Bronchopulmonary dysplasia Chronic lung disease of infancy that follows mechanical ventilation and oxygen therapy for acute respiratory distress after birth in premature newborns.

Ciliated Cells with hair-like structures (cilia) on the surface.

Cytopathology Cell damage.

Endocytosis Uptake of material into the cell by membrane-bound vesicles.

Endosome Membrane-bound vesicle formed during endocytosis.

Heterotypic Of different types.

Nasal mucosa Mucous membrane lining the nasal cavity.

Nasopharynx The portion of the pharynx extending from the posterior nares to the level of the soft palate.

Nim Neutralizing immunogenic site.

Otitus media Infection and inflammation of the middle ear space and ear drum.

Peak expiratory flow The maximum flow at the outset of forced expiration.

Rhinorrhoea The free discharge of a thin nasal mucus.

Sinusitis Inflammation of the sinus.

TBP TATA-binding protein, part of RNA polymerase II transcription system.

History

Rhinoviruses are the most common infectious agents of humans and most frequent cause of the common cold (acute nasopharyngitis), a mild disease of the upper respiratory tract. More recently, their role in acute exacerbations of asthma and other airway disease has been highlighted, implicating the virus in illnesses significantly more severe than the common cold. Hieroglyphs representing the cough and common cold date back to ancient Egypt. In the fifth century BC Hippocrates gave a description of the disease and in the first century Pliny the Elder suggested 'kissing the hairy muzzle of a mule' as therapy for colds. The common cold was also known among the ancient American Indian, Aztec, and Maya civilizations. It was not until first Walter Kruse and then Alphonse Donchez in the early part of the twentieth century demonstrated that viruses (filtered material from the nasal secretions from a cold sufferer) caused the common cold. The first isolations of human rhinovirus (HRV) were reported by two laboratories in the late 1950s: Price in 1956 and Pelon and co-workers in 1957. With advances in tissue culture techniques that matched temperature and pH conditions to those found in the nose, identification of serologically distinct rhinoviruses increased rapidly such that by 1987 100 serotypes had been identified (**Table 1**). Efforts in the 1960s and 1970s to develop vaccines based on inactivated or attenuated viruses were unsuccessful due to the large number of rhinovirus serotypes and ineffective mucosal immunization. Lack of a practical small animal model for rhinovirus infection has meant that experimental human challenge models have been used to study virus pathogenesis. Although it has been long recognized that rhinovirus infections are the most frequent cause of the common cold, recent epidemiologic studies using sensitive polymerase chain reaction (PCR) techniques and data from human studies has highlighted the importance of rhinoviruses as precipitants of serious respiratory illnesses. This is especially evident in the context of persons suffering chronic airway diseases such as asthma and chronic obstructive pulmonary disease (COPD).

Taxonomy and Classification

The family *Picornaviridae* (pico = small + RNA) contains three genera of human pathogens that are structurally and genetically closely related: enterovirus, parechovirus, and rhinovirus. Rhinoviruses have been isolated from humans and cattle, with HRVs comprising by far the largest group. The HRV genus currently consists of 102 serotypes (HRV-1A to HRV-1B and HRV-2 to HRV-100, Hanks). Designation of serotypes is based on antibody neutralization, with absence of cross-reactivity of polyclonal antisera with defined serotypes constituting designation of a distinct serotype. (It should be noted that extensive serotyping has not been performed since the 1980s and several rhinovirus isolates await classification and may represent new serotypes.) The three bovine rhinoviruses (BRV-1–3) also await classification. All serotypes (except HRV-87) segregate into two genetic clusters or species based on nucleotide sequence across the VP4/VP2 interval: human rhinovirus A (HRV-A; 76 serotypes) and human rhinovirus B (HRV-B; 25 serotypes). Analysis of nucleotide sequences from HRV87 demonstrated that it is an enterovirus, most closely related to human enterovirus 68 (species D). The rhinovirus genus can also be

Table 1 Species[a] and receptor binding[b] grouping of human rhinovirus serotypes (excluding HRV-87)

Human rhinovirus A	Human rhinovirus B
1A, **1B**, **2**, 7, 8, 9, 10, 11, 12, 13, 15, 16, 18, 19, 20, 21, 22, 23, 24, 25, 28, **29**, **30**, **31**, 32, 33, 34, 36, 38, 39, 40, 41, 43, **44**, 45, 46, **47**, **49**, 50, 51, 53, 54, 55, 56, 57, 58, 59, 60, 61, **62**, 63, 64, 65, 66, 67, 68, 71, 73, 74, 75, 76, 77, 78, 80, 81, 82, 85, 88, 89, 90, 94, 95, 96, 98, 100	3, 4, 5, 6, 14, 17, 26, 27, 35, 37, 42, 48, 52, 69, 70, 72, 79, 83, 84, 86, 91, 92, 93, 97, 99

[a]Species classification is based on genetic clustering of capsid (VP4/VP2) gene nucleotide sequences.
[b]Viruses shown in bold type bind to the LDL receptor (minor group); the remainder bind to ICAM-1 (major group).

classified into two groups according to receptor tropism, with approximately 90% of HRV (major receptor group) exploiting the intercellular adhesion molecule 1 (ICAM-1, CD54) for cell binding. The remainder (minor receptor group) use members of the low-density lipoprotein (LDL) receptor family. HRV-87 uses an as yet unknown sialoprotein for cell-surface attachment. The rhinovirus genus can also be divided into two groups according to the variability in susceptibility to capsid-binding drugs. The pattern of susceptibility has served as an alternative method of classification of HRV serotypes into two groups, A and B.

Virion Structure and Physical Properties

Rhinoviruses, typical of the family *Picornaviridae*, are small (approximately 30 nm, molecular mass of 8.5×10^6 kDa) icosahedral particles (**Figure 1**) composed of 60 copies of each of the four capsid proteins VP1–VP4 with molecular masses of 32, 29, 26, and 7 kDa, respectively. The capsid proteins are symmetrically arranged into protomers which contain one copy of VP1, VP3, and a precursor (VP0) in which VP2 and VP4 are covalently linked. Protomers, arranged around a fivefold axis, form pentamers and 12 pentamers form the icosahedral capsid shell. Capsid precursors encapsidate viral genomic RNA to form 150S provirions. Maturation cleavage of VP0 to VP2 and VP4 is the final step of assembly and yields infectious mature virions. VP1, VP2, and VP3 structurally constitute most of the capsid. They are similar in structure and have eight-stranded, antiparallel β-barrel motifs differing mainly in the loops and elaborations which join or project from the β-strands. VP1 is the most external and dominant structural protein and contains most of the motifs known to interact with cellular receptors and neutralize monoclonal antibodies. VP4 is smaller, has an extended structure, and lies at the RNA–capsid interface in close association with the RNA core and functions as an anchor to the virus capsid. A deep cleft, called the canyon, surrounds the fivefold axes of icosahedral symmetry and encloses the ICAM-1 binding site in the major receptor group viruses. Amino acids at the base of the canyon are more conserved than those on the protruding rim of the canyon and surface of the virion, which are more prone to substitutions and contain the binding sites for neutralizing

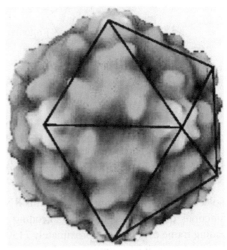

Figure 1 Human rhinovirus 14 solved by cryoelectron microscopy and image reconstruction. The fivefold axis of symmetry is superimposed on the image. Courtesy of The Big Picture Book of Viruses.

antibody. Beneath this canyon, within VP1, lies a pore that leads to a hydrophobic pocket occupied by a pocket factor that is likely to be a fatty acid. The minor group LDL receptor binds to the star-shaped dome on the fivefold axis of the virion.

Rhinoviruses have a buoyant density in CsCl of 1.38–1.42. The property that distinguishes them from the closely related enteroviruses is their acid lability with inactivation occurring below pH 6. In contrast most rhinoviruses are thermostable, surviving for days at 20–37 °C. The ability to survive for extended periods of time in the environment is likely to be an important factor in their spread. Several serotypes (3–12, 15, 18, and 19) are relatively stable at 50 °C for 1 h. The lack of a lipid membrane enables rhinoviruses to resist 20% ether, 5% chloroform, and sodium deoxycholate solutions. Alcohol/phenol disinfectants are effective virucidal agents.

Properties of the Rhinovirus Genome

The nonenveloped virion encapsidates a genome composed of a single-stranded positive-(messenger) sense

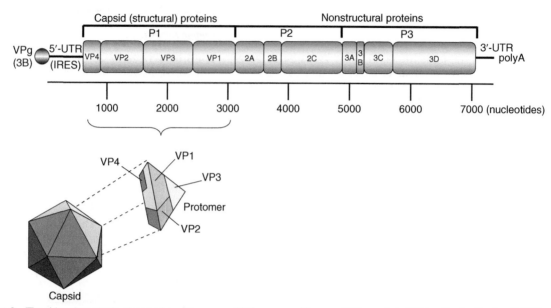

Figure 2 The rhinovirus single-stranded positive-sense RNA genome. The small VPg protein (3B) is attached to the 5′-UTR which encodes a type I internal ribosome entry site (IRES). The genome is polyadenylated (polyA) at the 3′ terminus. The single polyprotein encoded by the genome is cleaved by proteases to yield individual capsid and nonstructural proteins.

RNA molecule of 7100–7400 nucleotides. This RNA molecule functions directly as a message, encoding a single open reading frame containing approximately 2150 codons flanked at both termini by untranslated regions (UTRs) (**Figure 2**). At the 5′ terminus the 600-nucleotide-long UTR is covalently linked to a small, virus-encoded protein, VPg which initiates viral RNA synthesis. The UTRs have important secondary and tertiary structures; the first 100 nucleotides of the 5′-UTR forms a clover leaf structure that binds viral and host proteins forming a nucleoprotein complex required for viral RNA replication. The RNA molecule is directly translated from a type I internal ribosome entry site (IRES) also located in the 5′-UTR which directs recruitment of host-cell ribosomes and cap-independent translation of viral proteins. Downstream of the 5′-UTR is the capsid-coding region (P1), followed by the nonstructural protein encoding regions P2 and P3. The 3′ terminus of the genome contains a short (approximately 40 nucleotides) UTR and terminates with a poly-A tail. The single ~250 kDa polyprotein encoded by the rhinovirus genome is processed both during and after translation into mature viral proteins by a sequence of cleavages executed by virus-encoded proteases.

Properties of Rhinovirus Proteins

The rhinovirus proteins are numbered 1A(VP4), 1B(VP2), 1C(VP3), 1D(VP1), 2A, 2B, 2C, 3A, 3B, 3C, 3D, according to their physical location in the unprocessed polyprotein. The polyprotein is proteolytically cleaved to yield four capsid (structural) proteins and ten nonstructural

proteins: seven mature proteins and three intermediate proteins with functions distinct from their cleavage products (2BC, 3AB, and 3CD^{pro}). Three of the products of polyprotein processing function as proteases (^{pro}) while 3D^{pol} is the virally encoded RNA-dependent RNA polymerase. All of the nonstructural proteins are required for replication of the viral RNA. In addition, some nonstructural proteins alter host-cell function. The VPg protein (3B) acts as a primer for the initiation of RNA synthesis. Proteins 2A^{pro} and 3C^{pro} are cysteine proteases involved in processing the viral polyprotein. The first cleavage is catalyzed by 2A^{pro} which cleaves only at tyrosine–glycine bonds and performs the primary cleavage between the capsid and nonstructural precursors at the junction of the C terminus of VP1 and its own N terminus releasing P1. The 2A^{pro} also mediates shutdown of host-cell translation by cleaving cellular eIF-4G, a key factor in cap-dependent translation. The 3C^{pro} catalyzes most of the subsequent cleavage events on the picornaviral polyprotein and along with the 3CD^{pro} cleaves the polyprotein at glutamine–glycine bonds. Rhinovirus 3C^{pro} may also play a role in virus-induced shutoff of host-cell transcription (by RNA polymerase II) by cleavage of the transcription factor TBP. It is thought that 3C enters the nucleus via a nuclear localization signal within the 3CD precursor. Experiments with the 2B protein of enteroviruses indicate that this viral protein is a 'viroporin' increasing plasma membrane permeability and inhibiting secretory pathways. The 3A protein may also modulate the secretory functions of cells affecting surface expression of host major histocompatibility complex (MHC) class I.

Life Cycle

Entry, Replication, and Assembly

The major group HRVs utilize ICAM-1 to attach to cells. ICAM-1 is a cell-surface glycoprotein and a member of the immunoglobulin (Ig) protein superfamily. Once bound to the receptor the viral particle is internalized by receptor-mediated endocytosis. Replication of rhinoviruses takes place in the cytoplasm of host cells. Uncoating and release of the viral RNA into the cytoplasm occurs after acidification of the late endosome. Acidification triggers conformational changes in the capsid centered on the fivefold axis, where a channel through the capsid and the endosomal membrane opens allowing RNA release. The positive-(message) sense RNA genome is translated into a single large polyprotein from the IRES located in the 5′-UTR of the rhinovirus genome. The IRES forms a complex secondary structure which can direct ribosomes to the polyprotein start AUG, thus initiating cap-independent translation. This allows the synthesis of viral proteins while cap-dependent translation of cellular proteins is shut off. The polyprotein is processed into functionally active proteins through a sequence of cleavages performed by virus-encoded proteases (described in the previous section). The cloverleaf secondary structure of the 5′-UTR in the viral genome binds viral (3C or 3CD precursor) and host (poly(A)-binding protein) proteins to form a nucleoprotein complex required for RNA replication, which is catalyzed by newly synthesized 3D^{pol} (viral RNA-dependent RNA polymerase), the most highly conserved polypeptide among members of the family *Picornaviridae*. Initially primed by the terminally bound VPg protein, the viral RNA polymerase uses the genomic positive-sense RNA as a template for synthesizing negative-sense copies which in turn act as templates for positive-sense RNA synthesis. Some newly synthesized positive-sense RNA copies act as messages, whereas others are packaged into virus particles. The viral polymerase has a mutation rate of one every 2200 bases (approximately four mutations per transcript) and is therefore at the threshold for genetic maintenance. This characteristic in conjunction with the ability to undergo viral recombination is probably a significant reason why rhinoviruses are such efficient pathogens of humans.

There is still much not known about the assembly of virus particles. Capsid assembly is via the precursor 5S protomers and 14S pentamers already described and takes place in association with membranes. RNA is thought to be packaged into pre-formed 80S capsids although the molecular mechanism by which this process occurs is not well understood. Maturation to yield infectious virus relies on cleavage of VP0 into VP2 and VP4. Productive infection induces apoptosis (programmed cell death) and cell lysis facilitating release of virus from the cytoplasm.

Host Range, Propagation, and Detection

HRVs exhibit a high degree of species specificity due to the inability to bind nonhuman ICAM-1 on the cell surface. In addition, there appears to be a block to viral replication in nonpermissive cells. As a result efficient growth occurs only in human and some primate cells. An attempt to adapt a serotype for a mouse infection model had limited success and currently no small-animal HRV infection model has been reported. Nonhuman cells can be made permissive for infection if manipulated to express human ICAM-1 on the cell surface. Primary cells such as human embryonic kidney, bronchial epithelial, tonsil, and continuous human cell lines such as HeLa, H292, and HEP-2 can support growth of HRVs. The most commonly used cells for rhinovirus growth are the WI-38 strain and the MRC-5 strain of diploid fibroblasts, foetal tonsil cells, and HRV-sensitive HeLa (e.g., Ohio HeLa). Growth of virus in cell monolayers is usually detected by the appearance of cytopathic effect (CPE), which initially appears as foci of rounded up cells. HRVs can be plaqued on a number of cell lines with most techniques employing a semisolid overlay. Many HRV serotypes, particularly group B members, do not grow well in tissue culture. Nevertheless virus culture in susceptible cell lines has been the 'gold standard' for laboratory diagnosis of respiratory virus infections. However tissue culture techniques are generally laborious, time consuming, and insensitive when compared with more recent PCR-based assays. For this RNA is extracted from potentially infected samples and copied to cDNA by reverse transcription. PCR using HRV-specific primers targeting conserved viral sequences, such as the 5′-UTR, is then performed to determine the presence of viral genetic material in the original sample. PCR techniques have advanced further with the development of quantitative real-time PCR (qRT-PCR). This technique is more sensitive than conventional PCR and enables the number of viral RNA copies in a sample to be measured. In addition to direct detection of HRV by culture or PCR, antiviral antibodies can be measured by serological methods such as enzyme-linked immunosorbent assay (ELISA). Serological assays are diagnostically useful only when the HRV serotype is already known (i.e., for research purposes such as experimental human infections).

Serological Relationship and Antigenic Variability

With over 100 immunologically distinct serotypes currently recognized HRVs exhibit remarkable antigenic variability. The existence of a large number of HRV serotypes is in contrast to two other medically important picornaviruses, the polioviruses (three serotypes) and hepatitis A virus (a single serotype). While the development of virus-specific neutralizing antibody correlates with protection from disease, anti-HRV antibodies are highly serotype specific, rarely exhibiting cross-serotype neutralizing activity. Several serotypes can be grouped on the basis of low-level immunological cross-reactivity with hyperimmune rabbit serum (HRV-36, -58, and -89, for example), but it is not known whether this plays any role in cross-serotype protection. Mutagenesis studies have identified four neutralizing immunogenic sites along the edge of the capsid canyon. Nim-1a and Nim-1b on VP1 are located above the canyon, and Nim-2 on VP2 and Nim-3 on VP3 are positioned below. Structural analyses of neutralizing antibodies complexed with virus indicate that effective neutralizing activity depends on bivalent antibody binding that both blocks receptor interaction and stabilizes the virus capsid. Typically the most effective neutralizing antibodies bind with high affinity and span the canyon receptor site. In contrast to antibody responses, T-cell responses may be cross-reactive against numerous HRV serotypes, with the major T-cell epitopes buried within the viral capsid where amino acid sequences are more conserved.

Epidemiology

The common cold is almost certainly the commonest illness affecting mankind, occurring in all populations and ages throughout the year. The illness that results from infection is a major cause of morbidity and in turn lost productivity through absenteeism from work or school. Infection rates are highest among infants and children who may be infected up to 12 times a year. Infection rates decrease with age with adults infected on average 2 to 5 times per year. Infections exhibit a seasonal pattern and are more prevalent in autumn and in late spring. It is clear that school attendance is a major contributing factor to seasonality of infection. HRVs cause between 35% and 60% of common colds. While cold exposure does not seem to be a contributing factor to susceptibility to HRV infection, factors such as age and family structure are clearly important. Infections increase significantly from the second year of life, peak around the age of 6, and decline thereafter. The family unit is a major site for spread of HRV in modern societies. Most often an infected child introduces the infection into the family with other siblings and the mother most at risk of secondary infection, presumably because of increased exposure. Schools and day-care centers are also sites of high transmission due to overcrowding, low immunity, and the unhygienic habits of children. Rhinoviruses have also been shown to spread among university students and boarding school residents. HRVs also cause a significant number of afebrile respiratory illnesses in military populations. All populations are affected and observations indicate that multiple HRV serotypes circulate within a population at any given time, and prevalent serotypes change from year to year.

Pathogenesis of Rhinovirus-Induced Disease

Transmission

Two routes are likely to be important for person to person spread of rhinovirus infection via virus-contaminated respiratory secretions: direct hand–surface–hand contact and aerosol inhalation. Rhinoviruses are able to survive on environmental surfaces for several hours at ambient temperature. HRVs were recovered from up to 90% of hands of persons with a cold and from a range of environmental objects such as door knobs, dolls, cups, and glasses. Transfer of virus through touching such objects occurs in seconds. Subsequent rubbing of the nose or eyes with infected hands can result in direct inoculation. Despite compelling evidence supporting direct transmission, demonstrating this in natural circumstances has been less convincing. In contrast there is good evidence suggesting inhalation of aerosols is the major route of HRV infection.

The incubation period preceding virus shedding is 1–4 days, usually 2–3 days. Virus in nasal secretions peaks 2–4 days post infection and remains high for 7–10 days, although low levels may persist for as long as several weeks. Atopic asthmatic subjects may have impaired virus clearance and increased virus load, factors that correlate with increased severity of illness. High virus titers in nasal secretions, increased symptoms, time spent in contact, and social factors such as crowding and poor hygiene contribute to increased transmission of virus.

Pathogenesis and Clinical Features

The nose is the main portal for HRV entry into the body and the primary site of replication is the epithelial surface of nasal mucosa. The virus is then transported to the posterior nasopharynx by ciliated epithelial cells. Clinical signs of illness are generally limited to common cold-like symptoms. HRV replication may also occur in the lower airways and this may actually be a common occurrence following infection of the upper airways. Unlike influenza or adenovirus infections HRV infection produces little, if any cytopathology of the nasal mucous membrane. The absence of histopathology in infected nasal mucosa initially led to the suggestion that mediators of inflammation produced by infected cells in the airway are responsible for cold symptoms. HRV infection *in vitro* and *in vivo* induces production of numerous pro-inflammatory and immune mediators including interferons (IFN-α/β, IFN-λ), chemokines that attract neutrophils (CXCL8/IL-8, CXCL5/ENA-78, CXCL1/GROα), esoinophils

(Eotaxin/CCL10, CCL5/RANTES) or lymphocytes (CCL5/ RANTES, CXCL10/IP-10), pro-inflammatory cytokines (IL-1β, IL-2, IL-4, IL-11, IL-12, IL-13, IL-16, IFN-γ, and TNFα), growth and differentiation factors (IL-6, G-CSF, GM-CSF, IL-11), cell adhesion molecules ICAM-1 and vascular cell adhesion molecule (VCAM), and respiratory mucins. The presence of an array of pro-inflammatory mediators is supportive of an immune rather than cytopathic mechanism of rhinovirus-induced illness (**Figure 3**).

Rhinovirus infections are usually relatively trivial, producing symptoms of the common cold including rhinorrhoea, sneezing, nasal discharge and obstruction, coughing, and sore throat. Fever and malaise are less commonly seen than in other respiratory virus infections. Sleep patterns are often disrupted affecting mood and mental functioning. Symptoms appear after a 24–48 h incubation period, peak 2–3 days later, and last for 5–7 days in total, but may persist for up to 2–4 weeks.

Severity of symptoms resulting from HRV infections is highly variable ranging from a barely apparent illness to a non-influenza flu-like disease. The most common complications associated with infection of the upper respiratory tract in children are acute otitis media and sinusitis. Rhinoviruses can also infect the lower respiratory tract and thereby account for lower respiratory symptoms and can cause serious and debilitating disease, particularly in young children, the elderly, the immunocompromised, and patients with chronic disorders such as cystic fibrosis and bronchopulmonary dysplasia. In patients hospitalized with respiratory problems rhinovirus infection has been associated with pneumonia in infants, wheezing in asthmatic children, exacerbations of chronic bronchitis, asthma and COPD, and congestive heart failure in older adults. HRV infection is the most frequent causative agent of asthma exacerbations. Recent studies have demonstrated that 80–85% of asthma exacerbations in children are associated with respiratory virus infections, with rhinoviruses

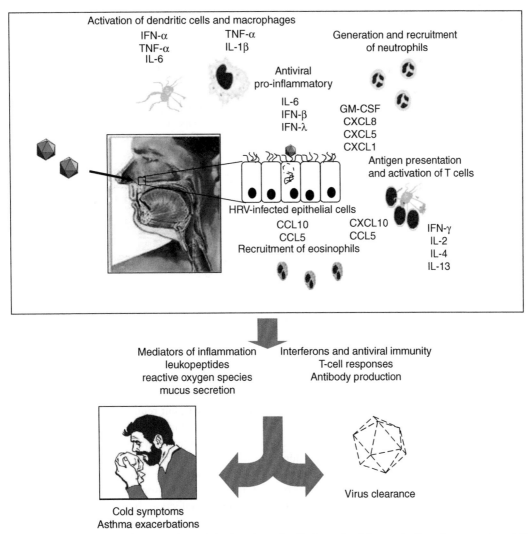

Figure 3 Mechanism of rhinovirus-induced illness. Infection of nasal epithelium stimulates production of a range of pro-inflammatory mediators causing immunopathology usually associated with cold symptoms, or exacerbations of asthma in susceptible individuals.

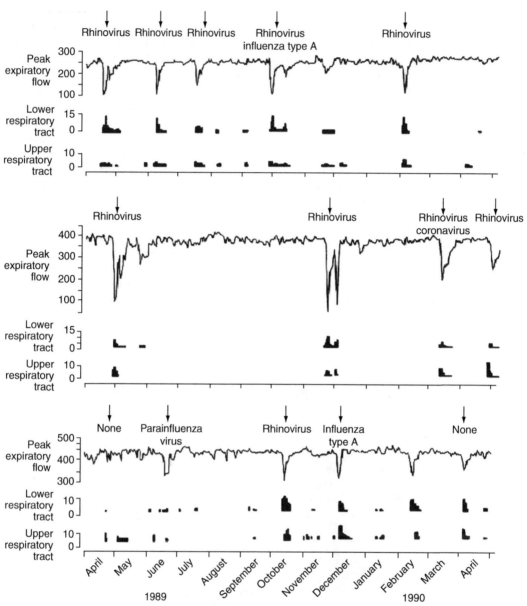

Figure 4 Association of marked reductions in lung function (peak expiratory flow) and exacerbations of lower respiratory tract symptoms with rhinovirus infection for three asthmatic children. Reproduced from SL Johnston, PK Pattemore, G Sanderson, *et al.* (1995) Community study of role of viral infections in exacerbations of asthma in 9–11-year-old children. *British Medical Journal* 310(6989): 1225–1229, with permission from BMJ Publishing Group.

accounting for two-thirds of these infections or 50% of all exacerbations (**Figure 4**).

Immune Response and Immunity

Serum antibody specific to the infecting HRV develops between 7 and 14 days after inoculation, but initially antibody-free volunteers may take up to 21 days to be detected. Virus-specific IgG and IgA antibodies remain low for the first week post infection, peaking approximately a week later. The dominant serum antibody response to infection is IgG1, followed by IgG3, IgG4, and IgG2; IgA1 is the dominant IgA subclass. IgG antibodies stay at high levels for at least a year, while IgA levels decline slowly, but remain detectable for the same period. IgA is the dominant immunoglobulin in nasal secretions, becoming detectable 2 weeks post inoculation, peaking 1 week later. Serum and secretory antibody persist for several years after infection, although levels decline. Given that HRV-specific antibodies appear relatively late in the infection, humoral immunity is likely to be not essential for recovery from viral illness but may be involved in final viral clearance. Preexisting antibodies are likely to be important in protection from reinfection with the same serotype. Mechanisms of antibody mediated virus inactivation might include virus aggregation and complement activation, blocking receptor binding and stabilization of capsid to prevent uncoating.

Cellular immunity is also activated following HRV infection. In contrast to the highly serotype-specific humoral response, virus-specific lymphocytes may be activated by several serotypes indicating shared viral epitopes, but their role in subsequent protection is not known.

Prevention and Control

Currently there are no effective strategies for prevention or treatment of rhinovirus common colds. The large number of serotypes and lack of heterotypic humoral immunity is a major issue precluding the use of conventional vaccine approaches. Vaccine enhancement of virus-specific cell-mediated immunity may be a more promising approach since T-cell epitopes are more conserved. The lack of a vaccine or specific therapies and the commonness of the illness have resulted in the emergence of numerous nonspecific therapies for the common cold. These include ascorbic acid, zinc gluconate, echinacea, and inhalation of hot humidified air. The efficacy of any nonspecific measure in prevention or treatment of the cold is yet to be generally accepted. Most work has been invested into the development of chemotherapeutic approaches. These include pharmacological antiviral agents that indirectly inhibit virus replication such as IFN-α. Studies demonstrated that IFN-α was effective in preventing the onset of cold symptoms when administered prophylactically. However it had little to no effect when given after infection and was often associated with various side effects. A large number of compounds designed to inhibit virus uncoating and/or cell binding and entry have been studied. So far an effective drug free of side effects is

yet to emerge from this research. One such drug, Pleconaril, was submitted for approval to market as a treatment for the common cold in adults. Evidence showed that Pleconaril reduced the duration of cold symptoms if taken within the first 24 h of a cold. Unfortunately, the drug was not approved due to interactions in test subjects with the oral contraceptive and associated side effects. Another approach has involved blocking virus binding to cells using a soluble form of the receptor. A number of reports have demonstrated that soluble ICAM-1 inactivates the virus and is effective at inhibiting viral entry. Despite encouraging results with soluble ICAM-1 no development is currently ongoing for these agents due to problems with formulation and delivery.

See also: Common Cold Viruses.

Further Reading

Contoli M, Message SD, Laza-Stanca V, *et al.* (2006) Role of deficient type III interferon-lambda production in asthma exacerbations. *Nature Medicine* 12(9): 1023–1026.

Couch RB (2001) Rhinoviruses. In: Knipe DM, Howely PM, Griffin DE, *et al.* (eds.) *Fields Virology,* 4th edn., pp. 777–797. Philadelphia, PA: Lippincott Williams and Wilkins.

Edwards ME, Kebadze T, Johnson MW, and Johnston SL (2006) New treatment regimes for virus-induced exacerbations of asthma. *Pulmonary Pharmacology and Therapeutics* 19: 320–334.

Heikkinen T and Jarvinen A (2003) The common cold. *Lancet* 361(9351): 51–59.

Johnston SL, Patterson PK, Sanderson G, *et al.* (1995) Community study of role of viral infections in exacerbations of asthma in 9–11-year-old children. *British Medical Journal* 310(6989): 1225–1229.

Papadopoulos NG and Johnston SL (2004) Rhinoviruses. In: Zuckerman AJ, Bantavala JR, Griffiths PD,, and Schoub BD (eds.) *Principles and Practice of Clinical Virology,* 5th edn., pp. 361–377. West Sussex, England: Wiley.

Wark PA, Johnston SL, Bucchieri F, *et al.* (2005) Asthmatic bronchial epithelial cells have a deficient innate immune response to infection with rhinovirus. *Journal of Experimental Medicine* 201(6): 937–947.

Rotaviruses

J Angel and M A Franco, Pontificia Universidad Javeriana, Bogota, Republic of Colombia
H B Greenberg, Stanford University School of Medicine and Veterans Affairs Palo Alto Health Care System, Palo Alto, CA, USA

Glossary

Antigenemia Presence of viral antigen in blood.
CFTR Cystic fibrosis transmembrane conductance regulator, a chloride channel localized in the apical membrane of epithelial cells implicated in secretory diarrhea.
Genotype Specific genetic makeup of one or more viral genes determined by sequence comparison.

Intussusception Pathological event in which the intestine acutely invaginates upon itself and becomes obstructed, followed by local necrosis of gut tissue.
Serotype Significant differences in the antigenic composition of the neutralizing antigens, VP4 and VP7 in the case of rotavirus.
Transcytosis Active transport by which polymeric IgA and IgM antibodies are transported from the basolateral to the lumen of the intestine by the polymeric Ig receptor.

Introduction

Using electron microscopy, rotaviruses were discovered as the etiological agents of epizootic diarrhea of infant mice (EDIM) in 1963 and of calf scours in 1969. Using this same technique, Ruth Bishop identified a rotavirus (RV) in intestinal biopsies of children with diarrhea in 1973. Since then, rotaviruses have been recognized as the most important cause of severe gastroenteritis in children worldwide and an important pathogen of the young of many animals.

Notwithstanding that the overall global mortality from childhood diarrhea decreased in the last 20 years, recent studies suggest that the proportion of hospitalizations attributable to RV-induced diarrhea may have increased during the same time period. For this reason, the burden of RV-related deaths was recently revised, and it is estimated that RV causes around 611 000 childhood deaths every year. More than 80% of these deaths occur in developing countries of sub-Saharan Africa, and South Asia. Worldwide, it is estimated that nearly every child under 5 years of age will have an episode of RV diarrhea,

one in five will require medical attention, one in 65 will be hospitalized, and approximately one in 293 will die from RV disease. Although deaths due to RV are rare in developed countries, the incidence of viral infection is the same as in developing countries and health costs associated with RV disease are considerable. In the United States, for example, it has been estimated that 58 000–70 000 rotavirus-associated hospitalizations occur each year and cost-effectiveness studies clearly justify the use of RV vaccines in that country.

Rotaviruses are very well adapted to their host: they replicate very efficiently, sterilizing immunity is not developed and, despite an important host range restriction, many animal hosts exist (**Table 1**). These characteristics help to explain the high viral prevalence, and suggest that the prevention of severe disease is an appropriate goal for vaccination.

Morphology

Rotaviruses were given their name because, when examined by classical electron microscopy, they appear as wheel (*rota*)-shaped, 70 nm particles. However, by cryoelectron microscopy (a method that permits visualization of the viral spikes), the viral diameter is 100 nm (**Figure 1**). Using this method, the virus particle has been shown to be formed by three concentric layers of proteins: the core comprises viral structural protein 2 (VP2), the RNA-dependent RNA polymerase (VP1), guanyl tranferase (VP3), and the viral genome (**Figure 1**), the intermediate layer is formed by structural protein VP6, the most abundant and most antigenic viral protein, and the external layer comprises 780 copies of glycoprotein VP7 and 60 viral spikes formed by VP4. The surface of the virion has three types of pores that penetrate into the interior of the capsid. These channels

Table 1 Virus-associated factors that contribute to high viral prevalence and reinfections

Characteristic	Comments
Natural infection does not generate sterilizing immunity	Goals of vaccination are to decrease severe disease but not to prevent infection
Multiple animal hosts exist	Eradication does not seem feasible
Short incubation period (1–2 days)	Does not allow time for the recall of high levels of immune effector mechanisms
The entry cell is the same as the cell used for viral replication	Does not allow time for the recall of high levels of immune effector mechanisms
Virus is excreted in high quantities (up to 10^{11} pfu g^{-1} of feces)	High levels of viral dissemination in the environment
Up to 30% of children excrete antigen up to 57 days after onset of diarrhea	High level of viral dissemination
High rate of viral mutation and gene reassortment	May permit the virus to evade the immune system. Currently unproven
Over 50% of infections are asymptomatic	RV well adapted to the human host

Reprinted from Franco MA, Angel J, and Greenberg HB (2006) Immunity and correlates of protection for rotavirus vaccines. *Vaccine*, 24: 2718–2731, with permission from Elsevier.

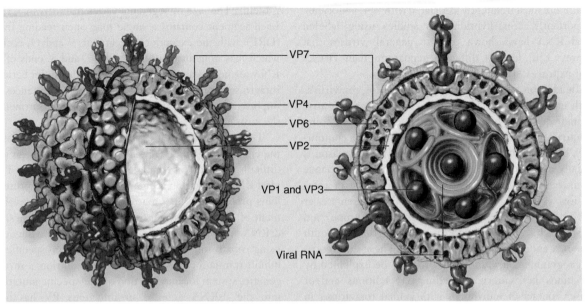

Figure 1 An artist's reconstruction based on cryoelectron microscopy studies of an RV particle. Shown are the seven structural proteins, and the viral RNA. Reproduced with permission from Andrew Swift, Swift Illustration.

seem to be important during viral replication, allowing exchange of compounds in aqueous solution to the inside of the capsid and the export of nascent RNA transcripts.

Several RV structural proteins and nonstructural proteins (NSPs) have been crystallized, permitting the initiation of detailed molecular studies of viral physiology. By this method, the viral spikes have been shown to consist of VP4 trimers, the structure of which rearranges upon trypsin cleavage (a process that enhances viral infection) and probably again on entry into the cell. These changes resemble the conformational transitions of membrane fusion proteins of enveloped viruses. The crystal structure of the viral hemaglutinin VP8 (VP4 is cleaved by trypsin into VP8 and VP5) that contains several virus-neutralizing epitopes has also been determined. Details of the characteristics and function of the viral proteins are described elsewhere in this encyclopedia.

Classification and Epidemiology

Rotaviruses are classified in the genus *Rotavirus* of the family *Reoviridae* that comprises icosahedral, nonenveloped viruses with segmented, double-stranded RNA (dsRNA) genomes. Based primarily on epitopes in VP6, rotaviruses are classified serologically into seven groups (A–G). These serologically distinct groups are also very distinct genetically and genome segment reassortment does not occur between serogroups. According to current taxonomic classification, serogroups A–E each correspond to a different RV species. Serogroups F and G are currently regarded as tentative species. Most human pathogens fall into groups

A, B, and C. The information presented in this chapter is mostly limited to group A rotaviruses which are, by far, the most common cause of severe diarrhea in humans. Among group A rotaviruses, antigenic differences in VP6 have also been identified and used to establish viral subgroups, primarily for epidemiological studies. Serotypes within each serogroup are defined by epitopes in VP7 (glycoprotein, G types) and VP4 (protease, P types) that induce neutralizing antibodies. As the genes encoding these two proteins segregate separately during genome segment reassortment, a binary serotyping system has been developed to identify isolates.

Genotypes, determined by nucleic acid sequence similarity of genes encoding VP7 and VP4, and serotypes, determined by antigenic similarity in VP4 or VP7, as tested by neutralization assays, are generally equivalent for VP7. Currently, 15 G types have been described. G1, G2, G3, G4, and G9 constitute more than 92% of all G serotypes of humans detected globally and appear to be equally virulent. For VP4, there is no direct relationship between genotypes and serotypes and, therefore, a dual system P classification is in use (P genotype numbers are denoted in brackets and P serotypes without brackets). At least 23 P genotypes P[1]–P[23] and 14 serotypes have been described. More than 91% of circulating human RV strains express the P[8] and P[4] genotypes. These genotypes correspond to two subtypes of P1 serotype (P1A and P1B, respectively) that share some cross-reactive epitopes.

Overall, strain variability is less than would be expected from a random association of G and P genotypes since human RV strains belonging to G1, G3, and G4 serotypes are preferentially associated with P[8], while G2 serotype strains are most frequently associated with P[4] genotypes. Importantly, cross-hybridization studies using labeled viral RNA have shown that, in general, viruses that express P[8] form a different genogroup than viruses that express P[4].

In addition to these more prevalent strains, rotaviruses with unusual serotypes currently circulate and can arise sporadically in developed and particularly in developing countries. Several serotypes may coexist within a community, but, in temperate climates especially, each season is usually dominated by a single serotype that may change from season to season. The global distribution of rotaviruses varies over continents: G1P[8] represents over 70% of RV infections in North America, Europe, and Australia, but only about 30% of the infections in South America and Asia, and 23% in Africa. These differences in geographic distribution can probably be explained by variations in sanitary and climatic conditions and/or closer contact of individuals with animal rotaviruses in areas with more RV diversity.

Animal and human group A rotaviruses can undergo genome segment reassortment *in vitro* and *in vivo*. Reassortment originates in cells simultaneously infected with two different rotaviruses and results in progeny viruses that have a combination of genes from each parental strain. In several cases, human rotaviruses have been found that have genes of animal RV origin, adding a further dimension to strain diversity. However, rotaviruses have an important host range restriction in that, in general, humans are infected only with human rotaviruses. This restriction has been exploited for the development of several viral vaccines.

In the temperate zones of the world (mostly developed countries), RV infection occurs primarily during epidemic peaks in the cooler months of the year. A yearly wave of rotaviral illness spreads over the United States; it begins in the southwest in November and terminates in the northeast in March. A similar phenomenon has recently been reported to occur in Europe. This pattern is not seen in countries within 10° of latitude from the Equator (mostly developing countries) where epidemics occur year-round. No clear explanation is available for these temporal patterns of viral prevalence.

Rotaviruses are highly contagious and spread easily but, unlike certain human bacterial infections that occur disproportionately in developing countries, the prevalence of RV infection is the same in developed and developing countries, implying that sanitation and hygiene are not effective measures for disease control.

The Viral Genome and Viral Replication

The RV genome comprises 11 dsRNA segments that code for six structural proteins and five or six nonstructural proteins. The size of segments varies from 0.6 to 3.3 kbp. Each segment contains a single long open reading frame (ORF), with the exception of segments 9 and 11, each of which may contain two ORFs. The 5′ and 3′ ends of the RNA segments have noncoding regions that differ between rotaviruses from groups A, B, and C. These sequences are important in transcription, replication, and reassortment of the virus genome.

The viral RNA itself is not infectious. For this reason, the engineering of recombinant rotaviruses has been very difficult, and this has impeded functional analysis of the viral RNA noncoding sequences and of the viral proteins. This problem has been partially solved by the development of a cell-free system that supports the synthesis of dsRNA from exogenous mRNA, and by gene silencing using small interfering RNA (siRNA) to specifically inhibit translation of viral proteins. In addition, a reverse genetics system for introduction of site-specific mutations into the dsRNA genome of infectious RV has been recently developed (see *recommend readings*). Evaluation of the utility of this method is eagerly awaited by scientists in the field.

Rotaviruses are highly variable. Three mechanisms for generating genetic diversity have been identified: point mutation, genome segment reassortment, and recombination. Rotaviruses have high rate of mutation and it has been estimated that, on average, at least one mutation occurs during each genome replication. Reassortment of genome segments also occurs at high frequency during mixed infections with two or more rotaviruses, both *in vitro* and *in vivo*. Natural reassortment *in vivo* appears to influence the serotypic diversity in humans, especially in less developed countries (see below). Recombination and related rearrangements of viral RNA segments (e.g., partial gene duplication or deletions) probably play a minor role in generating viral diversity but may be important in longer-term viral evolution.

RV entry into host cells is a multistep process and several molecules have been identified as RV receptors or co-receptors. However, the process has been shown to vary in different viral strains. For example, for several animal RV strains, the first binding step involves the interaction of VP8 with sialic acid, while some human RV strains appear to bind initially to GM1 ganglioside. As a second step, RV binds to the integrin α2β1 in an interaction mediated by the integrin-binding motif DGE in VP5. In addition to these two interactions, integrins αvβ3 and αxβ2, and the heat shock protein hsp70, have also been shown to be involved at a later step of rotavirus cell entry. It seems that the association of some of these molecules with rafts is important for viral entry.

Although it was initially proposed that rotaviruses enter by direct penetration, current models favor the hypothesis that virus entry is by endocytosis. Inside the cell, VP5 seems to induce a size-selective membrane permeabilization of the putative viral endosome that facilitates the transit of Ca^{2+} from the vesicle. When Ca^{2+} concentrations in the endosome are lowered, a disassembly of VP4 and VP7 is postulated to occur. This event permeabilizes the membrane of the endosome and the viral transciptase (viral particles without VP4 and VP7) gains access to the cytoplasm and begins to synthesize viral mRNAs. The mRNAs produced by the transcriptase are exact copies of each genome segment, with a $5'$-terminal type 1 methylated cap structure and without a $3'$-terminal poly(A) sequences.

The viral mRNAs are translated, giving rise to the structural and nonstructural proteins necessary to complete the viral replication cycle. NSP3 is reported to shut off the synthesis of cellular proteins and induces the preferential translation of viral proteins. These proteins accumulate in the cytoplasm in an electron dense region called the viroplasm, where the viral genome is replicated and the assembly of progeny double-layered particles takes place. The mechanism by which one viral particle assembles with each and only one of the 11 RNA segments is unknown. Synthesis of the dsRNAs occurs following the packaging of viral mRNAs into intermediate precursors of double-layered particles.

Assembled double-layered particles interact with NSP4, that has been synthesized by ribosomes associated with the endoplasmic reticulum (ER), and bud into the ER lumen. In this organelle, the double-layered particles acquire a transient lipid membrane. Then, in a very poorly understood mechanism (probably related to the high Ca^{2+} levels of the ER), the viral particles acquire VP7 and lose the transient enveloping membrane, giving rise to the triple-layered particle. Recent experiments suggest that VP4 is acquired by the viral particle in a compartment outside the ER.

The physiological mechanism of exit of the mature triple layer viral particle from the cell is unknown. In polarized Caco-2 cells (intestinal epithelial cells derived from a human colon adenocarcinoma), RV is released before cell death using a vesicle-associated vectorial transport system to the apical pole. However, rotaviruses are lytic viruses, and could also exit the cell after cell lysis. The mechanism of cell death induced by RV is not completely understood. Results in polarized Caco-2 cells and *in vivo* studies in mice suggest that it is by viral induced cell apoptosis.

Pathogenesis

Important viral antigenemia and some level of viremia are observed in the initial phase of RV-induced diarrhea in children and animals. In mice, extraintestinal viral replication occurs commonly during homologous and some heterologous infections. Also in this model, the level and location of extraintestinal replication varies between RV strains and replication can occur in several leukocytes subsets. However, the clinical relevance of these findings is still unclear and, in children and in animals, the bulk of RV replication most likely occurs in the mature villus tip cells of the small bowel.

RV-induced diarrhea probably occurs by multiple mechanisms that vary, depending on the animal species analyzed (**Table 2**). Pathological findings in the small intestine of children with RV diarrhea include: shortening and atrophy of the intestinal villi, enterocyte vacuolization with distended cisternae of the endoplasmic reticulum, and mononuclear infiltration in the intestinal lamina propia. However, in children a direct relationship between the extent of histopathology and disease has not been demonstrated. This finding suggests that RV diarrhea can occur without important enterocyte death.

In pigs, RV infection induces an intestinal lactase deficiency and increased lactose in feces induces an osmotic diarrhea. Elevated levels of lactose are also observed in the feces of some RV infected children. Lactase deficiency could be due to RV-induced enterocyte destruction or to alteration in the synthesis or metabolism of disaccharidases. In mice, two mechanisms of diarrhea, which do not involve enterocyte destruction, have been identified. NSP4, and a derived peptide of NSP4, induce diarrhea in mouse pups but not adult animals, making it the first viral

Table 2 Mechanisms of RV-induced diarrhea (may vary according to the animal species studied)

Mechanism	Comments
Action of NSP4 as a toxin induces a secretory diarrhea	Only demonstrated in rodents. Non-CFTR mediated. Occurs early in infection prior to cell death
RV stimulates the enteric nervous system (ENS) inducing a secretory diarrhea and increased intestinal motility	Drugs that inhibit the ENS are useful to treat RV diarrhea. Occurs early in infection prior to cell death
Altered metabolism of disaccharidases and other enterocyte membrane proteins induces malabsorptive/osmotic diarrhea	Occurs early in infection prior to cell death
Enterocyte death contributes to malabsorptive/osmotic diarrhea	Late mechanism. In polarized intestinal epithelial cell lines and *in vivo* in murine enterocytes, RV infected cells seem to die by apoptosis

Reprinted from Franco MA, Angel J, and Greenberg HB (2006) Immunity an correlates of protection for rotavirus vaccines. *Vaccine*, 24: 2718–2731, with permission from Elsevier.

enterotoxin described. However, its role in RV-induced diarrhea in other species has not been characterized. Also in mice, RV has been shown to activate the intestinal autonomous neural system and increase the secretion of water and electrolytes, as well as the intestinal motility. Racecadotril, an inhibitor of the enteric nervous system, is somewhat efficacious in treating RV-induced diarrhea in children, suggesting that this mechanism plays at least some role in human diarrhea.

It is possible that the three mechanisms (malabsorption, NSP4 enterotoxicity, and enteric neural system stimulation) may play a major or minor role in the pathophysiology of RV-induced diarrhea, depending on the species and the time point after the onset of disease.

Diagnosis, Clinical Characteristics, and Treatment

Initial efforts to isolate wild-type rotaviruses in tissue culture were not very successful. For this reason, early clinical studies characterized rotaviruses by isolating viral RNA from feces and then analyzing the RNA by electrophoresis in polyacrylamide gels. Using this method, rotaviruses were classified depending on the pattern of migration of their RNA segments (electropherotypes). At present, this method seems of limited value because a relationship between electropherotypes and virulence or serotypes is not generally apparent. Currently, diagnosis is commonly conducted using commercial ELISAs that detect viral antigen (mostly VP6) in the feces. Rotavirus is shed in very large amounts making the ELISA a highly effective and accurate diagnostic assay. For epidemiological studies, human RV strains present in feces can be grown in cell culture in MA104 (African green monkey kidney) and Caco-2 cells using trypsin for enhancement of viral growth during the culture. Trypsin cleaves VP4 and increases infectivity in culture. Genotype characterization of RV strains is mainly by reverse transcription-polymerase chain reaction (RT-PCR). RV detection by electron microscopy is only conducted in research laboratories, especially when other viral pathogens are being investigated.

Rotaviruses are highly contagious since approximately 10^{11} particles per gram of feces are excreted, and they are very resistant to ambient conditions. In addition, viral excretion in most children lasts for up to 10 days and, in some children, may extend for 2 months after onset of infection. Rotaviruses are mainly transmitted by an oral–fecal route although, in some cases, a respiratory route has been suggested.

In developing countries, the peak incidence of RV disease occurs in children between 6 and 11 months of age. In contrast, in developed countries, the highest incidence is observed in older children (2 years old). This difference is probably related to differences in sanitation

in the different settings. Notwithstanding this variation, RV incidence is similar in both developing and developed countries but mortality is mainly observed in developing countries, presumably due to limited access to appropriate health care. The relative protection of infants younger than 2 months of age, which occurs worldwide, could be related to the presence of protective maternal antibodies. Up to 50% of adults caring for children with RV diarrhea can become infected and, of these, 50% develop disease which is generally mild.

The primary clinical syndrome caused by RV infection is acute gastroenteritis. After a short incubation period of 48 h or less, children frequently present with vomiting that lasts for 1–2 days. The vomiting is often accompanied with fever (37.9 °C or greater). Subsequently, or at the same time, a watery diarrhea appears and, if it is not treated, frequently induces dehydration. It is estimated that up to 50% of RV infections in children are asymptomatic but some of these may represent second or third exposures.

Children attending day care institutions are at high risk of developing RV-induced diarrhea. Although RV infections in neonatal care units have been classically described as asymptomatic, probably due to the presence of maternal antibodies, severe symptomatic outbreaks have also been described. RV strains that induce nosocomial infections in neonatal nurseries are generally different from those circulating in the community. RV infection can cause severe and prolonged disease in children with primary immunodeficiencies, some of whom develop a systemically disseminated infection. Acquired immunodeficiency also predisposes to severe RV disease in bone marrow- and liver-transplanted children. The role of RV-induced disease in immunosuppressed adults with HIV seems, at present, less important.

RV diarrhea is self-limited and treatment is aimed at reducing symptoms until the immune response resolves the infection. Children with mild diarrhea are treated by oral rehydration. Those presenting moderate to severe dehydration may require intravenous rehydration. In cases of severe disease, treatment with probiotics, preparations that contain antibodies against RV, Racecadotril (an inhibitor of the enteric nervous system), and Nitasoxanide (a drug of unknown mechanism of action) have been shown to accelerate resolution of the disease. However, it is not yet clear whether these interventions truly provide significant advantages to ill children.

Immune Response

Immunity to RV is incompletely understood and animal models have been important in the acquisition of our currently available knowledge. Pepsin and gastric acid seem to be important host defense factors against RV infection, since these factors inactivate rotaviruses in adult mice but not in suckling mice. In addition, the innate immune response and interferons, in particular, seem to mediate an antiviral effect, and viral mechanisms for evading this response involving NSP1 have recently been suggested. However, mice lacking T and B cells become chronically infected with RV, suggesting that the adaptive immune system is essential for viral elimination. Also, children lacking T and B cells, or only B cells have been shown to shed virus chronically.

Antibodies seem to be the principal mechanism that mediates protection against viral reinfection. In agreement with the fact that most viral replication occurs in the intestine, the localization of virus specific B cells in the intestine seems important for their capacity to mediate protection. It is postulated that local IgA antibodies can mediate expulsion of rotaviruses inside the enterocytes and exclusion (to avoid de novo infection of enterocytes) of rotaviruses in the gut lumen. Neutralizing antibodies to VP4 and/or VP7 can block enterocyte infection directly when present in the gut lumen (exclusion). In mice, anti-VP6 non-neutralizing polymeric IgA may bind virus VP6 during transcytosis from the basolateral membrane of enterocytes to the gut lumen and 'expulse it'. These antibodies may also inhibit RV transcription intracellularly. In addition, antibodies to NSP4 may block diarrhea, but not infection, by blocking the enterotoxic property of the molecule. However, the antiviral effects of antibodies against VP6 and NSP4 have only been shown to be protective in mice. In piglets, a model that is probably closer to humans than mice, the presence of antibodies against VP4 and/or VP7 seems necessary for protection.

Although local antibodies appear to be the principal mechanism that protects against viral infection, T cells also directly mediate antiviral immunity, at least in mice. CD4+ T cells are also essential for the development of more than 90% of the RV-specific intestinal IgA, and thus their presence seems critical for the establishment of protective long-term memory responses. Moreover, murine RV-specific CD8+ T cells are involved in the timely resolution of primary RV infection and can mediate short-term partial protection against reinfection.

In children, primary RV infections are generally the most severe, with severity decreasing as the number of reinfections increases. Complete protection against moderate-to-severe illness is achieved after two natural RV infections, whether symptomatic or asymptomatic. In agreement with the results of animal models mentioned previously, total serum RV IgA, induced by a primary infection, seems to be the best but imperfect correlate of protection against subsequent reinfections. Primary RV infection induces homotypic neutralizing antibodies to VP7 and VP4 and some level of heterotypic immunity, but the role in protection of these antibodies is still controversial. In this respect, it is noteworthy that an attenuated G1P[8] human RV vaccine has been shown

to induce excellent protection against severe diarrhea caused by P[8] rotaviruses, independently of their G type. This vaccine can also induce protection against G2P[4] rotaviruses, but this protection is somewhat lower than against the P[8] viruses. Altogether, these findings suggest a role for neutralizing antibodies directed against VP4 in protection. However, since, as mentioned previously, P[4] viruses belong to a separate genogroup from most P[8] viruses, differences in immunity to other non-neutralizing viral proteins could also be the explanation for the relatively lower protection rate induced by the vaccine against P[4] viruses.

The lack of understanding of RV immunity limits our capacity to develop new RV vaccines. Recent studies have tried to characterize RV-specific lymphocytes in humans to better understand human immunity. Due to the relative inaccessibility for study of the human intestinal immune tissue, cells involved in the RV immune response have been studied in peripheral blood. It is hypothesized that at least a fraction of these lymphocytes are recirculating to and from the intestine, and thus may reflect intestinal immunity. In blood of children with acute RV infection, plasmablasts and plasma cells (secreting mainly RV specific IgM) are found, and these express homing receptors, that allow them to return to the intestine. In the convalescence phase, RV-specific B cells are mainly memory cells, some of which express intestinal homing receptors. In addition, RV-specific CD4+ and CD8+ T cells have been characterized. In children and adults with acute infection, both types of T cells that secrete gamma interferon circulate, but in unexpectedly low frequencies. It is speculated that the limited induction of RV-specific T cells can be related to the occurrence of delayed viral clearance and symptomatic reinfections in a subset of individuals.

Viral Vaccines

The first commercially available RV vaccine was a simian-human reassortant tetravalent vaccine (RotaShield). Although this vaccine was highly effective, it was withdrawn from the market 1 year after its introduction due to its temporal association with low levels of intussusception (1 in 10 000 children). Two new RV vaccines have been recently licensed for use in many countries worldwide. These vaccines appear to be safe and not cause intussusception. The vaccine produced by Merck (RotaTeq^{TM}) contains mono-reassortants of a bovine virus with G1, G2, G3, G4, and P1A[8] human RV genes. The vaccine produced by GlaxoSmithKline (GSK, Rotarix) is a human-attenuated G1P1A[8] virus. In trials that involved over 60 000 infants, both of these vaccines have been shown to be safe and to provide over 70% protection against any RV diarrhea and over 98%

protection against severe RV infection. Importantly, both vaccines reduced the rates of all gastroenteritis-related hospitalizations of any cause by over 40%. Despite these encouraging results, it is still undetermined if these vaccines will work in very poor developing countries in Africa and Asia in which children can be malnourished and in which atypical RV strains may circulate frequently. Moreover, the intussusception associated with RotaShield was predominantly seen in children older than 2 months, and the children studied in the safety evaluation of the two new vaccines were mostly 2 months of age. Thus, the safety of the new RV vaccines in children of more than 2 months of age has not been fully established and the development of second-generation vaccines may be desirable. A promising strategy to drastically reduce the risk of intussusception is to administer the vaccine to neonates, in whom intussusception almost never occurs. Current studies in animal models are focused on the development of second generation nonreplicating RV vaccines, such as DNA vaccines, and recombinant RV proteins or virus-like particles.

Further Reading

Franco MA, Angel J, and Greenberg HB (2006) Immunity and correlates of protection for rotavirus vaccines. *Vaccine* 24(5): 2718–2731.

Franco MA and Greenberg HB (2002) Rotaviruses. In: Richman DD, Hayden FG,, and Whitley RJ (eds.) *Clinical Virology*, 2nd edn., pp. 743–762. Washington, DC: ASM Press.

Komoto S, Sasaki J, and Taniguchi K (2006) Reverse genetics system for introduction of site-specific mutations into the double-stranded RNA genome of infectious rotavirus. *Proceedings of the National Academy of Sciences, USA* 103(12): 4646–4651.

Rothman KJ, Young-Xu Y, and Arellano F (2006) Age dependence of the relation between reassortant rotavirus vaccine (RotaShield) and intussusception. *Journal of Infectious Diseases* 193(6): 898.

Ruiz-Palacios GM, Perez-Schael I, Velazquez FR, *et al.* (2006) Safety and efficacy of an attenuated vaccine against severe rotavirus gastroenteritis. *New England Journal of Medicine* 354(1): 11–22.

Santos N and Hoshino Y (2005) Global distribution of rotavirus serotypes/genotypes and its implication for the development and implementation of an effective rotavirus vaccine. *Reviews in Medical Virology* 15: 29–56.

Vesikari T, Matson DO, Dennehy P, *et al.* (2006) Safety and efficacy of a pentavalent human-bovine (WC3) reassortant rotavirus vaccine. *New England Journal of Medicine* 354(1): 23–33.

Rubella Virus

T K Frey, Georgia State University, Atlanta, GA, USA

Glossary

Birth defects Malformations or abnormalities developed during gestation that are apparent at, or soon after, delivery.

Congenital infection Infection of the fetus during gestation as a result of virus passage through the placenta.

Elimination program Vaccination program designed to eliminate 'indigenous' sources of a pathogen from a geographic region and thus restrict sources of the pathogen to imports from other regions.

Enveloped virion Virus particle with a lipid bilayer membrane, or envelope, surrounding the capsid or core. The envelope is usually derived from host cell membranes and contains virus-specified glycoproteins decorating its outer surface.

Icosahedral capsid In the virus particle, the proteinaceous shell surrounding the virus genome – in this case, with symmetry of an icosahedron (appears quasi-spherical or round in electron micrographs).

Live, attenuated vaccine A vaccine formulation using an infectious variant of the virus that has been attenuated or weakened by repeated passage in cell culture or alternate hosts. Such vaccines recapitulate the infection, including induction of a complete adaptive immune response, but do not cause disease.

Persistent infection Infection characterized by continued presence of the virus, often despite the induction of an adaptive immune response.

Plus-strand RNA virus Virus with a single-stranded RNA genome that is of messenger RNA sense and can be directly translated to produce virus-specified proteins.

Serodiagnosis Detection or diagnosis of infection through immune status, usually the presence of IgM antibodies or a rise in IgG antibodies in paired sera collected at the time of symptoms and convalescence (post-recovery).

Systemic infection Infection that spreads from local site entry via the lymphatic system and blood stream to one or more target internal organs or tissues.

Introduction

Rubella virus (RUBV) infection causes a benign disease known as rubella or German measles that can result in profound birth defects if contracted *in utero*. Norman Gregg, an Australian ophthalmologist, first reported the association of congenital cataracts as a consequence of gestational rubella in 1941, establishing RUBV as a major teratogen. The last major epidemic of rubella to impact the United States occurred in 1964–65, resulting in 20 000 congenital rubella syndrome (CRS) cases, and subsequently live, attenuated vaccines were developed and applied in the US, Canada, Japan, and several European countries by 1969. These programs have been successful in greatly reducing the incidence of both rubella and CRS in these countries, particularly the US, in which indigenous rubella was declared eliminated in 2004. Currently, ~50% of countries have national rubella vaccination programs, but the majority of the world's population is not covered and rubella thus remains a worldwide challenge.

Classification

RUBV is a member of the family *Togaviridae* and the only member of the genus *Rubivirus*. The other togavirus genus, *Alphavirus*, contains 26 members, all of which are arthropod-borne. In common with the alphaviruses, the rubella virion consists of a single-stranded, plus-sense genomic RNA contained within a quasi-spherical core or capsid, composed of a single virus-specified protein, C, which is surrounded by a lipid envelope in which are embedded two virus-specified glycoproteins, E1 and E2. Unlike alphaviruses, RUBV has no invertebrate vector and the only known natural reservoir is humans. RUBV also is antigenically distinct from the alphaviruses. Phylogenetic analysis of E1 gene nucleotide sequence of worldwide RUBV isolates has led the World Health Organization to propose a standardized taxonomy for RUBVs which consists of two clades, 1 and 2, and genotypes within each clade. Clade 1 contains seven genotypes and is distributed worldwide. Clade 2 contains three clades and appears to be restricted to Asia.

Host Range and Virus Propagation

RUBV has no known natural host other than humans. No reliable animal model exists for the study of RUBV pathogenesis. RUBV replicates in a number of laboratory cell culture lines; however, in most of these no cytopathic effects (CPEs) are routinely observed. Continuous cell lines commonly used to propagate RUBV include Vero (African green monkey kidney), RK-13 (rabbit kidney), and BHK-21 (baby hamster kidney). In all cell lines in which RUBV replicates, persistent infections are readily established and maintained, whether or not the cell line exhibits a functional interferon system, and persistent RUBV infection in cell culture cannot be cured by the inclusion of neutralizing antibodies in the culture medium because virus budding occurs at intracytoplasmic locations. Thus, RUBV is highly adapted for persisting infection.

Properties of the Virion

Rubella virions are 60–70 nm spherical particles composed of an electron-dense core separated from the lipid envelope by an electron-lucent zone. Rubella virions exhibit a marked degree of pleomorphism (**Figure 1**). The virion has a density of 1.18–1.19 g ml^{-1}, whereas isolated capsids have a density of 1.44 g ml^{-1}. The C protein (~34 kDa), which comprises the capsid, is present as disulfide-linked homodimers. Although presumed to be icosahedral, the symmetry of the RUBV capsid has not been solved.

The virion spikes are formed by two virion glycoproteins, E1 and E2. E1 has a molecular weight of 59 kDa whereas E2 is a heterogeneous species ranging from 44 to 50 kDa due to differential glycosylation. Both E1 and E2 appear to be primarily in the form of heterodimers which are easily disrupted by routine preparation techniques. The higher-order architecture of the virion spikes is entirely unclear. E1 is more exposed on the virion surface than is E2, contains both the viral hemagglutinin and receptor site, and is also immunodominant in terms of the humoral response.

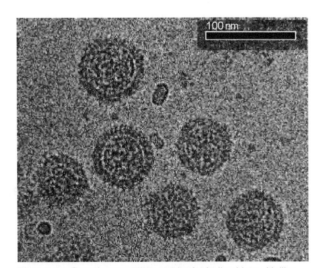

Figure 1   Cryoelectron micrograph of rubella virions. Unlike conventional negative staining, the virions have a uniform structure when visualized by this technique; however, pleomorphism of particle diameter and the gap between the core and envelope remains apparent. Courtesy of Tao Sun, Yumei Zhou, Michael Rossmann, and Teryl Frey (unpublished data).

Rubella virions are stable at physiological pH values and can be frozen at temperatures below −20 °C for years, without loss of infectivity. Live, attenuated vaccine virus is stored in lyophilized form. Rubella virions are susceptible to most commonly used inactivating agents, such as formaldehyde, UV light, and lipid solvents.

Genomic Organization

The RUBV genomic RNA is 9762 nucleotides in length and contains a 5′ terminal cap structure and a 3′ terminal poly(A) tract. A distinctive feature of the genomic RNA is that it contains 30% guanine residues and 39% cytosine residues, the highest G+C content of all RNA viruses. The genome contains two long, nonoverlapping open-reading frames (ORFs) plus untranslated regions (UTRs) at the 5′ and 3′ ends and between the ORF's (**Figure 2**). The 5′ proximal ORF, or nonstructural proteins ORF (NS-ORF), encodes a 2116-amino-acid product that is proteolytically cleaved into two products, 150 kDa (P150) and 90 kDa (P90), which are at the N- and C-termini of the ORF, respectively. The cleavage is mediated by a papain-like cysteine protease located at the C-terminus of P150. P150 and P90 are responsible for virus RNA replication. By computer-assisted comparisons with other viruses, P150 contains a domain predicted to have methyl/guanylyltransferase activity (responsible for forming the cap structure at the 5′ end of the genomic and subgenomic RNAs) in addition to the protease, whereas P90 contains both a helicase domain and an RNA-dependent RNA polymerase (or replicase) domain. The 3′ proximal ORF, or structural protein ORF (S-ORF), encodes a 1063-amino-acid product that is proteolytically processed into the virion proteins by a cell protease, signal endopeptidase. The order of the virion protein genes within the ORF is 5′ C-E2-E1 3′. The S-ORF is translated from a subgenomic RNA synthesized in infected cells and

containing the sequences from the start site through the 3′ end of the genome. An infectious clone for RUBV has been developed. An infectious clone is a cDNA copy of the viral RNA contained in a plasmid in which it is placed adjacent to an RNA polymerase promoter. Since RUBV has a plus-sense genome, *in vitro* transcripts from the plasmid will initiate virus replication following transfection into susceptible cells. The infectious clone allows for studies of the effects of site-directed mutagenesis on the RUBV genome.

Intracellular Replication Cycle

The receptor for RUBV on the surface of susceptible cells has not been identified. Following attachment to the receptor, the virus is taken into the cell by receptor-mediated endocytosis. In the reduced pH environment of the endocytic vesicle, fusion between the viral envelope and the vesicular membrane occurs, releasing the capsid and genomic RNA into the cytoplasm of the cell.

The genomic RNA is translated to produce the NS protein precursor which is cleaved into P150 and P90 (**Figure 3**). These proteins then use the genomic RNA as a template for synthesis of a genome-length, minus-sense RNA. The genome-length, minus-sense RNA is then used as the template for synthesis of both the genomic RNA and the subgenomic RNA. Synthesis of the subgenomic RNA is initiated by internal recognition of sequences on the genome-length, minus-sense RNA template. Host-cell proteins are likely involved in the replication process and, interestingly, recent evidence indicates that the C protein is as well. RNA synthesis is asymmetric in infected cells in that more of the plus-sense species than the minus-sense RNA is produced. The uncleaved NS protein precursor is active in minus-strand RNA synthesis, while the cleaved P150/P90 complex appears to be active in only plus-strand RNA synthesis. Thus the activity of the

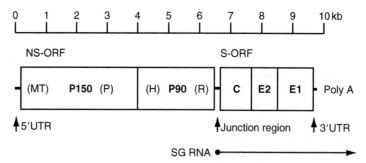

Figure 2 Coding strategy of the RUBV genome. Shown is a schematic representation of the RUBV genomic RNA with untranslated regions (UTRs) drawn as solid black lines and coding regions (ORFs) as open boxes (NS-ORF, nonstructural protein ORF; S-ORF, structural protein ORF). Within each ORF, the coding sequences for the proteins processed from the translation product of the ORF are delineated and, in addition, within the NS-ORF, the locations of motifs associated with the following activities are indicated: methyl/guanylyltransferase (MT), protease (P), helicase (H), and RNA-dependent RNA polymerase (R). The sequences encompassed by the subgenomic RNA (SG RNA) are also shown. The scale at the top of the diagram is in kilobases.

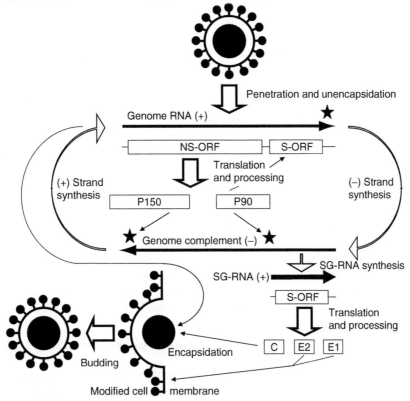

Figure 3 Replication strategy of RUBV. The plus-sense genome and subgenomic RNA are represented by solid black arrows indicating plus polarity; beneath each, the ORFs that they contain are shown as open boxes. The minus-sense genome RNA complement, represented as a dotted arrow, is used solely as a template for the two plus-sense RNA species. Putative *cis*-acting sequences on each RNA, which are recognized by the virus RNA-dependent RNA polymerase to initiate synthesis of complementary RNAs, are marked with stars. The general functions of the virus proteins are indicated by arrows (e.g., P150 and P90 functioning as the RNA-dependent RNA polymerase by interacting with *cis*-acting sequences on the viral RNA species and synthesizing complementary strands).

NS protease through mediating this cleavage is important in regulating plus- and minus-sense RNA synthesis. RUBV RNA synthesis occurs in cytopathic vacuoles of lysosomal origin, in infected cells.

In the structural protein ORF, E2 and E1 are immediately preceded by hydrophobic signal sequences that function to direct translation of secreted and membrane-associated proteins into the lumen of the endoplasmic reticulum (ER). Therefore, following translation of the C sequences within the ORF, the E2 signal sequence mediates association of the translation complex with the ER. C–E2 cleavage is mediated by signal endopeptidase, or signalase, which functions in the lumen of the ER to remove signal sequences from secreted and membrane-associated proteins; unlike the proteins of the alphaviruses, RUBV C protein does not have autocatalytic protease activity. Following cleavage, the E2 signal sequence remains associated with C. Similarly, the E1 signal sequence maintains the association of the translational complex with the ER, signalase mediates the E2–E1 cleavage, and the E1 signal sequence remains attached to E2. Soon after synthesis, heterodimerization of E2 and E1 occurs in the lumen of

the ER. The three-dimesional folding of E1 appears to be a complicated process requiring intramolecular disulfide-bond formation by all 20-Cys residues in the ectodomain of the protein. Both E1 and E2 acquire high-mannose glycans in the ER; E1 contains three potential glycosylation sites and E2 contains four and all appear to be utilized. The sites of O-glycosylation of the E2, which accounts for the size heterogeneity of E2, is not known. E1 contains an ER retention signal that is only overridden once conformational folding is complete, after which the E1–E2 heterodimer migrates to the Golgi. In the Golgi the N-glycans of both E2 and E1 are modified to complex form, although modification is not complete and the extent of modification on both proteins is heterogeneous. Modifications of the O-glycans on E2 also occur and E2 contains a Golgi retention signal, indicating that the Golgi is the preferred site of viral budding in infected cells. However, late in infection E1 and E2 migrate to the cell surface and budding can also occur at this site in some cell lines.

RUBV capsid morphogenesis occurs in association with cell membranes. The association of RUBV capsid protein with membranes is probably mediated by the E2 signal sequence, which is retained at the COOH terminus of C. In fact, C may associate with the E2–E1 heterodimer and migrate as a passenger on the cytoplasmic side of vesicles transporting E2–E1 from the ER to the Golgi and among the Golgi stacks. Unlike the alphaviruses, whose capsids accumulate in infected cells, RUBV capsids only become visible in association with deformed, thickened membranes that appear to be in the early process of budding. A putative encapsidation signal has been localized near the 5′ terminus of the genomic RNA. The C protein is phosphorylated and phosphorylation/dephosphorylation by cell enzymes is proposed as the regulator of the process by which the genome is unencapsidated following entry (phosphorylation) and encapsidated later in infection following replication (dephosphorylation). Interestingly, in cells in which the complete S-ORF is expressed in the absence of genomic RNA, virus-like particles form and are secreted and these have the same morphology and isopycnic density as do virions.

RUBV replicates in the cytoplasm of the infected cell. None of the virus proteins exhibit any involvement with the nucleus during infection and RUBV infection does not appear to inhibit cell macromolecular synthesis in any grossly detectable manner; however, perturbations of specific macromoleclar products and induction of specific genes may occur. Microsopically, RUBV-infected cells appear similar to uninfected cells; however, rearrangements of cellular cytoskeletal elements and organelles such as mitochondria have been reported. RUBV reportedly inhibits growth in primary human cell cultures in part due to an inhibition of mitosis; however, the virus has no reproducible effect on the growth of stable cell lines. In those cell lines which exhibit CPE (Vero and RK-13 cells), cell death is due to apoptosis.

Genetics and Evolution

The RUBV genome is extremely stable. Currently, the genomes of 19 independent strains of RUBV from eight genotypes, five in clade 1 and three in clade 2, have been sequenced in their entirety and all are nearly identical in terms of the size of the genome as well as the coding and noncoding regions within the genome. The only exceptions are 1–2 nucleotide deletions occasionally encountered in the junction region. Maximal observed distance at the nucleotide level is 5% among clade 1 viruses, 7.5% among clade 2 viruses, and 9% between viruses in the two clades. Across the 19 genomic sequences, 78% of the nucleotides are conserved, explaining the low level of variability. A unique feature of RUBV evolution is that changes to G and C are selected for, indicating an adaptive advantage of the high G+C content of the genome.

Because there are no known close relatives of RUBV, the origin of the virus prior to its introduction into the human population is unknown. Except for short stretches at the 5′ end of the genome and at the subgenomic promoter site, RUBV and the alphaviruses share no nucleotide homology. Thus these two genera are only distantly related. RUBV and the alphaviruses belong to the 'alphavirus-like superfamily' of plus-sense RNA viruses, which includes a large number of plant viruses as well as human hepatitis E virus, the sole member of the genus *Hepevirus*. Within this superfamily, computer-assisted phylogenetic analysis of the NS proteins indicates that RUBV is more closely related to hepatitis E virus than to the alphaviruses and this dissimilarity is borne out by differences in the order of motifs in the NS-ORF. Thus, it is hypothesized that the evolution of the togaviruses may have been more complicated than simple divergence from a common ancestor and probably involved recombination between progenitors of the current alphaviruses, RUBV, hepatitis E virus, and, possibly, certain plant viruses.

Serologic Relationships and Variability

RUBV is monotypic and immunological characterization of diverse strains, including both clade 1 and 2 viruses, has only revealed subtle antigenic differences which map to C or E2. As might be anticipated from the lack of serologic cross-reaction with the alphaviruses, there is no homology at the amino acid level between RUBV and alphaviruses within the virion proteins.

Epidemiology

Historically, RUBV was endemic worldwide. Over the past 35 years, vaccination programs have curtailed this distribution, as discussed below. Before the advent of vaccination programs, rubella was considered a disease of middle childhood in temperate zones, with seasonal peak occurrence in the spring and epidemics at 5–9-year intervals. However, in tropical zones the highest infection rates were in children under 5 years of age. RUBV is not as transmissible as is measles virus and even during epidemics, susceptibles are spared. Thus, infection of adolescents and young adults, the population at risk for CRS, in endemic areas is not uncommon.

Transmission and Tissue Tropism

RUBV is transmitted between individuals by aerosol. The epithelium of the buccal mucosa provides the initial site for virus replication and the mucosa of the upper respiratory tract and nasopharyngeal lymphoid tissue serve as portals of virus entry. The virus is then spread by local lymphatics, which seed regional lymph nodes where further virus replication occurs. After an incubation period of 7–9 days, virus appears in the blood. Viremia ceases with the onset of detectable rubella-specific antibody, shortly after the rash appears 2–3 weeks post infection. Patients are most infectious immediately preceeding and during the rash phase; virus generally disappears from nasopharyngeal secretions within 4 days of appearance of the rash. Congenitally infected infants shed virus for 3–6 months following birth and are a source of transmission during that period. Reinfection with RUBV occurs, usually without clinical illness or virus shedding. There are a small number of cases in which RUBV reinfection of pregnant women with well-documented immunity has resulted in CRS.

During pregnancy, placental tissues are very susceptible to infection. Placental infection results in scattered foci of necrotic syncytiotrophoblast and cytotrophoblast cells and evidence of damage to vascular endothelium. Following placental infection, virus can spread to the fetus but this does not always occur and RUBV is more often recovered from placental tissue than from fetal products of conception. Once fetal infection occurs, virus spreads throughout the fetus and almost any organ may be infected. Severe fetal damage is only associated with infection during the first trimester of pregnancy; the rate of CRS is >50%, 25%, and 10% when infection occurs during the first, second, and third months, respectively. This is due to a combination of an apparent decline in the efficiency of placental transfer after the first trimester and a reduction in the ability of the virus to inflict fetal damage after this time of gestational development.

Clinical Features of Infection

Rubella acquired in childhood or early adulthood is usually mild and it is estimated that up to 50% of rubella infections are clinically inapparent. Symptomatic rubella encompasses combinations of maculopapular rash, lymphadenopathy, low-grade fever, conjunctivitis, sore throat, and arthralgia. The rash is the most prominent feature and appears following an incubation period of 16–20 days. The rash begins as distinct pink maculopapules on the face that then spread over the trunk and distally onto the extremities. The maculopapules coalesce and the rash fades over several days. An associated posterior cervical and suboccipital lymphadenopathy is also characteristic. Infrequent complications include thrombocytopenia and post-infectious encephalitis. Acute polyarthralgia and arthritis following natural RUBV infections of adults are common and occur more frequently and with greater severity in women than in men. Joint involvement is usually transient; however, chronic arthritis, persisting or recurring over several years, has been reported.

The clinical manifestations of CRS apparent at birth vary widely, most frequently including thrombocytopenic purpura ('blueberry muffin syndrome'), intrauterine growth retardation, congenital heart disease (patent ductus arteriosus or pulmonary artery or valvular stenosis), psychomotor retardation, eye defects (cataract, glaucoma, retinopathy), hearing loss, and hepatomegaly and/or splenomegaly. Nearly 80% of CRS children show some type of neural involvement, particularly neurosensory hearing loss.

Most clinical manifestations of congenital rubella are evident at or shortly following birth and some are transient. However, recognition of retinopathy, hearing loss, and mental retardation may be delayed for several years in some cases. Progressive consequences of congenital rubella have become increasingly appreciated as CRS children from the 1964 epidemic have been followed longitudinally. These predominantly involve endocrine dysfunction (diabetes mellitus, which ultimately affects 40% of CRS patients, and thyroid dysfunction). A rare, fatal neurodegenerative disease, progressive rubella panencephalitis (PRP), described in CRS patients, bears superficial resemblance to subacute sclerosing panencephalitis associated with measles virus. Subsequently, PRP cases have been reported in individuals infected postnatally.

Pathogenesis, Pathology, and Histopathology

There is limited information on the pathogenesis of uncomplicated rubella because of the benign nature of the illness. With respect to the complications that can accompany acute rubella, the postinfectious encephalitis is thought to be autoimmune in nature since RUBV cannot be isolated from cerebrospinal fluid or brain at autopsy. Interestingly, however, extensive inflammation and demyelination are not observed. In a few cases of rubella arthritis, the presence of RUBV in synovial fluid and/or cells has been demonstrated and therefore it is assumed that virus persistence is involved. However, considering the age and sex factors in the incidence of arthritis, it seems likely that immunopathological mechanisms also play a role. In one study, human leukocyte antigen (HLA) class II haplotypes predisposing adult women to arthritis and arthralgia following rubella vaccination were found to also correlate with predisposition to arthritis and arthralgia regardless of vaccination status.

Following fetal infection, virus can be isolated from practically every organ of abortuses or infants who die soon after birth. However, only 1 in 10^3 to 1 in 10^5 cells are infected and it is not known how such a low infection rate leads to the profound birth defects exhibited in CRS. Affected organs are routinely small for gestational age and contain reduced numbers of cells. Considering the inhibitory effect of RUBV on primary cells, it is thought that virus infection early in organogenesis inhibits cell division, leading to both retardation and alteration in organ development. Virus persistence continues after birth, as evidenced by virus shedding, which generally ceases within 6 months of age. Whether virus persistence continues beyond cessation of shedding and plays a role in the delayed and progressive manifestations of CRS is not known.

Histologically, affected organs of CRS patients show a limited number of well-recognized malformations, with noninflammatory histopathology predominating. Particularly apparent are vascular lesions and focal destruction in tissue bordering these lesions. These lesions are likely to be due to virus replication in the vascular endothelium and damage to neighboring tissue may play a role in the pathogenesis of CRS. The neuropathology of CRS is of interest not only because of the defects manifest shortly after birth, but also because some CRS patients develop schizophrenia-like symptoms later in life. CRS brains are generally free of gross morphological malformations, with a common tendency toward microcephaly. Vascular damage, leptomeningitis, decreased number of oligodendroglial cells, and alteration of white matter are observed. Recently, magnetic resonance imaging of a group of CRS adults with schizophrenia-like symptoms revealed specifically reduced cortical gray matter and enlargement of the ventricles, which were not previously observed aspects of CRS-induced neuropathology. Interestingly, the comparative finding that non-CRS schizophrenia patients exhibit a pattern of brain dysmorphosis similar to that found in CRS patients with schizophrenia-like symptoms supports the hypothesis that schizophrenia is developmental in nature (there is some evidence for a viral trigger to schizophrenia).

Immune Response and Serodiagnosis

Following acute infection, anti-RUBV IgM antibodies are detectable at the time of rash onset and for a month or two afterwards, so that serodiagnostic testing for the presence of IgM is the current primary means for diagnosis of acute RUBV infection; in the succeeding weeks anti-RUBV antibodies in all immunoglobulin classes appear. The dominant early and persistent IgG response is in the IgG_1 subclass and antibodies of this class persist indefinitely after natural infection of otherwise healthy individuals. The majority of the antibody response is directed to the E1 glycoprotein, with proportionally lesser amounts of the response directed at E2 or C. Although neutralizing and complement-fixing antibodies are induced as well, the classical assay for the presence of anti-RUBV antibodies has been hemagglutination inhibition (HAI) and the current standard level of 10 IU ml^{-1} is based on an HAI titer of roughly 8. Because of the importance of serodiagnostic testing for rubella, a worldwide commercial market for rubella tests exists and a number of commercial

laboratories offer such kits, most of which are based on latex agglutination or enzyme immunoassay.

RUBV-specific cellular immune responses are measurable within 1–2 weeks of onset of illness. Major histocompatibility complex (MHC)-restricted CD4+ epitopes have been mapped to all three of the virus structural proteins; however, CD8+ epitopes have thus far only been mapped to the C protein. HLA class I and II alleles both positively and negatively associated with antibody and lymphoproliferative responses following rubella vaccination have recently been determined.

Following fetal infection, the fetus produces IgM antibody, detectable at 18–20 weeks of gestation, and maternal IgG antibody crosses the placenta. Both types of antibody exhibit virus-neutralizing activity *in vitro*; however, neither is sufficient to resolve virus infection during gestation. As discussed above, the intracellular maturation of virus probably shields it from antibody. After birth, the presence of IgM or a lack of decline of IgG titer are both considered diagnostic of fetal infection. CRS infants exhibit various degrees of impairment in the cellular immune response to RUBV and it is thus a deficiency in this arm of the immune response that allows the virus to persist. Considering the cellular immune deficiency in CRS infants, it is curious that detectable virus persistence ends relatively shortly after birth. The means by which virus persistence is cleared under these conditions is not understood.

Diagnosis

The common symptoms of acute rubella, lymphadenopathy, erythematous rash, and low-grade fever, are nonspecific and easily confused with illnesses caused by other common pathogens. A definitive diagnosis of rubella requires detection of the presence of IgM antibodies or a rise in IgG antibodies in paired acute-phase and convalescent-phase serum samples. Virus is also readily isolated from saliva or nasopharyngeal washings at the time of rash onset. Reverse transcription-polymerase chain reaction (RT-PCR) assays have been developed to detect virus in saliva, blood, or urine. Generally, virus isolation is only done to collect specimens for molecular epidemiological analysis. Diagnosis of acute rubella is of utmost importance during early pregnancy. There is no intervention for congenital rubella other than abortion; however, as discussed above, maternal infection does not always lead to CRS, resulting in an extremely difficult decision. RT-PCR can be used to detect virus RNA in amniotic fluid or chorionic villi, but is rarely employed. Diagnosis of CRS in a newborn is initially made on the basis of symptoms and confirmed in the laboratory by serological testing for the presence of IgM antibodies, by lack of decrease of IgG antibodies in serum specimens, or by detection of virus or virus RNA. As stated above, CRS infants shed virus and therefore are a source of contagion.

In countries with vaccination programs, the need for detection of acute rubella is rare. However, serodiagnosis for determination of immune status is routine for pre-pregnancy planning, employment in medical facilities and, in some states in the US, to obtain a marriage license. Serodiagnosis can also be used in lieu of proof of vaccination, which is required for school enrollment. Individuals found to be seronegative are subsequently vaccinated, which is done postpartum in the case of a woman who is pregnant at the time of testing.

Prevention and Control of Rubella

As discussed above live, attenuated vaccines were developed and placed in use by 1970. The vaccine used in most countries is the RA 27/3 vaccine. In Japan, five live, attenuated vaccine strains were developed and are currently in use. Additionally, at least one Chinese vaccine strain is currently in use in China.

Attenuated RUBV vaccines cause subclinical infection with transient viremia in susceptible patients. Natural transmission of vaccine virus has not been reported. The RA27/3 vaccine strain produces seroconversion in greater than 95% of recipients. Vaccine-induced titers are lower than those induced by natural infection but appear to last indefinitely. The RUBV vaccine is generally administered to children in trivalent form with the measles- and mumps-attenuated vaccines (MMR) but inclusion of the recently licensed varicella vaccine in a tetravalent vaccine is being strongly considered.

The RUBV vaccines have been among the most successful in terms of induction of immunity with an absence of side effects. However, two issues have arisen concerning rubella vaccination. The first is that the vaccine virus can cross the placenta and infect the fetus. However, US and Israel registries of deliveries to women inadvertently vaccinated during early pregnancy revealed no reported congenital abnormalities. Similar findings were reported in subsequent studies conducted in other countries in conjunction with mass vaccination campaigns. Nevertheless, vaccination during pregnancy is contraindicated and is deferred until postpartum. Second, is the occurrence of arthralgia and arthritis following vaccination. Joint complications are nonexistent in children with the currently used rubella vaccines; however, transient arthralgia and arthritis is reasonably common among adult female vaccinees. There have also been reports of chronic arthritis and related neurological involvement following vaccination of adult women. Although these complications are consistent

with complications that can accompany natural rubella in adult females, recent studies have shown that the incidence of such vaccine-related complications is low and cannot be statistically differentiated from the incidence of similar symptoms in control, unvaccinated populations.

Since the inception of rubella vaccination in 1969, the US has employed a strategy of universal vaccination at 15 months of age augmented with vaccination of sero-negative 'at-risk' individuals (women planning pregnancies, healthcare workers) which was successful in bringing the incidence of rubella and CRS to low levels by 1988. A resurgence of rubella and CRS that occurred between 1989 and 1991 among foci of unvaccinated individuals led, in part, to administration of a second dose of MMR vaccine when the recipients were between 5 and 10 years of age. After 2000, the incidence of rubella fell to fewer than 25 cases per year and in 2004 and it was concluded that indigenous rubella had been eliminated from the US. Vaccination programs have also been in place in Europe and Japan since the development of live, attenuated vaccines; however, developing countries were slower to institute rubella vaccination programs. However, efforts among developing countries have accelerated since 2000, particularly in conjunction with ongoing measles elimination efforts, and currently roughly 50% of countries worldwide have national rubella vaccine programs. The World Health Organization Regions of the Americas and Europe have set goals for elimination of rubella and CRS by 2010.

Despite the recent increase in intensity of rubella vaccination efforts worldwide, most of Asia and Africa are not currently included and thus well over half of the world's population is not covered. The cost of the vaccine, the general mildness of the disease, and the nature of national public health infrastructures are deterrents to vaccination programs in developing countries. Moreover, estimates of CRS incidence are difficult to obtain because the three hallmark symptoms of CRS, deafness, blindness, and mental retardation, are not uniformly present and are not readily diagnosable in newborns. Surveys in developing countries show that the rate of CRS in developing countries is the same as that in developed countries prior to vaccination and a recent economic analysis concluded that the cost/benefit ratio for rubella vaccination was similar to that for hepatitis B vaccination, a pathogen that is universally recognized to impart a societal load. Nevertheless, the success of worldwide rubella vaccination appears dependent on piggy-backing on global measles vaccination programs. In addition to its efforts to initiate rubella vaccination programs in developing regions, the WHO established a global Measles–Rubella Surveillance Network in 2003. Interestingly, rubella vaccination and the concomitant reduction in rubella simplifies measles surveillance which requires diagnosis of rubella because of the similarity of symptoms of the two diseases. A major modification in measles/rubella vaccination may be forth-coming in the form of aerosolized vaccines. Aerosol administration mimics the natural route by which these two viruses are contracted and preliminary studies show that aerosolized vaccine uptake and efficacy is as good as or better than the current injection route. Use of aero-solized vaccines would reduce vaccination costs by elim-inating needles and the concomitant need for trained personnel for administration. Finally, it is emphasized that rubella reduction in developing countries imparts benefit to developed countries, in which most rubella out-breaks are due to importation, by decreasing such outbreaks and thus easing control efforts. However, discontinuation of rubella vaccination in developed countries would require eradication.

Future

Because of its clinical similarity to any of a diverse group of clinical diseases, RUBV will remain a fascinating path-ogen. As an example, the incidence of diabetes in CRS patients is the best statistically direct association between a specific human virus and a specific autoimmune disease. The mechanism of viral involvement, if any, in each of these diseases is not fully understood. Elucidating the mechanism of RUBV-induced birth defects could also pro-vide understanding into teratogenesis by other infectious agents. Unfortunately, our present understanding of disease mechanisms in the RUBV-related syndromes is hindered by the lack of a suitable animal model system that fully mimics the infection seen in humans, making development of an animal model a research priority. RUBV is taxonomically unique and appears to have evolved as a recombinational

hybrid of distantly related ancestor viruses. Thus, investi-gation of the molecular biology of RUBV likely will reveal novel replication strategies and yield insight into virus evolution. The greatest challenge concerning RUBV is the current and forthcoming elimination efforts in most regions of the world.

See also: Hepatitis E Virus; Measles Virus; Togaviruses: General Features.

Further Reading

Best JM, Castillo-Solorzano C, Spika JS, *et al.* (2005) Reducing the global burden of congenital rubella syndrome: Report of the World Health Organization steering committee on research related to measles and rubella vaccines and vaccination, June 2004. *International Journal of Infectious Diseases* 192: 1890–1897.
Frey TK (1994) Molecular biology of RUBV. *Advances in Virus Research* 44: 69–160.
Hobman TC and Chantler JK (2007) RUBV. In: Knipe DM and Howley PM (eds.) *Fields Virology*, 5th edn., pp. 1069–1100. Philadelphia: Lippincott Williams and Wilkins.
Law LJ, Ilkow CS, Tzeng WP, *et al.* (2006) Analyses of phosphorylation events in the RUBV capsid protein: Role in early replication events. *Journal of Virology* 80: 6917–6925.
Ovsyannikova IG, Jacobson RM, Vierkant RA, Jacobsen SJ, Pankratz VS, and Poland GA (2005) Human leukocyte antigen class II alleles and rubella-specific humoral and cell-mediated immunity following measles–mumps–rubella-II vaccination. *International Journal of Infectious Diseases* 191: 515–519.
Plotkin SA (2006) The history of rubella and rubella vaccination leading to elimination. *Clinical Infectious Diseases* 43(supplement 3): S164–S168.
Reef SE, Frey TK, Theall K, *et al.* (2002) The changing epidemiology of rubella in the 1990s: On the verge of elimination and new challenges for control and prevention. *JAMA* 28(7): 464–472.
Tzeng WP, Matthews JD, and Frey TK (2006) Analysis of RUBV capsid protein-mediated enhancement of replicon replication and mutant rescue. *Journal of Virology* 80: 3966–3974.
Zhou Y, Ushijima H, and Frey TK (2007) Genomic analysis of diverse RUBV isolates. *Journal of General Virology* 88: 932–941.

Togaviruses: General Features

S C Weaver, University of Texas Medical Branch, Galveston, TX, USA
W B Klimstra and K D Ryman, Louisiana State University Health Sciences Center, Shreveport, LA, USA

Glossary

Alphavirus A virus in the genus *Alphavirus.*
Arbovirus A virus transmitted to vertebrates by hematophagous (blood-feeding) insects.
Endemic A disease constantly present in a community in a defined geographic region.
Enzootic A disease constantly present in an animal community in a defined geographic region.

Epidemic Outbreak of human disease above the normal (endemic) incidence.
Epizootic Outbreak of disease in animals above the normal (enzootic) incidence.
Vector An arthropod (mosquito in the case of most alphaviruses) that transmits an arbovirus.
Zoonotic A human disease whose causative agent is maintained in populations of wild animals.

Introduction and History

The *Togaviridae* is a family of enveloped, single-stranded, plus-strand RNA viruses that occur nearly worldwide. The family includes the genus *Alphavirus*, a group of zoonotic viruses maintained primarily in rodents, primates, and birds by mosquito vectors. Human disease occurs when people intrude on enzootic transmission habitats and are bitten by infected mosquitoes, or when the virus emerges to cause epizootics and epidemics. The other genus in the family *Togaviridae* is *Rubivirus*, with Rubella virus, the etiologic agent of 3-day measles (German measles), as its only member.

The first togaviruses to be isolated were the alphaviruses Western equine encephalitis virus (WEEV) and Eastern equine encephalitis virus (EEEV) in 1930 (although EEEV was not described until 1933), followed by Venezuelan equine encephalitis virus (VEEV) in 1938. Serologic tests using hemagglutination inhibition (HI) later indicated that these three viruses were antigenically related, and in 1954 Casals and Brown designated two groups of arboviruses: 'Group A' included WEEV, EEEV, and VEEV, Semliki Forest virus (SFV), and Sindbis virus (SINV), while 'Group B' is now known to include scores of flaviviruses. The HI test also indicated degrees of relatedness within viruses of Group A, with cross-reactions between EEEV and VEEV stronger than reactions between these viruses and WEEV, SFV, or SINV. These interrelationships, which formed the basis for the definitions of the antigenic complexes of alphaviruses, have generally stood the test of time, and are reflected in the phylogenetic relationships described below. Other assays including complement fixation (CF) and neutralization (NT) tests were used in some cases to define relationships on a finer scale. The introduction of the kinetic HI test later allowed further discrimination of certain alphaviruses, such as the antigenic varieties within the VEE complex and between North American and South American EEEV strains. The serological interrelationships among the alphaviruses were later determined to reflect the envelope glycoproteins in the case of HI and NT, and a mixture of structural and nonstructural proteins in the case of CF.

For some time, the *Togaviridae* included four genera: *Alphavirus, Rubivirus, Flavivirus,* and *Pestivirus.* Not until the morphology, RNA genome organizations and coding strategies, as well as the protein and nucleotide sequences were determined for representatives was it recognized that the former two genera differ dramatically from the latter two. The flaviviruses and pestiviruses were then placed into a distinct family, the *Flaviviridae* (now with three genera), and the *Alphavirus* and *Rubivirus* genera were retained in the family *Togaviridae.*

Structure, Systematics, and Evolution

The basis for grouping the alphaviruses and Rubella virus into the *Togaviridae* is that they have very similar genome organizations and coding strategies, as well as primary sequence homology that can be detected in short motifs in the nonstructural protein genes (**Figure 1**). Alphavirus virions have been visualized at high resolution using cryoelectron microscopy. The E1 envelope glycoprotein domain that lies outside of the lipid

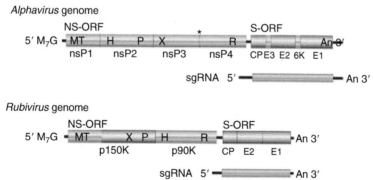

Figure 1 Togavirus genomic coding strategies. Shown are comparative schematic representations of the alphavirus and rubivirus genomic RNAs with untranslated regions represented as solid black lines and open reading frames (ORFs) as open boxes (NS-ORF, nonstructural protein ORF; S-ORF, structural protein ORF). Within each ORF, the coding sequences for the proteins processed from the translation product of the ORF are delineated. The asterisk between nsP3 and nsP4 in the alphavirus NS-ORF indicates the stop codon present in some alphaviruses that must be translationally read through to produce a precursor containing nsP4. Additionally, within the NS-ORFs, the locations of motifs associated with the following activities are indicated: MT, methyltransferase; P, protease; H, helicase; X, unknown function; and R, replicase. The sequences encompassed by the subgenomic RNA (sgRNA) are also shown. Reproduced from Weaver SC, Frey TK, Huang HV, *et al.* (2005) *Togaviridae.* In: Fauquet CM, Mayo MA, Maniloff J, Desselberger U, and Ball LA (eds.) *Virus Taxonomy: Eighth Report of the International Committee on Taxonomy of Viruses,* pp. 999–1008. San Diego, CA: Elsevier Academic Press, with permission from Elsevier.

envelope has been crystallized and its structure solved to atomic resolution. The folds of the alphavirus E1 protein are very similar to those of the flavivirus envelope protein, indicating that these proteins are homologous (share a common ancestral gene) and that the togaviruses and flaviviruses share a distant, common ancestor, at least for the E1/E protein genes which, due to their extensive divergence, cannot be detected from the nucleotide or amino acid sequences.

Alphavirus virions are about 70 nm in diameter; the nucleocapsid, which forms in the cytoplasm of infected cells, includes one molecule of genomic RNA and 240 copies of the capsid protein arranged in hexons and pentons in a $T = 4$ lattice. This icosahedral structure dictates the arrangement of the envelope proteins in the virion. Outside of the plasma membrane-derived lipid envelope, trimeric envelope spikes on the surface of the virion are composed of E1/E2 heterodimers, with the E2 protein most exposed and believed to interact with cellular receptors. The Rubella virion appears as a spherical particle, 60–70 nm in diameter, in electron micrographs. Rubella virus differs from alphaviruses in that the electron translucent zone between the nucleocapsid and envelope proteins is wider and the rubiviruses have a $T = 3$ icosahedral symmetry.

The alphaviruses and rubiviruses are quite distantly related and both share sequence homology with several taxa of plant viruses, some of which are transmitted by insects. These relationships suggest that the ancestor of these viruses was an insect virus that underwent a process called modular evolution that led to several genome rearrangements, including segmentation.

Before the era of molecular genetics, the alphaviruses were grouped into several antigenic complexes based on cross-reactivity in serologic assays including HI and CF (but generally not plaque reduction neutralization; PRNT) (**Table 1**). Within some of these complexes, the VEE complex, for example, differentiation of antigenic subtypes and varieties, some of which have fundamental and critical epidemiological and virulence differences, was accomplished using specialized forms of HI and, in some cases, PRNT. Direct genetic evidence of homology among the alphaviruses, and later between the alphaviruses, rubella virus, and some plant viruses, came first from direct protein sequencing, followed by nucleotide sequencing. Eventually, nucleotide sequencing largely replaced the serologic tests for determining relationships among the alphaviruses, although the latter remain useful from an epidemiological standpoint.

Nearly complete phylogenetic trees can now be constructed from homologous E1 envelope glycoprotein gene nucleotide or deduced amino acid sequences (**Figure 2**). These trees largely agree with the original antigenic groupings, with the exception of Middelburg virus, which

genetically belongs within the SF complex. The relationships of the New World members of the WEE antigenic complex have more complex relationships when the nonstructural protein genes are analyzed; these viruses group more closely with EEEV than with the Old World SINV-like members of the WEE complex or with the New World member, Aura virus. These relationships reflect an ancient recombination event between a SINV-like ancestor and a virus closely related to an ancestor of EEEV (**Figure 2**). The recombinant ancestor later gave rise to the WEE, Highlands J, and Fort Morgan virus ancestors.

Most estimates for the rate of RNA sequence evolution among alphaviruses are on the order of 10^4 substitutions per nucleotide per year, similar to those of other arboviruses and lower than those of most vertebrate viruses that do not use arthropods as vectors. These low rates may reflect constraints imposed by alternate replication on disparate hosts, as well as by persistent infection of mosquito vectors. However, the timescale for evolution of the togaviruses and alphaviruses is difficult to determine from sequence data because the ability of phylogenetic methods to compensate for sequential substitutions of the same nucleotides or amino acids is unknown.

Phylogenetic studies of alphaviruses generally point to purifying selection as dominating their evolution, presumably because most mutations are deleterious, especially when efficient replication in widely divergent hosts (mosquitoes and vertebrates) is required. Experimental evolutionary studies employing cell culture model systems also indicate that most adaptive mutations are host cell specific, supporting the hypothesis that the alternating host replication cycle constrains adaptation to new hosts by alphaviruses. The mobility of reservoir hosts appears to influence patterns of alphavirus evolution and their phylogeography. Viruses that use avian hosts, such as EEEV, WEEV, SINV, and Highlands J virus, tend to evolve within a relatively small number of sustained lineages that have very wide geographic distributions. For example, some lineages of WEEV have been sampled from California to Argentina. The efficient dispersal of these viruses by their highly mobile reservoir hosts presumably allows competition among different sympatric lineages to limit virus diversity. In contrast, alphaviruses that use hosts with more limited mobility, such as VEE complex viruses that rely on rodents and other small mammals, tend to exhibit more genetic diversity and lineages confined to smaller, nonoverlapping geographic regions.

Transovarial transmission from infected adult females to their offspring has been documented for a few alphaviruses, but it is not known whether this is important for maintenance of these viruses in nature. Persistent infection of vertebrate hosts also appears to be rare and is not known to be involved in long-term maintenance of

Table 1 Members of the genus *Alphavirus*

Antigenic complex	Virus	Antigenic subtype	Antigenic variety	Clinical syndrome in humans	Distribution
Barmah Forest	Barmah Forest virus (BFV)			Febrile illness, rash, arthritis	Australia
Eastern equine encephalitis (EEE)	Eastern equine encephalitis virus (EEEV)	I–IV		Febrile illness, encephalitis (none recognized in Latin America)	North, Central, South America
Middelburg	Middelburg virus (MIDV)			None recognized	Africa
Ndumu	Ndumu virus (NDUV)			None recognized	Africa
Semliki Forest	Semliki Forest virus (SFV)			Febrile illness	Africa
	Chikungunya virus (CHIKV)			Febrile illness, rash, arthritis	Africa
	O'nyong-nyong virus (ONNV)			Febrile illness, rash, arthritis	Africa
	Getah virus (GETV)			None recognized	Asia
	Bebaru virus (BEBV)			None recognized	Malaysia
	Ross River virus (RRV)	Sagiyama		Febrile illness, rash, arthritis	Australia, Oceania
	Mayaro virus (MAYV)			Febrile illness, rash, arthritis	South and Central America, Trinidad
	Una virus (UNAV)			None recognized	South America
Venezuelan equine encephalitis (VEE)	Venezuelan equine encephalitis virus (VEEV)	I	AB	Febrile illness, encephalitis	North, Central, South America
			C	Febrile illness, encephalitis	South America
			D	Febrile illness, encephalitis	South America, Panama
			E	Febrile illness, encephalitis	Central America, Mexico
	Mosso das Pedras virus (MDPV)		F		
	Everglades virus (EVEV)			Febrile illness, encephalitis	Florida (USA)
	Mucambo virus (MUCV)	III	A	Febrile illness, myalgia	South America, Trinidad
			C	Unknown	Peru
			D	Febrile illness	Peru
	Tonate virus (TONV)	III	B	Febrile illness, encephalitis	Brazil, Colorado (USA)
	Pixuna virus (PIXV)			Febrile illness, myalgia	Brazil
	Cabassou virus (CABV)			None recognized	French Guiana
	Rio Negro virus (RNV)			Febrile illness, myalgia	Argentina
Western equine encephalitis	Sindbis virus (SINV)			Febrile illness, rash, arthritis	Africa, Europe, Asia, Australia
		Babanki		Febrile illness, rash, arthritis	Africa
		Ockelbo		Febrile illness, rash, arthritis	Europe
		Kyzylagach		None recognized	Azerbaijan, China
	Whataroa virus (WHAV)			None recognized	New Zealand
	Aura virus (AURAV)			None recognized	South America
	Western equine encephalitis virus (WEEV)	Several		Febrile illness, encephalitis	Western North, South America
	Highlands J virus (HJV)				Eastern North America
	Fort Morgan virus (FMV)	Buggy Creek		None recognized	Western North America
Trocara	Trocara virus (TROV)				South America
Salmon pancreas disease	Salmon pancreas disease virus (SPDV)			Pancreatic disease (salmon)	Atlantic Ocean and tributaries
	Sleeping disease virus (SDV)			Sleeping disease (trout)	Worldwide
Southern elephant seal virus	Southern elephant seal virus (SESV)			None recognized	Australia

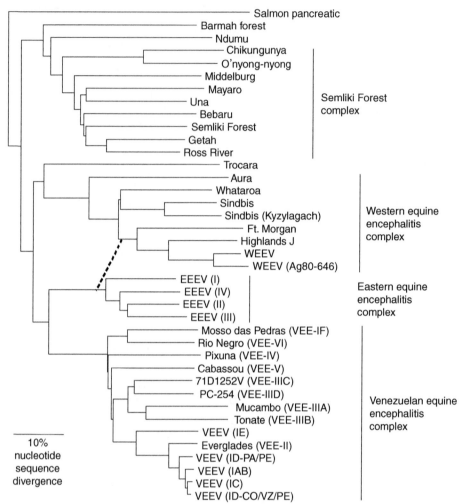

Figure 2 Phylogenetic tree of all alphavirus species except southern elephant seal virus (the homologous sequence region is not available), and selected subtypes and variants, generated from partial E1 envelope glycoprotein gene sequences using the neighbor joining program with the HKY distance formula. Antigenic complexes are shown on the right. The dashed line indicates the ancestral recombination event that led to Highlands J, Fort Morgan, and Western equine encephalitis viruses. Rubella virus cannot be included in this analysis because there is no detectable primary sequence homology with alphavirus structural protein sequences.

alphaviruses. However, mechanisms for the overwintering of alphaviruses in temperate regions, which has been suggested by several genetic studies, remain enigmatic and could include transovarial transmission and/or persistent infection of reservoir hosts.

Compared to the alphaviruses, rubella virus is relatively conserved genetically, with only one serotype described. However, phylogenetic analyses indicate the existence of at least two genotypes, with genotype I isolates predominant in Europe, Japan, and the Western Hemisphere, and the more diverse genotype II isolated in Asia and Europe. There is considerable geographic overlap between these genotypes and subgenotypes, presumably reflecting the efficient dispersal of Rubella virus by infected people.

Diseases

Most of the alphaviruses cause febrile disease in humans and/or domestic animals. However, a few alphaviruses have not been associated with any disease, including Aura, Trocara, Middelburg, Ndumu, Ft. Morgan, and Una viruses. The most severe alphaviral feature, encephalitis, is caused by the New World viruses EEEV, VEEV, and WEEV. In humans, apparent:inapparent infection rates range from very low for EEEV (*c.* 1:23) to *c.* 10:1 for VEEV. However, mortality rates in apparent human infections are inversely correlated with these ratios, with *c.* 50% for EEEV and less than 1% for VEEV. In equids, most infections are apparent, with high mortality rates (*c.* ≥50%) for all three viruses. Any of these viruses can also cause disease in a wide range of other domesticated and wild animals, with EEEV documented as the etiologic agent of severe disease in pigs, deer, emus, turkeys, pheasants, cranes, and other birds. Everglades virus is also known to cause neurologic disease in humans, and Highlands J virus has caused documented disease in domestic birds and in a horse.

Several of the Old World alphaviruses including Chikungunya (CHIKV), O'nyong nyong (ONNV), Ross River, and Barmah Forest viruses cause an arthralgic disease syndrome often accompanied by rash. Mayaro virus (MAYV), another member of the SF complex that was probably introduced into South America from the Old World, is the exception to the relationship between hemispheric distributions and disease syndromes. The arthralgic disease caused by these alphaviruses can be highly incapacitating and chronic, with affected persons unable to work or function normally for several months or longer.

Rubella virus is the etiologic agent of rubella, also known as German or 3-day measles, a generally benign infection. Occasionally, more serious complications such as arthritis, thrombocytopenia purpura, and encephalitis can occur. Congenital transmission to the fetus during the first trimester of pregnancy can lead to serious birth defects that comprise congenital rubella syndrome. Congenitally infected children suffer a variety of autoimmune and psychiatric disorders in later life, including a fatal neurodegenerative disease known as progressive rubella panencephalitis. Rubella has been largely controlled through vaccination in most developed countries, although it remains endemic worldwide.

Transmission Cycles

All alphaviruses are zoonotic, and the vast majority have transmission cycles involving mosquito vectors and avian or mammalian reservoir and/or amplification hosts. Exceptions include the fish viruses, sleeping disease virus, and salmon pancreatic disease virus; southern elephant seal virus was isolated from lice and may use these insects as mechanical, rather than biological, vectors, although transmission has not been documented. The mosquito-borne alphaviruses often have relatively narrow vector ranges, relying on one or a few principal mosquito vectors (**Figure 3**). Spillover to humans and domesticated animals results in epidemics and epizootics, with the affected animals (including humans) usually not generating sufficient viremia to participate in the transmission cycle (i.e., acting only as dead-end hosts). VEEV temporarily adapts via mutation to utilize equids as highly efficient amplification hosts (with high viremias), resulting in

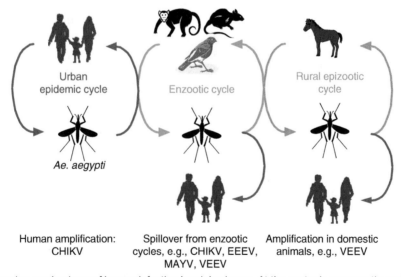

Human amplification: CHIKV

Spillover from enzootic cycles, e.g., CHIKV, EEEV, MAYV, VEEV

Amplification in domestic animals, e.g., VEEV

Figure 3 Cartoon showing mechanisms of human infection by alphaviruses. At the center is an enzootic cycle, typically involving avian, rodent, or nonhuman primates as amplification and/or reservoir hosts and mosquito vectors. Humans become infected via direct spillover when they enter enzootic habitats and/or when amplification results in high levels of circulation. Transmission to humans may involve the enzootic vector or bridge vectors with broader host preferences. Right panel: Secondary amplification involving domestic animals can increase circulation around humans, increasing their chance of infection via spillover. In the case of VEEV, mutations that enhance equine viremia are needed for secondary equine amplification. Left panel: CHIKV can use humans for amplification, resulting in urban epidemic cycles and massive outbreaks. Expanded form of virus abbreviations is provided in **Table 1**. Reproduced from Weaver SC (2005) Host range, amplification and arboviral disease emergence. *Archives of Virology* 19(supplement): 33–44, with permission from Springer-Verlag.

hundreds to several thousands of horses, donkeys, and mules affected during epizootics, and increased spillover to humans that results in epidemics of similar proportions. CHIKV and ONNV cause major epidemics by using humans as amplification hosts and, as vectors, mosquitoes that live in close association with humans, such as *Aedes aegypti, Ae. albopictus* (CHIKV), and *Anopheles* spp. (ONNV). Some alphaviruses, including EEEV, probably use secondary ('bridge') vectors during epidemics and epizootics because the primary mosquito vector (e.g., *Culiseta melanura* for EEEV) has a very narrow host range limited mainly to the animals serving as the reservoir hosts (**Figure 3**).

The infection of mosquito vectors by alphaviruses begins with the ingestion of a blood meal from a viremic vertebrate host. Susceptibility and minimum infectious doses for alphavirus infection of mosquitoes vary dramatically. Following the passage of ingested blood into the posterior midgut of the alimentary tract during feeding, infection of epithelial digestive cells occurs, presumably before the deposition of the peritrophic matrix around the blood meal, which begins with hours of feeding. Recent studies indicate that typical VEEV infections begin with fewer than 100 of the approximately 10 000 epithelial cells becoming infected, and thus the initial midgut infection may represent a bottleneck in alphavirus populations. After replication in the midgut epithelial cells, alphaviruses bud principally from the basal plasma membrane and somehow traverse the basal lamina to enter the hemocoel, or open body cavity of the mosquito. Then, transported by the hemolymph, the virus has access to many internal organs including the salivary glands, where replication leads to virus shedding into the saliva. Upon a subsequent blood meal from a naive host, transmission can occur via saliva deposited extravascularly during probing to locate a blood vessel, or intravascularly during engorgement. The amount of virus transmitted during blood feeding also varies widely, but rarely exceeds 100 infectious units of VEEV, again representing a bottleneck for virus populations. The extrinsic incubation period from an infectious blood meal to transmission by bite can occur in as little as 3 days, depending on the virus, mosquito, and temperature of incubation. However, mosquitoes generally do not re-feed until egg development and oviposition has occurred, which can require a week or more.

The sites of initial alphavirus replication in the vertebrate host are generally known only from studies using subcutaneous or intradermal needle inoculations, rather than by mosquito feeding, and can include Langerhans cells, dendritic cells, dermal macrophages, and fibroblasts in the skin. Because virus is also deposited intravascularly during mosquito feeding, other sites could be important in natural infections. Secondary replication and amplification sites also vary, including lymph nodes, spleen, myocytes, chondrocytes, osteoblasts, and neurons.

Rubella virus is transmitted via the respiratory route among infected humans, with no vector involvement. Transplacental transmission can result in severe complications and sequelae.

Alphaviruses of Greatest Medical and Veterinary Importance

The majority of alphaviruses can cause at least mild disease in humans, and most exceptions are lesser-known viruses that have not been well studied epidemiologically. Recent studies of 'dengue-like' illness in several locations have revealed that several alphaviruses such as VEEV, MAYV, and CHIKV account for a significant number of cases diagnosed clinically as dengue. Proper serological testing or virus detection is needed to accurately determine the cause of many tropical fevers that present with nonspecific 'flu-like' signs and symptoms. Brief descriptions of the most important alphaviruses follow.

Chikungunya Virus

CHIKV is probably the most important alphaviral pathogen worldwide, although it rarely causes fatal disease. CHIKV, named after a local Makonde word meaning 'that which bends up', refers to the characteristic posture assumed by patients suffering severe joint pains. The virus probably occurs in most of sub-Saharan Africa, as well as in India, Southeast Asia, Indonesia, and the Philippines. In Africa, a sylvan transmission cycle between wild primates and arboreal *Aedes* spp. mosquitoes has been characterized, and the virus probably occupies a niche similar to that of the flavivirus, yellow fever virus. In Asia and nearby islands, and recently on islands off the eastern coast of Africa in the Indian Ocean, urban and suburban CHIKV epidemics usually have been associated with *Ae. aegypti* and/or *Ae. albopictus* transmission among human amplification hosts. Explosive epidemics have affected hundreds of thousands to millions of people, and many cases are probably unrecognized because CHIKV infection is difficult to distinguish clinically from dengue. Because CHIKV infection of humans is sporadic, and no reservoir hosts or sylvatic vectors are known from Asia, it is not known whether the virus is zoonotic outside of Africa, where it is believed to have originated. Although CHIKV historically has been regarded as a nonfatal human pathogen, recent fatal cases on islands off the eastern coast of Africa in the Indian Ocean indicate a possible increase in virulence, although improved surveillance is an alternative explanation.

Eastern Equine Encephalitis Virus

In human cases, North American strains of EEEV are the most virulent of the alphaviruses with case–fatality rates generally exceeding 50%. Fortunately, only 220 confirmed cases occurred in the US from 1964 to 2004. A wide variety of domesticated mammals and birds also suffer fatal infections in North America. In South and Central America, EEEV is widespread and equine outbreaks are common, but human EEE is rare, probably due to lower human virulence in the genetically distinct strains that occur there. Attack rates in North America tend to be highest in young children and the elderly.

Transmission cycles of EEEV in North America involve *Culiseta melanura* as the principal enzootic mosquito vector, and passerine birds as reservoir hosts in hardwood swamp habitats. Bridge vectors in the genera *Aedes*, *Coquillettidia*, and *Culex* may be responsible for most transmission to humans and domestic animals. Foci occur in swamps along the eastern seaboard and the coast of the Gulf of Mexico, but have also been documented as far west as Texas and the Dakotas. In South and Central America, the ecology and epidemiology of EEEV are poorly understood. Isolates from mosquitoes suggest that the most important enzootic vectors are members of the subgenus *Culex* (*Melanoconion*), which are also enzootic vectors of most of the VEE complex viruses. Reservoir hosts are not well understood, but may include mammals or birds.

Mayaro Virus

Mayaro virus has been isolated from persons suffering from an arthralgia with rash in Surinam, French Guiana, Colombia, Panama, Brazil, Peru, and Bolivia, and probably occurs in lowland tropical forests throughout much of South America. As are infections with many other alphaviruses, clinical diagnosis of MAYV infection is unlikely and many cases are misdiagnosed as dengue. Sporadic and focal infections usually occur in people living near or working in tropical forests, and forest-dwelling mosquitoes in the genus *Haemagogus* are probably the principal vectors. Wild primates probably serve as reservoir hosts. Mayaro virus activity is often detected during investigations of outbreaks of sylvan yellow fever, probably because both viruses share the same mosquito vectors.

Mayaro virus infection is characterized by a sudden onset of fever, headache, myalgia, chills, and arthralgia, sometimes accompanied by dizziness, photophobia, retro-orbital pain, nausea, vomiting, and diarrhea. Though not known to be fatal, the arthralgia may be severe, may persist for up to 2 months, and usually affects the wrists, ankles, and toes, and less commonly the elbows and knees. Approximately two-thirds of patients develop a fine maculopapular rash on the trunk and extremities.

O'nyong-nyong Virus

ONNV, a close relative of CHIKV, derives its name from the description by the Acholi tribe, meaning 'joint breaker'. The virus was first isolated and characterized in 1959 during an epidemic involving *c.* 2 million people in Uganda, Kenya, Tanzania, Mozambique, Malawi, and Senegal. Since that epidemic ended in 1962, only a single major epidemic (1996, in the Rakai, Mbarara, and Masaka districts of southwestern Uganda and bordering Bukoba district of northern Tanzania) and a few sporadic reports of virus isolation have been reported. ONNV causes an arthralgia-rash syndrome that can persist for months, and all age groups are affected. Epidemic transmission involves *Anopheles funestus* and *An. gambiae* mosquitoes, which also transmit malaria parasites in Africa. ONNV is the only known alphavirus with *Anopheles* spp. vectors.

Ross River Virus

Ross River virus (RRV) infection has been recognized in Australia since 1928 as associated with epidemic polyarthritis. The disease there may involve up to thousands of people annually, and occurs mainly during the summer and autumn as sporadic cases and small outbreaks, usually among vacationers and other persons living or traveling in rural areas. RRV is maintained in Australia primarily among marsupials and other wild vertebrates, with *Culex annulirostris* and *Aedes vigilax* and other mosquitoes serving as vectors. Human cases and explosive epidemics also have been documented in islands of the South Pacific. Epidemiologic studies implicated *Ae. polynesiensis* as a vector and suggested that humans may have served as amplification hosts.

Following 3–21 days of incubation, disease begins suddenly with headache, malaise, myalgia, and joint pain. Joints may be swollen and tender. Multiple joints are involved; the most commonly affected are the ankles, fingers, knees, and wrists. Pain and loss of function usually last for several weeks, but some patients have persistent or recurrent arthralgia and arthritis for up to a year. About one-half of epidemic polyarthritis patients develop a maculopapular rash, usually lasting 5–10 days; 30–50% also have low-grade fever. Persons 20–50 years of age are most commonly affected, and the incidence is higher in females. Viremia is transient and may precede the onset of arthritis. The skin rash and joint swelling may be due to a local cell-mediated immune response rather than to immune complexes or complement-mediated reaction. The synovial exudate contains no detectable virus and consists almost entirely of mononuclear leukocytes.

Venezuelan Equine Encephalitis Virus

VEE was recognized first in Venezuela in 1936. The etiologic agent, VEEV, has caused explosive equine epizootics and epidemics in many regions of the Americas. The last major epidemic in northern Venezuela and Colombia in 1995 involved approximately 100 000 persons. VEEV strains use two distinct transmission cycles: enzootic, and epidemic or epizootic. The enzootic cycles generally rely on small rodent reservoir hosts and mosquito vectors in the subgenus *Culex* (*Melanoconion*), and occur in tropical forest and swamp habitats from Florida to Argentina. These viruses and subtypes are generally avirulent for equids, but are pathogenic for humans and can cause fatal disease. In contrast, epidemic or epizootic VEEV (subtypes IAB, IC) are virulent for both equids and humans, but have only temporary, unstable transmission cycles involving *Aedes* and *Psorophora* spp. mosquitoes, which transmit the virus among equids circulating high levels of viremia (**Figure 3**). People generally become infected by mosquitoes that previously engorged on viremic equids. VEE outbreaks are believed to occur following mutations of enzootic subtype ID viruses, which result in the transformation to an equid-virulent, IAB or IC subtype.

Following an incubation period of 1–4 days, symptoms of human VEE include fever, lethargy, headache, chills, dizziness, body aches, nausea, vomiting, and/or prostration. Symptoms usually subside after several days, but may recrudesce. Disease occurs in all age groups and both sexes, but severe neurologic signs, including convulsions and seizures, occur primarily in children (4–14% of pediatric cases) and usually late in the illness. Case–fatality rates are estimated at 0.5%.

Western Equine Encephalitis Virus

WEEV was first isolated from a horse brain in the Central Valley of California during a major epizootic in 1930. Like EEEV, WEEV was not established as an etiological agent of human disease until 1938. Later, WEEV was identified nearly throughout the Americas including the eastern US, but more detailed antigenic and genetic studies eventually elucidated other members of the WEE antigenic complex including Highlands J virus in eastern North America and Fort Morgan virus in the central United States. The distribution of WEEV is now believed to include western North America through Central and South America to Argentina. Virus strains from this wide range are remarkably conserved genetically, suggesting efficient transport by birds during migrations. Antigenically and genetically distinct WEEV subtypes with more limited distributions in South America have also been identified, and some are less virulent in murine models. All of these WEEV-related New World viruses are believed to have descended from an ancient, recombinant alphavirus that obtained its nonstructural and capsid protein genes from an EEEV-like ancestor and its envelope glycoprotein genes from an ancestor of SINV.

In the western US, WEEV is transmitted primarily in agricultural habitats by *Culex tarsalis* mosquitoes among passerine birds, principally sparrows and house finches. A secondary cycle involving *Aedes* spp. mosquitoes and lagomorphs has also been described in central California, and *Aedes* mosquitoes have been implicated as equine epizootic vectors in Argentina. Human infections with WEEV range from inapparent (the vast majority) to a flu-like syndrome to life-threatening encephalitis and meningitis. Symptomatic infection typically includes a sudden onset with fever, headache, nausea, vomiting, anorexia, and malaise, followed by cognitive symptoms, weakness, and meningeal involvement. Young children tend to be affected more severely than adults, and 5–30% suffer permanent neurologic sequelae. The overall human case–fatality rate is about 3%. WEEV also causes encephalitis in equids, with case–fatality rates of 10–50%. Despite a history of producing epidemics with thousands of human cases, WEEV has apparently declined as a human pathogen since the 1970s, probably due in part to irrigation, mosquito control, and culturally reduced human exposure to mosquitoes.

Alphavirus Pathogenesis

Detailed pathogenesis studies of alphavirus infections have been performed for only a few members of the genus. Although they do not normally cause encephalitis in humans or domestic animals, SINV and SFV have served as models for other alphaviruses because they can cause encephalitis in young mice yet require lower levels of biocontainment than the human-virulent members of the genus. In the experimental encephalitis model these viruses cause apoptotic death of neurons after intracerebral inoculation. Studies with these and other aphaviruses described below indicate that the type 1 interferon response is critical for the initial control of infection, and that humoral immunity is most important for clearance of primary infection and for protection against subsequent infections. Cell-mediated immunity has been regarded as less important, and elimination of alphaviruses from the central nervous system is thought to occur via noncytolytic mechanisms.

Among the highly human-pathogenic alphaviruses, VEEV pathogenesis has received the most attention. The murine model produces uniformly fatal encephalitis following all routes of infection. Following subcutaneous infection, dendritic cells are believed to be infected in the dermis, followed by migration to the draining lymph node where high levels of replication result in viremia and lymphodepletion. Also associated with infection is a vigorous innate immune response that may contribute to neuroinvasion and/or febrile illness. VEEV typically invades the central nervous system via olfactory neurons.

Encephalitis develops by day 5–7, when the virus has been cleared from the periphery by the adaptive immune response. However, VEEV continues to replicate to high titers in the brain and paralysis is quickly followed by death. Clinical encephalitis probably results from both virus- and immune-mediated neuronal cell death.

The pathogenesis of EEEV is poorly understood, but appears to differ fundamentally from that of VEEV in the murine model; EEEV also produces a biphasic disease, but the initial phase involves replication in fibroblasts, osteoblasts, and skeletal muscle myocytes. Invasion of the central nervous system probably occurs by a vascular route. Hamsters appear to more accurately reproduce the vascular component of EEE, which is prominent in human infections.

Among the alphaviruses that cause rash/arthralgia syndromes, only RRV has received much study as an etiological agent. In the murine model, initial targets of subcutaneous infection are similar to those of EEEV, including bone, joint, and skeletal muscle, with severe associated inflammation involving macrophages, natural killer cells, and CD4+ and CD8+ T lymphocytes. Recent studies with mice deficient in T lymphocytes indicate that the adaptive immune response does not play a critical role in the development of arthritic disease.

Diagnosis and Treatment

Diagnosis of alphavirus infections is rare because clinical signs and symptoms are similar to those caused by many other viral pathogens, including dengue and influenza viruses. Definitive diagnosis generally requires virus isolation from blood taken during the first 2–4 days of illness, or serologic confirmation as described below. Most alphaviruses can be isolated by intracerebral inoculation of newborn mice (usually fatal), and cause cytopathic effects in cells of a variety of mammalian and avian lines. Serodiagnosis can be made by detecting a fourfold or greater change in antibody titers in acute-phase and convalescent-phase serum samples drawn 1–3 weeks apart, using an enzyme-linked immunosorbent assay (ELISA), immunofluorescence, hemagglutination inhibition, CF, or NT. Detection of antiviral immunoglobulin M (IgM) using ELISA has more recently been applied for this purpose and is now the standard assay.

Treatment of most alphavirus infections is symptomatic and supportive. Anticonvulsive therapy may be effective in severe cases of encephalitis, especially in children. Lymphoid depletion caused by VEEV may lead to bacterial infection of the gastrointestinal tract, and antibiotic therapy should be considered in severe cases. Pneumonia secondary to VEE and EEE also is common. Neurologic sequelae occur following severe EEE, VEE, and WEE, including headache, amnesia, anxiety, and motor impairment.

Control of Disease

As is the case for many other arboviruses, control of alphaviral diseases relies upon interruption of transmission by mosquito vectors, and sometimes on vaccination of amplification hosts such as equids in the case of VEE. Mosquito vector control during epidemics and epizootics usually relies upon aerial application of insecticides such as malathion, optimally applied soon after floodwater species emerge from the aquatic immature stages, prior to dispersal, extrinsic infection, and transmission. People present during epidemics should avoid exposure to mosquitoes through limitation of outdoor activities and the use of repellents containing the active ingredient meta-N,N-diethyl toluamide (DEET) or picaridin. Persons entering sylvatic or swamp habitats where enzootic EEEV or VEEV circulate in the Americas, as well as forests of Africa enzootic for CHIKV, should also take these precautions. The diel periodicity of mosquito vectors should also be considered when planning outdoor activities and control measures. For example *Haemagogus* mosquitoes, the principal vectors of MAYV, feed during the daytime in forested neotropical habitats, and bed nets and window screens therefore do not effectively protect people. *Aedes aegypti*, an important urban vector of CHIKV, readily enters and rests in homes, and outdoor applications of adulticides are largely ineffective in controlling epidemics.

See also: Japanese Encephalitis Virus; Rubella Virus; Tick-Borne Encephalitis Viruses.

Further Reading

Calisher CH and Karabatsos N (1988) Arbovirus serogroups: Definition and geographic distribution. In: Monath TP (ed.) *The Arboviruses: Epidemiology and Ecology*, vol. 1, pp. 19–57. Boca Raton, FL: CRC Press.

Casals J and Brown LV (1954) Hemagglutination with arthropod-borne viruses. *Journal of Experimental Medicine* 99(5): 429–449.

Griffin DE (2001) Alphaviruses. In: Knipe DM and Howley (eds.) *Fields Virology*, 4th edn., pp. 917–962. New York: Lippincott Williams and Wilkins.

Powers AM, Brault AC, Shirako Y, et al. (2001) Evolutionary relationships and systematics of the alphaviruses. *Journal of Virology* 75(21): 10118–10131.

Strauss JH and Strauss EG (1994) The alphaviruses: Gene expression, replication, and evolution. *Microbiology Reviews* 58(3): 491–562.

Weaver SC (2005) Host range, amplification and arboviral disease emergence. *Archives of Virology* 19(supplement): 33–44.

Weaver SC and Barrett AD (2004) Transmission cycles, host range, evolution and emergence of arboviral disease. *Nature Reviews Microbiology* 2(10): 789–801.

Weaver SC, Frey TK, Huang HV, et al. (2005) *Togaviridae*. In: Fauquet CM, Mayo MA, Maniloff J, Desselberger U,, and Ball LA (eds.) *Virus Taxonomy: Eighth Report of the International Committee on Taxonomy of Viruses*, pp. 999–1008. San Diego, CA: Elsevier Academic Press.

Varicella-Zoster Virus: General Features

J I Cohen, National Institutes of Health, Bethesda, MD, USA

Published by Elsevier Ltd.

Glossary

Acantholysis Breakdown of a cell layer in the epidermis by separation of individual epidermal keratinocytes from their neighbors.
Dysesthesia Distortion of any sense, especially touch.

History

Descriptions of vesicular rashes characteristic of chickenpox (varicella) date back to the ninth century. In 1875, Steiner showed that chickenpox was an infectious agent by transmitting the disease from chickenpox vesicle fluid to previously uninfected people. Shingles (zoster) has been recognized since ancient times. In 1909, Von Bokay suggested that chickenpox and shingles were related infections, an idea that was confirmed experimentally in the 1920s and 1930s when children inoculated with fluid from zoster vesicles were shown to contract chickenpox. In 1943, Garland suggested that zoster was due to reactivation of varicella virus that remains latent in sensory nerve ganglia, and, in 1954, Hope–Simpson reaffirmed this hypothesis.

The viral agents of varicella and zoster were first cultivated by Weller in 1952 and shown on morphologic, cytopathic, and serologic criteria to be identical. In 1984, Straus and colleagues showed that viruses isolated during sequential episodes of chickenpox and zoster from the same patient had identical restriction endonuclease patterns, proving the concept of prolonged latent carriage of the virus. In 1983, Gilden showed that varicella-zoster virus (VZV) DNA is latent in human sensory ganglia and, Hyman and colleagues showed that VZV RNA is present in human trigeminal ganglia. In 1974, Takahashi developed a live attenuated VZV vaccine for prevention of varicella, and, in 2005, Oxman and colleagues showed that a high potency formulation of this vaccine is effective in reducing rates of zoster and postherpetic neuralgia.

Taxonomy and Classification

VZV (species *Human herpesvirus 3*) is a member of genus *Varicellovirus* in subfamuly *Alphaherpesvirus* of the family *Herpesviridae*. Other alphaherpesviruses that infect humans include herpes simplex viruses 1 and 2 (HSV-1 and HSV-2), and, rarely, B virus (a macaque herpesvirus).

All of these agents exhibit relatively short replicative cycles, destroy the infected cell, and establish latent infection in sensory ganglia.

Simian varicella virus (SVV) is the most closely related, well-characterized virus to VZV. Natural infection with SVV can cause a varicella-like illness in Old World monkeys; the virus establishes latency in trigeminal ganglia, and can spontaneously reactivate to cause a rash that can transmit the virus to naive animals. The complete sequence of SVV has been determined and the virus shares nearly an identical set of genes with VZV. SVV is not known to infect humans.

Geographic and Seasonal Distribution

Varicella and zoster infections occur worldwide. Over 90% of varicella occurs during childhood in industrialized countries located in the temperate zone, but infection is commonly delayed until adulthood in tropical regions. Zoster may occur less frequently in tropical areas, because of later acquisition of primary infection. Varicella infection is epidemic each winter and spring, while zoster occurs throughout the year, without a seasonal preference.

Host Range and Virus Propagation

The reservoir for VZV is limited to humans. The virus inherently grows poorly in nonhuman animals or cell lines. Myers and colleagues, however, developed a guinea pig animal model of VZV infection by adapting the virus for growth in guinea pig embryo cells *in vitro*. Inoculation of animals results in a self-limited viremic infection and the emergence of both humoral and cellular immunity. Latent VZV DNA has been demonstrated in dorsal root and trigeminal ganglia. Rats, cotton rats, and mice inoculated with VZV develop latent infection of dorsal root ganglia. Inoculation of VZV into fetal thymus–liver implants in severe combined immune deficiency (SCID) mice results in virus replication in T cells; inoculation of virus into subcutaneous fetal skin implants reproduces many of the histopathologic features of varicella. Intravenous inoculation of SCID mice with VZV-infected human T cells results in virus infection of human skin xenografts.

An alternative, but less ideal, animal model involves the common marmoset (*Callithrix jacchus*). VZV replicates in the lungs with a mild pneumonia and a subsequent humoral immune response. Inoculation of chimpanzees with VZV results in a transient rash containing viral DNA and evokes a modest humoral immune response. None of these animal models have, as yet, reproduced the disease pattern seen in humans, namely a vesicular rash and spontaneous reactivation from latency.

VZV is usually cultured in human fetal diploid lung cells in clinical laboratories. The virus has been cultivated in numerous other human cells including melanoma cells, primary human thyroid cells, astrocytes, Schwann cells, and neurons, and can be grown in some simian cells including primary African green monkey kidney cells and Vero cells, and in guinea pig embryo fibroblasts.

VZV is extremely cell associated. The titer of virus released into the cell culture supernatant is very low, and preparation of cell-free virus, by sonication or freeze–thawing cells, usually results in a marked drop in viral titer. Therefore, virus propagation is usually performed by passage of infected cells onto uninfected cell monolayers. VZV is detected by its cytopathic effect with refractile rounded cells that gradually detach from the monolayer, or by staining with fluorescein-labeled antibody.

Genetics

Several markers can be used to distinguish different strains of the virus. These include temperature sensitivity, plaque size, antiviral sensitivity, and restriction endonuclease cleavage patterns. The molecular basis for most of these strain differences is unknown, but viruses that are resistant to acyclovir usually have mutations in their thymidine kinase gene; other resistant strains have mutations in the DNA polymerase gene.

The genome of the prototypical laboratory strain VZV Dumas consists of 124 884 bp. The identification of many viral genes was made by analogy to HSV-1 genes with similar sequences and by genetic-complementation studies in which cell lines expressing selected VZV proteins were used to support the growth of HSV-1 mutants. Cosmids and bacterial artificial chromosomes (BACs) derived from VZV have been developed to allow targeted deletion, insertion, or site-directed point mutations in individual viral gene products. Using these systems, 22 viral genes have been shown to be dispensable, and 5 genes have been shown to be required, for virus replication in vitro. Recombinant VZV containing Epstein–Barr virus (EBV), hepatitis B virus, HIV, or HSV genes have been constructed.

Evolution

Comparison of the nucleotide and predicted amino acid sequences of VZV with HSV-1 and HSV-2 indicates that these viruses originated from a common ancestor. They share similar gene arrangements and only five genes of VZV do not appear to have HSV counterparts.

VZV is more distantly related to all other human herpesviruses, but many of the nonstructural proteins involved in viral replication have conserved elements and activities. Comparison of VZV, for example, with EBV shows that the majority of VZV genes are homologous with EBV. Three large blocks of genes are conserved, although rearranged within the two genomes.

VZV isolates have been classified into three different clades, corresponding to Japanese, European, and mosaic genotypes (combination of European and Japanese). Other investigators have proposed two clades: a Singapore/Japanese and a North American/European genotype.

Serologic Relationships and Variability

There is only one serotype of VZV. Antibodies detected by the complement-fixation test and virus-specific immunoglobulin M (IgM) antibodies decline rapidly after convalescence from varicella. Other, more sensitive serologic tests, including immune adherence hemagglutination (IAHA), fluorescence antibody to membrane antigen (FAMA), and enzyme-linked immunosorbent assay (ELISA), recognize antibodies that persist for life. VZV-specific antibodies are boosted by both recrudescent infection (zoster) and exposure to others with varicella.

Variability of VZV strains has been shown primarily by differences in restriction endonuclease patterns. Passage of individual strains in vitro eventually results in minor changes in restriction endonuclease patterns, predominantly through deletion or reiteration of small repeated elements scattered throughout the genome. Other than these sites, the genome sequence is remarkably stable. For example, the sequence of the thymidine kinase gene has been determined for several epidemiologically unrelated wild-type and acyclovir-resistant strains and found to possess >99% nucleotide and amino acid sequence identity.

Epidemiology

Varicella may occur after exposure of susceptible persons to chickenpox or herpes zoster. Over 95% of primary infections result in symptomatic chickenpox. Over 90% of individuals in temperate countries are infected with VZV before age 15.

Zoster is due to reactivation of VZV in patients who have had prior chickenpox; some of these patients may not recall the primary infection. Zoster is not clearly related to exposure to chickenpox or to other cases of zoster. About 10–20% of individuals ultimately develop herpes zoster – the risk of which rises steadily with age (**Figure 1**). Severely immunocompromised patients, such as those with the acquired immunodeficiency syndrome (AIDS),

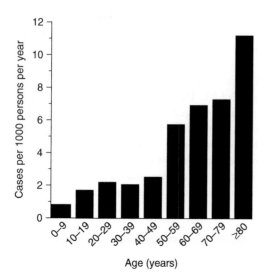

Figure 1 Incidence of herpes zoster. Reproduced from Kost RG and Straus SE (1996) Postherpetic neuralgia – pathogenesis, treatment, and prevention. *New England Journal of Medicine* 335: 32–42, with permission from Massachusetts Medical Society.

have a particularly high incidence of zoster. Recurrent zoster is uncommon; less than 4% of patients experience a second episode. Asymptomatic viremia has been detected in bone marrow transplant recipients and has been followed by recovery of cell-mediated immunity.

Transmission and Tissue Tropism

VZV is transmitted by the respiratory route. VZV has been detected by polymerase chain reaction (PCR) in room air from patients with varicella or zoster. Intimate, rather than casual, contact is important for transmission. Chickenpox is highly contagious; about 60–90% of susceptible household contacts become infected. Herpes zoster is less contagious than chickenpox. Only 20–30% of susceptible contacts develop varicella. Patients with varicella are infectious from two days before the onset of the rash until all the lesions have crusted.

Primary infection with VZV results in viral replication in the upper respiratory tract and oropharynx with lesions present on the respiratory mucosa. T cells subsequently becomes infected and transmit virus to the skin. Virus has been detected by PCR in the oropharynx and virus has been cultured from the blood early during varicella. Virus infection of epidermal cells in the skin is thought to be initially limited by interferon; later T cells trafficking in the skin may become infected and disseminate the virus to various organs throughout the body including the nervous system. During latency, VZV DNA can be detected in ganglia of the cranial nerves (e.g., trigeminal ganglia), dorsal roots (e.g., thoracic and trigeminal

ganglia), and autonomic nervous system (e.g., celiac and vagus nerve) by PCR. Using *in situ* hybridization, VZV has been detected predominantly, if not exclusively, in neurons. During latency, only 6 of the 70 known viral genes are expressed.

Zoster is due to reactivation of virus in the sensory ganglia. The factors leading to its reactivation are not known, but are associated with neural injury and cellular immune impairment. Reactivated virus spreads down the sensory nerve to the skin, where the resulting vesicles are typically confined to a single dermatome. Viremia and subsequent cutaneous or visceral dissemination of lesions may occur in zoster, especially in immunocompromised patients.

Pathogenicity

Passage of wild-type VZV in cell culture by Takahashi in 1974 led to attenuation of the virus and changes in its temperature sensitivity and infectivity for certain cell lines. The resulting Oka vaccine strain has nucleotide polymorphisms at 31 sites. Comparison of the complete nucleotide sequence of the Oka vaccine strain with its parental virus shows 42 nucleotide and 20 amino acid differences. Multiple nucleotide changes in several genes are responsible for attenuation of the vaccine for growth in skin. The Oka vaccine strain can be distinguished from wild-type strains by differences in restriction endonuclease patterns.

Clinical Features of Infection

The incubation period for chickenpox is 2 weeks, with a range of 10–21 days. The disease begins with fever and malaise, followed by a generalized vesicular rash (**Figure 2(b)**). Lesions tend to appear first on the head and trunk and then spread to the extremities. New lesions usually follow viremic waves for 3–5 days and, in the normal host, most lesions are crusted and healed by 2 weeks. Lesions in different stages coexist in an individual. The disease is usually self-limited in the normal host.

Complications of varicella are more common in neonates, children with malnutrition, immunocompromised patients (e.g., malignancy or immunosuppressive therapy), pregnant women, and older adults. These complications include bacterial superinfection of the skin, pneumonia, hepatitis, encephalitis, thrombocytopenia, and purpura fulminans. Reye syndrome occurs in rare children who take aspirin to treat varicella fevers. Prior to the widespread use of the varicella vaccine in the USA, there were about 3–4 million cases of varicella each year

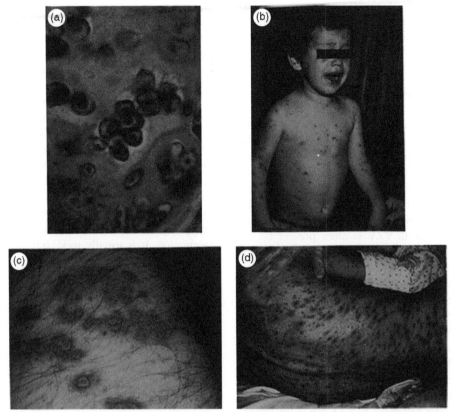

Figure 2 Histopathology and clinical findings of varicella-zoster virus infections. (a) Eosinophilic intranuclear inclusions from a skin biopsy in a patient with herpes zoster (original magnification ×400). (b) Chickenpox in a child. (c) Localized zoster in an adult. (d) Disseminated zoster in a patient with chronic lymphocytic leukemia. Reproduced from Straus SE, Ostrove JM, Inchauspe G, *et al.* (1988) Varicella-zoster virus infections: Biology, natural history, treatment, and prevention. *Annals of Internal Medicine* 108: 221–237, with permission from American College of Physicians.

with about 100 deaths; however, the number of cases has dropped sharply and death from varicella in the USA is very rare.

Zoster usually presents with pain and dysesthesias 1–4 days before the onset of the vesicular rash. The rash is usually painful and confined to a single dermatome (**Figure 2(c)**), but may involve several adjacent dermatomes. Fever and malaise often accompany the rash. Vesicles often are pustular by day 4 and become crusted by day 10 in the normal host.

Postherpetic neuralgia (PHN), manifested by pain lasting for weeks to several years in the area of the initial rash, is the most common and disconcerting complication of zoster in the normal host. Less common complications include encephalitis, myelitis, the Ramsay–Hunt syndrome (lesions in the ear canal, with auditory and facial nerve involvement), ophthalmoplegia, facial weakness, and pneumonitis. Immunocompromised patients with zoster are more likely to develop disseminated disease (**Figure 2(d)**) with neurologic, ocular, or visceral involvement. Patients with AIDS have a high frequency of zoster and may develop recurrent or chronic disease with verrucous, hyperkeratotic skin lesions.

Pathology and Histology

Varicella lesions are readily recognized in the skin and mucous membranes. However, similar lesions also occur in the mucosa of the respiratory and gastrointestinal tracts, liver, spleen, and any tissue, and remain unrecognized except in severe cases. With severe disease, there is inflammatory infiltration of the small vessels of most organs. Zoster causes inflammation and necrosis of the sensory ganglia and its nerves, and skin lesions that are histopathologically identical to those seen with varicella.

Cutaneous lesions due to VZV begin with infection of capillary endothelial cells followed by direct spread to epidermal epithelial cells. The epidermis becomes edematous with acantholysis and vesicle formation. Mononuclear cells infiltrate the small vessels of the dermis. Initially, vesicles contain clear fluid with cell-free virus, but later the vesicles become cloudy and contain neutrophils, macrophages, interferon, and other cellular and humoral components of the inflammatory response pathways. Subsequently, the vesicles dry leaving a crust that heals usually without scarring.

Cells infected with VZV show eosinophilic intranuclear inclusions with multinucleate giant cell formation (**Figure 2(a)**). These changes are not specific for VZV, as they are seen with HSV and cytomegalovirus infections.

Immune Response

Infection with VZV elicits both a humoral and cellular immune response. The ability of VZV immune globulin (VZIG) to attenuate or prevent infection in exposed children (see the next section) indicates that virus-specific antibody is important in protection from primary infection. The presence of VZV-specific immunoglobulin G (IgG) does not correlate, however, with protection from zoster. Antibody to VZV is often present by the time the rash of varicella first appears. Virus-specific IgM, IgG, and IgA are present within 5 days of symptomatic disease; however, only IgG persists for life. Antibodies to viral glycoproteins gE, gB, gH, and the immediate-early 62 protein (IE62) have been detected during acute infection, and the titers of antibodies to these proteins are boosted during recurrent infection. The mere presence of antibody to VZV glycoproteins in children with leukemia who had received live varicella vaccine is not adequate to prevent breakthrough varicella or zoster.

Cellular immune responses to VZV are more important in recovery from acute varicella infection and for prevention of, and recovery from, zoster. The level of cellular immunity correlates with disease severity during acute varicella. Cytotoxic T cells that lyse virus-infected cells are present by 2–3 days after the onset of the rash of varicella. Cell-mediated immunity, as measured by lymphocyte proliferative response, is directed against cells expressing glycoproteins gE, gB, gH, gI, and gC, the IE4, IE62, and IE63 proteins, and other viral proteins. Interferon is present in VZV vesicles.

Most varicella infections result in lifelong immunity to reinfection. Second episodes of varicella are rare; these individuals tend to have reduced humoral and cellular immunity to VZV at the time of the second infection. Zoster is associated with a reduction in cellular immunity to VZV that, in the normal host, is partially restored in response to this recurrent infection. Recurrent zoster is uncommon, except in severely immune-deficient patients, such as those with AIDS.

Prevention and Control

Prevention of varicella can be achieved by restricting exposure or by resorting to either immunoglobulin prophylaxis or vaccination with live, attenuated virus. If given within 4 days of exposure to the virus, VZIG prevents or attenuates varicella in seronegative persons. The preparation has no effect in modifying zoster. VZIG is recommended for individuals (1) with recent, close contact to patients with varicella or zoster, (2) who are susceptible to varicella, and (3) who fall in a high-risk category. The latter include premature or certain newborn infants, pregnant women, and patients with congenital or acquired cellular immunodeficiencies. Supplies of VZIG are currently very limited in the USA and VariZIG, prepared from high-titer human immune serum, has replaced VZIG.

The live, attenuated varicella vaccine (Oka strain) was licensed in the USA in 1995 and is recommended for vaccination of healthy children and adults. Most children develop adequate humoral and cellular immunity to varicella after a single dose of vaccine; an additional dose enhances the degree of immunity and is recommended for susceptible children and adults. A rash may follow vaccination. It is usually mild, but can be severe if the vaccine is given to patients experiencing periods of profound cellular immune impairment. The live vaccine virus establishes neural latency and can reactivate. Thus, zoster has been reported in vaccinees, especially those who are immunocompromised, but the rate appears to be no higher than that following natural infection. Vaccination may be used for postexposure prophylaxis.

A high-titer formulation of the Oka vaccine virus was licensed in the USA in 2006. It reduced the frequency of zoster and PHN by 51% and 67%, respectively, in healthy persons ≥60 years old. The most common side effects were mild injection-site reactions; no significant severe adverse reactions were attributed to the vaccine.

Patients with varicella or zoster should be isolated from susceptible persons until all lesions have crusted. This is particularly important for hospital workers and immune-deficient patients.

Acyclovir and leukocyte interferon have been used in the treatment of varicella and zoster in immunocompromised patients. Interferon proved to be an inadequate and impractical therapy. Acyclovir is the current treatment of choice for selected infections. It results in a shorter duration of symptoms and decreased visceral dissemination of varicella or zoster in the immunocompromised host. Acyclovir also prevents spread of trigeminal zoster to the eye and modestly shortens the duration of varicella and zoster symptoms in the normal host. Analogs of acyclovir, such as famciclovir and valaciclovir, result in higher levels of antiviral activity than oral acyclovir and have been licensed for oral therapy of zoster in the USA. Acyclovir-resistant strains of VZV have been reported in patients with AIDS; these infections are best treated with foscarnet. Corticosteroids, when used early during zoster, reduce acute pain. Herpes zoster, particularly in elderly patients, may lead to prolonged and severe PHN. Treatment of PHN is difficult and often unsatisfactory, but many patients experience improvement with gabapentin, pregabalin, or tricyclic antidepressant drugs like amitriptyline.

Future Perspectives

Widespread vaccination of children with the attenuated, live varicella vaccine has reduced the incidence and severity of varicella. Use of a high-titer live varicella vaccine was shown to lower the incidence of zoster and postherpetic neuralgia in the elderly. Further research is needed into the mechanisms of VZV latency and reactivation as well as identification of which viral proteins are critical for protection from varicella and zoster. Since the live varicella vaccine can reactivate to cause zoster and since breakthrough cases of varicella continue to occur in vaccinated persons, further knowledge of VZV latency and immunity should lead to safer and more effective vaccines against varicella and herpes zoster.

See also: Herpesviruses: Latency.

Further Reading

Cohen JI, Brunell PA, Straus SE, and Krause PR (1999) Recent advances in varicella-zoster virus infection. *Annals of Internal Medicine* 130: 922–932.

Cohen JI, Straus SE, and Arvin AM (2007) Varicella-zoster virus: Replication, pathogenesis, and management. In: Knipe DM, Howley PM, Griffin DE, et al. (eds.) *Fields Virology,* 5th edn, pp. 2773–2818. Philadelphia, PA: Lippincott Williams and Wilkins.

Gershon A and Arvin A (2000) *Varicella-Zoster Virus.* Cambridge: Cambridge University Press.

Gilden DH, Cohrs RJ, and Mahalingham R (2003) Clinical and molecular pathogenesis of varicella-zoster virus infection. *Viral Immunology* 16: 243–258.

Hambleton S and Gershon AA (2005) Preventing varicella-zoster disease. *Clinical Microbiology Reviews* 18: 70–80.

Heininger U and Seward JF (2006) Varicella. *Lancet* 368: 1365–1376.

Kimberlin D and Whitley R (2007) Varicella-zoster vaccine for the prevention of zoster. *New England Journal of Medicine* 356: 1338–1343.

Kost RG and Straus SE (1996) Postherpetic neuralgia – pathogenesis, treatment, and prevention. *New England Journal of Medicine* 335: 32–42.

Ku CC, Besser J, Abendroth A, Grose C, and Arvin AM (2005) Varicella-zoster virus pathogenesis and immunobiology: New concepts emerging from investigations with the SCIDhu mouse model. *Journal of Virology* 79: 2651–2658.

Mitchell BM, Bloom DC, Cohrs RJ, Gilden DH, and Kennedy PG (2003) Herpes simplex virus and varicella zoster latency in ganglia. *Journal of Neurovirology* 9: 194–204.

Oxman MN, Levin MJ, Johnson GR, et al. (2005) A vaccine to prevent herpes zoster and postherpetic neuralgia in older adults. *New England Journal of Medicine* 352: 2271–2284.

Straus SE, Ostrove JM, Inchauspe G, et al. (1988) Varicella-zoster virus infections: Biology, natural history, treatment, and prevention. *Annals of Internal Medicine* 108: 221–237.

HUMAN IMMUNODEFICIENCY VIRUSES

AIDS: Disease Manifestation

A Rapose, J East, M Sova, and W A O'Brien, University of Texas Medical Branch – Galveston, Galveston, TX, USA

Introduction

Human immunodeficiency virus (HIV) infection has had a staggering global impact despite its emergence only 25 years ago. It is estimated that there were around 40 million people in the world living with HIV infection in the year 2006; there were approximately 4.5 million new cases, and 3 million individuals died of acquired immunodeficiency syndrome (AIDS). Since the introduction of highly active antiretroviral therapy (HAART) in the USA and in western Europe, around 1996, there has been a significant reduction in mortality and morbidity among patients with HIV infection. The incidence of the three major opportunistic infections (OIs) associated with AIDS, namely *Pneumocystis carinii* (now called *Pneumocystis jiroveci*) pneumonia, *Mycobacterium avium complex* infection, and *Cytomegalovirus* infection is markedly reduced. Life expectancy for individuals with AIDS has increased from an estimated 4 years in 1997, to more than 24 years in 2004. Mortality rates for patients who are initiated on HAART appropriately are now comparable to populations successfully treated for other chronic conditions like diabetes. This paradigm shift has made OIs less common in populations able to access HAART. Cardiovascular disease, renal diseases, and malignancy are now the more common causes of death.

Since OIs commonly seen before the HAART era are rarely seen in patients with viral suppression, these are discussed only in passing, with citations referring to reviews or treatment guideline documents. This article focuses on clinical manifestations that pose problems in the management of HIV disease in the HAART era, including manifestations and consequences of HIV infection as well as toxic effects of treatment. There is overlap in these manifestations in that some HIV-related syndromes can be exacerbated by some antiretroviral medications. In addition, with prolonged survival, diseases associated with advancing age are becoming more prominent in HIV infection, most notably, the metabolic syndrome, which is associated with increased risk of morbidity and mortality from cardiovascular disease.

Opportunistic Infections and Malignancies Associated with HIV Infection

OIs and malignancies in patients with HIV infection emerge as a consequence of immune deficiency related to CD4+ T-lymphocyte depletion. A CD4+ T-lymphocyte count below 200 cells per mm^3 is defined as AIDS even in the absence of other diseases or symptoms since this represents such an increase in risk for OI and malignancy.

OIs and malignancies seen most commonly in HIV patients are listed in **Table 1**, and are discussed in detail in the 'AIDS surveillance case definition'. Although many of these diseases can occur in immunocompetent individuals, they are more common and often more severe in patients with AIDS. Detailed information regarding these diseases can be obtained from the website of the National Institutes of Health and the US National Library of Medicine.

Updated guidelines on the prevention of OIs in patients with HIV are available at 'Relevant website' section. While OIs are rarely seen in patients with viral suppression secondary to HAART, they may still be manifest on initial

Table 1 Common opportunistic diseases in AIDS

Fungal infections
Candidiasis
Pneumocystis jirovecii pneumonia
Cryptococcal meningitis
Disseminated histoplasmosis
Disseminated coccidioidomycosis
Mycobacterial infections
Mycobacterium tuberculosis
Mycobacterium avium complex
Mycobacterium kansasii
Viral infections
Herpes simplex virus (HSV)
Varicella zoster virus (VZV)
Cytomegalovirus (CMV)
Epstein–Barr virus (EBV-associated with oral hairy
 leukoplakia and lymphoma)
Human papilloma virus (HPV – associated with cervical
 dysplasia and ano-genital squamous cancers)
Human herpes virus-8 (HHV-8 – associated with Kaposi's
 sarcoma)
JC polyomavirus (JCPyV – associated with progressive
 multifocal leukoencephalopathy)
Bacterial infections
Salmonella septicemia
Listeriosis
Bartonella henselae (associated with bacillary angiomatosis)
Parasitic infections
Cerebral toxoplasmosis
Cryptosporidiosis
Isosporiasis
Malignancies
Kaposi's sarcoma (associated with HHV-8)
Primary CNS lymphoma
Other non-Hodgkin's lymphomas
Cervical cancer (associated with HPV)

presentation. *Pneumocystis jirovecii* infection remains an important and serious clinical manifestation as initial presentation of many HIV patients. Since HIV can be a sexually transmitted disease (STD), other STDs also occur and can pose problems in patients with AIDS. These have been recently reviewed by Jeanne Marrazzo. The differential diagnosis of oral lesions in HIV patients is vast; this has been reviewed by Baccaglini L *et al.* Eye involvement in patients with HIV infection in the era of HAART has been studied in the longitudinal study of ocular complications of AIDS (LSOCA) supported by the National Eye Institute.

Malignancies classically associated with HIV infection include Kaposi's sarcoma, primary brain lymphoma, and other non-Hodgkin's lymphomas. These have been reviewed by Mathew Cheung. While some of the AIDS-defining cancers are seen less frequently in patients on HAART, it should be noted that the incidence of anal squamous intraepithelial lesions and squamous cell carcinomas is increasing in HIV-positive individuals receiving HAART.

An important phenomenon to recognize is 'immune reconstitution inflammatory syndrome' (IRIS). Following initiation of HAART, recovery of the immune system can be associated with an apparent worsening of an HIV-associated OI or malignancy, or less commonly 'uncovering' of previously unrecognized and untreated diseases. Shingles (re-emergence of the chicken pox virus, *Varicella zoster virus*), other *Herpes* viruses, and mycobacterial infections are especially common in IRIS. With better global access to HAART, including Africa and Asia, an increasing number of cases of IRIS are being reported especially in areas with high prevalence of diseases like tuberculosis.

The Metabolic Syndrome in HIV-Infected Individuals

A constellation of laboratory and physical abnormalities, termed the metabolic syndrome, is associated with increased risk of cardiovascular morbidity and mortality (**Table 2**). This syndrome is seen in 24% of the US population overall; its prevalence is increasing in the US. The metabolic syndrome encompasses disturbances in glucose, insulin, and lipid metabolism, associated with abdominal obesity. The presence of the metabolic syndrome roughly doubles cardiovascular disease mortality. In other studies, the risk for cardiovascular disease with metabolic syndrome is even higher.

The metabolic syndrome may be even more common in HIV-infected individuals; there are many possible reasons. HIV infection on its own may exacerbate many of the manifestations of the metabolic syndrome, particularly elevation in serum triglycerides; this was seen in HIV-infected individuals prior to the advent of antiretroviral therapy.

Table 2   Universal classification of the metabolic syndrome, as defined by the International Diabetes Foundation (IDF)[41]

Characteristic	Measurement	
Waist circumference		
in women	>80 cm	(31.5 in)
in men	>94 cm	(37 in)
Triglycerides	>1.7 mmol l^{-1}	(>150 mg dl^{-1})
HDL	<1.29 mmol l^{-1}	(<50 mg dl^{-1})
Glucose	>5.6 mmol l^{-1}	(>100 mg dl^{-1})
Systolic blood pressure	>130 mm Hg	
or		
Diastolic blood pressure	>85 mm Hg	

In addition, many HIV-infected individuals smoke (50% vs. 25% in the US population overall), and many HIV-infected individuals have hypertension. The metabolic syndrome may be exacerbated by some of the drugs used to treat HIV infection, including thymidine analog reverse transcriptase inhibitors and some protease inhibitors; both tend to increase triglycerides and cholesterol, and may be associated with glucose intolerance.

There are several studies, however, that show a lower incidence of metabolic syndrome in HIV-infected individuals. In a cross-sectional study examining a cohort of 788 HIV-infected adults, metabolic syndrome prevalence was 14% by IDF criteria. Despite this low overall number, many patients in this study (49%) had at least two features of the metabolic syndrome but were not classified as having the metabolic syndrome, typically because waist circumference was not in the metabolic syndrome range. The metabolic syndrome was more common in those individuals currently receiving protease inhibitors. Although the formally defined metabolic syndrome may occur less commonly in HIV-infected individuals, components of this syndrome associated with increased risk of cardiovascular disease certainly are increased in HIV-infected individuals.

In contrast to the decreased risk of OIs seen in HIV-infected individuals who achieved virologic suppression, the metabolic syndrome and lipodystrophy (described below) appear to be more common in patients receiving HAART. The higher presence of cardiovascular disease risk factors and administration of drugs that may induce it, together with the increased survival from improved outcomes from antiretroviral therapy, make this syndrome an important one for primary care of HIV-infected individuals.

Management of the metabolic syndrome initially involves improvement in diet, increase in exercise, and avoidance of drugs that are more likely to cause the perturbation in lipid and glucose metabolism and girth. Unfortunately, switch from medications associated with higher risk of the metabolic syndrome to those that appear to be less toxic, typically, only result in minor, partial reversal of both laboratory abnormalities and abdominal fat accumulation.

HIV-Specific Diseases

Lipodystrophy

Lipodystrophy was identified and characterized by Carr and colleagues in 1998. In addition to laboratory abnormalities associated with the metabolic syndrome, there can also be subcutaneous lipodystrophy, which can involve either fat accumulation in the abdomen, neck and upper back, (**Figure 1**) or lipoatrophy, involving the extremities and the face; (**Figure 2**), and they can both be seen together. The lipoatrophy in the face is highly recognizable and can be stigmatizing. There is deepening of the nasolabial folds and loss of subcutaneous tissue in the temples and cheeks. Lipodystrophy has been associated with treatment with thymidine nucleoside analog-based (stavudine or zidovudine) regimens, and co-administration of a thymidine analog with some protease inhibitors may further accelerate fat loss. Studies investigating thymidine-sparing regimens

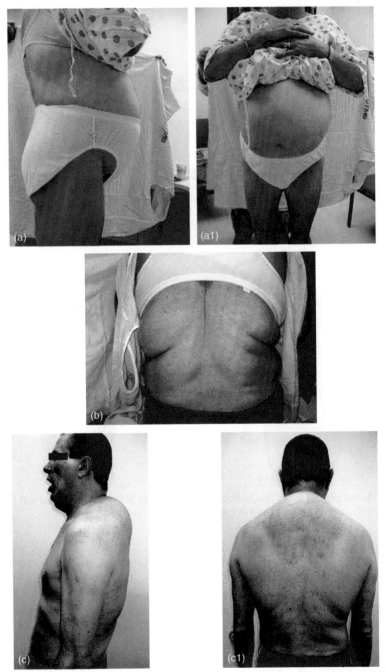

Figure 1 Lipodystrophy – fat accumulation. (a) Visceral fat accumulation, (b) flank fat accumulation, and (c) dorsal cervical fat-pad – 'Buffalo hump'.

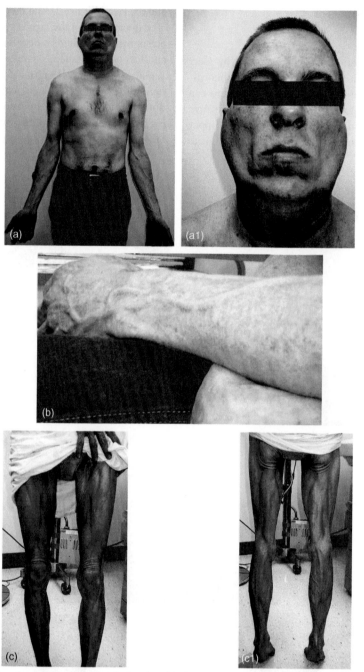

Figure 2 Lipodystrophy–lipoatrophy. (a) Facial lipodystrophy with deepening of the nasolabial fold and malar lipoatrophy, (b) partial fat atrophy with prominent veins, and (c) buttocks and leg wasting.

typically show normal limb fat mass and lower incidence of clinical lipoatrophy, even over prolonged follow-up.

Lipodystrophy is extremely difficult to manage, as specific treatments including rosiglitazone do not appear to be effective. Switching therapy from a thymidine analog to abacavir has shown modest improvement but not resolution of lipodystrophy. Recombinant growth hormone may increase subcutaneous fat but effects may not persist. Abacavir, lamivudine, and newer nucleotide reverse

transcriptase inhibitors (NRTIs) do not appear to be associated with development of lipodystrophy, and to prevent development of lipodystrophy, the older NRTIs are now commonly avoided. An exception is zidovudine, which may still retain activity in the presence of drug resistance mutations that render other drugs in this class ineffective. Nonetheless, toxicities of HIV medications are now of paramount importance since there appear to be many ways to effectively reduce viral load.

HIV and Kidney Disease

Kidney disease related to AIDS was described as early as 1984 in reports from New York and Florida. Since then, a wide spectrum of acute and chronic renal syndromes has been reported. HIV-associated kidney disease was initially thought to occur late in the course of the infection, but it is now known that the kidneys may be involved in all the stages of HIV disease including acute infection. Renal glomerular and tubular epithelial cells may be directly infected by HIV. Effective therapies for HIV infection and the associated OIs have led to improved patient survival, which in turn has resulted in an increased number of HIV-infected individuals who require renal replacement therapy. Antiretroviral treatment has also resulted in increased reports of drug-related nephrotoxicities. IRIS may also involve the kidneys. Mortality rates for kidney diseases in HIV-infected individuals are increasing, and there is evidence that HAART may slow or prevent progression.Appropriate screening for renal dysfunction and early intervention may reduce the incidence and progression of renal disease in patients with HIV infection.

Acute renal failure

Many of the causes of acute renal failure in HIV-infected patients are the same as for HIV-negative individuals, with a similar incidence of 5.9 cases per 100 patient-years. It is associated with a nearly sixfold increased risk of in-hospital mortality in HIV-infected patients. Factors associated with increased incidence in HIV-infected patients include advanced stage of HIV disease, exposure to antiretroviral therapy, and co-infection with hepatitis C virus. Pre-renal causes include hypovolemia, hypotension, or hypoalbuminemia. Intrinsic kidney diseases including acute tubular necrosis may occur secondary to hypotension, sepsis, or nephrotoxic drugs. Some agents used for treatment of OIs in HIV-infected patients, such as amphotericin B, aminoglycosides, foscarnet, and trimethoprim-sulphamethoxazole require careful renal monitoring. Post-renal etiologies in the setting of HIV may include outflow obstruction secondary to tumor, lymphadenopathy or fungus balls, and medication related nephrolithiasis as seen with the antiretroviral medications indinavir and atazanavir, and with sulfadiazine and acyclovir. Acute renal failure secondary to interstitial nephritis as a manifestation of IRIS has also been reported.

Chronic kidney disease

Three syndromes of chronic renal disease are associated with HIV infection: (1) HIV-associated nephropathy (HIV-AN), (2) HIV-associated immune complex disease (HIV-ICD), and (3) HIV-associated thrombotic microangiopathies. A kidney biopsy is required to make these diagnoses.

HIV-associated nephropathy

HIV-associated nephropathy (HIV-AN) is directly caused by HIV infection and is the most common form of chronic renal disease in HIV-infected patients. Although this syndrome has been reported in all stages of HIV disease including acute infection, advanced immunosuppression is strongly associated with HIV-AN risk. In one study, 83% of HIV-infected patients with microscopic albuminuria who were biopsied, had HIV-AN. The prevalence of HIV-AN is variable among different ethnic and racial groups suggesting that there may be genetic determinants of the disease. Casanova et al. did not find HIV-AN on biopsies in 26 Italian HIV-positive patients with renal disease. Also, none of 26 HIV-infected positive individuals with proteinuria were found to have HIV-AN in a study from Thailand by Praditpornsilpa et al. The majority of patients in the U.S. who have HIV-AN are African-American males (more than 85%). However, in one study on Ethiopian HIV patients, none of the patients fulfilled criteria for HIV-AN. This suggests that even among individuals with African heritage there may be genetic differences. Alternatively, factors other than race may play an important role in the epidemiology of this condition. Patients typically present with nephrotic syndrome in which large amounts of protein pass abnormally in the urine. However, peripheral edema, hypertension, and hematuria are often absent. Microalbuminuria is an early marker for HIV-AN and screening for microalbumniuria is recommended for early diagnosis of HIV-AN. Renal biopsy should be considered for HIV-seropositive African-American patients who present with microalbuminuria even if they have normal creatinine clearance. Classic HIV-AN is associated with focal and segmental glomerulosclerosis on histopathology. These patients can exhibit rapid progression to end-stage renal disease and prognosis is poor if left untreated. HAART may reduce the risk of development of HIV-AN and may also reduce progression of HIV-AN to end-stage renal disease, but this is controversial and antiretroviral therapy for patients with HIV-AN who do not otherwise have indications for treatment is not recommended. The best evidence for benefit of HAART in HIV-nephropathy is the reduction in incidence in the HAART era compared with earlier periods.

HIV-associated immune complex disease

HIV-associated immune complex disease (HIV-ICD) occurs less frequently than HIV-AN. There is a higher incidence in Caucasians. Four different categories have been described: (1) immune-complex mediated glomerulonephritis (with diffuse proliferative and crescentic forms), (2) IgA nephritis (with diffuse or segmental mesangial proliferation), (3) mixed sclerotic/inflammatory disease, and (4) lupus-like syndrome. The precise role of HIV infection in the pathogenesis of these entities has not been established, and glomerular inflammation may be due to the abnormal immune responses associated with HIV infection, or secondary to superinfections. The clinical presentation is often very different from HIV-AN. Patients present with hematuria and mild proteinuria. The course is more indolent, with low rates of progression to end-stage renal disease.

Thrombotic microangiopathy

Thrombotic microangiopathy in the setting of HIV infection is being increasingly recognized and has even been proposed as an AIDS-defining illness. It is seen more often in Caucasians as compared with African-Americans or Hispanics. Features include fever, diarrhea, hemolytic anemia, thrombocytopenia, renal failure, and neurological symptoms. Mortality rates are high even in the setting of aggressive treatment like plasma exchange and relapse is often seen in survivors. The pathogenesis of HIV-associated thrombotic microangiopathies is unknown.

Renal disease associated with HAART

In some cases, HAART can reverse or at least control nephropathy associated with HIV infection. However, many antiretroviral medications have been associated with renal toxicity including acute and chronic renal disease. The newer antiretroviral agents commonly in use are associated with few side effects. Adefovir was the first NRTI shown to have variable antiretroviral efficacy. However, it was highly nephrotoxic in doses (60–120 mg per day) used for treatment of HIV infection and for the first time an FDA advisory committee voted against the approval of an antiretroviral drug. It was subsequently used to treat hepatitis B infection, and appears to be safer at the lower dose. The follow-up NRTI tenofovir is associated with a modest decline in renal function, but this did not lead to greater rates of discontinuation of therapy. Also, in several large randomized trials, tenofovir did not show adverse effects on overall renal function. However as clinical use of tenofovir has widened, there have been reports of tenofovir-induced, acute renal failure, Fanconi's syndrome, renal tubular damage, and diabetes insipidus. The majority of cases have occurred in patients with underlying systemic or renal disease, or in patients taking other nephrotoxic agents including other antiretroviral agents like didanosine, lopinavir-ritonavir, or atazanavir. Patients receiving tenofovir should have creatinin clearance monitored closely. The protease inhibitor indinavir is associated with nephrolithiasis (the drug can crystallize in the urine) but cases of kidney stones associated with saquinavir, nelfinavir, and atazanavir often associated with dehydration have also been reported. The majority of medication-related, adverse events are reversible on discontinuation of the offending drug.

Although HAART can decrease the incidence of some HIV-related kidney diseases, the drugs used may cause renal problems on their own. Hence, patients should be carefully monitored clinically and by laboratory testing for microalbuminuria. A diagnosis of HIV-AN could be an indication for early initiation of HAART in an attempt to prevent further progression and potentially reverse renal disease. Other pathologies such as microangiopathy-associated renal disease carry a poor prognosis in spite of aggressive interventions. Long-term survival in patients on HAART will be associated with increased prevalence of metabolic alterations, diabetes, hypertension, and cardiovascular disease which in turn may be associated with increased secondary renal disease in these patients.

Neurologic Manifestations of HIV

Neurological complications of HIV infection are common, with more than 50% HIV patients ultimately developing some clinical manifestations. The spectrum of the disease is broad. Classical neurologic complications of HIV infection recognized in the 1980s include: (1) aseptic meningitis, (2) HIV-associated dementia (HAD), (3) vacuolar myelopathy, and (4) distal symmetric sensory polyneuropathy. More recently, neurologic manifestations are most commonly associated with the therapeutic agents used in HAART. The most dramatic neurologic manifestations occur in HIV patients not on HAART. These include manifestations secondary to opportunistic diseases like progressive multifocal leukoencephalopathy (PML), cerebral toxoplasmosis, cryptococcal meningitis, tuberculosis, and malignancies like CNS lymphomas.

Aseptic meningitis or encephalitis

Aseptic meningitis or encephalitis may be seen in up to 50–70% of patients who develop acute antiretroviral syndrome. Manifestations may recur during the course of the disease or as part of IRIS. As seen with other acute viral infections, symptoms are nonspecific and may consist of fever, headache, malaise, lymphadenopathy, and skin rash. Sometimes they may be severe enough to require hospitalization. Less common manifestations of early HIV infection include cranial nerve involvement (most commonly facial nerve), brachial plexus, and cauda equina syndromes, Guillian-Barré-like demyelinating polyneuropathy, mononeuritis multiplex, and radiculopathy.

HIV-associated dementia

HIV-associated dementia (HAD) is the most common neurological manifestation of chronic HIV infection and developed in 20–60% HIV patients before effective antiretroviral treatments became available; recently, the incidence of HAD has declined. However, the prolonged life span of individuals with HIV may ultimately lead to an increased prevalence of HAD. Even in the HAART era, HIV-related neuropsychologic deficits have significant influence on the lives of the HIV-infected patients, with rates of unemployment and dependence for activities of daily living being higher among these individuals. Minor forms of cognitive and motor abnormalities that do not progress to severe dementia are also seen. HAD manifests itself in the form of progressive impairment of attention, learning, memory, and motor skills, often accompanied by a variety of behavioral changes. In the early stages, symptoms include poor concentration, mental slowing, and apathy-mimicking depression. As the disease progresses, there is worsening memory loss, personality changes (either reduced emotion or increased irritability, or disinhibition), loss of fine motor control, tremors, slowing and unsteadiness of gait, urinary incontinence, generalized hyperreflexia, and cerebellar and frontal release signs. HAD is characterized by a waxing and waning course over months to years. Neuropsychologic testing is required to make the diagnosis and follow its progression. The effects of HAD on daily activities can be measured using standardized functional evaluations. Cerebrospinal fluid (CSF) levels of HIV RNA are strongly predictive of HIV-related cognitive disorders. Low peripheral CD4+ lymphocyte counts and high levels of HIV viral load in plasma may also predict future dementia. HAD should be a diagnosis of exclusion, meaning that other causes of cognitive impairment like depression, metabolic disorders, thyroid disorders, OIs and malignancies, and drugs should be excluded. Efavirenz, a nonnucleoside reverse transcriptase inhibitor, is associated with neuropsychiatric side effects including dizziness, confusion, impaired concentration, amnesia, hallucinations, and insomnia. Most of these symptoms occur early after initiation of efavirenz and tend to resolve within a few weeks of continued treatment. Delayed onset psychiatric symptoms have also been described. This is readily distinguished from classical HAD. Proximal muscle weakness without sensory changes suggests myopathy. Polymyositis characterized by myalgias and proximal muscle weakness can result from HIV infection itself, or secondary to zidovudine therapy.

Distal symmetric sensory polyneuropathy

Distal symmetric sensory polyneuropathy (DSPN) was recognized as a complication of HIV infection, but now is more commonly seen as a toxicity of some antiretroviral medications. In the pre-HAART era the prevalence rate was about 35% and at autopsy, 95% patients had sural nerve involvement. Low CD4+ lymphocyte counts and high viral load are significant risk factors for the development of DSPN. It is characterized by burning or aching pain, paresthesias, along with numbness or hyperpathia. It is seen more often in the lower extremities, starting in the toes and progressing proximally. On examination, there may be reduced sensation to pain, temperature, and vibration, along with reduced ankle reflexes. Strength is usually preserved. It is important to rule out other causes like diabetes, alcohol,

vitamin deficiencies, and drug related injury including HIV medications such as stavudine, didanosine, and the discontinued drug zalcitabine. Medications used to treat OIs such as the TB drug isoniazid can also cause neuropathy. Clinical presentation of neuropathy secondary to antiretroviral agents is similar to that of DSPN, though it is often more painful and may develop rapidly.

See also: Human Immunodeficiency Viruses: Antiretroviral Agents; Human Immunodeficiency Viruses: Origin; Human Immunodeficiency Viruses: Pathogenesis.

Further Reading

Baccaglini L, Atkinson JC, Patton LL, Glick M, Ficarra G, and Peterson DE (2007) Management of oral lesions in HIV-positive patients. *Oral Surgery Oral Medicine Oral Pathology Oral Radiology and Endodontics* 103(supplement): S50 e1–e23.

Carr A, Samaras K, Chisholm DJ, and Cooper DA (1998) Pathogenesis of HIV-1-protease inhibitor-associated peripheral lipodystrophy, hyperlipidaemia, and insulin resistance. *Lancet* 351(9119): 1881–1883.

Cheung MC, Pantanowitz L, and Dezube BJ (2005) AIDS-related malignancies: Emerging challenges in the era of highly active antiretroviral therapy. *Oncologist* 10(6): 412–426.

Cho ME and Kopp JB (2004) HIV and the kidney: A status report after 20 years. *Current HIV/AIDS Reports* 1(3): 109–115.

Daugas E, Rougier J-P, and Hill G (2005) HAART-related nephropathies in HIV-infected patients. *Kidney International* 67(2): 393–403.

Friis-Moller N, Reiss P, Sabin CA, et al. (2007) Class of antiretroviral drugs and the risk of myocardial infarction. *New England Journal of Medicine* 356(17): 1723–1735.

Kaplan JE, Hanson D, Dworkin MS, et al. (2000) Epidemiology of human immunodeficiency virus-associated opportunistic infections in the United States in the era of highly active antiretroviral therapy. *Clinical Infectious Diseases* 30(supplement 1): S5–S14.

Manji H and Miller R (2004) The neurology of HIV infection. *Journal of Neurology, Neurosurgery and Psychiatry* 75(supplement 1): i29–i35.

Marrazzo J (2007) Syphilis and other sexually transmitted diseases in HIV infection. *Topics in HIV Medicine* 15(1): 11–16.

Moyle GJ, Sabin CA, Cartledge J, et al. (2006) A randomized comparative trial of tenofovir DF or abacavir as replacement for a thymidine analogue in persons with lipoatrophy. *AIDS* 20(16): 2043–2050.

Palella FJ, Jr., Baker RK, Moorman AC, et al. (2006) Mortality in the highly active antiretroviral therapy era: Changing causes of death and disease in the HIV outpatient study. *Journal of Acquired Immune Deficiency Syndromes* 43(1): 27–34.

Roling J, Schmid H, Fischereder M, Draenert R, and Goebel FD (2006) HIV-associated renal diseases and highly active antiretroviral therapy-induced nephropathy. *Clinical Infectious Diseases* 42(10): 1488–1495.

Triant VA, Lee H, Hadigan C, and Grinspoon SK (2007) Increased acute myocardial infarction rates and cardiovascular risk factors among patients with HIV disease. *Journal of Clinical Endocrinology and Metabolism* 92: 2506–2512.

Weisberg LA (2001) Neurologic abnormalities in human immunodeficiency virus infection. *Southern Medical Journal* 94(3): 266–275.

Relevant Website

http://aidsinfo.nih.gov – Guidelines for the Use of Antiretroviral Agents in HIV-infected Adults and Adolescents.

AIDS: Global Epidemiology

P J Peters, P H Kilmarx, and T D Mastro, Centers for Disease Control and Prevention, Atlanta, GA, USA

Published by Elsevier Ltd.

Glossary

Adult prevalence Prevalence among the proportion of the population 15–49 years old (adults of reproductive age).

Antenatal Occurring before birth.

Concentrated epidemic HIV prevalence consistently over 5% in at least one defined subpopulation but below 1% in pregnant women. Implies that the epidemic is not established in the general population.

Generalized epidemic HIV prevalence consistently over 1% in pregnant women, a sentinel population used to assess trends in HIV prevalence and to estimate the adult HIV prevalence. Implies that sexual networking in the general population is sufficient to sustain the epidemic independent of high-risk subpopulations.

Incidence Number of new cases arising in a given time period (usually 1 year).

Nosocomial Relating to a hospital.

Pandemic An epidemic over a wide geographic area that affects a large population.

Prevalence Number of cases in the population at a given time point divided by the total population (a proportion).

Brief History of HIV/AIDS

Although the first cases of acquired immune deficiency syndrome (AIDS) were recognized in the United States in 1981, phylogenetic analysis of human immunodeficiency virus (HIV) sequences suggest that HIV may have been initially transmitted to humans around 1930. By 1985, HIV had been identified in every region of the world and an estimated 1.5 million people were infected globally. Since then, unprecedented scientific advances have been made in the epidemiology, basic science, and treatment of this newly identified virus. Despite these advances, the global HIV pandemic has expanded rapidly. By 2007, an estimated 33.2 million people were living with HIV and greater than 20 million people had died of AIDS. AIDS is now the leading cause of death among people 15–59 years old and the world's most urgent public health challenge. The implementation of effective prevention strategies has proven challenging but there have been notable successes. In the US and Western Europe, extensive prevention programs in the 1980s reduced rates of infection among men who had sex with men, and systematic screening of blood donations since 1985 has virtually eliminated the risk of HIV transmission from blood transfusion. Several middle- and low-income countries have also had successful prevention initiatives. Prevention campaigns in Thailand and Uganda, for example, have resulted in substantial reductions in HIV prevalence since the 1990s. Unfortunately, in many parts of the world, stigma, discrimination, and denial about issues such as sexuality and drug use have hampered attempts to contain this epidemic.

Molecular Epidemiology

HIV is an extremely genetically diverse virus. There are three phylogenetically distinct groups of HIV-1 based on genomic sequencing, groups M (main), O (outlier), and N (non-M, non-O). Each group has likely evolved from independent cross-species transmission events of chimpanzee simian immunodeficiency virus (SIVcpz) to humans. HIV-1 group M has spread to every region of the world and caused the global AIDS pandemic. Group O infections are uncommon and limited to people living in or epidemiologically linked to Central Africa (especially Cameroon). Group N infections have only rarely been described in Cameroon.

HIV-2 is a distinct primate lentivirus related to HIV-1 that is both less pathogenic and less transmissible. HIV-2 evolved from the cross-species transmission of sooty mangabey SIV (SIVsm). HIV-2 is highly concentrated in the West African country of Guinea-Bissau where the adult prevalence has been estimated to be as high as 8–10%. A lower prevalence (<2%) is found in surrounding West African countries. HIV-2 has remained geographically isolated to West Africa and countries with strong links to the region (Portugal, India, Angola, Mozambique, and France). Dual infection with HIV-1 and HIV-2 has been described but the viruses do not appear to recombine with each other.

High rates of viral replication coupled with continuous mutation and recombination events have resulted in the rapid genetic diversification of HIV-1 group M viruses. M group strains have diversified into nine distinct subtypes (or clades) and over 34 circulating recombinant forms (CRFs). The number of described CRFs has grown rapidly and is cataloged at the Los Alamos HIV sequence database. There are also a variety of unique recombinant forms (URFs) that have only been identi-

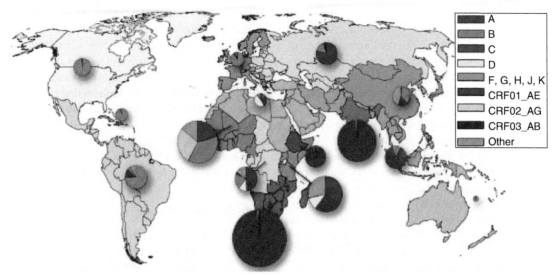

Figure 1   The global distribution of HIV-1 group M subtypes, 2004, by region. The world is subdivided into regions. Countries forming a region are shaded in the same color. Pie charts representing the distribution of HIV-1 subtypes and recombinants are superimposed on or connected by a line to the relevant region. The colors representing the different HIV-1 subtypes are indicated in the legend. The relative surface areas of the pie charts correspond to the relative number of individuals living with HIV in the region. Adapted from Hemelaar J, Gouws E, Ghys PD, and Osmanov S (2006) Global and regional distributions of HIV-1 genetic subtypes and recombinants in 2004. *AIDS* 20(16): W13–W23, with permission from Lippincott Williams and Wilkins.

fied in a single person or an epidemiologically linked pair. The precise implications of variation between HIV-1 subtypes on pathogenesis, transmission, drug resistance, and immune control are not well understood. However, HIV diagnostic tests (enzyme-linked immunosorbent assay (ELISA), polymerase chain reaction (PCR), Western blot) have been able to accurately detect the vast majority of emerging subtypes and CRFs.

The initial genetic diversification of HIV-1 group M viruses likely occurred in Central Africa where the greatest diversity and earliest cases of HIV-1 have been identified. Subsequently, HIV-1 subtypes have spread with a geographically heterogeneous distribution (**Figure 1**). Subtype C, the dominant subtype in Southern Africa, Ethiopia, and India, causes 50% of the HIV infections worldwide. The predominance of subtype C, especially in countries with high-prevalence epidemics driven by heterosexual sex, has led to speculation that it may have an increased fitness for transmission. Subtype A accounts for 12% of infections worldwide and has a broad geographic distribution. CRF01_AE and CRF02_AG are two additional recombinant viruses involving subtype A that are epidemiologically important in Southeast Asia and West Africa, respectively. The emergence of these CRFs has raised concern that recombination may contribute to the selection of viruses with increased fitness, immune escape, or transmissibility. Subtype B predominates in the Americas and Western Europe. Finally, URFs are important components of the epidemics in East Africa, Central Africa, and South America. Undoubtedly, some of these URFs will emerge as important CRFs in the future.

Table 1   Estimated per-act risk for acquisition of HIV, by exposure route

Exposure route	Risk per 100 exposures to an infected source[a]
Blood transfusion	90
Needle-sharing injection-drug use	0.67
Percutaneous needle stick	0.3
Receptive anal intercourse	0.5
Receptive penile-vaginal intercourse	0.1
Insertive anal intercourse	0.065
Insertive penile-vaginal intercourse	0.05
Receptive oral intercourse	0.01
Insertive oral intercourse	0.005
Mother-to-child transmission (without breast-feeding)	30
Breast-feeding for 18 months	15

[a]Estimates of risk for transmission from sexual exposure assumes no condom use.
Adapted from Smith DK, Grohskopf LA, Black RJ, *et al. (2005)* Antiretroviral postexposure prophylaxis after sexual, injection-drug use, or other nonoccupational exposure to HIV in the United States: Recommendations from the US Department of Health and Human Services. *MMWR Recommendations and Reports.* 54: 1–20 and Kourtis AP, Lee FK, Abrams EJ, Jamieson DJ, and Bulterys M (2007) Mother-to-child transmission of HIV-1: Timing and implications for prevention. *The Lancet Infectious Diseases* 6(11): 726–732.

Modes of Transmission

HIV can be transmitted by sexual contact, exposure to blood, and from mother to child with variable efficiency (**Table 1**). Although HIV has been isolated from a variety of body fluids, only blood, semen, genital fluids, and breast milk have been proven as sources of infection.

Unprotected sexual contact is the predominant mode of HIV transmission throughout the world. Despite a relatively low efficiency of transmission per sexual act, numerous factors can enhance transmission. Receptive anal intercourse often results in microtrauma to the rectal mucosa and therefore facilitates HIV transmission by exposing damaged mucosa to HIV-infected semen. Likewise, receptive vaginal intercourse probably transmits HIV (male-to-female) more efficiently than insertive vaginal intercourse. In general, concurrent sexual partners (and not simply the absolute number of partners) augment HIV's spread in a community. The probability of sexual transmission is also augmented by factors that affect the infectiousness of the source partner and the susceptibility of the recipient partner. A high HIV viral load, genital ulcerative disease (and other sexually transmitted diseases), and blood contact during sex (due to trauma or menstruation) can all increase the probability of transmission. Male circumcision reduces female-to-male transmission of HIV and may reduce male-to-female transmission to a lesser extent. Certain genetic factors can also decrease the probability of HIV transmission.

Among injection-drug users, HIV is transmitted by exposure to HIV-infected blood through shared contaminated needles and other injection equipment. Nosocomial transmission of HIV in hospitals from reuse of syringes and needles has also been documented and the risk of acquiring HIV from a transfusion with HIV-contaminated blood products approaches 100%.

Mother-to-child transmission can take place during pregnancy, labor and delivery, and during breast-feeding. The majority of transmissions (excluding breast-feeding) occur in the short interval during which the placenta detaches, labor occurs, and the infant passes through the birth canal. Overall rates of transmission are 15–40% without preventative interventions.

Epidemiology

An estimated 33.2 million people (2.5 million children) were living with HIV in 2007 (**Figure 2**), which is an increase of 4.2 million people since 2001. Every region of the world has had an increase in the number of people living with HIV from 2001 to 2007. The prevalence of HIV varies dramatically worldwide with a disproportionate number of infections in sub-Saharan Africa (**Figure 3**). Despite these statistics, there are some promising recent developments. The incidence of new HIV infections has peaked in many countries. There has also been a decline in the HIV prevalence among young women attending antenatal clinics (a sentinel population in generalized HIV epidemics) in several high-prevalence countries. These declines have correlated with reductions in high-risk sexual

behavior and increased condom usage. General trends should be interpreted cautiously, however, as even within countries there can be tremendous variability in the HIV epidemic. Improvements in surveillance techniques over time, which include expanding surveillance sites to antenatal clinics in rural areas and conducting population-based surveys, can also make trends difficult to interpret. Furthermore, the epidemics in countries with large populations, such as Nigeria, Ethiopia, Russia, India, and China (which together comprise 44% of the world's population), are still evolving and expanding in some populations.

Sub-Saharan Africa

HIV has caused a generalized epidemic in many parts of sub-Saharan Africa. In 2007, almost 22.5 million people were living with HIV in sub-Saharan Africa (68% of the global infections but only 11–12% of the world's population), and although considerable efforts have been made to improve access to anti-retrovirals in recent years, 1.6 million Africans still died of AIDS in 2007 (76% of the AIDS deaths worldwide). Within Africa, the distribution of HIV is heterogeneous. Although HIV originated in Central Africa, Southern Africa now has the highest HIV prevalence in the world. Conversely, many East African countries have seen declines in their HIV prevalence and most West African countries have maintained a relatively low HIV prevalence.

HIV arrived late in Southern Africa. In 1988, South Africa had an HIV prevalence of less than 1% and the epidemic was centered in East and Central Africa (**Figure 4**). Unfortunately in the ensuing years HIV spread to unprecedented levels. Swaziland now has the most intense HIV epidemic in the world with an estimated 1 in 4 (26%) adults living with HIV in 2007. Several other Southern African countries also had an HIV prevalence greater than 20% in 2005. Various social and biological factors have likely predisposed certain African countries to these massive HIV epidemics. High rates of men migrating for work, concurrent sex partners, and genital herpes, in addition to low rates of male circumcision and gender-based inequalities, combine to fuel the epidemic in this region.

From 2003 to 2005, the adult HIV prevalence has remained stable but high (19–24%) in Botswana, Lesotho, and Namibia and has continued to increase in South Africa from 18.6% (2003) to 18.8% (2005). This stability, however, masks extremely high rates of new infections that are being balanced by high rates of AIDS deaths (**Figure 5**). The impact of HIV in Southern Africa cannot be overstated. The average life expectancy in Botswana has dropped from 65 years (1985) to 34 years (2006) as a result of HIV. Denial continues to be a factor driving high rates of new infections as many people in the region believe that they are at low risk of infection. In a survey

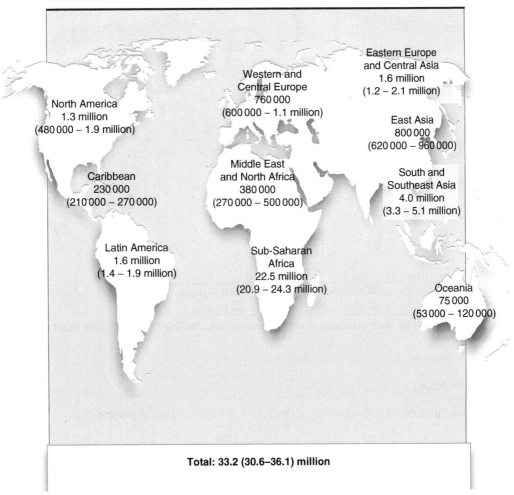

North America
1.3 million
(480 000 – 1.9 million)

Western and
Central Europe
760 000
(600 000 – 1.1 million)

Eastern Europe
and Central Asia
1.6 million
(1.2 – 2.1 million)

East Asia
800 000
(620 000 – 960 000)

Caribbean
230 000
(210 000 – 270 000)

Middle East
and North Africa
380 000
(270 000 – 500 000)

South and
Southeast Asia
4.0 million
(3.3 – 5.1 million)

Latin America
1.6 million
(1.4 – 1.9 million)

Sub-Saharan
Africa
22.5 million
(20.9 – 24.3 million)

Oceania
75 000
(53 000 – 120 000)

Total: 33.2 (30.6–36.1) million

Figure 2 Adults and children estimated to be living with HIV, 2007. Reproduced from UNAIDS/WHO (2007) AIDS Epidemic update: December 2007. http://www.unaids.org/en/HIV_data/2007Epiupdate/default.asp (accessed November 2007).

by Shisana *et al.* in 2005 in South Africa, 50% of people who tested HIV-positive stated that they had no risk of acquiring HIV.

East Africa was among the regions most severely affected by HIV in the early 1990s (**Figure 4**), but subsequently the HIV prevalence has dropped. Uganda's HIV epidemic was the first to stabilize and then fall sharply during the 1990s. Strong political leadership and major prevention campaigns have been credited with this success. Uganda's national adult HIV prevalence was still 6.7% in 2005, however, and new evidence of increasing infections in rural areas reinforces the need to adapt prevention campaigns to changes in the epidemic. Kenya provides another encouraging example of a serious HIV epidemic that has declined from a national prevalence of 10% in the late 1990s to 7% in 2003 and 6% in 2006. In Ethiopia, the prevalence of HIV has declined slowly in the capital city of Addis Ababa (4.7% in 2005) since the mid-1990s and has remained low in rural areas. A concerning trend has been a recent increase in the number of new infections in

rural parts of the country where 80% of the population lives. Halting the spread of HIV in rural communities will be one of the most important prevention priorities in East Africa.

Although the HIV prevalence in most of West Africa is comparatively low, HIV remains a serious problem in certain communities. The HIV epidemic in Côte d'Ivoire rapidly expanded in the 1980s and the adult prevalence has remained greater than 4% as of 2005. Fortunately, data from 2005 suggest a declining prevalence in the capital city of Abidjan as well as several other West African cities. As of 2005, an estimated 2.9 million people were living with HIV in Nigeria where the national prevalence is 4%. Within the country, there is considerable variation in rates of HIV for reasons not clear. In many low-prevalence West African countries, such as Senegal with a national prevalence of 1%, commercial sex work appears to be driving the epidemic. In Central Africa, incomplete data have hidden the exact nature of the HIV epidemic. Cameroon (5% national prevalence), the Central African Republic (11%), and

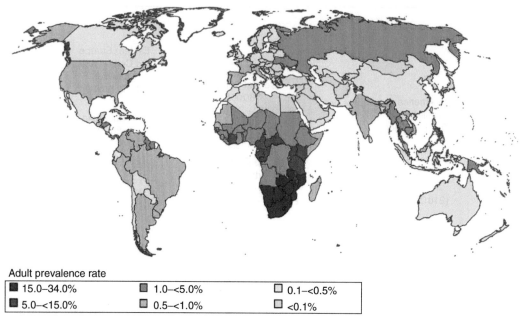

Figure 3   Adult prevalence of HIV, 2005. Reproduced with permission from UNAIDS/WHO (2006) 2006 report on the global AIDS epidemic. Geneva: UNAIDS.

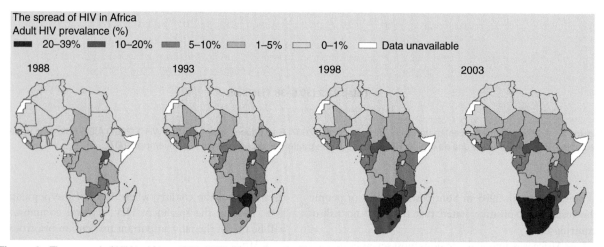

Figure 4   The spread of HIV in Africa, 1988–2003. Reproduced with permission from UNAIDS (2005) *AIDS in Africa: Three Scenarios to 2025*. Geneva: UNAIDS.

the Democratic Republic of the Congo (3%), however, all have significant epidemics based on estimates of prevalence from 2005.

Asia

The adult HIV prevalence is lower in Asian countries (**Figure 3**) than sub-Saharan Africa and concentrated in high-risk groups. The epidemic continues to spread considerably, however, with over 400 000 new infections and over 300 000 deaths in 2007.

The highest regional HIV prevalence has occurred in Southeast Asia where commercial sex work, sex between

men, and injection-drug use combine to fuel the epidemic. In Thailand and Cambodia, HIV spread rapidly in the late 1980s and early 1990s. Initial cases were seen in men who have sex with men and injection-drug users before spreading to female sex workers. HIV then spread to male clients who transmitted the virus to their wives and girlfriends. Extensive public education and prevention campaigns, however, have had some success in the region. Among young men in Thailand, increased knowledge of HIV and changes in sexual behavior, such as an increase in condom usage and a decrease in visits to sex workers, have correlated with reductions of the HIV prevalence in new military conscripts. Thailand's '100% Condom' campaign,

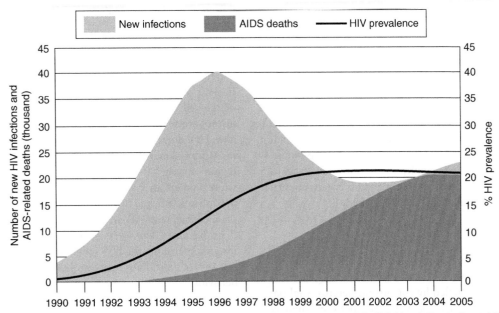

Figure 5 Estimated number of annual new infections and AIDS-related deaths among adults (15+) in relation to the stabilizing trend of estimated prevalence among adults (15–49), Lesotho, 1990–2005. Reproduced with permission from UNAIDS/WHO (2006) AIDS Epidemic Update: December 2006. Geneva: UNAIDS.

which educated sex workers and promoted condom use, has also decreased HIV transmission from female commercial sex workers to their clients. Encouragingly, the epidemics in Thailand and Cambodia have been declining since the 1990s.

India is experiencing a complex HIV epidemic. Although the precise number of HIV infections in India has been debated, the Indian National AIDS Control Organization estimates that 2.5 million people were living with HIV in 2006 (an adult HIV prevalence of 0.36%). The majority of infections in India result from unprotected heterosexual sex and a large proportion of women are getting infected by their regular partners who became infected during commercial sex. Fortunately, there is evidence of a reduction in the prevalence of HIV among women attending antenatal clinics in south India from 2000 to 2004 which has correlated with increased prevention efforts in several southern Indian states. HIV prevention targeting sex workers could have a dramatic effect on the epidemic but law enforcement barriers and stigma complicate these prevention efforts. Injection-drug use is the major risk factor for HIV in the northeast and has become increasingly important in several major cities (Chennai, Mumbai, New Delhi).

In China, the HIV epidemic has followed an unusual pattern by beginning in certain rural areas, then spreading to cities. HIV was first identified among injection-drug users in the Yunnan Province (near China's southwestern border) in 1989. In the mid-1990s, a major HIV outbreak occurred in paid plasma donors in China's rural east–central provinces (Henan). During plasma donation, blood is taken from the donor and using a technique called

apheresis the plasma is separated from the red blood cells. The red blood cells are then reinfused into the donor to prevent anemia. Reuse of tubing and mixing of red blood cells from multiple donors prior to reinfusion led to thousands of HIV infections in these paid donors. Since the mid-1990s, HIV has spread to all 31 of China's provinces and an estimated 650 000 people are living with HIV (0.05% prevalence in 2005). Although injection-drug use has been the predominant mode of transmission, sexual transmission has become increasingly important and accounted for an estimated 50% of new infections in 2005. China's response to its HIV epidemic was initially slow but has accelerated recently to incorporate evidence-based interventions from other countries (such as Australia's needle-exchange program and Thailand's condom campaign among sex workers).

Recently, the HIV epidemic has expanded among injection-drug users in several Asian countries, such as Pakistan, Afghanistan, Indonesia, and Malaysia. Given the overlap between injection-drug users and commercial sex workers, there is concern that the HIV epidemic could spread rapidly in these countries.

Eastern Europe and Central Asia

Until the late 1990s, the prevalence of HIV in Eastern Europe and Central Asia was extremely low. In the last decade, however, this region has experienced the fastest growing HIV epidemic and an estimated 1.7 million people are now living with HIV (over 90% of cases are in the Russian Federation and Ukraine). Injection drug use is the predominant method of HIV transmission but high rates of HIV are also emerging in the sex partners of injection drug users, female sex workers, and prisoners. Although the epidemic is still concentrated in high-risk groups in the Russian Federation and Ukraine, there is evidence that HIV is starting to spread into the general population. In the Ukraine, the proportion of people infected through heterosexual sex increased from an average of 14% from 1999–2003 to 35% in 2006. The Ukraine's HIV epidemic is also yet to peak despite an estimated adult HIV prevalence of 1.5% in 2005. The HIV epidemic is also starting to grow rapidly in the injection-drug user populations of several other Central Asian countries (Uzbekistan, Kazakhstan, and Tajikistan).

Caribbean

The HIV prevalence is high in many Caribbean countries where an estimated 1–4% of adults are living with HIV. The epidemic is fueled by concurrent heterosexual partners and commercial sex work. Sex between men is a hidden phenomenon but may account for 10% of cases. Since 2002, the adult HIV prevalence in urban areas of Haiti and the HIV prevalence among pregnant women in the Bahamas have declined, and these declines have correlated with high rates of condom use by sex workers.

Latin America

Brazil, the most populous country in Latin America, has 620 000 people living with HIV in 2005. In the 1990s, many experts predicted that Brazil's epidemic would rapidly accelerate. Brazil's sustained campaign, however, to promote sex education, condom use, harm reduction, and HIV testing, and to provide anti-retroviral therapy halted HIV's expansion. Overall, the adult prevalence has remained stable at 0.5%. The majority of HIV infections in South America is occurring among men who have sex with men and injection-drug users. Incarcerated men, in particular, are at high risk for infection. Recently, rates of HIV have also increased among poor women from unprotected heterosexual sex with injection-drug users and men who also have sex with men.

The countries of Central America have the highest estimated HIV prevalences (1–2.5% in 2005) in Latin America and the epidemics appear to be growing. Sex between men and commercial sex are the major risk factors, but there is evidence that the epidemics are generalizing. Mexico has a relatively low (0.3% in 2005) HIV prevalence, but increasing rates of infection in cities along the United States border are being driven by injection-drug use and commercial sex work.

North America

The total number of people living with HIV continues to grow in North America due to the combination of the life-prolonging anti-retroviral treatment (with a corresponding decline in AIDS deaths) and a steady rate of new infections. The main risk factors for HIV are estimated to be unsafe sex between men (44%), unprotected heterosexual sex (34%), and injection-drug use (17%). In the US, women are estimated to account for over 25% of the AIDS cases and minority populations have been disproportionately affected by the epidemic. The rate of new HIV infections in the US was seven times higher in African–American men than white men and 21 times higher among African–American women compared to white women. In Canada, aboriginal people are also disportionately affected by the epidemic. An estimated 250 000 people living with HIV in the United States are not aware of their diagnosis. This large group presents a major obstacle toward controlling the HIV epidemic since people who are unaware of their status may continue to engage in high-risk behaviors.

Western Europe

In the 1980s, HIV spread widely among men who had sex with men and injection-drug users in Western Europe. Subsequent prevention programs have had success in reducing the incidence of HIV in these risk groups although the HIV prevalence in injection-drug users in Southern Europe remains high. The major modes of HIV transmission are now unprotected heterosexual sex (56%), unsafe sex between men (35%), and injection drug use (8%). Although heterosexual transmission has emerged as an important mode of HIV transmission in Western Europe, there is no evidence of a generalized epidemic. In many Western European countries, including Belgium, Sweden, and the United Kingdom, immigrants from sub-Saharan Africa account for the majority of heterosexually acquired infections. Unprotected sex with injection-drug users or men who have sex with men represents the other major risk for heterosexual transmission.

Oceania

There is a serious HIV epidemic in Papua New Guinea with an estimated adult prevalence of 1.8% in 2005. High rates of concurrent sexual partners, transactional sex, and violence against women have allowed the epidemic to grow rapidly. Sex between men is the predominant mode of HIV transmission in Australia and New Zealand.

Middle East and North Africa

Uneven HIV surveillance makes it difficult to gauge the epidemics in this region. Sudan has a generalized epidemic with an HIV prevalence of 1.6% in 2005. High rates of HIV have also been observed in injection-drug users in Iran, Libya, Algeria, Egypt, Morocco, and Lebanon.

Global Response

The world was initially slow to recognize the severity of the HIV pandemic but global efforts have increased dramatically in recent years. Between 1996 and 2005, annual funding for AIDS in low- and middle-income countries increased from $300 million to $8.3 billion. This acceleration of the world's response was prompted by increased human rights advocacy from people living with HIV and a concern that AIDS could destabilize global economic systems and threaten global security. Although these increases in funding are impressive, an effective global response will depend on sustained growth in annual funding of effective prevention and treatment programs until the epidemic can be stopped.

HIV Prevention

Comprehensive and sustained prevention programs have been proven to reduce HIV transmission. Unfortunately, HIV prevention strategies have not reached the majority of people at high risk. The major challenge for prevention has been generating the political will and economic resources to effectively implement proven strategies that address issues such as sex, sexuality, and drug use.

Behavioral interventions to promote safer sexual behavior are essential to reduce HIV transmission. In Zimbabwe, sexual behavior change (increased condom use, delayed onset of sexual activity, and a reduction in sexual relations with nonregular partners) has contributed to declines in HIV prevalence. Successful behavioral interventions incorporate educational messages with prevention skills such as how to negotiate and use condoms and how to refuse sex. These interventions have been successfully implemented in school-based sex education classes, peer-led small group discussion groups, in the context of HIV counseling and testing, and as national structured interventions, such as Thailand's '100% Condom' program. For successful implementation, prevention programs must identify and engage high-risk populations.

Globally, an estimated 80% of people living with HIV are unaware of their status. Since people who are unaware that they are HIV-infected are more likely to continue transmitting HIV, an urgent priority is to increase access to HIV testing. Botswana has implemented a national, opt-out HIV-testing program in medical settings. Opt-out HIV testing has also been implemented in certain clinical settings in Kenya, Malawi, Uganda, and Zambia. In African countries with a high HIV prevalence a major risk factor for acquiring HIV is having a stable heterosexual partner who is HIV-infected (and often unaware of their status). Couples testing and counseling where both the male and female partners are counseled and HIV tested together has gained increased acceptance in certain African

countries (Rwanda, Zambia) as a prevention tool in this high risk population. Universal HIV testing could both reduce transmission of HIV among newly identified infections and reduce the stigma of HIV testing.

An effective HIV vaccine would be a major advance in HIV prevention and is the subject of intense research efforts. Several other biomedical strategies also have the potential to dramatically improve HIV prevention. Male circumcision reduces a man's risk of acquiring HIV heterosexually by 50–60%. Since the highest prevalence of HIV is in countries where men are uncircumcised, large-scale implementation of male circumcision has the potential to prevent millions of new infections if provided in a safe and culturally appropriate way. Herpes simplex virus type 2 (HSV-2) infection is the most common cause of genital ulcers and is associated with an increased risk of HIV transmission. Clinical trials are now evaluating whether antiviral prophylaxis (to suppress HSV-2) will reduce the rate of HIV transmission. Interventions under a woman's control such as barrier diaphragms and vaginal microbicides which incorporate anti-retroviral drugs to block HIV transmission are also being evaluated in clinical trials. Daily oral administration of anti-retroviral drugs to high-risk, HIV-negative individuals, a strategy called pre-exposure prophylaxis (PrEP), is also being assessed. Successful biomedical interventions must still be packaged with effective behavioral prevention strategies to avoid behavioral disinhibition (an increase in high-risk behavior driven by a perceived decrease in risk for HIV infection).

Prevention of mother-to-child transmission (PMTCT) strategies have almost eliminated pediatric HIV in high-income countries. Treating the HIV-infected mother with anti-retrovirals and replacing breast milk with formula reduces the rate of mother-to-child HIV transmission from as high as 41% to less than 2%. Even a single dose of nevirapine given to the mother in labor and to the infant at birth significantly decreases the rate of HIV transmission. Despite these effective prevention strategies, there are still an estimated 1800 new mother-to-child HIV infections per day. These pediatric infections are occurring predominantly in sub-Saharan Africa due to a lack of access to PMTCT services. Breast-feeding also presents a difficult problem in sub-Saharan Africa since substituting formula for breast milk results in higher mortality among both HIV-infected and HIV-negative infants born to HIV-infected mothers. Treating HIV-infected breast-feeding women and/or their children with anti-retrovirals to prevent breast milk transmission is an innovative strategy being investigated.

Treatment of drug addiction, education about safe injection practices, and access to clean needles are effective prevention strategies in injection-drug users. In hospitals, infection-control programs that prohibit the reuse of injection equipment are necessary to prevent

Table 2   Estimated number of people receiving anti-retroviral therapy, people needing anti-retroviral therapy, and percentage coverage in low- and middle-income countries according to region, Dec. 2003–Dec. 2006

Geographical region	Estimated number of people receiving antiretroviral therapy, Dec. 2006 (range)[a]	Estimated number of people needing antiretroviral therapy, 2006 (range)[a]	Antiretroviral therapy coverage, Dec. 2006 (range)[b]	Estimated number of people receiving antiretroviral therapy, Dec. 2005 (range)[a]	Estimated number of people receiving antiretroviral therapy, Dec. 2003 (range)[a]
Sub-Saharan Africa	1 340 000 (1 220 000–1 460 000)	4 800 000 (4 100 000–5 600 000)	28% (24–33%)	810 000 (730 000–890 000)	100 000 (75 000–125 000)
Latin America and the Caribbean	355 000 (315 000–395 000)	490 000 (370 000–640 000)	72% (55–96%)	315 000 (295 000–335 000)	210 000 (160 000–260 000)
East, South, and South-east Asia	280 000 (225 000–335 000)	1 500 000 (1 000 000–2 100 000)	19% (13–28%)	180 000 (150 000–210 000)	70 000 (52 000–88 000)
Europe and Central Asia	35 000 (33 000–37 000)	230 000 (160 000–320 000)	15% (11–22%)	21 000 (20 000–22 000)	15 000 (11 000–19 000)
North Africa and the Middle East	5000 (4000–6000)	77 000 (43 000–130 000)	6% (4–12%)	4000 (3 000–5000)	1000 (750–1250)
Total	2 015 000 (1 795 000–2 235 000)	7 100 000 (6 000 000–8 400 000)	28% (24–34%)	1 330 000 (1 200 000–1 460 000)	400 000 (300 000–500 000)

Note: Some numbers do not add up due to rounding.
[a]Data on children (when available) are included.
[b]The coverage estimate is based on the estimated numbers of people receiving and needing antiretroviral therapy.
Reproduced with permission from the World Health Organization. Data from World Health Organization (2007) Towards Universal Access. Scaling up Priority HIV/AIDS Interventions in the Health Sector. Progress Report, April 2007. Geneva: WHO.

nosocomial HIV transmission. Finally, maintaining the safety of the blood supply by screening voluntary donors for HIV risk factors, testing each unit of blood for HIV, and reducing unnecessary transfusions, is another critical intervention to prevent HIV transmission.

HIV Care and Treatment

HIV mortality dropped precipitously in high-income countries after the introduction of highly active anti-retroviral therapy (HAART) in 1996, but HAART remained unaffordable for many low- and middle-income countries. Brazil, however, made the pioneering decision to initiate a highly successful universal HIV treatment program which has inspired similar efforts in low-income countries. Since 2001, global financing for HIV care and treatment in low-income countries has increased mark-edly driven by funding from the Global Fund to Fight AIDS, Tuberculosis, and Malaria, the US President's Emergency Plan for AIDS Relief (PEPFAR), and the World Bank. By December 2006, over 2 million people living with HIV/AIDS were receiving treatment in low- and middle-income countries which represents 28% of the estimated 7.1 million people in need of treatment (**Table 2**). Treatment coverage remains strongest in Latin America (72%) driven by Brazil's leadership. The most encouraging improvements have been in sub-Saharan Africa where the number of people being treated has increased from 100 000 in 2003 to 1.3 million by December 2006. Sustained international funding from high-income countries and political will in low-income countries will be necessary to maintain high medication adherence, to monitor for drug toxicities and drug resistance, and to improve treatment regimens.

The HIV epidemic intersects with other important dis-eases. By weakening the immune system, HIV predisposes to opportunistic infections such as tuberculosis (TB). Globally, more than 21 million people are co-infected with TB and HIV. Although TB infection remains latent (neither contagious nor symptomatic) in most people without HIV, with TB/HIV co-infection the risk of progression to active, contagious disease increases 100-fold. TB and HIV synergistically worsen the burden of both diseases. The global TB incidence has increased, fueled by a rapid increase in HIV-associated TB in Africa. TB is also a leading cause of death among people living with HIV. Increased collaboration between TB-elimination and HIV-treatment programs is necessary to control both of these diseases.

Although there has been debate regarding the relative cost-effectiveness of prevention strategies compared to treatment programs, combined prevention and treatment strategies have synergistic benefits. Increased treatment access, for example, enhances awareness, reduces stigma,

and increases the use of HIV testing and counseling services. Increased HIV testing, in turn, identifies HIV-infected people who can be counseled to prevent further transmission and treated with HAART when indi-cated, which also decreases infectiousness. Only effective prevention programs can reduce the incidence of new infections and thereby reduce the number of people who will need treatment in the future.

Future Prospects

In the past 25 years, HIV has emerged as the world's most serious public health problem. Every region of the world has been affected by AIDS, but sub-Saharan Africa has been disproportionately affected. Recent successful efforts to provide HIV care and treatment in low-income countries must now be expanded and sustained. In addition, preven-tion programs need to expand in a similar manner into low-income countries. These prevention strategies must include evidence-based interventions such as safer sex education programs with access to condoms and HIV-testing and counseling services. These programs must also be able to incorporate new biomedical prevention techniques (such as male circumcision) without compromising existing effective prevention services. Most importantly, sustained financial and political commitments will be required from both high- and low-income countries to control the HIV pandemic.

See also: AIDS: Disease Manifestation; Human Immunode-ficiency Viruses: Antiretroviral Agents; Human Immunodefi-ciency Viruses: Origin.

Further Reading

Centers for Disease Control, Prevention (CDC) (2006) The Global HIV/AIDS Pandemic, 2006. *Morbidity Mortality Weekly Report* 55(31): 841–844.

Galvin SR and Cohen MS (2004) The role of sexually transmitted diseases in HIV transmission. *Nature Reviews Microbiology* 2(1): 33–42.

Global HIV Prevention Working Group (2006) New Approaches to HIV Prevention: Accelerating Research and Ensuring Future Access, Aug. 2006. http://www.kff.org/hivaids/hiv081506pkg.cfm (accessed August 2007).

Gupta K and Klasse PJ (2006) How do viral and host factors modulate the sexual transmission of HIV? Can transmission be blocked? *PLoS Medicine* 3(2): e79.

Hemelaar J, Gouws E, Ghys PD, and Osmanov S (2006) Global and regional distributions of HIV-1 genetic subtypes and recombinants in 2004. *AIDS* 20(16): W13–W23.

Kourtis AP, Lee FK, Abrams EJ, Jamieson DJ, and Bulterys M (2007) Mother-to-child transmission of HIV-1: Timing and implications for prevention. *Lancet Infectious Diseases* 6(11): 726–732.

Sawires SR, Dworkin SL, Fiamma A, Peacock D, Szekeres G, and Coates TJ (2007) Male circumcision and HIV/AIDS: Challenges and opportunities. *Lancet* 369(9562): 708–713.

Smith DK, Grohskopf LA, Black RJ, *et al.* (2005) Antiretroviral postexposure prophylaxis after sexual, injection-drug use, or other nonoccupational exposure to HIV in the United States: Recommendations from the US Department of Health and Human Services. *MMWR Recommendations and Reports* 54: 1–20.

UNAIDS (1998) Partners in Prevention: International Case Studies of Effective Health Promotion Practice in HIV/AIDS. http://data.unaids.org/Publications/IRC-pub01/JC093-PartnersInPrevention_en.pdf (accessed August 2007).

UNAIDS (2005) *AIDS in Africa: Three Scenarios to 2025.* Geneva: UNAIDS.

UNAIDS/WHO (2006) 2006 report on the global AIDS epidemic. http://www.unaids.org/en/HIV_data/2006GlobalReport/default.asp (accessed August 2007).

UNAIDS/WHO (2006) AIDS Epidemic Update: December 2006. http://www.unaids.org/en/HIV_data/epi2006/default.asp (accessed August 2007).

UNAIDS/WHO (2007) AIDS Epidemic update: December 2007. http://www.unaids.org/en/HIV_data/2007Epiupdate/default.asp (accessed November 2007).

Valdiserri RO, Ogden LL, and McCray E (2006) Accomplishments in HIV prevention science: Implications for stemming the epidemic. *Nature Medicine* 9(7): 881–886.

World Health Organization (2007) Towards Universal Access. Scaling up Priority HIV/AIDS Interventions in the Health Sector. Progress report, April 2007. http://www.who.int/hiv/mediacentre/universal_access_progress_report_en.pdf (accessed August 2007).

Relevant Website

http://www.hiv.lanl.gov – The Circulating Recombinant Forms (CRFs), HIV Sequence Database, Los Alamos National Laboratory.

Human Immunodeficiency Viruses: Antiretroviral Agents

A W Neuman and D C Liotta, Emory University, Atlanta, GA, USA

Glossary

Host cell A cell that has been infected by a virus.
Provirus A virus that has integrated itself into the DNA of a host cell.
Viral load A measure of the severity of a viral infection which is reported in nucleic acid copies per milliliter of blood.
Viral tropism The specificity of a virus for a particular host tissue.
Virion A single virus particle.

Introduction

In 2006, there were an estimated 39.5 million people worldwide living with human immunodeficiency virus (HIV). An estimated 4.3 million new infections arose in 2006, with 65% of those in sub-Saharan Africa. Acquired immune deficiency virus (AIDS)-related infections accounted for about 2.9 million deaths in 2006 and over 25 million deaths since the syndrome was first recognized in 1981. AIDS is now recognized as one of the most destructive pandemics in recorded history, and with no effective vaccine or cure, treatment of the disease relies on antiretroviral therapy.

The life cycle of HIV begins with the attachment of the virion to the target cell via CD4 binding followed by binding to co-receptor, CCR5 or CXCR4. The viral lipid membrane then fuses to the host cell membrane, allowing the viral core, encapsidating HIV RNA and enzymes, to enter the host cell cytoplasm. HIV RNA subsequently undergoes reverse transcription into DNA, a process mediated by reverse transcriptase. The viral DNA enters the host cell nucleus and is integrated into the cellular DNA by the enzyme integrase. At this point, the provirus may remain latent for up to several years. When the host cell receives a signal to become active, the proviral DNA is transcribed into mRNA. The mRNA is transported out of the nucleus and is translated into polyproteins. The polyproteins assemble to form an immature virus particle, which then buds out from the host cell. The enzyme protease cleaves these polyproteins into functional proteins, creating a mature virus.

Currently, 25 antiretroviral drugs are available, targeting three steps of the HIV life cycle: a fusion inhibitor, reverse transcriptase (RT) inhibitors (including two classes, nucleoside reverse transcriptase inhibitors (NRTIs) and non-nucleoside reverse transcriptase inhibitors (NNRTIs)), and protease inhibitors (PIs). Additional agents are being developed to target other steps in the viral life cycle. See **Table 1** for a list of antiretroviral drugs in development.

Most HIV patients are treated with highly active antiretroviral therapy (HAART), usually a combination of three antiretroviral agents. This treatment paradigm can often reduce a patient's viral load to below detectable levels for prolonged periods. The use of HAART over the past decade has led to significant declines in HIV-associated morbidity and mortality.

Table 1 HIV antiretroviral agents in clinical trials

Class	Name	Structure	Phase of development
Entry inhibitor (gp120-CD4)	BMS-378806		Phase I
Entry inhibitor (gp120-CD4)	TNX-355	Monoclonal antibody	Phase II
Entry inhibitor (CCR5)	Vicriviroc (SCH-D)		Phase II
Entry inhibitor (CCR5)	INCB9471	Structure not reported	Phase II
Entry inhibitor (CCR5)	PRO140	Monoclonal antibody	Phase I
Entry inhibitor (CCR5)	HGS004	Monoclonal antibody	Phase I
Entry inhibitor (CCR5)	AK602		Phase I
Entry inhibitor (CCR5)	TAK-652		Phase I
Entry inhibitor (CCR5)	TAK-220		Phase I
Fusion inhibitor	Suc-HSA	Succinylated human serum albumin	Phase I
Nucleoside reverse transcriptase inhibitor (NRTI)	Apricitabine (AVX754)		Phase II completed
NRTI	Racivir ±-FTC		Phase II completed

Continued

Table 1   Continued

Class	Name	Structure	Phase of development
NRTI	Elvucitabine		Phase II
NRTI	Alovudine		Phase II
NRTI	KP1461		Phase I
Non-nucleoside reverse transcriptase inhibitor (NNRTI)	BILR 355 BS		Phase II
NNRTI	Rilpivirine (TMC278)		Phase II
Integrase inhibitor	GS-9137		Phase II
Integrase inhibitor	GSK-364735	Structure not reported	Phase I
Protease inhibitor (PI)	PPL-100		Phase I
Maturation inhibitor	Bevirimat (PA-457)		Phase II

Entry Inhibitors

HIV entry into target cells is mediated by the envelope protein (Env), which is comprised of two glycoprotein subunits, the surface protein gp120 and transmembrane subunit gp41. Three distinct steps are required for the entry of HIV into host cells. First, the virus attaches to the cell surface via CD4 binding, changing the conformation of Env and exposing a co-receptor binding site on gp120, allowing the viral glycoprotein to bind to one of the co-receptors, CCR5 or CXCR4. The three gp41 glycoproteins in the trimeric envelope complex subsequently form a 6-helix bundle from interaction of the heptad repeat (HR-) 1 and HR2 domains present in the ectodomain of each subunit. The 6-helix bundle brings the viral and cellular membranes into close apposition and mediates their fusion. These three steps – attachment, co-receptor binding, and fusion – can be targeted by attachment inhibitors (including CD4 binding inhibitors), co-receptor binding inhibitors, and fusion inhibitors, respectively.

HIV entry inhibitors have recently exploded as potential therapeutic agents. The main reason for the great interest in this field is that entry inhibitors offer the opportunity to prevent infection of new target cells.

The CD4 receptor was identified in 1984 as the primary cellular receptor for HIV. Because gp120 is responsible for binding to the CD4 receptor on the surface of the host cell, the CD4–gp120 interaction is an attractive target for HIV therapy.

Several years after the discovery of CD4, it was determined that CD4 alone is insufficient to permit HIV infection. In 1996, CCR5 and CXCR4 were identified as the major co-receptors. It was determined that R5 tropic viruses, those which bind to CCR5, are involved in HIV transmission based on the discovery that CCR5Δ32 homozygotes are highly resistant to HIV infection. These individuals, mostly of northern European origin, have a 32 bp deletion in both copies of their CCR5 gene, which confers a recessive phenotype that is associated with resistance to HIV-1 infection and antibody production.

The CXCR4 and CCR5 co-receptors are appealing targets; however, their implementation will require viral phenotyping for co-receptor tropism. Patients infected with an X4 virus, for example, would need to be treated with a CXCR4-specific inhibitor.

Maraviroc is a small molecule which became the first-in-class CCR5 antagonist and the first oral entry inhibitor with its FDA approval in August 2007 (**Table 2**). Maraviroc monotherapy including twice-daily doses of 300 mg led to a viral load reduction of 1.6 $\log_{10}$ copies ml^{-1}. In phase III studies, twice as many patients taking maraviroc along with optimized combination therapy as those taking a placebo with combination therapy had an undetectable viral load (less than 40 copies ml^{-1}) after 48 weeks.

Several other attachment and co-receptor binding inhibitors are currently in development, and biological data have been reported for the drugs in more advanced stages. TNX-355 is a monoclonal antibody which inhibits

Table 2 FDA-approved HIV entry inhibitors

Name and structure	Dosing schedule[a]	Major toxicity[a]	Key mutations conferring resistance[b]
Acetyl-YTSLIHSLIEESQNQQEKN EQELLELDKWASLWNWF-amide Enfuvirtide (T-20, Fuzeon)	One subcutaneous injection of 90 mg b.i.d. into the upper arm, thigh, or abdomen	Injection site reactions (itching swelling, redness, pain or tenderness, hardened skin or bumps)	gp41 single point mutations between positions 36 and 45 gp41 double and triple point mutations between positions 36 and 45 gp41 mutations outside of positions 36–45 co-receptor tropism
Maraviroc (Selzentry)	One 300 mg tablet b.i.d.	Liver toxicity, cough, pyrexia, upper respiratory tract infections, rash, musculoskeletal symptoms, abdominal pain, dizziness	Changes in the V3 loop, including A316T, and A319A/S in the CC1/85 strain and a deletion in RU570[c]

[a]The Body: The Complete HIV/AIDS Resource. http://www.thebody.com (accessed October 2007).
[b]Stanford University HIV Drug resistance Database. http://hivdb.stanford.edu (accessed October 2007).
[c]Westby M, Smith-Burchnell C, Mori J, et al. (2007) Reduced maximal inhibition in phenotypic susceptibility assays indicates that viral strains resistant to the CCR5 antagonist maraviroc utilize inhibitor-bound receptor for entry. Journal of Virology 81: 2359–2371.

the interaction between gp120 and CD4. Intravenous infusion of $10\,mg\,kg^{-1}$ led to a viral load reduction of $1.33\,log_{10}$ copies ml^{-1}. Vicriviroc and INCB9471 are small-molecule antagonists of the CCR5 receptor. Twice-daily dosing of $50\,mg$ of vicriviroc resulted in a viral load reduction of $1.62\,log_{10}$ copies ml^{-1}. INCB9471 has recently been reported to show a $1.9\,log_{10}$ copies ml^{-1} viral load reduction with 14 days of monotherapy. Additionally, the viral load continued to drop for several days after discontinuation of therapy.

The field of fusion inhibitors is led by enfuvirtide, a biomimetic 36-amino acid peptide that was approved for use in March 2003 (**Table 2**). Enfuvirtide is based on the sequence of the HR2 region of gp41. When the drug binds to HR1, HR2 is unable to bind and fusion cannot occur.

Enfuvirtide was shown to block virus-mediated cell-to-cell fusion with an IC_{90} of $1.5\,ng\,ml^{-1}$. A 15-day monotherapy study, with patients receiving $100\,mg$ twice daily, resulted in an average plasma viral load reduction of $1.9\,log_{10}$ copies ml^{-1}. The main disadvantage of enfuvirtide is its dosing regimen consisting of twice-daily subcutaneous injections. Furthermore, due to the complexity of its 106-step chemical synthesis, enfuvirtide is the most expensive antiretroviral drug on the market. Because of these obstacles, enfuvirtide is generally prescribed to patients for whom other antiretroviral agents have failed.

Reverse Transcriptase Inhibitors

Since the identification in 1983 of HIV as the etiological agent of AIDS, HIV RT has been one of the major targets for the development of antiretroviral drugs. HIV RT is a heterodimeric, RNA-dependent DNA polymerase (RdDp) that contains two subunits: the p66 catalytic unit and the p51 structural unit. Two classes of antiretroviral agents inhibit RT. These include NRTIs, which compete with normal 2'-deoxynucleoside triphosphates, and NNRTIs, which are allosteric, noncompetitive inhibitors of RT.

NRTIs are synthetic analogs of natural nucleosides that are incorporated into a nascent viral DNA chain. Because the NRTIs lack a 3'-hydroxyl group, incoming nucleotides are unable to form new phosphodiester linkages, therefore halting DNA replication (chain termination). NRTIs are administered as prodrugs, which must be phosphorylated to the active triphosphate before being incorporated into the DNA by HIV RT. Since these compounds enter the cell via passive diffusion, the prodrugs must be sufficiently lipophilic to penetrate the cell membrane.

Because NRTIs inhibit DNA polymerase, they can also affect normal cells. The drugs show much higher affinity for HIV reverse transcriptase compared to most human DNA polymerases; however, mitochondrial DNA polymerase is significantly inhibited by NRTIs. Various side effects of NRTIs can be attributed to mitochondrial dysfunction, including polyneuropathy, myopathy, cardiomyopathy, pancreatitis, bone-marrow suppression, and lactic acidosis.

Zidovudine, commonly known as AZT, was the first HIV drug approved by the FDA. AZT is a thymidine analog with an azido group replacing the 3'-hydroxyl group.

The azido group not only prevents binding of subsequent nucleosides to the DNA chain but also increases the lipophilicity of AZT, allowing it to easily cross the cell membrane.

Since the approval of AZT in 1987, six other NRTIs have come into the market: didanosine (ddI), zalcitabine (ddC), stavudine (d4T), lamivudine (3TC), abacavir (ABC), and emtricitabine (FTC). Zalcitabine is no longer manufactured as of February 2006. Although each of the NRTIs works by competitive inhibition of RT, they have significantly different dosing, toxicity, and resistance profiles (**Table 3**).

Several more NRTIs are in clinical trials. Apricitabine demonstrated a $1.65\,log_{10}$ copies ml^{-1} viral load reduction after 10 days of $800\,mg$ b.i.d. monotherapy. Other compounds in early clinical trials have not released efficacy data.

Nucleotide analogs, another type of RT inhibitors, are also available. While several nucleotide analogs are approved to treat various viruses, only tenofovir is approved for the treatment of HIV. Tenofovir is an acyclic nucleoside phosphonate analog that displays increased efficacy owing to its ability to bypass the nucleoside kinase step of activation. Tenofovir and other nucleoside phosphonate analogs also show activity against a broad range of DNA viruses and retroviruses (**Table 3**).

NNRTIs, on the other hand, are noncompetitive inhibitors that bind to a hydrophobic pocket near the polymerase active site. NNRTIs inhibit HIV-1 RT by locking the active catalytic site in an inactive conformation. Despite their structural diversity, most NNRTIs assume a similar butterfly-like structure consisting of two hydrophobic wings connected to a central polar body. The wing portions of the molecules contain significant π-electron systems and can act as π-electron donors to aromatic side chains of RT residues around the NNRTI binding pocket. Although NNRTIs bind at a common site on RT, they differ with regard to the exact amino acids of the binding site with which they interact. Therefore, NNRTIs show differences in their pharmacology and pharmacokinetic profiles, interactions with other drugs, and safety and toxicity profiles.

Four NNRTIs are currently licensed for clinical use: nevirapine, delavirdine, efavirenz, and etravirine. Nevirapine, a dipyridodiazepinone derivative, has been shown to reduce perinatal HIV transmission by 47% compared to treatment with AZT. However, the compound can cause life-threatening liver toxicity. Therefore, it is generally

Table 3   FDA-approved reverse transcriptase inhibitors

Name and structure	Dosing schedule[b]	Major toxicity[b,c]	Key mutations conferring resistance[d]	Impact of monotherapy[e]
Zidovudine (AZT, Retrovir)	300 mg tablet b.i.d.	Pancreatitis; lactic acidosis; hepatomegaly; anemia; myopathy; neutropenia	Thymidine analog mutations (TAMs): M41L, D67N/G, K70R, L210W, T215F/Y, K219E/Q/N T215 revertants: T215C/D/E/S/I/V T69 insertion mutations Q151M complex usually in combination with V75I, F77L, F116Y	1.0 log$_{10}$ copies ml^{-1} decrease in viral load
Didanosine (ddI, Videx)	200 mg tablet b.i.d. or 250 mg powder b.i.d.	Pancreatitis; lactic acidosis; hepatomegaly; peripheral neuropathy; optic neuritis	L74V/I K65R TAMs: M41L, D67N/G, L210W, T215F/Y, K219E/Q/N M184V/I	0.8 log$_{10}$ copies ml^{-1} decrease in viral load
Zalcitabine (ddC, Hivid[a])	0.75 mg tablet t.i.d.	Pancreatitis; lactic acidosis; hepatomegaly; peripheral neuropathy; mouth and throat ulcers; neutropenia; stomatitis	T69A[f], L74V[g], K65R[h]	Less effective than either ddI or AZT
Stavudine (d4T, Zerit)	40 mg capsule b.i.d.	Pancreatitis; lactic acidosis; hepatomegaly; peripheral neuropathy; lipodystrophy; hyperlipidemia; rapidly progressive ascending neuromuscular weakness	TAMs: M41L, D67N/G, K70R, L210W, T215F/Y, K219E/Q/N T215 revertants: T215C/D/E/S/I/V T69 insertion mutations Q151M complex usually in combination with V75I, F77L, F116Y	0.8 log$_{10}$ copies ml^{-1} decrease in viral load
Lamivudine (3TC, Epivir)	300 mg tablet daily or 150 mg tablet b.i.d.	Lactic acidosis; hepatomegaly	M184V/I K65R Q151M complex usually in combination with V75I, F77L, F116Y TAMs: M41L, D67N/G, L210W, T215F/Y, K219E/Q/N	Limited monotherapy data available
Abacavir (ABC, Ziagen)	300 mg capsule b.i.d.	Hypersensitivity reaction which can be fatal	K65R L74V/I TAMs: M41L, D67N/G, L210W, T215F/Y, K219E/Q/N T69 insertion mutations	1.8 log$_{10}$ copies ml^{-1} decrease in viral load
Emtricitabine (FTC, Emtriva)	200 mg tablet q.d.	Lactic acidosis; hepatomegaly; hyperpigmentation	M184V/I K65R Q151M complex usually in combination with V75I, F77L, F116Y TAMs: M41L, D67N/G, L210W, T215F/Y	2.0 log$_{10}$ copies ml^{-1} decrease in viral load

Continued

Table 3   Continued

Name and structure	Dosing schedule[b]	Major toxicity[b,c]	Key mutations conferring resistance[d]	Impact of monotherapy[e]
Tenofovir (Viread)	300 mg capsule q.d.	Lactic acidosis; hepatomegaly; liver and kidney damage; reduction of bone mineral density	K61R TAMs: M41L, L210W, T215Y T215 revertants: T215C/D/E/S/I/V T69 insertion mutations	1.2 $\log_{10}$ copies ml^{-1} decrease in viral load
Nevirapine (Viramune)	200 mg capsule q.d. for first two weeks, then 200 mg b.i.d.	Skin rash; liver damage	K103N/S Y181C/I G190A/S/E Y188L/H/C	1.5 $\log_{10}$ copies ml^{-1} decrease in viral load[f]
Delavirdine (Rescriptor)	400 mg (two 200 mg tablets) t.i.d.	Skin rash; proteinuria; lipodystrophy	K103N/S Y181C/I P236L G190A/S/E	1.0 $\log_{10}$ copies ml^{-1} decrease in viral load[j]
Efavirenz (Sustiva, Stocrin)	600 mg capsule q.d.	Skin rash; depression and other psychiatric symptoms; high triglyceride levels	K103N/S ($\pm$ L100I, K101P, P225H, K238T/N) G190S/A/E Y188L/H/C Y191C/I	Limited monotherapy data available
Etravirine (Intelence)	200 mg (two 100 mg tablets) b.i.d.	Moderate to severe skin reactions	Three or more of the 13 specific NNRTI mutations: V90I, A98G, L100I, K101E/P, V106I, V179D/F, Y181C/I/V, G190A/S[k]	2.4 $\log_{10}$ copies ml^{-1} decrease in viral load[k]

---

[a]Zalcitabine is no longer manufactured as of February 2006.

[b]The Body: The Complete HIV/AIDS Resource. http://www.thebody.com (accessed October 2007).

[c]Painter GR, Almond MR, Mao S, and Liotta DC (2004) Biochemical and mechanistic basis for the activity of nucleoside analogue inhibitors of HIV reverse transcriptase. *Current Topics in Medicinal Chemistry* 4: 1035–1044.

[d]Stanford University HIV Drug Resistance Database. http://hivdb.stanford.edu (accessed October 2007).

[e]Sharma PL, Nurpeisov V, Hernandez-Santiago B, Beltran T, and Schinazi RF (2004) Nucleoside inhibitors of human immunodeficiency virus type 1 reverse transcriptase. *Current Topics in Medicinal Chemistry* 4: 895–919.

[f]Fitzgibbon JE, Howell RM, Haberzettl CA, Sperber SJ, Gocke DJ, and Dubin DT (1992) Human immunodeficiency virus type 1 *pol* gene mutations which cause decreased susceptibility to 2′,3′-dideoxycytidine. *Antimicrobial Agents and Chemotherapy* 36: 153–157.

[g]St. Clair MH, Martin JL, Tudor-Williams G, *et al.* (1991) Resistance to ddI and sensitivity to AZT induced by a mutation in HIV-1 reverse transcriptase. *Science* 253: 1557–1559.

[h]Gu Z, Gao Q, Fang H, *et al.* (1994) Identification of a mutation at codon 65 in the IKKK motif of reverse transcriptase that encodes human immunodeficiency virus resistance to 2′,3′-dideoxycytidine and 2′,3′-dideoxy-3′-thiacytidine. *Antimicrobial Agents and Chemotherapy* 38: 275–281.

[i]Lange JMA (2003) Efficacy and durability of nevirapine in antiretroviral drug naïve patients. *Journal of Acquired Immune Deficiency Syndromes* 34: S40–S52.

[j]Para MF, Meehan P, Holden-Wiltse JH, *et al.* (1999) ACTG 260: a randomized, phase I–II, dose-ranging trial of the anti-human immunodeficiency virus activity of delavirdine monotherapy. *Antimicrobial Agents and Chemotherapy* 43: 1373–1378.

[k]Madruga JV, Cahn P, Grinsztejn B, *et al.* (2007) Efficacy and safety of TMC125 (etravirine) in treatment-experienced HIV-1-infected patients in DUET-1: 24-Week results from a randomized, double-blind, placebo-controlled trial. *Lancet* 370: 29–38.

restricted to patients at lower risk for liver failure. Delavirdine is a bisheteroarylpiperazine derivative; it is not recommended as part of a first-line antiretroviral therapy program due to its inconvenient dosing regimen and lower efficacy compared to other NNRTIs. Efavirenz, a dihydrobenzoxazinone derivative, is the most commonly prescribed NNRTI due to its high efficacy, once-daily dosing, and relatively lower toxicity. Etravirine is second-generation NNRTI, a highly flexible diarylpyrimidine derivative with a higher genetic barrier to resistance than its precursors. It is the first NNRTI to demonstrate significant antiviral potency in patients with resistance to other NNRTIs.

Several other NNRTIs are currently in clinical trials and promise higher potency while eliciting fewer drug-resistant HIV strains. BILR 355 BS is a second-generation dipyridodiazepinone derivative that shows antiviral activity against a wide range of recombinant NNRTI-resistant viruses. Rilpivirine, like etravirine, is a diarylpyrimidine derivative. It shows a median viral load reduction of 1.20 $\log_{10}$ copies ml^{-1} regardless of dose.

Integrase Inhibitors

Following reverse transcription, HIV integrase mediates the integration of proviral cDNA by catalyzing two reactions. First, integrase mediates the endonucleolytic hydrolysis of the 3′ ends of the viral DNA. This 3′-processing step generates reactive nucleophilic hydroxyl groups. Integrase remains bound to the viral cDNA as a multimeric complex that bridges both ends of the viral DNA with intracellular particles called preintegration complexes (PICs). In the strand-transfer reaction, integrase mediates the nucleophilic attack of the viral 3′-hydroxyl cDNA across the major groove of the host DNA, resulting in a 5 bp stagger between the integrated viral and host DNA strands. The integration process is completed by DNA gap repair including a series of DNA polymerization, dinucleotide excision, and ligation reactions.

While integrase is essential for retroviral replication, there is no host-cell analog. Because integrase inhibitors do not interfere with normal cellular processes, they are an attractive target for antiretroviral agents. Integrase inhibitors were discovered as early as 1992, but not until 2007 was the first drug approved.

Raltegravir is a first-in-class integrase inhibitor that gained FDA approval in October 2007 (**Table 4**). Because it is the first integrase inhibitor on the market, raltegravir is efficacious even in patients with multidrug-resistant HIV. In phase III trials, raltegravir was found to reduce the HIV viral load to undetectable levels in nearly two-thirds of highly treatment-experienced patients after 16–24 weeks of combination therapy. While the initial approval is only for treatment-experienced patients, raltegravir may also prove to be an option for treatment-naive patients.

Two drugs in clinical trials, MK-0518 and GS-9137, and GSK364735 are shown in **Table 1**. GS-9137 is a dihydroquinoline carboxylic acid derivative which also acts by inhibition of strand transfer. GS-9137 displays a serum-free IC_{50} of 0.2 nM and has activity against viral strains resistant to NRTIs, NNRTIs, and protease inhibitors. A 10-day study in treatment-naive and treatment-experienced patients resulted in mean HIV RNA decreases of 1.91 $\log_{10}$ copies ml^{-1} in patients receiving 400 or 800 mg monotherapy, or 50 mg boosted with 100 mg of ritonavir.

Protease Inhibitors

HIV protease is an aspartyl proteinase responsible for cleaving the Gag and Gag-Pol polyproteins in a late stage of the viral life cycle. Because there is no corresponding aspartyl protease that cleaves the Gag polyprotein in mammalian cells, HIV protease has been a popular target for antiretroviral drug development.

HIV PIs are peptidomimetic products that prevent cleavage of Gag and Gag-Pol protein precursors, preventing virions from maturing and becoming infectious. PIs bind to the protease site with high affinity due to their structural similarity to the tetrahedral intermediate formed during hydrolytic cleavage of a peptide bond in

Table 4 FDA-approved integrase inhibitors

Name and structure	Dosing schedule[a]	Major toxicity[a]	Key mutations conferring resistance[b]
Raltegravir (Isentress)	One 400 mg tablet b.i.d.	Elevated levels of creatine phosphokinase (CPK) in muscles; diarrhea; nausea; headache	N155H, Q148K/R/H

[a]The Body: The Complete HIV/AIDS Resource. http://www.thebody.com (accessed January 2008).
[b]Markowitz M, Nguyen B-Y, Gotuzzo E, et al. (2007) Rapid and durable antiretroviral effect of the HIV-1 integrase inhibitor raltegravir as part of combination therapy in treatment-naïve patients with HIV-1 infection. *Journal of Acquired Immune Deficiency Syndromes* 46: 125–133.

the natural substrate. First-generation PIs have a hydroxy-ethylene core which acts as a nonhydrolyzable transition state isostere. These compounds bind in the protease active site in a manner that mimics the transition state formed during peptide cleavage.

Although many peptidomimetic inhibitors of HIV protease have been reported since the first one in 1990, researchers have faced challenges regarding the physico-chemical and pharmacokinetic properties of PIs. Many PIs exhibit poor bioavailability, a short plasma half-life, poor aqueous solubility, and high protein binding, and often require frequent dosing or high pill burden in order to achieve the necessary drug concentration. The newer PIs are starting to resolve these problems. The currently available PIs are shown in **Table 5**.

Saquinavir was the first HIV PI studied clinically; it was approved by the FDA in 1995. It was discovered as part of a strategy to find transition-state mimetics of the Phe-Pro peptide bond. The original formulation exhibited potent *in vitro* viral activity but very poor bioavailability in humans (3–5%). In 1997, the FDA approved a soft gelatin capsule formation that provided higher plasma levels and bioavailability.

Ritonavir was discovered as a result of efforts to design inhibitors based on the C_2-symmetric structure of HIV protease. It shows better bioavailability than saquinavir and also inhibits cytochrome P450-3A4, a liver enzyme that normally metabolizes PIs. Therefore, ritonavir is administered in combination with other PIs in order to enhance their pharmacokinetic profiles.

Indinavir resulted from a research program of mechanism-based drug design. The lead compounds preceding discovery of indinavir were modified to create smaller, less peptide-like structures with high water solubility and bioavailability. Nelfinavir was also discovered by rational design, which sought to maximize potency while improving on the pharmacokinetics of its predecessors.

An analysis of the molecular weight distribution of marketed drugs revealed that most drugs with acceptable pharmacokinetic profiles have molecular weights under 600 Da. Amprenavir therefore emerged from a program seeking to maintain high potency while reducing inhibitor size. This compound has a sulfonylated secondary amino hydroxyethyl core, with one of the sulfonyl oxygens playing a key structural role in binding to the enzyme. While amprenavir was the first FDA-approved PI for twice-daily dosing, the 1200 mg dose required by its poor aqueous solubility was very inconvenient, and amprenavir was later superseded by its prodrug fosamprenavir.

Lopinavir is a second-generation PI inhibitor based on the structure of ritonavir. It is potent against ritonavir-resistant virus and tenfold more potent than ritonavir in the presence of human serum. Because lopinavir is rapidly metabolized, it must be co-dosed with ritonavir in order to achieve good oral bioavailability.

Atazanavir, an azapeptide PI inhibitor, is the first PI approved for once-daily dosing. It also appears to have a reduced effect on cholesterol and triglyceride levels as compared to other PIs.

Because of the poor aqueous solubility of amprenavir, a more suitable analog was sought. Fosamprenavir, a phosphate ester prodrug of amprenavir, has excellent aqueous solubility due to the presence of the phosphate salt. Fosamprenavir is rapidly and extensively converted to amprenavir after oral administration and therefore maintains its positive pharmacokinetic profile.

Tipranavir, a nonpeptidic PI, shows excellent antiviral activity. However, its undesirable toxicity profile, including reports of hepatitis and hepatic failure, generally relegate this drug to salvage therapy for patients with resistance to other PIs.

Darunavir, the most recently approved PI, resulted from a drug discovery program aimed at replacing peptide segments of PIs with nonpeptidic isosteres – in particular, a bis-tetrahydrofuran system. The oxygen atoms in this portion of the molecule appear to form hydrogen bonds with aspartate residues in HIV protease. Because of these interactions, darunavir shows activity against a broad range of drug-resistant HIV strains.

Maturation Inhibitors

Recently, a new class of antiretroviral agents has been identified which blocks HIV-1 replication at a late step in the virus life cycle. PIs prevent the essential proteolytic processing of the Gag and Gag–Pol polyproteins, which leads to the structural maturation of the virus particle and activation of viral enzymes. Maturation inhibitors, on the other hand, act directly on the Gag protein by disrupting the conversion of the HIV capsid precursor p25 to the mature capsid protein p24. This results in the production of immature viral particles that have lost infectivity.

Bevirimat, also known as PA-457, is currently the only maturation inhibitor in clinical trials (**Table 1**). Bevirimat is a betulinic acid derivative, which exhibits a mean IC_{50} of 10.3 nM in assays using patient-derived WT virus isolates. The compound also retains a similar level of activity against a panel of virus isolates resistant to the three classes of drugs targeting the viral RT and PR enzymes. With an average 50% cytotoxicity value of 25 µM, the therapeutic index for bevirimat is *c.* 2500.

Combination Therapy

Antiretroviral agents are rarely used alone in treatment. Not only does monotherapy demonstrate inferior antiviral activity to combination therapy, but it also results in a

Table 5 FDA-approved protease inhibitors

Name and structure	Dosing schedule[a]	Major toxicity[a]	Key mutations conferring resistance[b]	Impact of monotherapy[c]
Saquinavir (Invirase)	Two 500 mg tablets b.i.d., boosted with ritonavir	Lipodistrophy; diabetes; increased bleeding in hemophiliacs; hyperlipidemia	G48V L90M ± G73S/C/T I184V I54V/T/L/M/A	0.7 $\log_{10}$ copies ml^{-1} decrease in viral load
Ritonavir (Norvir)	Generally used as a boosting agent for other PIs, 100–400 mg q.d. or b.i.d. Maximum approved dose is 600 mg b.i.d.	Lipodystrophy; diabetes; increased bleeding in hemophiliacs; pancreatitis; paresthesias; hyperlipidemia; hepatitis	V82A/T/F/S I84V V32I I54V/T/L/M[d]	Limited monotherapy data available
Indinavir (Crixivan)	400 mg capsule or 800 mg capsule b.i.d., boosted with ritonavir	Lipodystrophy; diabetes; increased bleeding in hemophiliacs; liver toxicity; kidney stones; jaundice; hyperlipidemia	V82A/T/F/S M46I/LI54V/T/M/L/A L90M	1.2 $\log_{10}$ copies ml^{-1} decrease in viral load[e]
Nelfinavir (Viracept)	Two 600 mg tablets b.i.d.	Lipodystrophy; diabetes; increased bleeding in hemophiliacs; hyperlipidemia	D30N±N88D/S L90M±M46I/ L I84V V82A/ T/F/S	1.5 $\log_{10}$ copies ml^{-1} decrease in viral load
Amprenavir (Agenerase)	24 50 mg capsules (1200 mg total) b.i.d.	Lipodystrophy; diabetes; increased bleeding in hemophiliacs; skin rash; oral paresthesias; hyperlipidemia		2.0 $\log_{10}$ copies ml^{-1} decrease in viral load[f]
Lopinavir (co-formulation with ritonavir is Kaletra)	Administered with ritonavir in a single tablet. Two 200/50 mg (lopinavir/ritonavir) tablets b.i.d. or four 200/50 mg q.d.	Lipodystrophy; diabetes; increased bleeding in hemophiliacs; liver damage; hyperlipidemia	V82A/T/F/S I54V/L/M/ A/T/SM46I/L I50V	1.9 $\log_{10}$ copies ml^{-1} decrease in viral load[g]

Continued

Table 5   Continued

Name and structure	Dosing schedule[a]	Major toxicity[a]	Key mutations conferring resistance[b]	Impact of monotherapy[c]
Atazanavir (Reyataz)	300 mg capsule or two 200 mg capsules q.d., boosted with ritonavir	Lipodystrophy; diabetes; increased bleeding in hemophiliacs; jaundice	I50L N88S/D V82A/T/F/S I84V	1.6 $\log_{10}$ copies ml^{-1} decrease in viral load[h]
Fosamprenavir (Lexiva)	Two 700 mg tablets q.d. or one 700 mg tablet b.i.d., boosted with ritonavir	Increased levels of cholesterol and triglycerides; lipodystrophy; diabetes; increased bleeding in hemophiliacs; skin rash	I50V I84V I54M/L/V/ T/A M46I/L	2.4 $\log_{10}$ copies ml^{-1} decrease in viral load[i]
Tipranavir (Aptivus)	Two 250 mg capsules b.i.d., boosted with ritonavir	Lipodystrophy; diabetes; increased bleeding in hemophiliacs; liver damage; cerebral hemorrhage; hyperlipidemia; skin rash	V82A/T/F/S/ M/L I84V/ A/C L90M M46I/L/V	1.6 $\log_{10}$ copies ml^{-1} decrease in viral load[j]
Darunavir (Prezista)	Two 300 mg tablets b.i.d., boosted with ritonavir	Lipodystrophy; diabetes; increased bleeding in hemophiliacs; skin rash; hyperlipidemia; hyperglycemia	I50V V82A/T/ F/S/M I8V/ A/C I47V/A	1.4 $\log_{10}$ copies ml^{-1} decrease in viral load[k]

[a]The Body: The Complete HIV/AIDS Resource. http://www.thebody.com (accessed October 2007).

[b]Stanford University HIV Drug Resistance Database. http://hivdb.stanford.edu (accessed October 2007).

[c]Eron JJ, Jr. (2000) HIV-1 protease inhibitors. *Clinical Infectious Diseases* 30(supplement 2): S160–S170.

[d]De Mendoza C and Soriano V (2004) Resistance to HIV protease inhibitors: Mechanisms and clinical consequences. *Current Drug Metabolism* 5: 321–328.

[e]Gulick RM, Mellors JW, Havlir D, *et al.* (1997) Treatment with indinavir, zidovudine, and lamivudine in adults with human immunodeficiency virus infection and prior antiretroviral therapy. *New England Journal of Medicine* 337: 734–739.

[f]Adkins JC and Faulds D (1998) Amprenavir. *Drugs* 55: 837–842.

[g]Oldfield V and Plosker GL (2006) Lopinavir/ritonavir: A review of its use in the management of HIV infection. *Drugs* 66: 1275–1299.

[h]Barreiro P, Rendón A, Rodríguez-Nóvoa S, and Soriano V (2005) Atazanavir: The advent of a new generation of more convenient protease inhibitors. *HIV clinical trials* 6: 50–61.

[i]Chapman TM, Plosker GL, and Perry CM (2004) Fosamprenavir: A review of its use in the management of antiretroviral therapy-naïve patients with HIV infection. *Drugs* 64: 2101–2124.

[j]Dong BJ and Cocohoba JM (2006) Tipranavir: A protease inhibitor for HIV salvage therapy. *Annals of Pharmacotherapy* 40: 1311–1321.

[k]Arastéh K, Clumeck N, Pozniak A, *et al.* (2005) TMC114/ritonavir substitution for protease inhibitor(s) in a non-suppressive antiretroviral regimen: A 14-day proof-of-principle trial. *AIDS* 19: 943–947.

rapid development of resistance. The most common antiretroviral regimens in treatment-naive patients generally contain two NRTIs along with one NNRTI or a single or ritonavir-boosted PI. Preferred regimens are shown below; patients who do not tolerate these combinations may try one of the alternative regimens. While these combinations are recommended by the Office of AIDS Research Advisory Council, each patient is encouraged to seek the optimal combination for his or her situation.

- Preferred
  - Atripla: efavirenz, tenofovir, emtricitabine
  - Atazanavir + ritonavir, tenofovir, emtricitabine
  - Fosamprenavir + ritonavir, tenofovir, emtricitabine
  - Lopinavir/ritonavir, tenofovir, emtricitabine
  - Efavirenz, zidovudine, lamivudine
  - Atazanavir + ritonavir, zidovudine, lamivudine
  - Fosamprenavir + ritonavir, zidovudine, lamivudine
  - Lopinavir/ritonavir, zidovudine, lamivudine

- Alternative
  - Nevirapine, abacavir, lamivudine
  - Atazanavir (unboosted), abacavir, lamivudine
  - Fosamprenavir (unboosted), abacavir, lamivudine
  - Fosamprenavir + ritonavir, abacavir, lamivudine
  - Lopinavir/ritonavir, abacavir, lamivudine
  - Nevirapine, didanosine, lamivudine
  - Atazanavir (unboosted), didanosine, lamivudine
  - Fosamprenavir (unboosted), didanosine, lamivudine
  - Fosamprenavir + ritonavir, didanosine, lamivudine
  - Lopinavir/ritonavir, didanosine, lamivudine

Conclusion

Significant progress in antiretroviral therapy has been made since AZT first hit the market in 1987. With 22 antiretroviral agents in four classes, patients have more choices than ever. Many of these new drugs also improve quality of life with more convenient dosing schedules and greatly improved tolerability.

Despite the important success of HAART, the evolution of many drug-resistant HIV strains has diminished the efficacy of antiretroviral therapy, and an ever-increasing number of patients have progressed to salvage therapy. An estimated 13% of adults receiving care in the USA exhibit resistance to all three drug classes, and 76% of patients show resistance to one or more drugs. Because so many individuals currently living with HIV infection are highly treatment experienced, there is a strong need for newer and more effective antiretroviral therapies.

See also: Human Immunodeficiency Viruses: Origin; Human Immunodeficiency Viruses: Pathogenesis.

Further Reading

Adkins JC and Faulds D (1998) Amprenavir. *Drugs* 55: 837–842.

Arastéh K, Clumeck N, Pozniak A, *et al.* (2005) TMC114/ritonavir substitution for protease inhibitor(s) in a non-suppressive antiretroviral regimen: A 14-day proof-of-principle trial. *AIDS* 19: 943–947.

Barreiro P, Rendón A, Rodríguez-Nóvoa S, and Soriano V (2005) Atazanavir: The advent of a new generation of more convenient protease inhibitors. *HIV Clinical Trials* 6: 50–61.

Castagna A, Biswas P, Beretta A, and Lazzarin A (2005) The appealing story of HIV entry inhibitors: From discovery of biological mechanisms to drug development. *Drugs* 65: 879–904.

Chapman TM, Plosker GL, and Perry CM (2004) Fosamprenavir: A review of its use in the management of antiretroviral therapy-naïve patients with HIV infection. *Drugs* 64: 2101–2124.

Chrusciel RA and Strohbach JW (2004) Non-peptidic HIV protease inhibitors. *Current Topics in Medicinal Chemistry* 4: 1097–1114.

De Clercq E (2004) Antiviral drugs in current clinical use. *Journal of Clinical Virology* 30: 115–133.

De Clercq E (2004) Non-nucleoside reverse transcriptase inhibitors (NNRTIs): Past, present, and future. *Chemistry and Biodiversity* 1: 44–64.

De Mendoza C and Soriano V (2004) Resistance to HIV protease inhibitors: Mechanisms and clinical consequences. *Current Drug Metabolism* 5: 321–328.

Dong BJ and Cocohoba JM (2006) Tipranavir: A protease inhibitor for HIV salvage therapy. *Annals of Pharmacotherapy* 40: 1311–1321.

Eron JJ, Jr. (2000) HIV-1 protease inhibitors. *Clinical Infectious Diseases* 30(supplement 2): S160–S170.

Fitzgibbon JE, Howell RM, Haberzettl CA, Sperber SJ, Gocke DJ, and Dubin DT (1992) Human immunodeficiency virus type 1 *pol* gene mutations which cause decreased susceptibility to 2′,3′-dideoxycytidine. *Antimicrobial Agents and Chemotherapy* 36: 153–157.

Gu Z, Gao Q, Fang H, *et al.* (1994) Identification of a mutation at codon 65 in the IKKK motif of reverse transcriptase that encodes human immunodeficiency virus resistance to 2′,3′-dideoxycytidine and 2′,3′-dideoxy-3′-thiacytidine. *Antimicrobial Agents and Chemotherapy* 38: 275–281.

Gulick RM, Mellors JW, Havlir D, *et al.* (1997) Treatment with indinavir, zidovudine, and lamivudine in adults with human immunodeficiency virus infection and prior antiretroviral therapy. *New England Journal of Medicine* 337: 734–739.

Lange JMA (2003) Efficacy and durability of nevirapine in antiretroviral drug naïve patients. *Journal of Acquired Immune Deficiency Syndromes* 34: S40–S52.

Madruga JV, Cahn P, Grinsztejn B, *et al.* (2007) Efficacy and safety of TMC125 (etravirine) in treatment-experienced HIV-1-infected patients in DUET-1: 24-Week results from a randomized, double-blind, placebo-controlled trial. *Lancet* 370: 29–38.

Markowitz M, Nguyen B-Y, Gotuzzo E, *et al.* (2007) Rapid and durable antiretroviral effect of the HIV-1 integrase inhibitor raltegravir as part of combination therapy in treatment-naïve patients with HIV-1 infection. *Journal of Acquired Immune Deficiency Syndromes* 46: 125–133.

Meadows DC and Gervay-Hague J (2006) Current developments in HIV chemotherapy. *ChemMedChem* 1: 16–29.

Office of AIDS Research Advisory Council (2006) Guidelines for the use of antiretroviral agents in HIV-1-infected adults and adolescents.

Oldfield V and Plosker GL (2006) Lopinavir/ritonavir: A review of its use in the management of HIV infection. *Drugs* 66: 1275–1299.

Painter GR, Almond MR, Mao S, and Liotta DC (2004) Biochemical and mechanistic basis for the activity of nucleoside analogue inhibitors of HIV reverse transcriptase. *Current Topics in Medicinal Chemistry* 4: 1035–1044.

Para MF, Meehan P, Holden-Wiltse JH, *et al.* (1999) ACTG 260: A randomized, phase I-II, dose-ranging trial of the anti-human immunodeficiency virus activity of delavirdine monotherapy. *Antimicrobial Agents and Chemotherapy* 43: 1373–1378.

Pereira CF and Paridaen JTML (2004) Anti-HIV drug development – an overview. *Current Pharmaceutical Design* 10: 4005–4037.

Piacenti FJ (2006) An update and review of antiretroviral therapy. *Pharmacotherapy* 26: 1111–1133.

Pommier Y, Johnson AA, and Marchand C (2005) Integrase inhibitors to treat HIV/AIDS. *Nature Reviews Drug Discovery* 4: 236–248.

Randolph JT and DeGoey DA (2004) Peptidomimetic inhibitors of HIV protease. *Current Topics in Medicinal Chemistry* 4: 1079–1095.

Sharma PL, Nurpeisov V, Hernandez-Santiago B, Beltran T, and Schinzai RF (2004) Nucleoside inhibitors of human immunodeficiency virus type 1 reverse transcriptase. *Current Topics in Medicinal Chemistry* 4: 895–919.

St. Clair MH, Martin JL, Tudor-Williams G, *et al.* (1991) Resistance to ddl and sensitivity to AZT induced by a mutation in HIV-1 reverse transcriptase. *Science* 253: 1557–1559.

Temesgen Z, Warnke D, and Kasten MJ (2006) Current status of antiretroviral therapy. *Expert Opinion in Pharmacotherapy* 7: 1541–1554.

Westby M, Smith-Burchnell C, Mori J, *et al.* (2007) Reduced maximal inhibition in phenotypic susceptibility assays indicates that viral strains resistant to the CCR5 antagonist maraviroc utilize inhibitor-bound receptor for entry. *Journal of Virology* 81: 2359–2371.

Relevant Websites

http://hivdb.stanford.edu – Stanford University HIV Drug Resistance Database.

http://www.thebody.com – The Body: The Complete HIV/AIDS Resource.

Human Immunodeficiency Viruses: Origin

F van Heuverswyn and M Peeters, University of Montpellier 1, Montpellier, France

Glossary

Circulating recombinant forms These forms represent recombinant HIV-1 genomes that have infected three of more persons who are not epidemiologically related.

Endemic A classification of an infectious disease that is maintained in the population without the need for external inputs.

Epidemic A classification of a disease that appears as new cases in a given human population, during a given period, at a rate that substantially exceeds what is expected, based on recent experience.

Neighbor-joining method This clustering method constructs trees by sequentially finding of pairs of operational taxonomic units (OTUs) or neighbors that minimize the total branch length at each stage of clustering OTUs starting with a starlike tree.

Pandemic An epidemic that spreads through human populations across a large region (for e.g., a continent), or even worldwide.

Phylogenetic tree A phylogenetic tree, also called evolutionary tree, is a graphical diagram, showing the evolutionary relationships among various biological species of other entities that are believed to have a common ancestor, comparable to a pedigree showing which genes or organisms are most closely related. In a phylogenetic tree, each node with descendants represents the most common ancestor of the descendants, and the edge lengths in most trees correspond to time estimates. External nodes are often called operational taxonomic units (OTUs), a generic term that can represent many types of comparable taxa. Internal nodes may be called hypothetical taxonomic units (HTUs) to emphasize that they are the hypohetical progenitors of OTUs.

Prevalence The prevalence of a disease in a statistical population is defined as the total number of cases of the disease in the population at a given time, or the number of cases in the population, divided by the number of individuals in the population.

Introduction

Infectious diseases have been an ever-present threat to mankind. A number of important pandemics and epidemics arose with the domestication of animals, such as influenza and tuberculosis. Whereas the cause of some of the historic pandemics, such as the bubonic plague (the Black Death) that killed at least 75 million people, have been successfully eradicated, many others still cause high mortality especially in developing countries. Emerging infectious diseases continue to represent a major threat to global health. As such, HIV/AIDS is one of the most important diseases to have emerged in the past century. When on 5 June 1981, a report was published, describing five young gay men infected with *Pneumocystis carinii* pneumonia (PCP), no one could have imagined that 25 years later, more than 40 million people all over the world would be infected with the human immunodeficiency virus (HIV), the cause of the acquired immunodeficiency syndrome (AIDS). With more than 25 million deaths, HIV/AIDS continues to be one of the most serious public health threats facing humankind in the twenty-first century.

It is important therefore to identify where HIV came from, whether a natural host reservoir exists and how it was introduced into the human population. Today it is well established that human immunodeficiency viruses HIV-1 and HIV-2 are the result of several cross-species transmissions from nonhuman primates to humans. West-Central African chimpanzees (*Pan troglodytes troglodytes*) are now recognized as the natural reservoir of the simian immunodeficiency viruses (SIVcpz*Ptt*), that are the ancestors of HIV-1. Similarly, HIV-2, which has remained largely restricted to west Africa, is the result of cross-species transmissions of SIVsmm from sooty mangabeys (*Cercocebus atys*).

Although it is clear now that HIV has a zoonotic origin, it remained for a long time less certain where, when, and how often these viruses entered the human population. In this article, we will describe in more detail the latest findings on the origin of HIV, more specifically of the three groups of HIV-1 (M, N, and O) and HIV-2.

Taxonomy, Classification, and Genomic Structure

Taxonomy

Human and *Simian immunodeficiency viruses* (HIV and SIV) belong to the genus *Lentivirus* of the family *Retroviridae*, characterized by their structure and replication mode. These viruses have two RNA genomes and rely on the reverse transcriptase (RT) enzyme to transcribe their genome from RNA into a DNA copy, which can then be integrated as a DNA provirus into the genomic DNA of the host cell. This replication cycle is common for all members of the family *Retroviridae*. As the name suggests, the genus *Lentivirus* consists of slow viruses, with a long incubation period. Five serogroups are recognized, each reflecting the vertebrate hosts with which they are associated (primates, sheep and goats, horses, cats, and cattle). A feature of the primate lentiviruses, HIV and SIV, is the use of a CD4 protein receptor and the absence of a dUTPase enzyme.

Classification

Classification of simian immunodeficiency viruses (SIVs)

SIVs isolated from different primate species are designated by a three-letter code, indicating their species of origin (e.g., SIVrcm from red-capped mangabey). When different subspecies of the same species are infected, the name of the subspecies is added to the virus designation, for example, SIVcpz*Ptt* and SIVcpz*Pts* to differentiate between the two subspecies of chimpanzees *P. t. troglodytes*

and *P. t. schweinfurthii*, respectively. For chimpanzee viruses, the known or suspected country of origin is often included; for example, SIVcpzCAM and SIVcpzGAB are isolates from Cameroon and Gabon, respectively.

Currently, serological evidence of SIV infection has been shown for 39 different primate species and SIV infection has been confirmed by sequence analysis in 32 (see **Table 1**). Overall, complete SIV genome sequences are available for 19 species. Importantly, 30 species of the 69 recognized Old World monkey and ape species in sub-Saharan Africa have not been tested yet or only very few have been tested. Knowing that the vast majority (90%) of the primate species tested are SIV infected, many of the remaining species would be expected to harbor additional SIV infections. Only Old World primates are infected with SIVs, and only those from the African continent; no SIVs have been identified in Asian primate species. It is important also to note that none of the African primates naturally infected with SIV develop disease.

Classification of human immunodeficiency viruses (HIVs)

AIDS can be caused by two related lentiviruses; human immunodeficiency virus types 1 and 2 (HIV-1 and HIV-2). On the basis of phylogenetic analyses of numerous isolates obtained from diverse geographic origins, HIV-1 is classified into three groups, M, N, and O. Group M (for Major) represents the vast majority of HIV-1 strains found worldwide and is responsible for the pandemic; group O (for Outlier) and N (non-M–non-O) remain restricted to West-Central Africa. Group M can be further subdivided into nine subtypes (A–D, F-H, J, K), circulating recombinant forms (CRFs, CRF01–CRF32), and unique recombinants. The geographic distribution of the different HIV-1 M variants is very heterogeneous and differs even from country to country. Compared to HIV-1, only a limited number of HIV-2 strains have been genetically characterized and eight groups (A–H) have been reported.

Genomic Structure

All primate lentiviruses have a common genomic structure, consisting of the long terminal repeats (LTRs), flanking both ends of the genome, three structural genes, *gag, pol,* and *env* and five accessory genes, *vif, vpr, tat, rev,* and *nef*. Some primate lentiviruses carry an additional accessory gene, *vpx* or *vpu,* in the region between *pol* and *env*. Based on this genomic organization, we can distinguish between three patterns (**Figure 1**): (1) SIVagm, SIVsyk, SIVmnd1, SIVlho, SIVsun, SIVcol, SIVtal, and SIVdeb display the basic structure with three major and five accessory genes; (2) SIVcpz, SIVgsn, SIVmus, SIVden, SIVmon, and also HIV-1 harbor an additional accessory gene, *vpu*; HIV-1 and SIVcpz differ from the

Table 1　Serological and/or molecular evidence for SIV infection in the African nonhuman primates

Genus	Species	Common name	SIV	Geographic distribution
Pan	troglodytes	Common chimpanzee	SIVcpz	West to East: Senegal to Tanzania
Gorilla	gorilla	Western gorilla	SIVgor[a]	Central: Cameroon, Gabon, Congo, Central Africa Republic
Colobus	guereza	Mantled guereza	SIVcol	Central: Nigeria to Ethiopia/Tanzania
Piliocolobus	badius	Western red colobus	SIVwrc[a]	West: Senegal to Ghana
Procolobus	verus	Olive colobus	SIVolc[a]	West: Sierra-Leone to Ghana
Lophocebus	albigena	Gray-cheeked managabey	?	Central: Nigeria to Uganda/Burundi
	aterrimus	Black crested mangabey	SIVbkm[a]	Central: Democratic Republic of Congo (DRC)
Papio	anubis	Olive baboon	?	West to East: Mali to Ethiopia
	cynocephalus	Yellow baboon	SIVagm-Ver[a]	Central: Angola to Tanzania
	ursinus	Chacma baboon	SIVagm-Ver[a]	South: southern Angola to Zambia
Cercocebus	atys	Sooty mangabey	SIVsmm	West: Senegal to Ghana
	torquatus	Red-capped mangabey	SIVrcm	West Central: Nigeria, Cameroon, Gabon
	agilis	Agile mangabey	SIVagi[a]	Central: northeast Gabon to northeast Congo
Mandrillus	sphinx	Mandrill	SIVmnd-1, SIVmnd-2	West Central: Cameroon (south of Sanaga) to Gabon, Congo
	leucophaeus	Drill	SIVdrl	West Central: southeast Nigeria to Cameroon (north of Sanaga)
Allenopithecus	nigroviridis	Allen's swamp monkey	?	Central: Congo
Miopithecus	talapoin	Angolan talapoin	SIVtal[a]	West Central: East coast of Angola into DRC
	ogouensis	Gabon talapoin	SIVtal	West Central: Cameroon (south of Sanaga)-Gabon
Erythrocebus	patas	Patas monkey	SIVagm-sab[a]	West to East: Senegal to Ethiopia, Tanzania
Chlorocebus	sabaeus	Green monkey	SIVagm-Sab	West: Senegal to Volta river in Burkina Faso
	aethiops	Grivet	SIVagm-Gri	East: Sudan, Erithrea, Ethiopia
	tantalus	Tantalus monkey	SIVagm-Tan	Central: Ghana to Uganda
	pygerythrus	Vervet monkey	SIVagm-Ver	South: South Africa to Somalia and Angola
Cercopithecus	diana	Diana monkey	?	West: Sierra-Leone to Ivory Coast
	nictitans	Greater spot-nosed monkey	SIVgsn	Central: forest blocks from West Africa to DRC
	mitis	Blue monkey	SIVblu[a]	East Central: East Congo to Rift-valley
	albogularis	Sykes's monkey	SIVsyk	East: Somalia to Eastern Cape
	mona	Mona monkey	SIVmon	West: Niger delta to Cameroon (north of Sanaga)
	campbelli	Campbell's mona	?	West: Gambia to Liberia
	pogonias	Crested mona	?	West Central: Cross River in Nigeria to Congo (east)
	denti	Dent's mona	SIVden	Central: south of Congo River
	cephus	Mustached guenon	SIVmus	West Central: Cameroon (south of Sanaga) to east of Congo River
	erythrotis	Red-eared monkey	SIVery[a]	West Central: Cross River in Nigeria to Sanaga in Cameroon, Bioko
	ascanius	Red-tailed monkey	SIVasc[a]	Central: South-East Congo to West Tanzania
	lhoest	l'Hoest monkey	SIVlho	Central: eastern Congo–Zaire to western Uganda
	solatus	Sun-tailed monkey	SIVsun	West Central: tropical forest of Gabon
	preussi	Preuss's monkey	SIVpre[a]	West Central: Cross river in Nigeria to Sanaga in Cameroon, Bioko
	hamlyni	Owl-faced monkey	?	Central: eastern DRC to Ruanda
	neglectus	de Brazza's monkey	SIVdeb	Central: Angola, Cameroon, Gabon to Uganda, western Kenya

[a]only partial sequences are available, ? only serological evidence for SIV infection.

other members of this group by the fact that *env* and *nef* genes are not overlapping; (3) SIVsmm, SIVrcm, SIVmnd2, SIVdrl, and SIVmac, and HIV-2 harbor a supplemental accessory gene, *vpx*. For the remaining SIVs, SIVolc, SIVwrc, SIVasc, SIVbkm, SIVery, SIVblu, SIVpre, SIVagi, and SIVgor, full-length sequences are not yet available.

Evolutionary History

HIV-2 and SIVsmm from Sooty Mangabeys

Shortly after the identification of HIV-1 as the cause of AIDS in 1983, the first SIV, SIVmac, was isolated from rhesus macaques (*Macaca mulatta*) at the New England Regional Primate Research Center (NERPRC).

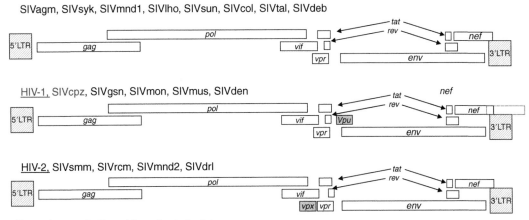

Figure 1 Genomic organization of the primate lentiviruses.

Retrospective research revealed that the newly identified SIV was introduced to the NERPRC by rhesus monkeys, previously housed at the California National Primate Research Center (CNPRC), where they survived an earlier (late 1960s) disease outbreak, characterized by immune suppression and opportunistic infections. A decade after the first outbreak, the story has been repeated in stump-nailed macaques (*Macaca arctoides*) in the same settings and 15 years later a lentivirus, called SIVstm, was isolated from frozen tissue from one of these monkeys. In both cases, the infected rhesus macaques had been in contact with healthy, but retrospectively shown SIVsmm seropositive sooty mangabeys at the CNPRC. The close phylogenetic relationship between SIVmac, SIVstm, and SIVsmm identified mangabeys as the plausible source of SIV in macaques. Since SIVmac induced a disease in rhesus macaques with remarkable similarity to human AIDS, a simian origin of HIV was soon suspected. The discovery in 1986 of HIV-2, the agent of AIDS in West Africa, and the remarkable high relatedness of HIV-2 with SIVsmm, naturally infecting sooty mangabeys in West Africa, reinforced this hypothesis.

In addition, the similarities in viral genome organization (the presence of *vpx*), the geographic coincidence of the natural range of sooty mangabeys and the epicenter of the HIV-2 epidemic in West Africa, as well as the fact that sooty mangabeys are frequently hunted for food or kept as pets, allowed the identification of SIVsmm from sooty mangabeys as the simian source of HIV-2.

HIV-1 and SIVcpz from Chimpanzees

The first SIVcpz strains, SIVcpzGAB1 and SIVcpzGAB2, were isolated from chimpanzees (*P. troglodytes*) in Gabon more than 15 years ago; of 50 wild-caught chimpanzees initially tested for SIVcpz infection, two (GAB1 and GAB2) harbored HIV-1 cross-reactive antibodies. Analysis of the SIVcpzGAB1 genome revealed the same genomic organization as HIV-1, including an accessory gene, named *vpu*, so far only identified in HIV-1. Furthermore, phylogenetic analysis indicated that SIVcpzGAB1 was more closely related to HIV-1 than to any other SIV. A few years later, a third positive chimpanzee, confiscated upon illegal importation into Belgium from the Democratic Republic of Congo (DRC, ex-Zaire), was identified among 43 other wild-caught chimpanzees. A virus, SIVcpzANT, was isolated and characterized, but this virus showed an unexpected high degree of divergence from the others. A fourth SIVcpz strain (SIVcpzUS) was obtained from a chimpanzee (Marilyn) housed in an American primate center and it was shown that SIVcpzUS was closely related to the SIVcpz strains from Gabon. Subspecies identification of the chimpanzee hosts revealed that the SIVcpzANT strain was isolated from a member of the *P.t. schweinfurtii* subspecies, whereas the other chimpanzees belonged to the *P.t. troglodytes* subspecies. These findings suggested two distinct SIVcpz lineages according to the host species: SIVcpz*Ptt*, from the West-Central African chimpanzees, and SIVcpz*Pts*, from eastern chimpanzees. HIV-1 strains are classified into three highly divergent clades, groups M, N, and O, each of which was more closely related to SIVcpz from *P. t. troglodytes* than to SIVcpz from *P. t. schweinfurthii*. These data pointed to the West-Central African subspecies, *P. t. troglodytes* as the natural reservoir of the ancestors of HIV-1.

Until recently, only a handful of complete or partial SIVcpz genomes have been derived. In addition to the four previously mentioned viruses, three other strains, SIVcpzCAM3, SIVcpzCAM5, and SIVcpzCAM13, have been identified in Cameroon and all clustered with the previously identified SIVcpz*Ptt* strains consistent with their species of origin. The discovery of HIV-1 group N in a Cameroonian patient in 1998 showed that HIV-1 N is closely related to SIVcpz*Ptt* in the envelope region of the viral genome, suggesting an ancient recombination event. This finding demonstrated the co-circulation of SIVcpz and

HIV-1 N viruses in the same geographic area and provided additional evidence that the western part of Central Africa is the likely site of origin of HIV-1.

However, the number of identified SIV strains in chimpanzees was low, compared to that of other naturally occurring SIV infections. The major problem in studying SIVcpz infection in chimpanzees is their endangered status and the fact that they live in isolated forest regions. All previously studied chimpanzees were among wild-caught but young and captive animals. They were initially captured as infants, mainly as a by-product of the bushmeat trade. Since the age of maturation of chimpanzees is around 9 for males and 10 for females, these infections were most probably the result of vertical transmission and do not reflect true prevalences among wild-living adult animals. Apparently, the frequency of vertical transmission is low among naturally infected primates, which can explain the low prevalence rates initially observed.

The recent development of noninvasive methods to detect and characterize SIVcpz in fecal and urine samples from wild ape populations boosted the search for new SIVcpz strains in the vast tropical forests of Central Africa. The first report of a full-length SIVcpz sequence obtained from a fecal sample, SIVcpzTAN1, was from a wild chimpanzee from the *P. t. schweinfurtii* subspecies in Gombe National Park, Tanzania. Subsequently, additional cases of SIVcpz*Pts* infections were documented in Tanzania (SIVcpzTAN2 to SIVcpzTAN5) and around Kisangani, northeastern DRC (SIVcpzDRC1). All the new SIVcpz*Pts* viruses formed a separate lineage with the initially described SIVcpzANT strain and suggest that the SIVcpz*Pts* strains are not at the origin of HIV-1 (**Figure 2**). A recent study in wild chimpanzee communities in southern Cameroon documented a prevalence of SIVcpz infection ranging from 4% to 35%, and identified 16 new SIVcpz*Ptt* strains. All of these newly identified viruses were found to fall within the radiation of SIVcpz*Ptt* strains from captive *P. t. troglodytes* apes, which also includes HIV-1 groups M and N, but not group O or SIVcpz*Pts* (**Figure 2**). The new SIVcpz*Ptt* viruses are characterized by high genetic diversity and SIVcpz*Ptt* strains were identified which are much more closely related to HIV-1 groups M and N than were any previously identified SIVcpz strains. Interestingly, the new SIVcpz*Ptt* viruses exhibited a significant geographic clustering and made it possible to trace the origins of present-day human AIDS viruses to geographically isolated chimpanzee communities in southern Cameroon.

HIV-1 and SIVgor from Gorillas

SIV infection has recently been described in western gorillas (*Gorilla gorilla*) in Cameroon. Surprisingly, the newly characterized gorilla viruses, termed SIVgor, formed a monophyletic group within the HIV-1/SIVcpz*Ptt* radiation, but in contrast to SIVcpz*Ptt*, they were most closely related to the HIV-1 group O lineage (**Figure 2**). However, the phylogenetic relationships between SIVcpz, SIVgor, and HIV-1 indicate that chimpanzees represent the original reservoir of SIVs now found in chimpanzees, gorillas, and humans. Given their herbivorous diet and peaceful coexistence with other primate species, especially chimpanzees, it remains a mystery by what route gorillas acquired SIVgor.

The data on SIV in wild chimpanzee and gorilla populations showed that distinct chimpanzee communities in southern Cameroon transmitted divergent SIVcpz to humans giving rise to HIV-1 groups M and N; and that chimpanzees transmitted HIV-1 group O-like viruses either to gorillas and humans independently, or first to gorillas which then transmitted the virus to humans. Additional studies are needed to determine if the other African great ape species, the eastern gorillas (*Gorilla berengei*) and the bonobo (*Pan paniscus*) harbor any SIV.

Cross-Species Transmission

Where?

HIV-1

Based on mitochondrial DNA sequences, common chimpanzees (*P. troglodytes*) are classified into four subspecies: *P. t. verus* in West Africa; *P. t. vellerosus*, restricted to a geographical area between the Cross River in Nigeria and the Sanaga River in Cameroon; *P. t. troglodytes* in southern Cameroon, Gabon, Equatorial Guinea, and the Republic of Congo; and *P. t. schweinfurtii* in the Democratic Republic of Congo, Uganda, Rwanda, and Tanzania. No evidence of SIV infection is found in *P. t. verus*, despite testing of more than 2000 chimpanzees, mostly captive animals exported to zoos or research centers in the US. Wild *P. t. vellerosus* apes have not been found to harbor SIVcpz, but only about 100 samples have been screened. The single reported SIV infection of *P. t. vellerosus*, SIVCAM4, was most probably the result of a cage transmission from a *P. t. troglodytes* ape, infected with SIVcpzCAM3. Since the three groups of HIV-1 (M, N, and O) all fall within the HIV-1/SIVcpz*Ptt*/SIVgor lineage, the cross-species transmissions giving rise to HIV-1 most likely occurred in western equatorial Africa. Furthermore, no human counterpart is found for SIVcpz*Pts* from *P. t. schweinfurtii*, which undermines the idea of a human-induced origin of HIV-1 by oral polio vaccine (OPV) programs in East-Central Africa in the late 1950s. It has been suggested that tissues derived from SIVcpz-infected chimpanzees, captured in the northeastern part of DRC were used for the polio vaccine production. However, this geographical region is situated in the middle of the *P. t. schweinfurtii* range and the characterization of a partial SIV genome (SIVcpzDRC1) from a wild chimpanzee in this region proved once more the inconsistency of the OPV theory (**Figure 2**).

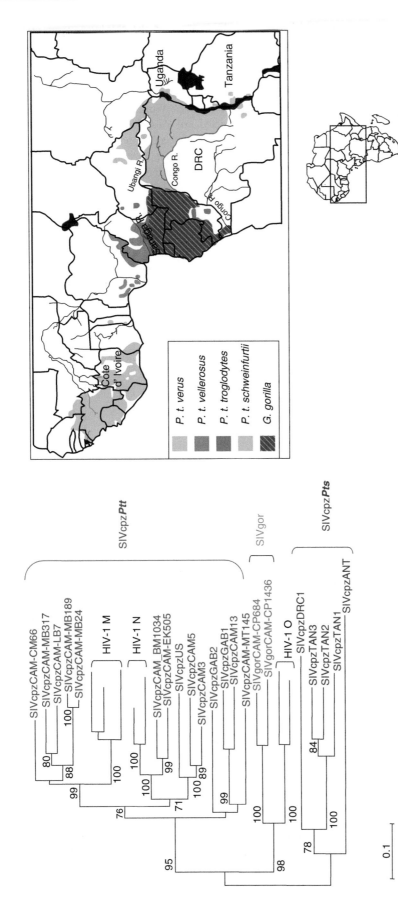

Figure 2. Natural range of chimpanzee subspecies and phylogeny of the HIV-1/SIVcpz/SIVgor lineage. The ranges of the four recognized chimpanzee subspecies are color-coded. The SIVcpz*Ptt* and SIVcpz*Pts* sequences in the phylogenetic tree are colored in red and blue, respectively, in accordance to the chimpanzee subspecies, illustrating that HIV-1 is more closely related to SIVcpz from West-Central African chimpanzees. The natural range for western gorillas (*Gorilla gorilla*) overlaps with the *P. t. troglodytes* range in West-Central Africa; SIVgor sequences are indicated in gray. The country of origin where SIVcpz strains were identified is indicated with a three-letter code: CAM for Cameroon, GAB for Gabon, TAN for Tanzania, DRC for the Democratic Republic of Congo, US for an animal in a primate center in the USA, and ANT for a captive animal in Antwerp, Belgium. This tree was derived by neighbor-joining analysis of partial *env/nef* nucleotide sequences. Horizontal branch lengths are drawn to scale.

The recent studies in wild chimpanzee communities in Cameroon, not only confirm the West-Central African origin of HIV-1, but also indicate that HIV-1 group M and N arose from geographically distinct chimpanzee populations. Phylogenetic analysis showed that all SIVcpz strains collected in southeast Cameroon formed a cluster with HIV-1 group M, whereas SIVcpz isolates from chimpanzee communities of a well-defined region in south-central Cameroon clustered with the nonpandemic HIV-1 group N. It is also interesting to note that there is an uneven dissemination of SIV infection among chimpanzee populations, with the absence of SIV infection in some of them and with major geographical elements, like rivers, that can serve as important barriers.

As discussed above, HIV-1 group N resulted from an ancestral recombination event between divergent lineages. The discovery of such a recombinant virus in a geographically isolated chimpanzee community in southern Cameroon shows that HIV-1 N was already a recombinant in its natural hosts prior to its transmission to humans.

The origin of the third group of HIV-1, group O, remained uncertain until the recent identification of HIV-1 group O-like viruses in two different wild-living gorilla populations, in southern Cameroon (SIVgor). So all three HIV-1 groups seem to have their seeds in West-Central Africa. While HIV-1 group O infections remained restricted to West-Central Africa (Cameroon, Nigeria, Gabon, Equatorial Guinea) and HIV-1 N to Cameroon only, HIV-1 group M strains have spread across Africa and all the other continents.

HIV-2

A close phylogenetic relatedness is also observed between SIVsmm from sooty mangabeys (*Cercocebus atys*) and HIV-2 in West Africa. Sooty mangabeys are indigenous to West Africa, from Senegal to Ivory Coast, coinciding with the endemic center of HIV-2 (**Figure 3**). Eight groups (A–H) of HIV-2 have been described so far, but only subtypes A and B are largely represented in the HIV-2 epidemic, with subtype A in the western part of

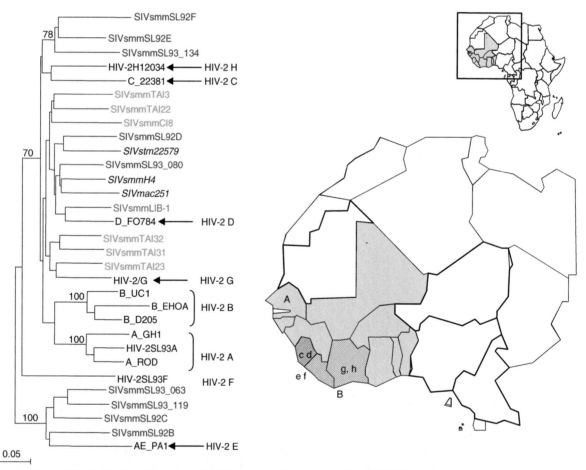

Figure 3 Geographic distribution of the different HIV-2 groups and phylogeny of the HIV-2/SIVsmm lineage. Countries where HIV-2 is endemic are colored in grey and overlap with the range of sooty mangabeys (*Cercocebus atys*) in West Africa. SIVsmm strains obtained from mangabeys in different regions are colored: green for Ivory Coast, blue for Sierra Leone, and pink for Liberia. SIVsmm strains isolated from mangabeys or macaques in US zoo's or primate centers are indicated in italic. This tree was derived by neighbor-joining analysis of partial *gag* nucleotide sequences from HIV-2 and SIVsmm sequences from West Africa. Horizontal branch lengths are drawn to scale.

West Africa (Senegal, Guinea-Bissau) and subtype B being predominant in Ivory Coast. The other subtypes have been documented in one or few individuals only. Except for groups G and H, groups C, D, E, and F were isolated in rural areas in Sierra Leone and Liberia and these viruses are more closely related to the SIVsmm strains obtained from sooty mangabeys found in the same area than to any other HIV-2 strains. This suggests that the different groups of HIV-2 must be the result of multiple independent cross-species transmissions of SIVsmm into the human population. Importantly, HIV-2 prevalence remains low and is even decreasing, since HIV-1 M is now predominating also in West Africa.

When?

It is clear now that each group of HIV-1 (M, N, and O) and HIV-2 (A–H) resulted from an independent cross-species transmission, followed by different viral evolution rates and possibly by one or more recombination events. HIV-1 group M can be further subdivided into subtypes, circulating recombinant forms and many unique recombinants, which had a heterogeneous geographical spread. The highest genetic diversity, in number of co-circulating subtypes and intrasubtype diversity has been observed in Central Africa, more precisely the western part of DRC, suggesting this region being the epicenter of HIV-1 M. Moreover, the earliest known HIV-1 virus, ZR59, isolated from an individual in Léopoldville (now Kinshasa) in 1959. The virus has been characterized as a member of HIV-1 M, subtype D. So, the common ancestor of this group should be dated prior to 1959. Molecular clock analyses estimated the date of the most recent common ancestor of HIV-1 group M around 1930 with a confidence interval of 1915–1941. A similar time frame is estimated for the origin of the HIV-1 group O radiation: 1920 with a range from 1931 to 1940. The oldest HIV-1 group O sample has been documented in a Norwegian sailor in 1964 infected in Cameroon (Douala), both groups show an exponential increase of the number of HIV infections during the twentieth century. However, the growth rate of HIV-1 group O ($r = 0.08$ [0.05–0.12]) is slower than the rate estimated for HIV-1 group M in Central Africa ($r = 0.17$). This is not surprising, considering the much lower prevalence of group O in Cameroon. Since the first identification of HIV-1 group N in 1998, about 10 group N infections have been described and all were from Cameroonian patients. The intra-group genetic diversity is significant lower for group N than for group M or O, which suggests a more recent introduction of the HIV-1 N lineage into the human population.

Similar analyses traced the origin of the pandemic HIV-2 groups A and B to be around 1940 with a confidence interval of ± 16 years, and around 1945 with a confidence interval of 1931–59, respectively.

How?

Although the precise conditions and circumstances of the SIVcpz and SIVsmm transmissions remain unknown, human exposure to blood or other secretions of infected primates, through hunting and butchering of primate bushmeat, represents the most plausible source for human infection. Also bites and other injuries caused by primates kept as pets can increase the probability of viral transmission. Direct evidence of human infection with other SIVs is not yet reported, but that retroviruses can jump from primates to humans has been documented for simian foamy viruses (SFV) and simian T-cell leukemia viruses (STLVs). For example, SFV infection has been detected in rural Central Africa among individuals who hunt monkeys and apes. The infection with SFV in an Asian man, who regularly visited an ancient temple, was most probably the result of a bite from a macaque. An analysis of the man's blood indicated the presence of an SFV strain similar to a strain from macaques living around the temple. So far, SFV has not been shown to cause disease in humans, but the long-term effects of SFV in humans are not yet known. These effects are well documented for SIV and its human counterpart HIV; the HIV-1 group M epidemic clearly illustrates the devastating results of a single cross-species transmission.

Other SIV Cross-Species Transmissions, Risk for Novel HIV?

A recent study on primate bushmeat in Cameroon revealed that about 10% is SIV infected and illustrates an ongoing exposure to a plethora of different SIVs. Today, 69 different nonhuman primate species are identified in Africa and for 32 species (47%) SIV infection could already be proved by genomic amplification of the virus. This means that, in addition to sooty mangabeys, chimpanzees, and possibly gorillas, at least 29 other primate species harbor SIV's, which poses a potential risk for transmission to humans, especially for those in direct contact with infected blood and tissues. Therefore, efforts to reduce exposure to SIV-infected primates should be a primary concern. However, the opposite is occuring; the bushmeat trade has increased significantly during the last few decades, especially through the development of the logging industry. As a consequence, roads are now penetrating the formerly isolated forest areas and create a free passage for transport of wood, bushmeat, people, and subsequently different pathogens. The surrounding villages change from modest, little communities to real trade centers, with up to several thousand inhabitants. In addition, human migration and social and economic networks support this industry. It is very likely that the estimated prevalence of SIV infection of wild monkey species is underestimated for three reasons: first, only half of the recognized species have been tested; second, for some species only a few monkeys were tested; and third, and the most important reason, the sensitivity of the available diagnostic tools, initially developed for HIV detection, may be inaccurate for the detection of divergent SIVs. The increasing magnitude of human exposure to SIVs, combined with socioeconomic changes, which favor the dissemination of a plausible SIV transmission into the human population, could be the basis of novel zoonoses that lead in turn to novel HIV epidemics.

It is important to note that there is more needed than transmission of a virus to initiate an epidemic. After the virus has crossed the species barrier, adaptation to the new host is necessary to be able to spread efficiently within a population. The pathogenic potential of the virus and host genetic differences between individuals, as well as between species, determine susceptibility or resistance to further disease progression. In addition, environmental, social, and demographic factors play a major role in the further spread of new viruses.

Evolution of SIVs in their Natural Primate Hosts: The Origin of SIVcpz

With the increasing number of full-length SIV sequences from different primate species it becomes clear that cross-species transmissions and subsequent recombinations have occurred frequently among primates lentiviruses. Cross-species transmissions among co-habiting species in the wild has been observed between African green monkeys and patas monkeys in West Africa; between African green monkeys and baboons in southern Africa; and between different *Cercopithecus* species in Central Africa, that is, greater spot-nosed guenons (*C. nictitans*) and moustached (*C. cephus*) monkeys in Cameroon.

One of the most striking examples of cross-species transmission, followed by recombination, is SIVcpz in chimpanzees. Chimpanzees are known to hunt other primates for food, such as red-capped mangabeys (*Cercocebus torquatus*), greater spot-nosed guenons (*Cercopithecus nictitans*), and colobus monkeys (*Colobinae*). The isolation and characterization of the SIV genomes from the former monkey species revealed an unexpected high level of similarity between some parts of the SIVcpz genome and SIVrcm and SIVgsn. The 5′ region of SIVcpz (*gag, pol, vif,* and *vpr*) is most similar to SIVrcm, except for the accessory gene *vpx*, which is characteristic for the SIVrcm lineage, but absent in the HIV-1 and SIVcpz strains. The 3′ region of SIVcpz (*vpu, env,* and *nef*) is closely related to SIVgsn. Furthermore, SIVgsn is the first reported monkey virus to encode a *vpu* gene, the accessory gene characteristic of the HIV-1/SIVcpz lineage. Most probably, the recombination of these monkey viruses occurred within chimpanzees and gave rise to the common ancestor of today's SIVcpz lineages, which in

turn were subsequently transmitted to humans. The cross-species transmission of this recombinant virus, or its progenitors, happened some time after the split of *P. t. verus* and *P. t. vellerosus* from the other subspecies, but possibly before the divergence between *P. t. troglodytes* and *P. t. schweinfurtii.*

The fact that gorillas are infected with an SIV from the SIVcpz lineage, represents a mystery, since only peaceful encounters have been documented among these sympatric apes. The evolutionary history of primate lentiviruses is complex and likely involved a series of consecutive interspecies transmissions, the timelines and directions of which remain to be deciphered.

Conclusion

We now have a clear picture of the origin of HIV and the seeds of the AIDS pandemic. SIVcpz, the progenitor of HIV-1, resulted from a recombination among ancestors of SIV lineages presently infecting red-capped mangabeys and *Cercopithecus* monkeys in West-Central Africa. HIV-1 groups M and O resulted from independent cross-species transmissions early in the twentieth century. The SIVcpz*Ptt* strains that gave rise to HIV-1 group M belonged to a viral lineage that persists today in *P. t. troglodytes* apes in south Cameroon. Most likely this virus was transmitted locally, but made its way to Kinshasa where the group M pandemic was spawned. HIV-1 group N, which has been identified in only a small number of AIDS patients from Cameroon, derived from a second SIVcpz*Ptt* lineage in south-central Cameroon and remained geographically more restricted. HIV-1 group O-related viruses are present in a second African great ape species, the western gorilla (*Gorilla gorilla*), but chimpanzees were the original reservoir of SIVgor.

Similarly, only HIV-2 group A and B play a major role in the HIV-2 epidemic, and most other groups (C–H) represent unique sequences found in a single patient. A possible explanation could be that some viruses were not able to adapt to the new host or that the environment was not suitable for epidemic spread.

Viral adaptation to the new host is one of the requirements for the generation of an epidemic, but also the interaction of sociocultural factors, such as deforestation, urbanization, and human migration, have been crucial in the emergence of the HIV-1 pandemic. While the origin of the HIV-1 and HIV-2 viruses has become clearer, important questions concerning pathogenicity and epidemic spread of certain SIV variants needs to be further elucidated.

See also: AIDS: Disease Manifestation; AIDS: Global Epidemiology; Human Immunodeficiency Viruses: Antiretroviral Agents; Human Immunodeficiency Viruses: Pathogenesis.

Further Reading

Aghokeng AF and Peeters M (2005) Simian immunodeficiency viruses (SIVs) in Africa. *Journal of Neurovirology* 11(supplement 1): 27–32.

Hahn BH, Shaw GM, De Cock KM, and Sharp PM (2000) AIDS as a zoonosis: Scientific and public health implications. *Science* 287: 607–614.

Keele BF, Van Heuverswyn F, Li Y, *et al.* (2006) Chimpanzee: Reservoirs of pandemic and nonpandemic HIV-1. *Science* 313: 523–526.

Korber B, Muldoon M, Theiler J, *et al.* (2000) Timing the ancestor of the HIV-1 pandemic strains. *Science* 288: 1789–1796.

Lemey P, Pybus OG, Rambaut A, *et al.* (2004) The molecular population genetics of HIV-1 group O. *Genetics* 167: 1059–1068.

Santiago ML, Range F, Keele BF, *et al.* (2005) Simian immunodeficiency virus infection in free-ranging sooty mangabeys (*Cercocebus atys atys*) from the Tai Forest, Cote d'Ivoire: Implications for the origin of epidemic human immunodeficiency virus type 2. *Journal of Virology* 79: 12515–12527.

Sharp PM, Shaw GM, and Hahn BH (2005) Simian immunodeficiency virus infection of chimpanzees. *Journal of Virology* 79: 3891–3902.

VandeWoude S and Apetrei C (2006) Going wild: Lessons from naturally occurring T-lymphotropic lentiviruses. *Clinical Microbiological Reviews* 19: 728–762.

Van Heuverswyn F, Li Y, Neel C, *et al.* (2006) Human immunodeficiency viruses: SIV infection in wild gorillas. *Nature* 44: 164.

Worobey M, Santiago ML, Keele BF, *et al.* (2004) Origin of AIDS: Contaminated polio vaccine theory refuted. *Nature* 428: 820.

Human Immunodeficiency Viruses: Pathogenesis

N R Klatt, A Chahroudi, and G Silvestri, University of Pennsylvania School of Medicine, Philadelphia, PA, USA

Glossary

Apoptosis Programmed cell death.

Bystander cell death The death of HIV-uninfected cells.

CCR5 A G-protein-coupled, seven transmembrane spanning receptor for the chemokines RANTES (CCL5), MIP-1α (CCL3), and MIP-1β (CCL4) that is primarily expressed on T lymphocytes, dendritic cells, macrophages, and microglial cells.

CD4+ T lymphocytes (also called T-helper cells) Cells bearing CD4, a co-receptor of the T-cell receptor (TCR) complex, that recognize peptide antigens bound to MHC class II molecules and are important for both humoral and cellular immunity.

Cytotoxic T lymphocytes (CTLs) Cells that are capable of killing other cells. Most CTLs express CD8, a co-receptor of the TCR complex, and recognize antigenic peptides from cytosolic pathogens, particularly viruses, that are bound to MHC class I molecules.

Generalized immune activation The activation of all lymphocyte subsets in HIV infection, leading to increased cell death.

Mucosal-associated lymphoid tissue (MALT) The system of lymphoid cells found in the epithelia and lamina propria of the body's mucosal sites, including the gastrointestinal tract, lungs, eyes, nose, and the female reproductive tract.

Neutralizing antibodies Antibodies that can limit the infectivity of a pathogen or the toxic effects of a toxin by binding to the receptor-binding site on the pathogen/toxin and thus block entry into the target cell.

Simian immunodeficiency virus (SIV) Like HIV it is a single-stranded, positive-sense, enveloped RNA virus that is classified as a member of the genus *Lentivirus* of the family *Retroviridae*. The virus infecting chimpanzees (SIV$_{cpz}$) is the origin of HIV-1 and the virus infecting sooty mangabeys (SIV$_{smm}$) is the origin of HIV-2.

Introduction

The AIDS pandemic, with an estimated 40 million individuals infected with the causative agent, human immunodeficiency virus (HIV), is without question one of the key medical challenges of modern times. Twenty-four years after the first identification of HIV, the situation in the fields of AIDS research, prevention, and treatment reflects several major advances as well as a number of areas where the progress has been slow or nonexistent (**Table 1**). While the #1 challenge (low rate of treatment in developing countries, particularly sub-Saharan Africa) is, in essence, a reflection of the sociopolitical climate arising from a lack of stability, development, and healthcare infrastructure in these countries, challenges #2 and #3 (absence of a preventative vaccine or a cure for HIV infection and AIDS) are a direct consequence of our incomplete understanding of the pathogenesis of HIV infection. Here we summarize the key advances that have improved our understanding of the mechanisms underlying the immunodeficiency that follows HIV infection.

While it is clear and universally accepted that HIV is the etiologic agent of AIDS and that the main

Table 1   Major achievements and remaining challenges in AIDS research

Major achievements in AIDS research:
1. Discovery and characterization of the etiologic agent.
2. Development of lab tests to monitor and prevent the infection via blood and blood products.
3. Definition of the origin of the epidemics.
4. Development of a large array of potent anti-HIV drugs, with consequent major reduction in mortality and MTCT in Western countries.

Major remaining challenges:
1. Abysmally low rate of treatment in developing countries.
2. Absence of a vaccine or a long-lasting microbicide.
3. Absence of a treatment that can eradicate infection.
4. Incomplete understanding of the pathogenesis of infection.

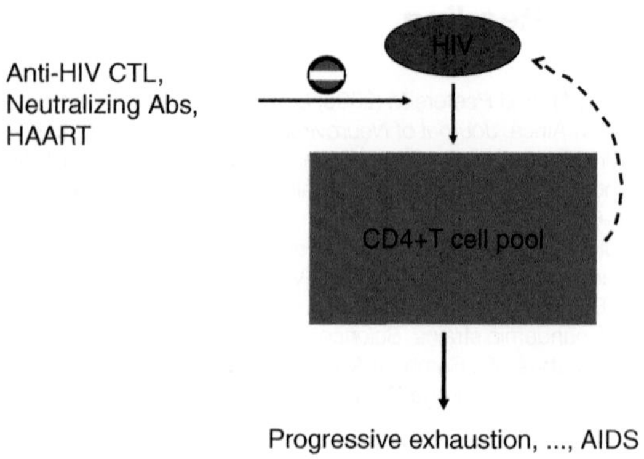

Anti-HIV CTL,
Neutralizing Abs,
HAART

CD4+T cell pool

Progressive exhaustion, ..., AIDS

Figure 1   The classical or virus-centric model of AIDS pathogenesis.

pathophysiologic assault during HIV infection is the development of a state of chronic, progressive, and ultimately fatal immunodeficiency, several questions remain regarding the exact sequence and cause of the pathogenic events that define the progression from HIV infection to the development of AIDS. In particular, the precise mechanisms that underlie the progressive and generalized CD4+ T-lymphocyte depletion that represents the most striking and consistent laboratory finding in HIV-infected individuals as well as the best predictor of progression to AIDS are still unclear. While it is well established that HIV infects and kills CD4+ T lymphocytes, it is not known to what extent this direct effect of the virus contributes to the overall *in vivo* loss of these cells when measured against a series of indirect mechanisms of CD4+ T-lymphocyte depletion that are related to the state of generalized immune activation associated with HIV infection. Understanding the mechanisms responsible for the HIV-associated CD4+ T-lymphocyte depletion is a matter of utmost importance, as it is likely that greater knowledge of the immunopathogenesis of AIDS will pave the way for the implementation of novel therapeutic strategies.

Direct Cytopathic Effect of HIV on Infected CD4+ T Lymphocytes

A series of crucial discoveries made between 1983 (when HIV was first identified and proposed as the etiologic agent of AIDS) and 1996 (when highly active antiretroviral therapy, HAART, became available) resulted in a model for the pathogenesis of HIV infection that explains a large number of experimental and clinical findings (**Figure 1**). This model is based primarily on the following observations: (1) after transmission of HIV through either the sexual or intravenous route, the virus infects (using the CD4 molecule as well as one of the chemokine receptors CCR5 or

CXCR4 as entry receptors) and then kills a subset of memory/activated CD4+ T lymphocytes; (2) the level of virus replication and the severity of CD4+ T-lymphocyte depletion are the key markers of disease progression from the initial asymptomatic phase of infection (lasting 2–15 years) to the phase characterized by constitutional symptoms and, eventually, the onset of opportunistic infections and cancer; (3) if HIV replication is controlled following the administration of antiviral drugs or spontaneously (in a small subset of HIV-infected individuals referred to as long-term nonprogressors, LTNP), the immunological damage induced by HIV is limited and survival improves dramatically. Collectively, these findings suggested that the pathogenesis of AIDS is mainly related to the direct, virus-mediated killing of CD4+ T lymphocytes that results in a slow but continuous erosion of the pool of these cells (**Figure 1**). This virus-centric model of AIDS pathogenesis was strengthened by the observations that HIV infection is associated with a high rate of virus turnover and a short lifespan of virus-infected cells. These studies were interpreted to mean that, in infected individuals, HIV kills large numbers of CD4+ T lymphocytes at a very fast pace, to the point that the compensatory drive to reconstitute the pool fails to maintain sufficient CD4+ T-lymphocyte numbers. Ultimately, this progressive depletion of CD4+ T lymphocytes results in the permanent loss of a key function of the human immune system, which in turn manifests itself as an increased susceptibility to opportunistic infections and neoplasms. It is important to note that, according to this model, the increased level of CD4+ T-lymphocyte proliferation that is consistently observed in HIV-infected patients is interpreted to be a homeostatic mechanism aimed at compensating for the loss of CD4+ T lymphocytes induced directly by HIV.

Further refinement of this model comes from studies defining the co-receptors used by HIV, in addition to CD4, to infect human cells. The main HIV co-receptor is the chemokine receptor CCR5 (CD195) that is used by the non-syncytium-inducing (NSI), macrophage-tropic viruses that are preferentially transmitted from person-to-person and represent the majority of strains found in infected patients. CCR5 is expressed in a relatively small fraction (approximately 10–15%) of circulating and lymph node CD4+ T lymphocytes that mainly display a memory phenotype (i.e., CD45RO+), but is present on a much larger fraction of mucosal-associated memory CD4+ T lymphocytes. This latter finding is particularly important as it may explain why CD4+ T lymphocytes may be more severely depleted in mucosal tissues than in peripheral blood and lymph nodes (see below). The second important HIV co-receptor is CXCR4 (CD184), that is used by syncytium-inducing (SI), T-lymphocyte tropic viruses that are found in a minority of HIV-infected individuals, usually during advanced stages of disease. Interestingly, CXCR4 is expressed primarily by naïve CD4+ T lymphocytes, thus potentially accounting for the relative preservation of naïve CD4+ T lymphocytes during the early stages of HIV infection. These data are important not only for their elucidation of potential targets for therapeutic interventions aimed at blocking HIV entry (e.g., CCR5 inhibitors), but also because they help to explain the finding that not all subsets of CD4+ T lymphocytes are equally sensitive to HIV infection, such that depletion of memory/activated CD4+ T lymphocytes is associated with infection with CCR5-tropic viruses, and depletion of naïve CD4+ T lymphocytes is associated with CXCR4-tropic viruses.

Indirect Mechanisms of Immunopathogenesis during HIV Infection

The virus-centric model of HIV/AIDS pathogenesis outlined in the previous section has the unquestionable advantage of being fairly straightforward while still encompassing several important observations. More recently, however, this model, at least in its simplest formulation, has been challenged by a series of new insights into the experimental data. First, the long period of time between virus transmission and the development of AIDS in which the level of CD4+ T lymphocytes appears to be in a quasi-steady state is not compatible with the kinetics of a typical viral infection that should rapidly and exponentially consume all available target cells. The original assumption was that the long duration of the disease process is due to the regenerative capacity of the CD4+ T-lymphocyte compartment that is able to at least partially (or temporarily) compensate for the virus-induced killing of these cells. However, it is now believed that it would be too striking of a coincidence that in the vast majority of patients the rate of killing by HIV happens to be just slightly faster than the rate of production of new CD4+ T lymphocytes (and never slower, in which patients would remain healthy, nor significantly faster, in which patients would die within days to weeks). It was then shown that the fraction of infected CD4+ T lymphocytes was remarkably low (i.e., 0.01–1%) at any given time during the course of infection, thus raising the question of why the immune system cannot simply ramp up the production of new CD4+ T lymphocytes to compensate for the relatively limited losses induced by direct viral infection and killing. The further observations that, in fact, the majority of CD4+ T lymphocytes that die *in vivo* in HIV-infected patients appear to be uninfected (termed bystander cell death) and that, when rates of cell turnover are measured *in vivo* in HIV-infected patients, both CD4+ and CD8+ T lymphocytes show similarly elevated rates of death, together support a pathogenic model, whereby nonviral (or indirect) factors are primarily responsible for HIV disease progression. It is important to note that the increased rate of death of uninfected CD4+ T lymphocytes clearly indicates that direct killing by HIV cannot be the only mechanism involved in the depletion of CD4+ T lymphocytes seen in HIV-infected patients.

Taken together, the above-mentioned observations suggest that the pathogenesis of the HIV-associated CD4+ T lymphocyte depletion is a complex phenomenon and that the host response to the virus must play a key role. In particular, it has been proposed that the presence of a chronic generalized immune activation that involves all lymphocyte subsets is an important driving force in the loss of CD4+ T lymphocytes that is associated with progression to AIDS. This concept of HIV infection having a general effect on the host immune system is confirmed by the fact that a large number of functional abnormalities involving virtually all other immune cell types are associated with HIV disease progression. Importantly, several clinical studies have shown that, in HIV-infected patients, disease progression correlates better with markers of immune activation than with viral load. In this perspective, the observation of the short *in vivo* lifespan of HIV-infected CD4+ T lymphocytes has been re-interpreted as the result of their heightened state of activation that dooms them to die (via activation-induced apoptosis) rather than as a consequence of direct infection. As such, the impact of HIV infection on the lifespan of infected CD4+ T lymphocytes may be less dramatic than was originally proposed and it has now been hypothesized that HIV, in essence, jumps from one activated cell (that is destined to die of apoptosis) to another without changing the fate of these infected cells. It could thus be conceived that the number of available activated CD4+ T lymphocytes dictates, independently, both the level of virus replication and the overall rate of CD4+ T lymphocyte death, and that these two factors are correlated with one another only because they reflect the prevailing level of immune activation.

Further key support for the immune activation hypothesis derives from studies of the nonpathogenic simian immunodeficiency virus (SIV) infections of natural hosts, such as sooty mangabeys (*Cercocebus atys*, SMs), African green monkeys (AGMs), mandrills, and numerous other nonhuman primate species. These natural SIV hosts are the origin of the human HIV epidemics through multiple episodes of cross-species transmission, with HIV-1 originating from the chimpanzee (*Pan troglodytes*) SIV_{cpz}, and HIV-2 originating from the SM SIV_{smm}. Naturally SIV-infected SMs are of interest also because SIV_{smm} is the source of the various rhesus macaque (*Macaca mulatta*)-adapted SIV_{mac} viruses (e.g., SIV_{mac239},

SIV_{mac251}) that are commonly used in laboratory studies of AIDS pathogenesis and vaccines. In natural SIV hosts, chronic high levels of virus replication and *in vivo* killing of CD4+ T lymphocytes are not associated with any signs of immunodeficiency in the setting of typically low levels of both immune activation and cellular immune responses to the virus. This phenotype suggests that natural SIV hosts have evolved to be disease-resistant without the acquisition of any special ability to control virus replication (via either immune or other mechanisms), but rather by an adaptation that attenuates the immune response to this retroviral infection (**Table 2**).

Interestingly, some recent findings may help to harmonize the classical (i.e., virus-centric) and immune activation models in that they support a more comprehensive model whereby the pathogenesis of HIV/AIDS involves both direct and indirect mechanisms (**Figure 2**). There are now thought to be two sequentially distinct phases in infection that involve very different pathogenic mechanisms. The first phase (acute infection) is characterized by a rapid, massive, directly HIV-mediated loss of memory CD4+ T lymphocytes that takes place mainly in mucosal tissues and may leave a profound scar on the overall function of the immune system. It is still unclear what

Table 2 Immunologic and virologic features of natural, nonpathogenic SIV infections vs. pathogenic HIV infection

	Natural SIVs	HIV
Chronic virus replication	Yes	Yes
Lack of immune control	Yes	Yes
Short lifespan of infected CD4+ T cells	Yes	Yes
Depletion of MALT CD4+ T cells	Yes	Yes
Systemic loss of CD4+ T cells	Rare	Yes
Generalized immune activation	No	Yes
Expression of CCR5 on CD4+ T cells	Low	High

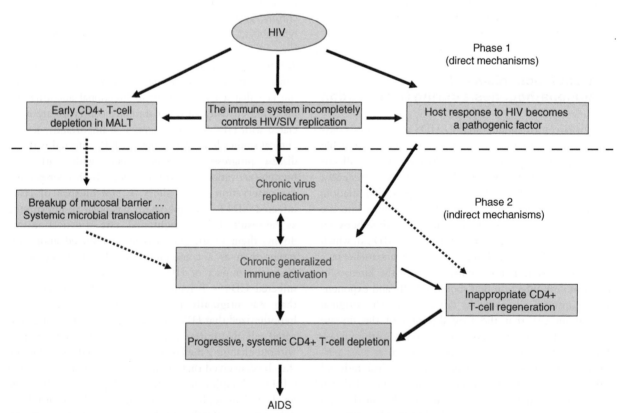

Figure 2 The biphasic model of AIDS pathogenesis. This model summarizes the key immunopathogenic events in acute and chronic infection that lead to progression to AIDS in HIV-infected individuals, taking into account both direct (virus-mediated) and indirect (immune activation-mediated) mechanisms.

determines the cessation of this brief early phase, although likely explanations include the consumption of available target cells and the generation of HIV-specific immune responses. The second phase (chronic infection) lasts typically for several years, and is characterized, in essence, by the immune system's struggle to both recover from the early injury (via activation of mechanisms of immune homeostasis) and control virus replication (via activation of humoral and cellular immune responses). Unfortunately, this latter endeavor proves almost always to be insurmountable as HIV is a pathogen of extraordinary genetic and structural plasticity allowing it to develop a series of highly effective strategies for immune evasion. The struggle of the second phase is characterized by the continuous generation of strong, though ultimately ineffective, immune responses to HIV, and by the attempt to maintain T-lymphocyte homeostasis in the face of massive T-lymphocyte loss due to both the direct effect of the HIV and bystander cell death. Sadly, this epic battle seems to end up inducing nothing but the very state of chronic immune activation that, as mentioned above, ultimately causes more damage than repair to the host immune system.

Determinants of HIV Transmission and Early Replication

A clearer understanding of the host and viral factors determining the likelihood of virus transmission upon exposure and/or the course of infection after transmission will likely provide useful information for the design of new strategies to prevent HIV infection and AIDS. However, while some host factors regulating the risk of infection and disease progression have been identified, predicting the natural course of the infection remains very difficult at the level of the individual patient. Among the host genetic factors that have been shown to induce resistance to HIV infection, a predominant role has been ascribed to the 32 bp deletion in the CCR5 gene seen in 1% of Caucasian individuals. This deletion results in a frameshift mutation that causes the CCR5 protein to be completely absent from the surface of all cells. Thus, individuals homozygous for the $\Delta 32$ allele are resistant to transmission of CCR5-tropic viral strains (the overwhelming majority of viruses involved in horizontal sexual transmission). Other genes whose polymorphisms have been associated with some effect on HIV disease progression include SDF-1, CX3CR-1, CCL3, and many others. The clinical consequence of these discoveries is that small molecule antagonists or a monoclonal antibody directed against CCR5 are increasingly recognized as promising strategies to prevent HIV transmission.

The search for host factors associated with more effective immune responses to HIV (and, in fact, the identification of any type of correlate of immune protection) has proved much more frustrating. As of early 2007, it is still unclear whether and to what extent the immune response to HIV is capable of inducing absolute (i.e., by preventing infection) or relative (i.e., by lowering virus replication) resistance to virus transmission and early dissemination. While stronger and/or broader T-lymphocyte responses to the virus have been associated with better course of disease, it is still unclear whether this apparently more effective immune response is cause or consequence of a more benign course of infection. Furthermore, the observation that natural SIV hosts, who are resistant to AIDS, show a low-level T-lymphocyte response to the virus and, more generally, an attenuated immune system activation clearly indicates that a strong host antiviral immune response is not necessary to lessen disease. While more studies are needed to fully elucidate the mechanisms underlying the lack of disease progression in natural SIV hosts, one clear message thus far is that co-evolution of SIV and its natural hosts have resulted in a happy equilibrium whereby the host immune function is preserved without any significant immune-mediated control of virus replication (**Table 2**).

Some recent advances in understanding what factors influence HIV-1 transmission come from recent studies of heterosexual transmission in Africa. One such study showed that the viruses that establish new infections encode an envelope surface glycoprotein (gp120) with a compact structure and reduced glycosylation that appears to be significantly more sensitive to antibody neutralization. To this end, it should be noted that the vast majority of gp120s isolated from patients with chronic HIV infection are resistant to neutralization by autologous sera. The implication of these findings for HIV vaccine development is significant, as they reveal a relative vulnerability of the HIV-Env glycoprotein in the very early phase of HIV infection. Also interesting is the finding that, in a cohort of discordant heterosexual partners (i.e., one HIV-infected and one HIV-uninfected) in Zambia, the sharing of HLA-B alleles is associated with a significant enhancement in the rate of transmission. This observation suggests that the foreign HLA molecules on virus-infected cells or the virus itself (acquired from the cell membrane) trigger protection against infection with a mechanism analogous to allogeneic transplant rejection; alternatively, transmission of viruses that have already escaped the cytotoxic T-lymphocyte (CTL) response may make infection more efficient in individuals with shared HLA alleles. While these reports shed some light on what type of adaptive immune response may control the spread of HIV infection, it is obvious that the virus appears to rapidly win the battle with the host immune system in the overwhelming majority of infected individuals.

When HIV first enters the body (most commonly via mucosal transmission but in certain instances through the bloodstream), the type and magnitude of the subsequent antiviral immune response is largely determined by

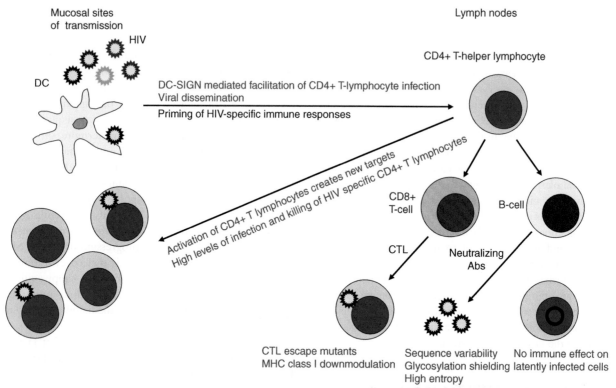

Figure 3   HIV transmission and generation of HIV-specific immune responses. HIV entry at mucosal sites is followed by capture by DCs that subsequently migrate to lymph nodes to present HIV antigens to CD4+ T-helper lymphocytes. In this process, DCs may also facilitate the infection of activated CD4+ T lymphocytes. CD4+ T lymphocytes help CD8+ T lymphocytes and B cells in mounting cellular and humoral anti-HIV immune responses. Legend in black indicates events of the HIV-specific immune response; legend in red indicates events leading to HIV immune evasion and dissemination.

immature dendritic cells (DCs), a cell type that is a component of the innate defense against mucosal penetration and widespread dissemination of many pathogens. Importantly, the role of DCs in the early events of HIV infection is complex and not always beneficial (**Figure 3**). On the one hand, DCs take up HIV-1 via C-type lectin binding receptors and migrate to the draining lymph node where they prime HIV-specific immune responses by presenting HIV antigens to CD4+ T lymphocytes. On the other hand, DCs may also contribute to early HIV dissemination throughout the body, due to their migratory potential and the fact that the DC–CD4+ T lymphocyte contact often results in productive infection of CD4+ T lymphocytes. While manipulation of the DC–T lymphocyte interaction may conceivably improve the host immune response to HIV, our limited understanding of the molecular mechanisms responsible for this interaction hampers the design of simple interventions aimed at blocking the early dissemination of HIV infection.

The Acute/Early Phase of HIV Infection

The acute phase of HIV infection is characterized by a peak of virus replication that occurs coincident with

a transient decline of circulating CD4+ T lymphocytes and the presence of a flu-like clinical syndrome. This acute infection lasts for approximately 2–3 weeks and ends at approximately the time of antibody seroconversion. Some recent elegant studies have highlighted the role of the mucosal-associated lymphoid tissue (MALT) in acute HIV infection. The MALT houses the majority of CD4+ T lymphocytes in the body, a large fraction of which express CCR5 and have an activated memory phenotype. A key feature of the early phases of HIV and SIV infections is the massive infection and depletion of MALT-associated CD4+CCR5+ memory T lymphocytes (**Figure 2**). HIV replication in activated CD4+CCR5+ memory T lymphocytes proceeds relatively unchecked for 2–3 weeks after transmission, resulting in large-scale depletion of these cells. During early pathogenic SIV infection of Asian macaques (i.e., non-natural hosts), up to 60% of memory CD4+ T lymphocytes in the intestinal lamina propria contain SIV-RNA at the peak of infection (day 10) and the majority of these cells are eliminated by day 14. Importantly, though, the best predictor of rapid disease progression may not be the extent of the early CD4+ T lymphocyte depletion from mucosal sites, but rather the ability to reconstitute the pool of memory CD4+ T lymphocytes in the MALT. MALT-associated memory

CD4+ T lymphocytes are an integral component of the mucosal immunological barrier against invading pathogens, and it is likely that their massive (and potentially irreversible) depletion may significantly affect the proper function of the mucosal barrier. This setting then allows for the emergence of numerous subclinical infections, thus inducing further microenvironment destruction and contributing to a state of chronic immune system activation (**Figure 2**). It should be noted, however, that to date the specific consequences of the early depletion of MALT-associated memory CD4+ T lymphocytes remain unknown, and it is still unclear why the opportunistic infections that are typical of full-blown AIDS do not appear until peripheral blood CD4+ T lymphocyte counts decline. Particularly puzzling is the observation that a rapid, severe, and persistent depletion of mucosal CD4+ T lymphocytes also occurs during nonpathogenic SIV infection of natural hosts such as SMs and AGMs (**Table 2**). However, in the context of the typically low levels of systemic and mucosal immune activation found in these species, no signs of mucosal immune dysfunction are observed, further emphasizing the potential protective role of an attenuated immune response during retroviral infection. Alternatively, it is possible that the early and rapid depletion of mucosal CD4+ T lymphocytes observed in pathogenic HIV/SIV infections simply reflects the systemic virus dissemination that is necessary to establish a chronically productive infection.

Generation of HIV-Specific Immune Responses and the Acute-to-Chronic Phase Transition

As mentioned above, the determinants of the relatively abrupt cessation of the early phase of HIV infection and the onset of the long chronic phase that occur at 2–3 weeks post infection are still poorly understood. However, several investigators have put forward the hypothesis that HIV-specific CTL responses as well as humoral responses directed against the virus envelope protein (i.e., neutralizing antibodies) play a central role in reducing the level of virus replication from its peak to set-point level. The evidence in favor of a significant role of CD8+ CTL-mediated responses reducing HIV replication include: (1) the temporal association between decline of viremia and emergence of cellular immune responses during primary HIV/SIV infection; (2) the increase in virus replication after experimental depletion of CD8+ T lymphocytes during pathogenic SIV infection of rhesus macaques; and (3) the observation that CTL escape mutations present in viruses transmitted between individuals with different HLA haplotypes are rapidly replaced by wild-type sequences. While CD8+ CTL-mediated responses play a significant role early on in protecting from unchecked HIV-1 replication and disease progression, their impact is ultimately limited by the extreme genetic variability of HIV that favors the emergence, during both acute and chronic infection, of viral escape mutants (**Figure 3**). The fact that HIV preferentially infects and kills HIV-specific memory CD4+ T lymphocytes (that are more likely to be activated, **Figure 3**) over memory T lymphocytes specific for other pathogens further complicates the situation, and results in a functional deficit in the anti-HIV response as compared to that directed against other pathogens. What must now be elucidated is whether preexisting, AIDS vaccine-induced HIV-specific CTLs will be more effective in controlling virus replication than those generated during natural infection. HIV-specific autologous neutralizing antibodies also exert potent and continuous selective pressure on the viral quasispecies. Unfortunately, HIV is able to escape antibody-mediated neutralization as efficiently as it does CTL control. A series of recent studies have clarified some of the mechanisms of HIV evasion from the humoral immune response (**Figure 3**). First, the envelope glycoprotein (Env) is highly variable, particularly in specific regions that form the surface of the virus. Second, the outer surface of gp120 is covered with a highly dynamic carbohydrate shield, in which glycans shift through point mutations to mask adjacent and distant epitopes. Third, conserved structural domains of Env are either sterically hindered or only transiently exposed. Fourth, receptor binding of Env is characterized by a high level of intrinsic entropy that makes it a moving target for antibody neutralization. The failure of both HIV-specific CTLs and neutralizing antibodies to completely suppress HIV replication during the transition between acute-to-chronic infection likely sets the stage for the following pathogenic events that are characterized by continuous, generalized immune activation in the face of chronic virus replication (**Figure 2**).

The Chronic Phase of Infection

Chronic HIV infection is a process lasting for several years that is characterized by a very slow decline of CD4+ T lymphocytes in peripheral blood, a small fraction of infected CD4+ T lymphocytes, and increased death rates of both CD4+ and CD8+ T lymphocytes. This last finding is related to the state of chronic, generalized immune activation that is now recognized as a major driving force behind CD4+ T lymphocyte depletion and a strong predictor of disease progression. The causes of the HIV-associated generalized immune activation are complex, and involve activation of T lymphocytes by specific antigens (e.g., HIV and a plethora of opportunistic pathogens), as well as bystander activation of T lymphocytes due to the presence of high levels of lymphotropic cytokines and other as yet poorly defined factors. But how does this increased immune activation induce CD4+ T lymphocyte depletion? First, CD4+ T lymphocyte activation provides new targets for HIV replication (that occurs preferentially in activated CD4+ T lymphocytes, **Figure 3**), thus creating an environment conducive to further virus-mediated damage to the immune system. Second, the increased T-lymphocyte turnover driven by this chronic immune activation (and, to some extent, by the increased compensatory homeostatic proliferation of T lymphocytes) results in chronic consumption of the pools of naïve and resting-memory cells, with a resultant relative expansion of short-lived effector CD4+ T lymphocytes. Third, the chronic activation and proliferation of T lymphocyte results in perturbations of cell-cycle control and an increased propensity to undergo activation-induced apoptosis. It is also possible that the HIV-associated immune activation is, at least in part, responsible for the changes in the lymph node architecture and thymic function that likely limit the proper reconstitution of the CD4+ T lymphocyte pool. It is hypothesized that depletion is unique to CD4+ T lymphocytes (and involves CD8+ T lymphocytes only in the very late stages of HIV disease) not only because these cells are targeted by HIV, but also because they are more sensitive to the deleterious effects of immune activation and/or are less efficiently regenerated.

Evidently, the assertion that chronic T-lymphocyte activation is a key pathogenic mechanism during HIV infection is in an apparent conflict with data suggesting that cellular immune responses to HIV/SIV infections may limit primary infection and/or disease progression. While T-lymphocyte responses to HIV likely play a protective role early on, T-lymphocyte immunity virtually always fails to control HIV infection due to the emergence of viral escape mutants. Once HIV-specific cellular immune responses are unable to control the virus, other mechanisms may determine the net effect that this ongoing T-lymphocyte activation has on the course of disease.

Is it possible that there is a direct connection between the early damage that HIV causes to the MALT-based pool of memory CD4+ T lymphocytes and the generation of the HIV-associated generalized immune activation? It is known that MALT-associated memory CD4+ T lymphocytes are an integral component of the mucosal immunological barrier that protects the host from both invading pathogens as well as commensal enteric bacteria that may also be recognized as pathogens if they cross the intestinal epithelium. It is likely that a massive depletion of these cells may affect the proper function of this mucosal barrier and thus may open the door to a series of subclinical infections (i.e., micro-invasion of the intestinal mucosa) that will, in turn, induce further micro-environment destruction and contribute to the generation of a state of chronic immune system activation (**Figure 2**). While this model delineates an interesting mechanistic link between direct and indirect (i.e., virus vs. immune

activation-mediated) mechanisms of HIV-associated CD4+ T-lymphocyte depletion, the specific consequences of the early depletion of MALT-associated memory CD4+ T lymphocytes are in fact unknown, and it remains unclear why the opportunistic infections that are typical of full-blown AIDS do not manifest until peripheral blood CD4+ T-lymphocyte counts decline.

Implications for HIV Therapy and Vaccine Development

As described above, AIDS pathogenesis likely recognizes two distinct phases, a brief acute phase dominated by the direct killing of large numbers of memory CD4+ T lymphocytes followed by a long chronic phase characterized by a slow attrition of the CD4+ T lymphocyte pool that is related mainly to the prevailing level of immune activation (**Figure 2**). However, many questions remain to be answered. First, a precise quantification of the relative contribution of the direct and indirect mechanisms of AIDS pathogenesis is still lacking. Second, we do not have a clear explanation as to why HIV appears to be so uniquely powerful in inducing a chronic state of immune activation (as opposed to other chronic viral infections), and why the HIV-induced immune activation is so disruptive of the immune system homeostasis. The fact that generalized immune activation follows HIV infection of humans, which is a very recent disease, but does not follow infections that date back many thousands or even millions of years (such as HCV infection of humans or SIV infection of natural hosts), would suggest that attenuation of the immune response to a chronically replicating virus is the result of an advantageous evolutionary adaptation of the host immune system. Unfortunately, the mechanisms underlying the ability of natural hosts for SIV infection to avoid the chronic immune activation seen in HIV-infected humans are still poorly understood.

This biphasic model of AIDS pathogenesis provides a few important implications for HIV therapy and vaccine design. In terms of therapy, an important observation is that a complete recovery of the mucosal CD4+ T-lymphocyte system is unlikely with the currently available antiretroviral drugs even in the presence of prolonged viral suppression. As such, additional immune-based interventions, in particular using CD4+ T-lymphocyte tropic cytokines (e.g., IL-2, IL-7) as well as factors promoting the CD4+ T-lymphocyte repopulation of the MALT, may be useful to improve the immune system recovery from the severe and persistent damages inflicted during the early phase of the infection. In addition, given the well-recognized pathogenic role of the generalized immune activation during the chronic infection, it is conceivable that, in many HIV-infected patients, immune-based interventions aimed at reducing immune activation, preserving proper cell-cycle control, and preventing excessive levels of bystander cell death may restore the overall CD4+ T-lymphocyte homeostasis. Among these potentially interesting new interventions are those that interfere directly with the signaling pathways involved in establishing the generalized immune activation or cell-cycle dysregulation (i.e., toll-like receptors, cytokine receptors, nuclear factor kappa B (NF-κB), cell cycle-dependent kinases) and those that improve the regeneration and/or the differentiation of T lymphocytes (i.e., cytokines and growth factors). Finally, a clearer understanding of the reason(s) why SIV infection is nonpathogenic in natural hosts (and, in particular, how virus replication can proceed in the absence of immune system damage and chronic immune activation) will likely also reveal further immune-based therapies to delay progression of disease.

Advances in the understanding of the early events of HIV transmission, with special emphasis on the immunogenic vulnerabilities of Env and the correlates of immune protection at the mucosal level, may lead to the development of vaccine and microbicide strategies that can limit the acute HIV-induced damage. In terms of vaccine development, the main implication of the accumulated pathogenesis research is that there may be only a short window of opportunity to control this rapidly disseminating virus that produces such extensive damage to the host immune system. This premise is especially disheartening for CTL-based vaccines that, in order to be effective, will have to induce a persistently high level of mucosa-associated, long-lived, HIV-specific memory CD8+ T lymphocytes that can rapidly proliferate and differentiate into effectors in the event of viral infection. Recent findings are more encouraging for a vaccine that aims to induce a high titer of broadly neutralizing antibodies, particularly if one considers that structural bottlenecks seem to be required for the virus to be efficiently transmitted to a new host in certain settings. In addition, it should be noted that even a vaccine that is only partially effective in containing the early viral dissemination (and resultant immune system damage) may end up having a significant impact on shaping the course of disease.

In summary, there have been many advances in the field of HIV immunopathogenesis over the past 24 years, but there is much that remains to be elucidated, particularly at the mechanistic level. It is critical that, with the help of new and highly sophisticated tools of analyses, we endeavor to more fully understand the dynamic interaction between HIV and the host immune system in order to eradicate this disease.

See also: AIDS: Disease Manifestation; AIDS: Global Epidemiology; Human Immunodeficiency Viruses: Antiretroviral Agents; Human Immunodeficiency Viruses: Origin.

Further Reading

Gordon S, Pandrea I, Dunham R, Apetrei C, and Silvestri G (2005) The call of the wild: What can be learned from studies of SIV infection of natural hosts? In: Leitner T, Foley B, Hahn B, *et al.* (eds.) *HIV Sequence Compendium 2005*, pp. 2–29. Los Alamos, NC: Theoretical Biology and Biophysics Group.

Grossman Z, Meier-Schellersheim M, Paul WE, and Picker LJ (2006) Pathogenesis of HIV infection: What the virus spares is as important as what it destroys. *Nature Medicine* 12(3): 289–295.

Guatelli JC, Siliciano RF, Kuritzkes DR, and Richman DD (2002) Human immunodeficiency virus. In: Richman DD, Whitley RJ, and Hayden FG (eds.) *Clinical Virology*, 2nd edn., pp. 685–730. Washington: ASM Press.

Lederman MM, Penn-Nicholson A, Cho M, and Mosier D (2006) Biology of CCR5 and its role in HIV infection and treatment. *JAMA* 296(7): 815–826.

EXOTIC VIRUS INFECTIONS

Bunyaviruses: Unassigned

C H Calisher, Colorado State University, Fort Collins, CO, USA

Glossary

Arbovirus A virus transmitted to vertebrates by hematophagous (blood-feeding) insects.
Arthralgia Joint pain.
Myalgia Muscle pain.
Orthobunyavirus, hantavirus, phlebovirus, nairovirus, tospovirus Any virus in the genus *Orthobunyavirus, Hantavirus, Phlebovirus, Nairovirus,* or *Tospovirus.*
Polyarthritis Simultaneous inflammation of several joints.
Taxon A taxonomic category or group, such as a phylum, order, family, genus, or species.
Unassigned bunyavirus A virus placed in a family *Bunyaviridae* but not in a genus within that family.
Unclassified A virus not yet placed in a taxon.
Ungrouped A virus not yet shown to be related to any other virus.
Viremia Virus in the blood.

Introduction

Although most viruses in the family *Bunyaviridae* have been placed in one of the five established genera (*Orthobunyavirus, Phlebovirus, Nairovirus, Hantavirus,* or *Tospovirus*), some have not. The original studies of all these viruses were done by serologic or other methods and were meant only to determine whether a virus was a newly recognized one or simply an additional isolate of a known virus. When two or more viruses were shown to be related antigenically, they were considered members of a 'group', nothing more. However, when results of further molecular studies provided definitive genetic information, it became possible to place a virus, or a group of viruses, in a particular taxon. Still other viruses, for which we lack data that would allow placement in a genus, were shown by electron microscopy (morphology of the virus and morphogenesis), or by other physical or biochemical characteristics to be analogous to recognized members of the family *Bunyaviridae* and so were placed in the family as 'unassigned' members. Many of these viruses are known to be related to each other and so are assigned to groups of unassigned virus and the rest are considered as ungrouped and unassigned. The unassigned viruses of the family *Bunyaviridae* (i.e., 'bunyaviruses') are listed in **Table 1**.

Certain of these viruses cause human illness but have not been adequately characterized nor, with few exceptions, have their epidemiologies been studied methodically and we do not have information regarding their prevalences.

Bhanja Virus

This virus, first isolated from *Haemaphysalis intermedia*, was collected from a paralyzed goat in India. It was subsequently isolated from ticks of other species collected in Senegal, Central African Republic, Nigeria, Cameroon, Somalia, Armenia, Bulgaria, Croatia (former Yugoslavia), and Italy. Infection of a laboratory worker provided the first evidence that this virus is pathogenic for humans. The patient had a mild illness characterized by myalgias and arthralgias, moderate frontal headache, slight photophobia, slight elevation of temperature, all lasting less than 2 days. Subsequently, a few additional human infections, including one fatal case, were recorded. Clearly, this virus is widespread geographically and its significance underreported.

Kasokero Virus

Kasokero virus was first isolated from the bloods of Egyptian rousette bats (*Rousettus aegyptiacus*) in Uganda. It subsequently was isolated from bloods of three people working in the laboratory at the time the bats and the virus were being manipulated and from the blood of a

Table 1 Unassigned viruses in the family *Bunyaviridae*

Group	Viruses
Bhanja	Bhanja, Forecariah, Kismayo
Kaisodi	Kaisodi, Lanjan, Silverwater
Mapputta	Gan Gan, Mapputta, Maprik, Trubanaman
Tanga	Okola, Tanga
Resistencia	Antequera, Barranqueras, Resistencia
Upolu	Aransas Bay, Upolu
Yogue	Kasokero, Yogue

Ungrouped: Bangui, Belem, Belmont, Bobaya, Caddo Canyon, Chim, Enseada, Keterah (= Issyk-Kul), Kowanyama, Lone Star, Pacora, Para, Razdan, Salanga, Santarem, Sunday Canyon, Tai, Tamdy, Tataguine, Wanowrie, Witwatersrand, Yacaaba.

driver who only occasionally entered the laboratory, suggesting the possibility of aerosol transmission of the virus. Patients suffered from fever, headache, abdominal pain, diarrhea, and from some or all of nausea, abdominal pain, chest pain, hyperactive reflexes, coughing, and severe myalgias and arthralgias, lasting 5–14 days, but followed by complete recovery.

Tataguine Virus

Tataguine virus was first isolated from mosquitoes aspirated from dwelling places near Tataguine, Senegal, and subsequently from mosquitoes collected in Nigeria, Central African Republic, Burkina Faso, Cameroon, and Senegal. Clinical manifestations of Tataguine virus infection in humans are mild, characterized by fever and rash, and can be confused with malaria and fevers of unknown origin in West Africa. When active surveillance for this virus was done in Nigeria and Senegal, it was found to be one of the most prevalent viruses in blood samples taken from febrile humans.

Wanowrie Virus

Wanowrie virus, first isolated from *Hyalmomma marginatum* ticks in India, has been isolated from other ticks in Egypt and Iran and from mosquitoes in India. It has also been isolated from the brain of a child in Sri Lanka, suggesting that further studies of this ungrouped pathogen are warranted.

Keterah Virus (Also Known As Issyk-Kul Virus)

This virus was first isolated from *Argas pusillus* ticks collected from bats in Malaysia and from the bloods of those bats (*Scotophilus temmencki*), and has been isolated from ticks and mosquitoes that had fed on infected bats. It was subsequently isolated from pooled brain, liver, spleen, and kidney tissues of other bats in Kyrgyzstan and Tadzhikistan. The virus also was isolated from a staff member of a virology institute in Tadzhikistan who had contracted the infection during field work with bats. Sporadic human cases of this disease have been recognized for more than 20 years in central Asia, particularly in Tadzhikistan, and in Malaysia, and the virus may occur in parts of Iran, Afghanistan, India, and Pakistan. The nonfatal illness caused by this virus is characterized by fever, headache, and myalgias, which are sufficiently nonspecific to be generally undiagnosed or mistaken for diseases caused by other pathogens.

Experimental infections of African green monkeys (*Cercopithecus aethiops*), golden hamsters (*Mesocrictus auratus*), and laboratory mice with the Issyk-Kul strain of this virus demonstrated virus in blood and organs of all animals. Histological studies revealed inflammatory and dystrophic changes in the central nervous system, lungs, liver, and kidneys and pronounced morphological changes in the spleen. The virus is pantropic, causing generalized infection in all animals, irrespective of the route of infection. In monkeys, asymptomatic infection was accompanied by marked organ damages and viremia.

Other Unassigned Orthobunyaviruses Causing Disease in Humans

Gan Gan virus, isolated thus far only from Australian mosquitoes, has been associated with a few cases of acute epidemic polyarthritis-like illness, and may be confused with other viruses causing this syndrome in Australia, such as Ross River virus and Barmah Forest viruses (*Togaviridae, Alphavirus*). Similarly, Trubanaman virus, also isolated only from Australian mosquitoes, is suspected of being pathogenic. These viruses may employ marsupials as principal vertebrate hosts. Finally, Tamdy virus, isolated from *Hyalomma* spp. ticks in Uzbekistan and Turkmenistan, also has been shown to be a human pathogen. Clearly, many more studies are needed, if we are to understand the natural cycles of these viruses, and their prevalences in humans and in wild animals.

Further Reading

Calisher CH and Goodpasture HC (1975) Human infection with Bhanja virus. *American Journal of Tropical Medicine and Hygiene* 24: 1040–1042.

Dandawate CN, Shah KV, and D'Lima LV (1970) Wanowrie virus: A new arbovirus isolated from *Hyalomma marginatum isaaci*. *Indian Journal of Medical Research* 58: 985–989.

Fagbami AH, Monath TP, Tomori O, Lee VH, and Fabiyi A (1972) Studies on Tataguine infection in Nigeria. *Tropical and Geographic Medicine* 24: 298–302.

Fauquet CM, Mayo MA, Maniloff J, Desselberger U,, and Ball LA (eds.) (2005) *Virus Taxonomy: Eighth Report of the International Committee on Taxonomy of Viruses*, pp. 713–714. San Diego, CA: Elsevier Academic Press.

Kalunda M, Mukwaya LG, Mukuye A, et al. (1986) Kasokero virus: A new human pathogen from bats (*Rousettus aegyptiacus*) in Uganda. *American Journal of Tropical Medicine and Hygiene* 35: 387–392.

L'vov DK, Sidorova GA, Gromashevskii VL, Skvortsova TM, and Aristova VA (1984) Isolation of Tamdy virus (*Bunyaviridae*) pathogenic for man from natural sources in Central Asia, Kazakhstan and Transcaucasia (in Russian). *Voprosy Virusologii* 29: 487–490.

L'vov DK, Terskikh II, Abramova LN, Savosina NS, Skvortsova TM, and Gromashevskii VL (1991) An experimental infection caused by the Issyk-Kul arbovirus (in Russian). *Meditsinskaia Parazitologiia I Parazitarnye Bolezni* 4: 15–16.

Mackenzie JS, Lindsay MD, Coelen RJ, Broom AK, Hall RA, and Smith DW (1994) Arboviruses causing human disease in the Australasian zoogeographic region. *Archives of Virology* 136: 447–467.

Moore DL, Causey OR, Carey DE, et al. (1975) Arthropod-borne viral infections of man in Nigeria, 1964–1970. *Annals of Tropical Medicine and Parasitology* 69: 49–64.

Pavri KM, Anandarajah M, Hermon YE, Nayar M, Wikramsinghe MR, and Dandawate CN (1976) Isolation of Wanowrie virus from brain of a fatal human case from Sri Lanka. *Indian Journal of Medical Research* 64: 557–561.

Cowpox Virus

M Bennett, University of Liverpool, Liverpool, UK
G L Smith, Imperial College London, London, UK
D Baxby, University of Liverpool, Liverpool, UK

History

The first published account of cowpox in man and cattle is probably that of Edward Jenner in his *Inquiry* published in 1798, although others, such as Benjamin Jesty, performed immunization of humans with cowpox material earlier. Jenner described the clinical signs of cowpox in both hosts, and how infection in man with *Variolae vaccinae* ('known by the name of the cowpox') provided protection against smallpox. At that time, smallpox was responsible for between 200 000 and 600 000 deaths each year in Europe and about 10% of all deaths in children. Jenner's discovery, despite the concern of some over the consequences of inoculating bovine material into man, soon led to the establishment of smallpox vaccination schemes around the world. However, not until Pasteur's work *c.* 100 years later was the principle of immunization used again. In fact, it was Pasteur who suggested that all such immunizations be called vaccines in honor of Jenner's work.

Although Jenner's first vaccines probably came indirectly from cattle, later vaccine material was often derived from horses, and the origin(s) of modern vaccinia virus (VACV) the smallpox vaccine, remain unknown. That cowpox virus (CPXV) and VACV are different was first published in 1939, since when further biological and genetic studies have confirmed that VACV represents a species in its own right, and is not simply a mutant of CPXV or a recombinant of variola virus (VARV) and CPVX.

Even Jenner seems to have had difficulty finding cowpox cases, and CPXV is not endemic in cattle. Rather, it is endemic in rodents, and cattle and man are merely accidental hosts. The domestic cat is the animal diagnosed most frequently with clinical cowpox in Europe.

Taxonomy and Classification

CPXV represents the species *Cowpox virus*, a member of the genus *Orthopoxvirus* in the family *Poxviridae*, and the international reference strain, Brighton Red, was isolated from farm workers in contact with infected cattle in 1937. CPXV can be differentiated from other orthopoxviruses (OPVs) by a combination of biological tests, including the ability to produce hemorrhagic pocks on chorioallantoic membranes, the production of A-type inclusions (ATIs) in infected cells, and its ceiling temperature for growth (40 °C, the highest temperature at which the virus will replicate), by minor antigenic differences, by restriction enzyme digestion of the entire genome, particularly with *Hin*dIII, by sequencing of certain genes, and by polymerase chain reaction (PCR). There is considerably more variation between some CPXV isolates than between strains of other OPV species, such that some CPXV-strains might be reclassified as separate species rather than strains of the same species. This variation is seen in biological properties (e.g., ceiling temperature of growth, and possibly virulence in different hosts) and genome (restriction enzyme fragment polymorphism, gene content, and nucleotide sequence). It is not yet known whether these differences reflect variation in geographic range or reservoir host.

Properties of the Virion

CPXV has a typical OPV morphology, and is indistinguishable from VACV by electron microscopy. Virions are brick shaped, approximately 300 nm × 200 nm × 200 nm in size, and are enveloped. There are two types of virion. The simpler form, termed intracellular mature virus (IMV), consists of a biconcave core, and within each concavity lies a lateral body. The whole is surrounded by a lipid membrane, and an outer layer of protein. The core contains DNA and proteins, many of which are virus-encoded enzymes. The second form is called extracellular enveloped virus (EEV), and these virions are surrounded by an additional lipid envelope that is fragile and is derived from either the *trans*-Golgi network or endosomes.

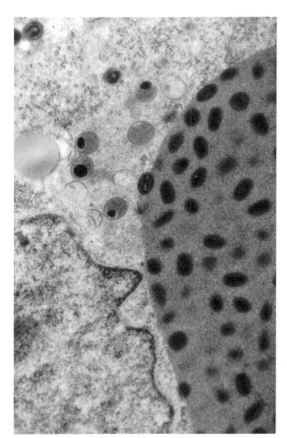

Figure 1 A CPXV-infected cell, showing intracytoplasmic virion synthesis and an ATI containing intracellular mature virions.

The life history of CPXV within the cell is very similar to that of VACV, except that intracellular nonenveloped, yet infectious, virions can become incorporated into large intracytoplasmic ATIs (**Figure 1**). It is thought that these inclusions help protect the virus after cell lysis, and so are important in survival in the environment and spread from animal to animal. In contrast, EEV is more important for spread within individual hosts.

Properties of the Genome

The genome consists of linear, double-stranded DNA with covalently linked inverted repeats at the termini. The CPXV genome is the largest of all the OPV genomes and for strain Brighton Red is 224 501 bp. Restriction endonuclease mapping and nucleotide sequencing demonstrated that the middle portion of the CPXV genome (approximately 100 kbp) is highly conserved between OPVs, but more variation occurs toward either end. Digestion with *Hin*dIII usually differentiates CPXVs from other known OPVs, but isolates, particularly geographically distinct strains, do vary in profile, and digestion of genomic DNA with other enzymes often reveals

much greater differences between strains. However, overall the genome is fundamentally very stable. The main exception to this is the deletion of 32–39 kbp of DNA from the right end of the genome and its replacement by DNA from the left end: these terminal transpositions are the cause of the 1% white pocks observed on infected chorioallantoic membranes. The size of the transposed fragment varies (5–50 kbp) but the net effect is a change in the length of the inverted terminal repeat (ITR), the duplication of some genes, and the loss of others.

The nucleotide sequences of two CPXV genomes, and of particular genes for a much greater number of isolates, have been determined. CPXV not only has the largest OPV genome, but it also encodes the greatest number of complete protein-coding open reading frames (ORFs) and has relatively few genes that are broken by mutation into fragments. Such broken ORFs are more common in other OPVs such as VARV, camelpox virus (CMLV), and taterapox virus (TAPV). These observations suggest that CPXV might be closest in its genetic complement to the ancestral poxvirus from which OPVs have evolved. PCR-based diagnostic methods are now used to distinguish CPXV from other OPVs.

Properties of Proteins

The genome of CPXV Brighton Red is predicted to encode more than 200 proteins. Like other OPVs, the proteins encoded in the central part of the genome are mostly essential for virus replication, and in this region 89 genes have counterparts in all sequenced chordopoxviruses. Generally, these CPXV proteins are very closely related to their counterparts in VACV, VARV, and other OPVs. This is certainly true for the proteins that are present in the infectious virion, and the finding that the proteins on the surface of IMV and EEV are very closely related provides a plausible explanation why VACV and CPXV were effective vaccines against smallpox. In contrast, genes located toward the genome termini are nonessential for virus replication in cell culture and these include approximately half of all CPXV genes. Notably, CPXV encodes many genes that are not found in VACV strains.

Interest has focused on proteins concerned with immune modulation, and these are encoded mostly near the left and right ends of the genome. Experimentation has demonstrated that several of these genes (or their orthologs in VACV) are associated with virulence in accidental hosts, but their functions in natural rodent hosts may be more subtle. Possibly their role in natural infection, where clinical disease is not seen and presumably not relevant to transmission, is to moderate the host's immune response, ensuring efficient contact between individuals and therefore transmission.

Other proteins expressed by CPXV but not VACV have been studied, such as those affecting the ability to grow on Chinese hamster ovary (CHO) cells and produce ATIs. Growth of CPXV in CHO cells is dependent on production of a 77 kDa protein and the insertion of the gene encoding this protein into VACV enables that virus to replicate in CHO cells. Formation of ATIs involves the production of two late proteins. One, of 160 kDa, is the major component of the inclusion itself. The other is required for occlusion of virions into the ATI.

A red pock character is associated with the *crmA* gene, which encodes a 38 kDa protein that is one of the most abundant early gene products and a serine protease inhibitor that inhibits apoptosis and the cleavage of pro-interleukin (IL)-1β to IL-1β. This gene is lost in the frequent deletion mutants referred to above. The essential difference between the wild-type and mutant white pock is the greater hemorrhage in the former and the massive leukocyte infiltration in the latter. Although a protein with 93% amino acid sequence identity is encoded by VACV strain Western Reserve, pocks formed by this virus are white irrespective of whether or not the protein (B13) is expressed.

Physical Properties

Little work has been done directly on the physical properties of CPXV, which are usually assumed to be similar to those of VACV and ectromelia virus (ECTV). The outer lipid envelope of extracellular forms of CPXV is labile and readily lost by mechanical stress, but is not essential for virus infectivity because its removal releases an infectious IMV particle. The virus is generally very hardy, and can survive for months in dry scab material at room temperature, and indefinitely at −70 °C. It is inactivated by moist heat at 60 °C for 10 min, and by hypochlorites, phenolics, and detergents, but less effectively by alcohols. The significance of survival in the environment to the epidemiology of cowpox is unknown. The transmission dynamics of natural infections suggest that most transmission is direct. However, in populations of rodents on small islands, infection occurs as small epidemics followed by apparent extinction: whether these epidemics result from immigration of infected individuals, or survival of the virus in the environment with rare reintroduction into naive populations, has not been resolved.

Replication

The mechanisms of DNA replication and temporally regulated transcription and translation of CPXV mRNA are assumed to be very similar to those in VACV. Virus replication takes place in the cytoplasm, and virus assembly occurs in areas known as B-type inclusions. Like VACV, CPXV virions can leave the cell as IMV by lysis of the cell membrane, or as EEV by exocytosis following fusion between the outer membrane of intracellular enveloped virus (IEV) and the plasma membrane. CPXV differs from VACV in that its genome also encodes for large proteinaceous inclusions known as ATIs, into which virions are incorporated (**Figure 1**). These inclusions are released by cell lysis, and are thought to act as protective packets that aid survival of the virus outside of the animal and therefore increase the chance of spread to another host on fomites.

Geographic and Seasonal Distribution

CPXV has been isolated, or detected by PCR and sequencing, throughout much of Northern Europe and as far east as Kazakhstan. Although cases of human and feline cowpox may be seen at any time of year, infection is most common in the late summer and autumn, which probably reflects increased infection in the reservoir hosts, which in turn reflects increased numbers of hosts at that time of year.

Host Range and Propagation

CPXV has a wide host range both *in vivo* and *in vitro*. It has been isolated from cattle, humans, domestic cats (perhaps the most common source of human infection), dogs, a horse, and a variety of zoo animals including cheetahs, ocelots, panthers, lynx, lions, pumas, jaguars, anteaters, elephants, rhinoceroses, and okapis. All of these are, however, accidental hosts, and the virus circulates mainly in wild rodents. The main reservoir hosts appear to be voles (*Clethrionomys* spp. and *Microtus* spp.) and wood mice (*Apodemus* spp.) throughout the virus' range. House mice (*Mus musculus*) and rats (*Rattus norvegicus*) are infected rarely and are probably accidental hosts (explaining the limited geographic range of the virus), although they may, like cats, act as liaison hosts and transmit the infection onward to man. Other rodents may also act as reservoirs toward the eastern range of the virus. CPXV has been isolated from wild susliks and gerbils (*Rhombomys* spp., *Citellus* spp., and *Meriones* spp.) in Turkmenia. Guinea pigs and rabbits have been infected experimentally with CPXV.

CPXV can be isolated and propagated on the chorioallantoic membrane of hens' eggs, but, unlike VACV, it does not grow in feather follicles of adult chickens. It can be propagated in a variety of cell cultures derived from human, simian, bovine, feline, murine, and rabbit tissues.

Genetics

CPXV produces red hemorrhagic pocks on the chorioallantoic membrane with about 1% white pock mutants.

The virus that produces the white pocks breeds true and the change in pock character reflects deletion and transposition events near the termini of the genome. White pock mutants are better able to grow on arginine-deprived cells than is the parent virus. Other properties that are inherited independently, and vary between individual strains, include production of the hemagglutinin, incorporation of virions into ATIs, resistance to heat inactivation, ceiling temperature for growth, and virulence for newborn mice and chick embryos. OPVs undergo genetic recombination in dual-infected cells, for example producing hybrids of CPXV and VARV.

Evolution

The genetic relationships of CPXV and other OPVs have been studied by bioinformatics. Nucleotide sequencing demonstrated that the OPVs are very closely related as a whole (although the North American OPVs appear more distantly related), but each species can be readily differentiated by biological properties and genome structure. Bioinformatic analyses demonstrated that the two CPXV genomes sequenced are quite divergent and it was proposed they should be reclassified as separate species. As noted above, the presence of the greatest number of intact genes and fewest broken genes suggests that CPXV is closest to the ancestral OPV. With the exception of terminal transposition events (see above), CPXV isolates are genetically stable *in vitro* and *in vivo*. Modern isolates often have near-identical restriction enzyme profiles to isolates made many years ago, and the Brighton Red strain behaves the same now as when first isolated over 60 years ago. However, isolates of CPXV do differ in restriction enzyme pattern and minor biological characteristics, and generally greater differences occur between geographically distinct isolates. Furthermore, the greatest variation appears to be seen among isolates in central Europe, and this may reflect a central European origin for CPXV and divergence as individual strains spread out into different host reservoirs and different geographical areas.

CPXV isolates are all clearly different from other OPVs, such as VACV and VARV, but the genome sequence of horsepox virus (from Central Asia) shows that it is intermediate between VACV and CPXV and shares some properties of each virus.

Serologic Relationships and Variability

Within the genus *Orthopoxvirus*, there is extensive antigenic cross-reactivity in all serologic tests, although minor differences can allow differentiation of species using monoclonal antibodies. No significant serologic differences have been reported among CPXV strains.

Epidemiology

CPXV is rarely isolated from cattle, and serologic surveys show that cattle are not the reservoir host. Most human infection cannot be traced to contact with infected cattle, but about half of the recent human cases in Britain were traced to contact with an infected cat. The domestic cat, although the species in which clinical cowpox is most frequently diagnosed in Europe, is not the reservoir host of CPXV either. Although cat-to-cat transmission can occur, antibody to CPXV is uncommon in surveys of healthy cats. There is no evidence that CPXV can become endemic in any of the zoo animals that have been infected, but with increasing reliance on zoo populations for the survival of many species, these outbreaks may cause conservation problems.

Rather, CPXV is endemic in rodent populations. Transmission has been studied in most detail in several populations of voles (*Clethrionomys glareolus* and *Microtus agrestis*) and wood mice (*Apodemus sylvaticus*) in northern England, where it has been used as a model system for investigating the ecology of endemic infections in wildlife populations. Transmission dynamics appear linked to host population dynamics, with the highest incidence of infections occurring in the autumn when population sizes are at their greatest. This is reflected in the highest incidence of infection in cats and human beings also at this time of year. Although cross-species transmission may occur, empirical evidence combined with mathematical models suggests that most transmission occurs among members of the same rodent species, even where two rodent host species share the same habitat.

Transmission and Tissue Tropism

Both natural rodent hosts and laboratory rodents can be infected with CPXV by the oral and respiratory routes as well as skin inoculation: natural hosts can often be infected with less virus than is required to infect cell culture, as is the case with ECTV where the lethal dose for some strains of mice may be less than one plaque-forming unit. However, it is not known how the virus is transmitted in the wild, and transmission has not occurred among laboratory-housed rodent hosts. This may be because a particular behavior, not elicited in the laboratory, is involved in transmission. Transmission rates in the wild can be very high, and longitudinal studies of naturally infected populations suggest that much transmission, although not all, is frequency, rather than density, dependent, which might itself suggest an important role for particular behaviors in transmission.

Among the occasional hosts of CPXV, the most frequent route of infection appears to be through the skin, probably through a cut or abrasion. Domestic cats, however, can be infected experimentally by oronasal inoculation, and limited respiratory spread sometimes occurs in domestic or zoo cat colonies.

Virus replication in cattle and man is mainly limited to the epidermis at the site of entry, and possibly also to draining lymph nodes. In cats, virus can be isolated not only from skin lesions but also from lymphoid, lung, and turbinate tissue. Skin inoculation of cats is followed by virus replication both at the site of entry and in draining lymph nodes, which leads to the development of a viremia, and virus can be isolated from the white cell fraction of blood, from the spleen, and other lymphoid organs. After about 7–10 days, virus can be detected in the epidermis, leading to the development of secondary skin lesions. The viremia in cats appears to last 1–8 days, and no virus has been isolated from cats after the skin lesions have healed, which may take 5–6 weeks.

Oral, nasal, and skin inoculation of various rodents with CPXV also causes systemic infection. Virus has been isolated from lung, kidney, liver, and lymph nodes of susliks and gerbils, and detected by PCR in a similar range of tissues, and the cellular fraction of blood from naturally and experimentally infected British wild rodents. Laboratory infection and studies of naturally infected wild voles and wood mice suggest that they remain infected for around 4 weeks before clearing the infection.

Virulence

It is not known whether different strains of CPXV vary in virulence for most accidental hosts, including man. In a small-scale experiment, no differences in the ability to cause infection or a primary lesion in domestic cats could be detected between the Brighton Red strain and isolates from a cheetah and a domestic cat. Differences in virulence of different strains do exist for newborn laboratory mice and chick embryos, but these differences are not associated with the ability to infect various accidental hosts and it is not known whether they have any significance in the maintenance of different strains of CPXV in different reservoir tests.

Wild-type CPXV outgrows the white pock mutants and is more virulent for laboratory animals.

Clinical Features of Infection

In cattle, CPXV causes teat lesions, but little apparent systemic disease. Human infection is characterized usually by a single skin lesion, often on a hand or the face. Spread of skin lesions in man is usually the result of direct transmission, for example, from hand to face, but multiple lesions may also occur if there is a preexisting skin condition. Cowpox in man is often accompanied by systemic signs such as nausea, fever, and lymphadenopathy, and children are often hospitalized. Death is rare, and usually the result of an underlying condition, such as immunodeficiency, which increases the severity of disease.

CPXV infection in domestic cats is usually a more severe disease than in cattle or man. There is often a history of a single primary lesion, especially on the head or a forelimb, but by the time the cat is presented for veterinary attention widespread skin lesions have usually developed. The primary lesions vary enormously in character, and secondary bacterial infection is common. The widespread secondary lesions first appear as small erythematous macules, which develop into papules and ulcers over several days. These scab over, and the cat usually recovers within 6–8 weeks. Cats may be slightly pyrexic in the early stages of the disease and some show signs of mild upper respiratory disease. More severe illness such as large nonhealing lesions or pneumonia usually, but not always, results from secondary bacterial infection or immunosuppression. In some zoo-kept cats, such as cheetahs, pneumonia is more common and is associated with a high mortality rate.

No obvious clinical signs are observed in either naturally or experimentally infected rodents (unless the experimental dose used is high). However, longitudinal studies of naturally infected wild voles and wood mice, at both the individual and population levels, as well as experimental infections, have shown an effect on rodent fecundity. Infected voles and mice delay reproduction compared to uninfected animals in the wild by perhaps a whole season.

Pathology and Histopathology

Skin lesions associated with cowpox in most accidental hosts are typical of those expected of an OPV infection, developing through papule, vesicle, pustule, ulcer, and healing stages, although macroscopic vesicles often ulcerate quickly because of abrasion or, in the case of domestic cats, because the epidermis is too thin in most areas to support a vesicle. Microscopic examination reveals hypertrophy and hyperplasia of infected cells, multilocular vesicle formation, large, intracytoplasmic eosinophilic inclusion bodies (ATIs) (**Figure 1**) in epithelial cells, and a vigorous polymorph infiltration of the dermis. Immunostaining demonstrates virus antigen in epithelial cells of the skin, hair follicles, and sebaceous glands, and in dermal macrophages.

Even in lungs and turbinates of cats from which large amounts of virus can be isolated, there are often no gross lesions, and microscopic lesions may be difficult to find. In cats showing clinical signs of pneumonia, there is often an interstitial pneumonia, and, again, eosinophilic inclusions can be seen in infected cells. The tonsils and lymph nodes of infected cats contain many large reactive follicles, and immunostaining may demonstrate antigen in macrophage-like cells. Some follicles have large necrotic centers, suggesting that virus replication is occurring here.

After 3 days of growth on the chorioallantoic membrane of 12 day chick embryos, CPXV causes hemorrhagic pocks approximately 2 mm in diameter, with a few (usually 1%) white pocks. Microscopically, the red pocks consist of ectodermal proliferation and hypertrophy with many cells containing ATIs, and extensive edema and hemorrhage into the mesoderm. The histopathology of white pocks is similar but consists of more inflammatory infiltration and no hemorrhage.

Immune Response

Relatively little is known about the immune response to CPXV in naturally infected hosts. Antibody can be detected by enzyme-linked immunosorbent assay (ELISA), immuno-fluorescence, virus neutralization (VN) (usually done with the IMV form of virus) with or without complement, complement-fixation, and hemagglutination-inhibition (HAI) tests. HAI antibody can be detected before VN antibody, and in cattle and cats begins to decline after about 6 months. HAI antibody is therefore more useful for the diagnosis of acute infections than VN antibody, and in epidemiological studies indicates more recent infection than VN antibody alone.

As in VACV and ECTV infections, cell-mediated immunity plays an important role in protection against CPXV disease, but less work has been published specifically on the cell-mediated immunity to CPXV. A possible delayed-type hypersensitivity response has been reported in cats.

Prevention and Control

Infection in man and domestic animals is relatively uncommon and so measures to prevent infection are generally not warranted. Vaccination against smallpox is no longer routine, and might not protect against the development of a skin lesion, but would reduce the severity of any systemic illness. VACV infection of cattle and man often causes lesions and disease similar to cowpox. VACV does not grow well in cats, and its efficacy as a vaccine (although not necessarily as a vaccine vector) in felids is uncertain, although it has been recommended for some zoo animals.

Although CPXV can cause quite severe disease in man, it does not appear to be very infectious. Human-to-human spread of cowpox has not been reported (in contrast to

VACV). Many human cases of cowpox have been traced to contact with infected cats, but we know of no cases of cat-to-human transmission after cowpox was diagnosed in the cat. Simple hygiene – washing hands after handling the cat, keeping the cat or scab material away from cuts and the eyes – seems adequate to prevent transmission to man, although special measures might be taken for the very young, elderly, or immunosuppressed. Similarly, if an outbreak occurs in cattle, the main route of spread among the cows is through milking equipment, and simple hygiene should suffice to control spread.

Future Perspectives

CPXV is one of several OPVs that have wildlife reservoirs; others include monkeypox virus, raccoonpox virus, and Californian volepox virus. Buffalopox virus is now regarded as a variant of VACV and may also have a wild animal reservoir in India. Occasionally, these and other OPVs may infect other, accidental, hosts, such as domestic animals: there are reports of uncharacterized OPVs being isolated from horses, for example, in Africa, North America, and Australia, and a recent report of raccoonpox virus infection in a cat in Canada. Study of the ecology of CPXV is therefore useful as a model for OPV maintenance in a wildlife reservoir host and the mechanisms of transmission from animals to man. It is also being studied in wild rodents as an ecological model of transmission of endemic infections, and the interactions between host and parasite dynamics.

See also: Adenoviruses: Pathogenesis; Smallpox and Monkeypox Viruses.

Further Reading

Baxby D, Bennett M, and Getty B (1994) Human cowpox; A review based on 54 cases, 1969–93. *British Journal of Dermatology* 131: 598–607.

Bennett M, Gaskell RM, and Baxby D (2005) Feline poxvirus infection. In: Greene C (ed.) *Infectious Diseases of the Dog and Cat,* 3rd edn., pp. 158–160. Philadelphia: WB Saunders.

Carslake D, Bennett M, Hazel S, Telfer S, and Begon M (2006) Inference of cowpox virus transmission rates between wild rodent host classes using space–time interaction. *Proceedings of the Royal Society Series B* 272: 775–782.

Essbauer S and Meyer H (2007) Genus *Orthopoxvirus*: Cowpox virus. In: Mercer AA, Schmidt A, and Weber O (eds.) *Poxviruses*, pp. 75–88. Basel: Birkhäuser Verlag.

Fenner F, Wittek R, and Dumbell KR (1989) *The Orthopoxviruses*. London: Academic Press.

Gubser C, Hué S, Kellam P, and Smith GL (2004) Poxvirus genomes: A phylogenetic analysis. *Journal of General Virology* 85: 105–117.

Moss B (2001) *Poxviridae*: The viruses and their replication. In: Fields BN, Knipe DM, Howley PM, *et al.* (eds.) *Virology*, 4th edn., pp. 2849–2883. Philadelphia: Lippincott-Raven Publishers.

Pickup DJ, Ink BS, Hu W, Ray OA, and Juklik WK (1986) Hemorrhage in lesions caused by cowpox virus is induced by a viral protein that is related to plasma protein inhibitors of serine proteases. *Proceedings of the National Academy of Sciences, USA* 83: 7698–7702.

Shchelkunov SN, Safronov PF, Totmenin AV, *et al.* (1998) The genomic sequence analysis of the left and right species-specific terminal region of a cowpox virus strain reveals unique sequences and a cluster of intact ORFs for immunomodulatory and host range proteins. *Virology* 243: 432–460.

Telfer S, Bennett M, Bown K, *et al.* (2002) The effects of cowpox virus on survival in natural rodent populations: Increases and decreases. *Journal of Animal Ecology* 71: 558–568.

Telfer S, Bennett M, Bown K, *et al.* (2005) Infection with cowpox virus decreases female maturation rates in wild populations of woodland rodents. *Oikos* 109: 317–322.

Tulman ER, Delhon G, Afonso CL, *et al.* (2006) Genome of horsepox virus. *Journal of Virology* 80: 9244–9258.

Relevant Website

http://www.poxvirus.org – Poxvirus Bioinformatics Research Center.

Crimean–Congo Hemorrhagic Fever Virus and Other Nairoviruses

C A Whitehouse, United States Army Medical Research Institute of Infectious Diseases, Frederick, MD, USA

Published by Elsevier Ltd.

Glossary

Argasid ticks Any member of the family *Argasidae*, which are soft-shelled; commonly called soft ticks.

Ecchymosis The escape of blood into the tissues from ruptured blood vessels.

Ixodid ticks Any member of the family *Ixodidae*, which have a hard outer covering called scutum; commonly referred to as hard ticks.

Petechiae Minute reddish or purplish spots containing blood that appear in the skin or mucous membrane, especially in some infectious diseases.

Introduction

The genus *Nairovirus* within the family *Bunyaviridae* includes 34 predominantly tick-borne viruses. These viruses are enveloped, with a tripartite negative-sense, single-stranded RNA genome. Among the members of this genus, the most important pathogens are the Crimean–Congo hemorrhagic fever virus (CCHFV), which causes severe and often fatal hemorrhagic fever in humans, Crimean–Congo hemorrhagic fever (CCHF), and Nairobi sheep disease virus (NSDV), which circulates in Africa and Asia and causes acute hemorrhagic gastroenteritis in sheep and goats.

CCHF was first recognized during a large outbreak among soldiers and agricultural workers in the mid-1940s in the Crimean peninsula but the etiologic agent was not isolated at that time. In 1956 a virus named Congo virus was isolated from a febrile patient in the Belgian Congo (now the Democratic Republic of the Congo) and it was later recognized that Congo virus was the same as Crimean hemorrhagic fever virus, isolated in 1967 from a patient with this disease in (now) Uzbekistan. The disease now occurs sporadically throughout much of Africa, Asia, and Europe and results in an approximately 30% case–fatality rate. CCHF is characterized by a sudden onset of high fever, chills, severe headache, dizziness, and back and abdominal pains. Additional symptoms can include nausea, vomiting, diarrhea, neuropsychiatric disorders, and cardiovascular changes. In severe cases, hemorrhagic manifestations, ranging from petechiae to large areas of ecchymosis, develop. Ixodid ticks of numerous genera serve both as vector and reservoir for CCHFV. Ticks in the genus *Hyalomma* are particularly important in the ecology of this virus and exposure to these ticks represents a major risk factor for contracting disease. Other important risk factors include direct contact with blood and/or body fluids from infected patients or animals. The highly pathogenic nature of CCHFV has restricted research on the virus to biosafety level 4 (BSL-4) laboratories and has led to the fear that it might be used as a bioweapon.

NSDV, which is an important cause of veterinary disease, was originally isolated from sheep from Nairobi, Kenya in 1910. Dugbe virus was originally isolated from adult male *Amblyomma variegatum* ticks collected from cattle in Ibadan, Nigeria in 1964. Both Dugbe and Ganjam viruses (a variant of NSDV) have been isolated repeatedly from ticks removed from domestic animals and have both caused febrile illnesses in humans. Most other nairoviruses have been isolated from ixodid ticks or from argasid ticks, which are ectoparasites of seabirds and other birds, and their medical or veterinary significance is not known.

History

Crimean–Congo Hemorrhagic Fever Virus

A disease now considered to be CCHF was described by a physician in the twelfth century from the region that is presently Tadzhikistan. The description was of a hemorrhagic disease with the presence of blood in the urine, rectum, gums, vomitus, sputum, and abdominal cavity. The disease was said to be caused by a louse or tick, which normally parasitizes a blackbird. The arthropod described may well have been larvae of a species of *Hyalomma* ticks, which are frequently found on blackbirds. CCHF has also been recognized for centuries under at least three names by the indigenous people of southern Uzbekistan: *khungribta* (blood taking), *khunymuny* (nose bleeding), or *karakhalak* (black death). Various other names, including acute infectious capillarotoxicosis and Uzbekistan hemorrhagic fever, have been used for centuries in Central Asia to refer to CCHF.

In modern times, CCHF (then known as Crimean hemorrhagic fever (CHF)) was first described as a clinical entity in 1944–45 when about 200 Soviet military personnel and civilian farmers were infected during an epidemic in war-torn Crimea. Shortly thereafter, a viral etiology was suggested by reproducing a febrile syndrome in psychiatric patients who were inoculated with a filterable agent from the blood of CHF patients. Further evidence of a viral etiology and of a suspected tick-borne route of infection was demonstrated by inducing a mild form of disease in healthy human volunteers after their inoculation with filtered suspensions of nymphal *H. marginatum* ticks. In 1967, the Russian virologist M. P. Chumakov and his colleagues at the Institute of Poliomyelitis and Viral Encephalitides in Moscow were the first to use newborn white mice for CHF virus isolation.

In 1956, Dr. Ghislaine Courtois at the Provincial Medical Laboratory in what was then Stanleyville, Belgian Congo, isolated a virus, referred to as Congo virus, from the blood of a 13-year-old boy who had fever, headache, nausea, vomiting, and generalized joint pains. Interestingly, a second isolation of the virus was made from the blood of Dr. Courtois, who subsequently became ill with symptoms similar to those of the boy. Subsequent work showed that Crimean hemorrhagic fever virus was antigenically indistinguishable from Congo virus and were in fact, the same virus, leading to the new name, Crimean–Congo hemorrhagic fever virus.

Other Important Members of the Genus *Nairovirus*

NSDV, an important cause of livestock disease, was originally isolated from sheep in Nairobi, Kenya in 1910. Dugbe virus was originally isolated from *A. variegatum* ticks from Ibadan, Nigeria in 1964. Ganjam virus (**Figure 1**), which is now considered to be a strain of NSDV, was originally isolated from *Haemaphysalis intermedia* ticks collected from goats in the Ganjam district of India in 1954. Most other nairoviruses were first isolated in the 1960s or 1970s from ticks parasitizing seabirds and other birds (**Table 1**).

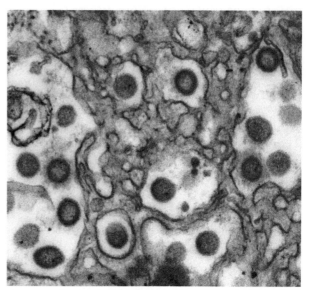

Figure 1   Electron micrograph of Ganjam virus. Photo courtesy of Frederick A. Murphy, Centers for Disease Control and Prevention, Atlanta, Georgia.

Taxonomy and Classification

According to the Eighth Report of the International Committee on the Taxonomy of Viruses, the species *Crimean–Congo hemorrhagic fever virus* is classified in the genus *Nairovirus*. There are seven recognized species in the genus, containing a total of 34 viruses, most of which are transmitted by either ixodid or argasid ticks (i.e., hard or soft ticks, respectively) (**Table 1**).

Geographical Distribution

The known distribution of CCHFV covers the greatest geographic range of any tick-borne virus and there are reports of viral isolation and/or disease from more than 30 countries in Africa, Asia, southeast Europe, and the Middle East. Evidence for its presence in France, Portugal, Egypt, and India is based only on limited serologic observations. Interestingly, after several decades of only serologic evidence of the existence of CCHFV in Turkey, a large outbreak of disease in that country began in 2002, is ongoing, and has resulted in more than 900 cases. This highlights the ability of CCHF to emerge in geographic regions that have previously been devoid of the disease.

Ecology and Epidemiology

As do other tick-borne zoonotic agents, CCHFV generally circulates in nature unnoticed in an enzootic tick-vertebrate-tick cycle. CCHFV has been isolated from numerous domestic and wild vertebrates, including cattle and goats,

Table 1 List of currently accepted species and other viruses within the genus *Nairovirus*[a]

Virus	Original source	Year of isolation	Abbreviation
Crimean–Congo hemorrhagic fever virus			
Crimean–Congo hemorrhagic fever virus	Human	1967	CCHFV
Hazara virus	*Ixodes* sp.	1964	HAZV
Khasan virus	*Haemaphysalis* sp.	1971	KHAV
Dera Ghazi Khan virus			
Dera Ghazi Khan	*Hyalomma* sp.	1966	DGKV
Abu Hammad virus	*Argas hermanni*	1971	AHV
Abu Mina virus	*Argas streptopelia*	1963	AMV
Kao Shuan virus	*Argas* sp.	1970	KSV
Pathum Thani virus	*Argas* sp.	1970	PTHV
Pretoria virus	*Argas* sp.	1970	PREV
Dugbe virus			
Dugbe virus	*Hyalomma* sp.	1966	DUGV
Nairobi sheep disease virus	Sheep	1910	NSDV
Ganjam virus[b]	*Haemaphysalis* sp.	1954	GANV
Hughes virus			
Hughes virus	*Ornithodoros* sp.	1962	HUGV
Farallon virus	*Carios capensis*	1964	FARV
Fraser Point virus	ND[c]	ND	FPV
Great Saltee virus	*Ornithodoros* sp.	1976	GRSV
Puffin Island virus	*Ornithodoros maritimus*	1979	PIV
Punta Salinas virus	*Ornithodoros* sp.	1967	PSV
Raza virus	*Carios denmarki*	1962	RAZAV
Sapphire II virus	*Argas cooley*	ND	SAPV
Soldado virus	*Ornithodoros* sp.	1963	SOLV
Zirqa virus	*Ornithodoros* sp.	1969	ZIRV
Qalyub virus			
Qalyub virus	*Ornithodoros erraticus*	1952	QYBV
Bakel virus	ND	ND	BAKV
Bandia virus	*Mastomys* sp.	1965	BDAV
Omo virus	*Mastomys* sp.	1971	OMOV
Sakhalin virus			
Sakhalin virus	*Ixodes* sp.	1969	SAKV
Avalon virus	*Ixodes* sp.	1972	AVAV
Clo Mor virus	*Ixodes* sp.	1973	CMV
Kachemak Bay virus	*Ixodes signatus*	1974	KBV
Taggert virus	*Ixodes* sp.	1972	TAGV
Tillamook virus	*Ixodes uriae*	1970	TILLV
Thiafora virus			
Thiafora virus	*Crocidura* sp. (shew)	1971	TFAV
Erve virus	*Crocidura russula* (shew)	1982	ERVEV

[a]Species names are in italics. Under each virus species name is listed other viruses of undetermined taxonomic status.
[b]Considered to be an Asian variant of NSDV.
[c]ND, not determined.

sheep, hares, hedgehogs, and even domestic dogs. Sera from wild mammals of several species have been shown to have antibodies to CCHFV and seroepidemiological studies have also detected antibodies to CCHFV in domestic cattle, horses, donkeys, sheep, goats, and pigs from various parts of Europe, Asia, and Africa. Interestingly, there has been only one report of antibody to CCHFV detected from a reptile, a tortoise from Tadzhikistan.

Although many domestic and wild vertebrates are infected with CCHFV, as evidenced by development of viremia and/or antibody response, birds, in general, appear to be refractory to infection with CCHFV. One interesting exception is ostriches, which become infected with CCHFV

and have been the source of several cases of CCHF associated with slaughtering ostriches in South Africa.

The natural cycle of CCHFV includes transovarial (i.e., passed through the eggs) and trans-stadial (i.e., passed directly from immature ticks to subsequent life stages) transmission among ticks in a tick–vertebrate–tick cycle. CCHFV has been isolated from ticks in at least 31 species. Viral isolations have been made from ticks of two species in the family *Argasidae* and from ticks of seven genera of the family *Ixodidae*. However, the virus appears to be most efficiently transmitted by ticks of the genus *Hyalomma* (**Figure 2**) and, in general, the known occurrence of CCHFV in Europe, Asia, and Africa coincides with the

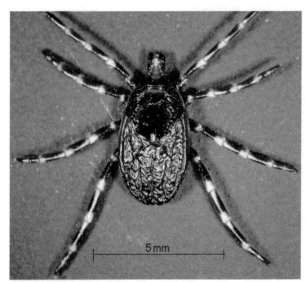

Figure 2 Dorsal view of a *Hyalomma marginatum marginatum* female tick. Photo courtesy of Dr. Zati Vatansever, Ankara University Faculty of Veterinary Medicine, Ankara, Turkey.

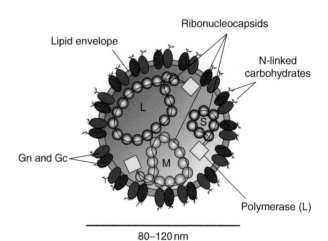

Figure 3 Schematic cross-section of a *Bunyaviridae* virion. The three RNA genome segments (S, M, and L) are complexed with nucleocapsid protein to form the ribonucleocapsids. The nucleocapsids and RNA-dependent RNA polymerase are packaged within a lipid envelope that contains the viral glycoproteins, Gn and Gc. Adapted from Schmaljohn CS and Hooper JW (2001) Bunyaviridae: The viruses and their replication. In: Knipe DM and Howley PM (eds.) *Fields Virology*, 4th edn., pp. 1447–1472. Philadelphia: Lippincott Williams and Wilkins, with permission from Lippincott Williams and Wilkins.

geographic distribution of these ticks. Although *Hyalomma* spp. ticks are considered the most important in the epidemiology of CCHF, the virus has been isolated from ticks in other genera (i.e., *Rhipicephalus, Boophilus, Dermacentor,* and *Ixodes* spp.) as well, which may contribute to its wide geographical distribution.

The principal vector of NSDV is the ixodid tick *Rhipicephalus appendiculatus*, which occurs throughout East and Central Africa. Most other nairoviruses have been isolated from ticks parasitizing birds and their ecology has not been well studied.

Properties of the Virion and Genome

The morphology and structure of the CCHFV virion was first described in the early 1970s from the brains of infected newborn mice. It is now known that CCHFV and nairoviruses in general, are typical of other members of the family *Bunyaviridae* in terms of their basic structure, morphogenesis, replication cycle, and physicochemical properties. Virions are spherical, approximately 100 nm in diameter, and have a host cell-derived lipid bilayered envelope approximately 5–7 nm thick, through which protrude glycoprotein spikes 8–10 nm in length (**Figure 3**). Virions of members of the family *Bunyaviridae* contain three structural proteins: two envelope glycoproteins (Gn and Gc (previously termed G2 and G1)), named in accordance with their relative proximity to the amino or carboxy terminus of the M segment-encoded polyprotein, respectively, and a nucleocapsid protein (N), plus a large polypeptide (L), which is the viron-associated RNA-dependent RNA polymerase (**Figure 3**).

The genome is typical of those of other members of the family and is composed of three negative-strand RNA segments, S, M, and L, encoding the N nucleocapsid, Gn and Gc glycoproteins, and the L polymerase, respectively. The RNA segments are complexed with N to form individual S, M, and L nucleocapsids, which appear to be circular or loosely helical. The M segment of nairoviruses is 30–50% larger than the M segments of members of other genera in the *Bunyaviridae* family and has a potential coding capacity of up to 240 kDa of protein. At least one of each of the S, M, and L ribonucleocapsids must be contained in a virion for infectivity; however, equal numbers of nucleocapsids may not always be packaged in mature virions. Recent data show that the N protein is targeted to the perinuclear region of infected cells in the absence of native RNA segments and that this targeting is actin filament dependent. The first 8–13 nucleotide bases at the 3′-termini of all three RNA segments have a sequence (3′-AGAGUUUCU-) that is conserved within viruses of the genus, with a complementary consensus sequence at the 5′-termini. Base-pairing of the terminal nucleotides is predicted to form stable panhandle structures and noncovalently closed circular RNAs, which have been directly observed by electron microscopy of RNA extracted from the bunyavirus *Uukuniemi Virus*.

The principal stages of the replication process for viruses in the *Bunyaviridae* are similar to those of many other enveloped viruses. The viral glycoproteins are believed to be responsible for recognition of receptor sites on susceptible cells. Viruses that attach to receptors on susceptible cells are internalized by endocytosis, and replication occurs in the cytoplasm. Virions mature by budding through endoplasmic reticulum into cytoplasmic vesicles in the Golgi region, which are presumed to fuse with the plasma membrane to release virus.

Recently, a reverse genetics system was developed for CCHFV. The development of such a system was a major step forward in efforts to understand the biology of the virus. Developing an infectious clone for CCHFV will allow for more extensive studies of its biology and pathogenesis, and may ultimately lead to better therapeutic and prophylactic measures against CCHFV infections.

Phylogenetic Relationships

Many early studies, based on serological testing, suggested that there are very few significant differences among strains of CCHFV. Recent data based on nucleic acid sequence analyses have revealed extensive genetic diversity. For example, analysis of the S RNA segment reveals the existence of seven distinct virus groups (i.e., genotypes) (**Figure 4**). These genotypes show a strong correlation with the geographical area of viral isolation. Furthermore, studies have discovered similar genotypes in distant geographical locations. Movement of

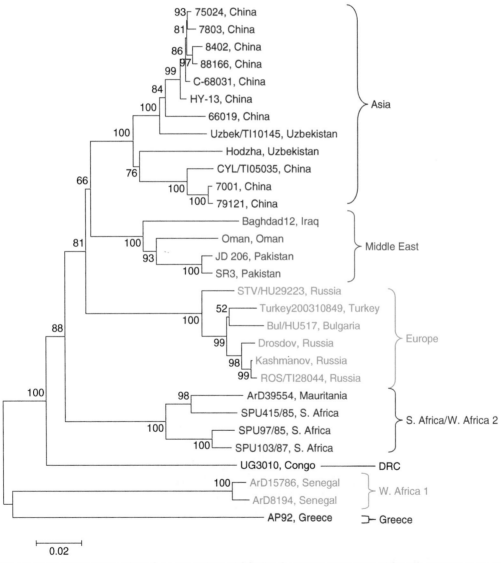

Figure 4 Phylogenetic relationships of the S segment RNA of CCHFV. Complete sequences of S segment RNA were aligned and analyzed by a neighbor-joining method with Kimura two-parameter distances by using MEGA software (version 3.1). The lengths of the horizontal branches are proportional to the number of nucleotide differences between taxa. Bootstrap values above 50%, obtained from 500 replicates of the analysis, are shown at the appropriate branch points. CCHFV strains are described as strain designation, country of origin. Scale = 2% divergence.

CCHFV-infected livestock or uninfected livestock carrying infected ticks may explain some of the movement of viral genetic lineages within diverse regions. Other explanations include the movement of virus via migratory animals or birds that are either infected or are carrying virus-infected ticks. It is interesting that the Greek strain AP92 differed greatly from other European strains, and therefore is in a group by itself (**Figure 4**). AP92 strain was originally isolated in Greece from a *Rhipicephalus bursa* tick and has not yet been associated with disease in humans.

Sequence information on the L RNA segment has lagged behind those of the S and M RNA segments; nevertheless, there is evidence that the S and L RNA segments have the same evolutionary history. Thus, essentially identical S and L tree topologies are seen when analyzing all the available segment sequences. This, however, is not the case for the M RNA segment. This is generally taken for evidence of RNA segment reassortment. RNA viruses with segmented genomes have the capacity to reassort their genomic segments into new, genetically distinct viruses if the two or more viruses co-infect the same target cell. Indeed, several examples of RNA segment reassortment have been documented among viruses of the family *Bunyaviridae*, including CCHFV. Furthermore, reassortment appears to be much more frequently observed among CCHFV M RNA segments than among S and L RNA segments.

Clinical Features

Except for newborn mice, humans appear to be the only host of CCHFV in which disease is manifested. In contrast to the inapparent infection in most other vertebrate hosts, human infection with CCHFV often results in severe hemorrhagic disease. The typical course of CCHF is noted by some authors as progressing through four distinct phases, that is, 'incubation', 'prehemorrhagic',

'hemorrhagic', and 'convalescence'; it is noteworthy that the duration and associated symptoms of these phases can vary greatly. In general, the incubation period after a tick bite can be as brief as 1–3 days, but can be much longer depending on several factors including route of exposure. After the incubation period, the prehemorrhagic period is characterized by sudden onset of fever, chills, severe headache, dizziness, photophobia, and back and abdominal pains. Additional symptoms such as nausea, vomiting, diarrhea, and an accompanying loss of appetite are common. Fever is often very high (39–41 °C) and can remain continually elevated for 5–12 days or may be biphasic. It is interesting that neuropsychiatric changes have been reported in some CCHF patients. These have included sharp changes in mood, with feelings of confusion and aggression and even some bouts of violent behavior. Cardiovascular changes can also be seen and include bradycardia and low blood pressure. In severe cases, 3–6 days after the onset of disease, hemorrhagic manifestations develop. These can range from petechiae to large areas of ecchymosis and often appear on the mucous membranes and skin, especially on the upper body and/or extremities (**Figure 5**). Bleeding in the form of melena, hematemesis, and epistaxis is also commonly seen by day 4 or 5 and can often be characterized by dark 'coffee grounds' vomitus and tarlike stools resulting from intestinal hemorrhages. Bleeding from other sites including the vagina, gingival bleeding, and, in the most severe cases, cerebral hemorrhage have been reported. About 50% of the patients develop hepatomegaly. Not surprisingly, poor prognosis is associated with cerebral hemorrhage and massive liver necrosis. Mortality rates for the various CCHF epidemics and outbreaks have varied greatly. The average mortality rate is often cited at 30–50%; however, rates as high as 72.7% and 80% have been reported from the United Arab Emirates and China, respectively. During the recent outbreak in Turkey, of the 500 cases reported to the Turkish Ministry

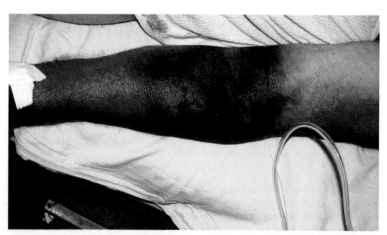

Figure 5   Ecchymosis seen on the arm of a CCHF patient. Photo courtesy of Dr. Miro Petrovec, University of Ljubljana, Slovenia.

of Health, 26 (5.2%) were fatal. Mortality rates of nosocomial infections are often much higher than those acquired naturally through tick bite. The exact reasons for this phenomenon are not known, but may simply relate to viral dose.

Pathogenesis

Because of the difficulties of working with CCHFV (e.g., the need for specialized containment laboratories) and the lack of an animal model of disease, the pathogenesis of CCHF is poorly understood. Capillary fragility is a common feature of CCHF, suggesting infection of the endothelium. This is surely where the alternative term 'capillary toxicosis', given to CCHF by the early Soviet workers, was derived. Localization of CCHFV in tissues by immunohistochemistry has shown that mononuclear phagocytes and endothelial cells are major sites of viral infection. Endothelial damage would account for the characteristic rash and contribute to hemostatic failure by stimulating platelet aggregation and degranulation, with consequent activation of the intrinsic coagulation cascade. Thrombocytopenia appears to be a consistent feature of CCHF infection and platelet counts can often be extremely low beginning at the early stage of illness in fatal cases.

Some have argued that the characteristic endothelial damage seen in CCHF is not necessarily the result of direct infection of the endothelial cells by CCHFV. Evidence is mounting that for viral hemorrhagic fever, caused by the Ebola virus, much of the cellular damage and resulting coagulopathy results from multiple host-induced mechanisms. These include massive apoptosis of lymphocytes both intravascularly and in lymphoid organs; induction of pro-inflammatory cytokines, including tumor necrosis factor (TNF)-α; and the dysregulation of the coagulation cascade leading to disseminated intravascular coagulation (DIC). Indeed, many of these same features are seen in CCHF, including DIC, vascular dysfunction, and shock. Clearly, more work needs to be done in this area to completely understand the pathogenesis of CCHF.

Diagnosis

A diagnosis of CCHF should be considered when severe flu-like symptoms with a sudden onset are seen in patients with a history of tick bite, travel to an endemic area, and/or exposure to blood or other tissues of livestock or human patients. Early diagnosis is essential, both for the outcome of the patient and because of the potential for nosocomial infections. The differential diagnosis should include rickettsiosis (tick-borne typhus or African

tick bite fever caused by *Rickettsia conorii* and *R. africae*, respectively), leptospirosis, and borreliosis (relapsing fever). Additionally, other infections, which present as hemorrhagic disease such as meningococcal infections, hantaviral hemorrhagic fever, malaria, yellow fever, dengue, Omsk hemorrhagic fever, and Kyasanur Forest disease should be considered. In Africa, Lassa fever and infection with the filoviruses, Ebola and Marburg, must also be included in the differential diagnosis.

The diagnosis of CCHF is confirmed by detecting viral nucleic acid by reverse transcription-polymerase chain reaction (RT-PCR), demonstration of viral antigen by enzyme-linked immunosorbent assay (ELISA), or isolation of the virus. Any attempts at isolating and culturing the virus should be performed only under BSL-4 containment. The traditional method and 'gold standard' for CCHFV isolation has been by intracranial or intraperitoneal inoculation of a sample into newborn mice. However, isolation in cell culture is far simpler and safer and provides a more rapid result. Virus can be isolated from blood and organ suspensions in a wide variety of susceptible cell lines including LLC-MK2, Vero, BHK-21, and SW-13 cells with maximal viral yields after 4–7 days of incubation. In some cases however, depending on the cell line and strain, the virus may induce little or no cytopathic effect (CPE). In these cases, the presence of virus can be identified by performing an immunofluorescence assay (IFA) with specific antibodies to CCHFV or by RT-PCR.

The neutralizing antibody response to CCHFV, as well as to other nairoviruses, is weak and difficult to demonstrate. Both IgG and IgM antibodies are detectable by IFA by about day 5 of illness and are present in the sera of survivors by day 9. The IgM antibody declines to undetectable levels by the fourth month after infection, and IgG titers may also begin to decline gradually at this time, but remain demonstrable for at least 5 years. An antibody response is rarely detectable in fatal cases and diagnosis is usually confirmed by isolating the virus from the serum or from liver biopsy specimens or by demonstrating the presence of CCHFV antigen by immunohistochemical techniques of paraffin-embedded liver sections or by IFA of liver impression smears.

Molecular-based diagnostic assays, such as RT-PCR, provide a useful complement to serodiagnosis and now often serve as the front-line tool both in the diagnosis of CCHF and in epidemiological studies of the disease.

Prevention and Control

Several groups of individuals are considered to be at risk of contracting CCHF – specifically, people from endemic areas who are liable to be fed upon by ticks, particularly *Hyalomma* spp. ticks. These include individuals who work outdoors, particularly those who work with large domestic animals. Exposures such as crushing infected ticks and butchering infected animals have also been a frequent source of CCHFV infection. Other groups who are at risk include those caring for CCHF patients. In fact, the risk of nosocomial infection in healthcare workers is well documented and can be extremely high, especially during the hemorrhagic period of disease.

Avoiding or minimizing exposure to the virus is the best means of preventing CCHF. Persons in high-risk occupations (i.e., slaughterhouse workers, veterinarians, sheep herders, etc.) should take every precaution to avoid exposure to virus-infected ticks or virus-contaminated animal blood or other tissues. For example, wearing gloves and limiting exposure of naked skin to fresh blood and other tissues of animals are effective practical control measures. Likewise, medical personnel who care for suspected CCHF patients should practice standard barrier-nursing techniques. Tick control may not be practical in many regions of the world where *Hyalomma* ticks are most prevalent. However, acaricide treatment of livestock in CCHFV-endemic areas is effective in reducing the population of infected ticks. Applying commercially available insect repellents (i.e., meta-*N,N*-diethyl toluamide (DEET)) to exposed skin and using clothes impregnated with permethrin can provide some protection against tick bites. As for other tick-borne viruses, inspecting one's body and clothes for ticks, and their prompt removal can minimize the risk of infection. An inactivated vaccine, prepared from the brains of infected suckling mice, was used in Eastern Europe and the former Soviet Union in the past, but no vaccines are currently available.

Treatment

Treatment options for CCHF are limited and primarily consist of supportive and replacement therapies. Standard treatment consists of monitoring patients with replacement of red blood cells, platelets, and other coagulation factors. Immunotherapy has been attempted by passive transfer of CCHF survivor convalescent plasma, but the efficacy of this treatment is not clear. There is currently no specific antiviral therapy for CCHF approved for use in humans by the US Food and Drug Administration. An antiviral drug, ribavirin, is effective against CCHFV in culture and has shown the most promise in treating CCHF patients over the years. However, for the best patient outcome, treatment should be started early, ideally, before day 5 of illness.

Disclaimer

The views, opinions, and findings contained herein are those of the author and should not be construed as an official Department of the Army position, policy, or decision unless so designated by other documentation.

See also: Orthobunyaviruses.

Further Reading

Flick R and Whitehouse CA (2005) Crimean–Congo hemorrhagic fever virus. *Current Molecular Medicine* 5: 753–760.

Hoogstraal H (1979) The epidemiology of tick-borne Crimean–Congo hemorrhagic fever in Asia, Europe, and Africa. *Journal of Medical Entomology* 15: 307–417.

Linthicum KJ and Bailey CL (1994) Ecology of Crimean–Congo hemorrhagic fever. In: Sonenshine DE and Mather TN (eds.) *Ecological Dynamics of Tick-Borne Zoonoses*, pp. 392–437. New York: Oxford University Press.

Montgomery E (1917) On a tick-borne gastro-enteritis of sheep and goats occurring in British East Africa. *Journal of Comparative Pathology and Therapy* 30: 28–57.

Schmaljohn CS and Hooper JW (2001) *Bunyaviridae:* The viruses and their replication. In: Knipe DM and Howley PM (eds.) *Fields Virology*, 4th edn., pp. 1447–1472. Philadelphia: Lippincott Williams and Wilkins.

Swanepoel R (1995) Nairovirus infections. In: Porterfield JS (ed.) *Exotic Viral Infections*, pp. 285–293. London: Chapman and Hall.

Watts DM, Ksiazek TG, Linthicum KJ, and Hoogstraal H (1989) Crimean–Congo hemorrhagic fever. In: Monath TP (ed.) *The Arboviruses: Epidemiology and Ecology*, vol. II, pp. 177–222. Boca Raton: CRC Press.

Whitehouse CA (2004) Crimean–Congo hemorrhagic fever. *Antiviral Research* 64: 145–160.

Dengue Viruses

D J Gubler, John A. Burns School of Medicine, Honolulu, HI, USA

Glossary

Arbovirus A virus transmitted to vertebrates by hematophagous (blood-feeding) arthropods.

Endemic A disease constantly present in a human population.

Extrinsic incubation The time between infection and becoming infectious.

Hyperendemicity The co-circulation of multiple dengue virus serotypes in the same population.

Vertical transmission Transmission of a virus from a female arthropod to her progeny.

History

Dengue fever is a very old disease; the earliest record of a dengue-like illness found to date is in a Chinese encyclopedia of disease symptoms and remedies, first published during the Chin Dynasty (AD 265–420) and formally edited in AD 610 (Tang Dynasty) and again in AD 992 during the Northern Sung Dynasty. There are reports of epidemics of dengue-like illnesses in the French West Indies in 1635 and in Panama in 1699. By the late 1700s, the disease had a worldwide distribution in the tropics, with epidemics of a clinically compatible disease occurring in 1779 in Batavia (Jakarta), Indonesia and Cairo, Egypt, and in 1780 in Philadelphia, Pennsylvania, USA. From the late 1700s to World War II, repeated epidemics of dengue-like illness occurred in most tropical and subtropical regions of the world at 10- to 30-year intervals. There is no documentation, however, that dengue viruses were responsible for all these epidemics because diagnosis was based only on clinical reports. Clinical descriptions of some early epidemics were compatible with chikungunya virus infection, which has a transmission cycle similar to that of the dengue viruses. It is likely that epidemic chikungunya did occur, but recent data show that the dengue viruses, not chikungunya virus, were responsible for the majority of epidemics in the past 50 years.

The virus etiology of dengue fever was not documented until 1943–44, when Japanese and American scientists simultaneously isolated the viruses from soldiers in the Pacific and Asian theaters during World War II. Albert Sabin isolated dengue viruses from soldiers who became ill in Calcutta (India), New Guinea, and Hawaii. The viruses from India, Hawaii, and one strain from New Guinea were antigenically similar, whereas three others from New Guinea were different. These viruses were called dengue 1 (DENV-1) and dengue 2 (DENV-2) and designated as prototype viruses (DENV-1, Hawaii, and DENV-2, New Guinea C). The Japanese virus, isolated by Susumu Hotta, was later shown to be DENV-1. Two more serotypes, called dengue 3 (DENV-3) and dengue 4 (DENV-4), were subsequently isolated by William McD. Hammon and his colleagues from children with hemorrhagic disease during an epidemic in Manila, Philippines, in 1956. Although thousands of dengue viruses have been isolated from different parts of the world since that time, all fit antigenically into the four serotype classification.

Many early workers suspected that dengue viruses were transmitted by mosquitoes, but actual transmission was first documented by H. Graham in 1903. In 1906, T. L. Bancroft demonstrated transmission by *Aedes aegypti*, later known to be the principal urban mosquito vector of dengue viruses. Subsequent studies in the Philippines, Indonesia, Japan, and the Pacific showed that *Aedes albopictus* and *Aedes polynesiensis* also were efficient secondary vectors for dengue viruses.

During and following World War II, *Ae. aegypti* greatly expanded its distribution in Asia, becoming the dominant day-biting mosquito in most Asian cities. Multiple dengue virus serotypes were also disseminated widely at that time. A dramatic increase in urbanization in the postwar years created ideal conditions for increased transmission of urban mosquito-borne diseases. These changes, plus an increased movement of people within and among countries of the region via airplane, resulted in increased movement of dengue viruses between population centers, increased frequency of epidemic activity, the development of hyperendemicity (co-circulation of multiple serotypes), and the emergence of epidemic dengue hemorrhagic fever/dengue shock syndrome (DHF/DSS) in many countries of Southeast Asia during the 1960s. By 1975, DHF/DSS was a leading cause of hospitalization and death among children in the region. During the 1980s and 1990s, epidemic DHF/DSS continued to expand geographically in Asia. In the 1970s DHF/DSS moved into the Pacific Islands after an absence of 25 years. In the Americas, where *Ae. aegypti* had been eradicated from many countries as a result of efforts to control yellow fever, increased epidemic dengue fever closely followed the reinfestation of countries by this mosquito in the 1970s, 1980s, and 1990s.

With the development of hyperendemicity, DHF/DSS has emerged as a global public health problem in the past 25 years. In 2007, dengue fever is the most important arbovirus disease of humans, with more than 2.5 billion people living in areas at risk for dengue in a belt around the tropics of the world (**Figure 1**). An estimated 100 million dengue infections and 500 thousand cases of DHF/DSS occur each year. The average case–fatality rate for DHF/DSS is 5%.

Taxonomy and Classification

Dengue viruses belong to the family *Flaviviridae*, genus *Flavivirus*. There are four serotypes: DENV-1, DENV-2, DENV-3, and DENV-4. They belong to a larger, heterogeneous group of viruses called arboviruses. This is an ecological classification, one which implies that transmission between vertebrate hosts, including humans, is dependent on hematophagous arthropod vectors.

As are other flaviviruses, dengue viruses are comprised of a single-stranded RNA genome surrounded by an icosahedral nucleocapsid. The latter is covered by a lipid envelope, which is derived from the host cell membrane from which the virus buds. The complete virion is about 50 nm in diameter. The mature virion contains three structural proteins as follows: the nucleocapsid core protein (C), a membrane associated protein (M), and the envelope protein (E). Functional domains responsible for virus neutralization, hemagglutination, fusion, and interaction with virus receptors are associated with the

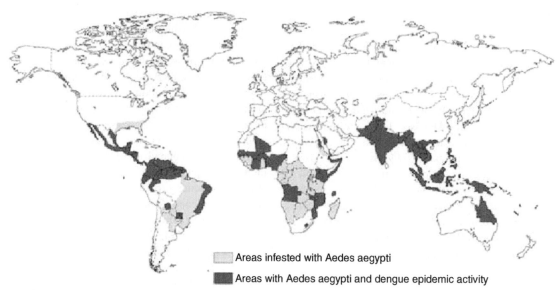

Figure 1   Global distribution of dengue fever and its principal epidemic mosquito vector, *Aedes aegypti, 2007.*

E protein. Epitope mapping has demonstrated three to four major antigenic sites.

Antigenically, the four dengue viruses make up a unique complex within the genus *Flavivirus*. Although the four dengue serotypes are antigenically distinct, there is evidence that serologic subcomplexes may exist within the group. For example, a close genetic relationship has been demonstrated between DENV-1 and DENV-3 and between DENV-2 and DENV-4. The sizes of the genomic open reading frames of DENV-1, DENV-2, DENV-3, and DENV-4 are 3392 to 3396, 3391, 3390, and 3387 amino acids, respectively, the shortest among the mosquito-borne flaviviruses. An amino acid sequence positional homology of 63–68% is observed among the DENV serotypes compared to 44–51% between DENVs and other flaviviruses such as yellow fever and West Nile.

There are 53 flaviviruses recognized by the International Committee on Taxonomy of Viruses (this classification considers dengue 1 virus with four serotypes instead of four distinct viruses), including the genus prototype, yellow fever virus, and Japanese encephalitis, Murray Valley encephalitis, St. Louis encephalitis, West Nile, Zika and other viruses, all of which are transmitted by mosquitoes. Another group of flaviviruses are tick-borne and include tick-borne encephalitis, Omsk hemorrhagic fever, and Kyasanur Forest disease viruses. A small number of flaviviruses have no known arthropod vector, and three have been isolated only from insects.

Geographic and Seasonal Distribution

Dengue viruses have a worldwide distribution in the tropics (**Figure 1**). The viruses are endemic in most urban

centers of the tropics, with transmission occurring year-round, and epidemics occurring every 3–6 years. It is well documented, however, that dengue viruses are maintained during interepidemic periods in most tropical areas and, although the risk of infection is lower than during epidemic periods, it is still substantial to unsuspecting visitors.

Peak transmission of dengue viruses usually is associated with periods of higher rainfall in most endemic countries. Factors influencing seasonal transmission patterns of dengue viruses are not well understood, but obviously include mosquito density, which may increase during the rainy season, especially in those areas where water level in larval habitats is dependent on rainfall. In areas where water in storage containers is not influenced by rainfall, however, other factors such as higher humidity and moderate ambient temperatures associated with the rainy season increase survival of infected mosquitoes, thus increasing the chances of secondary transmission to other persons. Virus strain and serotype, and herd immunity also influence transmission dynamics.

Host Range and Virus Propagation

There are only three known natural hosts for dengue viruses: *Aedes* mosquitoes, humans, and lower primates. Viremia in humans may last 2–12 days (average, 4–5 days) with titers ranging from undetectable to more than 10^8 mosquito infectious doses $50\,(MID_{50})$ ml^{-1}. Experimental evidence shows that several species of lower primates (chimpanzees, gibbons, and macaques) become infected and develop viremia titers high enough to infect mosquitoes, but do not develop illness. Viremia levels in lower primates are more transient, often lasting only 1–2 days if detectable, with titers seldom reaching $10^6 MID_{50} ml^{-1}$.

Dengue viruses are known to cause clinical illness and disease only in humans. Baby mice, which are used for the isolation and assay of many other arboviruses, may show no signs of illness after intracerebral inoculation with most unpassaged strains of dengue viruses. Experimentally, however, some strains can be adapted to produce illness and death in baby mice. SCID, $Rag^{2-1-8c-1}$ and AG129 mice have been used for pathogenesis studies.

Mosquitoes only of species of the genus *Aedes* appear to be natural hosts for dengue viruses. Species of the subgenus *Stegomyia* are the most important vectors in terms of human transmission, and include *Ae. (S.) aegypti*, the principal urban vector worldwide, *Ae. (S.) albopictus* (Asia, the Pacific, Americas, Africa, and Europe), *Ae. (S.) scutellaris* spp. (Pacific), and *Ae. (S.) africanus*, and *Ae. (S.) luteocephalus* (Africa). It is uncertain what role *Ae. Albopictus* plays in transmission in areas where it has been recently introduced. Species of the subgenera *Finlaya* (Asia) and *Diceromyia* (Africa) appear to be important mosquito hosts involved in forest maintenance cycles of these viruses. Two other species, *Ochlerotatus* (=*Aedes*) *(Gymnometopa) mediovittatus* (Caribbean) and *Oc.* (=*Aedes*) *(Protomacleaya) triseriatus* (North America), have been shown to be excellent experimental hosts of dengue viruses.

Low passage or unpassaged dengue viruses can be propagated with consistent results only in laboratory-reared mosquitoes and in mosquito cell lines. Mosquito species most commonly used for *in vivo* propagation include *Ae. aegypti*, *Ae. Albopictus*, and *Toxorhynchites* spp., all of which can be reared with ease in the laboratory. Only three mosquito cell lines show high susceptibility to dengue viruses: C6/36 from *Ae.albopictus*, AP-61 from *Ae. Pseudoscutellaris*, and TRA-284 from *Tx. amboinensis*.

Dengue viruses can also be propagated in baby mice (see above) and in several vertebrate cell lines. These all have lower susceptibility to infection than do mosquito cells however, and dengue viruses must be adapted to each system by serial passage before consistent results can be obtained. Mammalian cell lines commonly used include LLC-MK2 and VERO (monkey kidney), BHK-21 (baby hamster kidney), FRhL (fetal rhesus lung), and PDK (primary dog kidney).

Genetics

Laboratory and epidemiologic studies have documented that genetic variants of dengue viruses occur in nature. DENV-3 isolated during epidemics in Puerto Rico in 1963 and 1977, and in Tahiti in 1965 and 1969, are antigenically and biologically very similar to each other, but very different from Asian strains of the same serotype.

Similar antigenic differences were observed between Caribbean and Asian strains of DENV-4.

Oligonucleotide fingerprinting, restriction enzymes, primer extension sequencing, and nucleotide sequence comparison all have been used to study genetic variation among dengue viruses. In general, viruses circulating in the same geographic region during the same general time frame show genetic homogeneity, while differing from viruses of the same serotype from other regions. Because there is no good animal model for dengue however, it is not well understood how genetic variation influences phenotypic expression, in terms of clinical presentation or epidemic potential.

With increased transmission worldwide, dengue viruses have increased in diversity in recent years, most likely influencing both virulence and epidemic potential. This is supported by epidemiologic and virologic studies conducted in areas with sequential, but contrasting disease severity and transmission dynamics, such as Sri Lanka prior to and after the first DHF epidemic there in 1989. Other evidence includes the striking difference in replication characteristics between the South Pacific/American and the Southeast Asian subtypes of DENV-3 and DENV-2.

The number of genetic subtypes identified in each serotype varies with the method used, but more viruses have now been studied by partial nucleotide sequencing. Based on sequencing a 600 bp region of the envelope protein, which correlates well with sequencing the entire envelope protein, there are two distinct genotypes of DENV-1, four of DENV-2, four of DENV-3, and three of DENV-4. Of considerable epidemiologic interest is that there are currently two genotypes of DENV-2 circulating in the American region. One, designated American, has been in the Americas since at least 1952, whereas the second, designated Southeast Asia, was isolated for the first time from dengue patients in Jamaica in 1982 shortly after the 1981 Cuban epidemic of DHF/DSS. Analysis by restriction enzymes and primer extension sequencing has shown that the Jamaican virus is nearly identical to strains of DENV-2 isolated in Vietnam in 1987, suggesting that the DENV-2 virus causing the Cuban epidemic was introduced from Vietnam. This conclusion is supported by the fact that many Cubans were working in Vietnam on various aid projects during the late 1970s and early 1980s. The Southeast Asia genotype has subsequently become the predominant and most wide-spread strain of DENV-2 virus in the American region.

Although there have been increasingly frequent reports of intraserotypic recombination events among the dengue viruses, the data suggest that this has not been important in their evolution. However, with increased occurrence of the cocirculation of multiple serotypes in an area (hyperendemicity), there have been increased reports of concurrent infections with two serotypes. This will increase the probability that interserotypic recombination might occur.

Evolution

The two principal theories of flavivirus evolution are: (1) that the tick-borne and mosquito-borne flaviviruses evolved from viruses with no known vector and (2) that the tick-borne and no known vector viruses evolved from a common ancestor and the mosquito-borne viruses arose separately. The origin of dengue viruses is unknown. Their natural history, however, suggests a long association with mosquitoes, possibly prior to becoming adapted to lower primates and humans. Biologically, dengue viruses are highly adapted to their mosquito hosts, being maintained by vertical transmission (from female mosquito to her offspring) in those species responsible for the forest maintenance cycle, with periodic amplification in lower primates (**Figure 2**). Such forest cycles have been documented in Southeast Asia and Africa. At some point in the past, probably with the clearing of the forests and development of human settlements in Asia, these viruses moved out of the jungle and into a rural environment where they were, and still are, transmitted to humans by peri-domestic mosquitoes such as *Ae. albopictus*. Migration of people ultimately moved the viruses into the cities of the tropics where they became 'urbanized' and transmitted by the highly domesticated, urban *Ae. aegypti* mosquito, which had been spread around the world via sailing ships and increased commerce.

Because of the rather slow rate of change (genetic drift) of the dengue virus genome, viruses isolated over long periods of time in the same geographic region still show striking homogenicity. The greatest genetic difference between dengue virus strains was observed between DENV-2 and DENV-3 isolated from forest mosquitoes in Africa and Asia, respectively, and viruses of the same serotype isolated from humans or mosquitoes in nearby urban areas. This would suggest that there is little gene flow between the forest and urban cycles. On the other hand, both laboratory and field evidence suggest that significant genetic changes that influence epidemic potential do occur in nature (see above).

Serologic Relationships and Variability

Dengue viruses share common morphology, genomic structure, and antigenic determinants with 52 other flaviviruses. Serologic tests most frequently used to determine antigenic relationships have included the hemagglutination-inhibition (HI), complement fixation (CF), and the plaque reduction neutralization (PRNT) tests. Because all flaviviruses share common antigenic determinants, identification of individual family members using these tests is difficult. The dengue viruses make up one antigenic complex within the family *Flaviviridae*. They share complex-specific antigenic determinants on both structural and nonstructural proteins. Serotypes within the dengue virus complex are most accurately and easily identified with an indirect immunofluorescent antibody (IFA) assay using serotype-specific monoclonal antibodies which react with epitopes on the structural protein. They can also be readily identified using polymerase chain reaction (PCR).

Both antigenic and biologic variation among dengue viruses have been documented. As noted above, DENV-3 viruses isolated in the Caribbean and the South Pacific in the 1960s were found to be antigenically distinct from the prototype and Asian strains of DENV-3 using PRNT. They were also biologically unique in that they did not grow as well in baby mice and mosquitoes as did Asian strains. DENV-4 viruses isolated in the Caribbean after the introduction of this serotype into that region in 1981 were antigenically distinct from DENV-4 viruses from Asia.

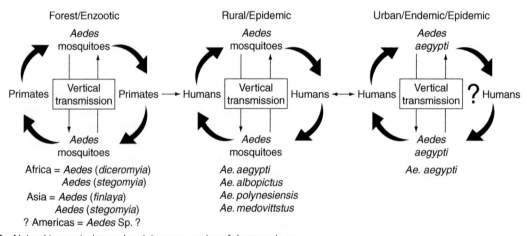

Figure 2   Natural transmission and maintenance cycles of dengue viruses.

Field and epidemiologic evidence for natural strain variation among dengue viruses is more circumstantial. When DENV-2 was introduced into the South and Central Pacific islands in 1971 after an absence of more than 25 years, epidemics occurred on numerous islands. Marked variation was observed in disease severity, viremia levels, and epidemic potential in epidemics on the various islands. This variation was observed with both DENV-1 and DENV-2 in the Pacific and with DENV-3 in Indonesia. Some DENV strains appeared naturally attenuated, causing mild illness with low viremia levels of short duration, whereas others caused explosive epidemics with severe hemorrhagic disease and high viremia levels. Factors that could influence epidemic transmission and disease severity, other than differences in the virus strain, were ruled out as a cause of this variation. Recent studies in the American region have shown that variation among strains of DENV-2 and DENV-4 has influenced epidemic transmission.

Epidemiology

Dengue viruses occur in nature in three basic maintenance cycles (**Figure 2**). The primitive forest cycle involves canopy-dwelling mosquitoes and lower primates. A rural cycle, primarily in Asia and the Pacific, involves peridomestic mosquitoes (*Ae. albopictus* and *Ae. scutellaris* Spp.) and humans. The urban cycle, which is the most important epidemiologically and in regard to public health and economic impact, involves the highly domesticated *Ae. aegypti* mosquito and humans. The viruses are maintained in most large urban centers of the tropics, with epidemics occurring at periodic intervals of 3–6 years.

A combination of increased urbanization in the tropics, changing life styles, and lack of effective mosquito control has made most tropical cities highly permissive for transmission of dengue viruses by *Ae. aegypti*. Increased air travel by humans provides the ideal mechanism to transport dengue viruses between population centers. As a result, in the past 25 years there has been a dramatic global increase in the movement of dengue viruses within and between regions, resulting in increased epidemic activity, development of hyperendemicity, and the geographic spread and increased incidence of the severe and fatal form of disease, DHF/DSS. Once observed only in Southeast Asia, epidemic DHF/DSS has spread to west Asia, the Peoples Republic of China, the Pacific islands, and the Americas in the past 25 years.

Factors responsible for the emergence and spread of the severe form of disease, DHF/DSS, are not fully understood. The changing disease pattern described above provides support for both principal hypotheses regarding the pathogenesis of DHF/DSS, secondary infection, and virus virulence. Thus, increased movement of viruses

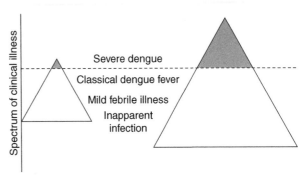

Figure 3 The iceberg concept of dengue/dengue hemorrhagic fever. The severe form of disease represents only the tip that protrudes from the water. As the incidence of infection increases, so too does the severe and fatal form of disease.

between population centers results in increased transmission and the development of hyperendemicity, which then increases the probability of a secondary infection, of a virulent virus emerging via genetic change or being imported from another area.

Increased transmission of multiple dengue serotypes raises the iceberg further out of the water, and increases the probability that severe disease will occur, regardless of whether the underlying cause is due to increased virulence, immune enhancement, or, more likely, a combination of both (**Figure 3**).

Dengue is primarily an urban disease. Most major epidemics of DHF/DSS occur in tropical urban centers where large and crowded human populations live in intimate contact with the principal mosquito vector, *Ae. aegypti*. This mosquito is a highly domesticated, day-biting species that lives and breeds in and around the home. High mosquito densities often occur in tropical cities because of water-storage practices and the accumulation of domestic trash. Primary larval habitats for *Ae. aegypti* include a variety of domestic water-storage containers such as clay jars and pots, metal drums, cement cisterns, and many other artificial containers found in the domestic environment that collect and hold rain water. The latter include, but are not limited to flower vases and pots, used automobile tires, buckets, bottles, cans, old machinery, etc.

Transmission and Tissue Tropism

Most dengue virus transmission is by the bite of an infective mosquito vector. Any of the four serotypes may cause high levels of viremia in humans ($\geq 10^8$ MID_{50} ml^{-1}) that lasts an average of 4–5 days (range, 2–12 days). If a competent mosquito vector takes a blood meal from a person during this viremic phase, virus is ingested with the blood meal and infects the cells of the mosquito mesenteron. After 8–12 days, depending on ambient temperature, the virus, and the mosquito, the virus will disseminate and infect other tissues, including the mosquito salivary glands. When the mosquito takes a subsequent blood meal, virus is injected into the person along with the salivary fluids. Dengue virus infection has no apparent effect on the mosquito, which is infected for life.

Ae. aegypti is a highly competent epidemic vector of dengue viruses. It lives in close association with humans because of its preference to lay eggs in artificial water-holding containers in the domestic environment, and to rest inside houses and feed on humans rather than other vertebrates. It has a nearly undetectable bite and is very restless in the sense that the slightest movement will make it interrupt feeding and fly away. It is not uncommon, therefore, to have a single mosquito bite several persons in the same room or general vicinity over a short period of time. If the mosquito is infective, all of the persons bitten may become infected.

In addition to transmitting the virus to humans or lower primates, the female mosquito may also transmit the virus vertically to her offspring through her eggs. Although the implications of vertical transmission are not fully understood, it is thought to be an important mechanism in the natural maintenance cycles of dengue viruses, especially in rural and forest settings.

The primary site of replication of dengue viruses after injection into humans by the feeding mosquito is believed to be dendritic cells. Other tissues from which these viruses have been isolated include phagocytic monocytes, liver, lungs, kidneys, lymph nodes, stomach, intestine, and brain, but it is not known to what extent the virus replicates in these tissues. Pathological changes similar to those observed in yellow fever, with focal central necrosis, have been observed in the liver of some patients who died of dengue virus infection. There is some evidence that the viruses also replicate in endothelial cells and possibly in bone marrow cells. Encephalopathy has been documented in dengue infection but whether dengue viruses cross the blood–brain barrier and replicate in the central nervous system is still open to question. Dengue viruses have been transmitted by blood transfusion and organ transplantation.

Pathogenicity

There is still some controversy about the pathogenesis of DHF/DSS. Evidence suggests that at least two pathogenetic mechanisms are associated with severe dengue infection. Classical DHF/DSS is characterized by a vascular leak syndrome which, if not corrected, may rapidly lead to hypovolemia, shock, and death. The underlying pathogenetic mechanism for this syndrome is thought to be an immune enhancement phenomenon whereby the infecting virus complexes with non-neutralizing dengue antibody, thus enhancing infection of mononuclear phago-

cytes. The latter produce vasoactive mediators, which are responsible for increased vascular permeability. Loss of plasma from the vascular compartment may range from mild and transient to severe and prolonged, the latter often resulting in irreversible shock and death. Although classical DSS is most commonly associated with secondary dengue infections, it has also been documented in primary infections, which suggest that subneutralizing levels of homologous antibody or other immune factors may also cause immune enhancement.

In vitro studies have shown that not all dengue viruses can be enhanced and that there are qualitative differences in the enhancing ability of antibody to dengue viruses. This raises the question as to whether dengue virus strains vary in their ability to stimulate production of enhancing antibody, whether this is associated with virulence, and, if so, how this relates to the immune enhancement hypothesis. Because an animal model is not available, no good data exist that demonstrate variation in virulence among dengue viruses. However, an accumulating body of both experimental and field data suggest the dengue viruses, like most other animal viruses, vary in their virulence and in their epidemic potential. When DENV-1 and DENV-2 viruses were introduced into the Pacific in the early 1970s after an absence of more than 25 years, some islands experienced explosive epidemics, with patients having high viremia levels and severe and fatal hemorrhagic disease, whereas other islands with similar ecology experienced only sporadic or silent transmission, with low or undetectable viremias and mild illnesses. Virus strain variation was the only logical explanation for these differences. Recent laboratory evidence suggests that a major Cuban epidemic of DHF/DSS in 1981, the first of its kind in the American Region, was caused by a DENV-2 introduced from Vietnam, which was genetically distinct from the original American DENV-2. Data from this epidemic support both the immune enhancement and virus virulence hypotheses, which are not mutually exclusive. The most consistent feature associated with the emergence of DHF/DSS in an area is the development of hyperendemicity. This increases the probability of secondary infection, which is thought to be associated with DHF/DSS. However, hyperendemicity is also associated with increased transmission and movement of viruses between population centers, which increases the probability of genetic change and introduction of virus strains that have greater epidemic potential or virulence (**Figure 4**).

Patients infected with dengue viruses may also experience severe and uncontrolled bleeding, usually from the upper gastrointestinal (GI) tract. This severe hemorrhagic disease may be associated with multiple organ failure, and is more difficult to manage than classical DHF/DSS. The underlying pathogenetic mechanism for this type of bleeding is clearly different from that of the vascular

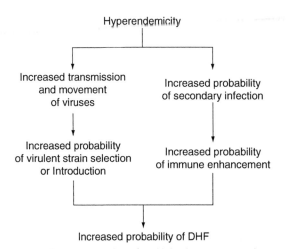

Figure 4 The cocirculation of multiple virus serotypes in a community (hyperendemicity) is the most important risk factor for the occurrence of dengue hemorrhagic fever and is compatible with the two principal hypotheses of pathogenesis, immune enhancement and virus strain variation.

Table 1 World Health Organization classification of dengue hemorrhagic fever

Grade I	Fever accompanied by nonspecific constitutional symptoms, with a positive tourniquet test and/or scattered petechiae as the only hemorrhagic manifestation
Grade II	The same as grade I, but with spontaneous hemorrhagic manifestations
Grade III	Circulatory failure manifested by rapid, weak pulse, narrowing of pulse pressure (20 mmHg or less), or hypotension
Grade IV	Profound shock with undetectable pulse and blood pressure

From Anonymous (1997) *Dengue Hemorrhagic Fever: Diagnosis, Treatment and Control*. Geneva: World Health Organization.

leak syndrome, and involves disseminated intravascular coagulation and thrombocytopenia.

A third type of severe and fatal dengue infection, which may or may not involve overt hemorrhagic disease, is encephalopathy. Although many patients with this syndrome present clinically as viral encephalitis, conclusive evidence that dengue viruses infect the central nervous system has not yet been documented. Available data suggest that neurologic symptoms may be secondary to cerebral hemorrhage, edema, or other indirect effects of dengue virus infection.

Clinical Features of Infection

Dengue infection causes a spectrum of illness in humans ranging from clinically inapparent to severe and fatal hemorrhagic disease with the latter representing only the tip of the iceberg (**Figure 3**). The incubation period may be as short as 3 days and as long as 14 days, but most often is 4–7 days. The majority of patients present with mild, nonspecific febrile illness, or with classical dengue fever. The latter is generally observed in older children and adults, and is characterized by sudden onset of fever, frontal headache, retroocular pain, and myalgias. Rash, joint pains, nausea and vomiting, and lymphadenopathy are common. The acute illness, which lasts for 3–7 days, is usually benign and self-limiting, but it can be very debilitating, and convalescence may be prolonged for several weeks.

The hemorrhagic form of disease, DHF/DSS, is most commonly observed in children under the age of 15 years, but it also occurs in adults in areas of lower endemicity. It is characterized by acute onset of fever and a variety of nonspecific signs and symptoms that may last 2–7 days.

During this stage of illness, DHF/DSS is difficult to distinguish from many other viral, bacterial, and protozoal infections. In children, upper respiratory symptoms caused by concurrent infection with other viruses or bacteria are not uncommon. The differential diagnosis should include other hemorrhagic fevers, hepatitis, leptospirosis, typhoid, malaria, measles, influenza, etc.

The critical stage in DHF/DSS occurs when the fever subsides to or below normal. At that time, the patient's condition may deteriorate rapidly with signs of circulatory failure, neurologic manifestations, shock and death if proper management is not implemented. Skin hemorrhages such as petechiae, easy bruising, bleeding at the sites of venepuncture, and purpura/ecchymoses are the most common hemorrhagic manifestations; GI hemorrhage may occur, usually after, but in some cases before, onset of shock.

The World Health Organization (WHO) has defined strict criteria for diagnosis of DHF/DSS, with four major clinical manifestations: high fever, hemorrhagic manifestations, hemoconcentration, and circulatory failure. WHO has classified DHF/DSS into four grades according to severity of illness: grades I and II represent the milder form of DHF and grades III and IV represent the more severe form, DSS (**Table 1**). Thrombocytopenia and hemoconcentration are constant features. However, there is some disagreement with the WHO case definition in that some patients may present with severe and uncontrollable upper GI bleeding with shock and death in the absence of hemoconcentration or other evidence of the vascular leak syndrome. These patients by the WHO criteria cannot be categorized as having DHF/DSS. In addition, hepatomegaly may not be a constant feature in all epidemics of DHF/DSS. The WHO is currently reevaluating the case definitions for dengue fever, DHF and DSS.

Dengue virus infection is associated with a variety of neurologic and psychiatric disorders, including headache, dizziness, hysteria, and depression. In addition, some patients present with clinical symptoms of viral encephalitis, but as noted above, there is no conclusive evidence that CNS infection occurs.

Treatment for DHF/DSS is symptomatic, and the prognosis of the disease depends on early recognition, initiation of corrective fluid replacement, and management of shock. Definitive diagnosis can only be made in the laboratory by serologic and/or virologic methods.

Pathology and Histopathology

The pathology of dengue virus infection is not well understood because systematic postmortem studies have not been done on patients representing all types of clinical presentations. The major pathophysiologic abnormality in classical DHF/DSS is an increase in vascular permeability which leads to leakage of plasma. Patients may have serous effusions in the pleural and abdominal cavities and a variable amount of hemorrhaging in most major organs. Studies have not revealed destructive inflammatory vascular lesions, but some swelling and occasional necrosis have been observed in endothelial cells.

Limited studies on patients with a fatal outcome have demonstrated focal necrosis of the hepatic cells, Councilman bodies, and hyaline necrosis of Kupffer cells in the liver. Changes in the kidney are suggestive of an immune complex type of glomerulonephritis. There is depression of bone marrow elements, which improve when the patient becomes afebrile. Biopsy studies of the skin rash have demonstrated perivascular edema with infiltration of lymphocytes and monocytes.

Immune Response

Persons infected with dengue viruses produce IgM and IgG antibodies, both of which appear 5–7 days after onset of illness in primary infections. The highest titers of IgM antibody are produced in primary dengue infections, but IgM antibody is also produced in secondary and tertiary infections. IgM antibody is transient and generally disappears 30–90 days after onset of illness in primary infections and after shorter periods in secondary and tertiary infections. IgG antibody, by contrast, persists for at least 60 years and probably for the life of the patient. In persons experiencing their first dengue or flavivirus infection, peak IgG titers are reached 14–21 days after onset of illness and seldom exceed 640–1280, although there are exceptions. In secondary infections, on the other hand, there is an immediate anamnestic IgG immune response to dengue complex-and/or flavivirus-specific antigenic determinants. In these patients, IgG antibody titers may exceed 20 480. Both IgM and IgG antibodies neutralize dengue viruses, and infection provides life-long immunity to that specific dengue virus serotype.

Both IgM and IgG antibodies to dengue viruses cross-react with other flavivirus antigens, including those of yellow fever, Japanese encephalitis, West Nile, and St. Louis encephalitis viruses. Cross-reactivity with viruses in the dengue complex is more extensive than with other flaviviruses, and makes interpretations of serologic results difficult. In patients with second and third flavivirus infections, original antigenic sin reactions are not uncommon. In geographic areas where several flaviviruses are endemic, therefore, definitive laboratory diagnosis can only be made by virus isolation or nucleic acid detection, and in patients with primary infection, by PRNT. Normally, a combination of laboratory (serologic and virologic), clinical, and epidemiologic data is used to make a diagnosis of dengue and other flavivirus infections.

Because IgG antibody persists for many years, its presence in a single serum sample is not diagnostic unless it occurs at high titer ($\geq$1280 by HI and PRNT, $\geq$256 by CF or $\geq$163 840 by IgG ELISA), which is considered presumptive evidence of a recent infection. Lower IgG titers simply indicate that the person has had a previous infection at some time in the past. Paired serum samples are required to confirm a current infection by demonstrating a fourfold or greater rise in IgG antibody. The presence of detectable IgM antibody in a singe serum sample is considered to be diagnostic for a recent infection because this isotype does not persist for long periods. The diagnosis is considered presumptive, and not confirmatory for a current infection, however, because IgM antibody may persist for 90 or more days.

Extensive work done in recent years has demonstrated that immunopathogenetic mechanisms play a major role in the pathophysiology of severe dengue infection. Generally, CD4+ and CD8+ T-cell responses are directed against multiple viral proteins. After primary infection, memory T cells proliferate in response to multiple dengue serotypes with both specific and cross-reactivities. After secondary infection, the T cell proliferation is of low-affinity and may be more cross-reactive to the first infecting virus serotype than the second, a phenomenon analogous to original antigenic sin seen in the antibody response.

Dengue virus infection results in the production of a number of chemokines, including IL-8, RANTES, MIP-1α, and MIP-β, which attract T cells and other inflammatory cells. Some, such as IL-8, are associated with plural effusions and may be important in inducing increased vascular permeability in patients with dengue infection.

There is accumulating evidence that cell-mediated immunity also plays a role in terminating dengue infections. Recent work suggests that dendritic cells (DCs) are likely the initial site of virus replication. Dengue virus infection stimulates DC maturation and activation, and production of TNF-α and INF-α. The DCs migrate to T-cell-rich lyphoid organs where T cells are activated, stimulating memory responses and releasing cytokines and chemokines. Circulating virus in the blood activates more T and B cells. During a second dengue infection, T-cell responses are likely to be dominated by a subset of specific memory T cells, which produce IFN δ and CD40L, resulting in greater DC activation, T cell stimulatory capacity, IL-12 release, increased secretion of TNF-α and IFNδ, as well as potential dysregulation of cytokine responses. As viremia is cleared, the cascade of events initiated by an early type 1 cytokine response may contribute to the pathogenesis of DHF. The cross-reactive T cells that have low affinity to the second infecting virus serotype (see above) may be ineffective in clearing viremia, thus permitting a higher virus load and more severe disease.

Prevention and Control of Dengue

The options available for prevention and control of DF/DHF are limited. Although currently not available, considerable progress has been made in recent years in development of a vaccine (for DF/DHF). Effective vaccination to prevent DF/DHF will likely require a tetravalent, live attenuated vaccine. Promising candidate attenuated vaccine viruses have been developed and have been evaluated in phase I and II trials.

Progress has also been made on developing second-generation, recombinant dengue vaccines by using cDNA infectious clone technology. At least three candidate chimeric vaccines have been constructed by inserting the PrM and E genes into the backbone of yellow fever 17D vaccine virus, into an attenuated DENV-2 (PDK-53) backbone and into an attenuated DENV-4 backbone. The yellow fever 17D chimeric vaccine is further along and appears promising after phase I safety trials. The other two, plus a subunit candidate vaccine, are still in the preclinical phase.

The development of other new technology vaccines is in its infancy. Despite the promising progress, it will likely be 5–7 or more years before an effective, safe, economical dengue vaccine is commercially available. Also very promising has been the rapid progress in developing antiviral drugs that can be used in treatment of dengue infection, and perhaps, even in prevention and control programs.

Currently, the only way to prevent dengue infection is to control the mosquito vector that transmits the virus. Unfortunately, our ability to control Ae. aegypti is limited. For more than 25 years, the recommended method of control was the use of ultralow volume (ULV) application of insecticides to kill adult mosquitoes. Field trials in Puerto Rico, Jamaica, and Venezuela, however, showed that this method was not effective in significantly reducing natural mosquito populations for any length of time. This supports epidemiologic observations that ULV has little or no impact on epidemic transmission of dengue viruses.

The only truly effective method of controlling Ae. aegypti is larval control, that is to eliminate or control the larval habitats where the mosquitioes lay their eggs. Most important larval habitats are found in the domestic environment, where most transmission occurs. To have sustainability of prevention and control programs, some responsibility for mosquito control should be transferred from government to citizen homeowners. For long-term sustainability, mosquito control programs must be community-based and integrated. Persons living in Ae. aegypti infested communities have to be educated to accept responsibility for their own health destiny by helping government agencies control the vector mosquitoes, and thus prevent epidemic DF/DHF/DSS.

Countries with endemic dengue should develop active, laboratory-based surveillance systems that can provide some degree of epidemic prediction. Finally, prevention of excess mortality associated with DHF/DSS can be achieved by educating physicians in endemic areas on clinical diagnosis and management of DHF/DSS. As demonstrated in countries such as Thailand, early recognition and proper management are the key to keeping DHF/DSS case–fatality rates low.

Future

Continued population growth and urbanization of the tropics, changing lifestyles, increased air travel and lack of effective mosquito control have been the most important factors responsible for the dramatic increased incidence and geographic expansion of DHF/DSS in the past 25 years. DF/DHF/DSS has become a global public health problem in the tropics and it is anticipated that this trend will continue unless something is done to reverse it. More effective integrated prevention and control strategies must be developed and implemented worldwide in the tropics. Ultimately, development of an economical, safe, and effective vaccine holds the greatest promise for sustainable prevention and control.

See also: Arboviruses; Flaviviruses: General Features.

Further Reading

Anonymous (1997) In: Dengue Haemorrhagic Fever: Diagnosis, Treatment and Control, 58 p. Geneva: World Health Organization.

Calisher CH, Shope RE, Brandt W, et al. (1989) Antigenic relationships among viruses of the genus Flavivirus (family Flaviviridae). Journal of General Virology 70: 37–43.

Gubler DJ (1989) Aedes aegypti and Aedes aegypti-borne disease control in the 1990's: Top down or bottom up. American Journal of Tropical Medicine and Hygiene 40: 571.

Gubler DJ (1998) Dengue and dengue hemorrhagic fever. Clinical Microbiology Reviews 11: 480–496.

Gubler DJ (2002) Epidemic dengue/dengue hemorrhagic fever as a public health, social and economic problem in the 21st century. Trends Microbiology 10: 100–103.

Gubler DJ and Kuno G (eds.) (1997) Dengue and Dengue Hemorrhagic Fever. Wallingford, UK: CAB International.

Gubler DJ, Kuno G, and Markoff L (2007) Flaviviruses. In: Knipe D and Howley P (eds.) *Fields Virology,* 5th edn., pp. 1153–1252. Philadelphia: Lippincott Williams and Wilkins.

PAHO (1994) *Dengue and Dengue Hemorrhagic Fever in the Americas: Guidelines for Prevention and Control,* No. 548. Washington, DC: Publicaciones Cientificas.

Phuong CX, Nhan NT, Kneen R, *et al.* (2004) Clinical diagnosis and assessment of severity of confirmed dengue infections in Vietnamese children: Is the World Health Organization classification system helpful? *Americal Journal of Tropical Medicine Hygiene* 70: 172–179.

Pugachev KV, Guirakhoo F, and Monath TP (2005) New developments in flavivirus vaccines with special attention to yellow fever. *Current Opinion Infectious Diseases* 18: 387–394.

Rico-Hesse R (2003) Microevolution and virulence of dengue viruses. *Advances in Virusus Research* 59: 315–341.

Thomas SJ, Strickman D, and Vaughn DW (2003) Dengue epidemiology: Virus epidemiology, ecology, and emergence. *Advances in Virusus Research* 61: 235–289.

Thongeharoen P (ed.) (1993) *Monograph on Dengue/Dengue Hemorrhagic Fever,* No. 22. New Delhi: World Health Organization.

Ebolavirus

K S Brown and A Silaghi, University of Manitoba, Winnipeg, MB, Canada
H Feldmann, National Microbiology Laboratory, Public Health Agency of Canada, Winnipeg, MB, Canada

History

Ebola virus (EBOV) first emerged as the causative agent of two major outbreaks of viral hemorrhagic fever (VHF) occurring almost simultaneously along the Ebola River in Democratic Republic of Congo (DRC, formerly Zaire) and Sudan in 1976 (see **Table 1**). Over 500 cases were reported, with case fatality rates (CFRs) of 88% and 53%, respectively. It was later recognized that these two outbreaks were caused by two distinct species of EBOV (*Zaire ebolavirus* and *Sudan ebolavirus*). In 1989, a novel virus, Reston ebolavirus (REBOV), was isolated from naturally infected cynomolgus macaques (*Macaca fascicularis*) imported from the Philippines into the United States. All shipments except one were traced to a single supplier in the Philippines; however, the actual origin of the virus and mode of contamination for the facility have never been ascertained. While pathogenic for naturally and experimentally infected monkeys, limited data indicate that REBOV may not be pathogenic for humans as animal caretakers were infected without producing clinical symptoms. In 1994, the first case of Ebola hemorrhagic fever (EHF) occurred in western Africa in the Tai Forest Reserve in Côte d'Ivoire (Ivory Coast). An ecologist was infected by performing a necropsy on a dead chimpanzee whose troop had lost several members to infection with Côte d'Ivoire ebolavirus (CIEBOV). A single seroconversion was later documented, suggesting another nonfatal human case in nearby Liberia. Zaire ebolavirus (ZEBOV) reemerged in Kikwit, DRC, in 1995, causing a large EHF outbreak with 81% CFR. Sudan ebolavirus (SEBOV) reemerged in 2000–01 in the Gulu District in northern Uganda. There were over 425 cases (53% CFR), making it the largest EHF epidemic documented so far. Starting in 1994, an endemic focus of ZEBOV activity became obvious in the northern boarder region of Gabon and the Republic of Congo (RC) with multiple small EHF outbreaks over the past decade. Most infections there have been associated with the hunting and handling of animal carcasses (mainly great apes). In addition, ZEBOV has virtually decimated the chimpanzee and gorilla populations in those areas. At least three laboratory exposures to EBOV have occurred; one in Russia (2004) was fatal.

Taxonomy and Classification

Filoviruses are classified in the order *Mononegavirales,* a large group of enveloped viruses containing nonsegmented, negative-sense (NNS) RNA genomes. The family *Filoviridae* is separated into two distinct genera, *Marburgvirus* and *Ebolavirus.* The genus *Ebolavirus* is subdivided into four species – *Zaire ebolavirus, Sudan ebolavirus, Côte d'Ivoire ebolavirus,* and *Reston ebolavirus.* Filoviruses are classified as maximum containment (biosafety level 4 (BSL-4)) agents as well as category A pathogens based on their generally high mortality rate, person-to-person transmission, potential aerosol infectivity, and absence of vaccines and chemotherapy.

Biological and Physical Properties of Virion

EBOV particles are pleomorphic, appearing as U-shaped, 6-shaped, circular forms, or as long filamentous, sometimes branched forms varying greatly in length (up to 14 000 nm), but have a uniform diameter of ~80 nm (see **Figures 1(a)** and **1(b)**). EBOV virions purified by ratezonal gradient centrifugation are bacilliform in outline and show an average length associated with peak infectivity of 970–1200 nm. Except for the differences in length, EBOVs seem to be very similar in morphology. Virions contain a helical ribonucleoprotein complex RNP or nucleocapsid roughly 50 nm in diameter bearing cross-striations with a periodicity of approximately 5 nm, and a

Table 1　Ebola hemorrhagic fever (EHF) outbreaks from 1976 to 2005

Ebola species	Year	Outbreak location (country)	Place of origin	Human cases (% case fatality rate)
Zaire ebolavirus	1976	Yambuku (DRC)	DRC	318 (88)
	1977	Tandala (DRC)	DRC	1 (100)
	1994	Ogooue-Invindo province (Gabon)	Gabon	51 (60)
	1995	Kikwit (DRC)	DRC	315 (79)
	1996	Mayibout (Gabon)	Gabon	37 (57)
	1996	Booue (Gabon); Johannesburg (South Africa)	Gabon	61 (74)
	2001–02	Ogooue-Invindo province (Gabon); Cuvette region (RC)	Gabon?[a]	124 (79)
	2002–03	Cuvette region (RC); Ogooue-Invindo province (Gabon)	RC?[a]	143 (90)
	2003	Mboma and Mbandza (RC)	RC	35 (83)
	2005	Etoumbi and Mbomo in Cuvette region (RC)	RC	12 (75)
	2007	Kampungu (DRC)	DRC	Ongoing
Sudan ebolavirus	1976	Nzara, Maridi, Tembura, Juba (Sudan)	Sudan	284 (53)
	1979	Nzara, Yambio (Sudan)	Sudan	34 (65)
	2000–01	Gulu District in Mbarrara, Masindi (Uganda)	Uganda	425 (53)
	2004	Yambio Country (Sudan)	Sudan	17 (41)
Côte d'Ivoire ebolavirus	1994	Tai Forest (Ivory Coast)	Ivory Coast	1 (0)
	1995	Liberia (Liberia)	Liberia?[a]	1 (0)
Reston ebolavirus	1989	Reston, Virginia (also Pennsylvania and Texas) (USA)	Philippines[b]	4 (0)[c]
	1992	Siena (Italy)	Philippines	0[d]
	1996	Alice, Texas (USA)	Philippines	0[d]

[a]Place of origin unconfirmed.

[b]Reston virus has only been traced to a single monkey-breeding facility in the city of Calamba, the Philippines, which was depopulated in 1996 and is no longer in operation.

[c]Mortality in monkeys was estimated at 82%.

[d]Only monkeys were infected in these outbreaks; no reported human cases.

DRC, Democratic Republic of the Congo; RC, Republic of the Congo.

dark, central axial space 20 nm in diameter running the length of the particle. The RNP complex is composed of the genomic RNA and the RNA-dependent RNA polymerase (L), nucleoprotein (NP), and virion proteins 35 and 30 (VP35 and VP30). A lipoprotein unit-membrane envelope derived from the host cell plasma membrane surrounds it. Spikes approximately 7–10 nm in length, spaced apart at ∼10 nm intervals, are visible on the virion surface and are formed by the viral glycoprotein (GP). Virus particles have a molecular weight of approximately 3–6×10^8 Da and a density in potassium tartrate of $1.14\ \mathrm{g\,cm^{-3}}$. Virus infectivity is quite stable at room temperature. Inactivation can be performed by ultraviolet (UV) light and γ-irradiation, 1% formalin, β-propiolactone, and brief exposure to phenolic disinfectants and lipid solvents, like deoxycholate and ether.

Properties of Genome

The EBOV genome consists of a molecule of linear, nonsegmented, negative-stranded RNA which is noninfectious,

not polyadenylated, and complementary to viral-specific messenger RNA. The genome amounts to *c.* 1.1% of the total virion. EBOV genomes are ∼19 kbp in length and fairly rich in adenosine and uridine residues. Genomes show a linear gene arrangement in the order 3′ leader–NP–VP35–VP40–GP–VP30–VP24–L–5′ trailer (see **Figure 1(b)**). All genes are flanked at their 3′ and 5′ ends by highly conserved transcriptional start (3′-CUnCnUn-UAAUU-5′) and termination signal sequences (3′-UAAUUCUUUUU-5), respectively, all of which contain the pentamer 3′-UAAUU-5′. Most genes are separated by intergenic sequences variable in length and nucleotide composition. A feature of all EBOV genomes is the fact that some intergenic regions overlap by the conserved pentamer (UAAUU) sequence. ZEBOV and SEBOV show three such overlaps within the intergenic sequences of VP35/VP40, GP/VP30, and VP24/L, whereas REBOV shows only two between VP35/VP40 and VP24/L. Extragenic leader and trailer sequences are present at the 3′ and 5′ genome ends. These sequences are complementary at their very extremities, showing the potential to form stem–loop structures. Phylogenetic analyses on the basis

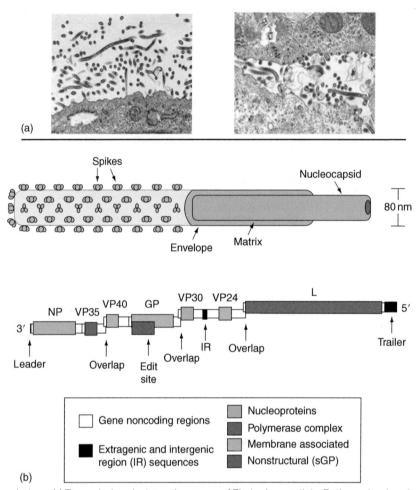

Figure 1 Particle morphology. (a) Transmission electron microscopy of Ebola virus particle. Both graphs show images of Vero E6 cells infected with Zaire ebolavirus. (b) Ebola virus particle structure and genome organization. The upper part provides a scheme of the virus particle separated into four components. The inner core consists of the nucleocapsid which is a structure formed by the single-stranded, negative-sense RNA genome associated with the two nucleoproteins (NP, VP30) and the polymerase complex (L and VP35). The matrix is built by the viral matrix protein VP40 and a minor component VP24. The envelope is derived from the infected cell during assembly/budding. The spikes consist of a homotrimer of the glycoprotein (GP).

of the GP gene of the different Ebola species show a 37–41% difference in their amino acid and nucleotide sequences. Analysis within one species shows remarkable genetic stability between strains (the variation in nucleotide sequences has been shown to be <7% and even <2% among distinct ZEBOV strains), unexpected for an RNA virus, but highly indicative that these viruses have reached a high degree of fitness to fill their respective niches.

Properties of Viral Proteins

Virions contain seven structural proteins with presumed identical functions for the different viruses (see **Table 2**). The electrophoretic mobility patterns of these proteins are characteristic for each species.

RNP Complex and Matrix Proteins

Four proteins are associated with the viral RNP complex: NP, L, VP30, and VP35 (see **Figure 1(b)**). These proteins are involved in the transcription and replication of the genome. NP and VP30 represent the major and minor nucleoproteins, respectively. They interact strongly with the genomic RNA molecule, and are both phosphoproteins. VP30 is also a zinc-binding protein that behaves as a transcriptional activator. The L and VP35 proteins form the polymerase complex. The L protein, like other L proteins of NNS RNA viruses, represents the RNA-dependent RNA polymerase. Motifs linked to RNA (template) binding, phosphodiester bonding (catalytic site), and ribonucleotide triphosphate binding have all been described. VP35 appears to behave in a mode similar to that of the phosphoproteins found in other NNS RNA viruses, acting as a cofactor

Table 2 Ebola virus proteins: functions and localization

Gene order[a]	Ebola virus proteins	Protein function (localization)
1	Nucleoprotein (NP)	Major nucleoprotein, RNA genome encapsidation (component of RNP complex)
2	Virion protein 35 (VP35)	Polymerase complex cofactor, type I interferon antagonist (component of RNP complex)
3	Virion protein 40 (VP40)	Matrix protein, virion assembly, and budding (membrane associated)
4 (primary)	Secreted glycoprotein (sGP) (nonstructural)	May have immunomodulatory role (secreted)
4 (secondary)	Glycoprotein (GP)	Receptor binding and membrane fusion (membrane associated)
5	Virion protein 30 (VP30)	Minor nucleoprotein, RNA binding, transcriptional activator (component of RNP complex)
6	Virion protein 24 (VP24)	Minor matrix protein, virion assembly, type I interferon antagonist (membrane associated)
7	Polymerase (L)	RNA-dependent RNA polymerase, enzymatic portion of polymerase complex (component of RNP complex)

[a]Gene order refers to 3'–5' gene arrangement as shown in **Figure 1(b)**.

that affects the mode of RNA synthesis (transcription vs replication). VP35 is also known to be a type I interferon (IFN) antagonist; it blocks IFN-α/β expression by inhibiting IFN regulatory factor 3 (IRF-3). VP40 functions as the viral matrix protein and represents the most abundant protein in the virion. It plays a number of roles in viral infection related to assembly and budding of the viral particles. The production of VP40 by itself is sufficient to initiate the budding process for the production of virus-like particles (VLPs); however, the production of these particles is greatly enhanced by the addition of GP and NP. Recent studies have shown that EBOV hijacks the cellular protein machinery in order to mediate assembly and budding from the cellular membranes. These functions have been associated with overlapping late domain sequences (PTAP and PPEY) found in VP40. Late domains interact with cellular proteins such as Tsg101 and Nedd4 and affect a late step in the budding process. VP24 is thought to be a secondary (minor) matrix protein that, unlike VP40, is only incorporated into virions in small amounts. It has an affinity for the plasma membrane and perinuclear region of infected cells. The precise role of VP24 in replication is unclear; however, VP24 is a known type I IFN antagonist. Unlike VP35, VP24 blocks the translocation of phosphorylated STAT1 into the nucleus, subverting the antiviral response. More recently, VP24 has been associated with adaptation in rodent hosts.

Glycoproteins

The structural GP is a type I transmembrane protein inserted into the membrane as a trimer (see **Figure 1(b)**). It functions in viral entry, influences pathogenesis, and acts as the major viral antigen. The GP gene shows two open reading frames (ORFs) encoding for the precursors of GP (pre-GP) and a nonstructural secreted glycoprotein

(pre-sGP), which is the primary product of this gene. Translation of pre-GP can only be achieved through mRNA editing, where one adenosine residue is added at a seven-uridine-stretch template sequence, resulting in a frameshift of the primary ORF. GP is cytotoxic when expressed at higher levels, leading to the hypothesis that mRNA editing may be evolutionarily related to the control of overexpression of this protein. The N-terminal ~300 amino acids of the pre-GP are identical to those of pre-sGP, but the C termini of each protein are unique. pre-GP is translocated to the endoplasmic reticulum (ER) by an N-terminal signal sequence, and anchored by an extremely short membrane-spanning sequence at the C-terminus. The protein is glycosylated in the ER and Golgi apparatus with both N-linked and O-linked glycans. Most of the O-linked glycans are located in a mucin-like region (rich in theronine, serine, and proline residues) located in the middle of the protein. pre-GP is then cleaved by a subtilisin/kexin-like convertase such as furin, leading to the formation of disulfide-bonded GP$_{1,2}$. The smaller C-terminal cleavage fragment GP$_2$ contains the transmembrane region that anchors GP to the membrane. Interestingly, proteolytic cleavage of pre-GP is not required for infectivity or for virulence, indicating that the uncleaved precursor can mediate receptor binding and fusion. The production of pre-sGP differentiates EBOV from Marburg viruses, which do not express this soluble protein. pre-sGP is also translocated into the ER, modified in the secretory (e.g., oligomerization, glycosylation) pathway, and cleaved by furin near the C-terminus to release a short peptide termed delta peptide. No biological properties have been attributed to delta peptide. Recent matrix-assisted laser desorption/ionization time-of-flight mass spectrometry (MALDI-TOF MS) analysis suggests that sGP forms a homodimer in a parallel orientation, held together by disulfide bonds between the most N-terminal and C-terminal cysteine residues. sGP circulates in the blood of acutely infected humans. Its exact function is still unknown; however, an interaction with the cellular and humoral host immune responses has been postulated. In contrast to GP which mediates endothelial cell (EC) activation and decreases EC barrier functions, sGP seems to have an anti-inflammatory role.

Viral Life Cycle

The viral life cycle consists of several events: binding/entry, uncoating, transcription, translation, genome replication, and packaging/budding (see **Figure 2**). EBOVs have selective tropism primarily for monocytes, macrophages, and dendritic cells (DCs), although other cell types such as fibroblasts, hepatocytes, and ECs can be infected. In contrast, lymphocytes generally do not support EBOV replication, which is believed to be due to the lack of expression of the viral receptor(s). Although several

molecules have been identified as possible viral receptors in various *in vitro* systems, it is not clear if any of the identified molecules are actually used *in vivo* or the degree of requirement for infection and disease. Folate receptor alpha was the first identified possible receptor but entry was also shown to occur in the absence of the molecule. C-type lectins such as DC-SIGN, DC-SIGNR, and hMGL were shown to be able to enhance binding but are not required for infection. Expression of members of the Tyro3 family converted the poorly susceptible Jurkat T cells into susceptible cells for particles pseudotyped with ZEBOV GP and enhanced ZEBOV infection. Receptor binding results in endocytosis into endosomes, possibly via clathrin-coated pits and caveolae although some studies suggest that they may not be necessary. Acidification of the endosomes is necessary for fusion of the viral and endosomal membranes, which is mediated by a region in GP$_2$. Proteolysis by cathepsins B and L in the acidic endosomes might be essential for infectivity.

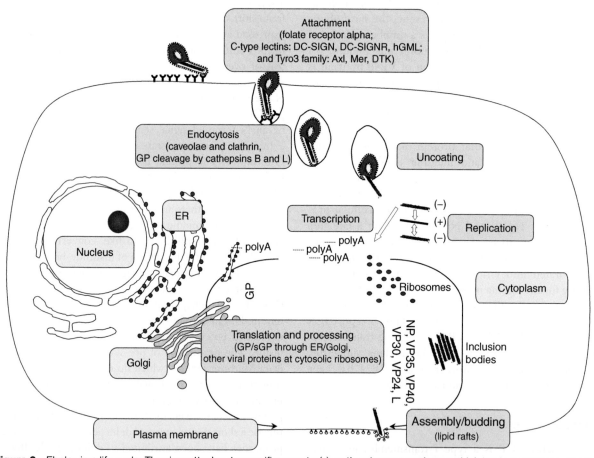

Figure 2 Ebola virus life cycle. The virus attaches to specific receptor(s) on the plasma membrane which leads to endocytosis via caveolae and clathrin-mediated pathways. The viral GP is cleaved in the endosome by cathepsins L and B. After uncoating, transcription and replication take place in the cytoplasm. All proteins except the GPs are translated on free ribosomes in the cytoplasm, while the glycoproteins are produced and modified in the ER and Golgi. Nucleocapsids formed in inclusion bodies interact with the matrix protein VP40 at the plasma membrane. Assembly and particle budding occurs at lipid rafts in the plasma membrane.

Transcription and genome replication seems to follow the general principles for *Mononegavirales*. There seems to be a gradual decrease in mRNA levels from 3′ to 5′ end of the genome. The encapsidated viral genome serves as the template for transcription, which in the case of EBOV requires the L proteins, VP35 and VP30. mRNA transcripts are monocistronic, capped, polyadenylated, and contain long noncoding regions at their 3′ and/or 5′ ends. Stem–loop structures at the 5′ ends of mRNA transcripts may affect transcript stability, ribosome binding, and translation. The switch from transcription to replication seems to be triggered by an accumulation of viral proteins, especially NP, in the cytoplasm. Large amounts of NP are localized in inclusion bodies to which other viral proteins are recruited. These inclusion bodies may function as sites of RNP complex formation.

Membrane/lipid rafts have been identified as platforms for the assembly of virions; GP trimers conveyed to the surface membrane have an affinity for these rafts that is associated with palmitoylation of the membrane-spanning anchor sequence. RNP complexes interact with VP40, which is deposited at the plasma membrane via the late retrograde endosomal pathway. Abolition of the late domains in VP40 blocks particle formation, but only partially affects viral replication, suggesting that other domains or proteins must be involved. VP24 is also associated with the plasma membrane and enhances particle formation, but a specific role in particle maturation has not been identified. GP trimers seem to interact with VP40 and/or VP24 to finalize the budding process.

Host Range and Experimental Models

Natural Hosts and Geographic Distribution

EBOVs typically infect humans and nonhuman primates (NHPs); ZEBOV and SEBOV appear to be the main causes of lethal infections in humans, and thus are of primary public health concern. EBOVs appear to be indigenous to the tropical rain forest regions of central Africa (with the exception of REBOV), as indicated by the geographic locations of known outbreaks and seroepidemiological studies. The discovery of REBOV in the Philippines suggests the presence of a filovirus in Asia. Many species have been discussed as possible natural hosts; however, no nonhuman vertebrate hosts or arthropod vectors have yet been definitely identified. Epidemiological data have suggested monkeys as a potential reservoir of filoviruses; however, the high pathogenicity of EBOV for NHPs does not generally support such a concept. Similarities in biological properties to other viral hemorrhagic fever agents, such as 'Old World' arenaviruses, favor a chronic infection of an animal that regulates survival of the viruses in nature. More recently, viral RNA and virus-specific antibodies could be detected in

African fruit bat species, suggesting that bats might be a reservoir for EBOV.

Experimental Models

Experimental hosts include monkeys (specifically rhesus and cynomolgus macaques), for which infection with ZEBOV is usually 100% lethal, guinea pigs (which show febrile responses 4–10 days after inoculation, but not uniform lethality), and newborn and immunocompromised mice when inoculated with wild-type virus. The resistance of the adult rodent models to EBOV infection has led to the production of guinea pig- and mouse-adapted ZEBOV strains (GPA-ZEBOV and MA-ZEBOV), produced through the serial passage of the virus through progressively older animals. These adapted strains are able to present uniform lethality in their respective hosts. MA-ZEBOV demonstrates reduced virulence in NHPs, whereas GPA-ZEBOV remains uniformly lethal in this model. Infected mice do not exhibit strong coagulation abnormalities (a hallmark of EBOV infection in humans and NHPs) and also slightly differ in other clinical symptoms. Mice, however, represent a good screening model for studies of antiviral and host immune responses. Infected guinea pigs do present coagulation defects that more closely resemble a human or an NHP infection. For growth in cell culture, primary monkey kidney cells and monkey kidney cell lines (e.g., Vero) are often used, but EBOV can replicate in many mammalian cell types including human ECs and monocytes/macrophages.

Clinical Features

Nonspecific, flu-like symptoms such as fever, chills, and malaise appear abruptly in infected individuals after an incubation period that ranges from 2 to 21 days, but on average lasts 4–10 days. Subsequently, multisystemic symptoms such as prostration, anorexia, vomiting, chest pain, and shortness of breath develop. Macropapular rash associated with varying degrees of erythema may also occur and is a valuable differential diagnostic feature. At the peak of the disease, vascular dysfunction signs appear ranging from petechiae, echymoses, and uncontrolled bleeding at venipuncture sites, to mucosal bleeding and diffuse coagulopathy. Massive blood loss is atypical, although it may happen in the gastrointestinal tract, and is not sufficient to lead to death. Fatal cases develop shock, multiorgan failure, and coma with death occurring between days 6 and 16. Survivors can have multiple sequelae such as hepatitis, myelitis, ocular disease, myalgia, asthenia, and psychosis. The mortality and severity of symptoms are viral species dependent, with ZEBOV causing 60–90% and SEBOV 50–60% lethality. Viremia in fatal cases can reach peak levels of 10^9 genomes ml^{-1}, while survivors have peak levels of about 10^7 genomes ml^{-1}. Viral antigen can be found systemically, although it is most abundant in the spleen and liver.

Diagnosis of EHF is based on the detection of virus-specific antibodies, virus particles, or particle components. The procedures are the same as for Marburg hemorrhagic fevers.

Pathogenicity

Most of the information available regarding pathogenicity is derived from ZEBOV infections in humans and animal models. Death seems to be the result of systemic shock due to vascular dysfunction, which is caused by a complex interaction of the immune system with vascular physiology. Three major processes – increase in vascular permeability, disseminated intravascular coagulation, and impaired

protective immunological responses – are the main events that lead to shock and death. The first two processes are the product of a series of events starting with infection of primary target cells (monocytes/macrophages (Mø) and DCs) and later leading to activation and decrease of barrier function of ECs, while the third is still being actively investigated (see **Figure 3**).

Infected Mø are strongly activated, secreting pro-inflammatory molecules such as interleukin 6(IL-6), tumor necrosis factor alpha (TNF)-α, IL-1β, nitric oxide (NO), and spread the infection systemically. In contrast, infection of DCs results in impaired activation, with no upregulation of co-stimulatory molecules such as major histocompatibility complexes (MHCs) I and II, CD80, CD86, and CD40. Early interaction with primary target cells is independent of virus replication and current models suggest that GP in the repetitive context of a particle is required for activation, possibly by binding

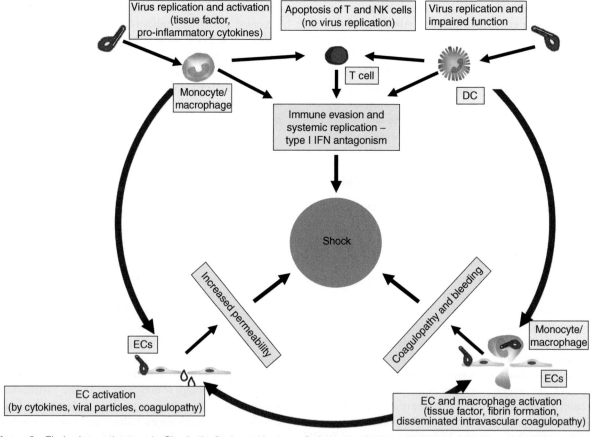

Figure 3 Ebola virus pathogenesis. Shock, the final event in severe/lethal cases, is caused by three processes, which influence each other: systemic viral replication and immune evasion, increase in vascular permeability, and coagulopathy. Infection of primary target cells such as monocytes/macrophages and DCs results in systemic spread of the virus and differential activation. Monocytes/macrophages are activated to produce pro-inflammatory cytokines and tissue factor (TF), while DC activation is impaired, leading to poor protective immune responses. Type I interferon responses are also inhibited by virus-encoded inhibitors (VP35 and VP24). Despite no infection of T- and natural killer (NK) cells, there is extensive apoptosis in those cell types. ECs are activated by pro-inflammatory cytokines and virus, which leads to increased permeability. TF expression induces coagulopathy, which is also able to increase inflammation.

and cross-linking cellular receptors. Activation of ECs by mediators such TNF-α and NO is believed to be the main cause for the decrease in EC barrier function. TNF-α, NO, and pro-inflammatory cytokines increase vascular permeability and EC surface adhesion molecule expression, which are necessary in extravasation of immune cells in inflamed tissue. Although these pro-inflammatory cytokines are an integral part of a normal, localized immune response by attracting and activating immune cells to the site of infection, in the context of a systemic and extensive response, they have a negative effect by inducing shock. ECs also serve as target cells and infection results in activation as indicated by upregulation of adhesion molecule expression followed by cytolysis. However, *in vivo* EC destruction can only be observed at the end stage of the disease.

Infection of Mø also results in the expression of tissue factor (TF), which can impair the anticoagulant–protein-C pathway by downmodulating thrombomodulin. TF is believed to be an important protein in the development of disseminated intravascular coagulopathy (DIC), as inhibition of TF delays death in NHPs and even protects 33% of the infected animals. TNF-α can also induce TF expression in ECs, which would further amplify coagulopathy and DIC. Coagulopathy is known to enhance inflammation, and this could lead to a vicious cycle where inflammation enhances coagulopathy, which in turn would amplify inflammation.

Rapid systemic viral replication is an integral part of the pathogenesis, as infection and even binding of particles results in not only Mø activation but also DC impairment. ZEBOV infection in humans and NHPs results in rapid massive viremia and high titers in various organs, especially spleen and liver. This correlates with an impaired innate and adaptive immune response. However, high viremia and lethality are only seen in guinea pigs and mice after host adaption or infection of various immune-deficient mice, suggesting that evasion of immune responses plays a pivotal role in pathogenesis. Mice lacking the IFN-α/β receptor or STAT1, the main signaling molecule in response to type I IFN, are extremely susceptible to ZEBOV. Treatment of NHPs with IFN-α did not protect the animals but delayed death, suggesting that type I IFN may be an important innate molecule in delaying viral replication. Interestingly, MA-ZEBOV is less sensitive to IFN-α treatment in murine macrophages compared to wild-type ZEBOV, and analysis of genomic mutations in GA- and MA-ZEBOV indicated that mutations in NP and VP24 are sufficient for a lethal phenotype. VP24 inhibits responses to interferon *in vitro*, but it is not clear yet if the mutations in the adapted strains are required for type I IFN evasion or other functions. ZEBOV is also able to inhibit IFN gene induction through VP35, and deletion of the region in VP35 involved in IFN antagonism results in a highly attenuated virus. Furthermore, comparative *in vitro* gene microarray analysis demonstrated a correlation between cytotoxicity and IFN antagonism, which was strongest with ZEBOV and weakest with REBOV.

Adaptive immune responses are also impaired during infection. As mentioned above, upregulation of co-stimulatory molecules is inhibited in DCs, which reduces activation of T cells. There is also a dramatic drop in number of T and natural killer (NK) cells despite the fact that lymphocytes do not support ZEBOV replication. It is believed that lymphopenia is caused by 'bystander' apoptosis, although the mechanism is not well understood. Activation of T cells could also be inhibited by treatment *in vitro* with a 17-amino-acid peptide present in GP$_2$, which has homology to a known immunosuppressive peptide in the retroviral Gag protein; yet there is no evidence that the complete ZEBOV GP has the same capabilities.

Treatment

The current treatment of EHF is strictly supportive, involving fluid and electrolyte replenishment and pain reduction. Due to the remote location of the outbreaks and limited resources available in the affected regions, treatment options have not been tested in patients. Several experimental treatment strategies have been successful in the rodent models, but failed in the NHP model, which is considered the most accurate in modeling human disease.

Therapeutic antibodies are still considered a short-term solution despite varying success in animal models and humans. Convalescent serum was used in a limited number of patients during the Kikwit 1995 ZEBOV outbreak but the success is a matter of dispute. Passive immunization with hyperimmune horse serum resulted in protection of hamadryl baboons, whereas it only delayed death in cynomolgus macaques. Monoclonal antibody treatment is successful in rodent models but has failed in preliminary NHP studies.

Currently the most feasible and promising approach relates to interference with coagulation using the recombinant nematode anticoagulant protein c2 (rNAPc2). Administration of the drug, which is already in clincial trials for other applications, as late as 24 h post infection resulted in 33% survival in the rhesus macaque model. Even more potent seems to be post-exposure treatment with a recombinant vesicular stomatitis virus (VSV) expressing the ZEBOV GP, which resulted in 50% protection when given 30 min post infection, but the mechanism of post-exposure protection is not yet understood. It is expected that approval of this attenuated replication-component vector will be difficult.

The recent advances in the understanding of EBOV pathogenesis and replication will open new avenues for intervention therapy. Novel antiviral strategies such as viral gene silencing through specific siRNA, cathepsin inhibition, and functional domain interference with small peptides showed promise in tissue culture and partially also in rodent models. Strategies targeting host responses are important alternative options and include anticytokine therapy and modulation of coagulation pathways. It should be noted that more classical approaches such as ribavirin treatment, which has been successfully used to treat other VHFs, are not indicated for EHF.

Vaccines

There are no approved vaccines against EBOV. Similar to therapeutic approaches, many initial vaccination strategies were successful in rodents but failed in NHPs. Nevertheless, there are several promising experimental strategies. Nonreplicating adenoviruses expressing the ZEBOV GP and NP were able to induce sterile immunity in cynomolgus macaques within 28 days or more post vaccination, either alone in a single shot approach or in combination with DNA priming and adenovirus boost. Although DNA priming is not necessary for protection of NHPs, it may be required to overcome the problem of preexisting immunity to human adenoviruses. DNA vaccination alone against EBOV is already in Phase I clinical trial, where it was shown to be safe and effective in inducing humoral and cellular immune responses.

Recombinant VSV expressing ZEBOV GP also induced sterile immunity when given 28 days prior to challenge of cynomolgus macaques, but was also able to protect 50% of rhesus macaques when administered 30 min post challenge. These results, together with the fact that prior immunity against the vector is extremely low, and the only target of neutralizing antibodies, VSV G protein, is removed from the vaccine vector, indicate that this platform may be successful in humans if licensing for the replication-competent vector can be achieved. Human parainfluenza virus-based vectors and VLPs are successful in protecting rodents, and preliminary results suggest that they even show efficacy in NHPs. Safety testing of vaccine vectors and the establishment of immune correlates is a priority for all these and future vaccine platforms.

Note: Investigation of an ongoing hemorrhagic fever outbreak in southwestern Uganda revealed what appears to be an additional distinct species of Ebola virus associated with this outbreak. Preliminary genome sequence analysis suggests the most closely related Ebola virus species would be the *Côte d'Ivoire ebolavirus*. Initial outbreak investigations suggest that infection with this newly discovered virus is associated with a lower case fatality than infections with

Zaire ebolavirus (60–90%) or Sudan ebolavirus (50–60%) (T. G. Ksiazek, Centers for Disease Control and Prevention, Atlanta, GA, United States, personal communication).

Acknowledgments

The Public Health Agency of Canada (PHAC), Canadian Institutes of Health Research (CIHR), and CBRNE (Chemical, Biological, Radiological & Nuclear) Research and Technology Initiative (CRTI), Canada, supported work on filoviruses at the National Microbiology Laboratory of the Public Health Agency of Canada.

See also: Marburg Virus.

Further Reading

Feldmann H, Geisbert TW, Jahrling PB, *et al.* (2005) *Filoviridae*. In: Fauquet CM, Mayo MA, Maniloff J, Desselberger U,, and Ball LA (eds.) *Virus Taxonomy: Eighth Report of the International Committee on Taxonomy of Viruses*, pp. 645–653. San Diego, CA: Elsevier Academic Press.

Feldmann H, Jones SM, Klenk HD, and Schnittler HJ (2003) Ebola virus: From discovery to vaccine. *Nature Reviews Immunology* 3: 677–685.

Feldmann H, Jones SM, Schnittler HJ, and Geisbert TW (2005) Therapy and prophylaxis of Ebola virus infections. *Current Opinion in Investigational Drugs* 6: 823–830.

Geisbert TW and Hensley LE (2004) Ebola virus: New insights into disease aetiopathology and possible therapeutic interventions. *Expert Reviews in Molecular Medicine* 6: 1–24.

Geisbert TW and Jahrling PB (2004) Exotic emerging viral diseases: Progress and challenges. *Nature Medicine* 10(supplement 12): S110–S121.

Hensley LE, Jones SM, Feldmann H, Jahrling PB, and Geisbert TW (2005) Ebola and Marburg viruses: Pathogenesis and development of countermeasures. *Current Molecular Medicine* 5: 761–772.

Hirsch M (ed.) (1999) *Journal of Infectious Diseases* 179(supplementum 1): S1–S288.

Jasenosky LD and Kawaoka Y (2004) Filovirus budding. *Virus Research* 106: 181–188.

Paragas J and Geibert TW (2006) Development of treatment strategies to combat Ebola and Marburg viruses. *Expert Reviews of Anti-Infective Therapy* 4: 67–76.

Pattyn SR (ed.) (1978) *Ebola Virus Hemorrhagic Fever*. Amsterdam: Elsevier/North-Holland Biomedical Press.

Reed DS and Mohamadzadeh M (2007) Status and challenges of filovirus vaccines. *Vaccine* 25: 1923–1934.

Sanchez A, Geisbert TW, and Feldmann H (2007) Marburg and Ebola viruses. In: Knipe DM, Howley PM Griffin DE, *et al.* (eds.) *Fields Virology*, 5th edn., pp. 1409–1448. Philadelphia: Kluwer/Lippincott Williams and Wilkins.

Walsh PD, Abernethy KA, Bermejo M, *et al.* (2003) Catastrophic ape decline in western equatorial Africa. *Nature* 422: 611–614.

Zaki SR and Goldsmith CS (1999) Pathologic features of filovirus infections in humans. *Current Topics in Microbiology and Immunology* 235: 97–116.

Filoviruses

G Olinger, USAMRIID, Fort Detrick, MD, USA

T W Geisbert, National Emerging Infectious Diseases Laboratories, Boston, MA, USA

L E Hensley, USAMRIID, Fort Detrick, MD, USA

Glossary

D-dimers Fibrinolysis is mediated by plasmin, which degrades fibrin clots into D-dimers. Clinically, D-dimers can be used to diagnose DIC.

Disseminated intravascular coagulation (DIC) An acquired syndrome characterized by inappropriate accelerated systemic activation of coagulation with fibrin deposition in the microvasculature and consumption of procoagulants and platelets.

Fibrin degradation products (FDPs) The protein fragments produced after digestion of fibrinogen or fibrin by plasmin. Typically, a hallmark of disseminated intravascular coagulation. Also, referred to as fibrin-split products.

RNAi The silencing of the expression of a selected gene by a homologous portion of double-stranded RNA. Also, referred to as RNA interference.

Tissue factor (TF) A procoagulant protein responsible for activation of the extrinsic coagulation pathways.

Introduction

In 1967, the first filovirus outbreak occurred in Germany and Yugoslavia among laboratory workers handling African green monkeys and/or tissues from contaminated monkeys imported from Uganda. The causative agent was identified as a new virus called Marburg virus (MARV). MARV re-emerged in 1975 in Johannesburg, South Africa, when a man who had recently returned from Zimbabwe became ill. The infection was spread to the man's traveling companion and a nurse at the hospital. While the man died of the disease, the other two cases recovered from the illness after receiving supportive care. The following year in 1976, a mysterious outbreak swept through several remote villages in Africa. The disease was rapidly fatal (318 cases; mortality rate 88%). Examination of samples revealed a previously unknown virus similar to that of the MARV. This virus was named Ebola after a local river in central Africa and became the second member of the family *Filoviridae*. Since 1976, there have been a number of outbreaks of both types of filoviruses. Isolation and characterization of the causative agents of the Ebola outbreaks resulted in the identification of a number of related viruses. Today *Filoviridae* forms a separate family within the order *Mononegavirales* and can be divided into two genera: *Marburgvirus* and *Ebolavirus*. The latter is composed of four distinct species with varying degrees of lethality in man, *Zaire ebolavirus* (~90% lethal), *Sudan ebolavirus* (~50 %), *Reston ebolavirus* (unknown lethality), and *Ivory Coast ebolavirus* (unknown lethality). In contrast, the MARV genus is composed of a single species, *Lake Victoria marburgvirus*. However, there have been a number of isolates of MARV identified with varying degrees of morbidity and mortality. The case–fatality (CF) rate from the most recent isolate, MARV-Angola, has been reported to be ~90%. Although there has been a tremendous amount of work performed on filoviruses, the source of these outbreaks remains undetermined and there remains no approved vaccine or therapeutic intervention.

Background

Ebola Virus History

Ebola virus (EBOV) was first discovered during near-simultaneous outbreaks in the former Zaire and Sudan. These outbreaks were due to serologically distinct viral species that would be designated ZEBOV and SEBOV, respectively. The CF was ~88% in the initial ZEBOV outbreak and ~53% in the SEBOV outbreak. The source of these outbreaks was never determined. These outbreaks were followed by several smaller outbreaks in the late 1970s. After an almost 20-year absence, a new EBOV outbreak was reported in 1989 in a colony of cynomolgus monkeys (*Macaca fascicularis*), imported from the Philippines to a holding facility in Reston (VA, USA). Although the Reston species appeared to be highly lethal in nonhuman primates (NHPs), no disease was reported in any of the documented human exposures. Although there have been a number of subsequent outbreaks of REBOV in NHP facilities both in and outside of the US, to date there have been no cases of human infections reported. Investigations traced the source of all REBOV outbreaks to a single export facility in the Philippines (Laguna Province); however, the original source and mechanism of entry into this facility remain unknown. In 1994, EBOV reemerged in Africa with the identification of a fourth species, ICEBOV, as well as the detection of ZEBOV for the first time in Gabon. The fourth species of EBOV, ICEBOV, was identified in Côte d'Ivoire following the exposure of a researcher during a necropsy to determine the cause of death of local chimpanzee populations. The source for the infection of the chimpanzees was undetermined. The outbreak in Gabon occurred in the Ogooue-Ivindo Province; a total of 51 cases and 31 deaths were documented (CF = 61%) in this outbreak.

The largest outbreak of EBOV occurred in 1995 in Kikwit, Democratic Republic of the Congo (DRC) (formerly Zaire). A total of 310 cases with 250 deaths (CF = 81%) were reported. Approximately one-fourth of all cases were reported among healthcare workers. This outbreak was quickly followed by two additional outbreaks that occurred in DRC and Gabon. Only one of the three primary cases identified could be linked to contact with a dead chimpanzee. A total of 31 cases with 21 deaths (CF = 68%) were documented. The second outbreak occurred as a series of unrelated cases in hunters during July and August 1996. Reminiscent of previous outbreaks (Gabon and Côte d'Ivoire), there were reports of several dead great apes (gorillas and chimpanzees) in the same area. A total of 60 cases with 45 deaths (CF = 75%) were reported. Interestingly, sequence analysis of the isolates from 1994 and 1996 differed by less than 0.1% in the glycoprotein and polymerase genes.

Ongoing, sporadic outbreaks of EBOV continue to be reported in central Africa. Most often, these outbreaks have been associated with infection of the great ape population. It is believed that these outbreaks are to blame for the widespread loss of these animals. It has been reported that the population of Western lowland gorillas has dropped by 50% and as much as 90% in some areas. Conservationists have stated that it will take decades for the populations of these animals to recover.

Marburg Virus History

MARV was first identified in 1967 during simultaneous outbreaks in Germany and Yugoslavia among laboratory workers handling African green monkeys and/or tissues from contaminated monkeys imported from Uganda. Secondary cases were reported among healthcare workers and family members. All secondary cases had direct contact with a primary case. A total of 32 cases and 7 deaths (CF = 21%) occurred during this outbreak. Over the next several decades MARV was associated with multiple sporadic and isolated cases among travelers and residents in southeast Africa.

From 1998 to 2000 a number of MARV cases were reported among young male workers at a gold mine in Durba, DRC. Cases were subsequently detected in the neighboring village. Although a few cases were detected among family members, secondary transmission appeared to be rare. Subsequent virological investigation revealed that these cases were due to multiple introductions of different strains

from an as-of-yet unidentified source. In total there were 154 cases with 128 deaths (CF = 83%) reported.

The largest and most deadly outbreak of MARV occurred in 2004–05 in the Uige Province of Angola. A total of 252 cases and 227 deaths (CF = 90%) were reported. Unlike previous outbreaks, a large number of the victims were children under the age of five. Virological analyses suggest that this isolate is very close to the strain from the original cases in 1967 in Europe. The reason for the increased virulence of the Angola isolate remains unclear.

Transmission

Both EBOV and MARV are transmitted by direct contact with the blood, secretions, organs, or other bodily fluids from infected persons, or infected animals. Many of the initial cases in outbreaks can be traced to the handling of infected animals, particularly chimpanzees and gorillas. Amplification has most often been associated with hospitals, where the virus is spread through nosocomial routes, or through burial ceremonies, where it is not uncommon for mourners to have direct contact with the deceased. While the modes of transmission have been well documented, the true source of these outbreaks and the reservoir for these viruses remain unclear. Although NHPs have been a source of infection for humans, the highly virulent nature of filoviruses in these animals suggests that they are not the reservoir. Different hypotheses have been developed to try to explain the origin of EBOV outbreaks. The presence of bats or contact with bat guano is often a common theme during outbreaks of both MARV and EBOV. Laboratory observation has shown that fruit and insectivorous bats experimentally infected with ZEBOV can support viral replication without apparent signs of illness. In a recent survey of small animals in Africa near areas of human or great ape EBOV outbreaks, asymptomatic infection of three species of fruit bats, *Hypsignathus monstrosus*, *Epomops franqueti*, and *Myonycteris torquata*, was reported. The exact ecology of EBOV and MARV remains to be determined and may include multiple natural reservoirs.

Virion Structure and Composition

Filoviruses are enveloped, nonsegmented, negative-strand RNA viruses. The virus envelope is derived from the lipid membrane envelope from the host cellular plasma membrane and therefore the lipid and protein composition reflect that of the infected cell. Filovirus virions have a characteristic thread-like, filamentous morphology (**Figure 1**). Pleomorphic virus structures ranging from straight tube-like structures, branched structures, and curved filaments shaped like a 6 (shepherd's crook), a U, or a circle. The diameter of filovirus virions are typically 80 nm, while the length can vary between 130 and 14 000 nm. The average length of a virus particle

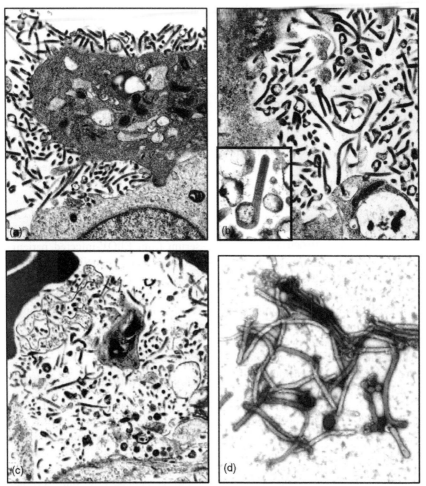

Figure 1 Electron micrographs of filoviruses. (a, b) Thin sections through Vero cells infected with MARV (Musoke strain). (c) Adrenal gland from a terminally ill mouse infected with mouse-adapted Ebola-Zaire. (d) Negative stain of Ebola-Reston virions recovered from serum of an experimentally infected NHP. Electron micrographs courtesy of Tom Geisbert and Densie Braun.

ranges from about 800 to 1000 nm with MARV being closer to 800 nm and EBOV closer to 1000 nm. Structurally, the virus particle is composed of seven viral proteins. The glycoprotein (GP), a type I transmembrane protein complex composed of two proteins, a $\sim$140 kDa GP_1 and $\sim$26 kDa GP_2. Normally, the two GP subunits are disulfide linked; however, when GP_1 is not disulfide-linked with GP_2, the GP_1 can be released in a soluble form from infected cells. Glycosylation, both N- and O-linked, provides approximately 50% of the GP mass. Complex cellular processing including glycosylation and proteolytic cleavage of the GP_1–GP_2 precursor protein leads to the generation of the GP_1–GP_2 heterotrimeric spikes in the virus envelope. GP_1 allows for receptor binding while GP_2 contains the fusion domain necessary for viral entry into the host cell. Surface projections of GP are dispersed evenly over the entire surface at 10 nm intervals. Functionally, the virus GP allows for attachment, receptor-mediated endocytosis, fusion with endocytotic vesicles, and release of the virion core into the host cell

cytoplasm. To date, no specific host cell receptor has been identified. A variety of putative receptors and cofactors have been identified including the asialoglycoprotein receptor, folate receptor-α, and C-type lectins. Given the wide cell tropism of the virus, or the receptors are likely either constitutively expressed proteins, that involve multiple proteins with conserved binding domains, or involve cofactors that facilitate virus entry. Viral particles may gain entry into the cell by co-opting common phagocytic pathways leading to a nonspecific entry mechanism.

The remaining six viral proteins are found within the virion, underlying the host-derived membrane. The viral protein 40 (VP40) functions as a matrix protein, and is essential for efficient viral assembly and budding. VP24 has been demonstrated to participate in the spontaneous formation of the nucleoprotein complex. Similar to VP40, studies indicate that VP24 behaves as a minor matrix protein. The nucleoprotein (NP) and VP30, VP35, polymerase (L) proteins, and the viral genomic RNA form the ribonucleoprotein complex. The nucleocapsids form a symmetrically helical filamentous structure underlying the viral envelope and the core structure has a striated appearance similar to that of rhabdoviruses. The L protein, the largest protein, functions as the virus-associated RNA-dependent RNA polymerase. VP30 functions as an EBOV-specific heterologous transcription activation factor that recognizes a secondary stem–loop structure during transcription. Similar to other transactivator factor proteins, VP30 exists in both phosphorylated and unphosphorylated forms within virions. In addition to their function as structural proteins, VP35 and VP24 have been shown to act as interferon antagonists.

Genome Organization and Expression

The linear genome is approximately 19 000 nt in length and consists of a single-stranded, negative-sense RNA (**Figure 2**). The genomic nucleic acid is not infectious. The genome contains highly conserved, transcription initiation and termination sites. Genomes contain intergenic sequence regions that vary in length, nucleotide sequences, and contain regions of gene overlap. While EBOV and MARV have a substantial degree of structural similarity in their respective genome organization, limited nucleotide sequence, homology is observed. Similar to the majority of other mononegaviruses, filovirus replication and transcription occurs in the cytoplasm of the infected cell. The viral-encoded RNA-dependent RNA polymerase generates full-length positive-sense antigenomes that serve as templates for the synthesis of the progeny negative-sense genomes. Filoviral subgenomic mRNAs are monocistronic and polyadenylated. A single genome contains seven genes that are arranged linearly. Monocistronic subgenomic mRNAs complementary to the viral RNA lead to the generation of seven filovirus proteins found within the virion. For both MARV and EBOV, each gene encodes a single polypeptide, except for the GP. The structural glycoprotein GP_1 and GP_2 are generated as a single precursor polypeptide that is cleaved by host cell pro-protein convertases to generate the two subunits of the final protein. EBOV is different from MARV in that an additional viral protein is generated; a nonstructural, soluble form of GP, referred to as secreted GP (sGP). sGP is translated from an mRNA that has undergone RNA editing. Interestingly, the majority of GP mRNA encodes for the sGP which has been detected in cell culture and serum from EBOV-infected patients. Both soluble GP_1 and sGP have been implicated in the pathogenesis of EBOV by acting as decoy proteins that sequester neutralizing antibodies during infection; however, the exact role of the soluble forms of GP remains to be elucidated.

Pathogenesis

Clinical Features/Presentation

The clinical manifestations of EBOV and MARV are often compared to that of severe sepsis or septic shock. Following a 2–21 day incubation period, cases often present with a variety of nonspecific symptoms including high fever, chills, malaise, and myalgia. As the disease progresses, there is evidence of multisystemic involvement, and

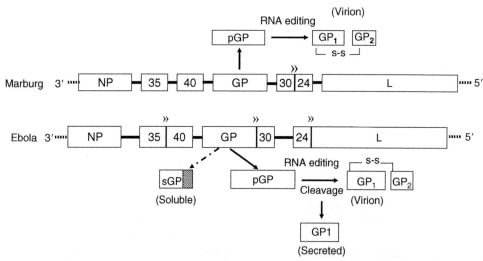

Figure 2 Filovirus genome organization and generation of glycoproteins. Linear, negative-sense, single-stranded, RNA monopartite genome, ~19 000 nt. Relative positions of the encoding regions for viral proteins depicted as boxes; NP, nucleoprotein; 35, VP35; 40, VP40; GP, glycoprotein; 30, VP30; 24, VP24; L, viral polymerase. Leader and trailer and intergenic regions (nontranscribed regions) shown as lines. Overlapping regions indicated by ≫ symbol. For Ebola, glycoprotein gene generates a soluble GP (sGP) and precursor GP (pGP). pGPs for Ebola and Marburg are cleaved by host-derived enzymes to generate a GP_1 and GP_2 subunit that are disulfide linked.

manifestations include prostration, anorexia, vomiting, nausea, abdominal pain, diarrhea, shortness of breath, hypotension, edema, confusion, maculopapular rash, and eventually coma. Patients normally progress rapidly with death occurring 6–9 days after the onset of symptoms. The development of petechiae, ecchymoses, mucosal hemorrhages, and uncontrolled bleeding at venipuncture sites are indicative of development of abnormalities in coagulation and fibrinolysis. Massive loss of blood is atypical and, when present, is largely restricted to the gastrointestinal tract. Fulminant infection typically evolves to shock, convulsions, and, in most cases, diffuse coagulopathy.

Animal Models

While only limited information is available for pathophysiology of human cases of EBOV or MARV, a lot has been learned from studies employing experimentally infected NHPs. Although the majority of studies in humans and NHPs to date have focused on ZEBOV, limited studies suggest that MARV may behave in a similar manner. EBOV and MARV are most often characterized by three common factors: development of lymphocyte apoptosis, aberrant production of pro-inflammatory cytokines, and the development of coagulation abnormalities. Sequential analysis of samples collected from ZEBOV-infected NHP shows early and prominent infection of monocyte/macrophages (MO/Φ) and dendritic cells (DCs). The importance of this selective targeting has been well documented. Infection of the MO/Φ not only facilitates distribution of virus to the spleen and lymph nodes but also triggers a cascade of events including the upregulation and production of the procoagulant protein tissue factor (TF) as well as a number of pro-inflammatory cytokines/chemokines and oxygen free radicals. *In vitro* studies of human MO/Φ have confirmed these observations. Similar to septic shock caused by bacterial pathogens, disease triggered by EBOV or MARV infection is thought to involve inappropriate or maladaptive host responses. It is likely that these responses are more important to the development of the observed pathology than any structural damage directly induced by viral replication. Infection of DC likely facilitates disease progression by hindering the ability of the host to orchestrate an effective immune response to clear the virus.

Although lymphocytes do not appear to be productively infected by filoviruses, the importance of their role in the development of the disease pathology cannot be understated. The loss of lymphocytes through apoptosis has been well documented. Flow cytometry demonstrated a striking loss of circulating CD8+ T cells and natural killer (NK) cells prior to or corresponding with the onset of symptoms. The exact mechanism(s) responsible for triggering this widespread loss of lymphocytes remains unclear. RNA analysis of peripheral blood mononuclear cells

(PBMCs) collected from NHPs has demonstrated the upregulation of a number of pro-apoptotic genes and anti-apoptotic genes.

Infection of MO/Φ also appears to be critical in the triggering and propagation of the coagulation abnormalities observed in filovirus infections. Recently, it was demonstrated that infection of MO/Φ *in vitro* or *in vivo* resulted in the upregulation of TF. Interestingly, this expression was observed only in infected cells, suggesting a direct correlation with the virus. Analysis of sera from infected animals revealed the presence of microparticles or small membrane vesicles with procoagulant and pro-inflammatory properties. Analysis of these microparticles showed that many of these expressed TF and may therefore have been derived from filovirus-infected MO/Φ.

The contribution of the endothelium as well as the infection of endothelium remains controversial. *In vitro* studies have demonstrated that endothelial cells are easily infected by either MARV or EBOV. However, analysis of tissues collected from human cases has produced conflicting results. Analysis of sequential tissues from NHP suggests that endothelial cells are not targeted until the later stages of disease. Electron microscopy examination of tissues showed activation of endothelial cells but no widespread damage to the vasculature. Analyses of clinical chemistries support this observation, with a drop in small molecular weight proteins but not total proteins. The cause for this vascular leakage is unclear and is likely multifactorial. Fibrin degradation products (FDPs), thrombin, reactive oxygen species, pro-inflammatory cytokines, as well as activation of the complement and kinin systems can all contribute to increased vascular permeability. Rapid increases in levels of D-dimers were observed in sera of EBOV-infected NHP with initial increases being detected before the onset of clinical symptoms. While the contributions of the complement and kinin systems in the development of EBOV and MARV pathogenesis are yet to be evaluated, the production of pro-inflammatory cytokines and oxygen free radicals has been well documented. In EBOV-infected NHP, IFN-α, interleukin-6 (IL-6), monocyte chemoattractant protein 1 (MCP-1), macrophage inflammatory protein (MIP)-1α, and MIP-1β were detected in sera at the early to mid-stages of disease. IFN-β, IFN-γ, IL-18, and TNF-α were also detected in sera but not until the later stages of disease.

In recent years, the importance of the interaction between coagulation and inflammation as a response to severe infection has become increasingly appreciated. In addition to driving upregulation of procoagulant proteins, inflammatory mediator, may inhibit fibrinolytic activity, and downregulate natural anticoagulant pathways, in particular, the protein C anticoagulant pathway. Uncontrolled activation of coagulation systems may lead to disseminated intravascular coagulation (DIC). DIC is a syndrome with both bleeding and thrombotic abnormalities characterized in part by the presence of histologically visible microthrombi in the microvasculature. These microthrombi may hamper tissue perfusion and thereby contribute to multiple organ dysfunction and high mortality rates. Before acute DIC can become apparent, there must be a sufficient stimulus to deplete or overwhelm the natural anticoagulant systems. During activation of the clotting system, the host regulates the process through the production and activation of a variety of inhibitors of the clotting system. In this process, however, the inhibitors are consumed, and if the rate of consumption exceeds the rate synthesized by liver parenchymal cells, plasma levels of inhibitors will decline. Analysis of tissue and sera from ZEBO-infected NHPs shows widespread fibrin deposition and marked decreases in plasma levels of protein C. The drops in protein C correlate with increase in D-dimers and disease progression.

Host Responses

The low sporadic disease incidence and remote locations of most outbreaks have led to limited careful study of the host responses to virus infection. Perturbations of the innate and acquired immune responses are consistent with fatal disease outcome. In a few studies patients that survived Ebola infections were reported to have generated a virus-specific immunoglobulin M (IgM) response and to have transient expression of pro-inflammatory cytokines. In sharp contrast, fatal EBOV cases have dysregulated cytokine expression levels, coagulation abnormalities, fibrin deposition, DIC, and evidence of cell death and the lack of an effective adaptive immune response. Through direct and indirect mechanisms, and pathways that are not clearly understood, the fatal cases are associated with the lack of B- or T-lymphocyte responses. Altered innate responses, both cellular and soluble, combined with early infection of MO/Φ and DC, likely impair the host's ability to initiate an appropriate adaptive immune response to clear filovirus-infected cells. Simultaneously, virus-induced or inappropriate host defenses lead to dysregulated innate immune responses. Filovirus proteins VP35 and VP24 interfere with and modulate these key immune pathways by inhibiting cellular antiviral defenses. Ultimately, these events result in immune dysregulation and uncontrolled explosive virus replication.

Animal models have offered some insight into protective immune responses. In EBOV infection in mice, early interferon responses are vital to controlling virus replication. In concert, EBOV-specific antibody and cellular responses help eliminate virus infection in this animal model. Protective filovirus vaccines have been shown to induce antibody and/or cellular responses that offer protection in rodents and NHPs. Therefore, an appropriate innate and adaptive immune response can offer immunity to both MARV and EBOV.

Treatment and Prevention

Currently, there are no approved therapies or vaccines for the treatment and/or prevention of EBOV and MARV. Control and treatment are limited to containment and basic supportive care. Suspected cases should be isolated from other patients and strict-barrier-nursing techniques implemented. Contact tracing and follow-up of people who may have been exposed through close contact with cases are essential. If not already implemented proper disinfection and handling of materials from infected patients must be initiated. Education of the community as to the presentation of the disease, the nature by which it is transmitted, and the sources by which patients are likely to come into contact with the virus are critical to preventing and containing future outbreaks.

Although there are no approved vaccines there has been considerable progress in the identification and successful testing of candidate vaccines in animal models. These platforms can be separated into several categories: replication-deficient platforms, replication-competent platforms, and virus-like particles (VLPs). The replication-deficient platforms are viral vectors such as adenovirus or Venezuelan equine encephalitis virus (VEEV) expressing filoviral proteins. The first successful strategy to protect NHP from EBOV employed a replication-deficient adenovirus expressing EBOV GP and NP. In this strategy, a DNA prime of GP and NP genes was followed by an adenovirus-expressing GP boost. Subsequent studies demonstrated protection using a single adenovirus GP vaccination 28 days before EBOV challenge. Questions have been raised about the durability of the replication-deficient strategies as well as the ability of these strategies to overcome any pre-existing immunity to the vaccine platform. Efficacy has also recently been demonstrated using a live-attenuated (replication-competent) vesicular stomatitis virus (VSV) expressing the GP of EBOV. Additional work demonstrated that by simply swapping out the EBOV GP for either the MARV or Lassa fever virus GP, this platform could provide full protection against lethal MARV or Lassa fever virus challenge, respectively. The VSV platform has the additional benefit in that it has been demonstrated to provide 100% protection against MARV when administered 30 min after MARV exposure and ~50% protection for EBOV when rapidly administered in an EBOV post-exposure setting. While it is likely that the replication-competent platforms may provide increased durability there is some concern about the safety of administration of any live vaccine. Therefore, additional studies are needed to fully evaluate the safety profile of this platform. Finally, filovirus-like particles generated by the co-expression of viral membrane proteins (GP and VP40) are currently being evaluated in NHPs. This strategy may be beneficial in that it will likely overcome the safety concern associated with the use of live-attenuated platforms and/or the issues of preexisting immunity. Consistent with other protein vaccines, there are concerns about the durability of the immunity, adjuvant choice, as well as the necessary dosing regimen to achieve long-lasting immunity.

In addition to the wealth of candidate vaccine platforms developed and tested over the last few years, there have also been a number of candidate therapeutics that been evaluated in animal models. These strategies have met with varying degrees of success and can be divided into two basic categories, those that directly target the virus and those that target the host and/or the disease manifestations in the host. Recently, investigators reported success using either antisense oligonucleotides or RNA interference (RNAi) corresponding to sequences in the viral genomic or mRNA *in vivo*. Additional studies will be needed to evaluate whether the antisense technology can provide any therapeutic value when used after exposure and whether the success of the RNAi strategies in guinea pig models will translate into the more stringent NHP models. Reduction in morbidity and mortality has also been observed using therapeutics targeting the clinical manifestations in the NHP models. Treatment of ZEBOV-infected NHP with a recombinant protein, recombinant nematode anticoagulant protein c2 (rNAPc2) that blocks the TF-mediated activation of the extrinsic pathway of blood coagulation, resulted in ~33% survival as well a substantial increase in the mean time to death. Interestingly, substantial reductions in plasma levels of IL-6, MCP-1, and viral load were noted in rNAPc2-treated animals. It is unknown if treatment with other anticoagulant strategies that block the intrinsic and/or common pathways may also offer comparable and/or improved therapeutic benefit.

Finally, it is important to mention therapeutic strategies that are yet to provide any survival benefit when tested in NHP models. Although type I IFNs have shown promise in the mouse model of EBOV infection, testing of IFN-α2 failed to protect NHPs against EBOV or MARV. In addition, *S*-adenosylhomocysteine, which had been hypothesized to protect mice against EBOV, at least in part through induction of a type I IFN response, also failed to protect NHP. Currently, alternative IFN therapies and formulations are under evaluation. It is unclear if these approaches will have any improved efficacy in NHPs. In addition, heparin, convalescent serum, and equine anti-EBOV immunoglobulin have been used to treat infections in humans and/or NHPs, but were inconsistent and appeared to be of little therapeutic value. While passive antibody treatment has been successful in mice, the benefit of antibody immunotherapy remains controversial. Although results in rodent models have been encouraging, initial studies in NHPs have not been as successful. Additional studies are needed to fully evaluate the utility of this therapeutic avenue.

Acknowledgments

Work on filoviruses at USAMRIID was supported by the Medical Chemical/Biological Defense Research Program, US Army Medical Research, and Material Command.

See also: Ebolavirus.

Further Reading

Bosio CM, Moore BD, Warfield KL, *et al.* (2004) Ebola and Marburg virus-like particles activate human myeloid dendritic cells. *Virology* 326: 280–287.

Feldmann H, Geisbert TW, Jahrling PB, *et al.* (2004) *Filoviridae*. In: Fauquet C, Mayo MA, Maniloff J, Desselberger U, and Ball LA (eds.) *Virus Taxonomy: Eighth Report of the International Committee on Taxonomy of Viruses,*, pp 645–653. San Diego, CA: Elsevier Academic Press.

Feldmann H, Volchkov VE, Volchkova VA, and Kenk HD (1999) The glycoproteins of Marburg and Ebola virus and their potential roles in pathogenesis. *Archives of Virology Supplementum* 15: 159–169.

Geisbert TW, Young HA, Jahrling PB, Davis KJ, Kagan E, and Hensley LE (2003) Mechanisms underlying coagulation abnormalities in Ebola hemorrhagic fever: Overexpression of tissue factor in primate monocytes/macrophages is a key event. *Journal of Infectious Diseases* 1(188): 1618–1629.

Grolla A, Lucht A, Dick D, Strong JE, and Feldmann H (2005) Laboratory diagnosis of Ebola and Marburg hemorrhagic fever. *Bulletin de la Société de Pathologie Exotique* 98(3): 205–209.

Harlieb B and Weissenhorn W (2006) Filovirus assembly and budding. *Virology* 344: 64–70.

Hensley LE, Jones SM, Feldmann H, Jahrling PB, and Geisbert TW (2005) Ebola and Marburg viruses: Pathogenesis and development of countermeasures. *Current Molecular Medicine* 5: 761–772.

Ignatyev GM (1999) Immune response to filovirus infections. *Current Topics in Microbiology and Immunology* 235: 205–217.

Jones SM, Feldmann H, Stroher U, *et al.* (2005) Live attenuated recombinant vaccine protects nonhuman primates against Ebola and Marburg viruses. *Nature Medicine* 11: 786–790.

Mohamadzadeh M, Chen L, Olinger GG, Pratt WD, and Schmaljohn AL (2006) Filoviruses and the balance of innate, adaptive, and inflammatory responses. *Viral Immunology* 19: 602–612.

Paragas J and Geisbert TW (2006) Development of treatment strategies to combat Ebola and Marburg viruses. *Expert Review Anti-Infective Therapy* 4: 67–76.

Peterson AT, Bauer JT, and Mills JN (2004) Ecologic and geographic distribution of filovirus disease. *Emerging Infectious Diseases* 10: 40–47.

Reed DS, Hensley LE, Geisbert JB, Jahrling PB, and Geisbert TW (2004) Depletion of peripheral blood T lymphocytes and NK cells during the course of Ebola hemorrhagic fever in cynomolgus macaques. *Viral Immunology* 17: 390–400.

Schnittler HJ and Feldmann H (1999) Molecular pathogenesis of filovirus infections: Role of macrophages and endothelial cells. *Current Topics in Microbiology and Immunology* 235: 175–204.

Theriault S, Groseth A, Artsob H, and Feldmann H (2005) The role of reverse genetics systems in determining filovirus pathogenicity. *Archives of Virology Supplementum* 19: 157–177.

Hantaviruses

A Vaheri, University of Helsinki, Helsinki, Finland

Glossary

Coevolution Evolution of a virus together with its rodent/insectivore host.
Hantavirus A virus in the genus *Hantavirus.*
Reassortant A virus having genome segments of two different viruses.
Robovirus A virus transmitted from rodents to other vertebrates without arthropods.
Sympatric Occupying the same or overlapping geographic areas without interbreeding.

Historical Introduction

Hantavirus infections are not new to humankind. The first description of a hemorrhagic fever with renal syndrome (HFRS)-like disease can be found in a Chinese medical account written in about AD 960 and the earliest definite description of HFRS comes from Far East Russian clinical records dating back to 1913. During World Wars I and II, HFRS became an important military problem; for example, 'field nephritis' in Flanders during World War I may well have been caused by a hantavirus. In Manchuria in the mid-1930s, 12 000 Japanese soldiers caught the disease and military researchers were investigating the cause of the disease, sometimes using prisoners of war in infection experiments. Finnish and German soldiers encountered an HFRS-like epidemic in Finnish Lapland in 1943–44. During the Korean conflict in 1950–53, the disease again gained much attention when about 3000 United Nations troops contracted it – since then known as Korean hemorrhagic fever – with a 5–10% case–fatality rate. The milder form of HFRS, nephropathia epidemica (NE), common in Fennoscandia (Scandinavia and Finland), was first described by Swedish authors in 1934. However, the infecting agent of HFRS remained unknown until 1976, when the Korean researcher Ho Wang Lee discovered that cryostat-sectioned lungs of striped field mice (*Apodemus agrarius*), trapped near the Hantaan river, contained virus-specific antigen reactive with HFRS-patient sera. By a similar approach, the causative agent of NE was demonstrated in 1980 in bank voles, *Clethryonomys glareolus*, trapped in Puumala, Finland. Another agent, this one from urban rats in Seoul, Korea, was also found to cause HFRS. In the early 1990s, a further distinct European human-pathogenic hantavirus was isolated from the yellow-necked mouse, *Apodemus flavicollis,*

near the village of Dobrava in Slovenia, and a few years later, the related, less pathogenic, Saaremaa virus from striped field mice on Saaremaa Island, Estonia. Thottapalayam virus from an insectivore (*Suncus murinus,* a shrew) in India, Prospect Hill virus from a meadow vole (Microtus *pennsylvanicus*) in USA, and Thailand virus from a bandicoot rat (*Bandicota indica*) already had been isolated in the early 1970s to the 1980s – they all apparently are nonpathogenic for humans.

Human disease had not been known to be caused by a hantavirus in the Americas until a cluster of acute respiratory distress syndrome cases with a high (60%) case–fatality rate in the Four Corners area of the American Southwest (where Arizona, Utah, Colorado, and New Mexico are contiguous) was recognized in May 1993. Subsequent studies led to the discovery of Sin Nombre virus and other hantaviruses that cause hantavirus pulmonary syndrome (HPS), all transmitted from sigmodontine rodents indigenous to the New World. An increasing number of pathogenic hantaviruses have been reported in South America, including Andes virus, which can be transmitted person to person, and which have high case–fatality rates. While only about 2000 HPS cases have been reported so far, approximately 150 000 HFRS cases are estimated to occur worldwide annually.

Virology

Hantaviruses are enveloped viruses with a tripartite negative-stranded RNA genome and belong to the genus *Hantavirus* of the large virus family *Bunyaviridae.* The 6.4 kb L (large) genome segment encodes the $\sim$250 kDa RNA polymerase, the $\sim$3.6 kb M (medium) segment, the two glycoproteins 68–76 kDa Gn and 52–58 kDa Gc (formerly known as G1 and G2), and the $\sim$1.7 kb S (small) segment the 50–54 kDa nucleocapsid protein (N). In addition, the S segment of hantaviruses carried by arvicolid and sigmodontine rodents has another overlapping (+1) open reading frame (ORF) named NSs, which has been shown to inhibit the interferon response. Viral messenger RNAs of the members of the *Bunyaviridae* are not polyadenylated and are truncated relative to the genomic RNAs at the 3′ termini. Messenger RNAs have 5′-methylated caps and 10–18 nontemplated nucleotides derived from host cell mRNAs. The termini of all three segments are highly conserved and complementary to each other, a feature that has assisted in cloning and discovery of new hantaviruses.

Unlike most other bunyaviruses, hantaviruses are not arthropod borne (arboviruses), but are rodent borne (roboviruses). Each hantavirus is primarily carried by a distinct rodent/insectivore species, although several host switches seem to have occurred during the tens of millions of years of their co-evolution with their carrier hosts. We now know that the genetic diversity of hantaviruses is generated by (1) genetic drift (accumulation of point mutations and insertions/deletions) leading to mixtures of closely related genetic variants, quasispecies; (2) genetic shift (reassortment of genome fragments within a given virus genotype/species); and (3) according to recent findings, also by homologous recombination, a mechanism not previously observed for negative-strand RNA viruses.

Ecology and Epidemiology

Hantavirus infections are prime examples of emerging and reemerging infections. As are most of these infections, hantaviral diseases are zoonoses. With the exception of the South American Andes virus, hantavirus infections are thought to be transmitted to humans primarily from aerosols of rodent excreta (feces, urine, saliva). Only some hantaviruses cause disease in humans. In Asia, Hantaan and Amur viruses, carried by *Apodemus* spp. mice, cause severe HFRS, and Seoul virus, carried by rats, a milder disease. In Europe, there are three major hantaviral pathogens: Puumala virus carried by bank voles causes NE; Dobrava virus, carried by yellow-necked mice, causes severe HFRS; and the genetically and antigenically closely related Saaremaa virus carried by striped field mice causes mild NE-like disease. There also are reports that Seoul virus, carried by rats (*Rattus norvegicus* and *Rattus rattus*), causes HFRS of moderate severity both in Europe and North America. In addition, European common voles (*Microtus arvalis* and *Microtus rossiaemeridionalis*) carry Tula hantavirus, which can asymptomatically infect humans. Topografov hantavirus isolated from Siberian lemmings (*Lemmus sibiricus*) has not been detected in North European lemmings (*Lemmus lemmus*), although it can replicate in them. Infections of hantaviruses in rodents are asymptomatic and, often, persistent.

Hantavirus infections are quite common in Europe. Puumala virus occurs in Northern Europe, European Russia, and parts of central-western Europe. Dobrava virus is found mainly in the Balkans and the neighboring Central European areas. Saaremaa virus has been detected in Eastern and Central Europe, and in Slovenia the two viruses Dobrava and Saaremaa occur sympatrically. Apart from infections of laboratory rats, Seoul virus has been detected in wild rats in France and in several city harbors. It is apparent that many parts of Europe, such as Britain, Poland, and Byelorussia, and most of Africa,

remain completely or relatively unstudied with regard to hantaviruses. This suggests either that HFRS is rare or nonexistent in these regions or is not generally recognized and is not diagnosed by local biomedical communities.

In Northern Europe, HFRS as well as the carrier rodents exhibit peaks in 3–4 year cycles, while in Central Europe the HFRS incidence follows the fluctuations of 'mast years', that is, the abundance of beech and oak seeds for the hantavirus-carrying rodents. In Central Europe, HFRS peaks in the summer whereas in Northern Europe most cases occur in late autumn and early winter, from November to January. Risk factors for acquiring hantavirus infections and HFRS include professions such as forestry, farming, and military, or activities such as camping, and the use of summer cottages. Cigarette smokers and males are more likely to be infected than are females. In the Americas, the increased precipitation during El Niño/Southern Oscillation in South and North America has been suggested as the main reason for the peaks in rodent population densities and for the consequent increased number of HPS cases.

Sigmodontine-borne hantaviruses circulating in North America (**Table 1**) form three phylogenetically distinct groups: those associated with *Peromyscus* spp. and *Reithrodontomys* spp. rodents, and the third carried by *Sigmodon* spp. and *Oryzomys* spp. rats. The first group carries both human pathogens (Sin Nombre virus, New York virus) and viruses not thus far associated with human disease (e.g., Blue River virus, Limestone Canyon virus). *Reithrodontomys*-borne viruses have not been shown to cause human disease. Hantaviruses discovered in South America are associated with several tribes of Sigmodontinae, mostly Oryzomyini-associated viruses, several of which are important human pathogens, including Andes, Lechiguanas, and Laguna Negra viruses. Results of phylogenetic analyses of South American hantaviruses suggest that several host-switching events have occurred during coevolution with their rodent hosts. The phylogenetic split between murine and sigmodontine rodents presumably dates to a divergence that occurred between subfamilies 30 million years ago, when the precursors of the sigmodontine rodents crossed the Bering Strait into the Americas. Notably, sigmodontine rodents are found only in the Americas and thus it is unlikely that HPS would occur in Eurasia, unless imported.

Clinical Picture and Pathogenesis

Amur, Dobrava, Hantaan, Seoul, Puumala, and Saaremaa viruses all cause HFRS but the infections differ considerably in severity. All are characterized by acute-onset, fever, headache, abdominal pains, backache, temporary renal insufficiency (first oliguria, proteinuria, and increase in serum creatinine, and then polyuria), and

Table 1   Hantavirus types

Virus	Host	Distribution (origin)	Disease
Murid-borne viruses	Mice and rats		
Hantaan (HTNV)[a]	Striped field mouse (*Apodemus agrarius*)	Asia (Korea)	HFRS
Da Bie Shan	Chinese white-bellied rat (*Niviventer confucianus*)	Asia (China)	NR
Seoul (SEOV)	Rat (*Rattus rattus, R. norvegicus*)	Worldwide (Korea)	HFRS
Dobrava (DOBV)	Yellow-necked mouse (*A. flavicollis*)	Europe (Slovenia)	HFRS
Saaremaa (SAAV)	Striped field mouse; western (*A. agrarius*)	Europe (Estonia)	HFRS
Thailand (THAIV)	Bandicoot rat (*Bandicota indica*)	Thailand (Thailand)	NR
Amur (AMRV)	Korean field mouse (*A. peninsulae*)	Asia (Far East Russia, China)	HFRS
Arvicolid-borne viruses	Voles and lemmings		
Puumala (PUUV)	Bank vole (*Clethrionomys glareolus*)	Europe (Finland)	HFRS
Hokkaido (HOKV)	Red bank vole (*C. rufocanus*)	Asia (Japan)	NR
Tula (TULV)	European common vole (*Microtus arvalis*)	Europe (Russia)	NR
Prospect Hill (PHV)	Meadow vole (*M. pennsylvanicus*)	North America (USA)	NR
Bloodland Lake (BLLV)	Prairie vole (*M. ochrogaster*)	North America (USA)	NR
Isla Vista (ISLAV)	Californian vole (*M. californicus*)	North America (USA)	NR
Khabarovsk (KHAV)	Reed vole (*M. fortis*)	Asia (Far East Russia)	NR
Topografov (TOPV)	Lemming (*Lemmus sibiricus*)	Siberia (Russia)	NR
Vladivostok (VLAV)	Reed vole (*M. fortis*)	Asia (Far East Russia)	NR
Sigmodontine borne	New World sigmodontine rodents		
Sin Nombre (SNV)	Deer mouse (*Peromyscus maniculatus*)	North America (USA)	HPS
Monongahela (MGLV)	Deer mouse (*P. maniculatus nubiterrae*)	North America (USA)	HPS
New York (NYV)	White-footed mouse (*P. leucopus*)	North America (USA)	HPS
Blue River (BRV)	White-footed mouse (*P. leucopus*)	North America (USA)	NR
Limestone Canyon (LCV)	Brush mouse (*P. boylii*)	North America (USA)	NR
Bayou (BAYV)	Rice rat (*Oryzomys palustris*)	North America (USA)	HPS
Black Creek Canal (BCCV)	Hispid cotton rat (*Sigmodon hispidus*)	North America (USA)	HPS
Muleshoe (MULV)	Hispid cotton rat (*S. hispidus*)	North America (USA)	NR
Andes (ANDV)	Long-tailed pygmy rice rat (*Oligoryzomys longicaudatus*)	South America (Argentina)	HPS
Lechiguanas (LECV)	Rice rat (*O. flavescence*)	South America (Argentina)	HPS
Oran (ORNV)	*O. longicaudatus*	South America (Argentina)	NR
Bermejo (BERV)	*O. chacoensis*	South America (Argentina)	NR
HU39694	Unknown	South America (Argentina)	HPS
Choclo (CHOV)	Pygmy rice rat (*O. fulvescens*)	Central America (Panama)	HPS
Calabazo	*Zygodontomys brevicauda*	Central America (Panama)	NR
Laguna Negra (LANV)	Vesper mouse (*Calomys laucha*)	South America (Paraguay)	HPS
Rio Mamore (RIOMV)	Small-eared pygmy rice rat (*O. microtis*)	South America (Bolivia)	NR
Caño Delgadito (CADV)	Cane mouse (*S. alstoni*)	South America (Venezuela)	NR
El Moro Canyon (ELMCV)	Western harvest mouse (*Reithrodontomys megalotis*)	North America (USA)	NR
Rio Segundo (RIOSV)	Mexican harvest mouse (*R. mexicanus*)	Central America (Costa Rica)	NR
Maciel (MACV)	Dark field mouse (*Necromys benefactus*)	South America (Argentina)	NR
Pergamino (PERV)	Grass field mouse (*Akodon azarae*)	South America (Argentina)	NR
Juquitiba	Unknown	South America (Brazil)	HPS
Araraquara	Unknown	South America (Brazil)	HPS
Castelo dos Sonhos	Unknown	South America (Brazil)	HPS
Insectivore-borne	Insectivores		
Thottapalayam (TPMV)	Asian house shrew (*Suncus murinus*)	Asia (India)	NR

Distinct hantavirus species listed in the 8th ICTV Report are shown in bold.
HFRS, hemorrhagic fever with renal syndrome; HPS, hantavirus pulmonary syndrome; NR, disease not recorded.
[a]Type species.

thrombocytopenia, but the extent of hemorrhages (hematuria, petechiae, internal hemorrhages), requirement for dialysis treatment, hypotension, and case–fatality rates are much higher in HFRS caused by Amur, Dobrava, or Hantaan viruses than in NE caused by Puumala or Saaremaa viruses. About a third of NE patients experience temporary visual disturbances (myopia), which is a very characteristic if not pathognomonic sign of the disease. Notably, the clinical consequences of all of the hantaviral pathogens in humans vary from none to fatal. Severe NE is associated with a certain haplotype, HLA-B8, DR3, DQ2 alleles, severe HPS with HLA-B35, and mild NE with HLA-B27. Yet, although Puumala virus infection is generally associated with mild HFRS, NE may have significant long-term consequences. A 5 year followup study demonstrated that 20% of NE patients had a somewhat increased systolic blood pressure and proteinuria. This is important, since the infection is so common in many areas of Europe. In addition, in some patients, Puumala virus infection may infect the pituitary gland and lead to mortality or at least to hypophyseal insufficiency requiring hormone-replacement therapy.

The pathogeneses of HFRS and HPS are poorly understood. However, it is known that β3 integrins can mediate the entry of pathogenic hantaviruses and that hantaviruses can regulate apoptosis. Also, there is evidence that increased capillary permeability is an essential component in the pathogenesis of both HFRS and HPS, although different target tissues, kidneys and lungs, respectively, are affected in the two diseases. HFRS and HPS patients show activation of tumor necrosis factor α (TNF-α) in the plasma and tissues and high levels of urinary secretion of the pro-inflammatory cytokine interleukin 6 (IL-6) are seen in NE. Studies with a monkey model mimicking human Puumala virus infection and HPS-like disease in Andes virus-infected Syrian hamsters may assist in elucidating the mechanism of pathogenesis.

HPS is characterized by pulmonary edema but death often results from cardiac failure; thus the term hantavirus cardiopulmonary syndrome (HCPS) has been proposed for the disease. HFRS and HPS, although primarily targeted at kidneys and lungs, respectively, share a number of clinical features, such as capillary leakage, TNF-α, and thrombocytopenia; notably, hemorrhages and alterations in renal function occur also in HPS and pulmonary involvement is not rare in HFRS.

Of the four structural proteins, both in humoral and cellular immunity, the nucleocapsid protein appears to be the principal immunogen. Cytotoxic T-lymphocyte responses are seen in both HFRS and HPS and may be important for both protective immunity and pathogenesis in hantavirus infections.

Diagnostics and Prevention

The diagnosis of acute hantavirus infection is primarily based on serology. Both immunofluorescence tests and enzyme immunoassays are widely used for detection of specific IgM or low-avidity IgG antibodies, characteristics of acute infection. In addition, immunochromatographic 5 min IgM-antibody tests have been developed. Hantaviruses show extensive serological cross-reactivity, especially within each of the three virus subgroups (murid, arvicolid, and sigmodontine borne; **Table 1**), but for accurate typing, neutralization tests are needed. For example, in Paraguay, a considerable seroprevalence of

hantavirus antibodies, as high as 40%, is noted in people without a history of HPS. Average seroprevalences in Finland and Sweden suggest that only 10–25% of Puumala virus infections are diagnosed; thus, most infections either are subclinical or are mild or atypical and remain undiagnosed.

Viral RNA usually can be detected in the blood of HPS patients using polymerase chain reaction with samples collected during the first week of illness, which is useful because it also identifies the infecting virus genotype. The same is true for severe forms of HFRS but in the case of Puumala virus infections, viral RNA cannot be regularly detected in the blood or urine of NE patients.

Vaccines against hantaviral infections have been used for years in China and Korea, but not in Europe or the Americas. No specific therapy is used in Europe, but both ribavirin and interferon-α have been administered in trials in China. A major problem is that at the time the patients are hospitalized, the rate of virus replication is declining, so that reduction of virus replication no longer is necessary for the patient. Thus, prevention of hantaviral infections continues to rely on reduced contact with excreta from infected rodents.

See also: Bunyaviruses: General Features; Human Eye Infections; Zoonoses.

Further Reading

Brummer-Korvenkontio M, Vapalahti O, Henttonen H, Koskela P, Kuusisto P, and Vaheri A (1999) Epidemiological study of nephropathia epidemica in Finland 1989–96. *Scandinavian Journal of Infectious Diseases* 31: 427–435.

Calisher CH (ed.) (1990) *Hemorrhagic Fever with Renal Syndrome, Tick and Mosquito-Borne Viruses: Archives of Virology, Supplementum 1*, pp. 1–347. Vienna: Springer.

Fauquet CM, Mayo MA, Maniloff J, Desselberger U,, and Ball LA (eds.) (2005) *Virus Taxonomy: Eighth Report of the International Committee on Taxonomy of Viruses, Bunyaviridae, Hantavirus*, pp. 704–707. San Diego, CA: Elsevier Academic Press.

Kallio-Kokko H, Uzcategui N, Vapalahti O, and Vaheri A (2005) Viral zoonoses in Europe. *FEMS Microbiology Reviews* 29: 1051–1077.

Kaukinen P, Vaheri A, and Plyusnin A (2005) Hantavirus nucleocapsid protein: A multifunctional molecule with both housekeeping and ambassadorial duties. *Archives of Virology* 150: 1693–1713.

Khaiboullina SF, Morzunov SP, and St. Jeor SC (2005) Hantaviruses: Molecular biology, evolution and pathogenesis. *Current Molecular Medicine* 5: 773–790.

Kukkonen SKJ, Vaheri A, and Plyusnin A (2005) L protein, the RNA-dependent RNA polymerase of hantaviruses. *Archives of Virology* 150: 533–555.

Maes P, Clement J, Gavrilovskaya I, and Van Ranst M (2004) Hantaviruses: Immunology, treatment, and prevention. *Viral Immunology* 17: 481–497.

Muranyi W, Bahr U, Zeier M, and van der Woude FJ (2005) Hantavirus infection. *Journal of the American Society of Nephrology* 16: 3669–3679.

Peters CJ and Khan AS (2002) Hantavirus pulmonary syndrome: The new American hemorrhagic fever. *Clinical Infectious Diseases* 34: 1224–1230.

Pini N (2004) Hantavirus pulmonary syndrome in Latin America. *Current Opinion in Infectious Diseases* 17: 427–431.

Plyusnin A (2002) Genetics of hantaviruses: Implications to taxonomy (review). *Archives of Virology* 147: 665–682.

Schmaljohn CS and Nichol ST (eds.) (2001) Hantaviruses. *Current Topics in Microbiology and Immunology* 256: 1–191.

Terajima M, Vapalahti O, Van Epps HL, Vaheri A, and Ennis FA (2004) Immune response to Puumala virus infection and the pathogenesis of nephropathia epidemica. *Microbes and Infection* 6: 238–245.

Vapalahti O, Mustonen J, Lundkvist Å, Henttonen H, Plyusnin A, and Vaheri A (2003) Hantavirus infections in Europe. *Lancet Infectious Diseases* 3: 653–661.

Henipaviruses

B T Eaton and L-F Wang, Australian Animal Health Laboratory, Geelong, VIC, Australia

History

The first henipavirus was isolated in 1994 following an outbreak of acute respiratory disease in a stable in Brisbane, Australia. In less than 3 weeks, 21 of 30 horses became infected and 14 either died or were euthanized. Two people who worked at the stable also became infected and one died. The virus responsible was a previously undescribed paramyxovirus, subsequently called Hendra virus (HeV) after the suburb where the outbreak occurred. In the subsequent decade, HeV was identified as the cause of equine deaths at four separate locations in Queensland, spilling over on two occasions to cause single human infections, one of which was fatal. In the latter instance, the patient succumbed to encephalitis over a year after infection during the necropsy of HeV-infected horses. Initial serological evidence suggested that fruit bats (flying foxes) in the genus *Pteropus* were reservoir hosts and in 1996, HeV was isolated from several Australian flying fox species.

The second member of the genus, Nipah virus (NiV), emerged in 1998–99 in Perak State, Peninsular Malaysia, as the cause of an outbreak of respiratory and encephalitic disease of low morbidity and mortality in pigs. The virus spread to humans causing febrile encephalitis among pig farmers and those who had direct contact with pigs. The epidemic moved south to the intensive pig-farming areas of Negeri Sembilan in December 1998 and was only brought under control by the imposition of movement restrictions and the culling of over 1 million pigs. Two hundred and sixty-five human cases of encephalitis were documented with 105 deaths. A cluster of 11 cases with one death occurred among abattoir workers in Singapore. NiV was subsequently isolated from the urine of Malaysian flying foxes in 2002. NiV re-emerged in Bangladesh and an adjoining area of India (West Bengal) in 2001, and since then outbreaks of encephalitis caused by the virus have re-occurred in Bangladesh almost every year, with case–fatality rates approaching 75%.

Taxonomy and Classification

The full-length genome sequence of HeV revealed it to be a member of the family *Paramyxoviridae*, subfamily *Paramyxovirinae*, but one with unique genetic features that precluded its classification in the genera *Morbillivirus, Respirovirus,* or *Rubulavirus,* the three genera established in the subfamily at that time. Complete genome sequencing of NiV revealed a high degree of similarity to HeV and, in 2002, the genus *Henipavirus* was created to accommodate these novel paramyxoviruses. The genus *Henipavirus* is now one of five genera in the subfamily *Paramyxovirinae* (**Figure 1**).

Several molecular features distinguish henipaviruses from other paramyxoviruses. First, the genome length of NiV and HeV at 18 246 and 18 234 nt, respectively, is approximately 15% larger than most other paramyxoviruses. It is not the extra length *per se* that is unique to henipaviruses. The unclassified paramyxoviruses J virus and Beilong virus have genomes over 19 000 nt in length. The novel henipavirus genomic feature is the length of the noncoding regions at the 3' end of five of the six genes, which in most cases are 3–13 times longer than their *Paramyxovirinae* counterparts. The function of these regions is unknown. A second unique feature of henipaviruses commensurate with their status in a separate genus within the family *Paramyxoviridae* is the presence of 3' and 5' genomic terminal sequences 12 nt in length, that differ from all other paramyxoviruses and contain the genus-specific promoter elements for replication and transcription.

Molecular Biology

Although the genomes of henipaviruses, respiroviruses, and morbilliviruses are organized in an identical manner and, with the exception of the P protein, virus-encoded proteins in each genus are similar in size, analyses have revealed

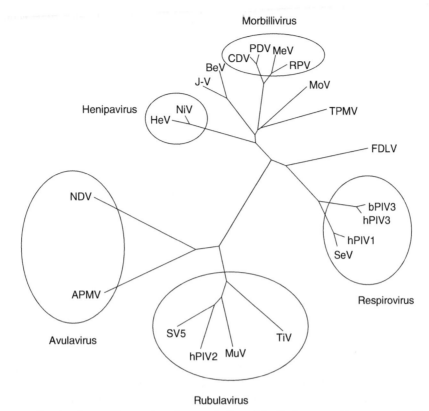

Figure 1 Classification of henipaviruses. The number of genera in the subfamily *Paramyxovirinae* was raised in 2002 from three (*Respirovirus*, *Morbillivirus*, and *Rubulavirus*) to five by the addition of two new genera, *Avulavirus* and *Henipavirus*. The phylogenetic tree shown here is based on an alignment of the deduced amino acid sequence of the L gene of selected family members using the neigbor-joining method. Viruses are grouped according to genus and abbreviated as follows. *Avulavirus* genus: APMV (avian paramyxovirus), NDV (Newcastle disease virus); *Respirovirus* genus: SeV (Sendai virus), hPIV1 (human parainfluenzavirus 1), hPIV3 (human parainfluenzavirus 3), bPIV3 (bovine parainfluenzavirus 3); *Morbillivirus* genus: MeV (measles virus), CDV (canine distemper virus), RPV (rinderpest virus), PDV (phocine distemper virus); *Henipavirus* genus: HeV (Hendra virus), NiV (Nipah virus); *Rubulavirus* genus: hPIV2 (human parainfluenzavirus 2), MuV (mumps virus), SV5 (simian parainfluenzavirus 5), TiV (Tioman virus); and unclassified viruses: MoV (Mossman virus), BeV (Beilong virus), FDLV (Fer-de-lance virus), TPMV (Tupaia paramyxovirus), and J-V (J virus).

striking differences between some henipavirus proteins and their respirovirus and morbillivirus counterparts.

The attachment glycoproteins of paramyxoviruses are designated as hemagglutin-neuraminidase (HN), hemagglutinin (H), or glycoprotein (G) on the basis of their capacity to agglutinate red blood cells and remove sialic acid from carbohydrate moieties. The HN-positive status of respiroviruses, avulaviruses, and the vast majority of rubulaviruses reflects their use of sialic acids as cell surface receptors. In contrast, morbilliviruses and henipaviruses bind to cells using sialic acid-independent mechanisms. SLAM (signaling lymphocyte-activation molecule) is regarded as a universal morbillivirus receptor and ephrin B2 has been identified as a functional receptor for both HeV and NiV. Ephrin B2 is a member of a family of cell surface glycoprotein ligands that bind to surface-expressed tyrosine kinases known as Eph receptors. Binding of ephrins to Eph receptors leads to bidirectional signaling and cell-to-cell communication. The widespread distribution of ephrin B2 among mammals may help explain the extensive host range

of henipaviruses (see below). Like the fusion protein of all other paramyxoviruses, the henipavirus F protein is activated by proteolytic cleavage of a precursor F_0 protein. Henipaviruses invariably generate systemic infections and most paramyxoviruses which do so synthesize F proteins which are cleaved at a multibasic cleavage site by furin, a cellular protease located in the *trans*-Golgi network. Surprisingly, the cleavage site of both HeV and NiV is a single basic amino acid, arginine and lysine, respectively. What is more, that basic residue and the amino acids in the vicinity of it are not required for proteolytic cleavage. A second unique feature of henipavirus F proteins is the presence of an endocytosis consensus motif YXXφ (where Y is tyrosine, X is any amino acid, and φ is an amino acid with a bulky hydrophobic group) in the cytoplasmic tail of the protein. Endocytosis is required for F protein cleavage activation, an observation consistent with the fact that cathepsin L, a lysosomal cysteine protease that lacks a distinctive cleavage recognition site, is responsible for cleavage of the HeV F protein.

In paramyxoviruses, mechanisms to inhibit the antiviral effects of interferon are encoded by the P gene, which generates multiple proteins (P, V, W, and C in henipaviruses) by means of internal translation initiation sites, overlapping reading frames, and a transcription process in which nontemplated G nucleotides are inserted at a conserved editing site, resulting in a reading frameshift during translation. Insertions of one and two G residues generate transcripts which encode the V and W proteins, respectively. Whereas the henipavirus V protein resembles that of other paramyxoviruses in having a conserved cysteine-rich C-terminal domain, the henipavirus W protein is unusual because the C-terminal domain is significantly longer than that of most *Paramyxovirinae*, where translation of the encoding P gene transcript terminates soon after the editing site.

Host Range and Viral Propagation

HeV and NiV replicate in a variety of mammalian cell lines. The rate of replication, the size of syncytia generated, and the location of nuclei in syncytia vary depending on cell type and virus species. Infected Vero cell monolayers yield titers in excess of 10^8 infectious virions per milliliter. The broad host range of henipaviruses has been corroborated by experiments in which cells infected with vaccinia virus recombinants and expressing henipavirus cell attachment (G) and fusion (F) proteins on the surface fuse with cells from a gamut of vertebrate sources. Susceptibility to virus infection and virus glycoprotein-mediated fusion *in vitro* are reflected in the wide range of mammalian hosts sensitive to virus infection *in vivo*. The host range of henipaviruses is considered uncommon for paramyxoviruses, which usually adopt a narrow host range. In addition to bats, NiV has been shown to infect animals in six other mammalian orders. Although the widespread distribution of ephrin B2 in vertebrates provides an explanation for the diverse host range of henipaviruses, there are mammalian species such as mice which express functional ephrin B2, shown to bind henipaviruses, but remain resistant to infection with HeV and NiV.

Serologic Relationships

NiV was initially described as Hendra-like on the basis of its reactivity with anti-HeV antibodies, a similarity corroborated by complete genome sequencing. No serological relationship between henipaviruses and other paramyxoviruses has been confirmed. The close serological relationship of HeV and NiV makes it difficult to identify antibodies to each virus and determine the virus species circulating in specific geographical areas. A four- to eightfold difference between homologous and heterologous neutralization titers is the basis upon which antibody specificity has been determined.

Four neutralizing epitopes have been mapped on the globular head of the HeV G protein. Two discontinuous epitopes are located on the base of the head and two on the top, in locations resembling those identified as neutralizing sites in other paramyxoviruses. The amino acid homology between HeV and NiV is relatively high at one of the discontinuous epitopes but decreases significantly at the other three sites.

Geographical Distribution

HeV has been isolated from horses, humans, and flying foxes in Australia and NiV from humans, pigs, and flying foxes in Malaysia, Bangladesh, and Cambodia. NiV has also been isolated from fruit partially eaten by flying foxes in Malaysia, and NiV RNA has been detected in human patients and bats in India and Thailand, respectively. Comparative neutralization studies using Australian bat sera confirm that HeV populates the southern domain of the henipavirus distribution. Conversely, Malaysian and Indonesian sera preferentially neutralize NiV, rather than HeV. Equivalent neutralization titers to both HeV and NiV suggest that a related virus may be circulating in the Cambodian bat population. The geographic distribution of *Pteropus* species which range from the east coast of Africa, through the Indian subcontinent and Southeast Asia, north to Okinawa and south to Australia, suggests that henipaviruses may also be found in flying fox populations in geographically more diverse locations.

Evolution and Genetics

Genetically diverse populations of NiV circulate in Southeast Asia. In Malaysia, three closely related lineages of NiV have been identified. A number of identical isolates from humans and pigs during the major outbreak in the pig-farming communities in central Malaysia in 1999 constitute the first lineage. A 1999 isolate from the initial focus of infection in northern Malaysia is the sole representative of a second lineage and NiV isolated from the urine of flying foxes on Tioman Island off the east coast of peninsular Malaysia constitutes the third lineage, one that is genetically closer to viruses isolated during the major outbreak. It has been suggested that there may have been two bat-to-pig spillover events in Malaysia, only one of which caused significant transmission to humans. However, the role played by virus evolution in pigs, particularly during the period following introduction into the pig population in 1998 and prior to the major outbreak in 1999, remains uncertain.

Unlike the Malaysian isolates which displayed an overall sequence divergence of less than 1%, regardless of source,

NiV isolates from human patients in Bangladesh in 2004 differed from the Malaysian isolates by approximately 7% in the protein-coding regions and up to 25% in the non-coding regions. The heterogeneity of Bangladesh isolates suggested multiple spillovers of NiV from flying foxes into the human population. A further evolutionary lineage situated between the NiV-Malaysia isolates and NiV-Bangladesh isolates appears to exist in Cambodia.

The paucity of HeV isolates has restricted speculation on the evolution of this henipavirus in Australia. Partial sequencing suggests that viruses isolated from equine and human sources during the initial outbreak in Brisbane in 1994 and from flying foxes two years later were identical.

Epidemiology and Transmission

Human henipavirus infections in Australia and Malaysia occurred as a result of transmission of the viruses from flying foxes via horses and pigs, respectively. In contrast, NiV may have been directly transmitted to humans in Bangladesh, where it is believed that date palm juice contaminated with bat secretions constituted a potential transmission route. The mode of transmission from bats to spillover hosts in Australia and Malaysia is not known. It has been suggested that horses and pigs may have been infected by HeV and NiV through masticated fruit pulp spat out by flying foxes or by flying fox urine which contaminated pastures or pig sties. Alternatively, the source of virus may have been infected fetal tissues or fluids, a suggestion based on the fact that HeV outbreaks occurred during the birthing period of some species of flying fox, the isolation of HeV from a pregnant flying fox and its fetus, and the transplacental transmission of HeV in experimental infections.

HeV has been transmitted from horse to man on four occasions. The source of the virus may have been the saliva of infected horses, the nasal discharge commonly found at the terminal stages of the disease, or a wide range of infected tissues made accessible by necropsy. The paucity of virus in the bronchi or bronchioles of infected horses suggests transmission of HeV to either man or horse by aerosol is highly unlikely and experimental infection has confirmed the poor transmissibility of HeV in horses.

Risk factors for human infection by NiV in Malaysia were contact with pigs or fresh pig products and because the virus was present in a wide range of organs, the greatest likelihood arose for those in direct contact with sick or dying pigs on farms during farrowing or slaughtering or in abattoirs. NiV is readily observed in the respiratory epithelium of naturally and experimentally infected pigs, a feature suggesting that the virus probably spread to humans and within the pig population by aerosol or by direct contact with oropharyngeal or nasal secretions. Although NiV was present in the urine and respiratory secretions of patients, human-to-human transmission in Malaysia was extremely rare. In contrast, in Bangladesh, epidemiologic evidence indicates spread of the virus from person to person.

Tissue Tropism

Henipaviruses cause systemic infections displaying a predilection for vascular endothelial cells. The identification of ephrin B2 as a henipavirus receptor not only provides an explanation for the diverse host range of these viruses, but also helps to explain the observed systemic distribution of viral antigen particularly in arterial endothelial cells and smooth muscle. Ephrin B2 is found in arteries, arterioles, and capillaries in multiple tissues and organs but is absent from venous components of the vasculature. It is also found in arterial smooth muscle. Ephrins play critical roles in axonal guidance during vertebrate embryonic development and ephrin B2 is expressed on neurons. The availability of ephrin B2 or other receptors, the requirement for co-receptors, or the differing capacities of cells to support the production of infectious virus may determine whether henipaviruses act as respiratory or neurological pathogens.

Pathogenicity

The outcome of henipavirus infections can range from high mortality, as seen with HeV in horses and NiV in humans, through low mortality and morbidity, best exemplified by NiV in pigs, to asymptomatic as observed in flying foxes. The highly virulent nature of henipaviruses in humans and the lack of therapeutic modalities have led to the classification of HeV and NiV as Biosafety Level 4 (BSL4) pathogens. Experimental infections reveal that henipaviruses are infectious following either oronasal or parenteral administration. Figures for the minimum lethal dose of henipaviruses are known only for NiV in golden hamsters (*Mesocricetus auratus*) where the LD_{50} was 270 plaque-forming units (pfu) and 47 000 pfu following intraperitoneal and intranasal administration, respectively.

Clinical Features of Infection

Henipaviruses display either predominantly respiratory or neurological tropisms depending on the host. In natural infections of horses and young pigs with HeV and NiV, respectively, and in experimental infections of cats with either virus, respiratory symptoms predominate. Neurological symptoms were also observed in a proportion of HeV-infected horses. Experimental infection of horses and cats is usually fatal, with death or euthanasia occurring 5–10 days post infection. Following natural infection of horses, however, the observations during the initial outbreak indicated that some animals displayed respiratory symptoms but survived and others responded to infection asymptomatically. HeV-induced respiratory disease in horses may be accompanied by facial swelling and ataxia and *in extremis*, a copious frothy nasal discharge. Natural infection of pigs with NiV is usually asymptomatic, an outcome also observed after experimental administration of NiV by the ocular and oronasal route. When symptoms are present, they vary according to the age of the pig. Young animals present primarily with respiratory symptoms. Older animals display increased salivation and nasal discharge and on occasion develop neurological signs such as trembling, muscle spasms, and an uncoordinated gait. In Malaysia, pigs displaying symptoms of NiV infection, such as nasal discharge and rapid and labored respiration, had a harsh and nonproductive cough, which gave rise to the name 'barking-pig-disease'.

In contrast, NiV infection in humans is usually associated with severe acute encephalitis and although a proportion of cases presented with respiratory disease, particularly in Bangladesh, the majority displayed fever, headache, drowsiness, dizziness, myalgia, vomiting, and a reduced level of consciousness. Clinical signs such as the absence of reflexes and the irregular twitching of muscles or parts of muscles and an abnormal doll's eye reflex are indicative of brainstem and upper cervical spinal cord dysfunction. In the Malaysian outbreak, 105 of 256 patients died, a mortality rate of 41%. However, this figure reduces to *c.* 30% when individuals who experienced either a mild or asymptomatic infection are taken into account. In Bangladesh, 66 of 90 patients died in outbreaks in 2001, 2003, and 2004, giving a combined case–fatality rate of approximately 70%. Whereas HeV or NiV infection of cats presents a model of respiratory infection, the clinical and pathological features observed in NiV-infected hamsters resemble those found in human cases of encephalitis.

Both HeV and NiV can cause prolonged infection in humans before manifesting as causes of severe neurological disease. In Malaysia, NiV persisted in a proportion of patients (*c.* 10%) who either recovered from encephalitis or who had experienced an asymptomatic infection. Such cases of relapsed and late-onset encephalitis respectively presented from months to years after the initial infection. Only four cases of human HeV infection have been recorded. Two displayed influenza-like symptoms and one died. A third, fatal case of encephalitis occurred over a year after a self-limiting episode of meningitis, attributed to HeV infection.

Pathology and Histopathology

The respiratory disease caused by HeV in horses is characterized by pulmonary edema and congestion. Viral antigen is found in endothelial cells in a range of organs including lungs, lymph nodes, kidneys, spleen, bladder, and meninges, and virus can be recovered from a number of internal organs, including lung, and from saliva and urine. Young pigs infected with NiV present primarily with respiratory symptoms caused by tracheitis and bronchial and interstitial pneumonia. After experimental infection by the ocular and oronasal routes, virus replication occurs in the oropharynx and spreads to the respiratory tract and lymphoid tissues before appearing in the trigeminal ganglion and neural tissue. Viral antigen is found, particularly in clinically affected animals, in both lungs and meninges and virus is recovered from a range of tissues including tonsil, nasal, and throat swabs and lung. Detection of NiV in the urine of infected pigs is uncommon.

The primary site of replication and dynamics of henipavirus spread in humans are unknown but the distribution and time of appearance of lesions throughout the vasculature and in the brain in NiV encephalitis suggest that hematogenous spread delivers the virus from primary to secondary sites of replication in widely dispersed vascular endothelial cells. Inflammation of blood vessels, particularly small arteries, arterioles, and capillaries, occurs in most organs but is prominent in brain, lung, heart, and kidney. The interval between maximum vasculitis in the brain and parenchymal infection in NiV encephalitis suggests that infection of neurons occurs as a result of vascular damage and that neurological impairment may be due, not only to the effects of ischemia and infarction, but also viral infection of neurons. Although NiV antigen is found infrequently in epithelial cells of the bronchi and kidney, replication in such locations may play a role in virus dissemination. Recent outbreaks of NiV in Bangladesh strongly suggest human to human transmission.

No disease syndromes associated with henipaviruses have been documented in wild flying fox populations. Nor does HeV cause clinical disease in experimentally infected flying foxes and only a proportion of infected bats respond with sporadic vasculitis in the lung, spleen, meninges, kidney, and gastrointestinal tract. The mode of henipavirus transmission between flying foxes is unknown but the presence of virus in the placenta and transmission without apparent harm to the fetus in experimentally infected bats suggests that horizontal transmission is feasible.

Immune Response

Adaptive

In susceptible nonpteropid species, henipaviruses elicit strong humoral immune responses. No studies have been made of cellular responses to henipavirus infection. Antibodies to P, N, and M proteins are evident in Western blots and anti-F and anti-G antibodies are readily detected by enzyme linked immunosorbent assay (ELISA), using both traditional and bead-based formats, and by immune precipitation. In contrast to the consistent antibody response in susceptible, nonvolant species, in flying foxes there appears to be little direct correlation between detectable virus replication and the appearance of antiviral antibody. Antibody production is irregular and of uncertain longevity.

Anti-NiV antibodies were present in a majority of patients with clinical NiV encephalitis and IgM antibodies occurred more frequently than IgG antibodies in both serum and cerebrospinal fluid (CSF). The appearance of specific IgM antibodies in serum preceded their appearance in the CSF, a sequence consistent with viremia preceding central nervous system infection.

Innate

Henipaviruses inhibit both interferon (IFN) induction and IFN signaling. In the induction phase, the detection of viral double-stranded (ds)RNA by both RNA helicase enzymes and Toll-like receptor 3 (TLR3) leads to the transcription of IFN. Henipaviruses inhibit this process in a number of ways. The V protein, like that of other paramyxoviruses, blocks the activity of the helicase sensor in the cytoplasm but does not inhibit the TLR3 pathway. In contrast, in a process unique to paramyxoviruses and by virtue of the nuclear localization signal in its C-terminal domain, the W protein inhibits IFN induction by blocking a late nuclear step in the activation process which is shared by both helicase and TLR3 pathways.

In the IFN signaling pathway, IFN binds to cell surface receptors in a paracrine manner and initiates a sequence of reactions that leads to activation of members of a family of proteins called signal transducers and activators of transcription (STAT). STAT proteins activate transcription of hundreds of genes some of whose products inhibit virus replication. In a strategy unique to paramyxoviruses, henipaviruses inhibit IFN signaling by sequestering STAT proteins in high molecular weight complexes. The V and P proteins bind STAT proteins in the cytoplasm, whereas the W protein co-localizes with STAT in the nucleus. The extra length of the henipavirus P gene compared with that of other *Paramyxovirinae* results in the encoded P, V, and W proteins having an N-terminal extension of *c.* 100 amino acids compared with their morbillivirus and respirovirus counterparts. This domain appears to provide henipaviruses with a multifaceted anti-IFN signaling activity.

Prevention and Control

Therapeutic options for treatment of infections caused by henipaviruses are limited and currently use of ribavirin appears to be the only recourse. The drug inhibits replication of HeV in cells in culture, and in an open-label study of 194 patients during the NiV outbreak in Malaysia, its use resulted in a 35% reduction in mortality. Duration of ventilation and total hospital stay were both significantly shorter in those receiving ribavirin. Human monoclonal antibodies to the henipavirus G protein also appear to have therapeutic potential. Antibodies which react with the soluble G protein of HeV have been generated from naive recombinant human antibody libraries and they neutralize both HeV and NiV *in vitro*.

A number of promising strategies to develop henipavirus vaccines are being explored. NiV F and G glycoproteins expressed from vaccinia virus elicit neutralizing antibodies in both mice and hamsters and in the latter both anti-F and anti-G antibodies protected from a lethal NiV challenge, although they did not prevent virus replication. Murine anti-F and anti-G antisera also inhibited membrane fusion mediated by F and G glycoproteins expressed in cell culture. More importantly, because of the attractiveness of a subunit compared with a recombinant vaccine, purified soluble HeV and NiV G proteins elicit potent neutralizing antibody responses in rabbits. Antibodies neutralized both HeV and NiV in cell culture and displayed a slightly higher titer against the homologous virus.

A further therapeutic option relies on the fact that henipavirus F_1 glycoproteins have α-helical heptad repeat (HR) domains proximal to the fusion peptide and transmembrane domain at the N- and C-terminal of the protein, respectively. HR domains form a trimer-of-hairpins structure during the fusion of virus and cell membranes. Peptides corresponding to the N- and C-terminal HR domains of HeV and NiV form trimer-of-hairpins structures *in vitro*. Addition of exogenous peptide from either HR domain blocks formation of the trimer-of-hairpins, inhibits cell fusion mediated by vaccinia virus-expressed F and G proteins, and prevents virus infection of cells in culture.

Future Perspectives

The presence of HeV or NiV in flying foxes throughout Australia, Southeast Asia, and part of the Indian subcontinent suggests that the distribution of henipaviruses may parallel that of pteropid species, which range from Madagascar to the South Pacific. Although the factors responsible for the emergence of henipaviruses have not been clearly elucidated, the destruction of native habitats, a process which is unlikely to abate, forces flying foxes into contact with man as they seek food in areas frequented by humans. Although documented outbreaks of disease caused by henipaviruses are relatively infrequent, lack of knowledge of the modes of transmission between fruit bats and from fruit bats to spillover hosts, the high infectivity of the viruses for certain species, their broad species tropism, and their zoonotic potential will ensure that further work on henipaviruses remains a priority.

See also: Measles Virus; Mumps Virus.

Further Reading

Eaton BT, Broder CC, Middleton D, and Wang LF (2006) Hendra and Nipah viruses: Different and dangerous. *Nature Reviews Microbiology* 4: 23–35.

Eaton BT, Mackenzie JS, and Wang LF (2006) Henipaviruses. In: Knipe DM and Howley PM (eds.) *Fields Virology,* 5th edn., pp. 1587–1600. Philadelphia: Lippincott Williams and Wilkins.

Field HF, Mackenzie JS, and Daszak P (2007) Henipaviruses: Emerging paramyxoviruses associated with fruit bats. *Current Topics in Microbiology and Immunology* 315: 133–160.

Hyatt AD, Zaki SR, Goldsmith CS, Wise TG, and Hengstberger SG (2001) Ultrastructure of Hendra virus and Nipah virus. *Microbes and Infection* 3: 297–306.

Lamb RA and Parks GD (2006) *Paramyxoviridae*: The viruses and their replication. In: Knipe DM and Howley PM (eds.) *Fields Virology,* 5th edn., pp. 1449–1496. Philadelphia: Lippincott Williams and Wilkins.

Wong KT, Grosjean I, Brisson C, *et al.* (2003) A golden hamster model for human acute Nipah virus infection. *American Journal of Pathology* 163: 2127–2137.

Wong KT, Shieh WJ, Zaki SR, and Tan CT (2002) Nipah virus infection, an emerging paramyxoviral zoonosis. *Springer Seminars in Immunopathology* 24: 215–228.

Human T-Cell Leukemia Viruses: General Features

M Yoshida, University of Tokyo, Chiba, Japan

Glossary

pX region HTLV sequence between the env and 3′ LTR, encoding Tax, Rex and other small regulatory proteins.
Rex Trans-modulator of viral RNA splicing and transport.
Tax Pleiotropic regulator activating viral and cellular replication interacting with cellular transcription factors, tumor suppressor proteins, and cell cycle checkpoints.

Introduction

Human T-cell leukemia virus 1 (HTLV-1) is the first established tumorigenic retrovirus of humans; exogenous to humans this virus is classified as the species *Human T-cell leukemia virus,* in *Deltaretroviridae,* within the family *Retroviridae.* HTLV-1 infection is associated with leukemia and neural disease, adult T-cell leukemia (ATL) and HTLV-1-associated myelopathy/tropical spastic paraparesis (HAM/TSP), respectively. The genomic structure of the virus with genes for nonstructural proteins established a distinct viral genus that includes *Bovine leukemia virus.* HTLV-1 has no oncogene, but nevertheless transforms T cells rather efficiently and is identified as the etiologic agent of ATL. HTLV-1 has unique regulatory proteins, Tax and Rex, and Tax has been identified as a critical molecule not only in regulation of viral replication but also in induction of ATL.

History and Classification

After long and enormous efforts to identify a retrovirus in human tumors, HTLV was described in T-cell lines as a convincing human retrovirus. The first report of the virus (HTLV) was from a patient with Mycosis (MF) in the US, and another (adult T-cell leukemia virus (ATLV)) was from a patient with ATL in Japan. Subsequently, the MF case was characterized as ATL and the two isolates were established to be the same following a comparison of their genomes.

A prototypical retroviral genome contains the *gag, pol,* and *env* genes encoding the virion proteins including core proteins, reverse transcriptase, and surface glycoprotein, respectively. Acute leukemia viruses generally have an oncogene acquired from cellular genes that substitutes a part of the *gag, pol,* and *env* sequences. In contrast to these genomes, HTLV has additional genes in an extra pX region between *env* and the 3′ LTR (LTR – long terminal repeat). This unique genomic structure classified HTLV as a member of a distinct genus of the *Retroviridae,* which includes HTLV-1, and-2, bovine leukemia virus (BLV), and simian T-cell leukemia viruses (STLV-1, -2, and -3). HTLV-2 was isolated from a patient with hairy T-cell leukemia and its genome similarity to the type 1 is about 60%.

STLVs have been isolated from various species of Old World nonhuman primates, including the Japanese macaque, African green monkey, pig-tailed macaque, gorilla, and chimpanzee. Their genomes share 90–95% homology.

BLV infects and replicates in B cells of cows and sheep and induces B-cell lymphoma.

Geographic Distribution

Geographic Clustering

HTLV-1 carriers are defined by virus-specific antibodies. Nationwide surveys in Japan revealed the following: almost all ATL and HAM/TSP patients are infected with HTLV-1, 5–15% of adults in southwestern Japan are infected with HTLV-1 but this percentage is less in other areas of Japan. Worldwide, virus carriers are localized in the Caribbean islands and South America, Central Africa, and Papua New Guinea and the Solomon Islands. The prevalence of asymptomatic, seropositive adults varies significantly from district to district and even from village to village within these endemic areas. The unique clustering of virus infection in such remote areas is considered to reflect its mode of transmission and familial close contact such as sexual relations and breastfeeding. The presence of ATL and HAM/TSP is overlapping and clustered with HTLV-1 infection. Although some patients with ATL and healthy HTLV-1-infected carriers are found in nonendemic areas, they have frequently moved from an endemic area.

HTLV-2 is endemic in South America and is also detected in populations infected with HIV. STLVs are distributed in Old World monkeys in various areas, but not in New World monkeys. Although viruses were isolated from most species of Old World monkeys, some colonies are found to be virus-free even in the same geographic area.

Age-Dependent Infection

The frequency of HTLV-1 carriers increases with age after 20, reaching a maximum between 40 and 60 years of age. The prevalence is slightly (1.6 times) higher in females than in males, which is attributed to sexual transmission.

Familial aggregation

Familial aggregation of the HTLV-1 infection is apparent. If a mother is HTLV-1 positive, her children are frequently positive. This aggregation is due to viral transmission from husband to wife and mother to her children.

Host Range and Transmission

Receptor, Infection, and Transformation

The receptor for HTLV-1 infection is a glucose transporter, Glut-1, which is ubiquitously expressed on most cell types. Glut-1 is required for viral binding and infection, but it alone is not sufficient to understand preferential infection of CD4+ T cells *in vivo*. Cell-free viral particles of HTLV-1 released from established cell lines show extremely low infectivity *in vitro*, and co-cultivation with virus-producing cells is generally used to establish infection. A variety of cell types are infected including human T and B lymphocytes, fibroblasts, and epithelial cells, as well as cells from monkeys, rats, rabbits, and hamsters, but curiously not cells from mice. These cells infected by co-cultivation contain multiple integrated proviral copies of complete and defective genomes. Only T cells of the CD4+ phenotype are immortalized upon infection *in vitro*.

Despite the broad cell type host range *in vitro*, the cells infected *in vivo* are T cells. HTLV-1 infects both T cells with CD4+ and CD8+ phenotypes, although preferentially those of the CD4+ phenotype, but ATL cells are exclusively CD4+ T cells. Inoculation of infected cells can establish infection in rats, rabbits, and mice providing animal models for studies of the virus.

Natural Transmission

HTLV-1 is transmitted through (1) nursing of infants by infected mothers, (2) sexual contact, and (3) blood transfusion.

Mother to child. About 30% of the children born to seropositive mothers were seropositive. Infected T cells in breast milk are a source of transmissible virus. This mode of transmission was initially suggested by epidemiological studies and then direct evidence was obtained through cessation of breastfeeding by seropositive mothers that drastically reduced the seropositive rates in their children.

Sexual transmission. Wives with seropositive husbands are usually seropositive. Conversely, the husbands of seropositive wives show the same frequency of seropositivity as those in the region under study, indicating transmission occurs from husband to wife but not vice versa. Infected T cells in semen are thought to mediate transmission. This pathway may explain the higher (1.6 times) prevalence in females than in males, and is in sharp contrast to HIV infection. Infection in adulthood is not thought to be linked to subsequent ATL.

Blood transfusion. Transfusion of fresh and total blood transmits HTLV-1 into 60–70% of the recipients. The transfer of infected cells is critical for transmission. This mode of transmission does not lead to ATL, but does to HAM/TSP.

Zoonotic infections with retroviruses endemic in most Old World primates are described in people living in central African forests who have had contact with blood and body fluids of wild nonhuman primates. Such interspecies infection may explain the unique similarities between HTLVs and STLVs.

Genetics and Replication

Genome

The virion is spherical, enveloped with a membrane similar to that of the host cell and contains RNA genomes, core proteins, and reverse transcriptase, and envelope glycoproteins on the surface (**Figure 1**). The RNA

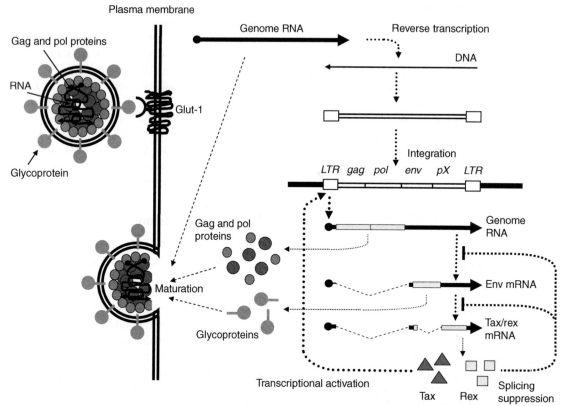

Figure 1 Replication cycle of HTLV. HTLV-1 binds to glucose transporter (Glut-1) and the genomic RNA is transcribed into complementary DNA by reverse transcriptase. The circularized proviral DNA is finally integrated into host chromosomal DNA establishing infection. The integrated provirus is transcribed into genomic RNA and expression of the viral proteins is regulated by Tax and Rex at transcriptional and splicing level making the expression transient. Genomic RNA and virion proteins mature at specific sites under plasma membrane and bud as the matured particles.

genome is copied into a 'proviral' DNA upon infection and analysis of the retroviral genome is generally performed with the integrated proviral genome.

The integrated HTLV-1 proviral genome is 9032 bp long and its organization is LTR-*gag-pol-env*-pX-LTR. The pX sequence contains multiple overlapping genes encoding for the regulatory factors for the viral replication, but none of them has any homology to cellular genes. The major regulatory factors are p40^{tax} and p27^{rex}. Alternative splicing of the pX sequence also expresses various proteins such as p12(I), p10(I), p11(V).

Antisense viral transcripts from the pX region code for HBZ proteins (HTLV-1 bZIP with a leucine zipper motif), which represent additional regulatory proteins, and also function at the RNA level.

Replication with Feedback Regulation

Reverse transcription and integration

Upon infection, the viral RNA genome is reverse-transcribed into complementary DNA (cDNA) by viral reverse transcriptase in the virion and further copied into double-stranded DNA, defined as 'proviral DNA'. The

proviral DNA is integrated into the host cell DNA establishing the viral infection.

Transcription and splicing

RNA transcription from the 5′ LTR to 3′ LTR generates the viral genomic RNA, and this step represents a potential regulatory stage of the viral replication cycle. HTLV genomic RNA serves as an mRNA for Gag and Pol proteins, but has to be spliced to express other viral proteins: into a 4.2 kbp (singly spliced) env mRNA for Env expression, and into a 2.1 kbp (doubly spliced) mRNA for the regulatory proteins, Tax and Rex (**Figure 1**). Various alternative splicing events also take place to express alternative proteins.

Genomic transcription depends on cellular factors that respond to 21 bp enhancers in the HTLV LTR, but initial transcriptional activity is weak. The low levels of viral transcripts are fully spliced into Tax/Rex mRNA. The Tax thus produced *trans*-activates transcription further enhancing viral transcription to produce more Tax/Rex mRNA. This *trans*-activation is mediated by Tax binding to a transcriptional factor, cAMP-responsive element binding protein (CREB) that responds to the 21 bp enhancers in the LTR. To express the virion proteins, Gag, Pol, and Env, the accumulated Rex protein specifically suppresses splicing of the viral RNA, and thus upregulates expression of unspliced genomic RNA and singly spliced *env* mRNA. In return, this Rex regulation reduces the level of spliced Tax/Rex mRNA, resulting in a lower level of Tax and ultimately reducing viral transcription. The combination of Tax and Rex functions exerts a feedback control on viral expression, making viral expression transient and resulting in the escape of infected cells from host immune surveillance. This feedback mechanism is unique to HTLV among oncogenic retroviruses and explains why HTLV is so repressed in expression and replication.

HTLV replication has also been reported to be regulated by small proteins such as p12(I), p10(I), p11(V), that are expressed by alternative splicing of the pX sequence. The regulatory mechanisms are not well understood but seem to be important for *in vivo* viral replication.

Maturation and budding

Genomic and *env* RNAs are efficiently accumulated by Rex and thus virion proteins, Gag, Pol, and Env, are transiently expressed. These virion proteins and genomic RNA come together and assemble at specific sites under the plasma membrane, finally budding by being enveloped with cellular membrane. The molecular mechanisms of these processes are not well characterized.

Variability and Evolution

The retroviral genome is rather labile in general since the reverse transcription process has no proofreading mechanism. In sharp contrast to HIV for example, however, the HTLV genome is highly stable and conserved among isolates from Japan, the Caribbean, and Africa. The viral isolates from Papua New Guinea may vary somewhat more but are still 90–95% homologous. This stable property is a reflection of an HTLV survival strategy that replicates the viral genome through infected cell replication rather than virus replication.

It has been suggested that HTLV and STLV are transmitted across species. Each of the isolates from various monkeys (STLV-1, -2, and -3) and humans (HTLV-1 and -2) are highly homologous and their variability is sometimes higher within the species than among species. Such unusual genomic conservation under different conditions is also well explained by a viral survival strategy through proliferation of infected cells.

Pathogenicity

Adult T-Cell Leukemia

Clinical features

Symptoms of ATL are variable and frequently complicated by skin lesions, enlargement of lymph node, liver and/or spleen, and infiltration of leukemic cells into various organs. Patients usually have antibodies to HTLV-1 proteins, show an increased level of serum lactate dehydrogenase (LDH), and most suffer from hypercalcemia.

The onset of ATL is observed in individuals between 20 and 70 years of age, the highest frequency being observed in people in their 40s and 50s. The male/female ratio of ATL incidence is 1.4/1.

Smoldering, chronic, acute forms of ATL and a lymphoma type have been recognized. Patients with smoldering ATL have a few or several percent of morphologically abnormal T cells in their peripheral blood, but do not show signs of severe illness for a long period. Patients with chronic ATL have rather high levels of HTLV-1-infected leukemic cells, but can maintain stable phenotypes for a certain period of time. Acute ATL is aggressive and resistant to any treatment; consequently, most patients die within one-half year of its onset.

Leukemic cells are exclusively CD4+ T cells with usually a highly lobulated nucleus. Leukemic cells generally have one complete integrated copy of an HTLV-1 provirus in their genome. Less frequently two copies are found, sometimes with defective forms. The site of integration is clonal in a given ATL patient, but different among patients. Leukemic cells carry aberrant chromosomes, frequently with multiple abnormalities, and express a high level of IL-2Ralpha, PTHrP, IL-1alpha, but no common abnormality has been described.

Etiology of ATL

An etiologic linkage of HTLV-1 with ATL is apparent from the observations: (1) ATL and HTLV-1 show identical geographic distribution, (2) almost all ATL patients are infected with HTLV-1, (3) leukemic cells are all infected with HTLV-1 but a vast majority of normal T cells are not, (4) leukemic cells are clonally integrated with an HTLV-1 provirus indicating their origin from a single infected cell, and (5) infection by HTLV-1 can immortalize T cells *in vitro* and the phenotypes of immortalized T cells are similar to those of leukemic cells.

There are approximately 1 million carriers of HTLV-1 in Japan. About 2–5% of all carriers of HTLV-1 are thought to develop ATL during their lifetime. While the vast majority of cases of ATL are associated with HTLV-1 infection, a form of ATL 'unrelated to HTLV-1 infection' has been described. The etiologic factor of these cases has not been identified.

Molecular mechanism of leukemogenesis

ATL cells have clonally integrated HTLV-1 proviruses; however, no common site for integration was observed among ATL patients. In this respect, HTLV-1 differs from animal chronic leukemia viruses, wherein integration was commonly adjacent to a proto-oncogene for its activation. Thus, the Tax protein has been focused on as a critical transforming protein.

Tax protein

Tax is able to transform fibroblasts and immortalize CD4+ T cells *in vitro*, and can induce tumors in transgenic mice. Tax exerts pleiotropic effects including (1) transcriptional activation of specific genes, (2) transcriptional repression of some other specific genes, (3) functional inactivation of tumor suppressor proteins, and (4) attenuation of cell-cycle checkpoints (**Table 1**). Cooperation of these pleiotropic functions is thought to contribute to ATL induction.

Transcriptional activation. Tax activates HTLV-1 genome transcription, which in turn is regulated by an enhancer binding protein, cyclic AMP-responsive element binding (CREB) protein. CREB has to be phosphorylated for active transcription, while Tax binds to CREB and activates it without a phosphorylation signal leading to a constitutively active protein. Similarly, Tax binds to other enhancer binding proteins such as nuclear factor kappa B (NF-κB) and serum responsive factor (SRF) and activates many specific cellular genes including IL-2Ralpha, IL-6, c-fos, and Bcl-x. NF-κB is alternatively activated by Tax through activation of IκB kinase (IKK) which disrupts inactive IκB–NF-κB complexes. The genes finally activated are linked to enhancement of cell proliferation or suppression of apoptosis.

Transcriptional repression. Tax also binds to transcription factors, CBP and P300, which interact with various enhancer binding proteins. The binding of Tax to CBP or p300 interferes with their interaction with the corresponding enhancer binding protein unless Tax is able to bind to enhancer binding protein, and consequently inhibits formation of a transcriptional initiation complex. The targets include p53-dependent transcription, DNA polymerase beta, p18ink4, Bax, and many others. The

genes eventually repressed are linked to downregulation of p53-dependent stress responses, DNA repair and apoptosis.

Functional inactivation of tumor suppressor proteins. Tax directly binds to or modifies some tumor suppressor proteins and inactivates their negative regulation of the cell cycle. RB, APC, and p53 are targets. (a) Tax binds to and inactivates p16ink4 and p15ink4, which normally inhibit CDK4 and maintain an active RB pathway; consequently, Tax activates CDK4 which results in inactivation of RB and promotes cells to move from G1 arrest into S phase. Tax is also reported to bind directly to CDK4 to activate kinase activity. (b) Tax also binds to another tumor suppressor protein, hDlg, through its PDZ domain and inactivates its growth-retarding signal through APC and β-catenin. An abnormality in this pathway has been shown to play a critical role in colorectal tumors. (c) Tax inactivates p53 through phosphorylation and complex formation of p53–p300. Inactivation of the p53 pathway implies suppression of DNA repair resulting in the frequent fixation of mutations.

Attenuation of cell-cycle checkpoints. Check and review mechanisms for genomic processes before entering the next phase of the cell cycle is important to avoid genetic fixation of mutations. Tax interacts with hMad-1 and Chek-1 and attenuates the S- and G2-checkpoint functions. Tax also binds to Ran and Ran-binding protein and induces centrosome fragmentation and aneuploidy. These properties would explain a higher mutation rate in Tax-positive cells and may be the basis for why ATL cells have highly frequent choromosomal abnormalities.

Collectively, it has been proposed that these pleiotropic effects of Tax cooperate for abnormal cell proliferation. Significance of the Tax roles are twofold: (1) enhancing

Table 1   Typical examples of pleiotropic Tax effects on cellular activities

Category/primary target	Targeted gene or process	Targeted cellular activity
Transcriptional activation		
CREB–CBP	HTLV-1 provirus	Viral replication/activation
	Unidentified	Transformation/activation
NF-κB-p300 and IKK-IκB	IL-2Ralpha, IL-6	Proliferation/activation
	Bcl-X	Apoptosis/suppression
SRF-CBP	c-Fos	Transformation/activation
Transcriptional repression		
p300–p53	p53-dependent transcription	Stress response/Suppression
	p18ink4	Proliferation/activation
CBP	DNA polymerase beta	DNA repair/suppression
	Bax	Apoptosis/suppression
Tumor suppressor protein		
p16ink4-CDK4	RB signaling	Cell cycle/promotion
p15ink4-CDK4		
hDLG-APC	APC signaling	Proliferation/activation
Kinase-p53	p53 signaling	Stress response/suppression
Checkpoint		
hMad-1	G2 checkpoint	Fidelity/suppression
Check-1	S, G2 checkpoint	Fidelity/suppression

proviral replication and (2) promoting cells into leukemo-genesis. Infected T cells are abnormally stimulated to proliferate through transcriptional activation/repression and inactivation of tumor suppressor proteins. Concomitantly, attenuation of cell-cycle checkpoints, reduction of DNA repair, and apoptosis would result in more mutations and their fixation, eventually leading to the leukemogenesis. In this respect, the pleiotropic effects of Tax may be equivalent to a multistep process for tumor formation.

Paradox in the leukemogenic mechanism

Tax plays a central role in the induction of ATL. Even its functional similarity to transforming proteins of DNA tumor viruses has been pointed out. However, it remains to be answered: (1) Why HTLV-1 transformation is selective for CD4+ T cells? and (2) Why ATL cells *in vivo* maintain tumor phenotypes in the absence of Tax? Tax/Rex mRNA is expressed only in a small percentage of tumor cells even using highly sensitive RT-PCR assays, yet tumor phenotypes are maintained in all ATL cells. The simplest answer for the latter question may be that Tax was critical for induction of tumors, but after establishment of tumors Tax is no longer required. If this is the case, what is the mechanism to maintain the tumor phenotypes?

An antisense gene, HTLV basic leucine zipper (HBZ) protein, may account for the paradox. This gene is transcribed from the pX region and codes for a DNA-binding protein with a bZIP domain. HBZ is able to moderately enhance T-cell proliferation *in vitro* and counteracts Tax *trans*-activation through dimer formation with other bZIP proteins. The antisense transcripts also operate at the RNA level. An exciting aspect of HBZ is that the antisense transcript is expressed in almost all ATL cases tested so far. It is therefore proposed to play a role after Tax *in vivo*. Tax is a potent antigenic protein; thus, its downregulation may make sense for tumor cell to escape from immune responses.

HAM/TSP and other diseases

Clinical features

HTLV-1 also induces a slowly progressive myelopathy known in tropical zones as tropical spastic paraparesis (TSP) and, in endemic areas of Japan, as HTLV-1-associated myelopathy (HAM). The unique phenotypes of HAM/TSP are chronic, symmetrical, bilateral involvement of the pyramidal tracts, at mainly the thoracic level of the spinal cord, and include progressive spastic paresis with spastic bladder and minimal sensory deficits. HTLV-1-infected T cells infiltrate into the spinal fluid and cord.

Most patients with HAM/TSP have much higher titers of HTLV-1 antibodies than those of asymptomatic carriers or ATL patients. This might be associated with particular types of human leukocyte antigens (HLAs). Despite their strong immunological responses to HTLV-1 infection, most HAM/TSP patients have larger populations of infected cells than do HTLV-1 carriers.

Etiology and other features

In endemic Japanese, all HAM/TSP patients are infected with HTLV-1. After screening for seropositive blood, the incidence of HAM/TSP has greatly decreased, clearly indicating that HTLV-1 is an etiologic agent of HAM/TSP. In contrast, TSP patients in the tropical areas are not always infected with HTLV-1, but the etiology in these cases is unknown. Indirect immunological reaction has been proposed as a pathogenic mechanism, but further studies are required.

The two HTLV-1-associated diseases, HAM/TSP and ATL, are mutually exclusive. The reason for this phenomenon is not well understood, but the route of primary viral infection may affect the pathogenic course: mucosal exposure to HTLV-1 for ATL, while primary infection of peripheral blood for HAM/TSP.

HTLV-1 infection is also proposed to be associated with some other diseases including uveitis, chronic lung disease, monoclonal gammopathy, and rheumatoid arthritis, but further systematic studies are required.

Prevention and Control of Infection

Transfusion of seropositive blood transmits HTLV-1 to two-thirds of the recipients. With the introduction of HTLV-1 screening systems in blood banks, viral transmission through transfusion has been greatly reduced. Application of these systems to populations in all endemic areas is critical to prevent HTLV-1 infection.

The major, natural route of viral transmission is from mother to child via infected T cells in breast milk. In Nagasaki City, Japan, pregnant women are tested for HTLV-1 antibodies by consent and those who are seropositive are recommended to avoid breastfeeding. A trial of this approach resulted in a drastic reduction in the incidence of seropositive children, from about 30% to just a few percent. The early success of this trial provides direct evidence for viral transmission through milk and suggests the possibility of eliminating ATL in the next few generations. Unfortunately, not all of children of seropositive mothers who did not breastfeed remained seronegative.

Future

Studies on HTLV-1 infection linked to ATL and HAM/TSP have progressed, but several very basic questions are still not answered: Why does only a small fraction of the infected population develop ATL or HAM/TSP? Why are ATL and HAM/TSP mutually exclusive? Why are only CD4+ T cells transformed into leukemic cells? What is required for ATL induction in addition to Tax? On the other hand, HTLV-1 transmission is now preventable in certain countries. However, it may not be feasible everywhere in the world. For example, cessation of breastfeeding might result in more serious problems in children in certain environments. So, original questions should be asked: Is a vaccine possible for complete eradication of the HTLV-1? Is vaccination possible for preventing disease development after infection?

Modern technologies developed in conjunction with genome research are now becoming available and make it possible to revisit these questions utilizing new appraoches.

See also: Human Immunodeficiency Viruses: Origin; Human Immunodeficiency Viruses: Pathogenesis; Human T-Cell Leukemia Viruses: Human Disease.

Further Reading

Gallo RC (2002) Human retroviruses after 20 years: A perspective from the past and prospects for their future control. *Immunological Reviews* 185: 236–265.

Matsuoka M and Jeang KT (2005) Human T-cell leukemia virus type I at age 25: A progress report. *Cancer Research* 65: 4467–4470.

Yoshida M (2001) Multiple viral strategies of HTLV-1 for dysregulation of cell growth control. *Annual Review of Immunology* 19: 475–496.

Yoshida M (2005) Discovery of HTLV-1, the first human retrovirus, its unique regulatory mechanisms and insights into pathogenesis. *Oncogene* 24: 5931–5937.

Japanese Encephalitis Virus

A D T Barrett, University of Texas Medical Branch, Galveston, TX, USA

Glossary

Arbovirus Virus which replicates in hematophagous insects and which then may be transmitted to vertebrates.
Flavivirus Any virus in the genus *Flavivirus*, family *Flaviviridae*.
Japanese encephalitis Disease caused by Japanese encephalitis virus.
Viremia Multiplication of virus in the blood of animals.

Introduction

Japanese encephalitis (JE) is a rural, zoonotic viral disease and is a major public health problem in many Asian countries. It is the most important of the arthropod-borne virus encephalitides and has replaced polioviruses as the major cause of human epidemic encephalitis in some parts of the world. Although a disease resembling JE was described in the late nineteenth century, the virus causing it, Japanese encephalitis virus (JEV), was first isolated in Japan in 1935. This prototype strain is known as Nakayama. Originally, JEV was termed 'Japanese B encephalitis virus' and was classified on the basis of antigenic characteristics as a member of the group B arboviruses. Subsequently it was reclassified as JEV in the family *Togaviridae*, before being reclassified as a member of the family *Flaviviridae* (species *Japanese encephalitis virus*). The virus is transmitted between vertebrate hosts by mosquitoes. Humans, as are most vertebrates, are 'dead-end' hosts, due to production of a low viremia, such that mosquitoes cannot be infected while feeding. JE is characterized by infection of the central nervous system. There are at least 50 000 clinical cases of JE reported each year but it is thought that the actual number is much higher. The majority of cases occur in children below the age of 10 years. The case–fatality rate is 15–25% and up to 70% of those who survive infection develop neurological sequelae. In addition, JE is the most important flavivirus disease of livestock. Horses and pigs are considered to be of veterinary importance. Horses become encephalitic and are dead-end hosts, whereas JEV can induce abortion in pigs, which are considered a major amplifying host.

Virus

Japanese encephalitis virus is a species in the genus *Flavivirus*, family *Flaviviridae*. The genus contains approximately 70 viruses. JEV is a member of the JEV complex, viruses that are closely related on the basis of cross-reactivity in neutralization tests and at the nucleotide level. The JEV complex includes Cacipacore, JEV, Koutango, Kunjin, Murray Valley encephalitis, St. Louis encephalitis, Usutu, West Nile, and Yaounde viruses. JEV replicates in a wide range of cell cultures derived from various animals and mosquitoes. Monkey kidney-derived Vero and LLC-MK2 cells usually are used for infectivity titrations, and these cell lines as well as C6-36 cells from *Aedes albopictus* mosquitoes usually are used to grow the virus.

Physical Properties

JEV virions are approximately 50 nm in diameter, icosahedral in shape, and have a lipid envelope. The envelope is derived from the host cell. Infectivity is lost after treatment with heat, detergents, lipid solvents, or acidic pH. Lipid solvents (e.g., ether and chloroform) and ionic detergents (e.g., sodium dodecyl sulfate) inactivate both infectivity and hemagglutination activity, while the milder nonionic detergents (e.g., nonidet P40, triton X-100, or X-113) only destroy infectivity. The sedimentation coefficient of the virion is approximately 200S and it sediments at a density of 1.20–1.23 g cm^{-3} in potassium tartrate-glycerol or sucrose gradients.

Virions contain three structural proteins. The small capsid (C) protein surrounds the genome of the virus and the envelope contains two proteins known as envelope (E) and membrane (M). The E protein is the viral hemagglutinin (i.e., the protein that binds to red blood cells) and contains most of the epitopes recognized by neutralizing antibodies. The E protein is the major virion protein and has one glycosylation site, at residue 154. Two types of virions are recognized; mature extracellular virions containing M protein, and immature intracellular virions containing precursor M (prM) protein, which is proteolytically cleaved during maturation to yield M protein. The genome comprises one positive-sense, single-stranded RNA molecule of *c.* 11 000 nt and is infectious. The 5′ terminus of the genome possesses a type I cap (m-^{7}GpppAmp) followed by the conserved dinucleotide AG. There is no terminal poly(A) tract at the 3′ terminus. The gene order is C-prM-E-NS1-NS2A-NS2B-NS3-NS4A-NS4B-NS5. There are 95 nucleotides in the 5′ noncoding region, and the single open reading frame has 10 296 nucleotides. The 3′ noncoding region is variable in length, depending on the strain.

In addition to the mature virion, two additional physical entities have been described, namely the slowly sedimenting hemagglutinin and soluble complement-fixing antigen. The former is associated with immature particles and the latter with secreted NS1 protein.

Replication Cycle

The replication cycle involves virion binding to cell receptor(s), mediated by the viral E protein. Uptake of the virion into cells is via receptor-mediated endocytosis followed by pH-dependent membrane fusion to release the virus nucleocapsid into the cytoplasm. The input virus does not contain viral RNA-dependent RNA polymerase. Thus, the positive-sense genomic RNA is translated to generate the

nonstructural proteins required for replication of the virus, including the RNA-dependent RNA polymerase. RNA replication is associated with membranes and begins with transcription of the input genomic RNA to synthesize complementary negative-sense strands, which are then used as templates to transcribe positive-sense genomic RNA. The genomic RNA is synthesized by a semiconservative mechanism involving replicative intermediates (i.e., containing double-stranded regions as well as nascent single-stranded molecules) and replicative forms (i.e., duplex RNA molecules). Synthesis of negative-sense RNA continues throughout the replication cycle. All viral proteins are produced as a single polyprotein that is co- and post-translationally processed by cellular proteases and by the viral NS2B-NS3 serine protease to generate individual structural and nonstructural proteins. In addition to the three structural proteins C, prM, and E, seven nonstructural (NS) proteins are found in virus-infected cells: NS1, NS2A, NS2B, NS3, NS4A, NS4B, and NS5. Few of the nonstructural proteins have been studied in detail. NS3 is a multifunctional protein whose N-terminal one-third forms the viral serine proteinase complex together with NS2B. The C-terminal portion of NS3 contains an RNA helicase domain involved in RNA replication, as well as an RNA triphosphatase activity involved in the formation of the 5′ terminal cap structure of the viral RNA. Two enzymatic activities have been assigned to NS5: the RNA-dependent RNA polymerase and the methyltransferase activity necessary for methylation of the 5′ cap structure. NS1 is an unusual nonstructural protein as it is glycosylated at two sites: residues 130 and 207. The functions of NS2A, NS4A, and NS4B are poorly understood, but current evidence suggests that NS2A, NS2B, NS4A, and NS5 are all part of the replication complex, and that NS1 is involved in RNA synthesis and virus assembly. The function in NS4B is not clear but may be an interferon antagonist. Other studies suggest that NS5 is involved in this function.

Virions are first observed in the rough endoplasmic reticulum, which is believed to be the site of virus assembly (i.e., interaction of genomic positive-sense RNA molecules with structural proteins C, prM, and E). Progeny virions assemble by budding through intracellular membranes into cytoplasmic vesicles. These immature virions (i.e., containing prM (which is thought to act as a chaperone) rather than M protein) are then transported through the membrane systems of the host secretory pathway to the cell surface where exocytosis occurs. Shortly before virion release, the prM protein is cleaved by furin or a furin-like cellular protease to generate mature virions that contain M protein. Immature virions have low infectivity compared to mature virions. Host-cell macromolecular synthesis is not shut-off during virus replication and is not decreased until cytopathic effect is evident late in the infection process.

Geographic Distribution

JEV is found throughout much of Asia. It is epidemic in temperate regions of Asia (e.g., Japan, Taiwan, People's Republic of China, Korea, eastern Russia, northern Vietnam, northern Thailand, Burma, Nepal, Sri Lanka, and India) and endemic in tropical regions (e.g., Malaysia, Indonesia, southern Vietnam, southern Thailand, and the Philippines). JE was not described in Australia until 1995, when cases of JE were reported on the island of Badu in the Torres Strait. The first human case of JE was reported on mainland Australia in 1998. This recent introduction into the Torres Straits and northern Australia is thought to be due to wind-blown mosquitoes.

Epidemiology

JE is reported in nearly all Asian countries. It is endemic in tropical areas of Asia and epidemic in temperate regions of Asia. Endemicity in tropical areas is thought to be due to the availability of mosquito vectors throughout the year, while there is seasonal incidence in temperate climates. Specifically, the disease is reported annually with seasonal (peaking in June and July during the rainy season) and age (mainly children between the ages of 1 and 15 but peaking in those 3–5 years of age) distributions. Some endemic countries that utilize childhood immunization have seen the age distribution of cases move toward older children and adults. Human infections are related to increased vector densities associated with rainfall or with irrigation practices. It is estimated that 3 billion people live in JE endemic areas. Of this population, approximately 700 million are children under the age of 15 years with an annual birth cohort of 70 million per year. The disease incidence varies greatly between countries, ranging from <10 to >100 per 100 000 population. On the basis of these figures, it is estimated that there are approximately 175 000 cases of JE per year, of which approximately 50 000 have clinical encephalitis. Only 1 in 1000 JEV infections are symptomatic. The estimated case–fatality rate is 25% (5–40% have been reported), and approximately 45% (plus reports of up to 70%) of surviving patients have neurological and/or psychiatric sequelae. These include neurological and psychomotor retardation, motor deficits, convulsions, memory impairment, optic nerve atrophy, limb paralysis, parkinsonism, and also psychological and behavioral disorders. Much of the information on neurological sequelae comes from case reports rather than detailed studies incorporating controls. Nonetheless, it appears that a large proportion of patients with neurological sequelae do recover completely over time.

The effect of concurrent infection with human immunodeficiency virus on JEV infection is unknown and there are few reports of JEV infection of pregnant women, given that the virus predominantly causes disease in children. However, there are reports from India that JEV infection can cause abortion during the first two trimesters of pregnancy.

JE appears to be age related, with the majority of patients being children and the elderly tending to have encephalitis. It is thought that this is due to the high prevalence of antibody in adults. All evidence indicates that there is one serotype of JEV and that infection provides lifelong protection from reinfection against all known antigenic and genetic variants of the virus.

Swine are important amplifying hosts of JEV. Infected pigs develop viremias sufficient to infect mosquitoes that subsequently feed on them. Importantly, adult pigs do not show clinical signs of JE. In terms of veterinary disease, infection of pregnant sows results in abortion and stillbirth due to transplacental infection and causes aspermia in boars. Infected equids can succumb to JE and cattle seroconvert; however, both are considered dead-end hosts.

Molecular Epidemiology

Strain variation has been recognized for many years. Initially antigenic variation was detected with polyclonal antisera in neutralization, complement fixation, agar gel diffusion, and hemagglutination inhibition tests and subsequently with monoclonal antibodies. Overall, two major immunotypes of JEV have been differentiated: Nakayama and Beijing-1/JaGAr-01. Other antigenically distinct groups of strains have been identified, including those from northern Thailand and Malaysia, while studies with monoclonal antibodies suggested that at least five antigenic groups could be identified. Oligonucleotide mapping provided the first evidence for genetic variation among strains of JEV. Subsequent studies used direct nucleotide sequencing of portions of the genome to identify four genotypes (genetic clusters) of JEV. Genotype I includes isolates from Cambodia and northern Thailand; genotype II includes isolates from Indonesia, southern Thailand, and Malaysia; and genotype III includes isolates from temperate regions of Asia (Japan, China, Taiwan, India, Nepal, Sri Lanka, and the Philippines). Subsequent studies showed that isolates from Japan, Korea, and India clustered within genotype III. Genotype IV includes certain isolates from Indonesia. Interestingly, recent studies have shown that during the past 25 years, genotype I is replacing genotype III in China, Japan, Korea, and Vietnam.

Overall, molecular epidemiologic studies of JEV have identified at least five antigenic groups and four genotypes. The relationship of the antigenic groups to the genotypes is not clear at present. The practical significance of these differences has been the subject of much debate. In particular, should strains from one or more antigenic groups/genotypes be included in vaccines to give effective protection against all JEV strains found in nature (see below)? Also, there is very little information on the molecular basis of neurovirulence of JEV or on biological differences between genotypes of JEV (see below). However, it is noteworthy that JEV isolates from Thailand can be distinguished genetically: isolates from northern Thailand are of genotype I while isolates from southern Thailand are of genotype II. The incidence of encephalitis in humans in northern Thailand is 12.2 per 100 000 while it is only 0.3 per 100 000 in southern Thailand. There are many potential explanations for this situation, but genetic differences between the viruses may contribute to these epidemiologic differences. Finally, the entire genome of a number of strains of JEV has been sequenced, including representatives of all four genotypes.

Pathogenicity and Virulence

Vertebrates of many species are susceptible to JEV. The virus is lethal for newborn mice and rats by all routes of inoculation. As the animals get older, age-related resistance to disease is observed following inoculation by peripheral routes, while adult mice are still susceptible following direct inoculation of virus into the brain, that is, neuroinvasiveness decreases with age while the virus is still neurovirulent for all ages of mice. The virus causes a lethal disease in primates inoculated intracerebrally, while some strains are lethal also by intranasal inoculation; peripheral inoculation of JEV causes only asymptomatic infection.

In nature, the virus readily infects individuals of a large number of vertebrate and invertebrate species. Many vertebrates are considered 'dead-end' hosts. Horses and humans develop encephalitis, and swine have inapparent infections, while the virus causes aspermia in boars and stillbirth or abortion in pregnant swine. Persistent infections have been reported in experimental infection of pregnant mice and virus has been passed vertically to offspring.

Although it is known that the virus appears in the blood before invading the central nervous system, the host and viral determinants of disease are poorly understood. It is not known whether the virus directly crosses the blood–brain barrier or uses the olfactory nerve route to invade the brain, nor is it known why the virus targets particular regions of the brain. The cell receptor for the virus has not been identified.

Strains of the virus differ in neuroinvasiveness and this appears to be related to the level of viremia, but the exact molecular determinants of JEV that control neuroinvasion have not been identified. However, studies on the attenuated vaccine strain SA14-14-2 have shown that the E protein is a major determinant of neurovirulence in the mouse model, with residue 138 dominant, and residues 107, 176, and 279 also contributing to neurovirulence.

Clinical Symptoms

Following the bite of a JEV-infected mosquito, there is an incubation period of 4–16 days before clinical symptoms are observed. These take the form of a febrile illness with headache, aseptic meningitis, or encephalitis. The most important form of the disease is acute meningomyeloencephalitis. Onset is rapid, with 1–4 days of fever, headache, chills, drowsiness, mental confusion, stupor, anorexia, nausea and vomiting. Subsequently, patients show symptoms of nuchal rigidity, photophobia, tremors, involuntary movements, focal motor nerve impairment involving the central and peripheral nervous systems, or coma. Generalized motor seizures are seen in children. Examination of the cerebrospinal fluids of patients may provide indicators of infection, including one or more of increased pressure, increased concentration of protein, an increased number of lymphocytes, anti-JEV IgM antibody, and virus. Fatal cases usually have respiratory complications, seizures, virus in cerebrospinal fluid, and low levels of anti-JEV IgM antibody. Pathological examination of brain tissue from fatal cases and imaging studies of patients show that infection of neurons is widespread in the central nervous system, although the thalamus, basal ganglia, and anterior horns of the spinal cord appear to be particularly involved. Microscopic lesions include perivascular inflammation, neuronal degeneration, and necrosis, rather than apoptosis. Nonfatal cases recover in 1 to 2 weeks. However, neurological and/or psychiatric sequelae are seen in a large proportion of patients who survive the acute disease (see the section titled 'Epidemiology').

Diagnosis

The virus is rarely isolated from peripheral blood during the acute stage of the disease in humans. This is thought to be due to a combination of a low viremia and clinical symptoms of the disease, which are not normally seen until after the virus has invaded the central nervous system by which time the viremia has finished. Virus can be isolated from cerebrospinal fluid early in the course of acute encephalitis, but this is consistent with a poor prognosis. Most virus isolates have been obtained from brains of patients at autopsy, or from mosquito pools. Viral antigen can also be detected by immunohistochemical techniques applied to neurons of patients at autopsy.

Many procedures have been used to detect serum antibodies against JEV: hemagglutination-inhibition, complement fixation, immunofluoresence, and enzyme-linked immunosorbent assay (ELISA). It is necessary to show at least a fourfold increase or decrease in titers of antibody to JEV between paired serum samples for any of these tests to be used to make a presumptive diagnosis of JE. Such a 'presumptive' diagnosis is required because of the extensive serological cross-reactions with antibodies against other flaviviruses, and all such serodiagnoses must be confirmed by neutralization tests. Many other flaviviruses overlap geographically with JEV, including the dengue and West Nile viruses, and can result in misinterpretation of test results. Detection of IgM antibodies is considered a relatively (JE complex-specific) specific test for JEV infection and is the serologic method of choice. An IgM-capture ELISA is usually used to detect IgM antibody to JEV in blood or cerebrospinal fluid within 7 days of onset of clinical symptoms. Recently, a dot-blot IgM assay has become available. Detection of IgM antibody in cerebrospinal fluid is associated with clinical JE and is predictive of a poor outcome.

Transmission

The virus is transmitted between vertebrate hosts by mosquitoes. The natural cycle involves rice-field-breeding mosquitoes and domestic pigs or wading ardeids (e.g., egrets and herons). The most important vector is *Culex tritaeniorhynchus*, found in most parts of Asia and which breeds in water pools and flooded rice fields. The virus also has been demonstrated to infect mosquitoes of other species, including *Cx. fuscocephala*, *Cx. gelidus*, *Cx. pipiens*, *Cx. bitaeniorhynchus*, *Cx. epidesmus*, *Cx. vishnui*, *Mansonia uniformis*, *M. bonneae/dives*, *Aedes curtipes*, *Ae. albopictus*, *Armigeres obturans*, *Anopheles hyrcanus*, and *An. barbirostris*. In temperate regions, the 'JE season' is considered to start in April–June with detection of virus in mosquitoes; this peaks in July. During July and August, virus is detected with increasing frequency in pig and bird amplifying hosts. The 'season' usually ends in September–October. Human infections are concurrent with the increased frequency in amplifying hosts. The exact timing of the 'JE season' will vary depending on geographic location in Asia, rainfall, and migration of birds. It is not clear how JEV survives between 'JE seasons' in temperate areas. There is no evidence that JE epidemics follow heavy rains, major floods, etc.; intervals between outbreaks vary from 2 to 15 years. There is evidence to support vertical transmission by *Culex* and *Aedes* spp. mosquitoes, sexual transmission between male and female mosquitoes, and a potential role for migratory birds in long-distance movement of JEV. However, none of these possibilities has been conclusively demonstrated.

Culex tritaeniorhynchus preferentially feeds on animals other than humans. Consequently, high seroprevalence rates are seen in a wide range of animals including dogs, ducks, chickens, cattle, bats, water buffaloes, donkeys, monkeys, snakes, and frogs. The role, if any, that these animals play in the ecology of JEV is not known. However, birds and pigs are considered to be the major viremic amplifying hosts of the virus. Among birds, ducks, chickens, water hens, egrets, and herons seroconvert.

Swine are important amplifying hosts in the epidemiology of the virus. Infected pigs develop sufficiently high viremias to infect mosquitoes. Importantly, adult pigs do not show clinical signs of JEV infection.

Infected equids can succumb to JE, while cattle seroconvert; however, both are considered dead-end hosts as viremias are too low to infect mosquitoes.

Treatment

There are no antiviral treatments to control flavivirus infections; rather, supportive therapy is the norm.

Control

As with most mosquito-borne diseases, transmission of JEV can be blocked by mosquito control measures. In addition, immunization of pigs, a major vertebrate amplifying host, blocks the transmission cycle. However, given that JE is usually found in rural areas, human immunization is the method of choice. Although vaccination is used to control JE, socioeconomic development of Asian countries is also contributing to control. Smaller areas of rice fields, centralized pig production, use of agricultural pesticides, and reduction of the rural population at the expense of increased urbanization have all contributed to a decrease in cases of JE.

There are licensed vaccines available to control JE. Inactivated vaccines are based on strains Nakayama, Beijing-1, or P3. The former two are based on formalin-inactivated mouse brain preparations that are semipurified to remove brain materials while strain P3 is also formalin-inactivated, but grown in primary hamster kidney cell cultures in the People's Republic of China. Inactivated mouse brain-derived vaccines are approved by the World Health Organization for international use. The above vaccines require two doses given on days 0 and 7–28 to induce protective immunity with a booster dose at 1 year, and subsequently every 3–4 years to maintain immunity. Initial formalin-inactivated mouse brain vaccines were based on strain Nakayama; however, in 1989, this strain was replaced with strain Beijing-1 in most markets because the latter is antigenically closer to recent Japanese isolates of JEV, a high potency being retained following purification, and immunogenicity is superior to that of strain Nakayama. This resulted in a vaccine that required a dose equivalent to half that needed for strain Nakayama vaccines. Inactivated vaccines are manufactured in India, Japan, Republic of Korea, People's Republic of China, Thailand, Taiwan, and Vietnam. The mouse-brain inactivated vaccine has been reported to cause occasional adverse events (estimated to be one in a million doses), including allergic mucocutaneous reactions. The majority of the reactions take place after the second or subsequent dose of vaccine. There were a number of adverse events reported during the period 1989–92 of which 15% were hospitalized and two-thirds required medical treatment. In addition, there have been occasional reported cases of acute disseminated encephalomyelitis since 1983. Studies to date suggest there is no reduced seroconversion rate or an increase in adverse events when mouse brain-derived JE vaccine is given simultaneously with vaccines against measles, DPT, and polio. Due to the adverse events, consideration is being given in Japan to employ an inactivated vaccine produced in Vero cells, and this second-generation vaccine is undergoing clinical trials to demonstrate noninferiority of immunogenicity compared to the mouse brain product.

There are no contraindications to the use of this vaccine, other than a history of hypersensitivity reactions to previous doses. However, vaccination is not recommended during pregnancy and pregnant women are only vaccinated when at high risk of exposure to the infection. Mouse brain-derived vaccine has been given safely in various states of immunodeficiency, including HIV infection.

There is also a live Japanese encephalitis vaccine based on strain SA14-14-2 grown in primary hamster kidney cell culture. Until recently, this vaccine was only licensed for use in the People's Republic of China. However, the World Health Organization has now developed criteria for the production of the vaccine, and it is now licensed in Nepal, India, and Republic of Korea, and clinical trials are being undertaken in Sri Lanka, the Philippines, Thailand, and Indonesia. This vaccine appears to be very efficacious and over 300 million doses of this vaccine have been administered in the People's Republic of China since 1988 with no known reports of serious adverse events.

The success of human vaccination has been demonstrated by the decrease in the number of cases in Japan. Prior to 1966, there were 1000–5000 cases per year with mortality up to 50%. Following the introduction of vaccination, the number of cases has steadily decreased to the point where fewer than 10 cases have been reported each year during the 1990s. A similar situation has taken place in the Republic of Korea and Taiwan, and all three countries have reported a shift from cases in children to cases in adults, particularly in the elderly. Since the vast majority of JE cases are children, vaccination has focused on children.

Vaccination is used to reduce the incidence of abortions in JEV-infected pigs. A live vaccine has been used in the People's Republic of China to protect horses.

The mechanism of protective immunity is poorly understood for most flaviviruses, although production of neutralizing antibodies ($\geq$1:10) appears to correlate with immunity. Most neutralizing antibodies recognize epitopes of the E protein. Significantly, in passively immunized mice, detectable neutralizing antibodies will protect against a wild-type challenge administered by the intracerebral route. Cell-mediated immunity, in particular T-cell epitopes, have been mapped to nonstructural proteins, in particular NS3.

See also: Flaviviruses: General Features.

Further Reading

Burke DS and Leake CJ (1988) Japanese encephalitis. In: Monath TP (ed.) *The Arboviruses: Epidemiology and Ecology,* vol. 3, pp. 63–92. Boca Raton, FL: CRC Press.

Burke DS, Tingpalapong M, Ward GS, Andre R, and Leake CJ (1986) Intense transmission of Japanese encephalitis to pigs in a region free of epidemic encephalitis. *Japanese Encephalitis and Haemorrhagic Renal Syndrome Bulletin* 1: 17–26.

Chen W-R, Tesh RB, and Rico-Hesse R (1990) Genetic variation of Japanese encephalitis virus in nature. *Journal of General Virology* 71: 2915–2922.

Halstead HB and Jacobson J (2003) Japanese encephalitis. *Advances in Virus Research* 61: 103–138.

Halstead SB and Tsai TF (2004) Japanese encephalitis vaccines. In: Plotkin SA and Orenstein WA (eds.) *Vaccines,* 4th edn., pp. 919–958. Philadelphia: W B Saunders.

Huang C (1982) Studies of Japanese encephalitis in China. *Advances in Virus Research* 27: 72–100.

Mackenzie JS, Deubel V, and Barrett ADT (eds.) (2002) *Japanese Encephalitis and West Nile Viruses, Vol. 267: Current Topics in Microbiology and Immunology,* pp. 1–416. Vienna: Springer.

Mackenzie JS, Gubler DJ, and Petersen LR (2004) Emerging flaviviruses: The spread and resurgence of Japanese encephalitis, West Nile and dengue viruses. *Nature Medicine* 10(supplement): S98–S109.

Solomon T (2003) Recent advances in Japanese encephalitis. *Journal of Neurovirology* 9: 274–283.

Solomon T and Winter PM (2004) Neurovirulence and host factors in flavivirus encephalitis – Evidence from clinical epidemiology. *Archives of Virology Supplement* 18: 161–170.

Lassa, Junin, Machupo and Guanarito Viruses

J B McCormick, University of Texas, School of Public Health, Brownsville, TX, USA

This article is reproduced from the previous edition, volume 2, pp 887–897, © 1999, Elsevier Ltd., with an update by the Editor.

History

Lymphocytic choriomeningitis (LCM) virus, the first identified arenavirus, was isolated by Lillie and Armstrong in 1933 from the cerebrospinal fluid of a patient suspected of having St Louis encephalitis. The virus was again isolated in 1935 from patients with aseptic meningitis, and finally by Traub in 1935 from laboratory mice. More than 20 years passed before Junin virus, the next member of this taxon to be identified, was isolated from patients with Argentine hemorrhagic fever in 1957. Machupo virus from patients with Bolivian hemorrhagic fever was similarly identified in 1964. A third arenavirus from South America which is pathogenic for humans is Guanarito virus, isolated from patients in Venezuela in 1991. Yet another pathogenic arenavirus, Sabia virus, this time from Brazil, was isolated from a fatally ill individual. Several other arenaviruses have also recently been isolated from rodent species in South America, but none of these have yet been associated with human illness. Lassa virus was the first arenavirus isolated from Africa, in 1969, and remains the only arenavirus pathogenic for humans from Africa, although several other arenaviruses have also been identified from Africa. In total, 23 arenaviruses have been identified worldwide, but only six are known to be pathogenic for humans.

Classification

The 23 members in the *Arenavirus* genus of the *Arenaviridae* have traditionally been placed in categories of Old and New World arenaviruses (**Table 1**), based on geographic locations. More recently, Tacaribe complex viruses (in the Western hemisphere) have been more completely placed in phylogenetic relationship with each other based on a sequence of about 600+nucleotides in the nucleoprotein. The present information suggests three related groups: lineage A contains Pichinde, Parana, Flexal and Tamiami, Allpahuayo, Pirital, Whitewater Arroyo, and Bear Canyou viruses; lineage B contains Junin, Machupo, Amapari, Guanarito, Sabia, Cupixi, Chapare, and Tacaribe viruses; lineage C contains Latino and Oliveros viruses. More recently still, further genetic analysis has led to the suggestion that Pichinde and Oliveros viruses are most closely associated with Old World arenaviruses. The likelihood that arenaviruses and their rodent hosts have coevolved was suggested sometime ago, and now seems a possible hypothesis to begin to test through the parallel use of rodent genetics, alongside the understanding of the genetic relationships between arenaviruses.

Table 1 Arenaviruses: basic biological information

Virus	Human disease	Geographic distribution
LCM	Choriomeningitis	Europe, Asia, Western Hemisphere
Lassa	Lassa fever	West Africa
Mopeia	Human infection, no disease known	Southern Africa/Mozambique, Zimbabwe, Rep. of South Africa
Mobala	Human infection, no known disease	Central African Republic
Ippy	Unknown	Central African Republic
Lineage B[a]		
Cupixi	None	Brazil
Chapare	One human hemorrhagic fever	Bolivia
Junin	Argentine hemorrhagic fever	Argentina
Machupo	Bolivian hemorrhagic fever	Bolivia
Guanarito	Venezuelan hemorrhagic fever	Venezuela
Sabia	Hemorrhagic fever	Brazil
Amapari	None	Brazil
Tacaribe	None	Trinidad
Lineage A[a]		
Parana	None	Paraguay
Tamiami	None	Florida
Pichinde	None	Colombia
Flexal	None	Brazil
Pirital	None known	Venezuela
Whitewater Arroyo	None known	North America
Allpahuayo	None	Peru
Bear Canyou	None	California
Lineage C[a]		
Latino	None	Bolivia
Oliveros	None known	Argentina

[a]In current phylogenetic scheme suggested for Tacaribe complex viruses.

The six arenaviruses presently known to be pathogenic for humans (LCM, Lassa, Junin, Machupo, Guanarito, and Sabia viruses) will be the primary subjects of this article.

Properties of the Virion

The arenaviruses are enveloped, pleomorphic, membrane viruses ranging in diameter from 50 to 300 nm, with a mean diameter of 110–130 nm. The virion density in sucrose is 1.17 g ml^{-1}. They contain two segments of single-stranded RNA tightly associated with a nucleocapsid protein. This is enclosed in a membrane consisting of two glycosylated proteins (or in some cases a single glycosylated protein). The genome consists of two segments of single-stranded RNA both containing two genes encoded in an ambisense structure. The small RNA segments encode for the glycoprotein precursor (GPC) and for the nucleoprotein (NP). The NP and GPC genes are encoded in nonoverlapping reading frames with origins at the 3′ and 5′ ends of the molecule, respectively. The N gene is encoded by the 5′ half of the viral complementary RNA sequence corresponding to the 3′ half of the viral RNA molecule. The GPC gene is encoded by the 5′ half of the viral RNA molecule. Similarly, the large strand of RNA codes for the RNA-dependent viral RNA polymerase and a smaller ring-finger protein involved in replication. The arenaviruses are virtually indistinguishable from each other morphologically, and all share the characteristic granules noted in electron micrographs. These granules appear to be the results of the binding of the zinc-binding ring-finger protein of arenaviruses with the nuclear fraction of ribosomal proportion. The *nuclear ribosomal* protein (PO) appears in the virion, while other ribosomal proteins do not. This suggests that the granules, believed to be nonspecific inclusion of ribosomes into the virion, may rather be a specific process related to virion replication and assembly. These granules give rise to the family name *Arenaviridae*, derived from *arenos*, the Latin word for sand, based on their electron micrographic appearance as grains of sand.

Geographic and Seasonal Distribution

Junin, Machupo, and Guanarito viruses occur in Argentina, Bolivia, and Venezuela, respectively. Junin and Guanarito are endemic in their respective areas. Junin virus primarily infects workers during the corn harvesting season, by disturbance of the rodent host, *Calomys callosus*, which lives in the corn fields. Guanarito virus infection is endemic, and its epidemiology may resemble that of Lassa virus in Africa, which occurs throughout the year; however, insufficient data presently exist to confirm this impression. Machupo virus occurred in epidemic fashion in the 1960s in a circumscribed area of Bolivia. It was associated with the transient marked increase in the population of *Calomys*

rodents, which are normally field rodents but because of overpopulation moved into human dwellings in search of food. Elimination of the rodents in the towns stopped the epidemic, and few further cases have since been reported (though a few cases were reported in 1996). Chapare virus has been isolated from a human fatal hemorrhagic fever patient in Bolivia in 2004. No reservoir has been identified and nothing is known about its epidemiology or geographic distribution. Lassa virus infection is endemic in West Africa from Senegal to Cameroon and perhaps other areas not yet explored. There are increases in Lassa infection during the dry seasons, perhaps because of increased virus stability in lower humidity, but other, as yet unknown, factors may also be involved.

Host Range and Virus Propagation

All of the New World arenaviruses have rodent reservoir hosts with the exception of Tacaribe virus, which was isolated from bats in Trinidad (**Table 1**). A hallmark of the arenaviruses is their intimate biological relationship with rodents, resulting in lifetime infection and chronic virus excretion. Many arenaviruses have more than one rodent host, although usually a single species will predominate as the reservoir in nature.

The hosts of LCM virus (LCMV) have included *Mus* species and hamsters. Guinea pigs are also capable of transmitting the virus in laboratory settings. Machupo virus often renders its major natural host, *Calomys callosus*, essentially sterile by causing the young to die *in utero*. Machupo virus also induces a hemolytic anemia in its rodent host, with significant splenomegaly, often an important identifier of infected rodents in the field. The major rodent hosts for Junin virus are *Calomys* species. Transmission of Junin virus from rodent to rodent is generally horizontal, and not vertical, and is believed to occur through contaminated saliva and urine. The *Calomys* rodents are affected by the virus, with up to 50% fatality among infected suckling animals, and stunted growth in many others. Both Junin and Machupo viruses induce a humoral immune response when transmitted to their suckling natural rodent hosts, which may have neutralizing antibody in the face of persistent infection. Guanarito virus has been isolated from *Zygodontomys brevicauda*, though its detailed biology remains to be learned.

The only known reservoir of Lassa virus in West Africa is *Mastomys natalensis*, one of the most commonly occurring rodents in Africa. At least two species of *Mastomys* (diploid types with 32 and 38 chromosomes) inhabit West Africa, and both have been found to harbor the virus. All species are equally susceptible to silent persistent infection, as seen when LCMV infects mice. This presumably occurs as in LCM infection, from a selective deletion of the thymic T cell response to the virus. All of the arenaviruses pathogenic for humans will also infect and produce illness in a wide range of primates. However, it is not known whether such infections occur in nature, as is known for Ebola virus for example. In addition, human infection plays no biological role in the life cycle and ecology of the arenaviruses.

Virus Propagation

The original isolation of LCMV was made in suckling mice, which have been important in isolation and characterization of several of the arenaviruses. The arenaviruses are, however, easily cultivated in a wide variety of mammalian cell monolayers. The Vero E6 remains the cell of choice for primary isolation and cultivation, but arenaviruses also replicate in baby hamster kidney cells, as well as in a number of specialized cells such as continuous macrophage lines, endothelial cells, fibroblasts and a variety of mouse cell lines, with specific MHC markers used as targets for immunological studies. The infected cells may produce a cytopathic effect (CPE) beginning on days 4–7 of incubation. However, not all arenaviruses produce CPE, especially on primary isolation. For diagnosis, cells may be harvested after 48–72 h and assayed for antigen by immunofluorescent antibody (IFA) or ELISA. Virus plaquing techniques may also be used for the arenaviruses.

Genetics

While advances have been made in determining the genetic relationship between different arenaviruses (see Classification), the level of genetic variability within species of arenaviruses is not well characterized, though it must be added that little genetic data on field isolates exist on which to make this judgment. It would appear that the frequency of variability at the amino acid level, as judged by B cell epitope variability, is not high. Thus the variability in B cell epitopes among Lassa viruses isolated from humans or rodents over a 10-year period in a circumscribed area was not substantial, suggesting that B cell epitopes are under limited immune pressure in their rodent hosts. Knowledge of the epitopes recognized by T cells may be crucial for the development of recombinant Lassa virus vaccines. A human T-helper cell epitope, highly conserved between Old and New World arenaviruses, as well as HLA-A2-restricted CD8 T cell protective Lassa virus epitope have been described. The South American arenaviruses may be under both B and T cell immune pressure in their rodent hosts, though no data are available on this issue. Reassortment, demonstrated only in the laboratory, may also be a means of genetic variability, but its occurrence in nature and therefore its importance is unknown.

Evolution

The *Arenaviridae* are distributed over five continents and can be divided into three 'coevolutionary' groups: Lassa complex in Africa, LCM in North America, Europe, and South America, and the Tacaribe complex in South America. Today's arenaviruses probably descended from an ancestral virus which subsequently differentiated in parallel with the evolution of the Cricetid rodents persistently infected by arena viruses. It seems likely, therefore, that the present distribution and evolution of these viruses are directly related to the distribution and evolution of the earliest Cricetid rodents and their descendants, which now make up the natural hosts of most of this family of viruses (Tacaribe virus has a bat host). The coevolution of these viruses will undoubtedly continue and depend primarily on mutations, selected by the persistently infected host's immune pressure, and perhaps on reassortment in the rodent host.

Epidemiology

The fundamental determinant of the ecology of hemorrhagic fevers is the occurrence of persistent virus infection in rodents. Who becomes infected and what are the functions of the behavior of the persistently infected rodent, and the cultural and occupational patterns of human populations. The arenavirus hemorrhagic fevers are primarily rural and semirural diseases; however, some evidence exists that under certain conditions (poverty, overcrowding), their rodent reservoirs may also establish urban habits. The rodents infect the environment via urine, feces and saliva. Interactions between rodents and humans are peridomestic or in agricultural areas. However, details of the rodent population dynamics, behavior, and the natural history of the persistent virus infection in the feral rodent hosts are only poorly understood. The Old World arenaviruses, LCM and Lassa, produce persistent infection in their rodent hosts without significant detrimental effects. The South American viruses, in contrast, may cause illness and death in newborn rodents, or may induce persistence. The modes of transmission from rodents to humans are not precisely known. Direct contact by humans, with cuts and scratches on hands and feet, with articles and surfaces contaminated by virus may be a more important and consistent mode of transmission. Transmission through mucosal surfaces may also occur under some circumstances.

Lassa Fever

Lassa fever occurs in West Africa, but with a wide geographic area from Northern Nigeria to Guinea, encompassing perhaps 100 million population. At least two species of *Mastomys* occupy West Africa, and both have been found to harbor the virus. These rodents, especially the species with 32 chromosomes, are highly commensal with humans. The movement of *Mastomys* within a village is very limited, and their average lifespan is about 6 months, with little seasonal fluctuation in their breeding pattern. From 5% to as many as 70% have been found to be infected with virus in some village houses. Therefore, most virus transmission takes place in and around the homes. All age groups and both sexes are affected and antibody prevalence increases with age. Risk factors for human infection include contact with rodents, direct contact with ill persons infected with Lassa virus, presence of a large household rodent population, and human practices such as catching, cooking and eating rodents, and indiscriminant storage of food. In many endemic areas, Lassa fever is a common cause of hospitalization. The death rate in systematically studied, untreated hospitalized patients with Lassa fever is 16%, very similar to that described for Junin and Machupo infections. Nosocomial transmission occurs in Africa from contact with infected patients, or through improper use or sterilization of needles, sometimes leading to an outbreak. Person-to-person spread of Lassa virus in households is common, a unique characteristic of Lassa virus in relation to other arenaviruses (no data are yet available on Guanarito virus from Venezuela, or Sabia virus from Brazil), and is usually associated with direct contact or care of someone with a febrile illness, or possibly with sexual contact with the spouse during the incubation or convalescent phases of illness. Illness to infection ratios are 10–25% in some endemic areas of West Africa. Antibody prevalence ranges from less than 1% to over 40% in some villages.

Argentine Hemorrhagic Fever (AHF)

AHF, caused by Junin virus, was recognized in the 1950s in the northwestern part of the Buenos Aires Province in Argentina, an area of very fertile farmland and therefore of great economic importance. The total number of cases reported over a 30 year period is about 21 000. AHF is a seasonal disease with peak yearly incidence in May. The average number of cases from 1981 to 1986 was 360 per year. Although all ages and sexes are susceptible, nevertheless the major group affected is the male working population, explained by the habits of the rodent hosts for Junin virus, *Calomys musculinus* and *Calomys laucha*. These animals are not peridomestic, but rather occupy grain fields, and this is the major reason for the affected population of field workers. Infection also occurs infrequently in other rodents: *Mus musculus*, *Akodon azarae*, and *Oryzomys flavecens*. Transmission from rodent to rodent is horizontal, not vertical, and is thought to occur via contaminated saliva and urine. It is believed that the major routes of virus transmission from humans is through contact with

virus-infected dust and grain products and subsequent infection through cuts and abrasions on the skin, or through airborne dust generated primarily by killing and scattering of rodents during mechanized farming. The disease has spread over the 30 years or so since its recognition from an area of 16 000 km² and a quarter of a million persons to an area greater than 120 000 km² containing a population of over 1 million persons. Furthermore, the incidence in the older affected areas appears to wane after 5–10 years. Overall antibody prevalence is 12%, with a typical predominance in agricultural workers. One-third of the seropositive individuals have no history of typical illness, suggesting that the case: infection ratio is about 2:3. The incidence of AHF is now very low due to the extensive vaccination campaign in the endemic area.

Bolivian Hemorrhagic Fever (BHF)

The only known reservoir for the virus is *Callomys callosus*, a Cricetid rodent that is found in the highest density at the borders of tropical grassland and forest. The distribution of this rodent appears to include the eastern Bolivian plains, as well as northern Paraguay and adjacent areas of western Brazil. The disease was recognized in 1959, and by 1962 more than 1000 cases had been identified in a confined area of two provinces, with a 22% case fatality ratio. The largest known epidemic of BHF, involving several hundred cases, occurred in the town of San Joaquin in 1963 and 1964. This outbreak occurred because of a marked increase in the *Callomys* population, and the subsequent invasion of homes in the town by these rodents. Although the *Callomys* appears to be capable of living both in the areas surrounding the towns and in the towns themselves (where the most efficient transmission of virus would appear to occur), they favor a nonperidomestic habitat where contact with humans is much reduced. It appears that the situation in San Joaquin was unusual, and such an event has not been observed again after nearly 25 years. There has not appeared to be any increase in the geographic areas affected by BHF recently, and few cases have been reported.

Venezuelan Hemorrhagic Fever

The epidemiologic pattern of this disease has not yet been well characterized. In one survey the antibody prevalence in the population in the endemic area in central Venezuela was 2.6%. Guanarito virus was isolated from the cane rat *Zygodontomys brevicauda*. The occurrence of person-to-person transmission has not yet been demonstrated. The low frequency of infection in family contacts and lack of disease in hospital workers caring for patients suggest that person-to-person spread is uncommon. The pattern of infection includes all ages and sexes, suggesting that transmission occurs in and around houses, similar to Lassa fever and BHF and unlike AHF.

Transmission and Tissue Tropism

The primary mode of arenavirus transmission is from human contact with rodent urine or blood. This probably occurs primarily when individuals come into contact with surfaces or materials recently contaminated by rodent urine, or when they trap a rodent and handle the carcass. Some evidence suggests that rodent blood or urine might be aerosolized by machinery during mechanized harvesting of corn in Argentina, with consequent transmission of Junin virus to people working near the machinery; however, no detailed studies of specific risk factors exist. In Africa, the rodents are highly commensal and probably deposit virus-laden urine in many areas of the houses they inhabit. The people tend to walk barefooted, and, based on the epidemiologic pattern of somewhat sporadic infection in households, it seems likely that contact with infectious urine is the primary source of contamination. In addition, in parts of Africa people catch and eat rodents, putting them in direct contact with rodent tissue, blood and secretions during the preparation. Finally, for some of the viruses, particularly Lassa virus, there is person-to-person transmission primarily through contact with the blood or secretions of an infected, ill person. Whatever the mode of transmission, it would seem that the reticuloendothelial system is probably a primary target of replication of the arenaviruses, though they replicate well in many organs, including liver, adrenal gland, placenta, lung and many other organs.

Pathogenesis

The most common sites of initiation of human infection by the arenaviruses are not yet known, although they seem likely to be cuts and abrasions in the skin. Following the initiation of infection, all arenaviruses progress to generalized multiorgan infections, especially of the reticuloendothelial system. Thereafter, however, the pathogenesis of the different infections is variable. Cellular receptors for both New and Old world arenaviruses have recently been described.

Lassa fever

The 1–3 week incubation that follows infection suggests an unknown primary replication site, probably within the reticuloendothelial system. Route and titer of infecting dose may be important determinants of outcome, as may the virus strain. For example, death rates in nosocomial outbreaks where parenteral exposure is substantial are usually higher than community-acquired infections.

The degree of organ damage in fatal human infections is mild, which is sharply at variance with the clinical course and collapse of the patient. Indeed, there are few clues to the pathogenesis of Lassa fever in standard pathological studies. Liver damage is variable, with concomitant cellular injury, necrosis and regeneration. Nevertheless, serum aspartate aminotransferase (AST) levels over 150 iu ml^{-1} are correlated with poor outcome, and an ever-increasing level is also associated with increased risk of death. Alanine aminotransferase (ALT) is only marginally raised, and the ratio of AST:ALT in natural infections and in experimentally infected primates is as high as 11:1. Furthermore, prothrombin times, glucose and bilirubin levels are near normal, excluding biochemical hepatic failure. An increasing Lassa viremia is also associated with increasing case fatality. In addition to the liver, high virus titers occur in many other organs without significant pathologic or functional lesions, perhaps reflecting blood rather than parenchymal levels of virus.

Some patients develop severe pulmonary edema and adult respiratory distress syndrome, gross head and neck edema, pharyngeal stridor and hypovolemic shock. This pattern is consistent with edema due to capillary leakage, rather than cardiac failure and impaired venous return. Endothelial cell dysfunction has been demonstrated in primates experimentally infected by Lassa fever, in that there is apparently a marked decrease in prostacyclin production by endothelial cells. Loss of integrity of the capillary bed presumably causes the leakage of fluids and macromolecules into the extravascular spaces and the subsequent hemoconcentration, hypoalbuminemia, and hypovolemic shock. Proteinuria is common, occurring in two-thirds of patients.

Edema and bleeding may occur together or independently. Since there is a minimal disturbance of the intrinsic, and almost none of the extrinsic, coagulation system, and there is no increase in fibrinogen breakdown products, disseminated intravascular coagulation (DIC) is excluded. Furthermore, platelet and fibrinogen turnover in experimental primate infections are normal. Though platelet numbers are only moderately depressed, in severe disease platelet aggregation is almost completely abolished by a circulating inhibitor. The origin of this inhibitor is not known; however, it cannot be reproduced with viral material nor can it be blocked by antibodies to Lassa virus. In the platelet, it blocks dense granule and ATP release and thus abolishes the secondary wave of *in vitro* aggregation, while sparing the arachidonic acid metabolite-dependent primary wave. The inhibitor of platelet function also interferes with the generation of the FMLP-induced superoxide generation in polymorphonuclear leukocytes probably through a similar mechanism.

AHF and BHF

Despite the different degrees of bleeding, there are sufficient similarities between the course of disease in AHF, BHF, and Lassa fever to speculate that there exists a similar pathophysiologic pathway underlying all of the diseases. Organ function, other than the endothelial system, appears to remain intact, and the critical period of shock is brief, lasting only 24–48 h. Hepatitis is mild, and renal function is also well maintained. Bleeding is more pronounced with AHF and BHF than Lassa fever, but it is not the cause of shock and death. Capillary leakage is significant, with loss of protein and intravascular volume being much more pronounced than loss of red cells. Proteinuria is significant, and dehydration with hemoconcentration appears to be an important process. The shock is not associated with evidence of disseminated intravascular coagulation, and even though there are petechiae suggesting some direct endothelial damage, no clear evidence of virus replication in, and damage of, endothelium has been demonstrated. Thus, clinical observations suggest that vascular endothelial dysfunction may be the basis of subsequent circulatory failure in AHF and BHF. Persistent hypovolemic shock in the face of intravascular volume expanders suggests that it is due to the loss of endothelial function and leakage of fluid into extravascular spaces. This is supported by the tissue edema frequently observed, and more directly by the pulmonary edema which may result from vigorous fluid therapy of the shock. These events lead to irreversible shock and death in the most severely ill patients. Two other observations have been made in AHF: high levels of interferon in severely/fatally ill patients, and a decrease in complement. These are general phenomena observed in other severe infectious processes and are consistent with the events described above. Neither would dictate a substantially different pathophysiologic explanation of these diseases.

Clinical Features

Lassa Fever

Lassa fever begins after 7–18 days of incubation, with fever, headache, and malaise. Aching in the large joints, pain in the lower back, a nonproductive cough, severe headache, and sore throat are common. Many patients also develop severe retrosternal or epigastric pain. Vomiting and diarrhea occurs in 50–70% of patients. In more severely ill patients, complete prostration may occur by the 6th to 8th day of illness. Patients with Lassa fever appear toxic and anxious, and in the absence of shock, the skin is usually moist from diapheresis. There is an elevated respiratory rate and pulse. The systolic blood pressure may be low. There is no characteristic skin rash; petechiae and ecchymoses are rare, nor is jaundice a feature of Lassa fever. Conjunctivitis is common, but rare conjunctival hemorrhages portend a poor prognosis. Seventy percent of patients have pharyngitis, often exudative, but few if any petechiae, and ulcers are rare. Mucosal bleeding occurs in 15–20% of all patients, and although associated with severe disease it is almost never of a magnitude to produce shock by itself. Edema of the face and neck are commonly seen in severe disease. About 20% of patients have pleural or pericardial rubs heard late in disease at the beginning of convalescence. The abdomen may be diffusely tender. The ECG may be abnormal, primarily with elevated T waves, but without a characteristic pattern. Moderate or severe diffuse encephalopathy with or without general seizures is characteristic in severe disease. Severe Lassa fever can progress rapidly between the 6th and 10th day to *respiratory distress* with stridor due to laryngeal edema, central cyanosis, hypovolemic shock and clinical signs of encephalopathy, sometimes with coma and seizures. Tremors are often seen in the hours just before death. Acute, focal neurological signs rarely occur, with the exception of VIII nerve deafness seen in convalescence. Residual ataxia is common. Lassa fever is also a pediatric disease affecting all ages of children. The disease appears to be even more difficult to diagnose by clinical criteria in children than in adults because its manifestations are so general. In very young babies marked edema may be seen, associated with very severe disease. In older children the disease may manifest as a primary diarrheal disease or as pneumonia or simply as an unexplained prolonged fever. The case fatality in children is 12–14%.

The mean white count in early Lassa fever may be low or normal, with a relative lymphopenia, but late neutrophilia may supervene in severe disease. Proteinuria is very characteristic. A serum AST (SGOT) level of >150 iu ml^{-1} is associated with a case fatality of 50%, and there is a correlation between an ever-increasing level and an increased risk of death. A viremia of $>1 \times 10^3$ TCID$_{50}$ ml^{-1} is associated with an increasing case fatality. Both factors together carry a risk of death of 80%.

Pharyngitis, proteinuria, and retrosternal chest pain have a predictive value for Lassa fever in febrile hospitalized patients of 81% and a specificity of 89%. Likewise, a triad of pharyngitis, retrosternal chest pain, and proteinuria (in a febrile patient) correctly predicted Lassa fever 80% of the time (in an endemic area). Both triads have sensitivities of 50% for detecting cases of Lassa fever. Significant complications of Lassa fever include a two- to threefold increased risk of maternal death from infection in the third trimester, and a fetal/perinatal loss of 84% that does not seem to vary by trimester. Another significant complication is that of acute VIII nerve deafness, with nearly 30% of patients suffering an acute loss of hearing in one or both ears. Other complications which appear to occur much less frequently are uveitis, pericarditis, orchitis, pleural effusion and ascites.

AHF and BHF

These diseases have an insidious onset of malaise, fever, general myalgia, and anorexia. Lumbar pain, epigastric pain, retro-orbital pain, often with photophobia, and constipation occur commonly. Nausea and vomiting frequently occur. Temperature is high, reaching 40 °C or above. Unlike LCM and Lassa fever, AHF and BHF do not usually lead to respiratory symptoms and sore throat. On physical examination, patients appear toxic. Conjunctivitis, erythema of the face, neck, and thorax are prominent. Petechiae may be observed in the axillae by the 4th or 5th day of the illness. There may be a pharyngeal enanthem, but pharyngitis is uncommon. Relative bradycardia is often observed. The disease may begin to subside after 6 days of illness; if not, the second stage of illness supervenes, and most commonly manifests as epistaxis and/or hematemesis or acute neurological disease. The bleeding may be from mucosal surfaces or into the skin, with petechiae and hemorrhagic rash, with preceding increase in packed red cell volume. Pulmonary edema is common in severely ill patients. The appearance of intractable shock is a serious sign which becomes irreversible in some patients, and accounts for the majority of deaths from AHF and BHF. Fifty percent of AHF and BHF patients also have neurologic symptoms during the second stage of illness, such as tremors of the hands and tongue, progressing in some patients to delirium, oculogyrus, and strabismus.

A low white blood cell count (under $1000 \, \text{mm}^{-1}$) and a platelet count under 100 000 are invariable. Proteinuria is common and microscopic hematuria also occurs. Alterations in clotting functions are minor, and DIC is not a significant part of the diseases. Liver and renal function tests are only mildly abnormal.

Venezuelan Hemorrhagic Fever

Little information is available on the spectrum of disease caused by Guanarito virus infection. Hospitalized patients with severe diseases are febrile on admission, with prostration, headache, arthralgia, cough, sore throat, nausea/vomiting, diarrhea, and hemorrhage. The bleeding includes epistaxis, bleeding gums, menorrhagia, and melena. On physical examination, patients with severe disease appear toxic, and usually dehydrated. They are described as having one or more of a series of signs, including pharyngitis, conjunctivitis, cervical lymphadenopathy, facial edema, and petechiae. Thrombocytopenia and neutropenia are common at admission. Case fatality of a single group of 15 hospitalized patients was over 60%; however, the single serum survey available suggests that overall mortality:infection ratio is much lower.

Pathology and Histopathology

Lassa Fever

The most frequently and consistently observed microscopic lesions in fatal human Lassa fever are focal necrosis of the liver, adrenal glands, and spleen. The liver damage is variable in the degree of hepatocytic necrosis. The liver demonstrates cellular injury, necrosis, and regeneration, with any or all present at death. A substantial macrophage response occurs, with little if any lymphocytic inflammatory response. Nevertheless, fatal cases do not exhibit sufficient hepatic damage to implicate hepatic failure as a cause of death. Similarly, moderate splenic necrosis is a consistent finding, primarily involving the marginal zone of the periarteriolar lymphocytic sheath. Diffuse focal adrenocortical cellular necrosis has been less frequently observed. Although high virus titers occur in other organs, such as brain, ovary, pancreas, uterus, and placenta, no significant lesions have been found. Thus, few clues to the pathogenesis of Lassa fever are found in standard pathological studies. It is clear that the outcome in Lassa fever is associated with the degree of virus replication; nevertheless the effect of replication is not major tissue destruction, but a more subtle biological effect on vascular endothelium, and perhaps other key cells or organs.

AHF and BHF

AHF and BHF are typical hemorrhagic diseases and have very similar pathologic features, some of which differ from Lassa fever. Patients with AHF manifest a skin rash and petechiae, and gross examination of organs at necropsy also show petechiae on the organ surfaces. Ulcerations of the digestive tract have been described, but the bleeding is not massive. Microscopic examination shows a general alteration in endothelial cells, mild edema of the vascular walls, with capillary swelling, and perivascular hemorrhage. Large areas of intra-alveolar or bronchial hemorrhage are often seen with no evidence of inflammatory process. Pneumonia with necrotizing bronchitis or pulmonary emboli is observed in half of the fatal necropsied cases. Hemorrhage and a lymphocytic infiltrate have been observed in the pericardium, occasionally with interstitial myocarditis. The lymphnodes are enlarged and congested with reticular cell hyperplasia. Splenic hemorrhage is common. Medullary congestion with pericapsular and pelvic hemorrhages are frequently seen. Acute tubular necrosis occurs in about half of the fatal cases, but adrenal necrosis has not been reported.

Venezuelan Hemorrhagic Fever

Only a limited number of post-mortem dissections have been performed. Observations included pulmonary edema with diffuse hemorrhages in the parenchyma, and subpleural, focal hepatic hemorrhages with congestion and yellow discoloration, cardiomegally with epicardial hemorrhages, splenic and renal swelling, and bleeding into numerous cavities, including stomach, intestines, bladder, and uterus.

Immune Response

There is a brisk B cell response to Lassa virus, with a classic primary IgG and IgM antibody response to virus early in the illness. This event does not, however, coincide with virus clearance, and high viremia and high IgG and IgM titers often coexist in both humans and primates. Indeed, virus may persist in the serum and urine of humans for several months after infection, and possibly longer in occult sites, such as renal tissue. Neutralizing antibodies to Lassa virus are absent in the serum of patients at the beginning of convalescence, and in most people they are never detectable. In a minority of patients some low titer serum neutralizing activity may be observed several months after resolution of the disease. Passive protection with antibody to Lassa virus has been demonstrated in animals given selected antiserum at the time or soon after inoculation with virus, but clinical trials of human plasma given after onset of illness have shown little or no protective effect. Thus, the clearance of Lassa virus in acute infection appears to be less dependent of antibody formation, and presumably depends more on the cell immune response. This is supported by recent experience with experimental Lassa vaccines in primates. In recent studies of LCM infection there is clearly apoptosis of T cells and probably B cells during acute infection in the mouse model. Such a scenario must be entertained for acute Lassa infection, and could help explain the fulminant course in some patients. Such work will need to be performed in primate models or during studies of human disease in endemic areas. Neutralizing and complement fixing antibody to Junin and Machupo are usually detectable 3–4 weeks after the onset of illness. Indirect fluorescent antibodies may be detected at the end of the second week of illness. The efficacy of convalescent plasma has been demonstrated in the therapy of Junin infection (see Therapy). The effectiveness of the plasma has been demonstrated to be associated with the level of Junin virus-neutralizing antibodies. The IFA test is the most commonly performed test for diagnosis by antibody detection for AHF and BHF. Little data are available on Guanarito virus, which appear to induce an antibody response. However, more like AHF and BHF, antibodies to Guanarito virus seem to appear later in illness.

Prevention and Control

Rodent Control

The ideal method of prevention for these rodent-borne diseases is to prevent contact between rodents and humans. The effectiveness of this was shown in the outbreaks of BHF in the 1960s. However, the prospects of rodent control in preventing AHF are not so bright. The human–rodent encounter resulting in AHF occurs during the crop harvests, and with the present technology it is difficult to imagine how control of noncommensal feral rodents could be accomplished. The best choice may be better protection of the agricultural worker from contact with rodent secretions and blood. Similarly, the control of rodents as a broad approach to preventing Lassa fever is not realistic. The improvement of housing and food storage could reduce the domestic rodent population, but such changes are not easily made. Rodent trapping in an individual village where transmission is high has demonstrated as much as a fivefold reduction in the rate of virus transmission. However, such a program is only applicable in villages with exceptional transmission rates, and would certainly not be applicable to large areas.

Vaccines

The live attenuated Junin vaccine has now been shown to be not only effective but also has had a dramatic effect in reducing the number of cases of AHF seen each year in the endemic area. A vaccine against Lassa fever has been made by cloning and expressing the Lassa virus glycoprotein gene into vaccinia virus. This vaccine has proved highly successful in preventing severe disease and death in challenged monkeys. Only the glycoprotein gene is protective in the two species of monkeys thus far tested, and the basis of protection is not neutralizing antibody, which does not develop, but more likely the cell-mediated immune response. Vaccines using the glycoprotein vectored by VSV prevent disease and death in the non-human primates model.

Drug Prophylaxis

In the event of identifiable exposure to Lassa virus (and possibly other pathogenic arenaviruses) in a hospital or laboratory setting, the prophylactic use of orally administered ribavirin is recommended, although efficacy data are missing.

Therapy

Significant advances have been made in the therapy of Junin and Lassa virus infections since the early 1990s. Convalescent plasma is effective in the treatment of Junin virus during the first 8 days of illness, but not Lassa virus. Ribavirin is effective in reducing the viremia and mortality of Lassa fever particularly when given in the first week of illness.

Lassa Fever

Ribavirin can prevent death in Lassa fever when given at any point in the illness, but it is more effective when given early and intravenously. Thus, patients with risk factors for severe disease who were treated within the first 6 days of illness experienced a 5–9% case fatality. Those with the same risk factors, in whom treatment was initiated more than 6 days after the onset of illness, had a case fatality of 20–47%. Regardless, the case fatality was significantly less for ribavirin-treated patients in all categories than for either nontreated patients or for those treated with plasma alone. As such it seems reasonable to assume that it would also be an effective measure in the event of laboratory or hospital exposure to the disease. The pathogenesis of the infection is less reversible later in illness. Furthermore, patients treated with ribavirin had significant declines in viremia regardless of outcome, whereas patients who were untreated or treated with plasma and who died showed no decrease in viremia, consistent with the observation that outcome, and presumably the result of therapy, is closely related to the inhibition of virus replication. Therefore, patients coming late in disease will require more effective clinical management of physiologic dysfunction, and perhaps other drugs which may be used to stabilize the shock state sufficiently long to allow recovery and improve survival (see Pathogenesis).

AHF

A randomized trial of patients with AHF demonstrated that convalescent-phase plasma reduced the mortality from 16% to 1% in the patients who were treated in the first 8 days of illness. The efficacy of the plasma was directly related to the concentration of neutralizing antibodies of the plasma.

The success of this therapy was not without a price, however, which was the development of a late neurological syndrome in about 10% of cases. Thus far, there is no correlation between either the day of therapy or the dose of neutralizing antibodies given and the occurrence of late neurological syndrome. Passive antibody therapy depends on collection of plasma from persons known to have had the disease, testing the plasma (or screening the donor) for antibodies to blood-borne agents such as hepatitis, and proper storage until its use. In addition, the advent of the acquired immunodeficiency syndrome (AIDS) and the other diseases transmissible by blood products means that further screening is required before use.

BHF

Recent experience of successful treatment of two patients with intravenous ribavirin suggests that further efforts to evaluate the effectiveness of ribavirin in this disease will be worthwhile.

Future Perspectives

An important area of future research includes a more through understanding of the viral and host components of the virus-clearing and protective immune response in humans. A second area of substantial interest is the nature of the persistent infection in the rodent host. A more complete understanding of the pathogenesis of Lassa fever may provide insight not only to that disease, but to basic elements of how the host response may be detrimental as well as beneficial to the host. Finally, a more through comprehension of how to control the more widespread arenavirus diseases, either through vaccination, or preferably rodent control, is essential.

See also: Lymphocytic Choriomeningitis Virus: General Features.

Further Reading

Buchmeier MJ, Bowen MD, and Peters CJ (2001) Arenaviridae: The viruses and their replication. In: Knipe DM and Howley PM (eds.) *Fields Virology*, 4th edn., pp. 1635–1668. Philadelphia: Lippincott Williams and Wilkins.

Cajimat MNB and Fulhorst CF (2004) Phylogeny of the Venezuelan arenaviruses. *Virus Research* 102: 199–206.

Clegg JCS (2002) Molecular Phylogeny of the Arenaviruses. *Current Topics in Microbiology and Immunology* 262: 1–24.

Damonte EB and Coto CE (2002) Treatment of arenavirus infections: from basic studies to the challenge of antiviral therapy. *Advances in Virus Research* 58: 125–155.

Enria D, Mills JA, Flick R, *et al.* (2006) Arenavirus infections. In: Guerrant RL, Walker DH,, and Weller PF (eds.) *Tropical Infectious Diseases. Principles, Pathogens and Practice*, 2nd edn., pp. 734–755. Philadelphia, PA: Elsevier Churchill Livingstone.

Fisher-Hoch SP and McCormick JB (2004) Lassa fever vaccine. *Expert Review of Vaccines* 3: 189–197.

Gunther S and Lenz O (2004) Lassa virus. *Critical Reviews in Clinical Laboratory Sciences* 41: 339–390.

Kunz S, Borrow P, and Oldstone MBA (2002) Receptor structure, binding, and cell entry of arenaviruses. *Current Topics in Microbiology and Immunology* 262: 111–137.

McCormick JB, Webb PA, Scribner CL, *et al.* (1986) Lassa fever: Effective therapy with ribavirin. *New England Journal of Medicine* 314: 20.

McCormick JB, Webb PA, Krebs JW, Johnson KM, and Smith K (1986) A prospective study of the epidemiology and ecology of Lassa fever. *Journal of Infectious Diseases* 155: 437.

Rojek JM, Spiropoulou CF, and Kunz S (2006) Characterization of the cellular receptors for the South American hemorrhagic fever viruses Junin, Guanarito, and Machupo. *Virology* 349: 476–491.

Salazar-Bravo J, Ruedas LA, and Yates TL (2002) Mammalian Reservoirs of Arenaviruses. *Current Topics in Microbiology and Immunology* 262: 25–63.

Lymphocytic Choriomeningitis Virus: General Features

R M Welsh, University of Massachusetts Medical School, Worcester, MA, USA

History

Lymphocytic choriomeningitis virus (LCMV), of the family *Arenaviridae*, is an etiological agent for human acute aseptic meningitis and grippe-like infections and is maintained in nature by lifelong persistent infections of mice (*Mus musculus*). Three strains still being studied today were initially isolated in the USA in the 1930s. During an attempt to recover and passage virus from a suspected human case of St. Louis encephalitis, Armstrong and Lillie isolated LCMV (Armstrong strain) from a monkey that developed a lymphocytic choriomeningitis – hence the name. Traub then reported the isolation of a serologically indistinguishable virus contaminating his mouse colony (Traub strain), and Rivers and Scott isolated similar viruses from human meningitis patients (one being the WE strain). Subsequently, many other isolations from man and animals were made, and a clear cause–effect relationship between LCMV and about 8% of the US cases of human nonbacterial meningitis was established.

The LCMV infection of the mouse soon became an important model system for studying viral immunology. A distinguishing feature of the LCMV infection was that it established a long-term persistent infection in mice infected *in utero* or shortly after birth, whereas adult mice inoculated with LCMV either cleared the virus with lasting immunity or, in the case of an intracranial infection, died of a lethal meningoencephalitis (**Figure 1**). Antiviral antibody was difficult to detect in the persistently infected mice, and this led Burnet and Fenner to postulate that exposure to viral antigens before the maturation of the immune system resulted in mice becoming immunologically tolerant to LCMV and thus unable to clear the infection. This was one of the systems that provided the basis for Burnet's Nobel Prize-winning theories of immunological tolerance. Subsequent work by Oldstone and Dixon, however, demonstrated that persistently infected mice did make antiviral antibody, but it was difficult to detect because of excess viral antigen. The antiviral antibody traveled in the circulation complexed to virus and complement, and these circulating as well as tissue-bound immune complexes contributed to a progressive degenerative disease involving glomerulonephritis, arteritis, and chronic inflammatory lesions. In the acute infection both the clearance of the virus and the lethal meningoencephalitis were shown to be due mostly to the cytotoxic T lymphocyte (CTL) response. Antiviral CTLs were first demonstrated in the LCMV model, and Zinkernagel and Doherty used this model to demonstrate the Nobel Prize-winning concept of major histocompatibility complex (MHC) restriction in CTL recognition. Persistently infected mice were eventually shown to have split-tolerance to LCMV, in that, although they could mount an antibody response to LCMV, they could not

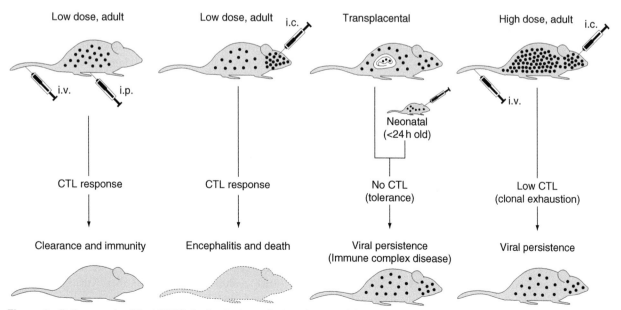

Figure 1 Pathogenesis of the LCMV infection is dependent on the age of the host, the route of infection, and the dose of the virus.

generate the LCMV-specific CTLs which were needed to clear the infection.

Taxonomy and Classification

LCMV is the prototype virus of the *Arenaviridae* family of RNA viruses, and, although it has some homology with all arenaviruses, it is most closely related to the African virus *Lassa* and is classified as an Old World arenavirus. Its ambisense genome consists of two single-stranded RNAs, each encoding two genes of opposite polarity and separated by intergenic regions with strong RNA secondary structure. The small S RNA $(1.1 \times 10^3 \, \text{kDa})$ in the virion encodes in the negative-sense a 63 kDa nucleoprotein (NP) and in the positive- or message-sense a 75 kDa cell-associated glycoprotein (GPC), which is cleaved into two virion glycoproteins, GP1 (44 kDa) and GP2 (35 kDa). The large L RNA $(2.3 \times 10^3 \, \text{kDa})$ in the virion encodes in the negative-sense a 200 kDa RNA-dependent RNA polymerase (L) and in the positive-sense a smaller 11 kDa zinc-binding protein (Z) which binds to the ribonucleoprotein complex and is involved in transcriptional regulation. LCMV replicates in the cytoplasm and buds from the plasma membrane, incorporating host lipids into the viral membrane. It is pleomorphic, with sizes reported from 50 to 300 nm. Some of the virions, which may or may not be infectious, contain ribosome-like structures, giving the virion the characteristic arenavirus appearance.

Geographic and Seasonal Distribution

LCMV infections of mice and man have been well established in Europe and in North and South America, but they are not well documented elsewhere. LCMV is considered an Old World arenavirus brought to the Americas by its host, *Mus musculus*. There is some evidence that human infections occur more commonly in the winter and spring.

Host Range and Viral Propagation

The natural host for LCMV is the mouse, but it can be transmitted to man, hamsters, guinea pigs, rats, dogs, swine, monkeys, chimpanzees, and chick embryos. It commonly causes long-term persistent infections in mice and hamsters, and this has provided a source for human infections. The receptor for LCMV is alpha-dystroglycan, and LCMV strains binding to this receptor at high affinity tend to disseminate *in vivo* more than those that bind at lower affinity. LCMV grows in a wide variety of tissues *in vivo* and in most cells tested in culture. For instance, LCMV has been propagated and plaque assayed in 3T3, baby hamster kidney (BHK), Detroit-98, HeLa, JLSV-9, L-929, MDBK, MDCK,

Vero, and vole cell lines. Vero, L-929, and BHK cells are most commonly used for plaque assays, and BHK cells have been the choice for most biochemical analyses because of the relatively high yields of virus ($c.$ 10^8 plaque-forming units (PFU) ml^{-1}) and the lack of secreted endogenous retrovirus contaminants. LCMV also grows in lymphocytes and macrophages, and the latter can be used as stimulator or target cells in T-cell proliferation or cytotoxicity assays, respectively.

Genetics

Like other single-stranded RNA viruses, LCMV mutates frequently, and these mutants vary in their tropism and disease-producing potential. A single passage of a cloned LCMV variant into mice will soon segregate into clear neurotropic and turbid viscerotropic plaque variants, which can be recovered from the brain and spleen, respectively. A single amino acid change in the LCMV glycoprotein (residue 260) can convert the immunostimulatory Armstrong strain of LCMV into an immunosuppressive (clone 13) variant, and these genotypes rapidly intraconvert during *in vivo* passage. Several strains of LCMV have been sequenced, and the highest level of sequence homology is at the 5′ and 3′ termini of the S and L virion RNA. These are presumed polymerasebinding sites well conserved throughout the arenavirus family. Different arenaviruses cross-interfere via a defective-interfering virus mechanism. The preservation of these polymerase-binding sites may allow for this heterotypic interference. The NP and GP of the Armstrong and WE strains share 90% amino acid homology.

The presence of two virion RNAs allows for highfrequency recombination due to reassortment of viral genomes. The technique of generating reassortants has led to the assignment of viral-encoded proteins to the appropriate RNA and has facilitated the mapping of genes required for disease-producing potential. The ease of producing reassortants in the laboratory suggests that they also occur in nature and probably play roles in enhancing the genetic diversity of arenaviruses.

Evolution

Arenaviruses do not show substantial sequence homology with any other virus group, but the homology within members of this family suggests a common origin for all arenaviruses. LCMV is most closely related to Lassa virus, which, like LCMV, has its origins in the Eastern Hemisphere. Each arenavirus favors a specific rodent host, and selective evolutionary pressure on these viruses must have been conferred by their adaptation to their respective hosts in forms that established persistent infections. Of interest is that LCMV and other arenaviruses undergo rapid evolution as they form persistent infections. These persistent infections *in vitro* and *in vivo* result in the extensive production of defective-interfering virus and of attenuated relatively noncytopathic plaque variants which may help in the maintenance of persistent infections by preventing virus-induced cell death.

Serological Relationships and Variability

Antisera to Lassa virus and to all members of the Tacaribe complex cross-react to some extent with LCMV by complement fixation and immunofluorescence assays but not at the level of viral neutralization. Few monoclonal antibodies show cross-reactivity between LCMV and other Tacaribe complex viruses, but several cross-react with the more closely related Lassa virus. Infection of guinea pigs with LCMV immunizes them against a lethal dose of Lassa virus. Different strains of LCMV are not easily distinguishable by antisera but can be distinguished by some monoclonal antibodies and molecular methods.

Epidemiology

Human LCMV infections occur without sexual bias and at all ages, but most frequently in the 20–30-year age group. A longitudinal study in the USA from 1941 to 1958 implicated LCMV infections in about 8% of patients diagnosed with suspected viral meningitis, and serological studies have suggested up to a 10–15% incidence of LCMV infection in the general population. Most of these infections are probably mild or subclinical. Laboratory infections with LCMV are relatively common, and several cases have occurred in laboratories working with the WE strain, which was re-isolated from one laboratory worker and identified serologically with monoclonal antibodies.

Transmission and Tissue Tropism

LCMV has been experimentally transferred to man by intramuscular injection, but the normal route of infection is probably via the respiratory tract after exposure to mouse secretions. LCMV is shed at high titer in mouse feces and urine and is probably not transmitted by arthropod vectors. Another source of infection is the Syrian hamster (*Mesocricetus auratus*), which, like the mouse, can harbor a long-term persistent infection. Several cases of LCMV in different geographic areas have been linked to a colony of persistently infected hamsters distributed throughout the USA. Recently, several patients developed severe LCMV infections after receiving transplanted organs from a deceased individual who had contracted LCMV from a pet hamster. Horizontal man-to-man transmission is rare, but LCMV can cross the placenta and infect the fetus.

Pathogenicity

LCMV strains appear to differ in their pathogenicity in man, but conclusive analyses of strain virulence differences in humans have not been carried out. Several human infections have occurred in laboratories working with the WE strain, and the WE strain has been reisolated from a laboratory worker with meningitis and clearly identified. There appear to be fewer (if any) anecdotal reports of human infection with the parent Armstrong strain. However, the more rapidly disseminating clone 13 variant of the Armstrong strain of LCMV has also been linked to human infection. The WE strain is much more virulent than the parent Armstrong strain in hamsters and guinea pigs, and reassortant analyses have mapped the ability to cause lethal infections in guinea pigs to the L RNA of the WE strain. The United States Centers for Disease Control recommends Biosafety Level 2 practices for most studies with LCMV in mice but Biosafety Level 3 practices for work with hamsters. This is based on the presumption that LCMV becomes more virulent for humans as it passes through hamsters. Although this has not been formally proven, this precaution would appear necessary due to the high number of clinical infections in individuals exposed to persistently infected hamsters.

LCMV has been used in a number of pathogenesis studies in mice. Viral strain variant differences exist in the encephalitis model, in which 'docile' or viscerotropic variants fail to kill mice, whereas 'aggressive' or more exclusively neurotropic variants do. However, a docile variant for one strain of mouse may be aggressive to another strain of mouse, and the susceptibility of mice to these variants seems to be linked to both MHC- and non-MHC genes. One reason for 'docility' is the immunosuppressive nature of some LCMV strains, particularly when inoculated into mice at high dose. Lethal encephalitis does not occur when the T-cell response is severely compromised. Immunosuppressive variants of LCMV tend to replicate to very high levels in the visceral organs. This high-dose antigen load can clonally exhaust the T cells by either driving them into apoptosis or into a functional anergy. This clonal exhaustion may limit the encephalitis but can result in a long-term persistent infection (**Figure 1**).

One interesting pathogenic feature of LCMV is its ability to cause a loss in cellular specialized or 'luxury' functions required not for cell survival but for homeostasis of the whole organism. Persistent LCMV infection results in reduced neurotransmitter enzyme activity in cultured neuroblastoma cells *in vitro* and reduced levels of growth and thyroid hormones in mice. Reduced growth hormone synthesis is associated with a runting syndrome in young infected mice. LCMV infects *in vivo* the cells that produce growth hormone and thyroid hormone and causes significant reductions in levels of mRNA encoding these hormones but not other hormones and proteins such as thyroid-stimulating hormone, actin, and collagen.

Clinical Features of Infection

The LCMV infection of man can be an inapparent or subclinical infection, or it can present as a nonmeningeal grippe-like ailment, an aseptic meningitis, or a more severe meningoencephalitis. The incubation period is 1–2 weeks or longer, and the disease may come in two or three waves. The grippal type is characterized by fever, malaise, lethargy, weakness, myalgia, arthralgia, fever, headache, photophobia, anorexia, and nausea. Some patients develop a rash, arthritis, parotitis, or orchitis. The grippal type is likely the most common form of the disease. The meningeal type is often preceded by the grippal type and presents with stiff neck, vomiting, irritability, and Brudzinski's and Kernig's signs. The meningoencephalomyelitic form, which is relatively rare, is associated with confusion, hallucinations, papilledema, and weakness progressing to paralysis. Patients usually recover without lasting sequelae. Death is very rare. There have been only nine fatal cases documented between 1942 and 1992, but two deaths were more recently seen in infected transplant recipients. There are also some reports of human transplacental infection, resulting in fetal abortion or malformation.

Pathology and Histopathology

LCMV can be recovered from the blood, cerebrospinal fluid (CSF), urine, and nasopharyngeal secretions during the human LCMV disease. Leukopenia is a common feature of the infection, but there is a pleocytosis in the CSF in the meningeal stages, and histological analyses of diseased brain tissue in lethal cases of LCMV have revealed meningeal perivascular inflammation and many lymphocytes and monocytes in the arachnoid. This is consistent with studies in the mouse which have demonstrated a lymphocytic infiltration of the meninges. Extensive studies in the mouse model of LCMV-induced acute meningoencephalitis have indicated that virus-specific MHC class I-restricted CD8+ CTLs are the major mediators of the lethal disease, and this may also be the mechanism for the human disease. The mouse model has also shown that antibody–virus–complement immune complexes can be pathological entities, and these could be involved in some of the human arthritic symptoms and the rash, when present.

Immune Response

Human cases of LCMV are characterized by a rise in antibody titer after infection, followed by lasting immunity. Little work has been done on human cellular immunity to infection. However, the LCMV infection of the mouse has provided the most extensive analyses of the cellular immune response to any virus disease. The infection is characterized by an early stage (1–5 days post infection) and later stage (6–10 days post infection). The early stage involves the log-phase replication of the virus and a variety of antigen-nonspecific responses including the liberation of type 1 interferon (IFN)-α and -β and tumor necrosis factor (TNF)-α, the activation and proliferation of natural killer (NK) cells, and a depression in bone marrow hematopoiesis. The type 1 IFN and probably some of the TNFα is directly and rapidly induced in cells by the LCMV infection. Type 1 IFN and IL-15 stimulate the activation and proliferation of NK cells, which substantially increase in number and accumulate in virus-infected tissue. There is initially a type 1 IFN-induced attrition of memory T cells and other cell types, resulting in a leukopenia. Depressed bone marrow function, which is likely due to the effects of inhibitory cytokines like IFN and TNFα and to the ability of activated NK cells to lyse or suppress hematopoietic precursor cells, may contribute to the leukopenia. Antibodies to IFN-α and -β (as well as γ) enhance the synthesis of LCMV, but antibodies to NK cells do not alter the course of the infection. During this early stage of infection there is a pronounced type 1 IFN-induced increase in class I MHC antigen expression throughout the body, an increase in the susceptibility of the cells to CTLs, and a decrease in their susceptibility to NK cells. IFN-mediated protection of uninfected and LCMV-infected target cells may make them resistant to surveillance by NK cells.

The second phase of the response is associated with the expansion of clones of virus-specific T and B cells, a decrease in the production of virus, an increase in the production of IFN-γ and interleukin (IL)-2, and an increase in the activation of macrophages. The major factor in the control of the LCMV infection and in the development of encephalitis and immunopathological lesions throughout the body is the generation of CD8+ CTLs, which can develop in CD4+ T-cell-depleted mice. CD4 T cells and CD40/CD40L interactions, however, seem to be needed for the maintenance of long-term memory CD8 T-cell responses. The IFN-induced upregulation of class I MHC antigens conditions cells in the host to be good targets for CD8+ T cells, which recognize viral peptides in the context of class I antigens. Many LCMV-encoded immunodominant and subdominant T-cell epitopes have been identified, and, in the context of synthetic peptides or vaccinia virus recombinants, they can immunize mice against LCMV.

LCMV infection is so profound at inducing CD8 T-cell responses in the mouse that over 20% of the CD8 T cells can remain LCMV-specific in the memory pool. This has enabled the LCMV infection to be very useful in the discovery and analysis of T-cell-dependent heterologous immunity, where T cells specific for one pathogen are recruited into the response to an unrelated pathogen and alter protective immunity and immunopathology. For example, a complex network of T-cell cross-reactivities between LCMV and vaccinia virus causes LCMV-immune mice to partially resist vaccinia virus infection, while at the same time developing severe T-cell-associated immunopathological lesions.

Antiviral antibody plays only a minor role in the acute LCMV infection and is not needed to clear the infection. However, in the absence of antibody, virus may eventually recrudesce in immune mice. In the absence of a CTL response, such as in congenitally infected mice, antibody–virus–complement immune complexes mediate the development of glomerulonephritis, arteritis, and other inflammatory lesions. Usually the LCMV infection *per se* is relatively mild, and it is the immune response to the virus that causes the damage in the infected mouse.

Prevention and Control of LCMV

LCMV has not been a sufficiently significant human pathogen to warrant special public health measures for its control. However, the disease can be reduced in frequency by ridding houses of mice, by ensuring that pet hamsters are not infected, and by adhering at least to Biosafety Level 2 procedures in the laboratory. Supportive therapy without antiviral chemotherapy is recommended for patients experiencing LCMV infection.

Future Perspectives

Studies with LCMV have in the past provided much of the conceptual basis for viral immunology and pathogenesis, including (1) the theory of immunological tolerance, (2) the concept of virus-induced immunopathology, (3) the analysis of immune complex disease, (4) the discovery of virus-specific CTLs and demonstration of their roles in viral clearance and immunopathology, (5)

the discovery of MHC restriction in T-cell recognition, (6) the discovery and analysis of NK cell activation and proliferation, (7) the concept that sublethal viral infections can abrogate specialized 'luxury' functions of cells and lead to metabolic disturbances, (8) the observation that high antigen loads can cause T-cell clonal exhaustion and lead to persistent infection, and (9) the phenomenon of T-cell-dependent heterologous immunity. In the future, the LCMV infection will likely continue to be an important model used for the development of vaccines directed against T-cell epitopes, for examining the clearance of virus by T-cell immunotherapy, for elucidating mechanisms of virus-induced immunosuppression and T-cell tolerance that contribute to persistent infections, for analyzing the regulatory roles of cytokines in the development of the NK-cell and T-cell responses, and for clarifying regulatory mechanisms of heterologous immunity. LCMV variants can produce in mice syndromes that very closely resemble acquired immunodeficiency syndrome (AIDS), and it is possible to manipulate this system to get a persistent infection without a CTL response at all, a persistent infection associated with immunosuppression, and a low-level CTL response, or an acute infection with a strong CTL response which clears the infection. Exploiting the biology of these systems should continue to provide basic concepts fundamental to viral immunology and pathogenesis.

See also: Lassa, Junin, Machupo and Guanarito Viruses.

Further Reading

Buchmeier MJ, Welsh RM, Dutko FJ, and Oldstone MB (1980) The virology and immunobiology of lymphocytic choriomeningitis virus infection. *Advances in Immunology* 30: 275–331.

Lehmann-Grube F (1986) Lymphocytic choriomeningitis virus. In: Braude AL, Davis CE,, and Fierer J (eds.) *Infectious Diseases and Medical Microbiology*, 1076pp. Philadelphia, PA: W.B. Saunders.

Oldstone MBA (2002) Biology and pathogenesis of lymphocytic choriomeningitis virus infection. *Current Topics in Microbiology and Immunology* 263: 83–117.

Sevilla N and de la Torre JC (2006) Arenavirus diversity and evolution: Quasispecies *in vivo*. *Current Topics in Microbiology and Immunology* 299: 315–335.

Welsh RM (1999) Lymphocytic choriomeningitis virus as a model for the study of cellular immunology. In: Cunningham MW and Fujinami RS (eds.) *Effects of Microbes on the Immune System*, pp. 280–312. Philadelphia, PA: Lippincott Williams and Wilkins.

Marburg Virus

D Falzarano, University of Manitoba, Winnipeg, MB, Canada
H Feldmann, Public Health Agency of Canada, Winnipeg, MB, Canada

History

In 1967 the first noted cases of a viral hemorrhagic fever (VHF) caused by a new family of viruses, the *Filoviridae*, occurred when laboratory workers in Germany contracted severe VHF after handling tissues from African green monkeys (*Cercopithecus aethiops*) imported from Uganda. Shortly after, two cases were identified in the former Yugoslavia, where a veterinarian was infected during the necropsy of a dead monkey. In total there were 32 cases, including six secondary infections and a single retrospective case. Overall, there were seven fatalities in the primary infections resulting in a case–fatality rate of 23%. The new virus was named Marburg virus (MARV) after the German city which had reported the first cases (see **Figure 1** for a map of all known occurrences of MARV).

Following these initial cases of Marburg hemorrhagic fever (MHF) there were only a small number of isolated cases noted until 1998. In 1975, three cases of MHF were reported in Johannesburg, South Africa. The index case, who did not survive, had traveled to Zimbabwe immediately before becoming ill. Shortly afterward, his travel companion and a nurse who cared for them also became ill but both later recovered. Cases of MHF also occurred in Kenya in 1980 and 1987. In 1980 the index case became ill in western Kenya and died in Nairobi where a physician also got infected but survived. In 1987, a fatal case occurred in the same region of western Kenya. The index cases in both 1980 and 1987 had traveled to the Mt. Elgon region, which is located close to Lake Victoria and was the source of the monkeys that initiated the original 1967 outbreak (trapped near Lake Kyogo, Uganda).

The first large community outbreak of MHF occurred in 1998 in central Africa. The community of Durba/Watsa, located in the northeastern region of the Democratic Republic of the Congo (DRC), had 149 cases with an 83% fatality rate. The response to this outbreak was limited due in part to the remote location and an ongoing conflict in the region. Sporadic cases continued after the end of the outbreak with most cases being linked either directly or indirectly to illegal mining in an underground gold mine. Typically, the index cases were gold miners who initiated multiple, short chains of human-to-human transmission within their families. The Durba outbreak was somewhat unusual compared to previous MARV and Ebola virus (EBOV) outbreaks in that it continued for almost 2 years, during which multiple distinct genetic lineages were found to be circulating, indicating several independent introductions of virus into the human population from the unknown natural reservoir.

To date, the largest outbreak of MHF occurred in the Uíge Province of Angola in 2004–05. At the conclusion of the outbreak, the Ministry of Health in Angola reported a total of 252 cases, including 227 deaths. This case–fatality rate of 90% is the highest observed during an MHF outbreak thus far and is more typical of past severe Ebola hemorrhagic fever (EHF) outbreaks. A large proportion of the cases were found among young children, which is unusual for filovirus outbreaks. The high case–fatality rate and fast progression of the disease were suggestive of a more virulent strain. In contrast to the Durba/Watsa outbreak, the viruses isolated from patients were highly conserved, indicating a single introduction with little evolution of the virus during the outbreak similar to what has been reported for previous EHF outbreaks. The most recent occurrence of MHF was in 2007 in Uganda, where there were three confirmed cases.

In addition to the initial outbreak and those that have occurred in the natural setting there have also been at least three laboratory-acquired infections of MARV since the mid-1980s, with one fatality occurring in Russia.

Taxonomy and Classification

All MARVs are classified as a single species, *Lake Victoria marburgvirus*, which comprise the genus *Marburgvirus*, family *Filoviridae*, within the order *Mononegavirales*. They share unique morphologic, physicochemical, genetic, and biological features with members of the genus *Ebolavirus*. Due to their high fatality rates, frequency of person-to-person transmission, the potential for aerosol infectivity, and the absence of vaccines and treatments, these viruses are considered to be 'biosafety level 4' (BCL-4) agents and have been placed on the 'category A' and 'select agent' list.

Virus Structure and Composition

Electron microscopy of MARV reveals distinctive pleomorphic filamentous particles (**Figure 2(a)**) that can appear in U-shaped, 6-shaped, or circular (torus) configurations, or as elongated filamentous forms of varying length (up to 14 000 nm). Filamentous particles may also form branched structures. The length of peak infectivity for MARV particles is between 790 and 860 nm with a uniform diameter of 80 nm for all particles. Virus particles contain a helical

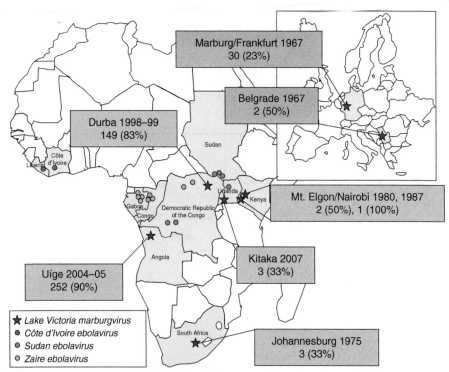

Figure 1 Location of known filovirus outbreaks. Countries that have experienced occurrences of filoviruses are indicated in yellow. For MARVs, the location of the outbreak is indicated by a red star. The main center (city/village) of the outbreak is indicated, along with the year of the outbreak, the number of cases, and the case–fatality rate (indicated in brackets). Incidents of the various EBOV species are also indicated.

ribonucleoprotein (RNP) complex, which contains the negative-sense viral RNA genome, the polymerase (L) protein, the nucleoprotein (NP), and viron protein (VP) 35 and 30. The RNP is surrounded by the matrix protein (VP40) and a closely apposed outer envelope derived from the host cell plasma membrane (**Figure 2(b)**). The surface of the particle has membrane-anchored protein spikes, made up by the virus glycoprotein (GP), which gives the virus particle a rough appearance. These spikes are approximately 7 nm in length and are spaced at approximately 10 nm intervals. Virus particles have a molecular weight of approximately $3-6 \times 10^8$ Da and a density of $1.14 \mathrm{~g~ml}^{-1}$ as determined by centrifugation in a potassium tartrate gradient; uniform, bacilliform particles have a sedimentation coefficient of 1300–1400 S. Virus infectivity is rather stable at room temperature. Inactivation can be performed by ultraviolet (UV) light or gamma irradiation, 1% formalin, β-propiolactone or brief exposure to phenolic disinfectants and lipid solvents, like deoxycholate and ether, as well as ionic detergents such as sodium dodecyl sulfate.

Genome Organization and Expression

The MARV genome consists of a single, linear molecule of negative-stranded RNA that is just over 19 000 bp in length. The genome is slightly larger than that of EBOV but is organized in a similar manner (**Figure 2(b)**). The MARV genome is noninfectious, rich in adenosine and uridine residues, not polyadenylated and complementary to viral-specific messenger RNA. Complete genome sequences are available from isolates covering six episodes of MHF (1967, 1975, 1980, 1987, 1999, and 2005). The genome amounts to 1.1% of the total virion weight with a sedimentation coefficient of 46 S (0.15 M NaCl, pH 7.4).

The genes are arranged in a linear fashion in the following order: 3′ leader; NP; viral structural protein (VP)-35; VP40; GP; VP30; VP24; polymerase (L); 5′ trailer (**Figure 2(b)**). All genes are flanked at their 3′ and 5′ ends by highly conserved transcriptional start and stop signal sequences that almost always include the pentamer 3′-UAAUU-5′. Most genes are separated by intergenic sequences that are variable in length and nucleotide composition. An unusual feature of the MARV genome is the presence of a gene overlap, between VP30 and VP24, a feature that is shared with EBOV, which have two or three gene overlaps (VP35–VP40, GP–VP30, and or VP24–L). Extragenic sequences that are complementary at their very extremities are present at the 3′ and 5′ end of the genome. This complementarity favors formation of a panhandle structure between the genomic termini, but it is unclear if such a structure can actually form due to co-transcriptional encapsidation. Both genomic ends are self-complementary and modeling suggests that almost identical hairpin-like

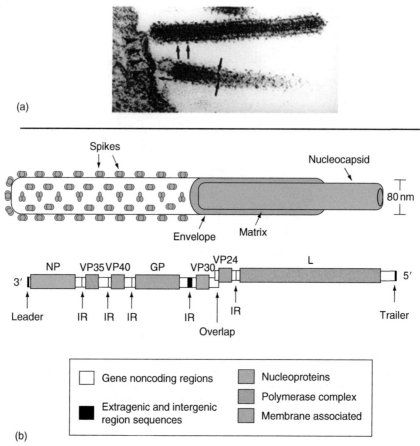

(a)

(b)

Figure 2 Virus particle morphology. (a) Transmission electron micrograph (negative stain) of MARV particles budding from an infected cell. The arrows indicate the glycoprotein spikes. (b) Schematic representation of the MARV particle structure (upper portion) and genome (lower portion) indicating open reading frames, noncoding regions, a single gene overlap (VP30/VP24), and intergenic regions (IRs).

Table 1   MARV proteins: Function(s) and localization

Gene order [a]	Marburg virus proteins	Protein function (localization)
1	Nucleoprotein (NP)	Major nucleoprotein, RNA genome encapsidation (component of RNP[b])
2	Virion protein 35 (VP35)	Polymerase complex cofactor, type I interferon antagonist (component of RNP)
3	Virion protein 40 (VP40)	Matrix protein, virion assembly and budding (membrane associated)
4	Glycoprotein (GP)	Receptor binding and membrane fusion (membrane associated)
5	Virion protein 30 (VP30)	Minor nucleoprotein (component of RNP)
6	Virion protein 24 (VP24)	Minor matrix protein, virion assembly (membrane associated)
7	Polymerase (L)	RNA-dependent RNA polymerase, enzymatic portion of polymerase complex (component of RNP)

[a]Gene order refers to 3′–5′ gene arrangement as shown in **Figure 2(b)**.
[b]Ribonucleoprotein complex.

structures are present at the 3′ ends of the genome and antigenome.

All of the MARV proteins are incorporated into the virus and are either part of the RNP complex or associated with the envelope. For a summary of protein functions, see **Table 1**. RNP-associated proteins are involved

in transcription and replication while envelope-associated proteins are primarily involved in assembly/budding or entry. NP and VP30 are phosphoproteins and are considered the major and minor nucleoproteins, respectively. They interact strongly with the genomic RNA molecule, forming the viral RNP complex, in combination with

VP35 and L which form the polymerase complex. EBOV VP30 is thought to be a transcriptional activator that is regulated by phosphorylation but MARV VP30 does not appear to function in this manner.

The polymerase complex transcribes and replicates the MARV genome. L is the RNA-dependent RNA polymerase and contains motifs that are linked to RNA (template), phosphodiester (catalytic site), and ribonucleotide triphosphate binding. MARV L is larger than EBOV L and while there are areas of conservation between the two, nearly 25% of the C-terminal quarter is not conserved, in addition to stretches of sequences that are totally unique to MARV L. VP35 is thought to act as an essential cofactor of L that affects the mode of RNA synthesis (transcription or replication) similar to that of the P proteins of other negative-stranded viruses. In addition, VP35 also acts as a linker between L and NP as well as having an antagonistic effect on the type I interferon pathway.

The surface of MARV particles is covered with spike structures (**Figures 2(a)** and **2(b)**) that are composed of the structural glycoprotein, GP, which is anchored in the membrane as a timer in a type I orientation. These spike proteins play a role in entry and are thought to influence pathogenesis. MARV GP is encoded in a single open reading frame in contrast to EBOV GP, which is encoded in two open reading frames and is only expressed after RNA editing. Sequence analysis of MARV GP genes indicates that a nucleotide sequence that corresponds to the editing region of EBOV GP genes is absent. MARV GP is processed similar to EBOV GP but in contrast to EBOV GP the glycans on MARV GP lack terminal sialic acids if propagated in specific cell lines. This may be caused by differences in processing as the protein is directed through the *trans*-Golgi apparatus.

VP40 functions as the matrix protein in combination with VP24, which acts as a minor matrix protein. VP40 is the most abundant protein in the virion; however, only small amounts of VP24 are incorporated into virus particles. Both VP40 and VP24 are hydrophobic, have an affinity for membranes, and are associated with the virion envelope. VP40 is essential for virus budding as it initiates and drives the envelopment of the RNP by the plasma membrane. The role of VP24 in the replication of MARV is still unclear and direct interactions with other virus proteins have not been described.

Replication

MARVs are thought to replicate in a similar manner to EBOV; however, most of the research on replication has been performed on EBOV. Only the NP, VP35, and L proteins are required for transcription and replication of MARV, in contrast to EBOV, which also requires VP30. This indicates that there may be differences in the factors required for transcription/replication. It also appears that there might be differences in receptor binding for MARV, which appear to have a higher affinity for asialoglycoprotein, whereas this interaction does not seem to be important for EBOV infection. For a detailed description of MARV replication, the reader is referred to the replication section of Zaire ebolovirus (*Filoviridae*) which is covered elsewhere in this encyclopedia.

Evolutionary Relationship between Viruses

MARV and EBOV are clearly related in sequence, morphology, and the general disease that they cause; however, it is also clear that they represent different genera of filoviruses. The nucleotide and amino acid differences between MARV and EBOV are both *c.* 55%. Phylogenetic analysis indicates that within MARV there are two distinct lineages of viruses (**Figure 3**) that show a diversity of up to 21%, with the 1987 isolate from Kenya (Ravn) being the most divergent from the rest. This distinct lineage was also seen again in the Durba/Watsa outbreak, along with other isolates that cover most, if not all, of the MARV repertoire.

The outbreak in 2005 in the Uíge Province of northern Angola was a surprise as the origins of all earlier outbreaks were linked directly to East Africa. What is somewhat surprising is that the Angola strain of MARV was less different (~7%) from the main group of East African MARV than one would expect given the large geographic separation (**Figure 3**). This suggests that the virus reservoir in these regions may not be substantially different. However, an index case was never identified, and thus the importation of the virus from East Africa cannot be ruled out. Given the length of the outbreak (from fall of 2004 to July 2005) it seemed possible that multiple introductions of MARV could be possible. However, remarkably few nucleotide differences were found among the Angolan clinical specimens (0–0.07%), which is consistent with a single introduction of virus into the human population, followed by person-to-person transmission with little accumulation of mutations. Typically, RNA viruses evolve rapidly due to positive selection in combination with the large number of errors that are made and cannot be corrected during replication (missing proof-reading activity of the polymerase). However, disease progression is so rapid that most individuals seem to die before an effective immune response can be mounted. Therefore, the positive selection of viruses may not occur.

Transmission and Host Range

The reservoir for MARV remains unknown, but its emergence in Angola extends the scope of the reservoir search

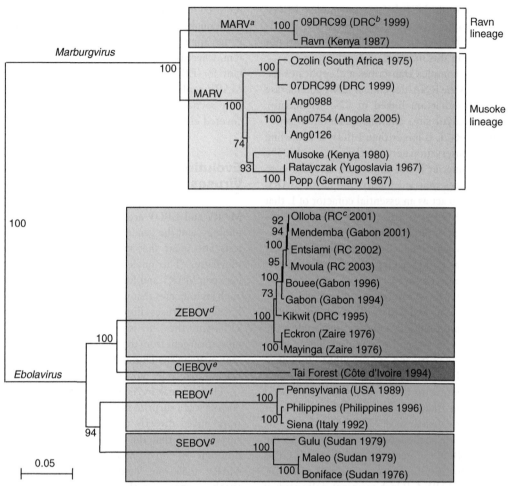

Figure 3 Phylogeny of the family *Filoviridae*. Neighbor-joining analysis of the nucleotide sequence of the GP gene of Marburg and Ebola virus isolates, indicating the two lineages of MARV and the different species of EBOV. Sequences were obtained from GenBank. Confidence values at branch point were obtained from 1000 bootstraps. The bar length equals 5% nucleotide difference. [a]MARV – *Lake Victoria marburgvirus*, [b]Democratic Republic of the Congo, [c]Republic of the Cango, [d]ZEBOV – *Zaire ebolavirus*, [e]CIEBOV – *Côte d'Ivore ebolavirus*, [f]REBOV – *Reston ebolavirus*, [g]SEBOV – *Sudan ebolavirus*.

beyond East Africa. Humans and nonhuman primates serve as natural hosts and it is unclear if other animals are infected. In Durba/Watsa, epidemiological data linked over 70% of the cases with mines or caves, suggesting that the natural reservoir could well be associated with such environments and that bats have been a favorable species for a reservoir. With the Angola outbreak, difficulties in surveillance and contact tracing, combined with the delay in the identification of the outbreak, led to poor epidemiological linkage of MARV cases and ultimately to a lack of success in identifying a point source or mounting any ecological study. Filovirus outbreaks in general are relatively rare events. If the natural reservoir of MARV is similar to that of EBOV, the emergence of MARV in western Africa should not be surprising, as the sites of multiple large EHF outbreaks are less than 500 miles away (**Figure 1**), including areas which have experienced almost yearly activity over the last decade.

EBOV has recently been linked to fruit bats in Gabon and the Republic of the Congo. It is thought that MHF outbreaks start with the rare introduction of the virus into the human population followed by waves of human-to-human transmission (usually through close contact with infected individuals or their body fluids), with little if any evolution of the virus during the course of the outbreak.

Clinical Features

MARVs cause severe hemorrhagic fever in both humans and nonhuman primates. The incubation period lasts from 2 to 21 days (average 4–10), after which there is a sudden onset of nonspecific flu-like symptoms that can include fever, chills, malaise, headache, and myalgia (**Figure 4**). This is followed 2–10 days later by the development of

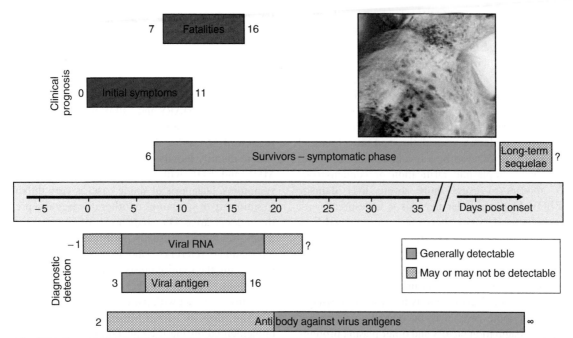

Figure 4 Clinical presentation and diagnostic window. The upper portion describes the appearance of clinical symptoms in humans. Also shown are the characteristic petechiae, seen here on the neck and upper body, of a nonhuman primate with MHF (inset). The lower portion illustrates the timeframe for the appearance of diagnostic targets (viral RNA, viral antigen, and host antibody response).

more severe symptoms that include systemic (i.e., prostration, anorexia), gastrointestinal (nausea, vomiting, abdominal pain, diarrhea), respiratory (chest pain, shortness of breath, cough), vascular (conjunctival injection, postural hypotension, edema), and neurologic (headache, confusion, coma) manifestations. The presence of a macropapular rash associated with varying degrees of erythema is also frequently observed and is a useful differential diagnostic.

In cases where coagulation abnormalities develop, hemorrhagic manifestations can include petechiae, ecchymoses, bleeding from venipuncture sites, mucosal bleeding (typically involving the gastrointestinal tract), and visceral hemorrhagic effusions. Patients that develop coagulation abnormalities usually have a bad prognosis. The late stages of the disease are characterized by the development of shock with convulsions, severe metabolic disturbances, and coagulopathy. The onset of shock, with or without obvious bleeding, leads to multiple organ failure with death typically occurring between days 7 and 16. Nonfatal cases have fever for approximately 5–9 days with improvement typically occurring around days 7–11 – the time that the humoral antibody response is noted (**Figure 4**). In patients who survive, convalescence is prolonged and is sometimes associated with myelitis, recurrent hepatitis, psychosis, or uveitis in addition to psycho-social difficulties integrating back into their community.

The mortality for MARV seems to average around 70–85% with the exception of the outbreak in Europe (only 23%). The reason for the large difference in mortality in the European versus the African cases is unknown

and may be the result of important host-genetic differences, genetic difference between virus strains, or the standard of care available to infected individuals.

Pathogenesis and Pathology

Clinical investigations of outbreaks of human MARV infections have provided most of the descriptive information on the pathology and pathogenesis of these viruses. However, studies in laboratory animals are much more comprehensive and consistent. Guinea pigs have been employed to study MHF. While guinea pigs have served as effective early screens for evaluating antiviral drugs and candidate vaccines, the disease pathogenesis seen in these animals is not nearly as representative of the human clinical picture as nonhuman primates are.

The different strains of MARV appear to have different levels of virulence. Initially, it appeared that MARV strains were more comparable to *Sudan ebolavirus*; however, virulence of the recently isolated Angola strain appears to be similar to *Zaire ebolavirus*. Most strains of MARV produce uniformly lethal infections in cynomolgus and rhesus macaques. Infections of macaques with the Angola strain appear to progress more rapidly than infections with other strains. For example, challenge of rhesus macaques by intramuscular injection with 1000 pfu of the Musoke or Angola strains produces a uniformly lethal infection, but death occurs within 10–12 days versus 6–8 days, respectively.

While the pathology of MARV is less extensively studied than that of EBOV, it appears to be similar. The pathological changes seen in patients fatally infected with any of the filoviruses include extensive necrosis of parenchymal cells of many organs, including the liver, spleen, kidney, and gonads with little infiltration in infected tissues. However, no single organ is sufficiently damaged to explain the fatal outcome. Infection of cells leads to intracytoplasmic vesiculation and mitochondrial swelling which is followed by a breakdown of organelles and terminal cytoplasmic rarification or condensation. MARV appears to cause more severe liver damage than EBOV. Hepatocellular necrosis is widespread with extremely high infectivity titers present in infected liver samples. Elevations in liver enzymes are prominent findings in most filovirus infections and the hepatocellular degeneration and necrosis observed during MARV infections is extensive. Liver function impairment could contribute to the overall pathogenesis because hemorrhagic tendencies in some cases may be related to decreased synthesis of coagulation factors and other plasma proteins as a result of hepatocellular necrosis. In the late stages of the disease, hemorrhage occurs in the gastrointestinal tract, pleural, pericardial, and peritoneal spaces, as well as the renal tubules with deposition of fibrin. Abnormalities in coagulation parameters include fibrin split products and prolonged prothrombin and partial thromboplastin times. Clinical and biochemical findings support anatomical observations of extensive liver involvement, renal damage, changes in vascular permeability, and activation of the clotting cascade.

Fluid distribution and platelet abnormalities indicate dysfunction of endothelial cells and platelets. In addition to direct vascular involvement in infected hosts, active host mediator molecules probably play a significant role in these disorders. Infected monocytes/macrophages are probably responsible for producing different proteases, peroxide, and other mediators, such as tumor necrosis factor alpha (TNF-α) that may have a negative effect on the infected host. The increased production of TNF-α can result in secondary activation of mediators with important protective as well as deleterious effects. For example, supernatants of MARV-infected monocytes/macrophages cultures are capable of increasing paraendothelial permeability, thus exacerbating the development of the shock syndrome seen in severe and lethal cases. The endothelium is also directly targeted by the virus and endothelial cells support cytolytic MARV replication in culture. The bleeding disorders observed during infection could be due to direct endothelial damage caused directly by virus replication or indirectly by cytokine-mediated processes. The combination of viral replication in endothelial cells and virus-induced mediator release from infected leukocytes may also promote a distinct pro-inflammatory phenotype of the endothelium that triggers, most likely via tissue factor, the coagulation cascade.

Diagnosis

Diagnostics for MARV and EBOV infections use the same principles. As these infections typically occur in isolated regions of Africa that do not have the diagnostic capabilities to identify filovirus infections, the initial diagnosis of MHF and EHF will most likely be based on clinical symptoms. Diagnosis of single cases is very difficult due to similarity of symptoms to other diseases also present in the endemic areas. Due to the rarity of filovirus infections, diagnostic testing is usually performed at national and/or international reference laboratories that are capable of performing the required tests under suitable containment conditions. During outbreaks, healthcare workers who have direct contact with patients are at high risk for infection and adequate barrier nursing precautions need to be implemented during the collection of samples and treatment of patients. Laboratory diagnosis is based on either detection of virus-specific antibodies, virus particles, or particle components. Inactivation of samples is necessary when testing is not done under BSL-4 conditions.

Currently, reverse transcriptase-polymerase chain reaction (RT-PCR) and antigen detection enzyme-linked immunosorbent assay (ELISA) are the primary test systems to diagnose acute infections; RT-PCR, however, is more sensitive than antigen detection ELISA. Viral antigen and/or nucleic acid can be detected in blood from 3 to 18 days post onset of symptoms (**Figure 4**). Most laboratories currently favor RT-PCR because of its sensitivity, specificity, and rapidity. RT-PCR is also readily used in a mobile lab setting and has proved to be accurate and effective in both MHF and EHF outbreaks. Due to the seriousness of a positive test for filoviruses, the diagnosis of index cases or of single imported cases should not be solely based on a single technology. Confirmation by an independent assay and/or laboratory should always be attempted.

Serological assays are second choice for acute diagnosis as patients often succumb to the disease before an antibody response is generated. Alternatively, immunohistochemistry, direct immunofluorescence on tissues, or electron microscopy can be used for diagnostics, but these methods lack sensitivity, are time consuming, or require expensive equipment. Virus isolation from clinical specimens in tissue culture and/or animals is easily achieved but takes time and requires BSL-4. Filoviruses grow well in a number of cell lines, including Vero and Vero E6, which are the most frequently used. The most commonly used laboratory animals for virus isolation are inbred guinea pig strains; however, it should be kept in mind that often several passages are required to obtain a lethal infection.

Treatment

The current treatment of MARV infections mainly involves supportive therapy, which is directed toward the maintenance of effective blood volume and electrolyte balance. Shock, cerebral edema, renal failure, coagulation disorders, and secondary bacterial infections may be life threatening and have to be managed. Most experimental treatment strategies have been studied for EBOV, but it is expected that several of these approaches would have similar effects on MARV.

Therapeutic antibodies are still considered a valuable short-term solution. This strategy might perhaps be more realistic for the treatment of MHF than EHF based on the observation that humoral responses seemed to be more effective against MARV. The use of recombinant nematode anticoagulant protein c2 (rNAPc2), which seems to be a promising approach for EBOV, did not result in a similar positive effect for MARV infections (Angola strain). Studies on novel antiviral strategies such as viral gene silencing through specific siRNA or functional domain interference with small peptides have been very limited for MARV. In contrast, more focus has been given to strategies targeting host responses. Treatment with TNF-α neutralizing antibodies has been partially successful in guinea pig models of MHF, but has yet to be evaluated in nonhuman primates. MARV-infected guinea pigs are partially protected by Desferal, an interleukin 1 (IL-1) and TNF-α antagonist. In a separate study, treatment of animals with IL-1 receptor antagonist (IL-1RA) or anti-TNF-α decreased the concentration of circulating TNF-α and allowed 50% survival.

As with EBOV, ribavirin is not indicated for MHF treatment. In general, it seems plausible that combination therapy for MHF and EHF will be superior over any single treatment form.

Prevention

Protective MARV vaccines would be extremely valuable for at-risk medical personnel, first responders, military personnel, researchers, and high-risk contact groups during outbreaks (such as family members). Past vaccine approaches were based on either inactivated virus preparations, which were of limited protective efficacy and considered unsafe, or subunit vaccines, which showed efficacy in the rodent but not nonhuman primate model. Protective efficacy in nonhuman primates could first be demonstrated with a system based on Venezuelan equine encephalitis virus replicons expressing the MARV GP and/or NP. Currently, the most promising vaccine approach seems to be a live-attenuated vector based on vesicular stomatits virus expressing the MARV GP (strain Musoke). The protective efficacy and safety of this vaccine vector has been demonstrated in two animal models, the guinea pig and nonhuman primate. Protective efficacy could also be achieved against challenge with heterologous MARV strains as well as homologous aerosol challenge. In addition, the vector showed astonishing efficacy in postexposure treatment of rhesus macaques; single, high-dose treatment 30 min after high-dose challenge protected all animals from lethal disease. Despite the success it remains questionable if a replication-competent vector will be granted approval for human use.

Acknowledgments

The Public Health Agency of Canada (PHAC), Canadian Institutes of Health Research (CIHR), and CBRNE (chemical, biological, radiological, and nuclear) Research and Technology Initiative (CRTI), Canada, supported work on filoviruses at the National Microbiology Laboratory of the Public Health Agency of Canada.

See also: Ebolavirus.

Further Reading

Bausch DG and Geisbert TW (2007) Development of vaccines for Marburg hemorrhagic fever. *Expert Reviews of Vaccines* 6: 57–74.

Bausch DG, Nichol ST, Muyembe-Tamfum JJ, *et al.* (2006) Marburg hemorrhagic fever associated with multiple genetic lineages of virus. *New England Journal of Medicine* 355: 909–919.

Becker S and Muhlberger E (1999) Co- and posttranslational modifications and functions of Marburg virus proteins. *Current Topics in Microbiology and Immunology* 235: 23–34.

Bray M and Paragas J (2002) Experimental therapy of filovirus infections. *Antiviral Research* 54: 1–17.

Feldmann H, Geisbert TW, Jahrling PB, *et al.* (2005) *Filoviridae*. In: Fauquet CM, Mayo MA, Maniloff J, Desselberger U,, and Ball LA (eds.) *Virus Taxonomy: Eighth Report of the International Committee on Taxonomy of Viruses*, pp. 645–653. San Diego, CA: Elsevier Academic Press.

Hensley LE, Jones SM, Feldmann H, Jahrling PB, and Geisbert TW (2005) Ebola and Marburg viruses: Pathogenesis and development of countermeasures. *Current Molecular Medicine* 5: 761–772.

Martini GA and Siegert R (eds.) (1971) *Marburg Virus Disease.* New York: Springer.

Mohamadzadeh M, Chen L, Olinger GG, Pratt WD, and Schmaljohn AL (2006) Filoviruses and the balance of innate, adaptive, and inflammatory responses. *Viral Immunology* 19: 602–612.

Paragas J and Geisbert TW (2006) Development of treatment strategies to combat Ebola and Marburg viruses. *Expert Reviews of Anti-Infective Therapy* 4: 67–76.

Sanchez A, Geisbert TW, and Feldmann H (2007) Marburg and Ebola viruses. In: Knipe DM, Howley PM, Griffin DE, *et al.* (eds.) *Fields Virology,* 5th edn., pp. 1409–1448. Philadelphia, PA: Lippincott Williams and Wilkins.

Siegert R, Shu HL, Slenczka W, Peters D, and Muller G (1967) On the etiology of an unknown human infection originating from monkeys. *Deutsche Medizinische Wochenschrift* 92: 2341–2343.

Slenczka WG (1999) The Marburg virus outbreak of 1967 and subsequent episodes. *Current Topics in Microbiology and Immunology* 235: 49–75.

Zaki SR and Goldsmith CS (1999) Pathologic features of filovirus infections in humans. *Current Topics in Microbiology and Immunology* 235: 97–116.

Orbiviruses

P P C Mertens, H Attoui, and P S Mellor, Institute for Animal Health, Pirbright, UK

Glossary

Arbovirus Viruses that are transmitted between their vertebrate host species, by insects or other arthropod vectors, replicating in both host and vector species.
Culicoides Blood-feeding dipterous insects also known as biting midges.
Ecchymosis Area of haemorrhage larger than petechiae.
Petechiae Pinpoint- to pinhead-sized red spots under the skin that are the result of small hemorrhages.

Introduction

The reoviruses (a term used here to indicate any member of the family *Reoviridae*) have genomes composed of 9–12 separate segments of linear double-stranded RNA (dsRNA), packaged as exactly one copy of each segment per icosahedral virion. The family *Reoviridae* contains a total of 12 established genera (*Orthoreovirus, Orbivirus, Cypovirus, Aquareovirus, Rotavirus, Coltivirus, Seadornavirus, Fijivirus, Phytoreovirus, Oryzavirus, Idnoreovirus,* and *Mycoreovirus*) as well as three proposed 'new' genera of viruses (*Mimoreovirus, Cardoreovirus,* and *Dinovernavirus*). Closely related reoviruses that infect the same cell can exchange genome segments by a process known as reassortment, generating new progeny virus strains. This ability to 'reassort' is regarded as a primary indication that different virus strains belong to the same virus species, within each of the genera of the *Reoviridae*. The largest genus *Orbivirus* contains 21 distinct virus species and 12 further unassigned viruses (**Table 1**), each of which has a ten-segmented dsRNA genome. The orbiviruses are transmitted between their vertebrate hosts by ticks or hematophagous insects (e.g., mosquitoes or biting midges (*Culicoides* spp.)) in which they also replicate, and they are therefore regarded as 'arthropod-borne viruses' or 'arboviruses'. Some orbiviruses cause severe diseases of domesticated and wild animals, including members of the species: *African horse sickness virus* (AHSV), *Bluetongue virus* (BTV), *Epizootic hemorrhagic disease virus* (EHDV), and *Equine encephalosis virus* (EEV). The prototype *Orbivirus* species, *Bluetongue virus,* has been extensively studied and provides a useful paradigm for other members of the genus.

Historical Overview

Bluetongue (BT) was originally recognized as a disease of sheep and cattle in South Africa in the late eighteenth century and was initially reported in the scientific literature, as 'malarial catarrhal fever'. In 1905, Spreull suggested the name 'bluetongue' to reflect a significant, although infrequent, clinical sign of the disease. He also showed that the agent was filterable and caused an inapparent infection in goats and cattle.

BT was initially regarded as a disease of ruminants that was exclusive to Africa. However, in 1943 an outbreak occurred in Cyprus, killing approximately 2500 sheep (70% mortality in infected animals), and it was suggested that less virulent strains had caused earlier but unrecognized outbreaks on the island. Subsequently outbreaks occurred in 1946, 1951, 1965, and 1977, and have continued sporadically to the present day. BT was recorded in the 1940s in Palestine and Turkey, and by 1950 was present in Israel. In 1948, an apparently new disease known as 'sore muzzle' was recognized in Texas and, in 1952, BTV serotype 10 was isolated from infected sheep in California. BTV serotypes 11, 17, 13, and 2 were subsequently isolated in New Mexico (1955), Wyoming (1962), Idaho/Florida (1967), and Florida (1983), respectively, and these types are now regarded as endemic in North America. More recently, BTV-1 was identified in Louisiana (2004), BTV-3 in Florida and Mississippi (1999–2006), and BTV types 5, 6, 14, 19, and 22 were isolated in Florida (2002–05). Several BTV serotypes are also present in Central and South America and, although less well characterized, these include BTV-1, 3, 4, 6, 8, 11, 12, 13, 14, and 17.

BT virus serotype 10 caused a single epizootic in Spain and Portugal in 1956, and was reported in West Pakistan in 1958 and 1960, and in India in 1961. The disease now occurs regularly and is regarded as endemic on the Indian subcontinent, involving many different serotypes. Although Australia was initially considered to be free of BT, in 1978 a virus that was collected in the Northern Territory (during 1976), was identified as BTV. Eight serotypes have subsequently been isolated in Australia (BTV-1, 3, 9, 15, 16, 20, 21, and 23). Initially outbreaks of BT in Europe were infrequent, involving a single virus strain on each occasion, and were generally short lived (4–5 years). However, since 1998, eight distinct BTV strains from six different serotypes (BTV-1, 2, 4, 8, 9, and 16) have invaded Europe, with new introductions almost every year, resulting in the deaths of >1.8 million animals.

Table 1 Species in the genus *Orbivirus*

Virus species (virus abbreviation)	Number of serotypes/strains	Vector species	Host species
African horse sickness virus (AHSV)	9 numbered serotypes (AHSV-1 to AHSV-9)	*Culicoides* spp. (biting midges)	Equids, dogs, elephants, camels, cattle, sheep, goats, humans (in special circumstances) predatory carnivores (by eating infected meat)
Bluetongue virus (BTV, *Orbivirus* type species)	24 numbered serotypes (BTV-1 to BTV-24)	*Culicoides* spp. (biting midges)	All ruminants, camelids and predatory carnivores (by eating infected meat)
Changuinola virus (CGLV)	12 named serotypes	Phlebotomines, culicine mosquitoes	Humans, rodents, sloths
Chenuda virus (CNUV)	7 named serotypes	Ticks	Seabirds
Chobar Gorge virus (CGV)	2 named serotypes	Ticks	Bats
Corriparta virus (CORV)	6 named serotypes/strains[a]	Culicine mosquitoes	Humans, rodents
Epizootic hemorrhagic disease virus (EHDV)	10 numbered or named serotypes/strains[a] (EHDV-1 to EHDV-8, EHDV 318, Ibaraki virus (atypical EHDV-2))	*Culicoides* spp. (biting midges)	Cattle, sheep, deer, camels, llamas, wild ruminants, marsupials
Equine encephalosis virus (EEV)	7 numbered serotypes (EEV-1 to EEV-7)	*Culicoides* spp. (biting midges)	Equids
Eubenangee virus (EUBV)	4 named serotypes	*Culicoides* spp., anopheline and culicine mosquitoes	Unknown hosts
Ieri virus (IERIV)	3 named serotypes	Mosquitoes	Birds
Great Island virus (GIV)	36 named serotypes/strains[a]	Argas, Ornithodoros, Ixodes ticks	Seabirds, rodents, humans
Lebombo virus (LEBV)	1 numbered serotype (LEBV-1)	Culicine mosquitoes	Humans, rodents
Orungo virus (ORUV)	4 numbered serotypes (ORUV-1 to ORUV-4)	Culicine mosquitoes	Humans, camels, cattle, goats, sheep, monkeys
Palyam virus (PALV)	13 named serotypes/strains[a]	*Culicoides* spp., culicine mosquitoes	Cattle, sheep
Peruvian horse sickness virus (PHSV)	1 numbered serotype (PHSV-1)	Mosquitoes	Horses
St. Croix River virus (SCRV)	1 numbered serotype (SCRV-1)	Ticks	Hosts unknown
Umatilla virus (UMAV)	4 named serotypes	Culicine mosquitoes	Birds
Wad Medani virus (WMV)	2 named serotypes	Boophilus, Rhipicephalus, Hyalomma, Argas ticks	Domesticated animals
Wallal virus (WALV)	3 serotypes/strains	*Culicoides* spp.	Marsupials
Warrego virus (WARV)	3 serotypes/strains	*Culicoides* spp., anopheline and culicine mosquitoes	Marsupials
Wongorr virus (WGRV)	8 serotypes/strains	*Culicoides* spp., mosquitoes	(Cattle, macropods)
Tentative species			
Andasibe virus (ANDV)		Mosquitoes	Unknown hosts
Codajas virus (COV)		Mosquitoes	Rodents
Ife virus (IFEV)		Mosquitoes	Rodents, birds, ruminants

Continued

Table 1 Continued

Virus species (virus abbreviation)	Number of serotypes/strains	Vector species	Host species
Itupiranga virus (ITUV)		Mosquitoes	Unknown hosts
Japanaut virus (JAPV)		Mosquitoes	Unknown hosts
Kammavanpettai virus (KMPV)		Unknown vectors	Birds
Lake Clarendon virus (LCV)		Ticks	Birds
Matucare virus (MATV)		Ticks	Unknown hosts
Tembe virus (TMEV)		Mosquitoes	Unknown hosts
Tracambe virus (TRV)		Mosquitoes	Unknown hosts
Yunnan orbivirus (YUOV)		Culex tritaeniorhyncus	Unknown hosts

[a]In some species the serological relationships between strains has not been fully determined. For more information concerning individual named types, see Mertens PPC, Duncan R, Attoui H, and Dermody TS (2005) *Reoviridae*. In: Fauquet CM, Mayo MA, Maniloff J, Desselberger U, and Ball LA (eds.) *Virus Taxonomy: Eighth Report of the International Committee on Taxonomy of Viruses*, pp. 466–483. San Diego, CA: Elsevier Academic Press.

African horse sickness (AHS) was recognized as early as 1780, during the early days of the European colonization and importation of horses into southern Africa, resulting in epizootics with high rates of mortality in infected animals. AHSV is only considered to be enzootic in sub-Saharan Africa but has caused occasional major epizootics, with very high levels of associated mortality in infected horses, in the Middle East, the Indian subcontinent, North Africa, and the Iberian Peninsula.

Epizootic hemorrhagic disease (EHD) has occurred as periodic outbreaks in the south-eastern United States since 1890, where it causes a fatal disease of deer known by 'back-woods men' as 'black tongue'. The New Jersey and South Dakota strains were isolated in 1955 and 1956, respectively, and a second serotype was isolated in the Canadian province of Alberta in 1962. EHDV has been isolated from a range of animal species including cattle (a possible 'reservoir' host). Ibaraki virus, which causes an acute febrile disease of cattle, was first recorded in Japan in 1959 and, although it is classified as EHDV serotype 2, it is regarded as atypical. There are also at least 5 serotypes of EHDV in Australia, which are known to infect cattle, buffalo, and deer without causing clinical disease. In 2006, outbreaks of the disease were recorded in cattle in Israel and Morocco.

Members of other orbivirus species are widely distributed around the world and have been isolated in Australia, North and South America, Africa, Asia, and Europe.

Host Range and Transmission

Orbiviruses are transmitted between their vertebrate hosts by a variety of hematophagous arthropods. BTV, AHSV, EHDV, and EEV are all transmitted by adult females of certain *Culicoides* species which bite the mammalian host in order to obtain proteins, prior to laying eggs. BTV is only enzootic in areas where these vectors are present and active for the majority of the year, thus maintaining a continuous infection cycle in the vector and vertebrate host species. Although there are in excess of 1000 species of *Culicoides* worldwide, only 17 have been connected with BTV and 11 are known to be capable of transmitting the virus. These are *C. sonorensis*, *C. imicola*, *C. fulvus*, *C. actoni*, *C. wadai*, *C. nubeculosus*, *C. dewulfi*, *C. brevitarsis*, *C. obsoletus*, *C. pulicaris*, and *C. insignis*. Many of the remaining *Culicoides* species may be refractory to infection, although environmental factors (particularly higher temperatures) can increase vector competence, even in species that are usually refractory. BTV vectors are most active between 18 and 29 °C, and are almost inactive below 10 °C or above 30 °C. The viral polymerase, which is responsible for all viral RNA synthesis, has a temperature optimum between 27 and 35 °C but is almost inactive below 15 °C. Relatively small rises in temperature within the range 15–30 °C can significantly increase both the activity of insect vectors, and the rate of virogenesis within infected individuals, significantly pincreasing their efficiency as vectors.

Infections caused by BTV and EHDV are normally restricted to domesticated and wild ruminants, although there is also evidence for BTV infection of shrews and some rodents. AHS is considered to be a disease primarily of horses and other equids. However, dogs infected with BTV (caused by a contaminated vaccine) developed a fatal viral pneumonia. AHSV infection of dogs (caused by ingestion of infected meat) can be fatal. BTV and AHSV infections have also been reported in large carnivores in Africa, and may significantly affect their numbers. The epidemiological significance of BTV or AHSV infection in dogs and other carnivores, caused by eating infected meat or by other routes, has not been fully assessed. It is unclear if they can develop a high level of viraemia, or can act as a source of infection to adult *Culicoides*. There is serological evidence that AHSV can infect elephants and isolates have occasionally been obtained from camels, cattle, sheep, and goats. Under unusual circumstances (involving inhalation of a freeze dried neurotropic vaccine strain), AHSV has also infected humans, causing encephalitis and retinitis. The potential risk to human health posed by consumption of AHSV infected meat has not yet been fully evaluated.

Orbiviruses can infect marsupials, humans, rodents, bats, monkeys, sloths, and particularly birds (*Great Island virus*, *Ieri virus*, and *Umatilla virus* species). Under experimental conditions, many orbiviruses can infect mice or embryonated chicken eggs, and these hosts are routinely used for virus isolation from infected tissue samples (e.g., blood) or from insect vectors. Adult mice can show high mortality levels when infected via a nasal route with some strains of AHSV. This may have relevance to the reported cases of AHSV in humans infected via the same route by neurotropic vaccine strains. Experimental animal systems can provide useful models for studies of the immune response to these viruses and for identification of virulence factors, as shown for members of the *Great Island virus* (GIV) and AHSV species.

Epidemiology and Disease

Infection with BTV, EHDV, or AHSV is accompanied by pyrexia and edema/inflammation, particularly around the face, mouth, and nose. BTV replicates in hematopoietic and lymphoid tissues, including the spleen, bone marrow, monocytes, macrophages, neutrophils, and draining lymphoid tissues. Infection of vascular endothelial cells causes vascular thrombosis and hemorrhages that vary from petechiae to ecchymosis and is accompanied by leakage of fluids, into surrounding tissues or the lungs (causing frothing). Clinical signs of BT may be severe, particularly in sheep and can include epithelial lesions or ulceration of the mouth, coronitis, degeneration of skeletal muscle, lameness, and vomiting, leading to pneumonia (which is frequently fatal), hemorrhages of the skin horn junction, torticollis (usually fatal), and occasionally to a cyanotic appearance of the tongue.

BT is effectively restricted to a band around the world between 53° N and 30° S, determined largely by the distribution of vector insects. Temperatures below 0 °C, when maintained for approximately 2 h or more, will kill adult *Culicoides*. Therefore, in those areas at relatively greater latitudes (which experience frosts), adult vectors may not be present or active in significant numbers throughout the entire year. Consequently, the virus may be absent, or maintained at only low levels in line with vector populations, for part of the year (usually in winter). However, in some areas there is evidence for a mechanism that allows the virus to persist through the winter (over-wintering). The exact nature of this mechanism is unknown; it has been suggested that it could involve persistent infection of either the mammalian host or larvae of vector insects, although over-wintering by these mechanisms has not been demonstrated. Seasonal variation in the incidence of disease is illustrated by the outbreaks of AHS in Spain, Portugal, and Morocco (1987–91), where cases were detected only in late summer and autumn, and by the outbreak of BT in northern Europe during the mid to late summer of 2006. The effects of high temperatures, together with relatively low humidity, may also be particularly significant in Africa, where it is evident that the Sahara represents at least a partial barrier to the spread of BT and other orbiviruses to the Mediterranean region.

The outbreaks of BTV in Europe (since 1998) collectively represent one of the clearest examples of disease distribution being affected by climate change. Increases in average temperatures in the region have been reflected by changes in the distribution of *C. imicola* (a major vector species) in southern Europe. This has not only allowed *C. imicola* to transmit BTV in new areas, it also generated a partial overlap with European populations of *C. obsoletus*, *C. pulicaris*, and *C. dewulfi* that are widespread across most of central and northern Europe, allowing the virus to be passed to at least one of these species as a new vector. The more northerly *Culicoides* species can clearly transmit the virus, particularly during the very warm summers that are now affecting much of Europe, as demonstrated by the outbreak of BTV-8 in the Netherlands, Belgium, Germany, France, and Luxemburg during the mid-to late summer of 2006, when record temperatures were experienced in the region. The whole of Europe must now be considered at risk to outbreaks of BT and some other orbivirus diseases that are transmitted by the same vectors (e.g., AHS or EHDV). This conclusion was confirmed by the further spread of BTV-8 and to the UK, Denmark, and Switzerland during 2007.

Although BTV and some of the other orbiviruses are widely distributed, not all serotypes of each virus species are present at each location. Introduction of orbiviruses (e.g., BTV or AHSV) into areas that are usually free of the disease, and which therefore contain immunologically naive populations of susceptible host species, can result in high mortality rates in infected animals. As an example, during the disease outbreak caused by BTV-8 in northern Europe during 2006, it was estimated that up to 50% of those sheep showing clinical signs of infection, eventually died from the disease. Although much smaller numbers of cattle showed clinical signs of infection, approximately 10–15% of these affected animals also died. Even the introduction of a new serotype of BTV into enzootic areas can result in disease in host animals that have neutralizing antibodies against the types already present.

The mortality rate caused by African horsesickness virus (AHSV) in naive horses is frequently cited as above 90%, making it the most lethal and most dangerous of the equine pathogens. The epidemiology of AHSV is discussed elsewhere in this encyclopedia.

BTV can cause a significant reduction in the productivity of domesticated animals in endemic areas. It has been estimated that annual losses in the USA are of the order of $120 million. Infectious BTV has been detected in bull semen and some early experiments (although not reproducible and therefore of uncertain significance) indicated the possibility of long-term persistence of virus and immunotolerance in cattle that were naturally infected *in utero*. Restrictions are imposed on the movement or importation of live animals or germ line materials (semen and ova) from infected areas, although the exact regulations, involving testing, quarantine periods, or even complete import/export bans differ from country to country. These barriers to trade, along with the associated surveillance and testing programs, also represent important causes of financial loss associated with outbreaks of orbivirus diseases.

Viral RNAS, Proteins, Virion Structure, and Properties

The structure, components, properties, and assembly of the BTV particle have been studied extensively by many techniques, including electron microscopy, cryoelectron microcopy, and X-ray crystallography.. The properties of the orbivirus particles and individual viral proteins described here are derived primarily from studies of BTV and AHSV.

Mature orbivirus particles are relatively featureless when viewed by negative-contrast electron microscopy (**Figure 1**). They are icosahedral, nonenveloped, approximately 90 nm in diameter and are composed of three layers

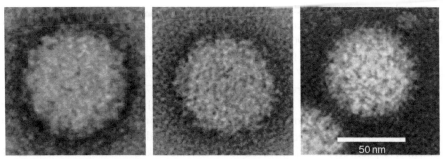

Figure 1 Electron micrographs of bluetongue virus serotype 1. Preparations of purified BTV-1 particles (strain – RSArrrr/01) were stained with 2% uranyl acetate: (left) virus particle, showing the relatively featureless surface structure; (center) infectious subviral particle (ISVP), in which outer capsid protein VP2 has been cleaved by treatment with chymotrypsin, showing some discontinuities in the outer capsid layer; (right) core particle, from which the entire outer capsid has been removed to reveal the structure of the VP7 (T13) core-surface layer and showing characteristic ring-shaped capsomeres.

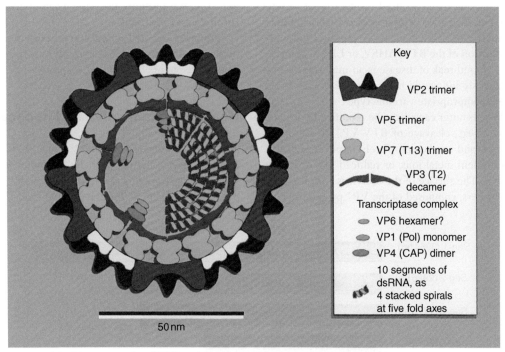

Figure 2 Diagram of the bluetongue virus (BTV) particle structure. A cross-section diagram of the orbivirus particle structure (viewed down a fivefold axis) was constructed using data from biochemical analyses, electron microscopy, cryoelectron microscopy and X-ray crystallography generated for bluetongue virus. Courtesy of P.P.C. Mertens and S. Archibald. Reproduced from Mertens PPC, Maan S, Samuel A, and Attoui H (2005) *Orbivirus, Reoviridae.* In: Fauquet CM, Mayo MA, Maniloff J, Desselberger U, and Ball LA (eds.) *Virus Taxonomy: Eighth Report of the International Committe on Taxonomy of Viruses*, pp. 466–483. San Diego, CA: Elsevier Academic Press, with permission from Elsevier.

of proteins, the subcore (VP3), the core-surface layer (VP7), and the outer capsid (VP2 and VP5) (**Figure 2**). Progeny orbivirus particles can leave infected cells by budding through the outer cell membrane, acquiring an envelope in the process, that can be lost soon after release. This may explain why unpurified virus is usually associated with cellular membranes and cell debris.

The buoyant densities of purified orbivirus particles in CsCl are $1.36\,\mathrm{g\,ml}^{-1}$ (intact virions) and $1.40\,\mathrm{g\,ml}^{-1}$ (cores). Virus infectivity is stable at pH 8–9 but virions exhibit a marked decrease in infectivity outside the pH range 6.5–10.2. This reflects the loss of outer capsid proteins at ~pH 6.5. Virus infectivity is abolished at pH 3.0, reflecting further disruption of the virus core. Viruses held *in vitro* at less than 15 °C in blood samples, serum, or albumin can remain infectious for decades, while virus infectivity is rapidly inactivated at 60 °C. Orbiviruses are relatively resistant to treatment with solvents, and nonionic detergents, or weak anionic detergents (such as sodium *N*-lauroyl sarcosine), although sensitivity varies with virus species.

However, strong anionic detergents such as sodium dodecyl sulfate (SDS) will disrupt the particle and destroy infectivity. Freezing reduces virus infectivity by ~90%, possibly due to particle disruption. However, once frozen, virus infectivity remains stable at −70 °C.

The orbivirus capsid contains seven structural proteins, arranged as three concentric capsid layers. The outer capsid layer of BTV and the related orbiviruses is composed of proteins VP2 and VP5 (encoded by genome segment 2 and segment 6, respectively). VP5 is involved in membrane penetration and can cause cell–cell fusion, while VP2 is primarily involved in cell attachment and is the major target for neutralizing antibodies generated by the infected host. VP2 is also the most variable of the virus proteins and the specificity of its interactions with these neutralizing antibodies (as determined by serum neutralization assays) can be used to identify 24 distinct BTV serotypes. The other orbivirus species also contain a variable number of distinct virus 'serotypes' (**Table 1**). The identification of the BTV, AHSV, or EHDV serotype involved in an outbreak of disease is an important aspect of virus diagnosis and would have direct relevance to the selection of an appropriate vaccine 'type'.

The orbivirus outer capsid can be modified by proteolytic enzymes (e.g., cleavage of BTV-VP2 by trypsin or chymotrypsin) and can be completely removed by treatment with divalent metal ions, or reduced pH, to release the virus core. The surface of the orbivirus core has ring-shaped capsomers, composed of the VP7 protein that are readily observed by electron microscopy (**Figure 1**) (hence orbivirus from Latin: *orbis*, meaning 'ring' or 'circle'). The BTV core is also infectious in its own right, for some mammalian cells, and particularly for adult *Culicoides* or *Culicoides* cell cultures, indicating that outer core protein VP7 can also mediate cell attachment and penetration in the absence of either VP2 or VP5. The core structural proteins are more conserved than those of the outer capsid and are serologically cross-reactive (e.g., by enzyme-linked immunosorbent assay (ELISA)) between different serotypes belonging to the same orbivirus species, but not between isolates from different species, providing a basis for serogroup-(virus-species-) specific assays. VP7 of BTV is particularly immunodominant and represents the major 'serogroup-specific' antigen detected in BTV-specific diagnostic assays, although the other core and nonstructural proteins also show virus-species/serotype-specific cross-reactions.

Orbivirus-infected cells also synthesize three nonstructural proteins (NS1, NS2, and NS3, encoded by BTV genome segments 5, 8, and 10, respectively).

Genome Organization and Replication

The BTV genome represents 12% and 19.5% of the total mass of intact orbivirus particles and cores, respectively. The genome segments range in size from 3954 to 822 bp (total of 19.2 kbp – **Figure 3**) and are identified as

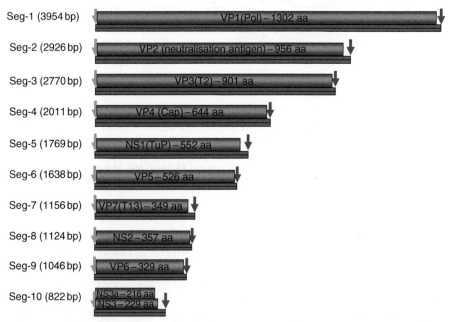

Figure 3 Organization of the BTV genome. The organization of the ten linear, dsRNA, genome segments of BTV-10. With the exception of Seg-10, each genome segment encodes a single viral protein. Seg-10 has two in-frame and functional initiation codons near to the upstream end of the segment (see http://www.iah.bbsrc.ac.uk/dsRNA_virus_proteins/BTV.htm). Like other members of the family, each AHSV genome segment contains conserved terminal sequences immediately adjacent to the upstream and downstream termini ((green arrow), 5'-GUUAAA..............ACUUAC-3' (red arrow) in the positive-sense strand) (see **Table 2**).

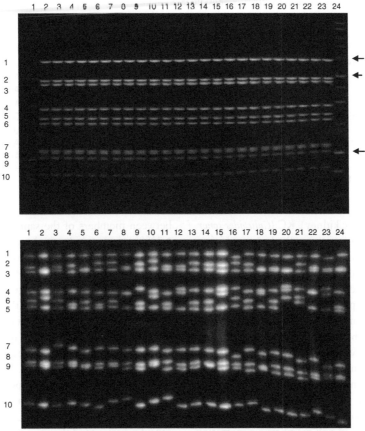

Figure 4 Electrophoretic analysis of BTV genomic dsRNAs. The genomic dsRNAs from the 24 reference strains of bluetongue viruses (BTV-1 to BTV-24: lanes 1–24) were analyzed by electrophoresis in a 1% agarose gel (top panel). Genome segments are referred to by numbers, in order of increasing electrophoretic mobility as indicated at the sides of gel. A consistent electropherotype was observed, which (despite similarities to that of some EHDV isolates) is different from the majority of other orbiviruses. The same set of dsRNAs were also analyzed by 11% polyacrylamide gel electrophoresis (PAGE) (bottom panel). Genome segments 5 and 6 migrate in a reverse order during PAGE, for most BTV isolates. Some of the more intense bands contain two genome segments which co-migrate. Differences were detected in the RNA migration pattern (PAGE-electropherotype) of each of the BTV isolates, which reflect variations in their primary nucleotide sequences.

'segments 1 to 10' (Seg-1 to Seg-10) in order of decreasing molecular weight and, hence, increasing electrophoretic mobility in 1% agarose gels. Different isolates belonging to the same orbivirus species usually have genome segments with a uniform size distribution, generating a uniform migration pattern (electropherotype) by agarose gel electrophoresis (AGE) (**Figure 4**), and this can be used to help identify individual virus species. However, variations in primary sequence often cause significant variations in migration patterns during polyacrylamide gel electrophoresis (PAGE) so that in most cases Seg-5 and Seg-6 of BTV migrate in the reverse order. This method can frequently be used to distinguish different virus strains or reassortants within the same virus species.

Orbivirus genome segments usually have a single major open reading frame (ORF) which is always on the same strand of the RNA (see **Table 2**). However, some ORFs can have more than one functional initiation site near to the 5′-end of the RNA, resulting in production of two

related proteins (e.g., segment 10 of BTV encoding NS3 and NS3a).

The 5′-untranslated regions (UTRs) of BTV type 10 genome segments range from 8 to 34 bp, while the 3′-UTR are 31–116 bp in length. For other BTV serotypes and other virus species, these lengths can vary. However, in general, the 5′-UTRs are shorter than the 3′-UTRs. The UTRs of almost all of the orbivirus genome segments that have been sequenced (**Table 2**) contain two conserved base pairs at each terminus (5′-GU... AC-3′, in the positive sense). The six terminal base pair sequences at both the 3′- and 5′-UTRs of the ten BTV genome segments are almost invariably conserved in different BTV isolates (**Table 2**). Other orbiviruses have terminal sequences which are comparable to, but not always the same as, those of BTV, although they may not be conserved in all ten genome segments.

Orbiviruses replicate in a variety of mammalian and insect cell lines, including BHK21 (baby hamster kidney),

Table 2   Conserved terminal sequences of orbivirus genome segments

Virus isolate	Conserved RNA termini (positive strand)
Bluetongue virus (BTV)	5'-GUUAAA..............................UUAC-3'
African horse sickness virus (AHSV)	5'-GUU $^A/_U$ A$^A/_U$..................AC$^A/_U$UAC-3'
Epizootic hemorrhagic disease virus (EHDV)	5'-GUUAAA.......................$^A/_G$CUUAC-3'
Great Island virus (BRDV)	5'-GUAAAA......................A$^A/_G$GAUAC-3'
Palyam virus (CHUV)	5'-GU $^A/_U$ AAA.....................$^A/_G$CUUAC-3'
Equine encephalosis virus (EEV)[a]	5'-GUUAAG..........................UGUUAC-3'
St. Croix River virus (SCRV)	5'-$^A/_G$UAAU$^G/_{A/U}$..........$^G/_{A/U}$$^C/_U$$^C/_A$UAC-3'
Peruvian horse sickness virus (PHRV)	5'-GUUAAAA..................$^A/_G$$^C/_G$$^A/_G$UAC-3'
Yunan orbivirus (YUOV)	5'-GUUAAAA...........................$^A/_G$UAC-3'

[a]Based on genome segment 10 (only) of the seven different serotypes.

Vero (African green monkey kidney), KC (*Culicoides sonorensis*), and C6/36 (*Aedes albopictus*) cells. Intact orbivirus particles bind to the host cell surface via their outer capsid proteins, leading to endocytosis and cell penetration. However, BTV core particles are also infectious, indicating that the core surface protein (VP7 of BTV) can also mediate cell attachment and entry. Cell-surface receptors for BTV have not yet been identified, although core particles can bind to glycosaminoglycans. VP2 is the BTV hemagglutinin (binds sialic acid residues) and (along with VP5, NS1, and NS3) appears to determine virulence of AHSV, which may reflect its role in cell entry and initiation of infection. VP5 can induce cell fusion, suggesting an involvement in cell membrane penetration (i.e., release from endosomes).

The details of cell infection and the intracellular replication cycle of BTV represent a paradigm for other orbiviruses and are discussed elsewhere in this encyclopedia.

Evolutionary Relationships among the Orbiviruses

Structural similarities, serological cross-reactions, and significant levels of nucleotide or amino acid sequence identities in specific genes or proteins clearly demonstrate that the different orbiviruses have a common ancestry. However, the members of distinct orbivirus species can be distinguished by a failure to cross-react in 'serogroup specific' serological assays, which target the more conserved core or nonstructural proteins (e.g., VP7). Different orbivirus species also show relatively large sequence differences even in their most conserved RNAs/proteins. These can be used to distinguish them and have been used to design species-specific primers for diagnostic reverse transcriptase-polymerase chain reaction (RT-PCR) assays. The nonstructural proteins and structural proteins of the orbivirus core are usually the most conserved components of each virus species (serogroup), while showing significantly higher levels of variation between different species. For example, the sub-core shell protein (VP3 of BTV) is very highly conserved

between members of the same orbivirus species (showing >73% amino acid identity between BTV strains) but shows significantly lower levels of conservation between virus species (serogroups 21.4% to 72%), reflecting more distant evolutionary relationships (**Figure 5**).

The protein components of the outermost capsid layer of the virus interact with the host defenses (including antibodies and cellular components of the mammalian immune system) and are therefore subjected to selective pressure, to change and avoid recognition. The outer surface components of different orbivirus species have also evolved to mediate transmission, cell attachment, and penetration in different host and vector species. Consequently, these outer capsid proteins (and the genome segments from which they are translated) usually show a greater degree of diversity within each species, than the protein components of the core or the nonstructural proteins.

In BTV, AHSV, or EHDV, the larger of the two outer capsid proteins (VP2 – encoded by genome segment 2) mediates cell attachment and is the major target for neutralizing antibodies. VP2 shows up to 27% amino acid sequence variation within a single serotype, while different BTV types can show as much as 73% variation in the sequence of this protein. Variations in the amino acid sequence of VP2 also reflect the serological relationships (cross-reactions) between different serotypes (**Figure 6**). The other orbivirus outer coat protein (VP5) can also influence serotype, although variations in the amino acid sequence of BTV VP5 show only a partial correlation with virus serotype. In some other orbiviruses (e.g., the Great Island viruses), it is the smaller outer capsid protein that exerts a greater influence over serotype. Despite its biological significance and at least partial control of cross-protection between different virus strains, the serotype of the virus currently has no formal taxonomic significance.

Within a single virus species, many of the genome segments also display sequence variations that reflect the geographic origin of the virus isolate (topotypes). For example, BTV and EHDV isolates can be divided into eastern and western groups, based on sequence comparisons of several genome segments/proteins (i.e., 'eastern' viruses

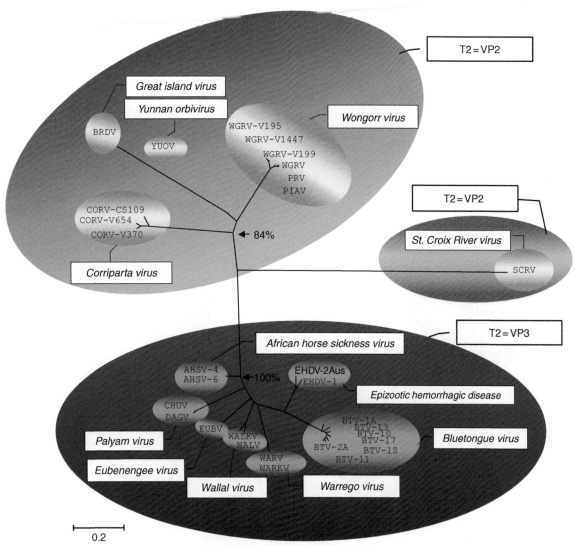

Figure 5 Phylogenetic comparison of sub-core shell (T2) proteins of different orbiviruses. Unrooted neighbor-joining tree showing relationships between the deduced amino acid sequences of the sub-core shell protein (T2) of different orbivirus species. This NJ tree was constructed using MEGA program version 3.1 and the p-distance algorithm based on partial sequences for VP3/VP2, as indicated (amino acids 393–548 relative to BTV-10 sequence). Similar trees were obtained with the Poisson correction and the gamma distance. Two major clusters of virus species were detected, one group with T2 proteins (VP2) encoded by genome segment 2 (supported by bootstrap values of >84%), and a second group with T2 protein (VP3) encoded by genome segment 3 (e.g., BTV and AHSV). These two groups appear to represent distinct evolutionary lineages. SCRV was the most divergent virus from either insect-borne or the other tick-borne orbiviruses and forms a separate small cluster.

from Australia, India, and Asia, and 'western' viruses from Africa and America). Since 1998, both eastern and western strains of BTV have invaded Europe, providing a potentially unique opportunity for these viruses to co-infect the same host and exchange (reassort) genome segments. Regional variations in VP2/Seg-2 and VP5/Seg-6 indicate that different BTV serotypes evolved before they became geographically dispersed, and then acquired further point mutations that distinguish these different topotypes. Sequence analyses of BTV Seg-2/VP2 provide rapid and reliable diagnostic methods to determine both the serotype and origin of individual isolates (molecular epidemiology).

However, VP7/genome segment 7 and NS3/genome segment 10 of BTV, EHDV, and AHSV show significant variations that do not appear to reflect virus serotype, or the geographic origins of the isolate. Indeed NS3 of AHSV is the second most variable of the viral proteins (after VP2), showing greater diversity than the smaller outer capsid protein VP5. As VP7 and NS3 can play roles in infection and virus release/dissemination that may be essential within the insect vector, it has been suggested that these proteins and genome segments might show variations that relate to the species or population of vector insects by which they are transmitted.

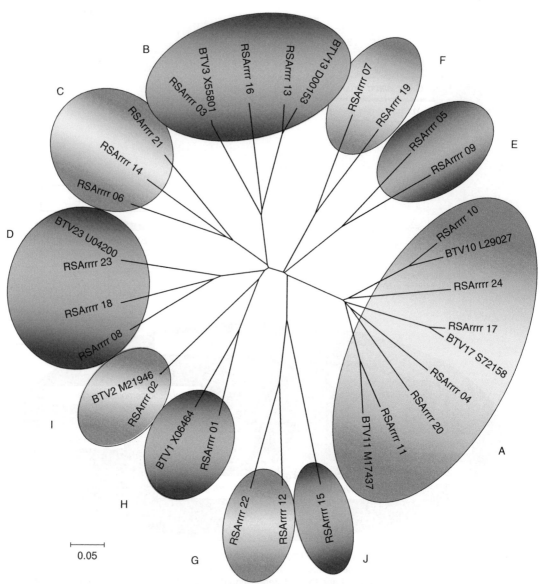

Figure 6 Phylogenetic relationships of bluetongue virus outer capsid protein VP2. Unrooted neighbor-joining tree showing the relationships between deduced amino acid sequences of VP2 (encoded by genome segment 2) from the 24 BTV serotypes. This NJ tree was constructed using MEGA program version 3.1 using the p-distance algorithm and the full-length VP2 sequences of the 24 BTV types. The different serotypes are distinct but show some relationships (green bubbles) that mirror the serological relatedness (cross-reactions) that are known to exist between different serotypes. These groupings are reflected in the nucleotide sequences of genome segment 2 and the ten distinct groups have previously been identified as nucleotypes A–J.

Orbiviruses of Humans

Orbiviruses and antibodies indicative of orbivirus infection have been isolated from and/or detected in humans. Changuinola virus (one of twelve 'named' serotypes within the *Changinola virus* species) was isolated in Panama from a human with a brief febrile illness. The virus has also been isolated from phlebotomine flies, and antibodies have been detected in rodents. Changuinola virus replicates in mosquito cells (C6/36) without producing CPE and is pathogenic for newborn mice or hamsters following intracerebral inoculation.

Kemerovo, Lipovnik, and Tribec viruses are among 36 tick-borne virus serotypes from the *Great island virus* species. These viruses were implicated as causes of a nonspecific fever, or neurological infection in the former USSR (Kemerovo) and Central Europe (Lipovnik and Tribec). More than 20 strains of Kemerovo virus were isolated in 1962 from patients with meningoencephalitis, and from *Ixodes persulcatus* ticks in the Kemerovo region of Russia. The virus was also isolated from birds and infects Vero or BHK-21 cells. Lipovnik and Tribec viruses may be involved in Central European encephalitis (CEE) and >50% of CEE patients had antibodies to Lipovnik virus.

The virus is also suspected in the etiology of some chronic neurological diseases including polyradiculoneuritis and multiple sclerosis. Antibodies against a Kemerovo-related virus have been detected in Oklahoma and Texas, in patients with Oklahoma tick fever. Sixgun City virus is one of seven tick-borne serotypes of the *Chenuda virus* species isolated from birds. Several Oklahoma tick fever patients also had antibodies to Sixgun City virus, although no virus was isolated.

Lebombo virus type 1 (the only serotype of the *Lebombo virus* species) was isolated in Ibadan, Nigeria, in 1968, from a child with fever. The virus replicates in C6/36 cells without CPE and lyses Vero and LLC-MK2 (Rhesus monkey kidney) cells. It is pathogenic for suckling mice and has also been isolated from rodents and mosquitoes (*Mansonia* and *Aedes* species) in Africa.

The *Orungo virus* species (ORV) contains four distinct serotypes (ORV-1 to ORV-4), transmitted by *Anopheles*, *Aedes*, and *Culex* mosquitoes. ORV is widely distributed in tropical Africa where it has been isolated from humans, camels, cattle, goats, sheep, monkeys, and mosquitoes. ORV was first isolated in Uganda during 1959 from the blood of a human patient with fever and diarrhoea, who developed weakness of the legs and generalized convulsion. The weakness progressed to flaccid paralysis. Only a few clinical cases were reported (involving fever, headache, myalgia, nausea, and vomiting), despite a high prevalence of virus infection and three deaths. ORV causes lethal encephalitis in suckling mice and hamsters. It also causes CPE and plaques in Vero and BHK-21 cells, and it replicates when inoculated into the thorax of adult *Aedes aegypti* mosquitoes. High rates of co-infection with yellow fever and Orungo viruses have been reported, reflecting their similar geographic distribution and transmission by Aedes mosquitoes, as the principal vectors.

See also: Reoviruses: General Features.

Further Reading

Anthony S, Jones H, Darpel KE, *et al.* (2007) A duplex RT-PCR assay for detection of genome segment 7 (VP7 gene) from 24 BTV serotypes. *Journal of Virological Methods* 141: 188–197.

Grimes JM, Burroughs JN, Gouet P, *et al.* (1998) The atomic structure of the bluetongue virus core. *Nature* 395: 470–478.

Maan S, Maan NS, Samuel AR, Rao S, Attoui H, and Mertens PPC (2006) Analysis and phylogenetic comparisons of full-length vp2 genes of the twenty-four bluetongue virus serotypes. *Journal of General Virology* 88: 621–630.

Mertens PPC and Attoui H (eds.) ReoID: Orbivirus reference collection. http://www.iah.bbsrc.ac.uk/dsRNA_virus_proteins/ReoID/viruses-at-iah.htm (accessed July 2007).

Mertens PPC, Attoui H, and Bamford DH (eds.) The RNAs and proteins of dsRNA viruses. http://www.iah.bbsrc.ac.uk/dsRNA_virus_proteins/ (accessed July 2007).

Mertens PPC and Diprose J (2004) The Bluetongue virus core: A nano-scale transcription machine. *Virus Research* 101: 29–43.

Mertens PPC, Duncan R, Attoui H, and Dermody TS (2005) *Reoviridae*. In: Fauquet CM, Mayo MA, Maniloff J, Desselberger U,, and Ball LA (eds.) *Virus Taxonomy: Eighth Report of the International Committee on Taxonomy of Viruses*, pp. 447–454. San Diego, CA: Elsevier Academic Press.

Mertens PPC, Maan NS, Prasad G, *et al.* (2007) The design of primers and use of RT-PCR assays for typing European BTV isolates: Differentiation of field and vaccine strains. *Journal of General Virology* 88: 621–630.

Mertens PPC, Maan S, Samuel A, and Attoui H (2005) Orbivirus, Reoviridae. In: Fauquet CM, Mayo MA, Maniloff J, Desselberger U,, and Ball LA (eds.) *Virus Taxonomy: Eighth Report of the International Committee on Taxonomy of Viruses*, pp. 466–483. San Diego, CA: Elsevier Academic Press.

Mertens PPC and Mellor PS (2003) Bluetongue. *State Veterinary Journal* 13: 18–25.

Mo CL, Thompson LH, Homan EJ, *et al.* (1994) Bluetongue virus isolations from vectors and ruminants in Central America and the Caribbean. Interamerican Bluetongue Team. *American Journal of Veterinary Research* 55: 211–215.

Owens RJ, Limn C, and Roy P (2004) Role of an arbovirus nonstructural protein in cellular pathogenesis and virus release. *Journal of Virology* 78: 6649–6656.

Purse BV, Mellor PS, Rogers DJ, Samuel AR, Mertens PPC, and Baylis M (2005) Climate change and the recent emergence of bluetongue in Europe. *Nature Reviews Microbiology* 3: 171–181.

Sellers RF (1980) Weather, host and vectors: Their interplay in the spread of insect-borne animal virus diseases. *Journal of Hygiene (Cambridge)* 85: 65–102.

Shaw AE, Monaghan P, Alpar HO, *et al.* (2007) Development and validation of a real-time RT-PCR assay to detect genome bluetongue virus segment 1. *Journal of Virological Methods*. 145: 115–126.

Relevant Websites

http://www.rcsb.org/pdb – Information concerning protein structures, RCSB Protein Data Bank.

http://viperdb.scripps.edu – Information concerning virus structure, virus particle explorer database(viperdb).

http://www.oie.int – OIE data on AHSV outbreaks, OIE homepage.

Orthobunyaviruses

C H Calisher, Colorado State University, Fort Collins, CO, USA

Glossary

Arbovirus A virus transmitted to vertebrates by hematophagous (blood-feeding) insects.
Orthobunyavirus A virus in the genus *Orthobunyavirus*.
Reassortant A virus having genomic RNAs of two different viruses.
Transovarial transmission Vertical transmission, from mother to offspring.
Sympatrically Occupying the same or overlapping geographic areas without interbreeding.
Teratogenic Causing malformations of an embryo or fetus.

Introduction

From the late 1950s and onward, Jordi Casals, Robert Shope and co-workers at the World Health Organization's Collaborating Centre for Arbovirus Reference and Research collected and studied the antigenic relationships among the many viruses that had been and were being collected by Rockefeller Institute workers investigating epidemics of yellow fever and other virus diseases. Through their meticulous studies, they were able to show that some of these viruses were related to each other serologically (antigenically) and formed 'groups' of viruses. However, at least one virus in each of certain groups reacted with antibody to at least one virus in another group or groups. This was confusing because a group logically comprises certain viruses and not others, else the 'others' would be considered in the group. Casals then proposed that these tenuously interrelated viruses formed a 'supergroup', the Bunyamwera supergroup, and suggested that there might be other supergroups to be found. Subsequently, many viruses were shown to have similarities antigenically, by size, morphogenetics, and morphology, and by molecular means, yet also could be distinguished by these methods, such that groups, supergroups, and, eventually, genera, were included in a family of viruses, the *Bunyaviridae* (named after *Bunyamwera virus*).

This family comprises five genera: *Orthobunyavirus, Nairovirus, Phlebovirus, Hantavirus,* and *Tospovirus*. Viruses of the first three are transmitted by hematophagous arthropods and infect vertebrates; hantaviruses are not known to be transmitted by arthropods but infect vertebrates; and tospoviruses are transmitted by plant-feeding thrips and do not infect vertebrates. Any virus in the family is 'a bunyavirus' so, to avoid confusion, the original genus name *Bunyavirus* was changed to *Orthobunyavirus*.

According to the International Committee on Taxonomy of Viruses, 48 species are recognized within the genus and these 48 species include 160 viruses, including various strains, plus three viruses that are, at this time, considered 'tentative species' (**Table 1**). As the current ICTV list is somewhat confusing (it lists strains and synonyms), **Table 1** provides a slightly modified list of species and viruses placed in genus *Orthobunyavirus*.

Many studies of the orthobunyavirus-type species (prototype), *Bunyamwera virus*, have yielded a commensurate amount of information. Much that is known about the orthobunyaviruses is known by extrapolation from studies of one or more viruses of the genus or of viruses in a particular group of viruses. However, whereas all orthobunyaviruses share some characteristics, they are distinct. The differences, which are relatively or seemingly trivial, may be biologically significant. For example, La Crosse and Snowshoe hare viruses share considerable RNA sequence similarities and are considered 'subtypes' or 'varieties' of the same virus. Their geographic ranges overlap and their natural cycles include being transmitted between small mammals by mosquitoes and they cause disease in humans, usually young humans. However, the small mammals they employ as principal vertebrate hosts for amplification differ (chipmunks [*Tamias* spp.] and squirrels [*Sciurus* spp.] for La Crosse virus, hares [*Lepus americanus*] for Snowshoe hare virus); their principal mosquito vectors differ (*Aedes triseriatus* for La Crosse virus, other *Aedes* spp. for Snowshoe hare virus); La Crosse virus is the primary cause of pediatric arboviral encephalitis in the US, Snowshoe hare virus is a rare cause of such infections; and La Crosse virus has been isolated as far south as Texas and Louisiana, Snowshoe hare virus has been found in Alaska, and in Canada in the Yukon and Northwest Territories, British Columbia, Alberta, Saskatchewan, Manitoba, Ontario and Quebec in Canada, but only as far south as Montana, Minnesota, Wisconsin, Ohio, Pennsylvania, New York and Massachusetts in the US. Clearly, differences between 'species' (a taxonomic term) and 'virus' (a nomenclatural term) may be confusing but they are epidemiologically and diagnostically relevant.

Most orthobunyaviruses were discovered during routine or epidemic surveillance efforts. Many have been isolated only once or, at most, a few times; some have

Table 1 Species and viruses[a] placed in the genus *Orthobunyavirus*

Species	Viruses
Acara virus	Acara, Moriche
Akabane virus	Akabane, Sabo, Tinaroo, Yaba-7
Alajuela virus	Alajuela, San Juan
Anopheles A virus	Anopheles A, Las Maloyas, Lukuni, Trombetas
Anopheles B virus	Anopheles B, Boraceia
Bakau virus	Bakau, Ketapang, Nola, Tanjong Rabok, Telok Forest
Batama virus	Batama
Benevides virus	Benevides
Bertioga virus	Bertioga, Cananeia, Guaratuba, Itimirim, Mirim
Bimiti virus	Bimiti
Botambi virus	Botambi
Bunyamwera virus	Batai, Birao, Bozo, Bunyamwera, Cache Valley, Fort Sherman, Germiston, Iaco, Ilesha, Lokern, Maguari, Mboke, Ngari, Northway, Playas, Potosi, Santa Rosa, Shokwe, Tensaw, Tlacotalpan, Tucunduba, Xingu
Bushbush virus	Benfica, Bushbush, Juan Diaz
Bwamba virus	Bwamba, Pongola
California encephalitis virus	California encephalitis, Inkoo, Jamestown Canyon, Keystone, La Crosse, Lumbo, Melao, San Angelo, Serra do Navio, Snowshoe hare, Tahyna, Trivitattus
Capim virus	Capim
Caraparu virus	Apeu, Bruconha, Caraparu, Ossa, Vinces
Catu virus	Catu
Estero Real virus	Estero Real
Gamboa virus	Gamboa, Pueblo Viejo
Guajara virus	Guajara
Guama virus	Ananindeua, Guama, Mahogany Hammock, Moju
Guaroa virus	Guaroa
Kairi virus	Kairi
Kaeng Khoi virus	Kaeng Khoi
Koongol virus	Koongol, Wongal
Madrid virus	Madrid
Main Drain virus	Main Drain
Manzanilla virus	Buttonwillow, Ingwavuma, Inini, Manzanilla, Mermet
Marituba virus	Gumbo Limbo, Marituba, Murutucu, Nepuyo, Restan
Minatitlan virus	Minatitlan, Palestina
M'Poko virus	M'Poko, Yaba-1
Nyando virus	Nyando, Eret-147
Olifantsvlei virus	Bobia, Dabakala, Olifantsvlei, Oubi
Oriboca virus	Itaqui, Oriboca
Oropouche virus	Facey's Paddock, Oropouche, Utinga, Utive
Patois virus	Abras, Babahoya, Pahayokee, Patois, Shark River
Sathuperi virus	Douglas, Sathuperi
Simbu virus	Simbu
Shamonda virus	Peaton, Sango, Shamonda

Continued

Table 1 Continued

Shuni virus	Aino, Kaikalur, Shuni
Tacaiuma virus	Tacaiuma, Virgin River
Tete virus	Bahig, Matruh, Tete, Tsuruse, Weldona
Thimiri virus	Thimiri
Timboteua virus	Timboteua
Turlock virus	Lednice, Turlock, Umbre
Wyeomyia virus	Anhembi, BeAr-328208 (unnamed), Macaua, Sororoca, Taiassui, Wyeomyia
Zegla virus	Zegla
Tentative species in the genus	
Leanyer, Mojui dos Campos, Termeil	

[a]The International Committee for Taxonomy of Viruses lists additional strains of certain of these viruses. Strain designations have been omitted from this list.

been isolated many times in a single location or a few times in many locations; some are isolated with considerable frequency; orthobunyaviruses are found worldwide. Most have not been associated with disease in humans, livestock, or wildlife but those that have been cause uncomplicated illnesses (fever, headache). However, certain orthobunyaviruses are recognized as the etiologic agents of severe disease, for example, the aforementioned La Crosse virus.

La Crosse Virus

In 1964, this virus was isolated from brain tissue of an encephalitic child from Minnesota who had died in 1960 in a hospital in nearby La Crosse, Wisconsin. Till then, the only recognized human pathogenic California serogroup virus in North America was California encephalitis virus, but La Crosse virus was soon shown to differ from that virus. Most infections are subclinical or cause mild illnesses, but the more severe infections can lead to illnesses characterized by frank encephalitis progressing to seizures with coma. The case–fatality rate is <1%, with neurological sequelae often requiring several years to resolve, if they do resolve and there are individual and social costs from the adverse effects on IQ and school performance. Short-term to long-term hospitalization costs can exceed $450 000. Since its recognition, La Crosse virus has been shown to cause childhood encephalitides each year. In the period 1964–2003, 3190 (a mean of 80 per year) human California group (mostly La Crosse virus infections) have been diagnosed in the US. In comparison, 4632 infections with St. Louis encephalitis (a flavivirus), 640 infections with Western equine encephalitis, and 215 infections with Eastern equine encephalitis (both togaviruses) occurred in the same period. Inapparent:apparent infection rates as high as 26:1 have been determined. Other California group viruses occasionally cause febrile illnesses with infrequent central nervous system involvement in Europe and North America.

Akabane Virus

Epizootics of congenital defects and abortion 'storms' had been observed in cattle, sheep, and goats in Japan and Australia since the 1930s, but an etiologic agent was not identified until 1959, when the orthobunyavirus Akabane virus was isolated from *Aedes vexans nipponii* and *Culex tritaeniorhynchus* mosquitoes in Japan; in Australia, the principal arthropod vector is the biting midge *Culicoides brevitarsis*. In other places, other vectors have been identified.

This virus now is known to occur widely in Africa and the Middle East and, wherever it occurs, has been responsible for malformations of the fetus. The range and severity of its effects are related to the stage of gestation at infection of the dam. In adult animals, infection is subclinical and preexisting immunity in the dam provides protection to the fetus, such that the presence of Akabane virus may go undetected in areas enzootic for the virus. When it does cause congenital malformations, they may present as increased incidence of abortions and premature births occurring during seasons when arthropods are most abundant. The principal malformations are hydranencephaly (congenital absence of the cerebral hemispheres in which the space in the cranium that they normally occupy is filled with fluid) and arthrogryposis (permanent fixation of a joint in a contracted position), but dystocia (slow or difficult labor or delivery) may occur, necessitating cesarian section to save the dam. Surviving offspring manifest various developmental deficits and do not thrive. Other orthobunyaviruses have been shown to be teratogenic and Cache Valley virus has been associated with congenital defects in ruminants and, perhaps, in humans.

Oropouche Virus

Another example of the variations among orthobunyaviruses is Oropouche virus, isolated in 1955 from a febrile forest worker in Trinidad. Since then, a great deal has been learned as a result of data accrued during numerous epidemics. Oropouche disease is not fatal, but patients suffer from a mélange of signs and symptoms, including abrupt onset, fever, headache, myalgias, arthralgias, anorexia, dizziness, chills, photophobia, and an assortment of other symptoms. The acute phase of illness lasts 2–5 days but recurrence of symptoms can occur in patients who resume strenuous activities prior to complete resolution of their illness. Repeated epidemics of thousands of cases of Oropouche disease have occurred in urban population centers throughout the Brazilian states of Para, Amapa, Amazonas, Tocantins, Maranhao, Rondonia, and Acre. Epidemics of Oropouche fever were also reported in Panama in 1989 and in the Amazon region of Peru in 1992 and 1994.

The principal vector is thought to be the biting midge *Culicoides paraensis*, although isolations of Oropouche virus have also been made from mosquitoes. During epidemics, transmission of Oropouche virus can be maintained in a vector-human cycle. Oropouche disease transmission does not occur year-round and investigators have shown that monkeys, sloths, and mosquitoes comprise a sylvatic maintenance cycle.

Reassortment

Among the many orthobunyaviruses causing uncomplicated febrile illness, the group C viruses are notable. These viruses (Apeu, Bruconha, Caraparu, Ossa, Vinces, Madrid, Gumbo Limbo, Marituba, Murutucu, Nepuyo, Restan, Itaqui, and Oriboca) are related one to another in various ways. They have been detected only in the Americas, from Florida to South America and have been isolated from mosquitoes, bats, rodents, marsupials, and humans. When the first group C viruses were isolated in Brazil in the 1950s antigenic analyses demonstrated complex patterns of relationships. That is, whereas pairs of group C viruses might be closely related by complement-fixation (CF) tests, they were not related, much less closely related, by hemagglutination-inhibition (HI) and neutralization (N) tests. Using CF tests, Apeu and Marituba, Caraparu and Itaqui, and Oriboca and Murutucu were shown to be related but Apeu and Itaqui, Oriboca and Caraparu, and Marituba and Murutucu were shown to be related by HI and N tests. Because these viruses occur sympatrically and are transmitted between vertebrate hosts by mosquitoes of the same species, it was thought that these results were an indication of a series of natural reassortments and that these viruses might serve as a model of viral evolution.

As detailed elsewhere in this volume, viruses of the family *Bunyaviridae* have tripartite genomes consisting of three RNA segments: designated small (S), medium (M) and large (L). The S segment encodes the nucleocapsid (N) protein and a nonstructural protein (NSs); the M segment encodes a polypeptide that is post-translationally cleaved to produce surface glycoproteins Gn and Gc, as well as a nonstructural protein (NSm); the L segment encodes a large protein containing the RNA-dependent RNA polymerase for replication and transcription of the genomic RNA segments. We now know that the group C viral CF antigen is the N protein and that the group C hemagglutinin is a surface glycoprotein, critical for virus attachment and, therefore, for neutralization. Recent molecular genetic studies of these viruses have corroborated earlier antigenic, ecologic, and genetic studies, and have shown that many of these viruses are genetic reassortants. That is, that they have various combinations of S, M, and L RNAs and that the various combinations lead to the various antigenic characteristics, patterns of cross-protection, and enzootic persistence in nature.

Naturally occurring reassortants of La Crosse virus and Patois group viruses have been documented; a Simbu group virus, Jatobal virus has been shown to contain the S RNA of Oropouche virus; Tinaroo and Akabane viruses are naturally occurring reassortants; and Ngari virus, a Bunyamwera group virus, is a reassortant comprising the S and L segments of Bunyamwera virus and the M segment from Batai virus. The Ngari virus strains (named Garissa virus at the time) had been isolated from human hemorrhagic fever patients, one in Kenya and one in Somalia, during a large outbreak of Rift Valley fever (Rift Valley fever virus is a phlebovirus) in East Africa. Thus, reassortment of orthobunyaviral RNAs produced a virus with characteristics atypical of Bunyamwera virus, which has not been associated with severe disease, and which mimic the clinical characteristics of Rift Valley fever. It is likely that other orthobunyaviruses will be shown to be reassortants, that reassortment is an on-going evolutionary process, and that reassortment will provide us with emerging diseases into the future.

Indeed, laboratory studies of experimental reassortants of La Crosse, Snowshoe hare, and other California group orthobunyaviruses have been useful in providing us with insights to understand the structure–function relationships of the various RNAs (neurovirulence or neuroinvasiveness and neuroattenuation map to the L RNA (which encodes the viral polymerase)). Lifelong infection of the arthropod vector, as well as transovarial transmission and venereal transmission, provide substantial opportunity for the virus to evolve by genetic drift or, under suitable circumstances of mixed infections, by segment reassortment. Orthobunyavirus reassortment, however, is limited to closely related viruses, reducing the possibility of unrestricted orthobunyaviral evolution.

Diagnosis and Treatment

Diagnosis of orthobunyavirus infections is by detection of viral RNA by PCR, as well as serologic assays including HI, CF, N, enzyme-linked immunosorbent assays, and immunofluoresence. Identification of orthobunyaviruses is by PCR, and the serologic assays mentioned above, the most specific of which is the N test. Treatment of illnesses caused by orthobunyaviruses is not needed for the more mild illnesses but when called for is merely symptomatic.

See also: Bunyaviruses: General Features.

Further Reading

Anderson CR, Spence L, Downs WG, and Aitken THG (1961) Oropouche virus: A new human disease agent from Trinidad, West Indies. *American Journal of Tropical Medicine and Hygiene* 10: 574–578.

Casals J (1963) New developments in the classification of arthropod-borne animal viruses. *Anais de Microbiologia* 11: 13–34.

Edwards JF, Karabatsos N, Collisson EW, and de la Concha Bermejillo A (1997) Ovine fetal malformations induced by *in utero* inoculation with Main Drain, San Angelo, and La Crosse viruses. *American Journal of Tropical Medicine and Hygiene* 56: 171–176.

Endres MJ, Griot C, Gonzalez-Scarano F, and Nathanson N (1991) Neuroattenuation of an avirulent bunyavirus variant maps to the L RNA segment. *Journal of Viology* 65: 5465–5470.

Fauquet CM, Mayo MA, Maniloff J, Desselberger U,, and Ball LA (eds.) (2005) *Virus Taxonomy: Eighth Report of the International Committee on Taxonomy of Viruses*, pp. 699–716. San Diego, CA: Elsevier Academic Press.

Gerrard SR, Li L, Barrett AD, and Nichol ST (2004) Ngari virus is a Bunyamwera virus reassortant that can be associated with large outbreaks of hemorrhagic fever in Africa. *Journal of Virology* 78: 8922–8926.

Hammon WMcD and Reeves WC (1952) California encephalitis virus, a newly described agent. Part I. Evidence of natural infection in man and other animals. *California Medicine* 77: 303–309.

Iroegbu CU and Pringle CR (1981) Genetic interactions among viruses of the Bunyamwera complex. *Journal of Virology* 37: 383–394.

Nunes MRT, Travassos da Rosa APA, Weaver SC, Tesh RB, and Vasconcelos PFC (2005) Molecular epidemiology of group C viruses (*Bunyaviridae, Orthobunyavirus*) isolated in the Americas. *Journal of Virology* 79: 10561–10570.

Saeed MF, Wang H, Suderman M, *et al.* (2001) Jatobal virus is a reassortant containing the small RNA of Oropouche virus. *Virus Research* 77: 25–30.

Shope RE and Causey OR (1962) Further studies on the serological relationships of group C arthropod-borne viruses and the association of these relationships to rapid identification of types. *American Journal of Tropical Medicine and Hygiene* 11: 283–290.

Thompson WH, Kalfayan B, and Anslow RO (1965) Isolation of California encephalitis group virus from a fatal human illness. *American Journal of Epidemiology* 81: 245–253.

Ushijima H, Clerx-van Haaster M, and Bishop DH (1981) Analyses of the Patois group bunyaviruses: Evidence for naturally occurring recombinant bunyaviruses and existence of viral coded nonstructural proteins induced in bunyavirus-infected cells. *Virology* 110: 318–332.

Watts DM, Pantuwatana S, DeFoliart GR, Yuill TM, and Thompson WH (1973) Transovarial transmission of La Crosse virus (California encephalitis group) in the mosquito *Aedes triseriatus*. *Science* 182: 1140–1141.

Relevant Website

http://www.cdc.gov – Centers for Disease Control and Prevention (accessed on 11 December 2006).

Severe Acute Respiratory Syndrome (SARS)

J S M Peiris and L L M Poon, The University of Hong Kong, Hong Kong, People's Republic of China

Glossary

Bioavailability A measurement of the proportion of the orally administered dose of a therapeutically active drug that reaches the systemic circulation and is available at the site of pathology.

Coryza A runny nose.

Desquamation Shedding of epithelialium.

Lymphopenia Reduction of lymphocytes in the circulating blood below the normal range for age.

Myalgia Muscle pain.

Pathognomonic Characteristic and diagnostic of a particular disease.

PEGylated An adjective for describing molecules conjugated with polyethylene glycol (PEG).

Radiological abnormalities Atypical findings observed by medical imaging procedures (e.g., chest X-ray).

History

From November 2002 to January 2003, cases of an unusually severe atypical pneumonia were being observed in Guangdong Province, China. The disease was characterized by the lack of response to conventional antibiotic therapy and the occurrence of clusters of cases within a family or healthcare setting. In retrospect, these were the first known cases of the disease that was later to be called severe acute respiratory syndrome (SARS). Through January, the numbers of cases of this unusual 'atypical pneumonia' continued to increase with examples of 'super-spreading incidents' that were to punctuate the course of the subsequent SARS epidemic. Between 16 November and 9 February, 305 cases were identified, one-third of them in healthcare workers (**Table 1**).

On 21 February 2003, a 65-year-old doctor working in a hospital in the city of Guangzhou, the provincial capital of Guangdong, arrived in Hong Kong and checked into Hotel M. He had treated patients with 'atypical pneumonia' in Guangzhou and had been ill himself since 15 February. His 1-day stay on the ninth floor at this hotel led to the infection of at least 17 other guests or visitors, some of whom traveled on to Hanoi, Toronto, Vancouver, Singapore, USA, Philippines, Guangzhou, and Australia. Five of these secondary cases initiated clusters of infection in Hanoi, Singapore, Toronto and two clusters of

infection within Hong Kong. This was the most significant single event in the global spread of SARS, and arguably the most dramatic known event in the global spread of any infectious disease. However, because the secondary cases had largely dispersed outside of Hong Kong, this cluster of cases remained 'invisible' until the epidemiological linkages were reconstructed in mid-March.

Between 26 February and 10 March, disease outbreaks were recognized in the Hanoi-French Hospital in Vietnam and in Prince of Wales Hospital in Hong Kong. Dr. Carlo Urbani, a World Health Organization (WHO) communicable diseases expert stationed in Vietnam, examined the first cases of the disease outbreak in Hanoi and provided WHO with the first case descriptions of this new disease. Later, Dr. Urbani was himself one of the victims who succumbed to this disease. On 12 March, the WHO issued a Global Health Alert regarding an atypical pneumonia that was a particular risk to healthcare workers. Subsequently, Singapore and Toronto also reported clusters of cases. On 15 March, the WHO issued a Travel Advisory. The new disease was named SARS and a preliminary case definition was provided. The WHO set up virtual networks of virologists, clinicians, and epidemiologists to rapidly collate, evaluate, and disseminate information about the new disease.

Within weeks, SARS had spread to affect 8096 patients in 29 countries across five continents with 744 fatalities, an overall case–fatality rate of 9.6%. Healthcare facilities served as a major amplifier of infection, constituting 21% of all reported cases.

By 21–24 March, the etiological agent of SARS was identified to be a novel coronavirus, subsequently termed SARS coronavirus (SARS CoV). Serological tests demonstrated that the human population had no prior evidence of infection with SARS CoV, indicating that this virus had newly emerged in humans and implying a likely zoonotic origin.

Early case detection and isolation of infected individuals reduced and interrupted SARS CoV transmission across the world. By 5 July 2003, the WHO announced that all chains of human transmission of SARS were broken and the outbreak was at an end. This was indeed a historic triumph for global public health. Although SARS was subsequently to re-emerge to cause limited human disease (and in one instance, limited human-to-human transmission) as a result of laboratory escapes and zoonotic transmission from the live game animal markets of Guangdong in December 2003–January 2004 (**Table 1**), the human outbreak of SARS had been controlled.

Table 1 A chronology of events in the emergence of SARS

Date	Key events
16 November 2002	45-year-old man in Foshan city, Guangdong Province, mainland China becomes ill with fever and respiratory symptoms and transmits the disease to four other relatives.
10 December 2002	35-year-old restaurant chef working in Shenzhen is admitted to Heyuan City People's Hospital. Transmits disease to eight healthcare workers.
January 2003	Pneumonia outbreaks in Guangzhou (capital city of Guangdong Province). These include number of healthcare workers infected through the care of patients with the disease.
11 February 2003	Guangdong health authorities report an outbreak of respiratory disease in Guangdong with 305 cases and five deaths, one-third of the cases being in healthcare workers caring for patients with the disease. Cases were reported from Foshan, Heyuan, Zhongshan, Jiangmen, Guangzhou, and Shenzhen municipalities of Guangdong Province.
21 February 2003	A 65-year-old doctor from Guangdong arrives and checks in at Hotel M in Hong Kong. His stay of 1 day at this hotel leads to the infection of at least 17 other guests or hotel visitors who initiate clusters of infection within Hong Kong, Vietnam, Singapore, and Toronto.
26 February 2003	A 48-year-old 'Hotel M contact' is admitted to Hanoi-French Hospital in Vietnam and is the source of an outbreak there. Seven healthcare workers were ill by 5 March.
1 March 2003	A 22-year-old 'Hotel M contact' is admitted to Tan Tock Seng Hospital, Singapore. She will pass on infection to 22 close contacts.
4 March 2003	A 26-year-old Hotel M contact admitted to Prince of Wales Hospital, Hong Kong. His illness is relatively mild and is not categorized as severe pneumonia. He transmits infection to 143 persons including 4 members of his family, 67 healthcare workers or medical students, and 30 other patients.
5 March 2003	A 78-year-old 'Hotel M contact' dies at home in Toronto, Canada. Four family members are infected. They are the source for the subsequent Toronto outbreak.
5–10 March 2003	Outbreaks are recognized in Hanoi and Hong Kong.
12 March 2003	WHO issues a Global Alert about atypical pneumonia in Guangdong, Hong Kong, and Vietnam that appears to place healthcare workers at high risk.
13–14 March 2003	Singapore and Toronto report clusters of atypical pneumonia. In retrospect, both groups have an epidemiological link to Hotel M. One of the doctors who had treated develops symptoms while traveling and is quarantined on arrival in Germany on 15 March.
15 March 2003	WHO has received reports of over 150 cases of this new disease, now named severe acute respiratory syndrome (SARS). An initial case definition is provided. Travel advisory issued.
17 March 2003	WHO multicenter laboratory network on SARS etiology and diagnosis is established.
21–24 March 2003	A novel coronavirus is identified in patients with SARS.
12 May 2003	The genome sequence of the SARS coronavirus is completed.
June 2003	A virus related to SARS CoV is detected in civets and other small mammals in live game-animal markets in Guangdong.
5 July 2003	Lack of further transmission in Taiwan, the last region to have SARS transmission, signals the end of the human SARS outbreak.
September 2003	Laboratory-acquired SARS coronavirus infection in Singapore.
December 2003–January 2004	Re-emergence of SARS infecting humans from animal markets in Guangdong. Laboratory-acquired SARS coronavirus infections in Taiwan.
February 2004	Laboratory-acquired SARS leads to community transmission in Beijing and Anhui in China.

Adapted from Peiris JSM, Guan Y, Poon LLM, Cheng VCC, Nicholls JM, and Yuen KY (2007) Severe acute respiratory syndrome (SARS). In: Scheld WM, Hooper DC, and Hughes JM (eds.) *Emerging Infections* 7, p. 23. Washington, DC: ASM Press, with permission from ASM Press.

Virology

SARS Virus

SARS coronavirus is a member of the genus *Coronavirus* within the family *Coronaviridae* and the order *Nidovirales*. Coronaviruses are classified on genetic and antigenic characteristics into three groups and SARS CoV is presently regarded as a group 2b coronavirus. It is an enveloped, positive-sense, single-stranded RNA virus with a genome size of approx 29.7 kbp. The virus particle is approximately 100–160 nm in diameter with a distinctive corona of petal-shaped spikes on the surface which is comprised of the spike glycoprotein (S). The S protein is in a trimeric form on the viral surface. It has an N-terminal variable subdomain (S1) which contains the motifs responsible for receptor binding. A more conserved subdomain (S2), which contains heptad repeats and a coiled-coil structure, is important in the membrane fusion process. The S1–S2 subdomains remain in a noncleaved form in the intact SARS CoV virion and cleavage is believed to occur within the endocytic vesicle during the viral entry process. The envelope also contains a transmembrane glycoprotein M and in much smaller amounts, an envelope (E) protein. The M protein is a triple-spanning membrane protein and has a key role in coronavirus assembly. The hemagglutinin-esterase (HE) glycoprotein, found in some group 2 coronaviruses, is absent in SARS CoV. The nucleocapsid protein (N) interacts with the viral genomic RNA to form the viral nucleocapsid. Viral replication complexes are believed to be localized within double-membraned vesicles or autophagosomes.

SARS CoV Genome

The genome of SARS CoV is that of a typical coronavirus. The viral genomic RNA has at least 14 open reading frames (ORFs) (**Figure 1**). The genome codes for 16 nonstructural proteins (nsp1–16), 5 structural proteins, and 7 accessory proteins. The genomic RNA encoding the replicase gene functions as mRNA to generate polyproteins 1a and 1ab. The translation of ORF1b is directed by a −1 ribosomal frameshift (RFS) signal that contains a nucleotide slippery sequence (5′-UUUAAAC-3′) and an RNA pseudoknot. By contrast, the structural and accessory proteins are products derived from subgenomic RNA (sgRNA 2–9) which are synthesized by discontinuous RNA transcription. Translated products from ORF2 (S), ORF4 (E), ORF5 (M), and ORF9a (N) are viral structural proteins as described above. Recently, it was reported that the protein encoded by the ORF3a, which is able to interact with S and contains ion channel activity, is also

a structural protein. However, the full function of this protein is yet to be determined.

The polyproteins 1a and 1ab generated from the replicase gene are cleaved by a papain-like proteinase (part of nsp3) and a 3C-like proteinase (nsp5) to generate 16 nonstructural proteins (**Figure 1(b)**). Nsp12 is a primer-dependent RNA-dependent RNA polymerase (RdRp), whereas nsp8 is a noncanonical RdRp (nsp8) synthesizing primers utilized by nsp12. In addition, eight nsp7 and eight nsp8 subunits are able to form a hexadecamer with a hollow, cylinder-like structure. RNA-binding studies and the overall architecture of this nsp7–nsp8 complex suggest that it might encircle RNA and confer processivity of nsp12. The nsp9 is a single-stranded RNA-binding protein and is able to interact with nsp8. The nsp13 is a helicase and unwinds duplex RNA (and DNA) in a 5′-to-3′ direction. The nsp3, nsp14, nsp15, and nsp16 have been shown to have ADP-ribose 1′-phosphatase, 5′-to-3′ exonuclease, endoribonuclease, and 2′-O-ribose methyltransferase activities, respectively. These four proteins are distantly related to cellular enzymes involved in RNA metabolism. These observations may be relevant to viral RNA processing. The nsp10 contains two zinc finger motifs and is suggested to be a regulator of vRNA synthesis. The biological functions of nsp1, nsp2, nsp4, nsp6,

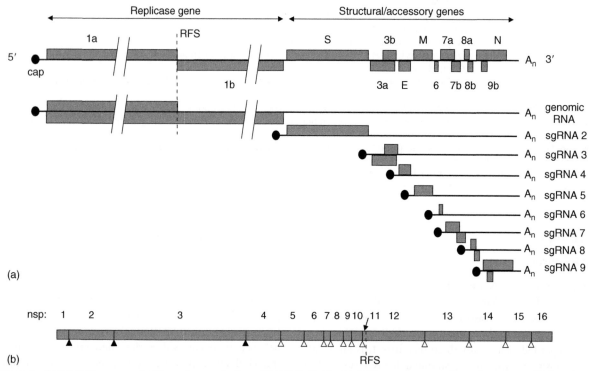

(a)

(b)

Figure 1 SARS CoV genome. (a) Genomic organization of SARS CoV. The 14 ORFs are expressed from the genome RNA and a nested set of subgenomic mRNA (sgRNA 2–9) that all have a common leader sequence derived from the 5′ end of the genome. The genomic RNA and all sgRNA contain a 5′ cap and a polyadenylated tail at the 3′ end. (b) Domain organization of the proteins for ORF1ab. Black and white arrow heads represent the sites cleaved by papain-like and 3C-like proteinases, respectively. The ribosomal frameshift (RFS) site is highlighted by a broken line.

and nsp11 are largely unknown. The nsp1 is reported to induce chemokine dysregulation and host mRNA degradation. The nsp2 is dispensable for virus replication. The nsp4 and nsp6 each contain a putative transmembrane domain.

Apart from the ORFs encoding the replicase and structural proteins, the viral genome contains additional ORFs that code for accessory proteins (3b, 6, 7a, 7b, 8a, 8b, and 9b). Genetically modified recombinant viruses without these accessory ORFs have been shown to be replication competent in cell cultures, indicating that the accessory ORFs may not be essential for virus replication *in vitro*. However, recombinant viruses with deletions in these regions are attenuated, suggesting that these proteins might have functions that are important for viral replication and pathogenesis *in vivo*. The accessory proteins from ORF3b and ORF7a induce apoptosis in transfected cells. There is also evidence suggesting that the 7a protein is incorporated into virions. The protein encoded in ORF6 has been shown to inhibit the nuclear import of STAT-1 and function as an interferon antagonist in infected cells. These properties might relate to virus virulence. Interestingly, comparative sequence analysis of SARS CoV isolated from palm civets (see below) and humans showed that all animal isolates contained a 29-nucleotide (nt) sequence which is absent from most human isolates obtained in the later phase of the SARS outbreak. As a result, the ORF8 in these human SARS CoVs encodes 8a and 8b proteins, whereas the corresponding ORF in the animal isolates encodes a single protein, known as the 8ab protein. These proteins from the animal and human ORF8 have differential binding affinities to various SARS CoV structural proteins. Furthermore, the expression of E can be downregulated by 8b but not 8a or 8ab in infected cells. These observations may suggest that the 29-nt deletion might modulate the replication or pathogenesis of the human SARS CoV. The crystal structure of the 9b protein suggests that it might be a lipid binding protein but its function is yet to be identified. Overall, these accessory proteins may play roles in viral replication and pathogenesis.

Ecology and Animal Reservoir

Until the end of January 2003, 39% of patients with SARS in Guangdong had handled, killed, or sold wild animals or prepared and served them as food. However, such risk factors were found in only 2–10% of cases from February to April 2003 when the virus had adapted to efficient human-to-human transmission. Thus, the early epidemiological evidence pointed to the live game animal trade as a potential source of the SARS CoV. SARS-like coronaviruses were identified in a number of small mammalian species sold in the live game animal markets in Guangdong, including the palm civet (*Paguma larvata*), raccoon dog (*Nyctereutes procyonides*), and the Chinese

ferret badger (*Melogale moschata*). A high proportion of individuals working in these markets were observed to have developed antibodies to SARS CoV, although none of them had a history of the disease. Viruses isolated from the re-emergent SARS cases in Guangdong in December 2003–January 2004 were more similar to those found in civets in these markets, rather than to viruses causing the global outbreak in early 2003. These observations strongly implicated the live game animal trade as the interface for interspecies transmission of a precursor animal SARS-like coronavirus to humans.

SARS CoV can be shed for weeks in experimentally infected palm civets but many of the other species appear to clear the virus rapidly. While civets in live animal markets were often observed to be positive for SARS-like coronavirus RNA, civets tested in the farms that supply these markets and those caught in the wild rarely have evidence of infection. Thus, palm civets were believed not likely to be the natural reservoir of the precursor SARS CoV (see below). More recently, group 2b coronaviruses related to SARS CoV have been identified in *Rhinolophus* bats in Hong Kong and mainland China. Such bats are also sold live in these game animal markets. It is now believed that these or related bat coronaviruses may be the precursor from which SARS CoV originated (see below).

Phylogeny

SARS CoV and the SARS-like civet and bat coronaviruses form a distinct phylogenetic subgroup (2b) within the group 2 coronaviruses (**Figure 2**). Genetic and phylogenetic analysis indicates that the viruses associated with the early phase of the human SARS outbreak are more closely related to the viruses found in palm civets and other small mammals in the live game animal markets in Guangdong. The genomes of viruses in the early phase of the human outbreak in 2003 were observed to be under strong positive selective pressure, suggesting that the virus was rapidly adapting in a new host. Furthermore, virus in civets was also found to be under strong positive selective pressure, supporting the view that civets were not the natural host of the precursor SARS-like coronavirus. The search for the precursor of SARS CoV led to the discovery of a number of novel coronaviruses in bats which are related to group 1 and group 2 coronaviruses. Some of these bat coronaviruses are genetically related to SARS CoV (group 2b) and are likely to be the direct or indirect precursor of SARS CoV (see below).

Interestingly, considered overall, the recently discovered group 1 and group 2 (including SARS CoV-like) bat coronaviruses appear to be in evolutionary stasis while many other mammalian coronaviruses still appear to be under evolutionary selection pressure, raising the intriguing possibility that bats may in fact be the precursors, not only of SARS CoV, but also of most other mammalian coronaviruses.

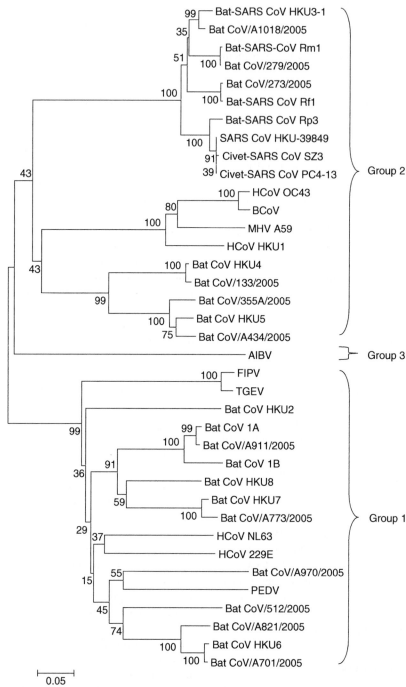

Figure 2 Phylogenetic analysis of RNA sequences coding for the RNA-dependent RNA polymerase (partial sequence). The phylogenetic tree was constructed by the neighbor-joining method and bootstrap values were determined with 1000 replicates. Human SARS CoV (GenBank accession AY278491.2), SARS CoVs isolated from palm civets in 2003 (AY304486.1) and 2004 (AY613948.1) and bat CoVs [Bat CoV 1A (DQ666337.1), Bat CoV 1B (DQ666338.1), Bat CoV HKU2 (DQ249235.1), Bat-SARS CoV HKU3–1 (DQ022305), Bat CoV HKU4 (DQ249214.1), Bat CoV HKU5 (DQ249217.1), Bat CoV HKU6 (DQ249224.1), Bat CoV HKU7 (DQ249226.1), Bat CoV HKU8 (DQ249228.1), Bat-SARS CoV Rp3 (DQ071615), Bat-SARS CoV Rm1 (DQ412043), Bat-SARS CoV Rf1 (DQ412042), Bat CoV/ A434/2005 (DQ648819.1), Bat CoV/A701/2005 (DQ648833.1), Bat CoV/A773/2005 (DQ648835.1) Bat CoV/A821/2005 (DQ648837.1), Bat CoV/A970/2005 (DQ648854.1) Bat CoV/A911/2005 (DQ648850.1), Bat CoV/A1018/2005 (DQ648795.1), Bat CoV/133/2005 (NC_008315), Bat CoV/273/2005 (DQ648856), Bat CoV/279/2005 (DQ648857), Bat CoV/355A/2005 (DQ648809.1), Bat CoV/512/2005 (DQ648858)] were aligned with references sequences as indicated. Reference sequences are: transmissible gastroenteritis virus, TGEV (DQ811789); HCoV 229E (AF304460); HCoV NL63 (AY567487); HCoV-OC43 (AY391777); HCoV-HKU1 (DQ415903 HKU1); porcine epidemic diarrhea virus, PEDV (AF353511); avian infectious bronchitis virus, AIBV (AY646283); mouse hepatitis virus, MHV (AY700211); bovine coronavirus, BCoV (AF220295); feline infectious peritonitis virus, FIPV (AY994055).

Virus Receptors

The functional receptor for SARS CoV on human cells is the angiotensin-converting enzyme 2 (ACE-2) which binds the receptor-binding motif (amino acid residues 424 to 494) of the SARS CoV spike (S) protein. While the human SARS CoV S protein binds efficiently to both human and civet ACE-2, the civet-like SARS CoV S protein binds efficiently to ACE-2 from civets but poorly to human ACE-2. The spike protein of the bat SARS-like coronavirus lacks the ACE-2 receptor-binding motif and is therefore unlikely to bind to human ACE-2.

These findings explain the increased human transmissibility of SARS CoV in the later stages of the SARS outbreak, the observation that human SARS CoV efficiently infects civets under experimental conditions, and the failure of civet SARS CoV or bat SARS-like CoV to replicate productively in primate (Vero-E6, FRhK4) cells that support replication of human SARS CoV. This finding also explains the poor virulence and transmissibility of re-emergent SARS in December 2003–January 2004 when humans are believed to have been infected with a civet-like SARS CoV.

Other cell-surface molecules such as L-SIGN, DC-SIGNR, DC-SIGN (CD209), and L-SECtin may serve as binding receptors but do not appear to be functional viral receptors in the absence of ACE-2. They may, however, promote cell-mediated transfer of the virus to other susceptible target cells. On the other hand, binding to L-SIGN appears to lead to proteasome-dependent viral degradation and it may function as a scavenger receptor (see below).

Human Disease

Transmission

Respiratory droplets are the major source of infectious virus for transmission of SARS. However, aerosol exposure has probably contributed to disease transmission, at least in some defined instances where aerosol-generating procedures (e.g., nebulizers, high-flow oxygen therapy, intubation) have been used. The unusual stability of SARS CoV also suggests that contaminated surfaces and fomites may contribute to disease spread. As SARS CoV is present in feces and urine (and possibly other body secretions), these body fluids may also play a part in disease transmission. The largest single outbreak of SARS at the Amoy Gardens apartment block in Hong Kong, where over 300 individuals were infected from a single index case, is believed to have been caused by aerosols generated from infected body secretions (e.g., feces).

The estimated incubation period for SARS is 2–14 days. During the 2003 outbreak, the majority of cases did not transmit disease at all and only a few patients accounted for a disproportionately large number of secondary cases. Host factors may have played a role in these super-spreading events but, in many cases, there was a unique combination of host factors and environmental circumstances that facilitated transmission. In contrast to the high transmission rates in these super-spreading events and within hospitals, there was less evidence of secondary transmission within the family or within households (e.g., 15% in Hong Kong). Notwithstanding the 'super-spreading phenomenon' that has characterized SARS, the basic reproduction number (Ro) of SARS is estimated to range from 2 to 4.

Seroepidemiological studies of contacts of SARS patients (both adults and children) have revealed that asymptomatic infection was uncommon. The absence of large numbers of asymptomatic transmitters and the paucity of transmission during the first 5 days of illness explain the success of the public health measures of aggressive case detection and isolation in interrupting transmission of human-adapted SARS CoV and the control of the global disease outbreak. These features of SARS have been attributed to the observation that, unlike many other acute viral respiratory infections, SARS transmission has mostly occurred only after the fifth day of illness. This is, in turn, probably related to the low viral load in the upper respiratory tract during the early phase of the illness (see below).

Clinical Features

As the clinical features of SARS are not pathognomonic, a contact history and virological evidence of infection are important for confirmatory diagnosis. SARS typically starts with myalgia and loose stools around the time of onset of fever without coryza or sore throat (seen in 70% of patients). The upper respiratory manifestations are less commonly observed. Radiological abnormalities have been observed in >60% of cases at initial presentation and preceded lower respiratory tract symptoms in approximately 41% of patients.

Children have had much milder illness than adults and mortality rates progressively increase with age. Some patients, particularly those with progressive lower respiratory tract involvement have had a watery diarrhea. Other extrapulmonary manifestations included hepatic dysfunction and a marked lymphopenia involving both B, T (CD4 and CD8 subsets), and natural killer (NK) cells. High serum levels of chemokines (interleukin 8 (IL-8), CCL2, and CCl10) and pro-inflammatory cytokines (IL-1, IL-6, IL-12) have been observed.

The overall case–fatality rate was 9.6% and the terminal events were severe respiratory failure associated with acute respiratory distress syndrome (ARDS) and multiple organ failure. Age, presence of co-morbidities, and viral load in the nasopharynx and serum during the first 5 days of illness correlated with an adverse prognosis.

Autopsy findings of those who died in the first 10 days of illness were diffuse alveolar damage, desquamation of pneumocytes, and hyaline membrane formation. Viral RNA was detected by quantitative polymerase chain reaction (PCR) at high copy number in the lung, intestine and lymph nodes, and at lower levels in spleen, liver, and kidney. In lung biopsy tissue or in autopsy tissue of patients dying in the first 10 days after disease onset, viral antigen and viral nucleic acid were demonstrated by immunohistochemistry and *in situ* hybridization methods respectively, in alveolar epithelial cells and to lesser extent in macrophages. A few unconfirmed studies have also reported the detection of virus particles or viral RNA in multiple organs but these findings require independent confirmation.

Laboratory Diagnosis

Highly sensitive and specific real-time PCR assays for detection of viral RNA remain the best choice for early SARS diagnosis. Viral RNA has been detected in respiratory specimens, feces, serum, and urine. Specimens from the lower respiratory tract such as endotracheal aspirates have higher viral load than those from the upper respiratory tract and are better diagnostic clinical specimens. As viral load is low during the first 5 days of disease, a negative PCR result from specimens collected at this time does not exclude the diagnosis. Testing multiple specimens improves the detection rate of SARS. Virus culture on Vero E6 or FRhK-4 cells and viral antigen detection tests are much less sensitive than reverse transcriptase PCR (RT-PCR) for detecting the virus. While viral RNA remains detectable in the respiratory secretions and feces for many weeks after the onset of illness, specimens rarely yield a virus isolate after the third week of illness.

Sero-conversion by immunofluoresence or neutralization occurs during the second week of illness and can provide reliable retrospective diagnosis. Enzyme-linked immunoassays using inactivated whole virus or recombinant antigens are convenient alternatives for serological screening, but any positive results must be confirmed by the more specific immunofluoresence or neutralization tests.

Pathogenesis

The primary mechanism of lung damage appears to be due to infection of type 1 and type 2 pneumocytes which are key target cells of the virus. Type 2 pneumocytes are important in the repair of lung injury and infection of these cells can potentially impair the regenerative responses of the lung and aggravate the respiratory impairment.

Whereas mice deficient in NK, T or B lymphocytes display similar kinetics of viral replication to normal mice, infection of mice with defects in the STAT1 signaling pathway results in more prolonged viral replication and more severe disease. These findings indicate the importance of innate immune responses in the control of infection, at least in the mouse. Infection of epithelial cells, macrophages, and myeloid dendritic cells fails to induce a type 1 interferon response although other interferon response genes are activated. Viral proteins expressed from ORF3b, ORF6, and the N gene have interferon antagonist effects *in vitro*. In contrast, macrophages and dendritic cells respond to infection *in vitro* with strong chemokine responses, including those (e.g., CCL10) that are elevated in the serum of SARS patients, and macrophage-chemoattractant chemokines (CCL2). This may explain the predominantly macrophage infiltrate in the lung.

There is evidence of viral replication within intestinal epithelial cells but there is minimal cellular infiltrate or disruption of intestinal architecture and the pathogenesis of diarrhoea in SARS remains unclear.

Treatment

As SARS emerged as a disease of unknown etiology, empirical therapeutic options were initially tested including broad spectrum antivirals and immunomodulators such as ribavirin, intravenous immune globulin, type 1 interferon, SARS convalescent plasma, and corticosteroids. However, in the absence of controlled clinical trials, no conclusions can be drawn on the efficacy of these interventions.

Anti-SARS CoV activity *in vitro* has been demonstrated for several therapeutics already in clinical use for other conditions, including lopinavir–nelfinavir, glycyrrhizin, baicalin, reserpine, and niclosamide. There are contradictory reports on the *in vitro* activity of ribavirin, interferon beta, and interferon alpha. In summary, taking into account bio-availability of these compounds and *in vitro* data, interferon alpha $n1/n3$, leukocytic interferon alpha, interferon beta and nelfinavir appear to be worthy of animal studies and randomized placebo-controlled clinical trials if SARS was to return.

A clinical trial of lopinavir 400 mg with ritonavir 100 mg orally every 12 h (added to an existing regimen of ribavirin and corticosteroid therapy) appeared to provide clinical benefit compared to historical controls. However, the lack of concurrent controls makes it difficult to draw conclusions. Similarly, a limited clinical trial of 13 patients using interferon alfacon-1 treatment showed a trend toward improved radiological and clinical outcomes, but without achieving statistical significance.

Studies in primate models have demonstrated prophylactic or therapeutic benefit from PEGylated recombinant interferon alpha-2b and from small interfering RNA therapy. More recently, screening of combinatorial chemical libraries *in vitro* has identified potential inhibitors of the viral protease, helicase, and spike protein-mediated entry.

Animal Models

Experimental SARS CoV infection leads to virus replication in a number of animal species including nonhuman primates (e.g., cynomolgous and rhesus macaques, African green monkeys, and marmoset monkeys), mice (BALB/c, C57/BL6), Golden Syrian hamsters, ferrets, and cats. Only some of these develop pathological lesions in the lungs (cynomolgous macaques, ferrets, hamsters, marmosets, aged BALB/C mice).

Interestingly, whereas SARS CoV replicates in the lung of both young and aged (12–14 months) BALB/c mice, only aged mice manifest clinical symptoms and histological evidence of lung pathology. This is reminiscent of disease in humans in which children have mild illness (see above). Furthermore, few animal models reproduce the gastrointestinal manifestations of the illness.

While the ideal animal model for understanding SARS pathogenesis is lacking, those that support viral replication (with or without clinical disease) are adequate for evaluating the efficacy of vaccines.

Vaccines and Immunity

A wide range of strategies have been explored for development of SARS vaccines. These have included: inactivated whole virus vaccines; subunit vaccines including baculovirus expressed S1 subdomain or the complete trimeric spike protein of the virus expressed in mammalian cells; DNA vaccines expressing S (full-length and fragments), N, M, or E proteins; and vectored vaccines based on modified vaccinia Ankara (MVA) virus, vesicular stomatitis virus, adenoviral vectors carrying S, M, or N proteins, and attenuated parainfluenza virus type 3 vectored vaccines carrying S, E, M, and N proteins. Neutralizing antibody responses and, where appropriate, cell-mediated immune responses have been measured as correlates of immunity. Some of these vaccines have been evaluated in experimental models by challenging with infectious SARS CoV.

Trials in hamsters of attenuated parainfluenza virus type 3-vectored vaccines individually expressing SARS CoV S, E, M, and N proteins have indicated that only the S protein construct elicits neutralizing antibody and protects against experimental challenge. Furthermore, passive transfer of serum containing S protein neutralizing antibody has been shown to be sufficient to induce protective immunity in mice. It is concluded that neutralizing antibody to the S protein is an important correlate

of protection. The receptor-binding determinant of the S1 subdomain is an immuno-dominant epitope and a critical determinant for virus neutralization.

As antibody can enhance rather than protect against the coronavirus disease feline infectious peritonitis, antibody-dependent enhancement has been a concern for SARS-Co vaccine development. However, no evidence of vaccine-enhanced disease has been observed to date, with two possible exceptions. There is a report that a modified vaccinia Ankara virus S protein vaccine has led to hepatitis in vaccinated ferrets but this has not been independently confirmed. There is also a report that S protein antibody elicited by a subunit vaccine enhances entry of pseudo-particles carrying S spike into lymphoblastoic cell lines which lack ACE-2 and are not normally permissive to infection. However, in the challenge experiments in hamsters, the vaccine did not induce protection and there is no evidence of disease enhancement.

Passive immunization with human monoclonal antibodies to the S protein has been successful at protecting mice and ferrets from experimental challenge by reducing viral load in the lung but not in the nasopharynx.

Most of these active and passive immunization studies have evaluated protection from challenge using the homologous human-adapted SARS CoV. However, a newly emergent SARS outbreak will probably arise from the animal reservoir and it is therefore important to investigate cross-protection against animal SARS-like CoV. As none of the civet or bat SARS CoV has yet been successfully grown *in vitro*, the cross-reactive neutralizing antibody response has been studied using lentiviruses pseudotyped with CoV S protein from a civet virus (SZ3), a civet-like virus causing re-emergent SARS in humans in December 2003 (GD03), and from a human SARS CoV (Urbani-strain) isolated from the major human SARS outbreak in 2003. The viruses pseudotyped with human Urbani virus S protein were neutralized by antibodies to the civet SARS-like virus but pseudotypes with the civet-like S protein were not neutralized by antibodies to the human SARS CoV (Urbani). On the contrary, antibody to the Urbani virus appeared to enhance the infectivity of the GD03 and SZ3 pseudotyped viruses. These findings appear to reflect receptor usage of these viruses as it has been shown that GD03 and SZ3 bind poorly to human ACE-2 (see above). The development of vaccines that can prevent re-emergence of SARV CoV from its zoonotic reservoir remains a challenge.

Conclusion: Will SARS Return?

Like many recent emerging infectious diseases that threaten human health, SARS was a zoonosis. The SARS CoV that was responsible for the global outbreak in 2003 was well adapted to bind to human ACE-2 and was efficiently transmitted human-to-human. Laboratories remain a potential source of infection from such viruses and, as occurred in February 2004, laboratory escape can lead to a community outbreak.

The SARS-like coronavirus found in civets (and other mammals) in live game-animal markets is very closely related to SARS CoV, but it binds inefficiently to the human ACE-2 receptor (see above). Consequently, when human infection with the civet SARS-like CoV occurred in December 2003–January 2004, there was no human-to-human transmission and clinical disease was mild. While SARS-like coronaviruses have been found in bats, they are genetically distinct to SARS CoV and the bat SARS-like CoV S protein appears unable to bind to human or civet ACE-2. Thus, it is likely that re-emergence of a virus capable of causing human disease from this source probably requires extensive adaptation in an intermediate host (e.g., small mammals such as civets). While it is difficult to assess the likelihood of SARS re-emergence, this possibility cannot be excluded.

The rapid expansion of the live game-animal trade and the development of large markets in southern China which house a diversity of wild and domestic animal species were probably important in facilitating the emergence of SARS CoV. It is therefore possible that, like Ebola, SARS may re-emerge at intervals in the future. However, a number of epidemiological characteristics of SARS (see above) should allow it to be contained by public health interventions, once the disease is diagnosed. Indeed, the chain of community transmission arising from a laboratory escape of SARS CoV in February 2004 was contained by such public health measures and community transmission was aborted. However, if the dynamics of transmission of a re-emergent virus are different, and particularly if transmission occurs earlier in the illness and there are more asymptomatic infections, the options for control and the ultimate consequences may be very different. It remains important, therefore, to understand better the ecological and viral factors that predispose to interspecies transmission and the emergence of animal viruses with efficient competence for transmission in humans. Attention should be directed toward the adaptation strategies and the ecological factors that

are important in determining interspecies transmission, rather than focus on the disease itself (i.e., SARS). Efforts to understand better the molecular basis for interspecies transmission that led to the genesis of SARS CoV will help us to prepare better for the next emerging infectious disease challenge; whether this comes from SARS CoV, avian influenza H5N1, or a yet unknown virus.

See also: Coronaviruses: General Features.

Further Reading

Chan JCK and Taam Wong VCW (2006) *Challenges of Severe Acute Respiratory Syndrome.* Singapore: Elsevier.

Cinatl J, Michaelis M, Hoever G, Preiser W, and Doerr HW (2005) Development of antiviral therapy for severe acute respiratory syndrome. *Antiviral Research* 66: 81.

de Haan CAM and Rottier PJM (2006) Hosting the severe acute respiratory syndrome coronavirus: Specific cell factors required for infection. *Cellular Microbiology* 8: 1211.

Gillim-Ross L and Subbarao K (2006) Emerging respiratory viruses: Challenges and vaccine strategies. *Clinical Microbiology Reviews* 19: 614.

Gorbalenya AE, Enjuanes L, Ziebuhr J, and Snijder EJ (2006) Nidovirales: Evolving the largest RNA virus genome. *Virus Research* 117: 17.

Li W, Wong SK, Li F, *et al.* (2006) Animal origins of the severe acute respiratory syndrome coronavirus: Insight from ACE-2 protein interactions. *Journal of Virology* 80: 4211.

May RM, McLean AR, Pattison J, and Weiss RA (2004) Emerging infections: What have we leant from SARS? *Philosophical Transactions of the Royal Society of London, Series B* 359: 1045.

Peiris JSM, Guan Y, Poon LLM, Cheng VCC, Nicholls JM, and Yuen KY (2007) Severe acute respiratory syndrome (SARS). In: Scheld WM, Hooper DC, and Hughes JM (eds.) *Emerging Infections 7*, p. 23. Washington, DC: ASM Press.

Peiris JSM, Yuen KY, Osterhaus ADME, and Stohr K (2003) The severe acute respiratory syndrome. *New England Journal of Medicine* 349: 2431.

Peiris M, Anderson L, Osterhaus A, Stohr K, and Yuen KY (2005) *Severe Acute Respiratory Syndrome.* Oxford: Blackwell.

Perlman S and Holmes KV (eds.) (2006) The *Nidoviruses*: Towards control of SARS and other nidovirus diseases. *Advances in Experimental Medicine and Biology*, vol. 581. 617pp. New York: Springer.

Stockman LJ, Bellamy R, and Garner P (2006) SARS: Systematic review of treatment effects. *PLoS Medicine* 3: e343.

World Health Organization(2003) A multicentre collaboration to investigate the cause of severe acute respiratory syndrome. *Lancet* 361: 1730.

World Health Organization, Western Pacific Region (2006) *SARS. How a Global Epidemic was Stopped.* Geneva: WHO Press.

Zhong NS and Zeng GQ (2003) Our strategies for fighting severe acute respiratory syndrome (SARS). *American Journal of Respiratory and Critical Care Medicine* 168: 7.

Smallpox and Monkeypox Viruses

S Parker, Saint Louis University School of Medicine, St. Louis, MO, USA
D A Schultz, Johns Hopkins University School of Medicine, Baltimore, MD, USA
H Meyer, Bundeswehr Institute of Microbiology, Munich, Germany
R M Buller, Saint Louis University School of Medicine, St. Louis, MO, USA

Glossary

Enanthem Eruptive lesion of mucous membranes.
Exanthem Eruptive lesion of skin.
Papule A small, solid, elevated lesion of the skin that is often inflammatory.
Pock A pustule on the body caused by an eruptive disease.
Pustule A small elevated pus-containing lesion of skin.
Vesicle A small cavity within the epidermis containing serous fluid.

Variola Virus

Smallpox is caused by variola major virus (VARV), which is a member of family *Poxviridae*, subfamily *Chordopoxviriniae*, genus *Orthopoxvirus*. VARV is a 200–250 nm brick-shaped enveloped virus with a double-stranded DNA genome of approximately 186 kbp. Compared with other orthopoxviruses, VARV exhibits gene conservation toward the center of the genome, with genetic variation increasing toward the termini. The genes in the terminal regions appear to encode virulence factors that differ among orthopoxviruses. Virus replication occurs in the cytoplasm of the host cell where intracellular mature virions (IMVs) and extracellular enveloped virions (EEVs) are produced. Humans are the only natural host of VARV, although monkeys can be infected when exposed to artificially high doses and baby mice and rabbits can briefly propagate the virus. For additional information regarding the replication and architecture of VARV, the reader is refered to the article on vaccinia virus in this encyclopedia. Vaccinia virus is an extensively studied orthopoxvirus that has many biological similarities to VARV.

History

Smallpox, so named to differentiate it from great-pox (*syphilis*), was described by Edward Jenner as "the most dreadful scourge of the human species." Although the exact number of deaths during Jenner's time is unknown, it is estimated to have been approximately 400 million in the twentieth century alone. Historically, smallpox has had a close association with humans. The origin of VARV remains unknown, but the dubious accolade probably goes to Egypt or India. Unmistakable descriptions of smallpox were documented in fourth-century China, seventh-century India, and tenth-century Mediterranean and southwestern Asia. Moreover, Egyptian mummies buried over 3000 years ago have skin lesions that are consistent with smallpox. Before the fifteenth century, smallpox was generally confined to the Eurasian landmass. However, European colonists introduced smallpox to the Americas, central and southern Africa, and Australia between the fifteenth and eighteenth centuries with devastating consequences, as indigenous populations were decimated with case–fatality rates approaching 90%. Smallpox enabled a handful of conquistadors such as Cortez and Pizarro to subjugate large parts of central and South America to Spanish rule, thereby permanently altering the future of these regions. This was not an isolated pattern.

By the end of the nineteenth century a milder and less lethal form of smallpox, named variola minor, became apparent. This virus was first documented in South Africa during 1904, but had been clinically apparent in the USA since 1896. Originally described as Amass (alastrim in South America), this virus eventually became recognized in Brazil during the 1960s and in Botswana, Ethiopia, and Somalia during the 1970s. The variola minor derivatives of variola major (classical smallpox) are believed to have originated in several places throughout the globe as the virus adapted to humans. The case–fatality rates for variola major were 16–30% and 1% for variola minor.

Clinical Features

Clinically, smallpox in an unvaccinated person has a 7–19 day incubation period from the time infection is established within the respiratory tract until the first symptoms of fever, malaise, headache, and backache occur, culminating in the start of the characteristic rash. The rash starts with papules, which sequentially transform into vesicles and then pustules; a majority of these lesions are located on the head and limbs (often confluent) compared to the trunk. The rash is typically centrifugal (head and limbs), but centripetal (trunk) rashes have been reported. Lesions are 0.5–1 cm in diameter and can spread over the entire body. Once pustules have dried, scabs will form which eventually desquamate during the following 2–3 week period. The resultant feature of these cutaneous lesions is the formation of the classic pock scar that is apparent on the skin of surviving patients.

Two clinical variations of smallpox have been identified. Flat-type smallpox is a rare form of the disease (about 6% in unvaccinated people), and is characterized by lesions that remain level with the skin. It was more frequently observed in children and usually resulted in death. Another variation of the disease is hemorrhagic smallpox (<2% in unvaccinated people), which occurred mainly in adults. Although this was a rare form of the disease, it also had a high mortality rate and is characterized by hemorrhages into the skin and/or mucous membranes early in the course of illness. Subconjuctival hemorrhages were most common as well as bleeding from the gums and other parts of the body.

Although smallpox is typically spread by respiratory droplets over a short distance, some examples of long-distance transmission are evident. One such case occurred in 1978 at the University of Birmingham, UK, where a woman who was vaccinated 12 years earlier died of smallpox. She is identified as the last human fatality of the disease. It is widely believed that VARV traveled up through an air duct that connected a smallpox virology laboratory to her work station. Other theories suggest that this woman was exposed by using the laboratory telephone or simply from laboratory personnel. Another case occurred in a hospital at Meschede, Germany in 1970. In this case, a recent returnee from Pakistan is believed to have initiated 19 other cases of smallpox on all levels of a large general hospital, despite being isolated for the 5 days of his stay. Factors that enabled VARV to travel long distances in the hospital were likely: a building design that facilitated strong rising air currents when it was heated, the patient's severe cough, and the humidity level in the hospital.

Variolation and Vaccination

Historically, it was understood that humans who survived an initial smallpox infection never developed the disease again. Furthermore, persons infected with VARV by cutaneous scratches suffered a less severe form of the disease. For these reasons, the practice of inoculating naive persons with pustular fluid collected from smallpox victims became a common practice; this type of inoculation was called variolation. Variolation usually induced a milder form of the disease, which was typified by a severe, local, cutaneous lesion at the site of variolation with smaller satellite cutaneous lesions; however, variolation sometimes led to generalized rashes with associated deaths. Variolation was likely developed in both India and China and was subsequently introduced to Egypt and the rest of Africa in the seventeenth century and Europe and its colonies in the eighteenth century.

By the end of the eighteenth century, variolation had been widely accepted throughout the world as a means to prevent smallpox. The widespread use of variolation in Great Britain and her North American colonies widely reduced the impact of the virus in the upper classes but not in the general population as a whole. Despite its successes, the mortality rate and the frequent development of classical smallpox in many patients, with associated disease transmission, meant that variolation was less than ideal. Fortunately, a solution emerged from the common observation that milkmaids were rarely susceptible to smallpox. This lack of susceptibility was widely attributed to a zoonotic disease, cowpox. Based on these observations, Edward Jenner inoculated a boy with cowpox virus and observed the child's resistance to smallpox. Over time, more children were inoculated, exposed, and subsequently resisted smallpox. By the beginning of the nineteenth century this method of vaccination (*vacca*, Latin for cow) had become accepted, as it afforded the same level of protection as variolation without the associated risks of mortality and transmissibility. In some countries (France in particular), vaccination was substituted with orthopoxviruses causing horsepox (a method called equination). Moreover, in a recent study it was found that the causative agent of horsepox is closely related to the vaccinia virus strains derived from the historic smallpox vaccine, supporting the hypothesis that horsepox, or close relatives, replaced cowpox virus as the preferred virus used for worldwide vaccination at some point in the mid-nineteenth century. By the 1950s, endemic smallpox had been eliminated from most industrial nations.

All smallpox vaccines used during the eradication campaign were prepared from vaccinia virus; however, this vaccine was not without complications. In some cases, atypically severe lesions developed, coupled with severe symptoms and occasionally death. The most common complications of vaccination were noted in persons with eczema, where the eczematous region became rapidly inflamed and necrotic with frequent spread of the virus to healthy tissue. Immunocompromised individuals also presented with complications because the vaccination site failed to heal and secondary lesions appeared and spread; this complication was typically fatal.

Smallpox Eradication

In May 1959 the World Health Assembly tasked the World Health Organization (WHO) with the goal of eradicating smallpox globally. Although this was not the first eradication program, it was the only successful one. Approximately 20 years later, in 1980, the WHO declared that smallpox had been eradicated from the world. Despite plans to destroy all stocks of the virus by the end of the twentieth century, none have been realized. Their preservation is due to the stated need (among others) to develop and evaluate antiviral agents, as VARV is a potential bio-weapon. The virus which once dominated the health of mankind is categorized as a bio-safety level (BSL)-4 agent, and virus collections are still kept officially in two BSL-4 WHO reference laboratories in the USA and Russia (as of 2007). Any work with live VARV has to be approved by a WHO advisory committee. The genome sequences of 45 VARV strains are freely available online (see the 'Relevant website' section).

Monkeypox Virus

Monkeypox virus (MPXV) is also a member of the genus *Orthopoxvirus*. The MPXV virion is consistent in structure with other orthopoxviruses, that is, a 200–250 nm brick-shaped, enveloped virus with characteristic surface tubules and a dumbbell-shaped core (**Figure 1(b)**). Its genome is approximately 199 kbp of double-stranded DNA. Orthopoxviruses have host specificities ranging from narrow (e.g., VARV and ectromelia virus) to broad (e.g., cowpox

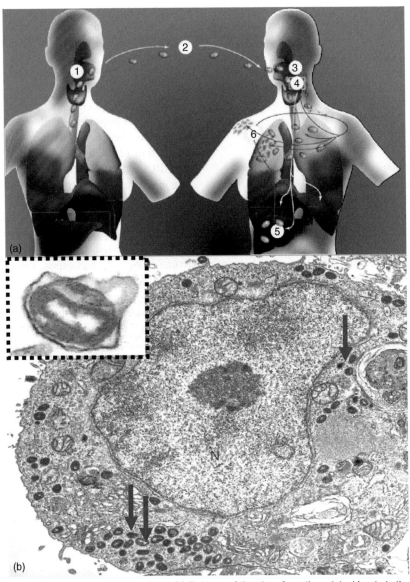

Figure 1 (a) Schematic of the natural life cycle of MPXV. (1) Release of the virus from the original host via the oropharyngeal mucosa. (2) Aerial dispersion of virus particles. (3) Seeding of the respiratory mucosa in a new host. (4) Initiation of replication and neutralization of the host's immune response. (5) Primary viremia and infection of internal organs and lymphatic system (white arrows). (6) Secondary viremia and development of exanthem and enanthem (red arrows). (b) A transmission electron micrograph (approximately ×10 000) of a BSC-1 cell infected with MPXV (red arrows). Virus replication occurs in the cytoplasm (not the nucleus, N). The inset image is an MPXV EEV particle (approximately ×165 000). Note the biconcave core and loose-fitting outer membrane. Adapted from Parker S, Nuara A, Buller RML, and Schultz DA (2007) Human monkeypox: An emerging zoonotic disease. *Future Microbiology* 2: 17–34, with permission from Future Medicine Ltd.

and vaccinia viruses), and the capability of MPXV to infect rodents, nonhuman primates, and humans places it in the latter group. MPXV and VARV cause similar diseases in humans, although they are distinct viruses.

History

MPXV was first isolated in 1958 from the vesiculo-pustular lesions found on infected cynomolgus macaques imported to the State Serum Institute of Copenhagen, Denmark. During the next few years, similar outbreaks were reported in monkey colonies in the USA and in a zoo in Rotterdam, The Netherlands. In the latter case, the first animals affected were giant anteaters from South America, but the disease spread to various species of apes and monkeys. The viruses isolated from these animals were found to be similar to each other and to represent a species of orthopoxvirus that had not been described previously. Currently, MPXV is classified as a BSL-3 agent for animal studies.

Human Monkeypox

MPXV remained primarily of academic interest throughout most of the 1960s. Attitudes changed radically when it was realized that MPXV could infect humans in known smallpox-free locales. This gave rise to concerns that MPXV could fill the niche vacated by VARV. However, a WHO-driven campaign suggested that this was unlikely. It was generally assumed that MPXV infections in humans had been occurring before VARV was expunged, but that they were masked under the guise of smallpox.

The most severe human MPXV infections have been reported in the Congo Basin area of Africa, whereas attenuated human infections have generally occurred in West African countries. Human infections usually result from handling MPXV-infected animals (bush-meat); however, cases of human-to-human transmission have been reported. In 2003, an MPXV outbreak occurred when MPXV-infected West African rodents were imported into the USA and thereafter infected native prairie dogs destined for sale in the pet industry. Human infections were initiated by several routes, which appeared to affect the clinical manifestations of the disease. No fatalities occurred, but the virus was of the less aggressive West African type (see below). Nevertheless, this incident demonstrated the ease with which MPXV can penetrate the interspecies barrier.

Clinical Features

MPXV-infected humans develop a skin rash and follow a disease course similar to that observed in smallpox victims (see above). However, some differences exist between smallpox and human monkeypox. First, humans infected with MPXV frequently present with severely swollen lymph nodes (lymphadenopathy of the neck, inguinal and axillary regions), which is not clinically apparent

with smallpox victims. Second, a hemorrhagic form of monkeypox has not been reported (however, it has been reported in some laboratory-housed African dormice infected with MPXV). Interestingly, humans infected with MPXV typically present with a rash similar to that observed in less severe cases of smallpox; to quantify this somewhat, approximately 58% of smallpox patients and 11% of human monkeypox (Congo Basin strain) cases had >100 pocks, respectively.

Epidemiology of Human Monkeypox

In humans, MPXV is a zoonotic infection that has limited capacity to transmit within the population. Between 1970 and 1979, only 47 cases of human monkeypox were reported in five African countries. Most (81%) of the cases were in the Democratic Republic of the Congo (DRC), and mathematical modeling experiments concluded that MPXV could not sustain itself in the unvaccinated human population without zoonotic amplification. Conversely, between 1970 and 2005, 2131 cases were reported in 12 countries. Most (94%) of the cases were in the DRC, and many were not confirmed in the laboratory. The majority of cases were reported in villages within, or close to, the tropical rainforest. African children were the most affected, with a 10% case–fatality rate. The reason for the upsurge, particularly in Africa, is unknown, but it has been suggested that a number of reported cases were actually cases of chickenpox, caused by varicella-zoster virus (a herpesvirus). A likely contributing factor is the cessation of smallpox vaccination by the WHO *c.* 1980, because recent vaccination with vaccinia virus is 85% effective at protecting against severe MPXV-induced disease. The broad host range of MPXV is also likely to permit additional species to become reservoirs or incidental hosts, thus increasing the exposure risk for humans.

Studies between 1981 and 1986 revealed that most human monkeypox cases occurred as single sporadic infections after contact with animals. The first-generation secondary attack rate in nonvaccinated household contacts was approximately 9% (compared to 58% with smallpox). The attack rate decreased over the second and third generations, and fourth generation attacks were very rare. That said, it has recently been reported that the transmissibility of MPXV is increasing in human hosts. Genetic changes that improve transmissibility to similar levels as those seen in VARV would be required for MPXV to infect humans in an endemic fashion.

Genetics

Although MPXV and VARV present similar disease profiles in humans, neither of the viruses is believed to have given rise to the other. Rather, both are considered to have arisen from a progenitor virus(es) similar to the cowpox virus lineage. MPXV isolates from West Africa are less virulent and less transmissible in human populations than isolates from the Congo Basin. Consistent with other orthopoxviruses, MPXV strains exhibit gene conservation toward the center of the genome, with variation increasing in frequency toward the termini, which encode for specific virulence genes. Genomic differences between strains have been mapped with restriction fragment length polymorphism studies and DNA sequencing techniques. Sequence analyses of strains from West Africa and the Congo Basin have revealed that isolates are approximately 95% identical to each other and approximately 96% identical to VARV. This value increases to 99% when comparing isolates from only West African or only the Congo Basin regions, allowing a separation into two groups or clades. The genomic sequences of eight MPXV strains are available online (see the 'Relevant website' section).

Ecology

The broad host range of MPXV and seroprevalence studies suggest that several animal species, rather than a single species, may act as reservoirs for MPXV in nature. In the latter part of the twentieth century, several field studies were conducted in the lowland tropical forests of the Congo Basin and West Africa; these studies revealed that MPXV can infect many animal species, including squirrels (*Funisciurus* spp. and *Heliosciurus* spp.) and nonhuman primates (such as *Cercopithecus* spp.). Species that are seropositive for MPXV antibodies have some similar and some dissimilar traits in relation to diet and habitat preference; approximately 40% are arboreal, 40% are semiterrestrial, and 20% are terrestrial. Therefore, MPXV infects species that inhabit all levels of the lowland tropical rainforest in the Congo Basin and West Africa. For a thorough discussion of this topic, the reader is directed to the article by Parker *et al.* listed in the 'Further reading' section.

New Hosts and Geographic Expansion

The interaction of MPXV with reservoir and incidental hosts is still poorly understood, as is the potential for virus transmission to humans within and outside its geographical range. Until the outbreak in the USA in 2003, MPXV had remained fairly localized to a handful of countries in central and West Africa, with the majority of cases detected in the DRC. The USA outbreak added to the breadth of host species capable of supporting MPXV replication, and demonstrated the potential of the virus to expand its geographical range. No human infections were attributed to the shipment of animals that entered the USA from Africa; rather, most patients had direct contact with infected native prairie dogs that had been housed with the imported African rodents. Subsequent to the USA outbreak, prairie dogs that were experimentally infected with MPXV were found to have ulcerative lesions on their lips, tongues, and buccal mucosa. High titer MPXV could be cultured from the nasal discharge and oropharynx

of these animals for up to 22 days post infection, indicating that transmission from prairie dogs was likely via the respiratory and mucocutaneous routes. The USA outbreak was caused by the less virulent West African strain, which probably made it easier to bring under control.

A more recent example (2005) of MPXV expanding its environs is found in 19 human monkeypox infections discovered in the previously MPXV-free country of Sudan. This outbreak occurred some 300 miles northeast of the edge of the tropical rainforest – the traditional home of the Congo Basin strain of MPXV. From experience with vaccinia virus, it would not be surprising if MPXV continues to adapt to new species. Such adaptation has already occurred with prairie dogs in the USA and is possibly the reason for the outbreak in Sudan.

Person-to-Person Transmission

MPXV and VARV transmission are likely similar. Human-to-human transmission can be separated into six steps, as demonstrated in **Figure 1**. Step 1: release of virions from lesions in the oropharyngeal mucosa and their aerosolization into the new host's breathing space. Step 2: virus particles, most likely in the EEV form, are transmitted by aerosols. Step 3: seeding of the new host's respiratory mucosa is initiated. Step 4: MPXV replication creates foci of infection and production of specific proteins to neutralize the immune response. Step 5: the primary viremia denotes successful virus replication and spread from the initial site(s) of infection to lymphoid tissues and internal organs. Step 6: the secondary viremia occurs when the virus moves from the infected lymphoid tissues and internal organs to the cornified and mucosal epithelium to cause the exanthem and enanthem, respectively. Transmissibility is dependent on the number of lesions in the host oropharyngeal mucosa, virus survivability in the face of the host immune response, and the ability of the virus to produce infectious virions for exhalation from the respiratory tract. As an explanation of the increased transmissibility of VARV over MPXV, it is likely that VARV produces more infectious virions in the respiratory mucosa than MPXV.

Treatment

Currently, the public health importance of human monkeypox is minor compared to that of VARV before the 1980s. However, MPXV is becoming a more common infection in central Africa, where there seems to be a rise in the number of transmission generations observed during outbreaks. MPXV could be controlled in the human population by vaccination against smallpox. However, considering the current poor transmissibility in human populations and zoonotic nature of MPXV, this would need to be weighed carefully against the adverse reactions expected from vaccination. As of 2007, two antiviral drugs with activity against orthopoxviruses are being evaluated in animal models.

Diagnostics

Historically, biological properties have been used to identify and differentiate orthopoxviruses. Growth characteristics in embryonated chick eggs were particularly useful during the smallpox eradication campaign. However, this approach is labor and time consuming and requires a high level of skill. Even today, electron microscopy is a first-line technique, but does not allow for differentiation between orthopoxvirus species. Real-time polymerase chain reaction (PCR) is now regarded as the technique of choice for species differentiation, and several protocols are available specifically to identify and differentiate VACV and MPXV from other poxviruses.

Future Perspectives

VARV has been exterminated from the world's human population and could only be reintroduced by artificial release of clandestinely stored stocks. Such an incident would have devastating ramifications. MPXV is of minor public health significance when compared to VARV, but human MPXV infections are increasing. Elimination of MPXV is not possible because, unlike VARV, the virus is likely to have several animal reservoirs. Lastly, the possibility that terrorist groups or rogue nations might bioengineer VARV or MPXV to enhance virulence and transmissibility is a potential threat. Since the molecular biology of both viruses (and other orthopoxviruses) is fairly well understood, genetic tinkering aimed at enhancing virulence is a possibility, although techniques to increase transmissibility are less well developed.

See also: Cowpox Virus; Poxviruses; Varicella-Zoster Virus: General Features.

Further Reading

Fenner F, Henderson DA, Arita I, Jezek Z, and Ladnyi ID (eds.) (1988) *Smallpox and Its Eradication.* Geneva, Switzerland: World Health Organization.

Jezek Z and Fenner F (1988) Human monkeypox. In: Melnick JL (ed.) *Monographs in Virology,* vol. 17. Basel, Switzerland: Karger.

Parker S, Nuara A, Buller RML, and Schultz DA (2007) Human monkeypox: An emerging zoonotic disease. *Future Microbiology* 2: 17–34.

Tulman ER, Delhon G, Afonso CL, *et al.* (2006) Genome of horsepox virus. *Journal of Virology* 80: 9244–9258.

Relevant Website

http://www.biovirus.org – Viral Bioinformatics Resource Center (VBRC).

St. Louis Encephalitis

W K Reisen, University of California, Davis, CA, USA

Glossary

Bridge vector Vector responsible for carrying virus from the primary cycle to tangential hosts such as humans.

Diapause Insect hibernation.

Gonotrophic cycle Recurrent cycle of blood feeding and egg laying by female mosquitoes.

Maintenance vector Vector responsible for transmission of virus among primary vertebrate host species.

Neuroinvasive Ability of virus to invade the central nervous system.

Vector competence Ability of an insect to become infected with and transmit a pathogen.

Viremia Concentration of virus within peripheral blood.

Viremogenic Ability to elicit an elevated viremia response.

History

St. Louis encephalitis virus (SLEV) probably has been present in the New World within its enzootic cycle for thousands of years. The arrival of European settlers in the 1600s and the extensive agricultural development that followed greatly altered the landscape by clearing and irrigating vast areas of North America and establishing extensive urban centers. These changes probably increased the abundance of peridomestic *Culex* mosquito species and avian hosts such as house finches and mourning doves, introduced new avian hosts such as house sparrows, intensified human–vector mosquito contact, and probably increased the incidence of human infection. However, diagnosis of diseases caused by arbovirus infections such as SLEV assuredly was confounded with other infections causing fever and central nervous system (CNS) disease during summer.

During the summer of 1933, a major encephalitis epidemic with more than 1000 clinical cases occurred in St. Louis, Missouri. These cases occurred during the middle of an exceptionally hot, dry summer and were concentrated within areas of the city adjacent to open storm water and sewage channels that produced a high abundance of *Culex* mosquitoes. A virus, later named St. Louis encephalitis virus, was isolated at autopsy from human brain specimens. Mouse protection assays using convalescent human sera demonstrated that SLEV differed from other viruses causing seasonal CNS disease, such as the equine encephalitides, poliomyelitis, and vesicular stomatitis. The epidemiological features of this epidemic included the late summer occurrence of cases (especially in persons over 50 years of age), exceptionally warm temperatures, and elevated *Culex* mosquito abundance associated with a poorly draining wastewater system. These features remain the hallmark of SLEV epidemics to date.

A multidisciplinary team of entomologists, vertebrate ecologists, epidemiologists, and microbiologists from the University of California subsequently investigated an SLEV epidemic in the Yakima Valley of Washington State during 1941 and 1942 and established the components of the summer transmission cycle, including wild birds as primary vertebrate hosts and *Culex* mosquitoes as vectors. The isolations of SLEV from *Culex tarsalis* and *Culex pipiens* mosquitoes were among the first isolations of any virus from mosquitoes and stimulated the redirection of mosquito control in North America from *Anopheles* malaria vectors and pestiferous *Aedes* to *Culex* encephalitis vectors.

Understanding the basic transmission cycle, an appreciation of the wide range of clinical symptoms, and the development of laboratory diagnostic procedures provided an expanding view of the public health significance of SLEV, with epidemics or clusters of cases recognized annually throughout the US. Wide geographic distribution and consistent annual transmission since 1933 has resulted in >1000 deaths, >10 000 cases of severe illness, and >1 000 000 mild or subclinical infections. The largest documented SLEV epidemic occurred during 1975 in the Ohio River drainage, with >2000 human cases documented. Other substantial human epidemics involving hundreds of cases have occurred in Missouri (1933, 1937), Texas (1954, 1956, 1964, 1966), Mississippi (1975), and Florida (1977, 1990). Smaller outbreaks have been recognized in California (1952), New Jersey (1962), and several other states plus Ontario (1975), Canada. Cases reported annually to the Centers for Disease Control and Prevention (CDC) since 1964 are shown in **Figure 1**.

Distribution

SLEV is distributed from southern Canada south through Argentina and from the west to the east coasts of North America and into the Caribbean Islands. Historically, human cases have been detected in Ontario and Manitoba, Canada, all of the continental US (except the New England States and South Carolina, **Figure 2**), Mexico, Panama, Brazil, Argentina, and Trinidad. The low number of human cases in Canada probably reflects the warm temperature requirements for SLEV replication in the mosquito host, whereas the low numbers of cases from tropical America may reflect inadequate laboratory diagnosis, the circulation of attenuated virus strains, and/or enzootic cycles involving mosquitoes that feed infrequently on humans. Support for this geographic distribution comes from laboratory-confirmed human cases, SLEV isolations

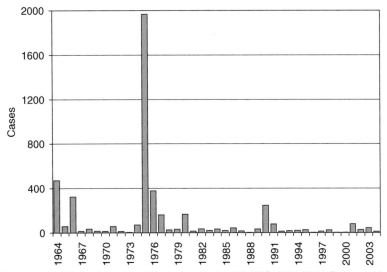

Figure 1 Number of clinical cases of St. Louis encephalitis reported to the US CDC, 1964–2004. Data provided by ArboNet, Center for Disease Control and Prevention, Ft. Collins, CO, USA.

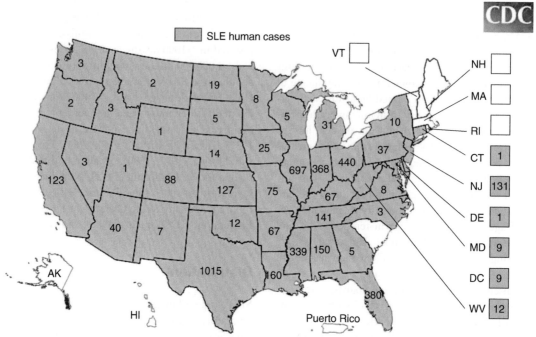

Figure 2 Distribution of human St. Louis encephalitis cases in the US, 1964–2004. Map provided by ArboNet, Center for Disease Control and Prevention, Ft. Collins, CO, USA.

from birds, mammals, and mosquitoes, and serological surveys of mammal and avian populations.

Classification

Taxonomically, SLEV is classified within the Japanese encephalitis virus (JEV) complex in the genus *Flavivirus* of the family *Flaviviridae*. Related viruses within this group include Japanese encephalitis, Murray Valley encephalitis, West Nile, and Usutu. SLEV consists of a positive-sense, single-stranded RNA enclosed within a capsid composed of a single polypeptide (C) and surrounded by an envelope containing one glycosylated (E) and one nonglycosylated (M) protein. Marked differences in the severity of SLEV epidemics stimulated interest in possible differences among isolates made over time and space. Detailed studies by the CDC during the 1980s clearly demonstrated geographic variation among 43 different SLEV isolates using oligonucleotide finger printing and virulence in model vertebrate hosts. These strains are grouped into six clusters: (1) east central and Atlantic USA, (2) Florida epidemic, (3) Florida enzootic, (4) eastern USA, (5) Central and South America with mixed virulence, and (6) South America with low virulence. Changes in virulence were attributed, in part, to differences in mosquito vector competence and were supported by the historical presence or absence of human cases. Subsequent genetic sequencing studies extended the

understanding of SLEV genetics and provided further insight into patterns of geographical variation. Sequences of the envelope gene from SLEV strains isolated in California from 1952 to 1995 varied temporally and spatially, but indicated regional persistence in the Central Valley for at least 25 years as well as sporadic introduction and extinction. Studies in Texas using a single-strand conformation polymorphism technique showed that multiple SLEV strains circulate concurrently and remain highly focal, whereas other strains amplify and disseminate aggressively during some summers, but then disappear. Further analyses of sequences from 62 isolates made throughout the known geographical range of SLEV indicated that there have been seven lineages that overlapped somewhat with the six groups the CDC defined previously using oligonucleotide fingerprinting: (1) western USA, (2) central and eastern USA and three isolates from Mexico and Central America, (3) one mosquito isolate from Argentina, (4) five isolates from Panama mosquitoes, (5) South American strains plus an isolate from Trinidad, (6) one Panama isolate from a chicken, and (7) two isolates from Argentina rodents. Collectively, these data indicated that SLEV strains vary markedly in virulence and that the frequency and intensity of epidemics in the US may be related to genetic selection by different host systems. Interestingly, transmission within the Neotropics appears to have given rise and/or allowed the persistence of less-virulent strains that rarely amplify to produce epidemic-level transmission, a scenario duplicated by West Nile virus in the Americas.

Host Range

Arthropods

Although a wide variety of mosquitoes occasionally have been found infected in nature, three avian-feeding species within the genus *Culex* appear to be the most frequently infected and important arthropod hosts: *C. pipiens* (including the subspecies *C. pipiens quinquefasciatus* at southern latitudes, *C. p. pipiens* at northern latitudes, and intergrades) in urban and periurban environments throughout North and South America, *C. tarsalis* in irrigated agricultural settings in western North America including northern Mexico, and *Culex nigripalpus* in the southeastern US, the Carribean, and parts of the Neotropics. Although these species feed predominantly on birds, they also feed on mammals including humans, and therefore function as both maintenance and bridge vectors. Other *Culex* species such as *stigmatosoma* in the west, *restuans* and *salinarius* in the east, and perhaps species in the subgenus *Melanoconion* in the Neotropics also may be important in local transmission. Ticks have been found naturally infected, but their role in virus epidemiology most likely is minimal.

Wild Birds

The importance of avian host species appears to be related to vector *Culex* host-selection patterns as well as to avian susceptibility to the virus. Species can be separated into those frequently, sporadically, and never found infected in nature, and these groupings are related directly to their nocturnal roosting/nesting behavior and the questing behavior of *Culex* vectors. Wild birds do not develop apparent illness following experimental infection, but their viremia response varies markedly, depending upon virus strain, bird species, and bird age. Titers sufficient to infect mosquitoes typically are limited to 1–5 days post-infection. Based on serological surveys during or after epidemics, peridomestic passerifoms (including house finches, house sparrows, cardinals, and blue jays) and columbiforms (including mourning oves and rock doves or domestic pigeons) seem to be infected most frequently. In house sparrows, SLEV strains isolated from *C. pipiens* complex mosquitoes from the central and eastern USA produced elevated viremias, whereas strains isolated from *C. tarsalis* from the western USA were weakly viremogenic. Although host competence studies have been limited, the adults of few bird species seem to develop elevated viremias. However, nestling house finches, house sparrows, and mourning doves produce high viremias that readily infect mosquitoes. Therefore, the nesting period of multibrooded species may be critical for virus amplification. Regardless of their viremia response, most experimentally infected birds produce antibody and, although titers typically decay rapidly, these birds remain protected for life.

Humans

Humans are incidental hosts and do not produce viremias sufficient to infect mosquitoes. Like most arboviruses that cause CNS disease, infection with SLEV does not result in a clear clinical picture in humans and most infections remain unrecognized, unless associated with an epidemic. When presented with such diverse symptoms, few physicians initially suspect SLEV, even in endemic areas. Most SLEV infections, especially in young or middle age groups, fail to produce clinical disease, and infected individuals rarely experience more than a mild malaise of short duration with spontaneous recovery.

Domestic Animals

Although frequently antibody positive during serosurveys, SLEV infection does not produce elevated viremias or cause clinical illness in domestic animals, including equines, porcines, bovines, or felines. In a single experiment, dogs (purebred beagles) produced a low-level viremia, with only two of eight dogs developing clinical illness. Similar to wild birds, immature fowl <1 month old (including chickens and ducks) consistently developed sufficient viremia to infect mosquitoes, but did not develop clinical illness. Adult chickens (>22 weeks old) usually failed to develop a detectable viremia, and along with immature birds, developed long-lasting antibodies.

Wild Mammals

The response of wild mammals to natural or experimental infection varies. Serosurveys occasionally have shown higher SLEV prevalence in mammals than in birds, but these data could be confounded because mammalian hosts typically live longer than avian hosts and therefore have a longer history of exposure. Rodents in the genera *Ammospermophilus* and *Dipodomys* were susceptible to infection after subcutaneous (s.c.) inoculation, whereas *Spermophilus, Rattus, Sigmodon,* and *Peromyscus* were refractory. Similarly varied were lagomorphs: *Lepus* was susceptible, whereas four species within *Sylvilagus* ranged from refractory to susceptible. Raccoons and skunks were refractory, whereas opossums and woodchucks were susceptible. Like birds, susceptible mammals produced an immediate viremic response that generally persisted for <1 week, and all species produced detectable antibodies regardless of their viremia response. SLEV frequently has been isolated from bats (*Tadarida, Myotis,* etc.), and many populations exhibit a high prevalence of neutralizing antibody. Overall, the role of mammalian infection in SLEV epidemiology is complex and difficult to interpret. All reputed *Culex* vectors feed most frequently on avian hosts, occasionally on large mammals and lagomorphs, rarely on rodents, and almost never on bats.

Pathogenicity

In humans, clinical disease due to SLEV infection may be divided into three syndromes in increasing order of severity: (1) 'Febrile headache' with fever, headache possibly associated with nausea or vomiting, and no CNS illness; (2) 'Aseptic meningitis' with high fever and stiff neck; and (3) 'Encephalitis' (including meningoencephalitis and encephalomyelitis) with high fever, altered consciousness, and/or neurological dysfunction. The onset of illness may be sudden (<4 days after infection) and acute, leading rapidly to encephalitis, or insidious, progressing gradually through all three syndromes. Symptoms may resolve spontaneously during any stage of the illness, with full recovery. Acute illness may be followed by 'convalescent fatigue syndrome' in <50% of patients, with complaints of general weakness, depression, and the inability to concentrate that generally resolve within 3 years. Other sequelae include headache, disturbances in gait, and memory loss.

Pathogensis in SLEV follows a course similar to other flaviviruses in the JEV complex. The extent of illness usually is dependent upon viremia level and duration. Virus replication occurs within the lymphatic system soon after infection, and resulting viremias reflect the balance between virus production and release by the lymphatic system and clearance mediated by phagocytes of the liver and spleen. The probability of CNS involvement is directly correlated with the extent and duration of the viremia, although the mechanism of neuroinvasion remains unclear. Movement from peripheral to central nervous tissue most likely is by passive transport through neuron cytoplasm and then by transport across associated membranes after cell lysis. CNS pathology consists of necrosis of neurons and glia cells and inflammatory changes. Inflammatory changes typically are most important in slowly progressing or sublethal CNS disease and sequelae. Viral clearance is dependent upon a functional immune system and the rapid production of neutralizing antibody, which usually appears within 7 days after infection.

Epidemiology

Transmission of SLEV is complex and requires that the virus replicate in and avoid the immune responses of alternating insect and vertebrate hosts under temperatures ranging from below 0 °C in diapausing mosquitoes to more than 40 °C in febrile avian hosts. Annual transmission activity may be divided into overwintering, vernal and/or summer amplification, and autumnal subsidence periods.

Overwintering

Three possible mechanisms may explain the persistence of SLEV at temperate latitudes; however, few supportive field data are available.

Persistence in mosquito populations

Three mechanisms may explain SLEV overwintering within vector mosquito populations. First, low-level vertical passage of SLEV from infected females to F1 progeny has been demonstrated repeatedly in laboratory experiments. Although not detected for SLEV in nature, vertical transmission has been documented for other viruses in the JEV complex, including JEV and West Nile virus (WNV). Second, *C. p. pipiens* females destined for diapause have been shown to take small blood meals during late summer and early fall without ovarian development. Two isolations of SLEV made from diapausing *C. p. pipiens* females collected resting during winter in Maryland were considered to have been infected by this mechanism, although infection by vertical transmission also was possible. Third, *Culex p. quinquefasciatus* and *C. nigripalpus* do not enter reproductive diapause, remain reproductively active throughout winter at southern latitudes and, depending upon ambient temperature, could maintain SLEV by continued, infrequent transmission among resident birds. Experimentally infected, reproductively active *C. p. quinquefasciatus* females have been shown to survive winter as gravid females and to then transmit SLEV to recipient birds throughout the following spring.

Persistence in vertebrate populations

SLEVs may also persist over winter within vertebrate host populations. Passeriform birds infrequently develop chronic infections that persist as long as a year following experimental infection. However, attempts to demonstrate natural relapse or to trigger relapse experimentally have not been successful. Flaviviruses, including SLEV, have also been isolated repeatedly from bats, and experimental infections in bats destined for hibernation have been maintained for 20 days at 10 °C. When returned to room temperature, SLEV was detected in the brown fat and at low levels in the blood. These data indicated that bats could function as an overwintering host. However, studies of mosquito host-selection patterns indicated that bats rarely, if ever, were fed upon by host-seeking mosquitoes.

Reintroduction of virus

An alternative hypothesis to local persistence involves annual or periodic reintroduction of virus into northern latitudes from southern refugia. Long-distance movement of SLEV has been indicated indirectly from genetic evidence as well as by the reappearance of SLEV after years of absence. Two possible hypotheses address reintroduction, but neither is well supported by field evidence. Many species of birds and some bats have long-distance annual migrations that could allow the transport of virus from foci active during winter in southern latitudes or south of the equator to receptive areas north of the equator during spring. These vertebrate migrations typically are very consistent in their summer and winter destinations, and this would allow the same or similar genetic strains to reappear each summer at the same locality. However, molecular genetic studies of North, Central, and South American isolates indicate that they are relatively distinct, thereby implying infrequent genetic exchange. In addition, migratory birds do not seem to be frequently involved in transmission because they infrequently are found positive for virus or antibody.

Amplification

Regardless of the persistence mechanism, summer enzootic amplification transmission in North America involves *Culex* mosquitoes and primarily birds in the orders Passeriformes and Columbiformes. Humans become infected tangentially to the primary cycle, do not develop viremias sufficient to infect mosquitoes, and are considered to be 'dead end' hosts (**Figure 3**). Transmission appears to be initiated after the *Culex* vectors resume blood-feeding and reproductive activity, and ambient temperatures warm sufficiently to allow the replication of virus in the mosquito host. Infection is acquired when a female *Culex* blood feeds on a viremic avian host. Virus imbibed within infectious blood meals taken in early in spring when ambient temperatures average <17 °C may lay dormant until warm conditions or changes in mosquito physiology stimulate replication. Under warm temperatures, virus replicates rapidly, disseminates within the mosquito during the ensuing extrinsic incubation period, and then may be transmitted by bite after the female oviposits and attempts to imbibe a subsequent blood meal. The duration of the extrinsic incubation period is temperature dependent and requires >10 days and perhaps two mosquito gonotrophic cycles when temperatures average 22 °C. In contrast, the viremia response in susceptible avian hosts typically is of short duration, lasting 2–4 days.

Four distinct transmission cycles of SLEV are defined by differences in the biology of the primary vector mosquito species and their distribution, and include: (1) rural North America, west of the Mississippi River transmitted by *C. tarsalis*; (2) rural and urban central and eastern North America transmitted by members of the *C. pipiens* complex; (3) Florida, Caribbean, and parts of Central America transmitted by *C. nigripalpus*; and (4) urban and rural South America transmitted by *C. pipiens* complex and mosquitoes of other taxa.

Subsidence

Intensity of enzootic transmission and occurrence of new human cases always subsides rapidly during autumn. Cool evening temperatures slow the replication of SLEV within infected mosquito hosts, decreasing the efficiency of transmission and, concurrently, the combination of cool water temperature and shortening days during larval development initiates reproductive diapause (*C. tarsalis*, *C. p. pipiens*) or quiescence (*C. p. quinquefasciatus*, *C. nigripalpus*) in vector females emerging during fall. The fall mosquito population declines in abundance and divides into newly emerged females that do not routinely blood-feed and survive the winter, and remnants of the summer population that continue reproductive activity, but fail to survive winter. The critical day length that triggers the

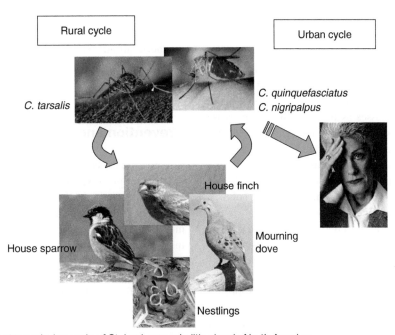

Figure 3 Amplification transmission cycle of St. Louis encephalitis virus in North America.

onset of diapause in *C. p. pipiens* may occur in late summer at northern latitudes, markedly shortening the SLEV transmission season. During warm days, however, females may become infected when taking partial blood meals from viremic birds, survive winter, and then transmit the virus after diapause is terminated by warm spring temperatures. *Culex p. quinquefasciatus* does not undergo diapause, so that reproductive activity may continue through winter, albeit at a rate slowed by winter temperatures. Populations exploiting underground storm water systems for resting or for larval development may be exposed to relatively warm temperatures throughout winter.

Risk Factors for Human Infection

Five factors have been associated with human risk of SLEV infection.

Residence

Clearly, place of residence markedly affects the risk of infection, with geographic regions in the southern USA having the greatest numbers of human cases and greatest incidence of disease (**Figure 2**). Based on experimental infection patterns in laboratory mice, virus strains from this geographical area also exhibit greater neurovirulence than strains from the western USA or South America. Because of mosquito abundance relative to humans and host-selection patterns, urban residents seem to be at greater risk for SLEV infection than rural residents. However, these conclusions may be confounded by protective immunity acquired early in life that may be greater among rural residents and by low apparent: inapparent case ratios that require a substantially large population to produce recognizable clusters of human cases.

Age

In the absence of acquired immunity, clinical illness and fatality rates, but not necessarily infection rates, increase dramatically with age. Infection seems to occur equally among different age classes as indicated by the increase in antibody as a function of age in endemic areas and by cohort seroconversion rates determined after epidemics in previously unexposed populations. For example, using data following the 1964 Houston (Texas) epidemic, seroprevalence rates remained similar among cohorts, whereas the case–incidence rates increased from 8.2 per 100 000 for the 0–9-year-old cohort to 13.5–27.6 for the 10–59-year-old cohorts and to 78.0 for the >60-year-old group; apparent to inapparent ratios decreased concomitantly from 1:806 to 1:490–1:239 and to 1:85, respectively. Case–fatality rates among 2288 cases reported to the CDC from 1971–83 increased from <6.7% for 0–64-year-old age classes to 9.5% for the 65–74-year-old class to 18% for the >75-year-old class.

Occupation

In the West, where SLE historically was a rural disease, infection risk was greatest among male agricultural workers who frequently lived in suboptimum housing and worked at night. However, infection patterns during recent urban outbreaks indicated that attack rates were highest among elderly women. These data indicated that there may be differences in risk related to vector species, with elderly women infected most readily during urban outbreaks associated with the *C. pipiens* complex, and men working outdoors at greatest risk during rural outbreaks associated with *C. tarsalis*.

Socioeconomic status

Historically, socioeconomic status has been related closely to the distribution of cases during urban epidemics. Homes and municipal drainage systems frequently were not well maintained in low-income neighborhoods, and this was related to the distribution of human cases, but not necessarily the occurrence of virus within the enzootic transmission cycle. TV and air conditioning ownership that brought people indoors during the evening *Culex* host-seeking period was found to reduce risk.

Weather

Climate variability affects temperature and precipitation patterns, mosquito abundance and survival, and therefore SLEV transmission. Annual temperature changes based on the El Niño/southern oscillation in the Pacific alter precipitation and temperature patterns over the Americas and cycle with varying intensity at 3–5 year intervals. These cycles alter storm tracks that affect mosquito and avian abundance, the intensity and frequency of rainfall events, and groundwater depth, all related to SLEV risk. Above-normal temperatures have been especially necessary for northern latitude SLEV epidemics, because elevated temperatures are required for effective SLEV replication within the mosquito host.

Prevention and Control

Effective vector control remains the only approach available to suppress summer virus amplification and prevent human infections. Best results are achieved using an integrated management approach that focuses on mosquito vector population suppression through habitat inspection and larviciding. Failure of larval management can be followed by emergency adult control focusing on reducing the force of transmission and preventing human infection. Protection of the human population by vaccination does not seem cost-effective or prudent, because there is no human-to-human transmission, few human infections produce disease, and infection rates remain relatively low, even during epidemics. However, if regional infection rates were to become high, thereby placing selected cohorts at high risk for disease, then selective vaccination may be warranted. There currently is no approved commercial vaccine for SLEV, although vaccination against other flaviviruses such as JEV may impart some protection. Control of avian hosts such as house sparrows and pigeons in urban situations could be done, but this approach is not generally acceptable to the public. Notification of the public of infection risk through the media and the wide scale use of personal protection through changes in behavior (staying indoors after sunset) and/or repellent application were credited with reducing the number of infections during the 1990 epidemic in Florida.

See also: Japanese Encephalitis Virus; Tick-Borne Encephalitis Viruses.

Further Reading

Day JF (2001) Predicting St. Louis encephalitis virus epidemics: Lessons from recent, and not so recent, outbreaks. *Annual Review of Entomology* 46: 111–138.

Kramer LD and Chandler LJ (2001) Phylogenetic analysis of the envelope gene of St. Louis encephalitis virus. *Archives of Virology* 146: 2341–2355.

Monath TP (1980) In: *St. Louis Encephalitis*, 680pp. Washington, DC: American Public Health Association.

Monath TP and Tsai TF (1987) St. Louis encephalitis: Lessons from the last decade. *American Journal of Tropical Medicine and Hygiene* 37: 40s–59s.

Reeves WC, Asman SM, Hardy JL, Milby MM, and Reisen WK (eds.) (1990) In: *Epidemiology and Control of Mosquito-Borne Arboviruses in California, 1943–1987*, 508pp. Sacramento, CA: California Mosquito and Vector Control Association.

Reisen WK (2003) Epidemiology of St. Louis encephalitis virus. In: Chambers TJ and Monath TP (eds.) *The Flaviviruses: Detection, Diagnosis and Vaccine Development*, pp. 139–183. San Diego, CA: Elsevier.

Tick-Borne Encephalitis Viruses

T S Gritsun and E A Gould, University of Reading, Reading, UK

Taxonomy, Nomenclature, and Phylogenetic Relationships

'Tick-borne encephalitis antigenic complex' was the original term for viruses now classified as the mammalian tick-borne flaviviruses. Together with the seabird-associated tick-borne flaviviruses they comprise one ecological group in the genus *Flavivirus*, family *Flaviviridae*. The genus contains two other groups, namely, the mosquito-borne flaviviruses and the flaviviruses with no known arthropod vectors. Other flaviviruses are referred to as nonclassified flaviviruses. The prototype TBEV is a human and animal pathogen. The earliest TBEV isolate, known as Russian Spring and Summer Encephalitis virus, was isolated in 1937 in far-East Asia. Currently, the TBEV (currently classified as virus species in the group of mammalian tick-borne flaviviruses) is subdivided into three subtypes, far-Eastern, Siberian, and West European reflecting their antigenic, phylogenetic, and geographic relationships. Other antigenically related but distinct tick-borne flaviviruses include Omsk hemorrhagic fever virus, Powassan virus (POWV), Langat virus, Kyasanur Forest disease virus, Alkhurma virus, Louping ill virus, Spanish sheep encephalomyelitis virus, Turkish sheep encephalomyelitis virus, and Greek goat encephalomyelitis virus. Each of them may cause encephalitis and/or hemorrhagic disease in humans, farmed, domestic, and wild animals. Other related mammalian tick-borne flaviviruses, not known to cause human or animal disease, include Royal Farm virus, Karshi virus, Gadgets Gully virus, and Kadam virus. The viruses associated primarily with seabirds and their ticks are Saumarez Reef virus, Meaban virus, and Tyuleniy (Three Arch) virus. They are not recognized pathogens but they show interesting geographic dispersion that reflects the flight patterns of the birds with which they are associated. The phylogenetic relationships between the TBEVs are illustrated in **Figure 1**.

Virions

Infectious (mature) virions are spherical particles (50 nm) with a relatively smooth surface and no distinct projections. They have an electron-dense core (30 nm) surrounded by a lipid membrane. The core consists of positive-polarity genomic RNA (~11 kbp) and capsid protein C (12K). The lipid membrane incorporates an envelope glycoprotein (E, 53K) and a membrane glycoprotein (M, 8K). The immature (intracellular) virions contain a precursor membrane protein (prM, 18K), the cleavage of which occurs in the secretory pathway during egress of virions from infected cells.

Virions sediment at about 200S and their buoyant density is $1.19 \, \text{g ml}^{-1}$, although there is significant heterogeneity among them. Electron micrographs frequently revealed virions in association with cellular membranes,

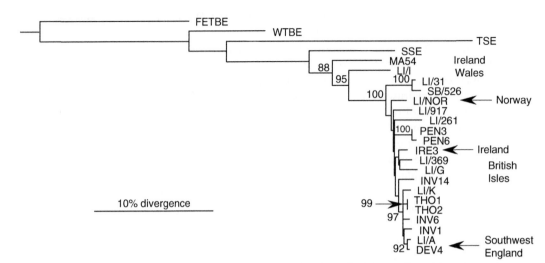

Figure 1 Maximum likelihood phylogenetic tree of the E gene from 24 tick-borne flaviviruses. Branch lengths are drawn to scale and all nodes supported by more than 75% bootstrap support are indicated. The tree is rooted with the sequence from FETBE virus, Sofjin (RSSE) strain. The three main populations of virus in the British Isles are indicated, along with those viruses secondarily introduced into Ireland and Norway, and the viruses found in the south-west of England. Reproduced from McGuire K, Holmes EC, Gao GF, Reid HW, and Gould EA (1998) Tracing the origins of Louping ill virus by molecular phylogenetic analysis. *Journal of General Virology* 79: 981–988.

probably explaining this heterogeneity. They are most stable at pH 8.0, although TBEV virions remain infectious in normal human gastric juice at pH 1.49–1.80. As with all enveloped viruses, infectivity of TBEVs decays rapidly at temperatures above 40 °C. Most flaviviruses agglutinate erythrocytes but a few nonagglutinating strains of TBEVs have been described. Most of the physical characteristics of the TBEVs were established using virus isolated from mammalian cells. However, after adaptation to ticks, they become less cytopathic for cultured cells and laboratory animals. These virions do not move toward the cathode in rocket immunoelectrophoresis and they have reduced hemagglutinating activity. These phenotypic characteristics may be reversed following re-adaptation to mammalian cells and host-selection of virions with a shifted net surface charge due to a single amino acid substitution in the E glycoprotein.

The E glycoprotein mediates virus binding to cellular receptors and thereby directly affects virus host range, virulence, and immunological properties by inducing protective antibodies. X-ray crystallography has revealed the E-protein ectodomain (N-terminal 395 amino acids) as homodimers folded in a 'head-to-tail' manner (**Figure 2(a)**) and orientated parallel to the membrane surface. It contains three structural domains, each based on β-sheets: the central domain I, the dimerization (fusion) domain II, and receptor domain III (dI, dII, and dIII in **Figure 2**). The C-terminal 101 residues of the E protein form a stem-anchor region consisting of two stem α-helices and two transmembrane α-helices that anchor the

E protein into the lipid bilayer (**Figure 3**). Domain II contains a hydrophobic fusion peptide consisting of 13 residues that is highly conserved between all flaviviruses. It is located on the tip of domain II and plays a central role in fusion of the virion membrane to cellular endosomal membranes resulting in release of virion RNA into the cytoplasm (**Figure 2**).

A three-dimensional image reconstruction of the virion surface reveals a protein shell composed of 90 E-dimers organized into a 'herringbone' configuration; three quasi-parallel E-dimer molecules make up the main structural asymmetric unit of the shell (**Figures 4(b)** and **4(c)**). The fivefold symmetry axes that appear as holes are generated by appropriate positioning of five domain IIIs and their lateral surface is accessible to cellular receptors and neutralizing antibodies. The M protein protrudes through holes formed between dimerization domains of E molecules. The transmembrane regions of the M and E proteins traverse the external but not the internal layer of the lipid membrane and there is no direct contact with the nucleocapsid (**Figure 3**).

In contrast with those of many other enveloped viruses, the flavivirus capsid is poorly organized and appears to be positioned randomly in the core. In solution, the capsid protein appears as dimer molecules with four helices (**Figure 5**). Two C-terminal helices fold into the positively charged interface interacting with viral RNA; the residues on the opposite side of these helices are hydrophobic and support dimerization. Two of the internal α-helices form capsid-dimers, are hydrophobic, and are required for contact with the virion membrane.

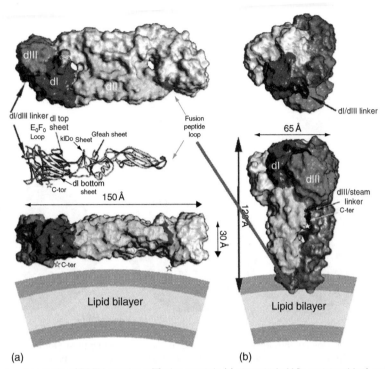

Figure 2 Three-dimensional analysis of TBEV envelope (E) glycoprotein (a) at neutral pH (in mature virion) and (b) acidic pH (postfusion conformation). The view from above and lateral view correspond to the top and bottom rows. Protein domains dI, dII, and dIII are colored in red, yellow, and blue, respectively. Ribbon diagram corresponds to the lateral view of the E protein. Reproduced from Bressanelli S, Stiasny K, Allison SL, *et al.* (2004) Structure of a flavivirus envelope glycoprotein in its low-pH-induced membrane fusion conformation. *EMBO Journal* 23: 728–738.

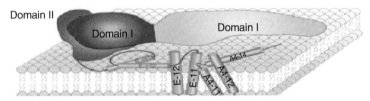

Figure 3 Schematic presentation of flavivirus structural glycoproteins E and M on the membrane surface. The coloring of the domains I, II, and III is as on **Figure 2**. Two α-helices of the stem-anchor region and two α-helices of the transmembrane domain of the E protein are depicted as blue- and colored cylinders. One α-helix of the stem region and two α-helices of the transmembrane domains of the M protein are depicted as orange-colored cylinders. Reproduced from Mukhopadhyay S, Kuhn RJ, and Rossmann MG (2005) A structural perspective of the flavivirus life cycle. *Nature Reviews Microbiology* 3: 13–22, with permission from Macmillan Magazines Limited.

TBEV Life Cycle

Virus Entry into the Cells

Cellular receptors for tick-borne flaviviruses

The virus life cycle commences with the attachment of virions to specific receptors on clathrin-coated pits on the cell surface. Flaviviruses infect a wide variety of primary and continuous cells, derived from mammalian, avian, and arthropod tissues. It is not yet clear if the different flaviviruses use similar or different cell surface receptors. Cellular heparan sulfate molecules are involved in TBEV attachment to cells. Nevertheless, cells that lack heparan sulfate are still sensitive to virus infection. For

TBEV, a number of different proteins have been associated with cell receptor activity, including the high-affinity laminin receptor and α1β3-integrin that also recognizes laminin as a natural ligand.

The E protein mediates attachment and entry of virions into cells

The immunoglobulin-like folding of the E-protein domain III implies that it is involved in cell attachment, mediated by high-affinity cellular receptors. The receptors on the surface of vertebrate and invertebrate cells are different and probably recognized by different residues on domain III. However, domains I and II on the surface of

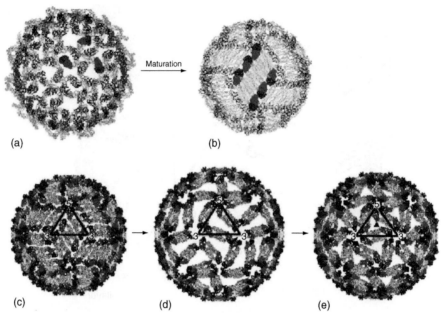

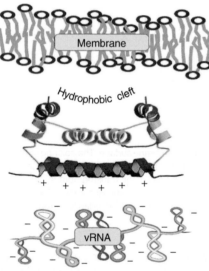

Figure 4 Different conformations of E protein during the transition from immature (a) into the mature (b) particles and during pH-dependent fusion of mature particles (c), through the putative intermediates T = 3 (d and e). Domains I, II, and III are depicted with the same colors as those on the **Figure 2**. Reproduced from Ma L, Jones CT, Groesch TD, Kuhn RJ, and Post CB (2004) Solution structure of Dengue virus capsid protein reveals another fold. *Proceedings of the National Academy of Sciences, USA* 101: 3414–3419, with permission from National Academy of Sciences USA.

Figure 5 Model for the molecular interactions of flavivirus capsid dimers with genome RNA and virion membrane. Reproduced from Ma L, Jones CT, Groesch TD, Kuhn RJ, and Post CB (2004) Solution structure of Dengue virus capsid protein reveals another fold. *Proceedings of the National Academy of Sciences, USA* 101: 3414–3419, with permission from National Academy of Sciences USA.

the E protein also appear to play a role in virus–cell interactions. Domain I carries N-linked carbohydrates, which are recognized by cell surface lectins. Domain II is enriched with patches of basic positively charged surface residues that have been shown to mediate virion attachment to the cellular, negatively charged, heparan sulfate; domains I and III might also contribute to this type of interaction.

Virus attachment to the cell receptors initiates receptor-mediated endocytosis, followed by fusion of virion and endosomal membranes (**Figures 4(c)–4(e)**). Exposure of the attached virus to the endosomal acid pH converts the herringbone configuration into a fusogenic structure resulting in particle expansion and eventually in the re-assembly of the E dimers into vertical trimers (**Figures 2** and **4**). It is believed that during this process domains I and II flex relative to each other, allowing domain II and the stem region to move toward the endosomal membrane facilitating trimerization of domain II; the fusion tripeptide is embedded into the target membrane followed by formation of a pre-fusion intermediate (**Figure 6**). Trimerization spreads from fusion peptides to domain I; meanwhile domain III rotates relative to domain II pushing the stem region back toward the fusion peptide. This refolding brings two membranes together, resulting in the formation of the 'hemifusion stalk' with only the proximal lipid leaflets fused. The 'zipping' up of stems followed by the migration of transmembrane domains eventually leads to fusion of the distal lipid outlets and formation of a fusion pore. In the final low-pH conformation, domains I and III appear to move to the tip of the vertical trimer whereas the fusion peptide becomes embedded in the membrane eventually being juxtaposed to the transmembrane

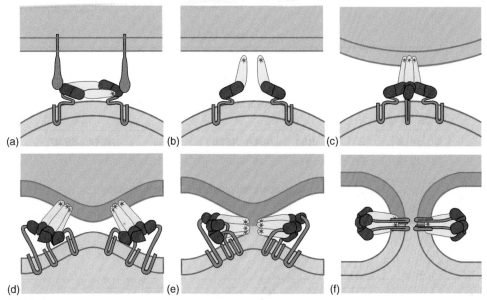

Figure 6 Tentative mechanism for the fusion of viral (brown) and endosomal (green) membranes mediated by the flavivirus E protein following interaction with cellular receptor (gray) (a). Acidic pH triggers the movement of domain II (with fusion peptide on the top) toward the endosomal membrane (b) with its subsequent trimerization and insertion into the endosomal membrane (c). Trimerization spread toward domains I and III (d) causing the C-terminal part of E protein to fold backwards toward the fusion peptide. The trimerization between stem-anchor and domain II (e) results in partial fusion (e) and eventually in the formation of a fusion pore (f). Reproduced with permission from Modis Y, Ogata S, Clements D, and Harrison SC (2005) Variable surface epitopes in the crystal structure of Dengue virus type 3 envelope glycoprotein. *Journal of Virology* 79: 1223–1231.

domains (**Figures 2(b)** and **6**). Five trimers form the fusion pore; the stem region appears to play an essential role in promoting and stabilizing trimer assembly. Although the E-protein domains shift and rotate during exposure to acidic pH, each retains the neutral-pH conformation, the essential feature of class II fusion molecules that do not require major molecular rearrangements at acidic pH.

Strategy of the TBEV Genome

Translation and processing of virus proteins

After uncoating, the RNA is translated into a polyprotein of ∼3400 residues from one open reading frame (ORF) that is co-translationally translocated and anchored in the endoplasmic reticulum (**Figure 7**). It is then processed by cellular signalases and viral serine protease producing three structural (capsid, prM, and E) and seven nonstructural (NS1 through NS5) proteins. The gene order, protein molecular masses, and their membrane localization are shown in **Figure 7**. Viral protease activity is provided by the N-terminal domain (∼180 residues) of the NS3 protein in association with cofactor activity of the NS2B protein that probably anchors the NS3 into the membrane. The ORF is flanked by 5′- and 3′-untranslated regions (UTRs; ∼ 130 and 700 bp, respectively) that contain signals essential to initiate translation and replication. The 5′-UTR preceding the ORF is capped by $m^7GpppAmpN_2$ and initiates virus translation *in vitro*

although an interactive effect from the 3′-UTR has also been demonstrated. Computer-assisted prediction has demonstrated folding of the 5′-UTR into a Y-shaped structure, conserved between all flaviviruses; mutations in this structure appear to impact on virus translation and replication. The translation of flavivirus proteins is probably carried out in specialized smooth membrane structures, called convoluted membranes, derived from proliferation of the rough endoplasmic reticulum in response to flavivirus infections.

Replication of viral RNA

The initiation of viral replication (synthesis of negative strand on positive strand from the 3′-UTR) requires direct interaction between the 5′- and 3′-UTRs resulting in the formation of a double-stranded RNA (dsRNA) stem and circularization of the virus genome. A terminal 3′ long stable hairpin (3′ LSH) structure has been revealed in the 3′-UTR that, together with the 5′-Y-shaped-structure and dsRNA circularization stem, forms a complex promoter required to initiate virus RNA replication. Additional predicted conserved secondary RNA structures in the 3′-UTR might function as replication enhancers, essential for efficient RNA synthesis and virus transmission. The synthesis of genome-size dsRNA (replicative form, RF) accomplishes the first stage of viral replication.

Flavivirus RNA replication is semiconservative and asymmetric, with an average of one nascent positive-

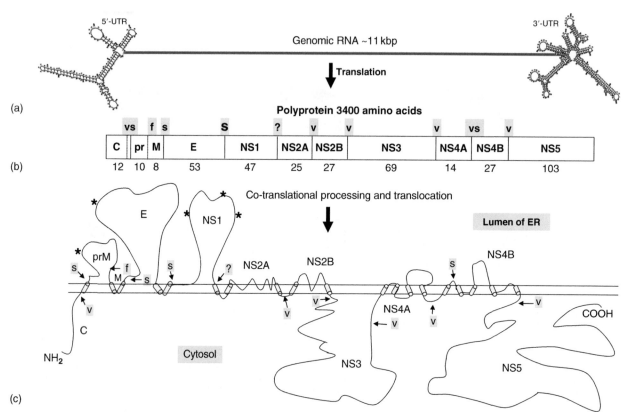

Figure 7 Genome strategy of TBEV. (a) Genomic RNA is presented as a solid line on the top; the 5'- and 3'-UTR are depicted in the predicted conformations according to Gritsun TS, Venugopal K, Zanotto PM, *et al.* (1997) Complete sequence of two tick-borne flaviviruses isolated from Siberia and the UK: Analysis and significance of the 5'- and 3'-UTRs. *Virus Research* 49: 27–39. (b) Translation and co-translational processing of flavivirus polyprotein. The flavivirus polyprotein is depicted as a bar, with specified individual proteins and their molecular masses (numbers below the bar). (c) Membrane topology of viral proteins in relation to the lumen of the ER and cytoplasm after the completion of co-translational processing and translocation. Adapted from Westaway EG, Mackenzie JM, and Khromykh AA (2003) Kunjin RNA replication and applications of Kunjin replicons. *Advances in Virus Research* 59: 99–140. Transmembrane domains are shown as cylinders. Glycosylation is indicated as (*). The polyprotein is processed by ER signalases (s) and viral-specific protease NS2B-NS3 (V). The cleavage of M from prM is carried out by the Golgi protease, furin (f) and cleavage between NS1 and NS2A is by an unknown (?) ER protease.

sense single-stranded RNA (ssRNA) molecule (genomic) per negative-sense template, with no free minus-strands and with 10–100 times excess of positive-strand relative to negative-strand RNA synthesis. The replicative intermediate presents a partially double-stranded RNA with nascent, and displaced, plus-sense ssRNA molecules undergoing elongation. Viral RNA capping of the 5'-UTR occurs on the displaced plus-strand RNA; the trifunctional NS3 and NS5 proteins provide nucleoside triphosphatase and guanylyl/methyltransferase activities, respectively.

Formation of the replication complex involves nonstructural proteins (**Figure 8**) most of which are bi- and even trifunctional. The C-terminal domain of NS5 protein acts as a viral RNA polymerase and the C-terminal domain of NS3 as a helicase; both NS5 and NS3 proteins interact with 3'-LSH to initiate virus replication. The functions of other nonstructural proteins are less precisely identified. The NS1 glycoprotein forms membrane-associated hexam-

ers that dissociate into dimers. This protein is translocated in the endoplasmic reticulum and secreted together with virions in mammalian but not in mosquito cells; its anchoring into the membranes is mediated by glycosyl-phosphatidylinositol. The NS1 protein induces the production of protective antibodies that also participate in complement-mediated lysis of infected cells, implying a role in immunopathology. The NS2A protein is found in association with the NS3 helicase domain, the NS5 protein, and the 3'-LSH. It may be involved in trafficking of viral RNA between the translation, replication, and virion assembly sites. The NS2B protein is a membrane-anchored cofactor of the serine proteinase, NS3. It also has membrane-permeability modulating activity possibly related to replication. The hydrophobic NS4A protein in conjunction with the NS1 protein probably anchors the polymerase complex to cell membranes and is involved in virus-induced membrane rearrangements that compartmentalize virus translation, replication, and assembly processes (**Figure 8**).

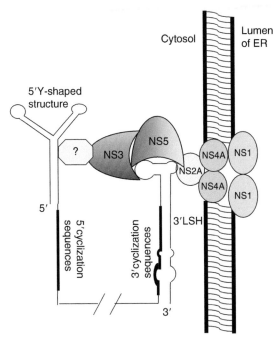

Figure 8 Representation of the assembly of the membrane-anchored polymerase complex. The conformations of 3'LSH and 5' Y-shaped structure are shown. This stage probably precedes the cyclization of the virus genome mediated by direct interaction between the inverted complementary 5'- and 3'-cyclization sequences (thick lines); this is followed by the initiation of minus-strand RNA synthesis. Adapted from Westaway EG, Mackenzie JM, and Khromykh AA (2002) Replication and gene function in Kunjin virus. *Current Topics in Microbiology and Immunology* 267: 323–351.

Replication of flavivirus RNA is associated with host membrane 75–100 nm vesicular packets enclosed in the second outer membrane and connected to convoluted membranes, the sites of virus translation. The vesicular packets proliferate in the perinuclear region in response to virus infection and are probably derived from the *trans*-Golgi network. The architecture of the replication complex in relation to vesicular packets and convoluted membranes is illustrated in **Figure 9**. The replicative forms and replication complexes are enclosed within vesicular packets, whereas nascent ssRNA is externally located. In addition, a variety of cellular proteins associates with the 5'-UTR, 3'-UTR, and the RNA polymerase; they probably facilitate assembly of the replication complex and trafficking of the viral RNA/polymerase into the appropriate cellular compartment for replication.

Assembly, Maturation, and Release of Virions

The sequence of molecular events during virion morphogenesis is not completely understood. On completion of post-translational processing, the prM and E proteins rapidly form heterodimeric complexes; the chaperone-like function of the prM protein is essential for correct folding of E protein. Heterodimers are rapidly assembled into immature particles or, in the absence of capsid, into virus-like particles that also accumulate during infection. Virion packaging is coupled with RNA replication; only actively replicating RNA is encapsidated. The orientation of structural proteins in the lipid membrane suggests that assembly is mediated by capsid budding through the endoplasmic reticulum. However, assembled virus capsids have never been visualized, neither have budding particles nor specific release mechanisms been identified.

Assembly of structural proteins in the viral lipid membrane initially results in the formation of immature (intracellular) virions that are noninfectious, resistant to acidic pH, and unable to be structurally rearranged prior to fusion. Image reconstruction has defined the different organization of E/prM proteins compared with E/M proteins on the surface of immature and mature virions, respectively (**Figure 4**). Sixty projections were identified on the surface of immature virions making them look larger (60 nm) in comparison with smooth 50 nm mature virus particles. Each spike is formed by three heterodimeric E/M molecules. In immature particles the E protein points away from the membrane with the fusion peptide at its extremity. Virion maturation is accompanied by cleavage of prM to M, mediated by the cellular protease furin in the *trans*-Golgi network at acidic pH, during the transportation of virions to the cell surface. PrM-to-M cleavage results in the dissociation of E/M trimeric spikes with the formation of E/E homodimers, probably following shift of the stem-transmembrane domain relative to the ectodomain. In mature particles, the E ectodomain lies on the virus membrane, with the fusion peptide embedded in the cavity between domains I and III of the neighboring dimer. Formation of the herringbone building unit and release of the glycosylated pre-peptide then follows. Eventually, *trans*-Golgi-derived vesicles packed with mature virions follow the host secretory pathway, fuse with the plasma membrane, and release mature virions.

Pathogenesis of TBEV

Incidence of Tick-Borne Encephalitis

Classical tick-borne encephalitis (TBE) is contracted by humans when they are fed upon by infected *Ixodes* spp. ticks. Forested areas across the Northern Hemisphere, with thick moist undergrowth and abundance of small wild animals, provide ideal habitats for ticks and for TBEV. Long-term survival of the virus occurs mainly in ticks, which remain infected throughout their 2–5-year life cycle. Efficient virus transmission between infected nymphs and noninfected larvae occurs on the forest animals when these ticks co-feed. There is no requirement

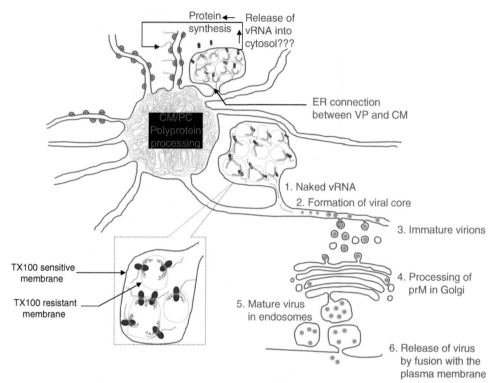

Figure 9 Proposed model of flavivirus replication in connection with cellular membranous structures. Translation of viral proteins is associated with CMs whereas replication is carried out within VPs. The dsRNA of RF in association with proteins of the polymerase complex (RC) is anchored to the internal leaflet of VP membrane whereas newly synthesized plus ssRNA is released from the RC. Reproduced with permission from Uchil PD and Satchidanandam V (2003) Architecture of the flaviviral replication complex. Protease, nuclease, and detergents reveal encasement within double-layered membrane compartments. *Journal of Biological Chemistry* 278: 24388–24398.

for viremia, since the virus can be transmitted to the larvae in animals that are not susceptible to the virus. Moreover, nonviremic transmission between the ticks can occur even on immune animals. Cells that migrate between the skin surface and local lymph nodes (e.g., dendritic cells) become infected and are then imbibed by the feeding noninfected larvae. Nonviremic transmission provides an efficient mechanism for long-term virus survival in the absence of overt disease. At the same time, susceptible animals such as sheep, goats, horses, pigs, dogs, grouse, and even humans may inadvertently become infected by ticks either in the forests or by ticks carried away from the forests. Under these circumstances the vertebrate host may become viremic and the virus may then be transmitted to a noninfected tick that subsequently transmits the virus to another vertebrate host when the infected tick feeds for a second time. Such situations arise on the sheep-rearing moorlands in the British Isles, Norway, Spain, Turkey, Greece, and other parts of Europe. In some situations sheep/goat and grouse populations may be severely affected.

The incidence of human TBE varies from year to year in different areas. The Urals and Siberia annually record the highest number of hospitalized cases. These numbers have risen from 700 to 1200 cases per year in the 1950s and 1960s to greater than 11 000 per year in the 1990s, following *Perestroika* and initial breakdown of the infrastructure. The incidence in Europe is lower but nonetheless significant, with about 3000 cases per year. Although it can affect people of all ages, the highest incidence occurs among the most active groups, that is, 17–40 year olds.

The incidence of clinical disease in endemic regions is dependent on the frequency of forest visits, the density of ticks in different years, the concentration of virus in ticks, and the virulence of circulating strains. Taking all these factors into account, it was estimated that one clinical case must occur for every 100 people bitten by ticks, and this correlates with the observation that in regions where more than 60% of ticks carry virus, about 1.4% of people develop TBE after being bitten.

Variety of Clinical Manifestations

TBEV is recognized as a dangerous human pathogen, causing a variety of clinical manifestations, although asymptomatic infections constitute about 70–95% of all TBEV infections. Symptoms include (1) mild or moderate fever with complete recovery of patients (about 90% of all clinical manifestations), (2) subacute encephalitis with nearly complete recovery or residual symptoms that may or may not disappear with time, (3) severe encephalitis associated with irreversible damage to the central nervous system (CNS), resulting in disability or death (about 4–8%), and (4) slow (months to decades) progressive or chronic encephalitis (1–2%).

Initially in the 1940–50s it was believed that the same virus produced encephalitis over the whole of Europe and Asia. However, with the improvement of serological diagnosis and the advent of phylogenetic analysis, three subtypes of TBEV were identified.

Human infections with far-Eastern TBEV subtype viruses produce the most severe form of CNS disorder, with a tendency for the patient to develop focal meningoencephalitis or polyencephalitis, and case–fatality rates between 20% and 40%. Siberian strains are often associated with high prevalence of the nonparalytic febrile form, with case–fatality rates rarely exceeding 6–8%. There is a tendency for some patients to develop chronic TBE, predominantly in association with Siberian TBEV strains. The disease produced by West European TBEV strains is biphasic, with fever during the first phase and neurological disorders of differing severity during the second phase, which occurs in 20–30% of patients, with a case–fatality rate of 1–2%. While Louping ill virus and the related Spanish, and Turkish/Greek viruses produce fatal encephalitis in animals, they are only rarely associated with disease in humans, probably primarily because of the lower (in comparison with TBEV) rates of human exposure to infected ticks.

Biphasic milk fever is an unusual form of TBE originally observed in western Russia mainly associated with the consumption of goat's milk. West European strains of TBEV were isolated from unpasteurized goat's milk and from patients. Later, similar outbreaks of biphasic milk fever were reported in central Europe and Siberia. The apparent difference in clinical manifestations of TBE contracted by tick-bite or by the alimentary route may be explained by differences in the type of immunological response.

Human Disease Produced by Other Tick-Borne Flaviviruses

POWV also produces encephalitic infections in humans although not on an epidemic scale. POWV circulates in Russia, the USA, and Canada, where it may cause human encephalitis with a high incidence of neurological sequelae and up to a 60% case–fatality rate. In North America POWV has diverged to produce a closely related deer tick virus (DTV) that has a predilection for different rodent species. Langat virus has been isolated in Malaysia and Thailand; there are no registered cases of human disease associated with this virus. However, when Langat virus was

used as a live, attenuated vaccine in human trials in Russia, one in 10 000 patients developed encephalitis.

Three tick-borne flaviviruses cause hemorrhagic disease rather than encephalitis in humans, namely Omsk hemorrhagic fever virus, Kyasanur Forest disease virus, and Alkhurma virus. As yet there is no explanation for these differences in virulence characteristics. Epidemic foci of Omsk hemorrhagic fever virus in the Omsk and Novosibirsk regions of western Siberia usually follow epizootics in muskrats (*Ondatra zibethica*) from which local hunters become infected by the virus when they handle infected animals. The most marked pathological signs of the disease are focal visceral hemorrhages in the mucus of the nose, gums, uterus, and lungs. Convalescence is usually uneventful without residual effects; fatal cases have been recorded, but rarely (0.5–3%).

Kyasanur Forest disease virus was first recognized in 1957 in India where it caused hemorrhagic disease among monkeys and humans, frequently with fatal outcome. It is believed that perturbation of regions of the forest for land development led to increased exposure of monkeys and humans to ticks carrying the virus. Subsequently, it has become evident that this virus circulates throughout western India and this may explain the close antigenic and genetic link with Alkhurma virus, which was isolated from fatal human cases of hemorrhagic fever in Saudi Arabia. Recent evidence has demonstrated the presence of Alkhurma virus in ticks associated with camels. Whether or not this or a closely related virus circulates in Africa remains to be determined.

Prevention and Control of TBE

Vaccination is the most efficient method available for preventing TBE in enzootic regions. Currently two inactivated vaccines are commercially available. The European vaccine has significantly reduced the annual incidence of TBE in Austria and Germany. A similar vaccine, based on a far-Eastern strain of TBEV, has been used successfully in Russia to immunize at-risk laboratory personnel. Other preventive measures routinely employed in TBE endemic areas are (1) education of residents in methods of avoiding tick-bites (when visiting tick-infested areas, wearing appropriate clothing, regularly inspect for feeding ticks, report tick-bite to medical authorities); (2) treat cats and dogs with acaricides; (3) clear thick, moist vegetation areas from around houses; and (4) spray acaricides in forested areas, close to habitation.

Human trials of a live, attenuated vaccine for Langat virus produced an unacceptably high incidence of TBE (1/10 000). However, these trials demonstrated the higher protection efficiency of live, attenuated vaccines in comparison with inactivated vaccines. Currently safer strategies to produce live, attenuated vaccine are being developed such as

(1) RNA- or DNA-based vaccines; (2) engineering TBEV mutants with multiple attenuating mutations or large deletions within their genomes, resulting in the loss of neuroinvasiveness; and (3) engineering chimeric yellow fever virus vaccine containing substituted TBEV E and M proteins.

Currently there are no safe, effective antivirals for TBEV infections, but there is promising progress in tests with small-interfering RNAs (siRNAs). These short molecules, ~21 nt long, bind to homologous regions of viral mRNA, thus interfering with the replication cycle. Another antiviral strategy with which rapid progress is being made is based on the design of molecules that can target specific regions within viral replicative enzymes. If the twentieth century was significant for its development of effective vaccines, the twenty-first century might be recognized for its development of effective antivirals.

See also: Japanese Encephalitis Virus; West Nile Virus.

Further Reading

Aberle JH, Aberle SW, Kofler RM, and Mandl CW (2005) Humoral and cellular immune response to RNA immunization with flavivirus replicons derived from tick-borne encephalitis virus. *Journal of Virology* 79: 15107–15113.

Anderson R (2003) Manipulation of cell surface macromolecules by flaviviruses. *Advances in Virus Research* 59: 229–274.

Bressanelli S, Stiasny K, Allison SL, *et al.* (2004) Structure of a flavivirus envelope glycoprotein in its low-pH-induced membrane fusion conformation. *EMBO Journal* 23: 728–738.

Gelpi E, Preusser M, Garzuly F, Holzmann H, Heinz FX, and Budka H (2005) Visualization of Central European tick-borne encephalitis infection in fatal human cases. *Journal of Neuropathology and Experimental Neurology* 64: 506–512.

Gritsun TS, Lashkevich VA, and Gould EA (2003) Tick-borne encephalitis. *Antiviral Research* 57: 129–146.

Gritsun TS, Nuttall PA, and Gould EA (2003) Tick-borne flaviviruses. *Advances in Virus Research* 61: 317–371.

Gritsun TS, Tuplin AK, and Gould EA (2006) Origin, evolution and function of flavivirus RNA in untranslated and coding regions: Implications for virus transmission. In: Kalitzky M and Borowski P (eds.) *Flaviviridae: Pathogenesis, Molecular Biology and Genetics*, pp. 47–99. Norwich, UK: Horizon Scientific Press.

Heinz FX and Allison SL (2003) Flavivirus structure and membrane fusion. *Advances in Virus Research* 59: 63–97.

Heinz FX, Stiasny K, and Allison SL (2004) The entry machinery of flaviviruses. *Archives of Virology Supplement* 18: 133–137.

Lindenbach BD and Rice CM (2001) *Flaviviridae*: The viruses and their replication. In: Knipe DM and Howley PM (eds.) *Fields Virology*, 4th edn., vol. 1, pp. 991–1042. London: Lippincott Williams and Wilkins.

Markoff L (2003) 5′- and 3′-noncoding regions in flavivirus RNA. *Advances in Virus Research* 59: 177–228.

Mukhopadhyay S, Kuhn RJ, and Rossmann MG (2005) A structural perspective of the flavivirus life cycle. *Nature Reviews Microbiology* 3: 13–22.

Rey FA, Heinz FX, Mandl C, Kunz C, and Harrison SC (1995) The envelope glycoprotein from tick-borne encephalitis virus at 2 Å resolution. *Nature* 375: 291–398.

Uchil PD and Sachidanandam V (2003) Architecture of the flaviviral replication complex. Protease, nuclease, and detergents reveal encasement within double-layered membrane compartments. *Journal of Biological Chemistry* 278: 24388–24398.

Westaway EG, Mackenzie JM, and Khromykh AA (2003) Kunjin RNA replication and applications of Kunjin replicons. *Advances in Virus Research* 59: 99–140.

Togaviruses Causing Rash and Fever

D W Smith, PathWest Laboratory Medicine WA, Nedlands, WA, Australia
J S Mackenzie, Curtin University of Technology, Shenton Park, WA, Australia
M D A Lindsay, Western Australian Department of Health, Mount Claremont, WA, Australia

Glossary

Analgesics Medications to relieve pain.

Arbovirus A virus transmitted to vertebrates by hematophagous (blood-feeding) insects and which replicates in the insect, as opposed to 'mechanical' transmission.

Arthritis Acute or chronic inflammation of one or more joints, usually accompanied by pain and stiffness, and sometimes swelling of the joint.

Fascia/fasciitis Fascia are bands or sheaths of connective tissues that support or connect parts of the body. Fasciitis is inflammation of these structures, most commonly the fascia of the sole of the foot and the wrist.

Maculopapular (referring to a rash) A mixture of flat red areas (macules) and small red raised spots (papules).

Nonsteroidal anti-inflammatory agents Medications used to relieve inflammation that are not corticosteroids, aspirin, or acetaminophen. Common ones include ibuprofen, naproxen, and indomethacin.

Sylvatic Involving wild animals.

Synovial Pertaining to the synovium, a thin membrane that lines joints and tendons and secretes synovial fluid.

Tenosynovitis Inflammation of tendons and the synovial membrane surrounding the tendon.

Teratogenic Causing malformations of an embryo or fetus.
Urticarial Characterized by pale or reddened irregular, elevated patches, and severe itching. An urticarial rash is also called 'hives'.

Introduction

Viruses of the family *Togaviridae* (togaviruses) are enveloped, positive-stranded RNA viruses of 60–70 nm diameter, and include viruses of two genera, *Alphavirus* and *Rubivirus*. The latter contains a single species, Rubella virus, a major cause of fever and rash internationally; it is discussed elsewhere in this series. Alphaviruses are distributed worldwide and cause illness in many hundreds of thousands of people each year. Clinical illness ranges from mild febrile illnesses to severe illnesses, such as encephalitis and hemorrhagic fever. One of the most common clinical manifestations of alphavirus infections is fever accompanied by rash and/or arthritis. The alphaviruses causing these illnesses are all closely related and belong to two major and one minor antigenic groups: the Semliki Forest virus (SFV) antigenic group (**Figure 1**), which includes SFV, Chikungunya virus

(CHIKV), O'nyong-nyong virus (ONNV), and Ross River virus (RRV); and the Sindbis virus (SINV) virus group (**Figure 2**), comprising SINV and Mayaro virus (MAYV). Barmah Forest virus (BFV) is in its own antigenic complex but is genetically linked to the SFV complex viruses. The diseases they cause are usually named after the virus, though an antigenic subtype of SINV is the cause of Ockelbo disease, Pogosta disease, and Karelian fever, while the disease due to RRV has been called epidemic polyarthritis in the past. All are mosquito-borne viruses, but with differences in their ecology and epidemiology. However, there are significant similarities in the clinical aspects of the diseases caused by these viruses, likely reflecting common pathogenic features.

Clinical Manifestations

Many infected individuals will develop clinical illness, and symptomatic to asymptomatic infection ratios have been estimated at 2:1 to 4:1 for CHIKV, ONNV, and MAYV disease, from 1:80 to 3:1 or higher for RRV infections in Australia, and 1:20 to 1:40 for Ockelbo and Pogosta diseases (**Table 1**).

Infections occur at all ages and in both sexes. The male to female ratio varies in different studies but there

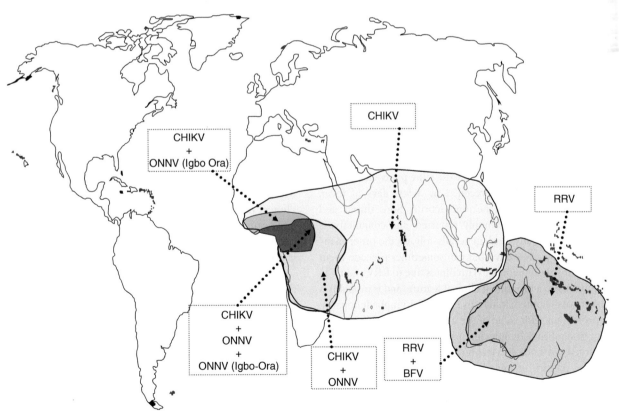

Figure 1 Geographical distribution of the major alphaviruses of the Semliki Forest virus antigenic complex that cause fever, rash, and arthritis in humans.

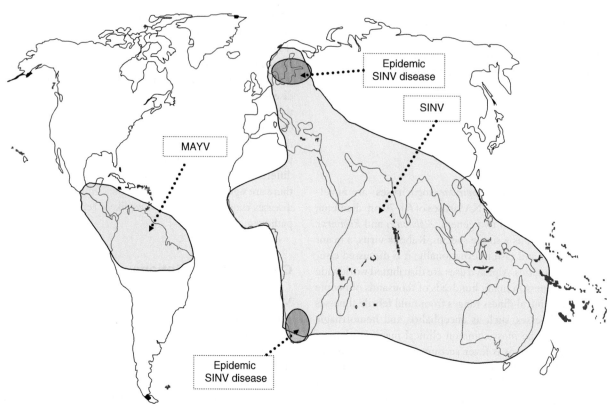

Figure 2 Geographical distribution of the major alphaviruses of the Sindbis virus antigenic complex that cause fever, rash, and arthritis in humans.

are no major gender effects on clinical illness. Infection of children in endemic areas or during epidemics occurs commonly, but clinical disease is less common and usually milder than in adults, and arthritis is rare in children.

Acute Infection

Clinical illness presents mainly as joint pains and muscle pains, accompanied by fever and/or rash in a varying proportion of cases.

Patients typically present with joint pains and muscle pains that are usually preceded by a few days of fever, at least in those who become febrile. Sore throat and headache are also commonly reported, and conjunctivitis occurs occasionally. Rash generally follows the other manifestations by a few days, but can sometimes precede them or appear simultaneously. With illness due to RRV and BFV, fatigue is also a prominent clinical feature, and is probably a feature of the other alphaviruses as well. Lymphadenopathy is prominent with some of the alphaviruses, CHIKV causing generalized lymphadenopathy and ONNV causing enlarged posterior cervical lymph nodes.

The pattern of joint involvement is consistent across this group of alphaviruses, commonly involving the ankles, knees, fingers, wrists, elbows, and shoulders. Several joints are involved and the joint involvement is usually symmetric. Other joints including the jaw and the

spine may also be affected and back pain is a common complaint. Pain is the most common feature, but most patients also have stiffness of the joints and, less frequently, swelling. The swelling can be due to effusion and/or synovial and soft tissue swelling. During recovery there is a gradual decline in both the number and severity of joint involvement. Inflammation of the fascia of the sole of the foot and the wrist is often reported with RRV and CHIKV infection. Pressure on nerves due to swelling of the fascia may cause tingling in the extremities. This is common with RRV, CHIKV, ONNV, and SINV disease. Muscle pain and tenderness is a prominent part of the clinical illness, usually involving the limbs and shoulders. This can sometimes be more troublesome than the joint pains and it is important to determine whether limb pain is arising from the joints or the muscles.

When rash occurs it is usually maculopapular and most florid on the face, trunk, and upper part of the limbs. However, it can involve the whole body surface, including the palms of the hands, the soles of the feet, and the scalp. Urticarial or vesicular rash occurs in some patients with SINV or BFV disease, but is rare in patients infected with the other viruses. Itchy rash is common with Pogosta disease and ONNV infection. Evidence from RRV and SINV studies suggests that the rashes probably result from presence of virus in the skin and the resulting local immune responses. The RRV rash shows a

Table 1 The clinical features of the major alphaviruses causing fever, rash, and arthritis in humans

	Chikungunya virus	O'nyong-nyong virus	Ross River virus	Barmah Forest virus	Sindbis virus (Pogosta)	Sindbis virus (Ockelbo)	Mayaro virus
Incubation period	3–12 days, usually 2–7 days	>8 days	3–21 days, usually 7–9 days	7–9 days	<7 days	<7 days	up to 12 days, usually 6–12 days
Fever	100%	Similar to CHIK	45–55%	50%	45%	40%	100%
Joint pains	80–100%	Similar to CHIK	95–100%	70–85%	95%	95%	50%
Arthritis (Joint stiffness/swelling)	Usually, soft tissue	Similar to CHIK	80–90%	30%	45%	60%	NI[a]
Fatigue	NI[a]	NI[a]	70–80%	80%	NI[a]	NI[a]	NI[a]
Rash	30–50% Maculopapular	30–50% Maculopapular, itchy; some vesicular	50–60% Maculopapular	50–100% Maculopapular; 10% vesicular, some urticarial	90%	95%	30%
Muscle pains	50%	Similar to CHIK	60–90%	70–80%	50%	NI[a]	75%
Tenderness of palms and soles, and/or fasciitis	20–30%	Similar to CHIK	50–60%	NI[a]	NI[a]	NI[a]	NI[a]
Backache	50%	Similar to CHIK	30–60%	NI[a]	NI[a]	NI[a]	NI[a]
Headache	50%	Similar to CHIK	Common	NI[a]	40%	NI[a]	100%
Lymphadenopathy	Generalized, common and prominent	Cervical, common and prominent	Common; generalized in 1–20%	Common; generalized in 5–10%	Not prominent	NI[a]	NI[a]
Severe illness/fatalities	Hemorrhagic disease, encephalitis, death	None reported	Possible meningitis/encephalitis	None reported	None reported	None reported	Hemorrhagic disease
Other	Conjunctivitis reported as common in some outbreaks. Severe congenital infections	Conjunctivitis common	Glomerulonephritis, asymptomatic congenital infections	None reported	None reported	None reported	None reported

[a]NI, no information.

monocytic infiltrate with presence of RRV antigen within epidermal cells, while the rare purpuric rashes are associated with cytotoxic T-cell responses and capillary leakage.

Gastrointestinal symptoms such as vomiting, abdominal pain, and diarrhea have been reported with RRV and CHIKV illness, particularly in children. Severe illness is rare, other than hemorrhagic disease resembling dengue that can occur following CHIKV infection.

In summary, the majority of infections with the arthritogenic alphaviruses are benign but temporarily debilitating. Fever and rash, if present, usually last less than a week and most patients recover fully within 4 weeks. Joint pains, muscle pains, and lethargy are the slowest to resolve.

Chronic Illness Following Infection

One of the features of alphavirus arthritis is the frequency of prolonged illness, especially persisting joint pains. For SINV, joint pain lasting more than 2 years has been reported for 50% of cases in Finland (i.e., Pogosta disease) and for 25% of cases in Sweden (i.e., Ockelbo disease). Persisting joint pain is also common in Russian cases (i.e., Karelian fever). Similarly, joint pains commonly persist for many months following acute CHIKV infection, and have been reported to follow MAYV infection. Most RRV patients return to full physical activity within 3–6 months, but some suffer from persisting disability due to joint pains, muscle pains, fatigue, and depression. One study found that joint pain persisted for more than 3 months in about 70% of patients. A separate prospective case-controlled study found that at 12 months after onset 90% of patients still had

joint pain, 80% had tiredness, 75% had joint stiffness, and 50% had muscle and/or tendon pain.

Infection in Pregnancy

Generally, infection in pregnancy has no special implications for the mother. RRV causes fetal and neonatal death in mice, but there is no evidence of this in humans. During outbreaks in the Pacific Islands possible congenital infection occurred in a small percentage of women, but there was no effect on length of gestation or fetal outcome, and no evidence of congenital malformation. In contrast, during the 2005 Indian Ocean outbreak of CHIKV, there was a 12% rate of transmission to the fetus, and most of these babies had either meningoencephalitis or a coagulation disorder.

Pathogenesis of Alphavirus Arthritis

The virus is introduced subcutaneously by a blood-feeding infected mosquito (**Table 2**) and initial replication probably occurs within subcutaneous tissue and local skeletal muscle. Little is known about the pathogenesis of the systemic manifestations of alphavirus infection, and interest has focused on the joint disease. RRV arthritis induces a predominantly monocytic inflammatory response in synovial fluid in humans. T-cell-derived interferon-γ has been found in joint fluid of RRV-infected humans, and is secreted by RRV-specific T cells of humans and mice. In animal models or *in vitro* a number of alphaviruses including RRV, BFV, CHIKV, and SINV infect synovial monocytes/macrophages and, in the case of RRV, can be found in synovial cells. A combination of release of inflammatory mediators from the infected monocytes/macrophages and

Table 2   Summary of the major ecological characteristics of the arthritogenic alphaviruses

Virus	Reservoir	Major vectors	Geographic distribution
Chikungunya virus	Nonhuman primates, possibly rodents	Africa (rural): *Aedes africanus*, *Ae. furcifer*, *Ae. luteocephalus*, *Ae. taylori*; Asia: *Ae. aegypti*, *Ae. albopictus*	Africa, Saudi Arabia, SE Asia, Philippines
O'nyong-nyong virus	Unknown	*Anopheles funestus*, *An. gambiae* (and related species)	Uganda, Kenya, Tanzania, Zaire, Malawi, Mozambique, Senegal, Zambia, Cameroon, and the Central African Republic; Igbo Ora variant in Nigeria, the Central African Republic, Côte d'Ivoire.
Ross River virus	Marsupials, especially macropods	*Culex annulirostris*, *Ae. vigilax*, *Ae. camptorhynchus*, *Ae. notoscriptus*, *Ae. sagax*	Australia, New Guinea, Irian Jaya, Pacific Islands
Barmah Forest virus	Marsupials, especially macropods	*Cx. annulirostris*, *Ae. vigilax*, *Ae. camptorhynchus*	Australia
Mayaro virus	Possibly wild vertebrates	*Haemagogus* spp.	Central America, northern South America, the Amazon Basin, Trinidad
Sindbis virus	Range of wild and domestic birds	Northern Europe: *Ae.* spp., *Culiseta* spp., *Culex* spp.; Africa: *Culex* spp., *Aedes* spp., *Mansonia* spp., *Cx. univittatus* (in South Africa); Australia: *Cx. annulirostris*	Southern and northeastern Africa, Scandinavia, Finland, Russia, Central and Eastern Europe, Asia, Southeast Asia, and Australia

the cytotoxic T-cell responses to viral antigens are the likely explanations for the synovial swelling, effusion, and joint pain experienced in acute alphavirus infection.

Attempts to isolate RRV from the joint fluid or tissues of patients with persisting joint disease following RRV infection have been unsuccessful, but RRV antigens have been detected within synovial fluid mononuclear cells. RRV RNA has been found within synovial tissue by polymerase chain reaction (PCR) and RRV can persist within macrophage cultures *in vitro* even in the presence of neutralizing antibodies. All this suggests that the chronic arthritis may result from a persistent, nonreplicative infection that induces an ongoing immune response to viral antigens.

There is also evidence that host factors are likely to influence outcomes. RRV joint disease in humans has been associated with HLA-DR7 positivity, which has a possible role in reducing the cytotoxic T-cell responses to the virus.

Diagnosis of Infection

A number of the alphaviruses produce a viremia detectable by culture or nucleic acid amplification during the early stages of infection, though most patients are not seen until after this period. Alphaviruses will grow in mosquito cells such as C6/36, AP-61, or TRA-284 incubated for 3–4 days at 28 °C, followed by blind passage to indicator cells, such as Vero, baby hamster kidney (BHK), or chick embryo cells that are incubated at 37 °C for a few days. The virus can be identified using monoclonal antibodies, by neutralization tests, or by amplification and characterization of viral nucleic acid using virus-specific primers, probes, or product sequencing.

Detection of viral RNA is significantly more sensitive than is culturing and has been used for detection of CHIKV, RRV, and SINV in blood, and occasionally from other clinical material. A variety of assays directed at NSP1 or E2 viral protein sequences have been used either in uniplex or multiplex formats and, more recently, DNA microarrays have been used for virus identification and characterization.

However, the culture and PCR-based methods are expensive, difficult to access, and negative in most cases. Therefore, diagnosis is almost exclusively done using serological tests. Most diagnostic testing uses the enzyme immunoassays (EIAs) or hemagglutination inhibition (HI) tests, with some use of indirect immunofluorescence antibody (IFA) assays. EIAs and IFA tests can be used to specifically detect either immunoglobulin G (IgG) or immunoglobulin M (IgM). HI will detect both IgG and IgM but is relatively insensitive for IgM detection. Neutralizing antibody titers are regarded as the most specific of the tests, but are confined to specialized laboratories.

IgM antibodies nearly always appear within 1 week of onset of illness, followed by a rise in IgG titer. It is characteristic of alphavirus infections that IgM persists for long periods of time. RRV IgM and BFV IgM usually persist for several months and sometimes years, independent of whether the patient has ongoing symptoms. Persisting IgM has also been documented for SINV and CHIKV, and is likely to be common to all the arthritogenic alphaviruses. Therefore detection of IgM does not, by itself, prove recent infection. That is best diagnosed either by seroconversion from IgG negative to IgG positive or by a fourfold or greater rise in rise in IgG titer between acute and convalescent samples tested in parallel.

False-positive IgM results may also occur occasionally and appear to be a problem particularly with EIA tests, but can occur with other tests as well. They are due to either a nonspecific reaction of the assay or to cross-reaction with IgM produced in response to infection with a related virus. For example, false-positive BFV IgM is occasionally seen in patients with genuine RRV IgM, incorrectly suggesting a dual infection. Cross-reacting antibodies are more likely to occur between closely related viruses, such as ONNV and CHIKV, or MAYV and SFV, but also occasionally occur with rubella or with infectious and noninfectious conditions that cause polyclonal B-cell activation.

Therefore, the proper interpretation of alphavirus serology requires a good clinical history of the illness and knowledge of the viruses to which the patient may have been exposed. Nevertheless, standard serological tests performed in the correct clinical context have proved to be very reliable.

Treatment of Alphavirus Infections

There is a very limited literature on the treatment of alphavirus arthritis. Rest and gentle exercise assist many patients, and nonsteroidal anti-inflammatory agents and simple analgesics are commonly used and provide substantial benefit for the musculoskeletal manifestations.

There are currently no specific antiviral agents available for the treatment of alphavirus infections, nor are there likely to be any in the near future. Drugs used for treatment of rheumatoid arthritis help some patients. Hydroxychloroquine has shown a benefit for patients with post-CHIKV arthritis in one small trial, and corticosteroids have been used for acute RRV arthritis, but most practitioners remain reluctant to use these agents until there are more data about long-term benefits and safety.

Barmah Forest Virus

BFV was first isolated from *Culex annulirostris* in southeast Australia in 1974, then from mosquitoes in other areas of eastern and northern Australia. Human cases were not reported until the 1980s in southeastern Australia, Queensland, the far north of Western Australia, and in the Northern Territory. The virus was subsequently found to be endemic in the tropical areas of northern Australia. Since then there has been appearance of human disease in new areas both within the tropical north and in the more southerly temperate areas where RRV is also active. BFV activity in new areas has been marked by human epidemics of varying size, after which it settles into an endemic pattern that is similar to, but not always coincident with, RRV activity. Human infections have now occurred throughout mainland Australia, with seasonality and incidence varying between regions.

BFV has been isolated from many of the same mosquito species that carry RRV. It is assumed that the same marsupial hosts are important in maintenance and amplification of the virus, but the full range of vertebrate hosts remains to be determined. BFV shows genetic homogeneity across Australia, suggesting that the same strain of BFV spreads widely across the country.

BFV disease has been reported in people aged 5–73 years old, although most cases of both BFV disease and RRV disease occur between the ages of 20 and 60 years. Clinically it is very similar to RRV disease, though joint involvement is less common and less severe, while rash is more common and more likely to be vesicular or urticarial.

Chronic illness occurs following BFV arthritis, but there are few data regarding this. Chronicity is less common after BFV infection than following RRV infection and probably occurs in about 10% of patients.

Chikungunya Virus

CHIKV disease was first recognized following an outbreak of arthritis in Tanzania in 1952, and shortly after was isolated from human serum as well as from *Aedes* spp. and *Culex* spp. mosquitoes. The name is a Swahili word meaning 'that which contorts (or bends up)' and refers to the severe joint pains and stiffness associated with this illness.

The virus is widespread across sub-Saharan Africa, Saudi Arabia, the Indian subcontinent, and Southeast Asia, especially the Philippines. Two major genetic lineages exist, of which one is restricted to West Africa. The other is further subdivided into Asian and East African sublineages. While there are some biological differences between these lineages, it is not known whether these have any specific pathogenic implications. There are data to suggest that genetic diversity may be seen among CHIKV strains responsible for individual outbreaks in Africa and in adjacent areas. For example, during the recent Indian Ocean outbreak, the virus was from the East African sublineage, but showed evolution during the course of the outbreak. The Asian sublineage shows a much greater genetic conservation.

In Africa, the virus shows low-level endemic activity in rural areas, where it is believed to be maintained in a cycle involving *Aedes* spp. mosquitoes, nonhuman primates, and, possibly, rodents. The role of nonhuman mammalian hosts in Asia is not known, though seropositive primates have been described. Occurrence of epidemic disease in Africa and Asia is associated with the rainy season and increases in numbers of *Aedes aegypti* and, in Asia, *Ae. albopictus*. Urban outbreaks may continue over 2 or more years, but cases then typically disappear for several years. *Mansonia* spp. and *Culex* spp. have also been implicated as potential vectors in laboratory studies.

Epidemics occur either due to reemergence of the virus in an area of prior activity once sufficient time has passed for a susceptible population to reestablish, or due to movement of the virus into areas without previous activity. They may involve up to half the population. There have been regular occurrences of epidemics in Africa, with the most recent being in Kinshasa in 1999/ 2000. In Asia a number of outbreaks occurred in the 1960s, followed by a relatively quiescent period in the 1970s, reemergence in Indonesia in 1982, further spread within Malaysia in 1988–89, reemergence in Thailand in 1995, and in Indonesia in 2001–03. The most recent outbreak began in late 2004 in southwestern Indian Ocean islands and subsequently spread over the next couple of years to affect several hundred thousand people in that region, with the largest number of cases on Réunion, the Seychelles, and in several areas of India. Subsequently, small numbers of cases were detected worldwide in travelers returning from epidemic areas.

CHIKV acute illness is more severe than that seen with the other alphaviruses, with fever that is more frequent and higher, worse joint pain, a greater incidence of severe disease, and occasional deaths. While most patients recover within a few days or weeks, chronic joint pains lasting months to years occur in about 10% of patients.

Hemorrhagic manifestations, including petechiae and gingival bleeding due to CHIKV infection, are well described but rare and can lead to a misdiagnosis of dengue. This is complicated by the fact that these two viruses may co-circulate and patients may be simultaneously infected by both. Fatalities in the past have been extremely rare and were reported to occur in the very young or in those with severe hemorrhagic disease, though it is not certain that the fatalities were due to CHIKV. In the recent Indian Ocean outbreak, a number of cases of CHIKV encephalitis and deaths have been reported. The latter have occurred in the elderly or those with co-morbidities.

Mayaro Virus

MAYV was first isolated from a forest worker in Trinidad in 1954, and is now known to be widely distributed in Central

America, northern South America, and the Amazon Basin. Transmission is primarily by forest-dwelling *Haemagogus* spp. mosquitoes, though *Mansonia venezuelensis* and *Ae. aegypti* are possible vectors. The virus is probably maintained in a sylvatic cycle between mosquitoes and wild vertebrates. There are two genotypes, one being widespread and the other found only in Brazil.

Occasional outbreaks and sporadic cases occur within the endemic areas following human contact with the forest environment. The illness is very similar to that caused by CHIKV, including hemorrhagic disease in some cases.

Una virus was initially classified as subtype of MAYV, but is now regarded as a separate species and has not been shown to cause human disease.

O'nyong-nyong Virus (Including Igbo-Ora Variant)

ONNV is closely related to CHIKV both virologically and clinically. The disease was first described in Uganda in 1959 and the name is a tribal word for painful joints. It was subsequently isolated from human serum and from mosquitoes. That epidemic eventually involved more than 2 million people in Uganda, Kenya, Tanzania, Zaire, Malawi, Mozambique, Senegal, and Zambia. Spread was thought to have occurred by movement of viremic humans. This virus has also been found in Cameroon and the Central African Republic. A variant called Igbo-Ora was later found in West Africa, in Nigeria, Central African Republic, and Côte d'Ivoire. ONNV disappeared for 35 years before reappearing in Uganda in 1996/1997, with subsequent cases in Kenya. Infections due to the major strain (i.e., not Igbo-Ora) have recently been reported from Côte d'Ivoire and Chad.

Transmission is by *Anopheles funestus* and *An. gambiae.* It is presumed that there is a nonhuman mammalian host to account for maintenance of the virus between epidemics, but it has not yet been identified.

The clinical illness is very similar to CHIKV disease, though fever is usually milder and there is prominent cervical lymphadenopathy. Joint pain persisting for several months has been noted, but the frequency is not known.

Ross River Virus

RRV was named after an area near Townsville in northeastern Australia, where it was first isolated from *Ae. vigilax* in 1966, from mosquitoes collected in 1959. It was isolated from the blood of a febrile child in 1973, then from a case of epidemic polyarthritis in 1979. It has since been found in Papua New Guinea, Irian Jaya, and the Solomon Islands. In 1979–80 an epidemic

occurred in various Pacific Islands involving over 50 000 cases, probably originating from a viremic air traveler from Australia.

Three genotypes of RRV have so far been described. Genotype 1 was present in Queensland in northeastern Australia until the mid-1970s, after which it disappeared. Genotype 2 has always been the major type on the east coast of Australia and is now the major current circulating type throughout Australia. Genotype 3 was the dominant type in the southwest of Australia until 1996, since which it has largely been replaced by genotype 2 virus. Pacific Islands isolates belong to genotype 2.

RRV is primarily maintained in a cycle between mosquitoes and vertebrate hosts. Two salt-marsh mosquitoes, *Ae. vigilax* and *Ae. camptorhynchus,* are important in northern and southern coastal areas of Australia, respectively. In some coastal and inland areas, transmission to humans occurs from several freshwater breeding species, especially *Cx. annulirostris* but also *Ae. sagax* and *Ae. normanensis,* as well as *Ae. camptorhynchus* breeding in brackish and freshwater. Other species, such as *Coquillettidia linealis* and *Ae. notoscriptus,* may play significant roles in urban environments.

The major vertebrate hosts for both maintenance and amplification of RRV are the macropod marsupials (kangaroos, wallabies, and euros). Horses and small marsupials, such as possums, may be important in periurban and urban areas. There is circumstantial evidence that RRV may survive for years in desiccation-resistant eggs of some *Aedes* spp.

RRV disease is reported every year in Australia, with between 2000 and 8000 notified cases per annum. In the tropical northern parts of the country most activity is seen during the wet season from December to May. Further south in temperate regions, human infections occur predominantly in late spring, summer, or autumn. In those seasons, rainfall or tidal inundation of coastal breeding sites coupled with warm temperatures leads to an increase in vector numbers. Major outbreaks in these areas occur every 2–4 years. In the arid inland regions of Australia occasional outbreaks occur following heavy rainfall with flooding.

RRV disease has been reported in people ranging in age from less than 1 year old to 88 years old, although most cases occur between the ages of 20 and 60 years. Clinical illness appears to be uncommon in children. The clinical illness is typical of these alphaviruses, though tenosynovitis and fasciitis are more common. Joint pains, muscle pains, and fatigue persist for months or years in 70–90% of patients.

Semliki Forest Virus

SFV was first isolated in 1942 from mosquitoes in Uganda and is distributed across sub-Saharan Africa. Serological surveys show that human infection is common in endemic areas, but it has only been associated with a single reported human outbreak of fever, headache, and joint pains that occurred in the Central African Republic in 1987.

Sindbis Virus (Including Ockelbo Virus)

SINV was first isolated from *Culex univittatus* at Sindbis in Egypt, and subsequently from a wide range of species of mosquitoes and vertebrates in Europe, the Middle East, Africa, India, Asia, the Philippines, and Australia. It was not until 1961 that it was isolated from the blood of a febrile human in Uganda, and then linked to human disease in South Africa in 1963.

SINV is the most widely distributed arbovirus causing human disease. It is found throughout southern and northeastern Africa, Northern, Central, and Eastern Europe, Asia, Southeast Asia, and Australia, but clinical disease is largely restricted to Sweden (Ockelbo disease), Norway (Ockelbo disease), Finland (Pogosta disease), Russia (Karelian fever), and South Africa. Clinical disease has only rarely been reported in Asia. Only isolated cases of illness in humans have been reported from Australia, although serological studies have indicated that human infections occur regularly.

Many species of birds and of other vertebrates have been shown to be capable of being infected with SINV, but disease has been identified only in humans. Mosquitoes feeding on birds appear to be the primary source of human infection. In Sweden the virus has been found primarily in the fieldfare (*Turdus pilaris*), redwing (*T. iliacu*), and song thrush (*T. philomelos*), and in Norway game birds also carry the virus. Transmission to humans is via *Aedes*, *Culiseta*, and *Culex* spp. in Sweden, Norway, and Finland. In Africa *Culex*, *Aedes*, and *Mansonia* spp. are important, with *Cx. univittatus* being the primary human vector in South Africa. In Australia, *Cx. annulirostris* is the dominant vector species, but it is also been isolated from *Aedes* spp. No maintenance cycles involving nonhuman vertebrates have been identified as yet in any country.

Two major lineages circulate: the Paleoarctic/Ethiopian and the Oriental/Australian. It is believed that migratory birds are responsible for the spread of the two lineages, though within each there is a genetic heterogeneity consistent with local adaptation and evolution of the virus. Studies in Australia have shown that there is also temporal evolution of the virus within a lineage, presumed to be due to periodic introduction of new variants by migratory birds. A third unique lineage has been identified in the southwest of that country.

The restricted distribution of human epidemics suggests that the Paleoarctic/Ethiopian lineage has a greater ability to cause disease than does the Oriental/Australian lineage. However, the ecology of SINV and the pathogenesis of disease are still poorly understood, so other factors may account for the unusual disease patterns.

Epidemics of Ockelbo disease and Pogosta disease occur during summer and autumn in northern Europe, coincident with the peak mosquito breeding period. Ockelbo occurs each year, while Pogosta disease has shown a consistent periodicity of 7 years since it was first recognized in 1974, the reasons for which are uncertain. Summer–autumn SINV epidemics have also been described in South Africa. Patients usually recover within a few weeks but chronic joint pains are common.

The Future

Alphavirus infections impose a substantial human health and economic burden, without any immediate prospect of antiviral therapy or vaccines. Further research is needed to understand the ecology and epidemiology of these viruses and the pathogenesis of disease.

See also: Arboviruses; Rubella Virus; Togaviruses: General Features; West Nile Virus.

Further Reading

Griffin DE (2001) Alphaviruses. In: Knipe DM and Howley PM (eds.) *Fields Virology*, 4th edn., pp. 917–962. Philadelphia, PA: Lippincott Williams and Wilkins.

Harley D, Sleigh A, and Ritchie S (2001) Ross River virus transmission, infection, and disease: A cross-disciplinary review. *Reviews in Clinical Microbiology* 14: 909–932.

Johnson BK (1989) O'nyong-nyong virus disease. In: Monath TP (ed.) *The Arboviruses: Epidemiology and Ecology*, vol. III, pp. 217–223. Boca Raton, FL: CRC Press.

Jupp PG and McIntosh BM (1989) Chikungunya virus disease. In: Monath TP (ed.) *The Arboviruses: Epidemiology and Ecology*, vol. II, pp. 137–157. Boca Raton, FL: CRC Press.

Kurkela S, Manni T, Myllynen J, Vaheri A, and Vapalahti O (2005) Clinical and laboratory manifestations of Sindbis virus infection: Prospective study, Finland, 2002–2003. *Journal of Infectious Diseases* 191: 1820–1829.

Laine M, Luukkainen R, and Toivanen A (2004) Sindbis virus and other alphaviruses as a cause of human arthritic disease. *Journal of Internal Medicine* 256: 457–471.

Mackenzie JS, Broom AK, Hall RA, et al. (1998) Arboviruses in the Australian region, 1990 to 1998. *Communicable Diseases Intelligence* 22: 93–100.

Niklasson B (1989) Sindbis and Sindbis-like viruses. In: Monath TP (ed.) *The Arboviruses: Epidemiology and Ecology*, vol. III, pp. 167–176. Boca Raton, FL: CRC Press.

Pinheiro FP and LeDuc JW (1989) Mayaro virus disease. In: Monath TP (ed.) *The Arboviruses: Epidemiology and Ecology*, vol. III, pp. 137–150. Boca Raton, FL: CRC Press.

Powers AM, Aguilar PV, Chandler LJ, et al. (2006) Genetic relationships among Mayaro and Una viruses suggest distinct patterns of transmission. *American Journal of Tropical Medicine and Hygiene* 75: 461–469.

Powers AM, Brault AC, Tesh RB, and Weaver SC (2000) Re-emergence of Chikungunya and O'nyong-nyong viruses: Evidence for distinct genetic lineages and distant evolutionary relationships. *Journal of General Virology* 81: 471–479.

Rulli NE, Suhrbier A, Hueston L, *et al.* (2005) Ross River virus: Molecular and cellular aspects of disease pathogenesis. *Pharmacology and Therapeutics* 107: 329–342.

Russell RC (2002) Ross River virus: Ecology and distribution. *Annual Reviews in Entomology* 47: 1–31.

Suhrbier A and Linn ML (2004) Clinical and pathological aspects of arthritis due to Ross River virus and other alphaviruses. *Current Opinions in Rheumatology* 16: 374–379.

Transmissible Spongiform Encephalopathies

E D Belay and L B Schonberger, Centers for Disease Control and Prevention, Atlanta, GA, USA

Glossary

Alleles Mutually exclusive forms of the same gene on homologous chromosomes.

Codon A sequence of three nucleotide bases in a gene that specifies an amino acid to be incorporated into a protein during its synthesis.

Encephalopathy Brain disease resulting from infectious agents such as prions.

Genetic polymorphism The regular occurrence in a population of two or more components of a gene with greater frequency than can be explained by recurrent mutation.

Mutation A permanent inheritable change in the genetic material of a host.

Prion Small, proteinaceous infectious particles that resist inactivation by procedures that affect nucleic acids; they are believed to be the causative agents of scrapie and other spongiform encephalopathies of animals and humans.

Prion protein A normal cellular version of the infectious prions encoded by the prion protein gene; its cellular function is not well understood.

Introduction

Prion diseases, also known as transmissible spongiform encephalopathies, constitute a group of fatal, human, and animal subacute neurodenerative diseases caused by an unconventional agent. Strong evidence indicates that their etiology and pathogenesis involve modification of a host-encoded normal cellular protein known as the prion protein (PrP^C). A unique hallmark of this group of diseases includes their sporadic occurrence without any apparent environmental source of infection or genetic association with prion protein gene mutations or as a result of disease transmission from infected humans and animals. Neuropathologically, most prion diseases manifest with widespread neuronal loss, spongiform lesions, and astrogliosis. Characteristically, no signs of inflammation are detected in pathologic samples. However, the presence of an abnormal, pathogenic prion protein, often called a scrapie prion protein (PrP^{Sc}) after the first recognized prion disease, scrapie, is demonstrable in the brain and often in other tissues of humans and animals affected by prion diseases. The incubation period of acquired forms of prion diseases is usually measured in years and sometimes in decades.

Etiologic Agent of Prion Diseases

Studies that characterized the causative agents of prion diseases initially focused on understanding the agents responsible for scrapie in sheep. This disease is the most common prion disease of animals and was first reported in the 1730s in England. Before the 1980s, prion diseases were widely believed to be caused by 'slow viruses' despite the fact that no viral particles or disease-specific nucleic acids were identified in association with scrapie transmission in laboratory animals. The scrapie agent could not be grown in cell culture, a feature that hampered research to characterize the agent. The successful transmission of scrapie to laboratory mice in 1961 contributed to overcoming this hurdle and greatly facilitated efforts to understand the nature of the agent. Quantitation of infectivitiy in a sample, however, still was tedious and required a year to complete.

Two distinctive properties of the scrapie agent led to the suspicion that the agent was devoid of nucleic acids and, thus, may not be a virus but primarily composed of a protein. These properties included (1) resistance of the scrapie agent to procedures, such as treatment with ultraviolet light and ionizing radiation, that normally inactivate other microorganisms, including viruses and (2) the reduction of the infectivity of the scrapie agent by procedures that denature or degrade proteins. The concept that the scrapie agent might replicate in the absence of nucleic acids or might just be a protein was postulated as early as the 1960s by Alper and colleagues, Pattison and Jones, and Griffith. In 1982, Prusiner and colleagues described the successful purification of a hydrophobic protein, the presence of which was required for scrapie transmission in laboratory animals. Prusiner introduced the term 'prion' to describe this protein by borrowing and mixing the first few letters from the descriptive phrase 'proteinaceous infectious' particle. Since then, additional evidence has accumulated indicating that prions may be acting alone in causing prion diseases. However, the critical steps in the production, propagation, and pathogenesis of this infectious protein remain unclear. As a result, the study of prions has become an important, relatively new area of biomedical investigation. Some critics of the prion hypothesis still believe that nucleic acids undetected by current methods may play a crucial role in the pathogenesis of prion diseases.

Prions appear to be composed largely or entirely of the abnormal protein designated as PrP^{Sc}. This protein is an abnormal conformer of a host-encoded cellular protein, PrP^{C}, which in humans is encoded by the prion protein gene located on the short arm of chromosome 20. PrP^{C} is a structural component of cell membranes of neurons and other tissues. Its normal function is poorly understood. However, it appears to be involved in supporting neuronal synaptic activity, copper binding, and neuroprotective functions by interacting with other cell-surface proteins.

The underlying pathophysiologic mechanism in the occurrence of prion diseases involves the biochemical conversion of PrP^{C} into the pathogenic PrP^{Sc}. This conversion occurs by a poorly defined post-translational autocatalytic process, possibly requiring the aid of cofactors such as proteins or nucleic acids. The initial instigating PrP^{Sc} molecule may originate from exogenous sources or within the brain from somatic or germline prion protein gene mutations. Knockout mice devoid of the prion protein gene are resistant to scrapie infection, indicating that the production of PrP^{C} is required for the generation and propagation of PrP^{Sc}. During its conversion, PrP^{Sc} acquires more β-sheet structure that renders it resistant to proteolytic enzymes, conventional disinfectants, and standard sterilization methods. A higher proportion of the tertiary structure of PrP^{C}, on the other hand, is composed of α-helices which make it more sensitive to denaturation by proteinase-K treatment. Removal of the neuroprotective functions of PrP^{C} as more of it becomes converted to the pathogenic PrP^{Sc} and accumulation of PrP^{Sc} in neurons have been suggested as major contributory factors in the underlying pathogenesis of prion diseases and widespread neuronal death.

Prion Diseases of Animals

Prion diseases of animals include scrapie in sheep, goats, and moufflon; bovine spongiform encephalopathy (BSE) in cattle; feline spongiform encephalopathy in domestic and zoo cats; ungulate spongiform encephalopathy in exotic zoo ruminants; chronic wasting disease (CWD) in deer, elk, and moose; and transmissible mink encephalopathy (TME) in mink (**Table 1**). Epidemiologic evidence

Table 1   Animal and human prion diseases

Type of prion disease	Affected host	Year first described or identified
Animal prion diseases		
Scrapie	Sheep and goats	1730s
Bovine spongiform encephalopathy	Cattle	1986
Chronic wasting disease	Deer, elk, and moose	1967
Transmissible mink encephalopathy[a]	Mink	1947
Feline spongiform encephalopathy[b]	Domestic and wild cats	1990
Ungulate spongiform encepahlopathy[b]	Exotic ruminants (e.g., kudu, nyala)	1986
Human prion diseases		
Kuru		1950s
Sporadic CJD		1920s
Iatrogenic CJD		1974[c]
Variant CJD		1996
Familial CJD		1924
Gerstmann–Sträussler–Scheinker syndrome		1936
Fatal familial insomnia		1986

[a]The last known outbreak of transmissible mink encephalopathy occurred in 1981 in Wisconsin.
[b]The known feline and ungulate spongiform encephalopathies are believed to have resulted from BSE transmission.
[c]The first report of iatrogenic CJD was in a recipient of cornea obtained from a CJD decedent; human pituitary growth hormone-associated CJD was first reported in 1985 and dura mater graft-associated CJD in 1987.
CJD, Creutzfeldt–Jakob disease.

indicates that feline and ungulate spongiform encephalopathies were caused by the BSE agent possibly transmitted via consumption of BSE-contaminated feed. Although strong evidence is lacking, speculations have persisted that scrapie in sheep may have been the original source of prion diseases in other animals, such as BSE and CWD.

TME occurred in outbreaks among ranched mink primarily in the US but also in Canada, Finland, Germany, and Russia. The last known outbreak of TME occurred in 1985 in Wisconsin. Nonepizootic cases of TME have not been reported.

Scrapie

Although scrapie was recognized as a distinct clinical entity of sheep over 250 years ago, many aspects of the disease including its natural origin in flocks and the precise means by which it usually spreads remain uncertain. Experimentally, the disease was first transmitted by intraocular inoculation of scrapie brain extracts. In the 1940s, more than 1500 sheep developed scrapie from receipt of a vaccine against louping ill virus that contained scrapie-contaminated lymphoid tissue.

Scrapie transmission may occur by different postulated mechanisms. A commonly cited source of transmission, for example, is the placenta and amniotic fluid of scrapie-infected ewes. These tissues are known to harbor the infectious agent and can cause scrapie when fed to sheep. They may contaminate pastures and barns that, in turn, may remain potentially infectious for years. Another possible source of spread is feces because prion replication occurs in gut lymphoid tissues after oral inoculation in sheep and goats. The importance of oral transmission is supported by experimental studies that detected prions in sheep tonsils examined early during the incubation period. Other poorly defined scrapie transmission mechanisms include (1) the vertical transfer of the scrapie agent and (2) the possible chance occurrence of scrapie caused by hypothesized rare, spontaneous changes in the animal's cellular prion protein.

Scrapie occurs endemically in many countries, including Europe and North America. Australia and New Zealand have sizable sheep populations but are generally recognized as free of the disease. To protect their 'scrapie free' status, these countries have established extensive safeguards to prevent the introduction of scrapie into their herds from imported animals.

The breed of sheep and polymorphisms of the prion protein gene can greatly influence susceptibility to scrapie. Experimental transmissions with scrapie-infected tissues, for example, have confirmed the differing susceptibility to scrapie of different breeds of sheep. Other studies of Suffolk sheep in the US indicated that susceptibility to scrapie was highly correlated with a polymorphism in the prion protein gene at codon 171 (glycine or arginine); the presence of arginine confers resistance to the disease.

Chronic Wasting Disease

Mule deer, white-tailed deer, and Rocky Mountain elk are the major known natural hosts for CWD. In 2005, a hunter-killed moose was confirmed with CWD in Colorado, suggesting that this member of the deer family too is a natural host. The disease was first identified as a fatal wasting syndrome of captive mule deer in the late 1960s in research facilities in Colorado. Subsequently, it was identified in mule deer in a research facility in Wyoming and then in captive elk in facilities in both Colorado and Wyoming. In 1977, CWD was first recognized as a spongiform encephalopathy.

In the early 1980s, the disease was recognized in free-ranging elk. By the mid-1990s, CWD was regarded as endemic in deer and elk in a contiguous area in northeastern Colorado and southeastern Wyoming. The known geographic extent of CWD has increased dramatically in the US since 1996. As of mid-2006, CWD in free-ranging cervids had been reported in 74 counties of 11 states, including Colorado, Kansas, Illinois, Nebraska, New Mexico, New York, South Dakota, Utah, West Virginia, Wisconsin, and Wyoming. In Canada, since 2001, CWD has been identified in wild deer and elk in Saskatchewan and since 2005 in several mule deer in Alberta.

Among cervids, CWD is most likely transmitted by direct animal contact or indirectly by exposure to a contaminated environment. Unlike other prion diseases, CWD is highly communicable in its natural host, particularly among captive cervids. In addition to becoming emaciated, animals with CWD characteristically develop polydipsia, polyuria, increased salivation, and difficulty in swallowing. These characteristics probably contribute to residual contamination of the environment that appears to be a very important source of transmission.

CWD does not appear to occur naturally outside the cervid family. It has been transmitted experimentally by intracerebral injection to laboratory mice, ferrets, mink, squirrel monkeys, goats, and cattle. However, experimental studies have not demonstrated transmission of CWD to cattle after oral challenge or after having cattle reside with infected deer herds.

No human cases of prion disease with strong evidence of a link with CWD have been identified despite several epidemiologic investigations of suspected cases. In addition, transgenic mice experiments indicate the existence of a significant species barrier against CWD transmission to humans. Nevertheless, concerns remain that this species barrier may not provide complete protection to humans against CWD and that the level and frequency of human exposures to CWD may increase with the spread of CWD in North America.

As a precaution, efforts to reduce human exposure to the CWD agent are generally recommended. Meat from depopulated CWD-infected captive cervids has not been allowed to enter the human food or animal feed supply. To minimize their risk of CWD exposure, hunters are encouraged to consult with their state wildlife agencies to identify areas where CWD occurs and to continue to follow advice provided by public health and wildlife agencies.

Bovine Spongiform Encephalopathy

Prion diseases became a focus of worldwide attention after a large outbreak of BSE in cattle emerged in the UK and spread to other countries. This attention increased dramatically when evidence accumulated indicating that the BSE agent was responsible for the occurrence of variant Creutzfeldt–Jakob disease (CJD) in humans. By far the largest number of BSE cases was reported from the UK, followed by other European countries.

Although BSE was first recognized in the UK in 1986; earlier cases probably occurred since the early 1980s. The number of UK BSE cases increased rapidly in the second half of the 1980s and early 1990s, peaked in 1992 with 37 280 confirmed cases, and has markedly declined since then (**Figure 1**). In 2005, the number of confirmed UK BSE cases had dropped to 225.

Clinically, the signs of BSE include neurologic dysfunction, including unsteady gait with falling and abnormal responses to touch and sound. In some animals, the onset of BSE can be insidious and subtle and may be difficult to recognize. During the early phase of the UK BSE outbreak, the public media introduced the popular term 'mad cow' disease to describe the strange disease causing fearful and aggressive behavior in some of the cattle infected with BSE.

Although the original source of the BSE outbreak is unknown, the two most accepted hypotheses are cross-species transmission of scrapie from sheep and the spontaneous occurrence of BSE in cattle. Data on the latter hypothesis may become available with increased detection and monitoring rates of atypical, as well as typical cases of BSE. According to the first hypothesis, transmission of scrapie to cattle occurred because of the practice of feeding cattle protein derived from rendered animal carcasses including those of scrapie-infected sheep. In the past, cattle feed rendering in the UK involved several treatment steps, including exposure of the feed to prolonged heating in the presence of a hydrocarbon solvent. Some researchers have suggested that omission of these steps in the late 1970s and early 1980s in the UK contributed to the emergence of BSE by allowing scrapie infectivity to survive the rendering process. Regardless of the origin of BSE, the epidemiologic evidence indicates that feeding cattle rendered BSE-infected carcasses greatly amplified the BSE outbreak. Several other factors may have contributed to the emergence of BSE in the UK, including a relatively high rate of endemic scrapie, a high population ratio of sheep to cattle, and the inclusion of rendered meat and bone meal at high rates in cattle feed.

Since the BSE outbreak was first detected, an estimated >2 million cattle have been infected with BSE in the UK. Approximately half of these BSE-infected cattle would have been slaughtered for human consumption, potentially exposing millions of UK residents. Beginning in 1988, UK animal and public health authorities implemented several protective measures to prevent further exposure of animals and humans to BSE-infected cattle products. The implementation of these measures, particularly animal feed bans, led to the dramatic decline in the UK BSE outbreak.

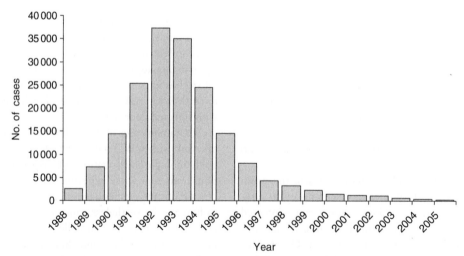

Figure 1 Bovine spongiform encephalopathy cases reported in the UK. BSE cases shown are by year of restriction: 442 BSE cases identified before 1988 are not included.

BSE was reported for the first time outside the UK in Ireland in 1989 and in Portugal and Switzerland in 1990. By August 2006, the number of countries that reported one or more BSE cases in native cattle increased to 25, including 21 countries in Europe. The four countries outside Europe that reported BSE cases are Canada, Israel, Japan, and the US. The BSE outbreak appears to be declining in most European countries, although some cases continue to occur.

In North America, BSE was first detected in 1993 in a cow that had been imported into Canada from the UK. Rendered cohorts of this cow may have been responsible for the 11 BSE cases subsequently identified during 2003–06 among cattle born in Canada; one of these cases was identified in Washington State but was later traced to a farm in Canada. At least six of these 11 BSE cases were born after the 1997 ruminant feed ban which was instituted to prevent BSE transmission among cattle. Because of the continued occurrence of new BSE infections after the 1997 ruminant feed ban, a specified risk material ban was recently instituted in Canada to further reduce cattle exposure to BSE by excluding potentially infectious nervous tissues from all animal feed. In 2005 and 2006, respectively, BSE was confirmed in an approximately 12-year-old cow born and raised in Texas and 10-year-old cow from Alabama. The source of BSE infection for these two cows remains unknown.

Because cattle carcasses were included in the production of animal feed, potential transmission of BSE to other animals was considered during the early phase of the BSE outbreak in the UK. BSE-like diseases were identified in zoo animals (ungulate spongiform encephalopathy) beginning in the late 1980s and in domestic cats (feline spongiform encephalopathy) beginning in 1990, indicating the potential for the BSE agent to cross the species barrier and spread to other animals. This development led to the establishment of enhanced CJD surveillance in the UK to monitor the possible transmission of BSE to humans.

Prion Diseases of Humans

Prion diseases of humans include kuru, CJD, variant CJD, Gerstmann–Sträussler–Scheinker syndrome (GSS), and fatal familial insomnia (FFI) (**Table 1**). Kuru is a fatal ataxic disease that was first described in the 1950s among the Fore tribe of the highlands of Papua New Guinea. In 1959, W. J. Hadlow described the similarity of the neuropathology of this disease with that of scrapie. In 1963, Gajdusek and colleagues successfully transmitted kuru by inoculating kuru brain tissue intracerebrally into chimpanzees, making this disease the first human prion disease to be successfully transmitted to experimental animals.

Kuru is the first epidemic human prion disease to be investigated. Since its investigation began in 1956, over 2700 cases have been documented. Strong epidemiologic evidence suggests that kuru spread among the Fore people by ritualistic endocannibalism. After this practice ended in the late 1950s, no children born after 1959 developed the disease and the number of new cases dramatically declined. Likely incubation periods of seven male cases recently reported by Collinge and colleagues ranged from 39 to 56 years and the incubation periods may have been up to 7 years longer. These male cases and four female cases had kuru from July 1996 to June 2004. The majority of these 11 kuru patients were reported to be heterozygous at the polymorphic codon 129 of the prion protein gene, a genotype associated with extended incubation periods and resistance to prion disease.

Creutzfeldt–Jakob Disease

CJD is the most common form of prion disease in humans. It was first recognized in the 1920s and bears the name of two German neurologists, Creutzfeldt and Jakob, who separately reported patients with rapidly progressive neurodegenerative diseases. Two of the patients initially reported by Jakob had the typical neuropathological features that we now recognize as CJD.

CJD is usually characterized by the onset of dementia, ataxia, or behavioral abnormalities. Later in the course of the illness, CJD patients commonly develop dysarthria, movement disorders such as myoclonus and tremors, and akinetic mutism. The presence of a characteristic electroencephalogram (EEG) finding of triphasic, periodic sharp wave complexes can be demonstrated with multiple testing in about 75% of patients. Elevated levels of 14-3-3 proteins in the cerebrospinal fluid (CSF) can also be demonstrated in most CJD patients. Elevated CSF 14-3-3 is a marker for rapid neuronal death and in the appropriate clinical context can often help in making a premortem diagnosis of CJD. This test is nonspecific, however, and may be elevated in other neurologic conditions that result in rapid neuronal death. More recently, magnetic resonant imaging (MRI) findings showing high intensity in the basal ganglia and cortical regions of the brain have been correlated with a CJD diagnosis. The median age of CJD patients at the time of death is 68 years with approximately 70% of cases occurring between 55 and 75 years of age. Typically, the disease progresses rapidly over a period of several weeks. Over 50% of the patients die within 6 months and 80% within 1 year of disease onset. A definitive diagnosis of CJD can only be made by histopathologic or immunodiagnostic testing of brain tissues obtained at autopsy or biopsy. Histopathologic examination of brain tissue demonstrates the hallmark triad of spongiform lesions, neuronal loss, and astrogliosis. Immunodiagnostic assays, such as immunohistochemistry and

Western blot testing, that show the presence of PrP^{Sc} confirm the CJD diagnosis.

Historically, three different forms of CJD have been reported: sporadic, iatrogenic, and familial CJD. Sporadic CJD occurs in the absence of outbreaks with no known environmental source of infection. Decades of research has not identified a specific source of infection for sporadic CJD that accounts for about 85% of patients. Spontaneous generation of the pathogenic prions was hypothesized as a cause for sporadic CJD, possibly resulting from random somatic mutations or errors during prion protein gene expression. Iatrogenic CJD, on the other hand, is associated with transmission of the CJD agent via medical interventions such as administration of contaminated human pituitary hormones and the use of contaminated dura mater grafts and neurosurgical equipment. Familial CJD has been associated with the presence of inheritable prion protein gene mutations. Beginning in the mid-1990s, the emergence of a variant form of CJD, linked with BSE transmission to humans, was reported. This newly emerged disease differs from other forms of CJD by the young age of affected patients and its clinical and pathologic features (**Table 2**).

Sporadic CJD is a heterogeneous disorder that can be further subdivided into five different subtypes based on the Western blot characteristics of protease-resistant fragment of PrP^{Sc} and the polymorphism at codon 129 of the host prion protein gene. These different subtypes correlate with characteristic clinical and neuropathologic phenotypes. The most common subtype is associated with a 21 kDa PrP^{Sc} fragment, designated type 1, and the presence of methionine at the polymorphic codon 129 of the prion protein gene.

Variant Creutzfeldt–Jakob Disease

In 1996, the identification of a cluster of young patients with a prion disease was reported in the UK as part of the CJD surveillance system that was established in response to concerns about the potential spread of BSE to humans. Because the patients' age and their clinical progression and neuropathologic profile were different from other endemic CJD patients, the term 'new variant CJD' was initially used to describe this emerging prion disease in humans. This term was later shortened to variant CJD. Since 1996, the number of variant CJD cases increased and strong scientific evidence indicated that variant CJD resulted from BSE transmission to humans. As of June 2007, a total of 202 variant CJD patients was reported worldwide, including 165 patients from the UK, 21 from France, four from Ireland, three from the US, two each from Netherlands and Portugal, and one each from Canada, Italy, Japan, Saudi Arabia, and Spain. At least seven of the non-UK variant CJD patients (two each from the US and Ireland, and one each from Canada, France, and Japan) were believed to have acquired variant CJD during their past residence or visit in the UK.

Variant CJD can be distinguished from the more common classic CJD by the clinical and laboratory findings (**Table 2**). The median age at death of variant CJD patients is 40 years younger than sporadic CJD patients (28 and 68 years, respectively), but their median illness duration is longer (14 and <6 months, respectively). Unlike classic CJD patients, variant CJD patients predominantly have psychiatric manifestations at onset with delayed appearance of frank neurologic signs and the typical 'pulvinar sign' on the MRI. The diagnostic EEG

Table 2 Clinical and pathologic characteristics distinguishing variant Creutzfeldt-Jakob disease (variant CJD) from classic CJD

Characteristic	Variant CJD	Classic CJD
Median age (range) at death (years)	28 (14–74)	68 (23–97)[a]
Median duration of illness (months)	13–14	4–5
Clinical presentation	Prominent psychiatric/behavioral symptoms, painful sensory symptoms, delayed neurologic signs	Dementia, early neurologic signs
Periodic sharp waves on electroencephalogram	Almost always absent	Often present
'Pulvinar sign' on magnetic resonance imaging[b]	Present in >75% of cases	Very rare or absent
Presence of 'florid plaques' on neuropathologic Sample	Present in great numbers	Rare or absent
Immunohistochemical analysis of brain tissue	Marked accumulation of PrP-res[c]	Variable accumulation
Presence of agent in lymphoid tissue	Readily detected	Not readily detected
Increased glycoform ratio on Western-blot analysis of PrP-res	Present	Not present
Genotype at codon 129 of prion protein	Methionine/valine[d]	Polymorphic

[a]US CJD surveillance data 1979–2001.
[b]Symmetrical high signal in the posterior thalamus relative to that of other deep and cortical gray matter.
[c]Protease-resistant prion protein.
[d]A patient with preclinical vCJD related to blood-borne transmission was heterozygous for methionine and valine.

finding that is common in classic CJD patients is very rare in patients with variant CJD. For unknown reasons, all variant CJD patients tested to date had methionine homozygosity in the prion protein gene at codon 129, which is polymorphic for methionine or valine. This homozygosity is present in approximately 35–40% of the general UK population. Similar to classic CJD, a definitive diagnosis of variant CJD requires laboratory testing of brain tissues. In addition to the spongiform lesion, neuronal loss, and astrogliosis typical of most prion diseases, the neuropathology in variant CJD patients is characterized by the presence of numerous 'florid plaques', consisting of amyloid deposits surrounded by a halo of spongiform lesions.

Studies in the UK have indicated the probable secondary person-to-person transmission of the variant CJD agent in three patients by blood collected up to 3.5 years before variant CJD onset in the donors. Because a large proportion of the UK population has potentially been exposed to the BSE agent, concerns still exist about additional secondary spread of the agent via blood products and possibly via contaminated surgical instruments.

Prion Diseases of Humans Associated with Genetic Mutations

One of the intriguing properties of prion diseases in humans is the fact that they can be both infectious and inheritable. The inherited or genetic forms of prion diseases are associated with insertion, deletion, or point mutations of the open reading frame of the prion protein gene. At least 24 different point mutations of the prion protein gene have been described in association with human prion diseases. These genetic prion diseases have widely varying clinical and neuropathologic manifestations. Historically, genetic forms of prion diseases, in part based on their phenotypical expression, were classified as familial CJD, GSS, and FFI. Beginning in 1989, many types of insertion mutations associated with markedly heterogeneous phenotypes have been reported in familial clusters.

In addition to influencing susceptibility to variant CJD, the polymorphism at codon 129 markedly influences the clinicopathologic phenotype of several inherited prion diseases. The most striking example of this influence is the phenotype associated with codon 178 mutation that substitutes aspartic acid with asparagine. Patients who have this mutation in combination with methionine on the mutant allele at codon 129 present with the FFI phenotype, whereas patients who have valine at codon 129 of the mutant allele present with the familial CJD phenotype. The codon 129 polymorphism may also influence the age at onset and duration of illness in some prion diseases.

Familial CJD

Patients with familial CJD generally have clinicopathologic phenotype similar to nongenetic forms of CJD. The disease has a dominant inheritance pattern and over half of affected family members carrying the mutation eventually die of CJD. Familial CJD has been reported among many family clusters from Canada, Europe, Japan, Israel, the US, and several Latin American countries. It is most frequently associated with a mutation substituting glutamic acid with lysine at codon 200 of the prion protein gene. Arguably, familial CJD associated with codon 200 mutation is the most common inheritable form of prion disease in humans. The largest familial cluster was reported among Jews of Libyan and Tunisian origin. About 14 other less-frequent mutations associated with familial CJD have been reported from many countries.

Gerstmann–Sträussler–Scheinker syndrome

The term GSS is used to describe a heterogeneous group of inherited human prion diseases that are characterized by a long duration of illness (median: ~5 years) and the presence of numerous PrP-amyloid plaques, primarily in the cerebellum. GSS carries the name of three physicians who in 1936 reported the disorder among patients spanning many generations of an Austrian family. The disease in this family was later shown to be associated with a mutation at codon 102 of the prion protein gene and may have been first identified as early as 1912.

At least 13 different types of prion protein gene mutations or a combination of mutations in at least 56 kindred or families have been reported in association with the GSS phenotype. Familial clusters with the GSS phenotype have been reported from Canada, Europe, Japan, Israel, Mexico, and the US. Many of the GSS mutations are associated with a greater degree of variability in the disease phenotype than other inherited forms of prion diseases. The most frequent GSS mutation results in leucine for proline substitution at codon 102 and is coupled with methionine at the polymorphic codon 129 of the mutant allele. Patients with this mutation commonly manifest with ataxia, dysarthria, movement disorders, and possibly dementia and akinetic mutism. The illness can last for up to 6 years in some patients with the GSS 102 mutation. In other forms of GSS, an illness duration exceeding 20 years has been reported.

Fatal familial insomnia

FFI is a human prion disease with predominant involvement of the thalamus, resulting in a clinical phenotype characterized often by intractable insomnia and autonomic nervous system dysfunction, including abnormalities in temperature regulation, increased heart rate, and hypertension. The neuropathologic lesions are more severe in the thalamus than other regions of the brain. FFI is primarily associated with a mutation at codon 178 of the prion protein gene resulting in a substitution of aspartic acid with asparagine in combination with methionine at the polymorphic codon 129 of the mutant allele.

Occasionally, sporadic FFI cases with no apparent mutation in the prion protein gene have been reported. FFI has been identified in Australia, Canada, Japan, the US, and several European countries.

Disclaimer

The findings and conclusions in this report are those of the authors and do not necessarily represent the views of the funding agency.

Further Reading

Belay ED, Maddox RA, Williams ES, Miller MW, Gambetti P, and Schonberger L (2004) Chronic wasting disease and potential transmission to humans. *Emerging Infectious Diseases* 10: 977–984.

Belay ED and Schonberger LB (2005) The public health impact of prion diseases. *Annual Review of Public Health* 26: 191–212.

Prusiner SB (1982) Novel proteinaceous infectious particles cause scrapie. *Science* 216: 136–144.

Prusiner SB (2003) *Prion Biology and Diseases,* 2nd edn., New York: Cold Spring Harbor Laboratory Press.

West Nile Virus

L D Kramer, Wadsworth Center, New York State Department of Health, Albany, NY, USA

Glossary

Bridge vector Competent mosquito vector that becomes infected following feeding on vertebrate hosts within the enzootic transmission cycle, and subsequently infects humans and other incidental hosts.

Enzootic A pathogen that is constantly present in an animal population, but usually only affects a small proportion of animals at any one time.

Epidemic Severe outbreak within a region or a group of humans.

Epizootic An outbreak of disease affecting many animals of one kind at the same time.

Extrinsic incubation period Period of time required for mosquito to transmit virus after ingesting infectious blood meal.

Neuroinvasive disease Disease caused by pathogen that infects nerve cells.

Nonviremic transmission Viral transmission to uninfected arthropod in the absence of detectable replication of virus in the vertebrate host.

Pathogenesis Origin and development of disease; more specifically the cellular events and reactions and other pathologic mechanisms occurring in the development of disease.

Phylogenetic analysis A method developed by biological systematists to reconstruct evolutionary genealogies of species based on nucleotide sequence relatedness.

Vertical transmission Viral transmission from adult female arthropod to her immediate progeny.

Viremia The presence of virus in the blood.

Zoonosis Also called zoonotic disease; refers to pathogens that can be transmitted from animals, whether wild or domesticated, to humans.

Classification

West Nile virus (WNV) is a member of the family *Flaviviridae*, genus *Flavivirus*, which is composed of approximately 70 members classified into 12 antigenic subgroups. The family *Flaviviridae* includes two additional genera, *Pestivirus* (including veterinary pathogens such as bovine viral diarrhea viruses) and *Hepacivirus* (including the human pathogen hepatitis C virus). WNV belongs to the Japanese encephalitis (JE) antigenic complex, which includes the human pathogens St. Louis encephalitis, Rocio, and Ilheus viruses in the Americas, Japanese encephalitis virus in Asia, Murray Valley encephalitis virus in Australia, and other viruses, most of them not associated with encephalitis.

History and Geographic Distribution

WNV was first isolated in 1937 from the blood of a febrile woman in the West Nile district of Uganda. The next evidence of activity occurred when WNV was isolated from mosquitoes and birds and identified as the etiologic agent in sick children in North Africa and the Middle East in the 1950s. West Nile neuroinvasive disease (WNND) was first recognized during an outbreak in elderly patients in Israel in 1957. In the 1960s, WN encephalitis in equines was recognized in Egypt and France. The largest outbreak of WN fever occurred in 1974 in Cape Province, South Africa, leading to approximately 10 000 cases. Increasing frequency of severe outbreaks began occurring in 1996 in humans and horses, largely in the Mediterranean Basin. The range of WNV expanded suddenly in 1999 with the introduction of the virus into the New York City area, although the mode of introduction is unknown. The virus became successfully established as it expanded its range westward to encompass the contiguous United States, northward into Canada in 2001, and southward beginning in 2002 into Mexico, Central America, the Caribbean and parts of South America. From 1999 to 2006, approximately 22 790 cases of WN disease were reported in the US. The largest epidemics of neuroinvasive disease caused by WNV in North America occurred in 2002 and 2003 in the US, when 2946 and 2866 cases, respectively, of WNND were identified. WNV disease also has been noted in Cuba and Argentina in addition to the US and Canada in the Western Hemisphere, but scant evidence of morbidity and mortality has been observed in tropical America. Possible reasons for the lack of overt disease in tropical America are cross-protection from other flaviviruses circulating in tropical regions, less virulent strains of WNV, less-competent arthropod and avian hosts than in temperate regions, and greater diversity of host species in the tropics.

Molecular Epidemiology

WNV is the most widely distributed flavivirus in the world (**Figure 1**). Isolates comprise two main lineages based on nucleotide sequence homology (**Figure 2**). Lineage 1 includes three clades: (1a) isolates from Africa, Asia, Europe, Middle East, North America, and Russia; (1b) isolates from Australia (Kunjin); (1c) most Indian isolates. The strain of WNV introduced into the US in 1999 has 99.7% homology in both nucleic acid and amino acid sequence

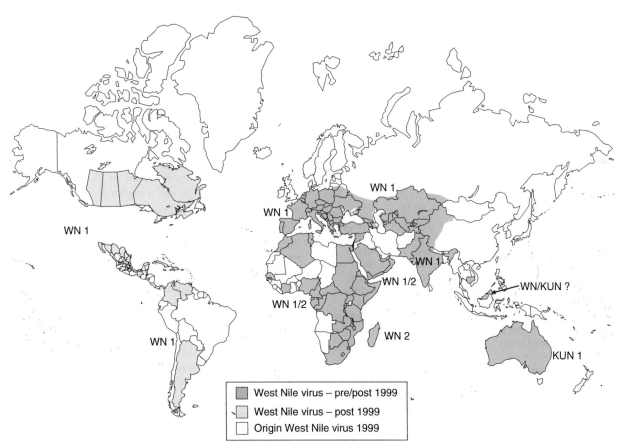

Figure 1 Global distribution of West Nile virus lineages 1 and 2. Areas in yellow have evidence of West Nile virus in the years (to 2006) following introduction of a lineage I (WN 1) virus strain in New York in 1999. This viral strain most likely originated in Israel, colored blue with yellow stripes. WN 1 viruses have been isolated from Africa, the Middle East, Europe, Russia, India, and North America. Isolations of lineage 2 WN viruses (WN 2) are found in Africa and the Middle East. Kunjin virus (KUN 1) is a subtype of lineage 1 isolated in Australia. A WN/KUN-like virus with a unique genotype (WN/KUN?) has been isolated from Sarawak, Malaysia. Modified from Scherret JH, Mackenzie JS, Hall RA, Duebel V, and Gould EA (2002) Phylogeny and molecular epidemiology of West Nile and Kunjin viruses. In: Mackenzie JS, Barrett ADT, and Duebel V (eds.) *Japanese Encephalitis and West Nile Viruses*, 379pp. Berlin, Heidelberg, and New York: Springer, with kind permission of Springer Science and Business Media.

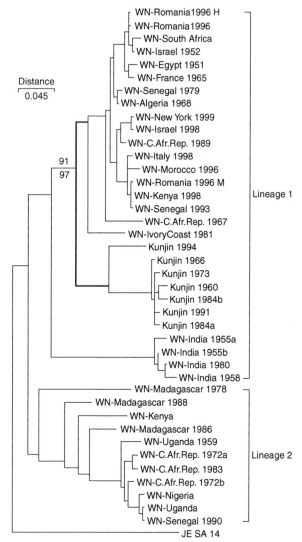

Distance
0.045

91
97

Lineage 1

Lineage 2

Figure 2 Phylogenetic tree based on E-glycoprotein nucleic acid sequence data (255 base pairs). The tree was constructed with the program MEGA by neighbor-joining with Kimura two-parameter distance (scale bar). Bootstrap confidence level (500 replicates) and a confidence probability value based on the standard error test were calculated using MEGA and are included on the tree (top and bottom values, respectively), illustrating support for the division between the lineage 1 WN virus group (not including the India isolates) and the KUN virus group. The best estimated length of the segment (bold line) separating these groups, in units of expected nucleotide substitutions per site, is 0.06928 and is statistically significantly positive ($P < 0.01$) by the likelihood ratio test (fastDNAml maximum likelihood program). An approximate 95% confidence interval for the true length of this segment is 0.03347, 0.10737. GenBank accession numbers can be found in Lanciotti RS, Roehrig JT, Deubel V, *et al.* (1999) Origin of the West Nile virus responsible for an outbreak of encephalitis in the northeastern United States. *Science* 286: 2333–2337, reproduced with permission.

with a 1998 Israeli goose isolate. Lineage 2 contains strains isolated in sub-Saharan Africa and Madagascar, and includes the prototype 1937 Ugandan isolate. Severe WNND in humans has been associated only with lineage

1 strains. The strain responsible for the South African WN fever outbreak in 1974 is in lineage 2. Comparison of isolates from lineage 1 indicates differences in virulence between North American and Afro-European strains, but the degree of difference varies with the specific avian host. Enhanced virulence of the North American strains appears to be partially correlated with envelope (E) protein glycosylation. Strains within lineage 2, while not associated with overt human outbreaks, also vary phenotypically with respect to virulence in animal models. Two potential new lineages have been identified recently; a lineage 3 virus was isolated from *Culex pipiens* in the Czech Republic (Rabensburg virus) in 1997 and 1999, and a lineage 4 virus isolated from *Dermacentor marginatus* ticks in Russia in 1998 (LEIV-Krnd88–190). Rabensburg virus showed 77–78% identity to lineage 1 and 2 WNV strains, 77% identity to strain LEIV-Krnd88–190, and 71–76% identity to other representatives of the JE antigenic complex.

Phylogenetic analyses of WNV isolates from the US indicate that the virus remains highly conserved genetically. A single conserved amino acid change in the E gene (V159A), first detected in 2001, occurred with increasing frequency from 2002 through 2004 throughout the US (**Figure 3**), and became the dominant genetic variant circulating throughout North America. This genotype, 'North American dominant', probably resulted from a random mutation that became fixed in the viral RNA of the originally introduced genotype, 'Eastern US' strain. The dominant genotype disseminates 2–4 days earlier following feeding, in *Culex* spp. mosquito vectors, effectively reducing the extrinsic incubation period and thereby increasing the reproductive ratio or R_0 of WNV. This reproductive advantage, and a higher viremia observed in some avian species, may have contributed to displacement of the Eastern US genotype. Temporal and spatial clustering of isolates suggest the occurrence in some cases of localized virus spread by mosquitoes or resident birds, and in others long-distance dispersal by migratory birds or possibly by human transport. Nonetheless, it is clear from the phylogenetic evidence based on US isolates that there was a single introduction of WNV into North America from the Old World. This is in contrast to WNV in Israel, where both lineage 1 and 2 strains are frequently introduced, most likely during bird migration.

The Virion and the Viral Genome

The West Nile virion is spherical, enveloped, approximately 50 nm in diameter, with relatively smooth surfaces and icosahedral symmetry (**Figure 4**). It contains a host-derived lipid bilayer surrounding a nucleocapsid that consists of the viral RNA complexed with multiple copies of the capsid protein. The viral genome is linear, positive-sense, single-stranded RNA, 11 029 bases in

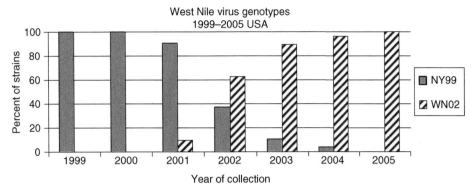

Figure 3 Prevalence of West Nile virus isolates in the United States characterized as Eastern US genotype (shaded box) and North American dominant genotype (striped box) from 2000 to 2005. Reproduced from Snapinn KW, Holmes EC, Young DS, Bernard KA, Kramer LD, and Ebel GD (2007) Declining growth rate of West Nile virus in North America. *Journal of Virology* 81(5): 2531–2534, with permission from American Society for Microbiology.

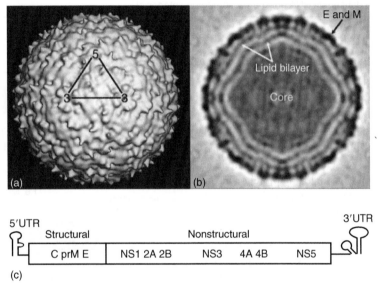

Figure 4 West Nile virion (a, b) and genome (c). WNV structure as reconstructed by cryo-EM. (a) A surface-shaded view with one asymmetric unit of the icosahedron indicated by the triangle. (b) Central section of the reconstruction, showing the concentric layers of mass density. (c) WNV genome, single-stranded positive-sense RNA, approximately 11 kb in length, consisting of a 5′ untranslated region (UTR), a single long open reading frame (ORF), and a 3′ UTR. The ORF encodes three structural and seven nonstructural proteins. (a, b) Modified from Mukhopadhyay S, Kim BS, Chipman PR, Rossmann MG, and Kuhn RJ (2003) Structure of West Nile virus. *Science* 302(5643): 248, as published in Kramer LD, Li J, and Shi PY (2007) West Nile virus: Highlights of recent advances. *Lancet Neurology* 6: 171–181, with permission from Science and Elsevier.

length. The 5′ noncoding region of WNV has a methylated type 1 cap (m^7GpppAmp); the 3′ noncoding region lacks a polyadenylated tail and in its place has a 5′-CU$_{OH}$-3′. These two regions contain conserved secondary structures critical to viral replication. The viral genome encodes three structural and seven nonstructural proteins in a single long open reading frame of 10 299 nt (nt 97–10 395), which is cleaved co- and post-translationally. The structural proteins (capsid (C), membrane (prM/M), and envelope (E)) are encoded at the 5′ end of the genome and the nonstructural proteins (NS1, NS2a, NS2b, NS3, NS4a, NS4b, and NS5) at the 3′ end. The E protein, the predominant protein of the virion,

plays a major role in viral assembly, receptor binding, and membrane fusion, and is the principal target for neutralizing antibody. The NS proteins are responsible for viral RNA replication but also may function in viral assembly and in evasion of the host immune response. The putative function and nucleotide positions of the viral proteins are listed in **Table 1**.

Replication

WNV is able to replicate in a great variety of vertebrate cells. Replication is a complex process mediated in a

Table 1 Functions and nucleotide positions of West Nile virus proteins

Viral protein	Function	Position in genome
Structural proteins		
C	Regulation of viral replication	97–465
(Pr)M	E folding and function	(466–7421) 742–966
E	Receptor binding	967–2469
	Membrane fusion	
	Viral assembly	
Nonstructural proteins (all NS proteins are required for viral replication)		
NS1	Early replication events (interaction with NS4A essential for replication)	2470–3525
NS2A[a]	Replication complex Interferon antagonist	3526–4218
NS2B[a]	Cofactor for viral protease Interferon antagonist assembly and release of virions	4219–4611
NS3	Serine protease	4612–6468
	NTPase and RTPase activity	
	RNA helicase Interferon antagonist	
NS4A[a]	Replication complex Interferon antagonist	6469–6915
NS4B[a]	Interferon antagonist Virion assembly	6916–7680
NS5	Methyl transferase	7681–10 395
	RNA dependent RNA polymerase Interferon antagonist	

[a]Functions not well characterized.

controlled fashion through sequential interactions among viral RNA, proteins and host factors (**Figure 5**). The virion initially binds to the cell receptor and then enters via receptor-mediated endocytosis. Glycosaminoglycans have been proposed as the putative receptors, although definitive proof is lacking. Following release of the nucleocapsid into the cytoplasm, the viral RNA is uncoated and translation proceeds, forming a single polyprotein which is cleaved into the ten viral proteins. Genomic plus-sense RNA is transcribed into complementary minus-sense RNA at the endoplasmic reticulum membranes, forming replication complexes, which in turn serve as templates for the synthesis of new plus-sense RNA. The process is asymmetric, yielding 10- to 100-fold excess plus strands. The plus-sense RNA is packaged by viral C protein to form the nucleocapsid that is enclosed in an envelope consisting of a host-derived lipid bilayer and viral prM/M and E proteins. prM is cleaved in the *trans*-Golgi network, while M remains inserted in the envelope of the virion. Mature virions are released from the infected cell by exocytosis beginning 10–12 h after infection.

Ecology

Vectors

WNV is a zoonosis maintained in an enzootic cycle, transmitted primarily between avian hosts and ornithophilic mosquito vectors (**Figure 6**). Mosquitoes of the genus *Culex* are the predominant vectors in the enzootic cycle throughout the range of the virus' distribution, although the particular species of *Culex* varies according to geographic location. In the northeast, *Culex pipiens* and *C. restuans* may be important enzootic catalysts in the

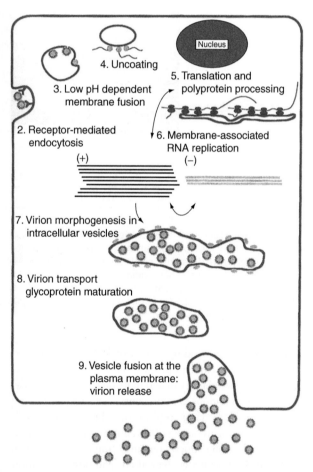

Figure 5 Flavivirus replication cycle. Highlights of the flaviviral replication cycle are diagrammed. Reproduced from Rice CM (1996) *Flaviviridae*: The viruses and their replication. In: Fields BN, Knipe DM, Howley PM, *et al*. (eds.) *Fields Virology*, 3rd edn., pp. 931–959. Philadelphia: Lippincott-Raven Publishers, with permission from Lippincott Williams and Wilkins.

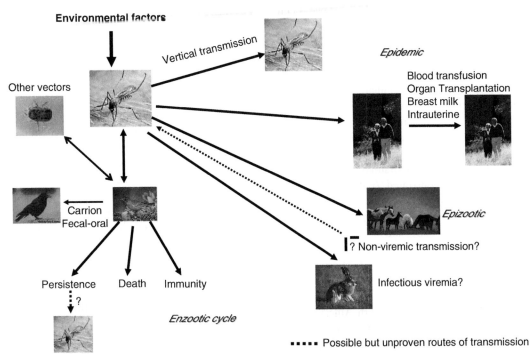

Figure 6 West Nile virus transmission cycle. The enzootic cycle is illustrated, as well as epidemic and epizootic hosts. Solid arrows indicate confirmed transmission pathways; dotted lines proposed pathways that have not been confirmed in nature.

spring, while the former, an urban species that reaches high densities in midsummer, also may be the critical vector to humans in the northeastern and north central US as well as in recent outbreaks in Europe and Israel. *C. quinquefasciatus*, a member of the *C. pipiens* complex, is the primary vector in the southern US and, presumably, Latin America. Another important vector in these locations is *C. nigripalpus*, while *C. tarsalis* is the predominant vector in rural areas of western states in the US. Other *Culex* spp., such as *C. univitattus* and *C. antennatus* (Europe and Africa), *C. vishnui complex* (India), and *C. annulirostris* (Australia) have been implicated in the transmission cycle.

Vector competence varies between species and within populations of individual species. The *C. pipiens* complex contains two genetically distinct forms, that is, *C. pipiens* form 'pipiens' and form 'molestus'. The two forms differ in physiology and behavior with obvious implications to their epidemiological importance. Form 'pipiens' is thought to be exclusively ornithophilic while the urban form 'molestus' will feed on mammals. The two forms have been shown to not interbreed in northern Europe, in contrast to US populations, which contain individuals with hybrid genetic signatures (*pipiens × molestus*). Such hybridization, which also has been noted in southern Europe, may generate bridge vectors, disposed to feed on both birds and mammals. Indeed, US populations of *C. pipiens*, as well as *C. nigripalpus* and *C. tarsalis*, have been demonstrated to shift their feeding from birds to mammals in the late summer and early fall, and therefore may

act as bridge vectors to infect equid and human hosts. It is likely that other species of bridge vectors also become involved since virus has been isolated from mosquitoes of approximately 75 species of 10 genera worldwide; but the relative importance of each species in transmission to birds or humans must take into account factors of vectorial capacity, including field infection rates and population density. Many mosquito species actually may be incidental vectors of little epidemiologic significance, but further research is required to determine their importance in the ecology and epidemiology of WNV in North America.

The mechanism(s) of WNV perpetuation over adverse seasons and years may vary by region and country, but possible mechanisms include continuous low-level virus transmission, reinitiation after reintroduction of virus by migratory birds from locations where virus is active year-round, vertical transmission to females about to enter reproductive diapause in winter, and recrudescence of low levels of virus in chronically infected birds when mosquitoes are active (**Figure 6**). Viral RNA and infectious virus have been detected in experimentally infected wild birds more than 6 weeks after inoculation. Virus has been isolated from diapausing adult *C. pipiens* in the eastern US in the winter, from vertically infected male and female *C. univitattus* in Kenya, and from *C. quinquefasciatus* larvae in California during the summer transmission season. Vertical transmission has been demonstrated in the laboratory at rates varying with the population of mosquitoes tested.

Alternate modes of vector transmission have been observed in the laboratory and/or field. Nonviremic transmission has been demonstrated in the laboratory, with low rates of infection in co-feeding mosquitoes. This mode of transmission may expand the enzootic transmission cycle to involve mammals and birds that generally mount viremias too low to infect feeding mosquitoes. WNV has been isolated repeatedly in Russia from soft ticks (*Argasidae*), but their role in the transmission cycle is not clear. In addition, soft ticks have been demonstrated to transmit virus in the laboratory, and nonviremic transmission has been demonstrated. *Ixodidae* (hard ticks) allow the virus to pass transstadially, but are incompetent vectors. Other arthropods have been suggested as alternative vectors, including dermanyssoid mites, swallow bugs, and hippoboscid flies.

Vertebrates: Birds

Birds of more than 300 species in North America have been reported infected with WNV, as determined by virus isolation or antibody, confirming their role as the primary vertebrate in the enzootic cycle. Feeding by infected mosquitoes is the most common route of infection, but transmission to birds also has been demonstrated by direct contact, presumably via the fecal–oral route since there is significant shedding of virus, and by ingestion of infected mosquitoes or of carrion by omnivorous birds such as corvids and raptors. Experimental studies indicate that birds vary significantly in susceptibility and response to infection. The hallmark of WNV activity in North America is the significant morbidity and mortality in a wide range of species, although bird deaths also have been noted in the Middle East and recently in eastern Europe. An Egyptian strain isolated in the 1950s from a sick pigeon (*Columba livia*) is virulent in experimentally infected hooded crows (*Corvus corone*) and house sparrows (*Passer domesticus*). Corvids, especially crows, magpies, and jays, appear to be the most highly susceptible to disease, with 100% of American crows (*Corvus brachyrhynchos*) becoming sick and dying after infection with low doses of WNV. Nonetheless, corvids do not appear to be the primary amplifying hosts in the enzootic transmission cycle. In the northeastern and mid-Atlantic US, the American robin (*Turdus migratorius*) appears to be highly preferred by the predominant vector *C. pipiens*. Disproportionate numbers of mosquito blood meals are taken from robins and they have high levels of IgG antibody to WNV, indicating their importance in the enzootic cycle. In the laboratory, robins have average host competence determined by susceptibility, number of days infectious, and level of viremia or mean infectiousness. High levels of WNV IgG have been detected in other birds as well, including cardinals and wrens, and in some locations, house sparrows.

Vertebrates: Other

Thirty species of mammals and occasionally other vertebrates including reptiles and amphibians have been found infected with WNV. Their role in the transmission cycle is less significant than that of birds because of their generally low levels of viremia, but some small mammals, such as rabbits and chipmunks, have been demonstrated in the laboratory to mount sufficiently high levels of virus in the blood to infect a small proportion of feeding *Culex* spp. mosquitoes. In the US and Mexico, farmed alligators raised at high temperatures in crowded conditions demonstrate significant mortality and mount high viremias. Transmission appears to occur directly between alligators, as well as through ingestion of uncooked infected horse meat. Enzootics in equines have occurred in the US, France, Italy, Morocco, and Israel. Unvaccinated equines develop infections ranging from asymptomatic to encephalitic disease, and demonstrate a case–fatality rate of approximately 25%. Because of their low viremias, they likely are incidental hosts in the transmission cycle.

Low levels of WNV antibody in domestic pets have been detected in serosurveys in the US and in the Highveld region of South Africa. In the laboratory, dogs and cats are readily infected with WNV, but dogs do not develop detectable viremia and peak titers in cats are too low to infect most mosquitoes. Cats also may become infected by the oral route following feeding on dead infected mice. Sera from wild-caught vertebrates after intensive activity in 2003 in the US also demonstrated high levels of infection in raccoons, Virginia opossums, fox squirrels, and eastern gray squirrels. It is unclear how much morbidity and mortality is associated with WNV in wild mammals, but occasional cases of overt disease have been reported. Some small mammals, such as chipmunks and rabbits, have been shown experimentally to mount viremias sufficient to infect mosquitoes.

Vertebrate Pathogenesis

Infected mosquitoes expectorate virus with their saliva mostly intradermally but also intravascularly while probing and feeding, and their salivary secretions contain potent pharmacologic compounds that affect viral pathogenesis. The initial site of viral replication in the vertebrate is thought to be subdural Langerhans' dendritic cells at the site of inoculation. Activated dendritic cells migrate to draining lymph nodes where the virus replicates further, antigen processing begins, and an early immune response may become evident. Virus enters the blood by way of the efferent lymphatics and thoracic duct, resulting in a viremia that carries the virus to the visceral organs of the body, and possibly facilitates virus crossing the blood–brain barrier. However, the mechanism for the latter is unknown and may occur via infected inflammatory cells, retrograde transport along peripheral nerve axons, replication in epithelial cells, or by another route. Neurons, the main target cell in the central nervous system, suffer pathology, as do bystander nerve cells. In addition, there is immune-mediated tissue damage.

Factors such as age, immune status, and genetic susceptibility of the host, strain of virus, dose of inoculum, and route of infection, affect pathogenesis of WNV. In the mouse, variations in a single gene, Flv, on chromosome 5, determine the rodent's susceptibility to WN disease, but not infection. Susceptibility has been mapped to the gene encoding the L1 isoform of the interferon-inducible, antiviral effector enzyme $2'-5'$-oligoadenylate synthetase. An intact immune system is critical to prevention of disease, and both humoral and cellular factors play a role in protection against disease. Neutralizing antibody is the principal means of viral clearance. Interferon-dependent innate immune responses are essential in limiting infection of WNV, as is the adaptive immune response. Complement, dendritic cells and chemokines probably also play roles in viral clearance. The mechanism by which infection is cleared from neurons appears to involve CD8+ T cells in the perforin-dependent class I major histocompatibility complex (MHC)-restricted system. Persistence of virus has been noted to occur in some vertebrates following natural and experimental infection, even in the presence of neutralizing antibody. Hamsters shed WNV in their urine for ≥ 8 months and virus can be isolated from their brains as long as 53 days after infection.

Clinical Disease

The range of symptoms associated with WNV infection extends from uncomplicated febrile illness to meningitis, neuropathies, muscle weakness, paralysis, and encephalitis. Symptoms generally become apparent 2–14 days after infection by mosquito bite, but 80% of infected individuals are asymptomatic. The majority of symptomatic patients present with flu-like symptoms, termed WN fever, which in the US has been associated with substantial morbidity. The duration of symptoms may be from days to months, and the patient may require hospitalization. WNND includes meningitis, encephalitis, and acute flaccid paralysis (AFP). From 1999 to 2007, 27 083 cases of WN disease were reported in the US, of which 57.3% were WN fever and 40.3% were WNND resulting in 1054 fatalities (3.9% of all, 9.7% of WNND) (**Table 2**). Given the proportion of symptomatic cases (~20%), approximately 135 415 individuals were infected with WNV over the 8-year period, and 8.1% of all infections were WNND. Males were more commonly infected than were females. Movement disorders, that is, dyskinesias, frequently characterized as parkinsonism are common. The constellation of fever, headache, and signs of meningeal irritation, cannot be easily discriminated from other flaviviral encephalitides. Patients with AFP experience loss of spinal anterior horn cells and have accompanying asymmetric weakness. Risk factors for WNND include age, diabetes, and possibly a history of hypertension or cardiovascular disease. The median age of WNND cases in the US since 1999 is 57 years (46 years for WNF), but there have been reports of WNND in children and AFP in young adults. Infection may persist in the central nervous system of immunologically compromised patients, leading to extended neurologic illness and sequelae. The mortality rate following WN encephalitis is greater than following WN meningitis. Immunosuppression, chronic renal disease, and hepatitis C infection have been recognized as risk factors for death after adjustment for age. Rare cases of hemorrhagic WNV disease have been noted.

The vast majority of human cases are transmitted by the bite of an infected mosquito. However, human-to-human transmission after blood transfusions, organ transplantation, and through mothers' milk have occurred in

Table 2 Human West Nile virus disease cases, United States, 1999–2005

Year	Total cases	WNND cases (% of total)	WNF cases (% of total)	Other clinical/unspecified	Fatalities (% of WNND cases)
1999	62	59	3	0	7
2000	21	19	2	0	2
2001	66	64	2	0	9
2002	4 156	2 946	1 160	50	284
2003	9 856	2 860	6 830	166	264
2004	2 539	1 142	1 269	128	100
2005	3 000	1 294	1 607	99	119
2006	4 269	1 459	2 616	194	177
2007	3 114	1 059	2 026	29	92
Total	27 083	10 902 (40.3%)	15 515 (57.3%)	666	1054 (3.9%/9.7%)

WNND, West Nile neurologic disease; WNF, West Nile fever.
Reported to CDC, as of 06 November 2007.

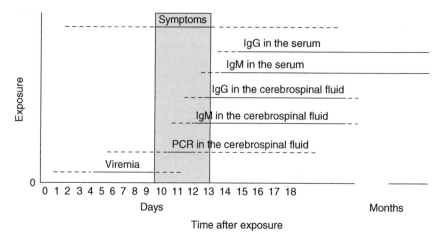

Figure 7   Schematic of virologic and serologic tests in West Nile virus encephalitis. Solid lines represent the more common results; broken lines represent reported ranges. The shaded box is an example of a typical patient. Reproduced from Gea-Banacloche J, Johnson RT, Bagic A, Butman JA, Murray PR, and Agrawal AG (2004) West Nile virus: Pathogenesis and therapeutic options. *Annals of Internal Medicine* 140: 545–553, with permission from American College of Physicians.

the US and there has been one instance of intrauterine transplacental transmission. High-throughput nucleic acid detection assays were developed and implemented by blood banks in response to transfusion transmission in order to protect the blood supply.

Diagnostics

Human

Studies of infected blood donors indicated the presence of WNV IgM and IgA at the earliest on day 3 and in all cases by day 8–9 after RNA was detected; IgG antibody appeared about 1 day later (**Figure 7**). The detection of IgM antibody in the cerebrospinal fluid (CSF) by a monoclonal antibody (MAb) capture enzyme-linked immunosorbent assay (MAC ELISA) in conjunction with evidence of neurologic symptoms has been accepted as diagnostic of WNV disease. Presence of IgM antibody in the serum alone is strongly suggestive of recent infection but not definitive due to persistence for at least 16 months (199 days in the CSF) in patients with WNND, and to some cross-reactivity with antibody to other flaviviruses. The plaque reduction neutralization test (PRNT) in Vero cell culture remains the gold standard in diagnosis of flavivirus infections because of the extensive cross-reactions complicating diagnosis. A fourfold rise in neutralizing antibody titer between paired acute-phase and convalescent-phase sera confirms WNV infection, as does a fourfold or greater titer to WNV compared to related flaviviruses. However, interpretation is complicated in individuals who have had prior infection with another flavivirus. Microsphere immuno assay (MIA) using recombinant E protein has equivalent sensitivity to ELISA. In primary flavivirus infection, the specificity of the MIA procedure is high

(>90%) compared to PRNT. However, as with PRNTs, the interpretation of WNV-E MIA is confounded when WNV is a secondary flavivirus infection. Sera from dengue (flavivirus) patients are highly likely to be positive in MIA procedures using recombinant WN E protein. Addition of WNV NS5 to a multiplex test panel increases specificity, since sera from patients with other past flavivirus infections are likely to be negative to WNV NS5 but reactive to WNV E. Serologic assays are more sensitive than detection of viral nucleic acid by reverse transcription-polymerase chain reaction (RT-PCR) once symptoms are evident because of the rapid clearance of virus by most individuals; however, detection of viral RNA is confirmatory.

Clinical findings also aid diagnosis. Neurologic symptoms indicate neuroinvasive disease. Electrophysiologic tests and magnetic resonance imaging (MRI) may be useful in cases of acute flaccid paralysis. Elevated lymphocyte counts and protein levels may be present in CSF during WNV infection. Epidemiological data also may be critical for diagnostic consideration because other flavivirus infections cause similar symptoms.

Surveillance Specimens

Submission of dead birds, particularly American crows, has provided an excellent sentinel system for WNV activity in the US, but depends upon participation by the public. In addition, over time this may not remain a reliable indicator of virus activity if selection for resistance to disease occurs. Tissues or swabs from dead birds and pooled mosquitoes are tested by real-time RT-PCR for viral nucleic acid, by cell culture procedures that detect live virus followed by confirmation using specific assays, and/or by procedures that detect viral antigen. High-throughput virus-specific molecular assays, such as real-time RT-PCR, have been developed to accommodate testing of large numbers of specimens in a timely manner. Rapid assays utilizing dip sticks to detect viral antigen also have been adopted for surveillance, but have low sensitivity. Detection of antibody in sera of live sentinel captive birds or wild-caught birds using an indirect or a competitive blocking ELISA, with confirmation by PRNT, generally has proven less useful as an early warning indicator of viral activity.

Prevention and Control

Vaccines and Therapeutics

Currently, the only available treatment for disease caused by WNV is supportive, given that no therapeutic treatment has shown consistent clinical efficacy. Therapeutic interventions include passive administration of high-titer immune immunoglobulin. MAb, in particular humanized MAb against WNV E protein, also has shown some benefit. Interferon offers promise based on animal models but may not be helpful in treating the late-stage central nervous system disease. Finally, antiviral therapy using small sequence-specific nucleic-acid-based molecules to suppress WNV replication in tissue culture is being evaluated but the timing and high dose required remain issues of concern. Targets of intervention include viral RNA polymerase, RNA helicase, or other viral replication enzymes. WNV replicon-based high-throughput screening assays have been developed to aid in discovery of compounds with potential antiviral activity.

Advances also have been made in development and implementation of effective vaccines. Protection has been demonstrated in equids following immunization with inactivated cell culture-derived virus (Ft. Dodge). Recombinant canarypox virus containing the prM and E genes of WNV also has been licensed for use in equids. Two recombinant live virus vaccines are in clinical trial in humans. One uses a yellow fever 17D strain infectious clone, with the original yellow fever virus prM and E genes replaced by attenuated WNV genes (Acambis' Chimerivax-WN), and another uses attenuated dengue virus 4 with deletions in the $3'$ end as the backbone (NIH/Macrogenics). Both live, attenuated and chimeric vaccines have the advantage of eliciting humoral and cellular responses in the host after a single dose. Other approaches include DNA vaccines that encode prM, E, or C; subunit vaccines of purified recombinant prM and E; and cross-reactive flaviviruses or WNV variants.

Public Health Measures

Reduction of WNV transmission currently relies on reduction of mosquito populations or minimizing contact between vectors and humans. Mosquito control agencies in the US have undertaken extensive larviciding to kill immature stages of mosquito vectors in the aquatic environment. Source reduction, that is, removal of standing water, also has proven helpful. Personal protection measures, for example, wearing loose clothing, use of repellents, particularly 'DEET' (*N,N*-diethyl-m-toluamide or *N,N*-diethly-3-methylbenamide), or use of window screens, reduce direct contact with mosquitoes. Community action groups have worked to increase awareness and educate the public.

Summary

The introduction of WNV to the US and its subsequent spread and successful establishment in the Western Hemisphere alerted the world to the impact of globalization on pathogen dissemination. The number of WNND cases in 2002 and 2003 represent the largest outbreak of neurologic diseases in North America. Future research undoubtedly will address development of efficacious therapeutics, effective vaccines, novel methods to control mosquitoes, and accurate risk prediction. Each of these is dependent upon solid basic research on WNV ecology, pathogenesis, and immunology.

See also: Dengue Viruses; Flaviviruses: General Features; Japanese Encephalitis Virus; Yellow Fever Virus.

Further Reading

Beasley DW (2005) Recent advances in the molecular biology of West Nile virus. *Current Molecular Medicine* 5: 835–850.

Brinton MA (2002) The molecular biology of West Nile Virus: A new invader of the Western Hemisphere. *Annual Review of Microbiology* 56: 371–402.

Davis CT, Ebel GD, Lanciotti RS, *et al.* (2005) Phylogenetic analysis of North American West Nile virus isolates, 2001–2004: Evidence for the emergence of a dominant genotype. *Virology* 25: 252–265.

Diamond MS (2005) Development of effective therapies against West Nile virus infection. *Expert Review of Anti-Infective Therapy* 3: 931–944.

Gea-Banacloche J, Johnson RT, Bagic A, Butman JA, Murray PR, and Agrawal AG (2004) West Nile virus: Pathogenesis and therapeutic options. *Annals of Internal Medicine* 140: 545–553.

Hayes CG (1989) West Nile fever. In: Monath TP (ed.) *The Arboviruses: Epidemiology and Ecology,* vol. V, ch. 49, pp. 59–88. Boca Raton, FL: CRC Press.

Hayes EB and Gubler DJ (2006) West Nile virus: Epidemiology and clinical features of an emerging epidemic in the United States. *Annual Review of Medicine* 57: 181–194.

Kramer LD, Li J, and Shi PY (2007) West Nile virus: Highlights of recent advances. *Lancet Neurology* 6(2): 171–181.

Lanciotti RS, Roehrig JT, Deubel V, *et al.* (1999) Origin of the West Nile virus responsible for an outbreak of encephalitis in the northeastern United States. *Science* 286: 2333–2337.

Monath TP and Heinz FX (1996) Flaviviruses. In: Fields BN, Knipe DM, Howley PM, *et al.* (eds.) *Fields Virology,* 3rd edn., pp. 961–1034. Philadelphia: Lippincott-Raven Publishers.

Mukhopadhyay S, Kim BS, Chipman PR, Rossmann MG, and Kuhn RJ (2003) Structure of West Nile virus. *Science* 302(5643): 248.

Rice CM (1996) *Flaviviridae*: The viruses and their replication. In: Fields BN, Knipe DM, Howley PM, *et al.* (eds.) *Fields Virology,* 3rd edn., pp. 931–959. Philadelphia: Lippincott-Raven Publishers.

Scherret JH, Mackenzie JS, Hall RA, Duebel V, and Gould EA (2002) Phylogeny and molecular epidemiology of West Nile and Kunjin viruses. In: Mackenzie JS, Barrett ADT, and Duebel V (eds.) *Japanese Encephalitis and West Nile Viruses*, 379pp. Berlin, Heidelberg, and New York: Springer.

Shi PY and Wong SJ (2003) Serologic diagnosis of West Nile virus infection. *Expert Review Molecular Diagnostics* 3: 733–741.

Smithburn KC, Hughes TP, Burke AW, *et al.* (1940) A neurotropic virus isolated from the blood of a native Ugandan. *American Journal of Tropical Medicine* 20: 471–492.

Snapinn KW, Holmes EC, Young DS, Bernard KA, Kramer LD, and Ebel GD (2007) Declining growth rate of West Nile virus in North America. *Journal of Virology* 81(5): 2531–2534.

Yellow Fever Virus

A A Marfin, Centers for Disease Control and Prevention, Atlanta, GA, USA
T P Monath, Kleiner Perkins Caufield and Byers, Menlo Park, CA, USA

Glossary

Aedes A genus of mosquitoes strongly involved in the transmission of yellow fever virus.

Aedes (Ae.) aegypti is a species belonging to the genus that breeds in close association with humans and is often responsible for epidemics of yellow fever.

Flavivirus A virus in the genus *Flavivirus*.

Genotype Genetic composition of an individual (virus), used to delineate relatedness of individuals.

Host A vertebrate species (including humans) infected by virus. An effective host is one that develops viremia sufficient to infect vectors and thus contributes to the virus transmission cycle.

Pathogenesis The process whereby virus infection proceeds in the host, leading to spread of the infection to vital organs and the development of damage to cells and tissues.

Transmission cycle The sequential infection of blood-feeding vectors and vertebrate hosts responsible for maintaining and amplifying virus in nature.

Vector An arthropod (e.g., mosquito or tick) capable of becoming actively infected by blood feeding and of subsequently transmitting virus to a vertebrate host.

Introduction

Yellow fever virus (YFV) is the prototype species of the virus family *Flaviviridae* (and of the genus *Flavivirus*), which includes approximately 70 single-stranded RNA viruses, most of which are transmitted by mosquitoes or ticks. Other viruses in this family include the four dengue viruses, West Nile virus, Japanese encephalitis virus, and tick-borne encephalitis viruses.

History

Yellow fever (YF) is the original 'viral hemorrhagic fever', a systemic illness characterized by high viremia; hepatic, renal, and myocardial injury; hemorrhage; and high lethality. Genetic sequence analysis reveals that YFV diverged from the ancestral flaviviral lineage, roughly 3000 years ago, earlier than did other mosquito-borne flaviviruses. The first description of epidemic hematemesis occurred in Mexico in 1648, which suggests that the virus and its mosquito vector, *Aedes aegypti*, were introduced from Africa with the slave trade. Furthermore, monkeys of New World species are more susceptible to lethal infection than are African monkeys, also suggesting that YFV was recently introduced. The West African and South American genotypes of YFV are more closely related to each other than to other genotypes, indicating the probable source of introduction. During the eighteenth and nineteenth centuries, YF epidemics affected coastal cities in the Americas and Europe; the disease was likely introduced via ships infested with YFV-infected mosquitoes. In the mid- and late nineteenth century, physicians, most notably Carlos Findlay, suggested that YFV was transmitted by mosquitoes. In 1900, Walter Reed and colleagues demonstrated that the agent was a filterable virus transmitted by *Ae. aegypti* mosquitoes. In 1927, YFV was isolated from a Ghanaian man; efforts to establish continuous direct passage in animals resulted in establishment of the Asibi strain. Isolation of the Asibi strain and a contemporary ('French') strain isolated in Dakar, Senegal, enabled development of quantitative methods that allowed more precise scientific studies, as well as two live, attenuated vaccines.

Taxonomy, Classification, and Variation

YFV is antigenically distinguished from all other flaviviruses by neutralization test, and all strains of YFV belong to a single serotype. Among flaviviruses, YFV is more closely related to Wesselsbron, Sepik, Edge Hill, Bouboui, Uganda S, Banzi, Jugra, Saboya, and Potiskum viruses.

Wild-type YFV is genetically stable compared to other RNA viruses, likely due to restrictions imposed by replication in vertebrate and invertebrate hosts and maintained by a high-fidelity RNA-dependent RNA polymerase. Despite this stability, genomic sequence analyses of structural and nonstructural genes and of YFV-specific repeat sequences have identified at least seven distinct genotypes. Analyses indicate YFV arose in Africa and divided into West and East African genotypes prior to introduction into the Americas. Currently, five African genotypes are recognized – West Africa I, West Africa II, East/Central Africa, East Africa, and Angola. South American YFV can be divided into two genotypes – South America I (in Brazil) and South America II (in the western part of the continent). These genotypes demonstrate a high degree of homology but can frequently be clustered by time periods, geography, and by predominant transmission patterns.

Properties of the Virion

YFV virions are small (40–60 nm diameter), spherical, and have short surface projections. The icosohedral nucleocapsid contains the single-stranded RNA genome and a single core protein (C protein), and is surrounded by a lipid bilayer. Viral infectivity is rapidly inactivated by heat (56 °C for 30 min), ultraviolet radiation, and lipid detergents.

Properties of the Genome

The YFV genome is comprised of a single strand of plus-sense (i.e., infectious) RNA that contains 10 862 nt and is composed of a 118-nt 5′ noncoding region (NCR) preceded by a type 1 cap structure, a single open reading frame (ORF) of 10 233 nt that encodes 11 viral proteins, and a 511-nt 3′ NCR without a polyadenylated tail. The 5′ and 3′ NCRs have conformational structure and complementary sequences that are important in cyclization of the viral genome during encapsidation and replication and which function as promoters during replication. Mutations or deletions in these regions affect replication and virulence. The 3′ NCR contains conserved consensus sequences which pair with 5′ NCR sequences during cyclization and serve as the common recognition site for the viral polymerase. Directly upstream from these sequences, the 3′ NCR forms a 3′ terminal hairpin structure and pseudoknots to serve as promoters for genomic replication.

Viral Proteins

The ORF encodes three structural proteins at the 5′ end (capsid (C), pre-membrane (preM), and envelope (E) proteins), followed downstream by 7 nonstructural (NS) proteins (NS1–NS2A–NS2B–NS3–NS4A–NS4B–NS5). The mature virion includes these three structural proteins, while the NS proteins are responsible for replication and polyprotein processing including cleavage of the polyprotein into proteins.

The C protein (MW ∼ 11 kDa) interacts with genomic RNA to form the virion nucleocapsid, anchors the nucleocapsid to the endoplamic reticulum, and provides signal sequence to the preM protein. The preM glycoprotein (∼27 kDa) forms an intracellular heterodimer to stabilize the E protein during exocytosis. During exocytosis, the preM protein is processed by a furin-like protease leaving a small M structural protein (∼8 kDa) anchored in the virus envelope of the extracellular virion. The M protein spans the viral membrane and has exposed antigenic domains that may induce a minor immunologic response. Abnormal preM/M cleavage may result in incorporation of preM into mature virions that later affect E protein conformation, inhibit fusion, and reduce infectivity.

The E protein (∼50 kDa) is the major surface structure glycoprotein. The three-dimensional configuration of the E protein forms three domains, is determined by disulfide bonding, and is critical for its role in cell tropism, membrane fusion, virulence, and immunity. Strain-, type-, and flavivirus group-specific epitopes are present in this glycoprotein. The hydrophobic C-terminus of this protein is anchored to the lipid bilayer of the viral envelope by a 170-Å-long rod. The C-terminus is connected by a flexible region to domain I, the central part of the molecule with up-and-down topology having eight antiparallel β-strands and containing the N-terminus. Inhibition of this flexible region results in decreased infectivity. Two long loops in domain II extend laterally and are responsible for dimerization. A conserved stretch of 14 amino acids in these loops is the fusion domain that allows internalization of the nucleocapsid into the infected cell. Domain III contains sites involved in binding cell receptors. Conformational neutralization determinants are scattered on the outer surface of all three domains.

The NS1 glycoprotein is involved in RNA replication through its interaction with NS4A and is both expressed on the cell surface and released extracellularly. The extracellular form contains virus-specific and cross-reactive epitopes. Antibodies to NS1 do not neutralize virus infectivity but do provide protective immunity by complement-mediated lysis and rapid clearance of cells with NS1 on the surface. NS1 is highly conserved across all YF strains. NS2A is a small protein (∼22 kDa) that interacts with NS3, NS5, and 3′ NCR sequences and plays an important role in RNA replication and in the assembly or release of virions. NS3 (∼70 kDa) and NS2B (∼14 kDa) interact to form a complex with important enzymatic functions, including serine protease (responsible for post-translational cleavage of virus polyprotein), RNA helicase, and RNA triphosphatase activities. Because of its critical functions, the NS3 gene sequence is also highly conserved. NS3 is also present in cell membranes, contains virus-specific T-cell epitopes that are targets for cytotoxic T-cells. The NS4A (~16 kDa) and NS4B (~27 kDa) proteins are membrane associated and play a role in regulating RNA replication. The NS5 protein (~103 kDa) is a highly conserved RNA-dependent RNA polymerase in virus replication and methyltransferase during 5' cap methylation.

Assembly and Replication

Assembly of these proteins into viral particles and subsequent exocytosis of mature virions occur in close association with the endoplasmic reticulum of secretory cells (e.g., mosquito salivary gland and various mammal exocrine and endocrine glands). Virion assembly occurs in concert with host cell secretory components and virions are released in secretory granules without significantly disturbing host cellular function or macromolecular synthesis.

After release, virions enter uninfected host cells by attaching to still-undefined receptors and are taken up in clathrin-coated vesicles. Following an acid-mediated change in the E protein that allows fusion of the virus with the host's endosomal membrane, nucleocapsids are released from the vesicles into the cytoplasm. The full-genome-length, plus-sense RNA is translated to make complementary minus strands that serve as templates for progeny plus strands. These plus strands serve as mRNAs for translation of structural and NS proteins including enzymes required for continued virus production and post-translational cleavage of the polyprotein; as templates for the transcription of new minus-sense strands; and as genomes of newly produced mature virions.

Molecular Determinants of Virulence

The entire genomes of the 17D and Asibi strains and of the French neurotropic vaccine and French viscerotropic strains have been sequenced and compared. Comparing sequences and different biological properties of these pairs allows insight into molecular determinants of virulence. Although some potentially important specific sequences have been identified, virulence is clearly multigenic and determined by nonstructural and structural genes. Most studies on these molecular determinants have employed mouse models. Because mice manifest neurotropism and not viscerotropism, such studies are of limited value in dissecting pathogenesis. More recent studies in hamsters susceptible to lethal hepatic dysfunction and necrosis resembling wild-type YFV may allow identifying genetic sequences associated with viscerotropism, but YFV strains

must be adapted by serial passage in hamsters before they elicit disease. Nonhuman primates are susceptible to wild-type YFV strains and develop a syndrome closely resembling that in humans.

The 17D and Asibi strains differ at four nucleotides in the 3' NCR and 20 amino acids in the coding region – eight in the E gene; four in the NS2A gene; two in the NS5 gene; and one each in the M, NS1, NS2B, NS3, NS4A, and NS4B genes.

Given the functional importance of E protein in attachment of YFV to and entry into the cell, one or more of the amino acid differences in this protein likely plays a role in attenuation. Mutations in three areas of E protein alter virulence properties – the tip of the fusion domain in domain II, the molecular hinge between domains I and II, and the portion of domain III containing the putative receptor ligand. Of the eight amino acids that distinguish E proteins of Asibi and 17D viruses four are nonconservative, suggesting that one or more may be responsible for attenuation. Three of these nonconservative changes occur in the hinge region and likely alter the acid-dependent change in E protein conformation required for virus entry. Of nonconservative mutations outside of the hinge region, two (E305 and E380) are located in domain III, which contains determinants involved in tropism and cell attachment. The mutation at amino acid E380 of YF 17D occurs in the putative integrin cell receptor. Studies of this region in other flaviviruses also suggest that mutations in the putative cell receptor-binding region of domain III play a role in determining neurovirulence.

Other studies emphasize the multigenic nature of virulence and suggest that one or more of the 11 amino acid changes in NS proteins, or base changes in the 3' NCR, may contribute to attenuation. Studies with other flaviviruses have shown that mutations in the NS proteins reduce neurovirulence, probably because NS proteins are critical to the virus replication mechanism. Eleven amino acid changes in the NS proteins of Asibi strain viruses occurred during derivation of the 17D vaccine strain. These changes in NS proteins may affect assembly or release of YFV particles, changes in the RNA helicase and triphosphatase enzymes for unwinding RNA during replication, and activity of the RNA-dependent RNA polymerase. Similarly, the 3' NCR terminal region is involved in folding of the stem–loop structure which serves as a critical promoter during replication. Changes in this sequence or the number of repeat sequences may alter the stem–loop region, interfere with virus replication, and contribute to attenuation.

Little is known about the determinants of YFV viscerotropism (the ability of YFV to replicate and damage non-neural tissue, such as the liver) principally because assessing this property in nonhuman primates is difficult. Because neuro- and viscerotropic properties may reside in distinct regions, one cannot conclude that attenuation of one correlates with attenuation of the other. However, the hinge region of the E protein contains residues implicated in both neurotropism and viscerotropism. Studies in golden hamsters, which develop disease resembling human YFV, suggest that domain III sites implicated as cell receptor ligands are responsible for hepatotropism.

Host Range and Virus Propagation

A highly conserved region in the domain III of the E protein contains an arginine-glycine-aspartic acid (RGD) motif and is the likely site of virus-cell attachment. Because of the broad host range of flaviviruses, the receptors are highly conserved structures found in chordate and arthropod phyla. YFV replicates and produces cytopathic changes and plaque formation in a wide variety of cell types including primary chick and duck embryo cells; continuous porcine, hamster, rabbit, and monkey kidney cell lines; and cells of human origin such as HeLa, KB, Chang liver, and SW-13. The virus replicates in Fc receptor-bearing macrophages and macrophage cell lines; replication is enhanced by antibody. Mosquito cell lines, especially AP-16 cells, are highly susceptible and often used for primary isolation or efficient laboratory propagation.

Virus isolation is accomplished by intrathoracic inoculation of *Toxorhynchites* or *Ae. aegypti* mosquitoes, inoculation of mosquito cell line cultures (i.e., AP61 and C6/36 cells), intracerebral inoculation of suckling mice or inoculation of specific nonhuman primates. Intrathoracic inoculation of mosquitoes is the most sensitive method. Because infected mosquitoes show no signs of infection, virus is demonstrated by immunofluorescence, subsequent passage to a susceptible host, or amplification of YFV RNA sequences by reverse transcriptase-polymerase chain reaction (RT-PCR). AP61 cells are more sensitive than other *in vitro* methods for primary isolation and show cytopathic effects within 5–7 days of inoculation. Immunofluorescence assays to identify viral antigens and RT-PCR to identify RNA sequences are positive before development of cytopathic effects.

Susceptible vertebrate hosts that show signs of infection include infant mice, which develop fatal encephalitis when infected by peripheral or intracerebral routes; mice greater than 8 days old develop fatal encephalitis only following intracerebral challenge. Nonhuman primates of many species develop fatal hepatitis resembling human disease. The only nonprimate species that develop lethal hepatitis following infection are the European hedgehog and the golden hamster. Antibodies to YFV have been found in a wide variety of field-collected wild vertebrates and wild animals such as rodents and bats. With the exception of opossums in South America, there is no support for a role of nonprimate species in the transmission cycle.

Geographic and Seasonal Distribution

YF occurs in tropical South America and sub-Saharan Africa, where the enzootic transmission cycle involves tree-hole-breeding mosquitoes and nonhuman primates. *Aedes aegypti*-infested regions of Central and North America, the Caribbean, and Southern Europe had periodic outbreaks through the early 1900s and are considered at risk, should the virus be reintroduced. Despite the prevalence of *Ae. aegypti* in tropical Asia, YFV has not appeared. Cross-protection by immunity to dengue viruses may decrease the probability that YFV can be transported from inaccessible, endemic parts of Africa and South America. Low vector competence of Asian populations of *Ae. aegypti* may be responsible for diminishing the risk of virus transmission. Areas at highest risk for reintroduction of virus and secondary spread by re-emerging *Ae. aegypti* include coastal regions and interior towns throughout equatorial South America, Panama, Central America, the West Indies, Mexico, and the southern United States. All are areas affected by YF in the past.

Breeding of many mosquito species that transmit YFV occurs in tree holes and is dependent on rainfall; consequently, transmission increases during tropical rainy seasons and decreases or stops during dry seasons. The peridomestic vector *Ae. aegypti* breeds in receptacles used by humans for water storage, and is less dependent on rainfall. Where this mosquito is involved in virus transmission, YF may occur in the dry season in both rural and urban areas. Temperature also influences YFV transmission rates; a few degrees increase may shorten the extrinsic incubation period (a period of viral replication in a recently infected mosquito prior to the mosquito being capable of transmitting virus to a host) by days, resulting in a significantly increased rate of transmission. Warm temperature also increases biting and reproductive rates of *Ae. aegypti*.

Disease Incidence

Official notifications of disease likely underestimate disease incidence and case–fatality rate, although underreporting occurs to variable degree. During the 20-year period ending in 2004, 28 264 cases and 7880 deaths were reported to the World Health Organization (WHO). In Africa, which accounted for 24 684 cases (87%), the annual incidence varied between 1 and 5104 cases, suggesting highly variable reporting. Despite inconsistent reporting, enzootic and endemic transmission was known to occur continuously in affected regions. During this period, Africa reported 5815 or 74% of the worldwide deaths due to YF, with a case–fatality rate of 24%. The frequency and intensity of epidemics in Africa are due to interhuman transmission by mosquito vectors present in high-density, high-human populations, and low immunization coverage. West Africa appears to be at highest risk of YF emergences, probably reflecting the role of domestic *Ae. aegypti* mosquito vectors. In South America, YF occurs in the Amazon region and contiguous areas. Between 1985 and 2004, 3580 cases and 2074 deaths (case–fatality rate 58%) were reported to WHO by South American countries. The annual incidence varies by country due to fluctuating epizootic activity. The incidence of YF in South America is roughly 20% of that of Africa, due to transmission by enzootic as opposed to epidemic vectors, lower densities of vectors, monkeys and human hosts, and relatively high vaccination coverage. The higher case–fatality rate in South America probably reflects the reporting of more severe cases there, and the fact that surveillance there is based on death reports and postmortem liver examination, although it remains possible that the South American genotype(s) is more virulent than those in Africa.

Epidemiology and Transmission Cycles

YFV is present at high titers in the blood of infected, susceptible hosts (humans and nonhuman primates) for several days, during which mosquito vectors collecting a blood meal may become infected. Virus replicates sequentially in the midgut epithelium, body, and salivary glands of the mosquito. The period between the infecting blood meal and the point at which sufficient replication allows transmission to a vertebrate host is the 'extrinsic incubation period'. This is a temperature-dependent process and takes roughly a week to complete.

Transmission cycles differ according to the hosts and vectors involved. Although the resulting clinical disease does not differ, recognizing the type of cycle is important for disease control. The 'urban cycle' involves humans as the viremic host and *Ae. aegypti* breeding in peridomestic, man-made containers that hold unpolluted water. The 'sylvatic cycle', the predominant pattern in equatorial rain forests of Africa and South America, involves transmission between nonhuman primates and tree-hole-breeding mosquito vectors. In Africa, a third cycle, the 'savanna cycle', is recognized in moist grasslands bordering the rain forests where *Aedes* mosquitoes other than *Ae. aegypti* feed on both humans and nonhuman primates. In all of these settings, the rate of transmission varies widely depending on the density of vectors and the presence of susceptible primates. Primates of many nonhuman species are susceptible to YFV infection. Most African primates produce viremias sufficient to infect mosquitoes without developing illness, whereas many South American primates develop lethal infections. Depletion of vertebrate hosts through natural immunization and death during epizootic waves is a factor in the cyclic appearance of YF activity. In many areas, with environmental pressures markedly reducing monkey populations, human beings serve as hosts in the YFV transmission cycle. No nonprimate species are involved in enzootic transmission.

The risk of nonimmune persons becoming infected is determined by geographic location, season, activities that lead to exposure, duration of exposure to mosquito bites, and the intensity of YFV transmission. Although reported cases of human disease are an important guide to YFV activity, reported numbers may be low due to a high level of immunity in the population or to insensitive surveillance. In areas where vaccination is widely practiced, YFV may circulate between monkeys and mosquitoes, with few human cases occurring.

The means of survival of YFV across long dry seasons, when sylvatic mosquito vectors are absent, remains in question. Transovarial transmission to *Aedes* and *Haemagogus* mosquito eggs, which survive desiccation in tree holes and hatch when the rains return, likely play a major role. Low-level horizontal transmission by drought-resistant vectors, and alternative horizontal and vertical transmission cycles involving ticks, are theorized mechanisms. Although persistent infection of experimentally infected nonhuman primates has been documented, infections in these hosts generally are not accompanied by viremia sufficiently high to infect vectors.

The most alarming future prospect involves the reemergence of urban transmission in South America and the spread to heavily populated, *Ae. aegypti*-infested areas currently free from disease, such as the coastal regions of South America, the Caribbean, and North America, and regions where the virus has never become established but which have susceptible human populations and competent mosquito vectors, such as the Middle East, coastal East Africa, the Indian subcontinent, Asia, and Australia. Alterations in human demography and behavior, in virus activity, and in the distribution of *Ae. aegypti* underlie the potential for epidemiological change. Such alterations include: (1) increasing urban populations; (2) changes in commerce, transportation, and communication that allow human population expansion into previously remote endemic zones; (3) reinvasion of South America by the peridomestic *Ae. aegypti*; (4) presence of efficient jungle vectors in degraded periurban habitats; (5) introduction of new competent *Aedes* species (e.g., *Ae. albopictus*) that may bridge the jungle and urban transmission cycles; (6) relaxation of regulations and of enforcement of vaccination certification for travelers; and (7) possibly climate change.

Laboratory-acquired infections were common in the pre-vaccine era and remain of concern today, particularly where unvaccinated clinical laboratory personnel encounter blood from patients in early stages of illness.

Some laboratory infections were probably acquired via bites of experimentally infected mosquitoes or of wild mosquitoes infected after feeding on experimental animals. Others resulted from direct contact with blood or aerosols of dried virus. The stability of YFV permits transmission within a short period after generation of an infectious aerosol.

Clinical Features

The broad clinical spectrum of YF includes abortive infection with nonspecific flu-like illness, and 'classic' YF – potentially lethal pansystemic disease with fever, jaundice, renal failure, and hemorrhage. Serosurveys to identify persons with asymptomatic infections estimate that only about 15–25% of infected persons develop classic YF. Diagnosis of sporadic cases without classic symptoms is difficult; as a result, often only cases of classic YF are notified, and deaths may be more frequently notified than cases. These features lead to an underestimate of morbidity and overestimate of case–fatality rate. The variability in clinical response to infection is multifactoral and includes intrinsic and acquired host resistance factors and differences in pathogenicity of virus strains.

Classic YF is a triphasic disease that begins with abrupt onset of fever, headache, myalgia, anorexia, and nausea 3–6 days after infection. This 'period of infection' is clinically nonspecific but corresponds to a viremic phase when a person is infectious to feeding mosquitoes. Fatal cases appear to have a longer duration of viremia than do survivors. After 3–4 days, a 'period of remission', lasting up to 48 h, begins with abatement of fever and symptoms. Cases of abortive infection simply recover at this stage. Because such cases remain anicteric with nonspecific symptoms, clinical diagnosis of YF is not possible. Roughly 15–25% of persons infected with YFV enter a 'period of intoxication', typically 3–5 days after onset, characterized by a moderate to severe disease characterized by jaundice, the return of fever, relative bradycardia, oliguria, hemetemesis, and other hemorrhagic diatheses. Virus disappears from blood and antibodies appear 7–10 days after infection. The subsequent course reflects dysfunction of the hepatic, renal, and cardiovascular systems. Central nervous system (CNS) signs include delirium, convulsions, and coma. In severe cases, the cerebrospinal fluid is under increased pressure and may contain elevated protein but no cells. No inflammatory changes have been found in brains of persons with severe illness; cerebral edema or metabolic factors apparently cause CNS signs. Between the fifth and tenth day of illness, the patient either dies or recovers rapidly. Terminal events are characterized by hypotension, shock, and respiratory distress.

Pathology and Pathogenesis

Two biological properties are inherent to all wild-type YFV strains: 'viscerotropism', the ability to cause viremia and subsequently to infect and damage liver, heart, and kidneys, and 'neurotropism', the ability to infect the brain parenchyma causing encephalitis. Wild-type YFV strains are predominantly viscerotropic in humans and in nonhuman primates. True YF viral encephalitis is rare; even after intracerebral inoculation of YFV, susceptible nonhuman primates die from hepatitis rather than from encephalitis.

The course of infection following inoculation of wild-type YFV has been partially investigated using nonhuman primates. Virus replicates at the site of skin inoculation and spreads to draining lymph nodes, then to central lymph nodes, and subsequently to visceral organs. Lymphoid cells are early viral replication sites, and in the liver Kupffer cells in the sinusoids are the gateway to subsequent hepatocyte infection. Results of prior research, primarily of dengue infections, makes clear that dendritic cells (DCs) play a primary role in the early stages of infection, and that these cells not only process viral antigens into immunogenic peptides and present them to T-cells, but also secrete a cascade of immunoregulatory cytokines that shape innate and adaptive immune responses.

In humans with viscerotropic disease, degeneration of hepatocytes occurs in the last phase of infection. In fatal cases, up to 100% of hepatocytes undergo coagulative necrosis characteristic of apoptosis. The mid-zone of the liver lobule is principally affected, with sparing of cells bordering the central vein and portal tracts. Viral antigen and viral RNA are demonstrable in cells undergoing pathological changes, suggesting that cytopathology is mediated by direct injury from virus replication and from accumulation of virions and viral protein in the endoplasmic reticulum. The reason for this peculiar distribution of hepatic injury is unknown; mid-zonal necrosis has been described in low-flow hypoxia, ATP depletion and oxidative stress of marginally oxygenated cells at the border between anoxic and normoxic cells. Eosinophilic degeneration with condensed nuclear chromatin (Councilman bodies), indicative of apoptosis, characterizes hepatocyte injury rather than the ballooning and rarefaction necrosis seen in hepatitis caused by other viruses. Inflammatory changes are minimal and persons who survive YF do not develop scarring or cirrhosis due to this infection. Eosinophilic degeneration without inflammation, along with fatty change of renal tubular epithelium, also characterizes renal pathology. Focal degeneration may be present in myocardial cells. Lymphoid follicles of lymph nodes and spleen show necrosis. The brain shows edema and petechial hemorrhage but viral invasion and encephalitis are rare. Decreased hepatic synthesis of clotting factors causes hemorrhagic manifestations.

The mediators of the profound shock of YF are unknown but cytokine dysregulation (systemic inflammatory response syndrome, SIRS) likely mediates this terminal stage as in other sepsis syndromes. The appearance of antibody and cellular responses coincides with onset of the 'period of intoxication', suggesting that immune clearance may be, in part, responsible for the cytokine storm events. Persons with fatal YF have elevated pro-inflammatory cytokines compared to persons with nonfatal cases of YF, resembling the profile seen in bacterial sepsis. Overall, these findings suggest that high levels of pro-inflammatory cytokines contribute to lethality.

Immune Responses

Prior to appearance of specific cytotoxic T-cells and immunoglobulins, innate immunity, comprised of natural killer (NK) cells, interferons (IFNs), and other pro-inflammatory cytokines, play a significant role in limiting viral replication during early infection. NK cells recognize and lyse cells displaying viral antigens; secrete IFN-α and pro-inflammatory cytokines that have direct antiviral activity; activate DCs and macrophages; and promote a Th1 adaptive immune response. YFV antigens directly activate DCs via type I IFN signal transduction and Toll-like receptors. Through Toll-like receptor activation, pro-inflammatory molecules (e.g., interleukins IL1-β, IL2, IL6, IL8, IL12) are expressed and further activate NK cells. This robust innate response to YFV likely underlies the rapid, strong, and durable adaptive responses to this virus. Flaviviruses have evolved weak mechanisms for avoiding these innate responses, including blocking the IFN signal transducer pathways by NS2A and NS4B. Those patients with a poor outcome may develop signs of a dysregulated pro-inflammatory cytokine response (SIRS).

Seven to ten days after infection, a specific immune response is detectable when immunoglobulin M (IgM; enzyme-linked immunosorbent assay, ELISA), hemagglutination-inhibiting, and neutralizing antibodies begin to appear. IgM antibodies peak during the second week and usually decline rapidly over the next 30–60 days while neutralizing antibody continues to increase. When YFV represents the patient's first flavivirus infection, the magnitude of the IgM response is significantly greater than in persons with prior flavivirus exposure. Although little is known about cytolytic antibodies against viral proteins on the surface of infected cells, antibody-dependent cell-mediated cytotoxicity (ADCC), and cytotoxic T-cells, these mechanisms, in addition to neutralizing antibody, presumably mediate clearance of primary infection. Based on immunologic studies of YFV vaccine recipients, neutralizing antibody generally peaks 4–6 weeks after infection but high titers of neutralizing antibodies persist for more than 10 years and provide complete protection against

disease on reexposure to the virus. No documented case of a second clinical YFV infection has ever been reported. Although initial antibody response to infection is YFV antigen specific, with affinity maturation, specificity declines and cross-reactions with other flaviviruses develop during the subsequent several week of the immune response. Persons with prior heterologous flavivirus immunity develop broadly cross-reactive antibody responses during YFV infections. Previous infection with flaviviruses, such as Zika, dengue, or Wesselsbron viruses, provides partial cross-protection against YFV and may ameliorate the clinical severity of YF.

Prevention and Control

Domestic control of *Ae. aegypti* mosquitoes remains important but is difficult to sustain. Currently, the most effective approach to control of YF is by immunizing persons living in or traveling to endemic areas. 17D vaccine is the only strain currently used for human immunization against YFV. It is a live, attenuated vaccine produced in embryonated chicken eggs. 17D vaccines are not biologically cloned and are heterogeneous mixtures of multiple virion subpopulations ('genetic swarms'); differences in plaque size, oligonucleotide fingerprints, and nucleotide sequences have been found but do not appear to affect safety or efficacy. Currently, manufacturers in seven countries market YFV 17D vaccine. Three manufacturers in Brazil, France, and Senegal produce large amounts of vaccine for the Expanded Programme of Immunization and for mass vaccination campaigns. As of 2006, annual global vaccine production was approximately 60 million doses. Monath *et al.* thoroughly review the development, immune response, and efficacy of the 17D vaccine strain.

As of 2006, over 400 million persons have been immunized with YFV vaccines. Over roughly 70 years of use, 17D vaccines have been acknowledged as one of the safest and most effective live vaccines in use. Recently, however, close scrutiny has been brought to bear as clinical and histopathological evidence has emerged linking 17D vaccines to severe and previously unrecognized adverse events, including viscerotropic disease closely resembling that caused by wild-type YFV. Although rare mutational events in 17D vaccine virus during replication in the host can alter pathogenicity, these recently reported serious adverse events were not associated with either mutations that change virulence or tropism of the virus or selection of virulent variants *in vivo*. Investigations suggest that host susceptibility, rather than a change in the virus, is responsible for these serious, adverse events. Advanced age and thymic disease appear to be risk factors for development of vaccine-associated viscerotropic disease. The incidence of this complication, which carries a case–fatality rate of approximately 50%, is believed to be 1:400 000.

Further Reading

Barrett ADT and Monath TP (2003) Epidemiology and ecology of yellow fever. *Advances in Virus Research* 61: 291–317.

Carter HR (1931) *Yellow Fever: An Epidemiological and Historical Study of Its Place of Origin.* Baltimore, MD: Williams and Wilkins.

Cordellier R (1991) The epidemiology of yellow fever in western Africa. *Bulletin of the World Health Organization* 69(1): 73–84.

Monath TP and Barrett ADT (2003) Pathogenesis and pathophysiology of yellow fever. *Advances in Virus Research* 60: 343–397.

Monath TP, Teuwen D, and Cetron M (in press) Yellow fever vaccine. In: Plotkin SA, Orenstein WA, and Offit PA (eds.) *Vaccines Expert Consult*, 5th edn. Philadelphia, PA: Saunders.

Strode GK (ed.) (1951) *Yellow Fever,* pp. 385–426. New York: McGraw-Hill.

TUMOR-ASSOCIATED VIRUSES

Adenoviruses: Malignant Transformation and Oncology

A S Turnell, The University of Birmingham, Birmingham, UK

Transforming and Oncogenic Properties of Human Adenoviruses

Human adenoviruses (Ads) are small, nonenveloped DNA viruses with linear, double-stranded genomes of about 35 kbp that are associated with a broad range of infections, but are most commonly linked with acute infections of the upper respiratory and gastrointestinal tracts. The clinical manifestations of an adenovirus infection are dependent on the adenovirus and the host cell type infected. The oncogenic capacity of adenovirus was first established by John Trentin and colleagues in 1962 when they showed that human adenovirus 12 (Ad12) was tumorigenic when injected into newborn hamsters. Adenovirus tumorigenicity was shown to be dependent upon various factors, such as virus serotype, virus dose, host age at infection time, and host genetic and immune status. Indeed, the tumorigenic potential of various adenoviruses was attributed to their ability to evade the host immune system, as nontumorigenic adenoviruses were shown to induce tumors in immunocompromised hosts. Adenovirus tumorigenicity in this regard is associated with nonproductive infections of human viruses in rodent cells. It is generally believed that a productive lytic infection in human cells precludes human adenoviruses from being tumorigenic in humans (see later). Consistent with the ability of nontumorigenic adenoviruses to promote tumors in nude mice, tissue culture studies later revealed that rodent cells could be transformed by both tumorigenic and nontumorigenic adenoviruses. Adenovirus serotypes have been classified into species (*Human adenovirus A* to *Human adenovirus F*) according to various criteria and correlated broadly with oncogenic potential (**Table 1**).

Transfection studies in primarily rodent, but also human, cells have revealed that various combinations of adenovirus DNA can transform primary cells in tissue culture, and this has greatly facilitated the study of the transformation properties of specific adenovirus genes. As with other DNA tumor viruses, the oncogenic properties of the various adenovirus genes become apparent when the mechanics of the productive lytic cycle are considered. Adenoviruses normally infect quiescent epithelial cells. In order to replicate the viral genome, the virus must first create a cellular environment conducive for DNA replication. It does this by reactivating the host cell cycle to create an S-phase-like environment. Additionally, it prevents the host cell from undergoing premature apoptosis, allowing for the assembly and production of progeny virions. Thus viral genes have evolved to circumvent the normal growth restrictions placed upon the cell. It is therefore perhaps no surprise that many viruses, in addition to adenovirus, target the tumor suppressor gene products pRB and p53 and proteins involved in DNA damage response/repair pathways (see later) to overcome normal cell cycle checkpoints. The focus of the rest of this article is a consideration of the biological functions of adenovirus-transforming genes.

Transforming and Immortalizing Properties of E1A

E1A expression is essential for a fully productive adenovirus infection and for adenovirus-mediated transformation. The Ad5 *E1A* gene encodes two major proteins of 289 and 243 amino acid residues (R) that differ only by an internal sequence of 46 residues present in the larger protein, namely, conserved region 3 (CR3), which is required specifically for adenovirus early gene expression during infection (**Figure 1**). As for E1A species from other Ad serotypes, the Ad5E1A 289R and 243R proteins possess transforming and immortalizing activity, although the smaller 243R protein is more efficient than the 289R protein in this regard. In isolation, however, E1A displays only poor transforming activity. This is due specifically to E1A's potent proapoptotic activity. E1A's transforming capacity only becomes apparent upon its expression with co-operating oncogenes such as adenovirus *E1B*, adenovirus *E4*, or activated, mutant $p21^{ras}$. Sequence comparisons of the largest E1A proteins of several adenovirus serotypes have identified four regions of sequence conservation, designated CR1, CR2, CR3, and CR4, which are largely responsible for many of E1A's biological activities, although the less well conserved N-terminal region also participates in E1A function (**Figure 1**). The transforming properties of E1A are mainly attributable to E1A's ability, through the reorchestration of host cell transcription programmes, to force quiescent cells to enter, and, for rodent cells at least, pass through the cell cycle; E1A does not promote mitosis in human cells. E1A also blocks cellular differentiation programmes.

The N-terminal region and CR1 of E1A promote transformation by targeting the transcriptional co-activators CBP and p300 (CBP/p300); E1A mutants unable to bind CBP/p300 are transformation defective. Specifically, E1A binding to CBP/p300 allows for quiescent G_0 rodent cells to enter the cell cycle and progress into S-phase. CBP and p300 are highly conserved lysine

Table 1   Classification and oncogenicity of human adenoviruses

Species	Serotype	Oncogenicity in rodents	Transformation in vitro
Human adenovirus A	12,18,31	High	+
Human adenovirus B	3, 7, 11, 14, 16, 21, 34, 35, 50	Moderate	+
Human adenovirus C	1, 2, 5, 6	Low or none	+
Human adenovirus D	8–10, 13, 15, 17, 19, 20, 22–30, 32, 33, 36–39, 42–49, 51	Low or none	+
Human adenovirus E	4	Low or none	+
Human adenovirus F	40, 41	Not reported	?

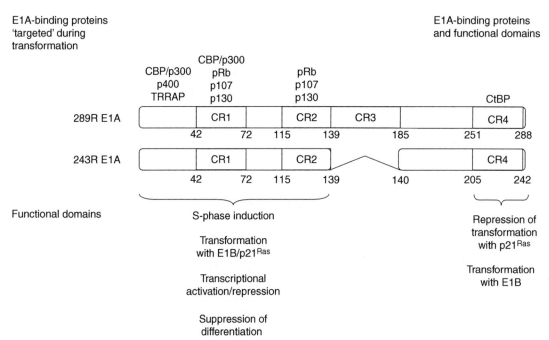

Figure 1   Linear depiction of the Ad5 243R and 289R E1A proteins. The regions conserved between serotypes are labeled as CR1, CR2, CR3, and CR4; amino acid ordinates show CR boundaries. The E1A-binding proteins considered important for E1A-mediated transformation are listed and their relative binding sites depicted. E1A regions important in cell cycle control and cellular transformation are also shown.

acetyltransferases. In this regard, the cellular activities of sequence-specific transcription factors such as p53, c-Myc, and NF-κB are all regulated by CBP/p300-acetyltransferase activity. CBP/p300 also acetylate the core histone proteins H2A, H2B, H3, and H4 to regulate transcription. It is as yet unclear, however, whether E1A utilizes CBP/p300 acetyltransferases during transformation to reprogram cellular transcription through altered acetylation, or, alternatively, promotes transformation by inhibiting CBP/p300 acetyltransferase activities. Indeed, E1A generally inhibits CBP/p300 transcription function in transient gene reporter assays. A model has been proposed, however, whereby E1A utilizes cellular acetyltransferases to alter cellular histone acetylation status, in order to stimulate E2F-regulated transcription programmes and induce S-phase. It is suggested that E1A first facilitates the demethylation of K9 of histone H3 to promote the release of repressor E2F

transcription factors from transcriptionally repressed promoters, whereupon it subsequently promotes the acetylation of K9 of histone H3 and the recruitment of activator E2F transcription factors to these promoter elements to activate transcription. The specific role played by CBP/p300 in the acetylation of K9 in this particular situation awaits clarification. Additionally, the ability of E1A to modulate CBP/p300 binding to transcription factors, independent of acetyltransferase activity, might also affect transforming activity. Theoretically, E1A could utilize other cellular acetyltransferases to promote G1–S progression. Specifically, it is possible that E1A could utilize the acetyltransferase P/CAF, to which it also binds, to regulate transcription programmes during transformation. Unfortunately, E1A point mutants have not yet been identified that unambiguously distinguish between CBP/p300 and P/CAF binding *in vivo*, such that the contribution of P/CAF in E1A-mediated transformation is unclear. It seems unlikely from the literature published thus far, however, that the interaction of other proteins with the N-terminal region of E1A spanning residues 4 and 25 is necessary to promote transformation.

Recent evidence suggests that the APC5 and APC7 components of the anaphase-promoting complex (APC/C) interact with CBP/p300 through protein interaction domains evolutionarily conserved in the N-terminal region, and CR1 ($Fx^D/_ExxxL$ motif) of E1A. E1A specifically targets APC/C-CBP/p300 complexes in order to promote the cellular transformation of rat embryo fibroblasts. Thus, exogenous expression of wild-type (w.t.) APC5 or APC7 suppresses the ability of E1A to cooperate with either E1B or activated $p21^{Ras}$ in the transformation process, whereas the expression of APC/C mutants unable to bind CBP/p300 does not suppress E1A-induced transformation. E1A also targets endogenous CBP/p300-APC/C complexes during transformation, such that RNAi-mediated knockdown of either APC5 and/or APC7 restores transforming activity to E1A species unable to bind CBP/p300, such as R2G.

Interestingly, the N-terminal region of E1A possesses additional transforming capacity. At limiting concentrations of E1A, it has been determined that residues 26–35 also promote transformation in cooperation with activated $p21^{Ras}$. It is yet to be established whether this region also cooperates with *E1B*, or other cellular or viral oncogenes, in transformation. It has been determined, however, that this region of E1A binds specifically to two cellular proteins, p400 and TRRAP, in order to promote transformation. p400 is a member of the SWI2/SNF2 chromatin-remodeling family, which associates specifically with TRRAP, the DNA helicases TAP54α/β, actin-like proteins, and the human homolog of the *Drosophila* enhancer of polycomb protein, EPc, while TRRAP is a Myc-binding protein and also a component of distinct GCN5/SAGA and Tip60/NuA4 acetyltransferase complexes. *In vitro* binding studies have indicated that E1A binds to p400 through a central region (residues 951–2048) of the protein, which also encompasses the SWI2/SNF2 homology domain and TAP54-binding site. Interestingly, E1A can also associate with p400 at a distinct C-terminal site *in vivo* (residues 2033–2484), through its interaction with TRRAP. Similar binding studies indicate that E1A binds TRRAP through residues 1360–2260. It has been determined that E1A utilizes p400 complexes to promote transformation, as co-expression of p400 fragments with E1A enhances E1A-dependent transformation. However, co-expression of a TRRAP fragment that binds E1A suppresses E1A-dependent transformation. Collectively, these data suggest that multiple and distinct E1A/p400/TRRAP complexes exist within cells which contribute differently to the transformation process. It has been proposed that during transformation E1A perturbs normal p400 and TRRAP function by forming E1A/p400 and E1A/TRRAP complexes with distinct subunit compositions to regulate chromatin structure and function.

The ability of CR1 and CR2 of E1A to promote cellular transformation resides in its capacity to interact with the protein product of the pRB tumor suppressor gene. Similar to its ability to bind CBP/p300, it has been established that E1A binding to pRB allows for quiescent G_0 rodent cells to enter the cell cycle and progress into S-phase; however, E1A must bind both CBP/p300 and pRB in order to promote mitosis in primary rodent cells. The integrity of the core DLxCxE motif in CR2 as well as CR1 is essential for E1A interaction with pRB and pRB family members p107 and p130. E1A binds specifically to the A and B pocket domains of these proteins. Like E1A's interaction with CBP and p300, any specific requirement for E1A binding to particular pRB family members during transformation is currently unknown. It has been proposed that E1A interaction with pRB and either p107 and/or p130 is important in driving quiescent cells into S-phase. In a temporally coordinated manner, E1A disrupts p130–E2F4 transcriptional repression complexes, allowing for chromatin remodeling, histone demethylation, and histone acetylation. E1A's ability to mimic cyclin-dependent kinase (CDK)-dependent phosphorylation of pRB through binding to pRB disrupts pRB–E2F1 complexes and allows the recruitment of activator E2Fs to promoters. This recruitment induces E2F-regulated genes important in S-phase induction, such as CDK2, CDC6, and cyclins E and A. The ability of E1A to disrupt pRB–E2F1 complexes also allows for E1A to overcome pRB-induced senescence programs initiated by CDK inhibitors, $p21^{CIP1/WAF1}$ and $p16^{INK4}$.

Interestingly, E1A has been found to reorganize, and associate with, PML-containing nuclear oncogenic bodies (PODs), nuclear structures implicated in regulating apoptosis, tumor suppression, antiviral responses, DNA repair, and transcriptional regulation. E1A recruitment to PODs is dependent on the pRB-interaction domain (pRB can be found associated with PODs). Whether E1A similarly associates with CBP in PODs is unclear. The precise requirement for E1A–POD interaction in the transformation process is unclear, though it is suspected that E1A might be associated with multiple POD functions.

E1A has been shown to target the CtBP family of transcriptional co-repressors through a conserved PxDLS motif located toward the C-terminal region of the protein. E1A's interaction with CtBP is believed to be important in the transformation process. The role of the region encoded by exon 2 in cellular immortalization and cellular transformation is, however, context dependent. In cooperation with exon 1, exon 2 enhances the E1A-dependent immortalization of rodent cells and E1A-dependent transformation with E1B, such that certain exon 2 deletion mutants have reduced immortalization/transformation capacities relative to w.t. 12S (243R) E1A. In contrast, exon 2 suppresses

12S E1A/p21^{Ras}-mediated immortalization and transformation, such that exon 2 deletion mutants enhance the E1A-dependent immortalization and transformation of primary cells in culture, and, moreover, their tumorigenicity and metastatic potential in nude mice. These differences in exon 2 functions presumably reside in the differential capacities of E1B and p21^{Ras} to activate/suppress cellular pathways involved in promoting immortalization and/or transformation.

It has been suggested that exon 2 promotes immortalization and transformation with E1B through its ability to complement exon 1 immortalization functions and evade Mortality stage 2 (crisis). It has also been proposed that the ability of exon 2, in the context of w.t. 12S E1A, to function as a tumor suppressor and suppress p21^{Ras}-mediated transformation resides in its ability to promote mesenchymal–epithelial cell transitions through the regulation of specific epithelial-promoting transcription programs. The ability of exon 2 mutants to promote hypertransformation, enhanced tumorigenicity and metastatic potential, relative to w.t. 12S E1A, of both epithelial and fibroblastic cells is believed to be mediated, in part, by the activation of the small Ras-related proteins, Rac and Cdc42, suggesting that w.t. 12S E1A may normally serve to suppress these pathways. The current literature suggests that the ability of exon 2 to regulate oncogenesis is mediated at least in part by its ability to bind to CtBP. A more thorough examination however of exon 2-binding proteins and exon 2 deletion mutants is required to determine whether E1A binding to CtBP accounts for all of these cellular phenotypes.

Oncogenicity of E1A

E1A from oncogenic serotypes specifically regulates pathways involved in immune regulation and contributes toward immune evasion – a major determinant of adenovirus oncogenicity. It is well established that E1A from the tumorigenic serotype, Ad12, downregulates the presentation of major histocompatibility complex class I (MHC-I) antigens in rodent cells, whereas E1A from the nontumorigenic serotype, Ad5, does not. MHC-I downregulation allows for adenovirus-infected cells to avoid clearance by cytotoxic T-lymphocytes (CTLs). A major difference between oncogenic and nononcogenic serotypes in this regard is in their ability to affect transcription mediated through the MHC-I enhancer sites R1 and R2. Oncogenic serotypes repress transcription mediated through the MHC-I enhancer by upregulating the transcriptional repressor COUP-TFII, which binds to the R2 site, while concomitantly reducing the level of NF-κB binding to the R1 site by reducing the level of phosphorylation of the p50 subunit of NF-κB. Nononcogenic serotypes do not upregulate COUP-TFII levels, and NF-κB binds to

the R1 site with high affinity. Oncogenic serotypes have also been shown to interfere with MHC-I presentation by downregulating components of the immune proteasome, such as LMP2 and LMP7, and downregulating the transporter proteins associated with antigen presentation, TAP1 and TAP2. A further feature of Ad12 E1A that facilitates immune evasion is that it does not produce immunological epitopes recognized by CTLs, whereas Ad5 E1A does. Ad12-infected cells are also resistant to natural killer cell lysis. These functions of E1A are largely attributed to an alanine-rich 20-residue spacer region present in Ad12 E1A between CR2 and CR3, which is not present in the nontumorigenic adenovirus serotypes. Other regions of Ad12 E1A do possess tumorigenic properties, but how these manifest mechanistically awaits further investigation.

Transforming Properties of Adenovirus E1B and E4 Regions

In the absence of cooperating oncogenes, such as *p21^{ras}*, *E1B*, or *E4*, *E1A* has little or no capacity to transform and immortalize embryonic human cells in tissue culture systems and only limited capacity to transform and immortalize embryonic rodent cells; E1A-immortalized clones tend to harbor mutations in the p53 tumor suppressor gene. Although the *E1B* and *E4* genes have no transforming capacity alone, they can cooperate with *E1A* in the transformation process through their ability to neutralize E1A-induced, p53-dependent and p53-independent, apoptosis. The biological properties of E1B and E4 proteins, in this regard, will be discussed in turn.

EIB-19K

The *E1B* gene expresses two principle proteins: E1B-19K and E1B-55K. E1B-19K was initially identified as a homolog of the cellular antiapoptotic protein, BCL-2. Despite sequence conservation between the two proteins, it is of interest to note that E1B-19K and BCL-2 differ in the methods they employ to neutralize the proapoptotic functions of BCL-2 family members BAX and BAK. Specifically, BCL-2 inhibits the activation of BAX/BAK by binding to BID and preventing its caspase-8 dependent cleavage to active tBID, which, under normal circumstances, promotes BAX/BAK heterooligomerization at mitochondrial membranes and the subsequent induction of apoptosis. E1B-19K, on the other hand, inhibits apoptosis by binding directly to tBID-activated BAX and/or BAK, preventing BAX/BAK heterooligomerization and the subsequent downstream events that lead to apoptosis (**Figure 2**). Significantly, the ability of E1A to induce p53-independent apoptosis relies, in part, upon its ability to specifically activate BAK/BAX. In this context, and akin to ultraviolet (UV)-induced DNA damage-induced apoptotic pathways, E1A can promote apoptosis by specifically downregulating the BCL-2 antiapoptotic family member MCL-1 through proteasomal-mediated degradation. MCL-1 normally serves to functionally inhibit BAK, but upon E1A-mediated degradation of MCL-1, BAK can activate apoptosis. In this regard, E1B-19K cooperates with E1A in the transformation process by inhibiting E1A-activated BAK (**Figure 2**).

E1B-55K and E4orf6

The Ad5 E1B-55K and 34K E4orf6 proteins functionally cooperate during viral infection to regulate p53, the MRE11-RAD50-NBS1 (MRN) complex (**Figure 3**), and potentially late-phase viral mRNA nuclear export and translation. For this reason, it is perhaps best to consider their roles in cellular transformation together. The current perception is that the independent, and combined, abilities of both E1B-55K and E4orf6 to repress

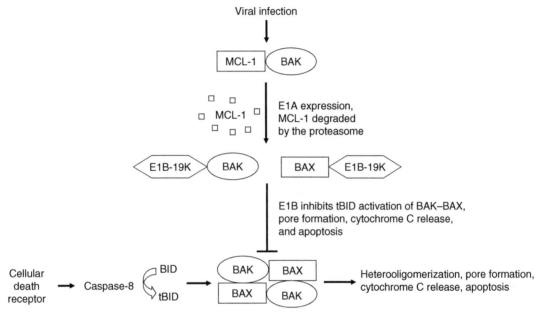

Figure 2 Role of E1B-19K in antiapoptotic signaling pathways. E1B-19K inhibits E1A-induced, p53-independent apoptosis by binding tBID-bound BAK and BAX, and specifically inhibiting the mitochondrial-release apoptosis pathway. See text for details.

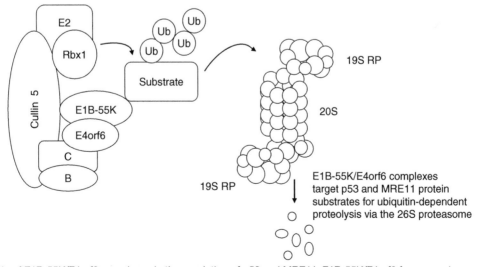

Figure 3 Role of E1B-55K/E4orf6 complexes in the regulation of p53 and MRE11. E1B-55K/E4orf6 form complexes with the Cullin 5-based E3 ubiquitin ligase to promote the poly-ubiquitylation, and hence 26S proteasomal-mediated destruction, of p53 and MRE11. See text for more detail. B, C, Elongin B, C; E2, ubiquitin conjugating enzyme; Ub, ubiquitin.

p53-transactivation of proapoptotic genes underlies their respective, and synergistic, capacities to co-operate with E1A in the transformation process. The requirement for E1B-55K and E4orf6 binding and regulation of the MRN complex in the transformation process awaits clarification.

Specifically, the central region of E1B-55K encompassing residues 250–310, and a small region around residue 180, bind to the N-terminal transactivation domain of p53, blocking co-activator recruitment and further inhibiting p53 transcription function through specific C-terminal transcriptional repression domains. In Ad5 E1A/E1B-55K transformed cells, E1B-55K and p53 are sequestered in cytoplasmic 'phase-dense' aggresome structures that also contain microfilaments, centrosomal proteins, hsp70, and WT1. The cytoplasmic location of E1B-55K is mediated in part by a leucine-rich nuclear export signal (NES) located between residues 83 and 93; the nuclear export of E1B-55K is dependent upon the CRM1 cellular export receptor. Significantly, mutation of the critical leucine residues in the E1B-55K NES potentiates E1A/E1B-mediated transformation through enhanced inhibition of p53 transactivation function and the accumulation of mutant E1B-55K and p53 in PODs. Consistent with a role for E1B-55K localized to PML-containing nuclear bodies in p53 repression and cellular transformation, it has been demonstrated through mutational studies that SUMOylation of K104 in E1B-55K not only promotes its recruitment to PML bodies, but augments p53 transcriptional repression and enhances cellular transformation. Other functions of E1B-55K might also contribute toward its transforming potential. Indeed, the Ad12 large E1B protein (equivalent to Ad5 E1B-55K) can extend the lifespan of human embryo fibroblasts, bypassing Mortality stage 1 through ALT maintenance of telomere length.

The C-terminal region of E4orf6 can, independently of E1B-55K, bind to the C-terminal oligomerization domain (residues 318–360) of p53 to repress specifically the p53 N-terminal transactivation function; E4orf6 disrupts p53 interaction with TFIID component TAFII31. In contrast to E1B-55K, however, E4orf6 also possesses an independent and distinct ability to relieve C-terminal p53 transcriptional repression through binding. Akin to E1B-55K, E4orf6 cooperates with E1A in the transformation of primary baby rat kidney (BRK) cells. E1A/E4orf6 transformants grow more slowly than E1A/E1B-55K transformants, but are essentially morphologically indistinguishable. As already indicated, E4orf6 will also synergize with E1B-55K, or E1B-55K and E1B-19K, to enhance the frequency of E1A-dependent transformation; E1A/E1B/E4orf6 mutants express lower levels of p53 than E1A/E1B and E1A/E4orf6 transformants. Interestingly, E1A/E1B/E4orf6 transformants arise more rapidly than E1A/E1B and E1A/E4orf6 transformants, and when injected subcutaneously into the nude mouse promote more rapid tumor formation. In support of the tumorigenic properties of the E4orf6

protein, it also converts human 293 cells from nontumorigenic to tumorigenic in nude mice. Interestingly, and in stark contrast to E1B-55K, E4orf6 does not cooperate with E1A and E1B-19K in the transformation process; in fact, E4orf6 suppresses E1A/E1B-19K mediated transformation. It has been suggested that the additional ability of E4orf6 to relieve p53 transcriptional repression contributes toward its ability to suppress transformation in this instance.

As indicated earlier, E1B-55K and E4orf6 also regulate the activity of the MRN complex. Functionally, the MRN complex is integral to both the ATM- and ATR-DNA damage response/repair signaling pathways initiated in response to ionizing and UV irradiation, respectively. It has been suggested that adenovirus circumvents these checkpoint controls through the ability of E1B-55K and E4orf6 to target the MRE11 component of the MRN complex for ubiquitin-mediated, proteasome-dependent degradation. Inactivation of MRE11 by E1B-55K and E4orf6 ensures, in the context of viral infection, that linear viral DNA is not concatemerized by double-strand break–repair pathways initiated by the MRN complex.

The functional cooperativity displayed by E1B-55K and E4orf6 is mediated through protein–protein interaction. It has been suggested that the N-terminal 55 residues of E4orf6 are required for its binding to E1B-55K, although others suggest that the amphipathic α-helical region toward the C-terminus governs the interaction; the central region of E1B-55K encompassing residues 262–326, and a region around residue 143, are required for interaction with E4orf6. Although the E4orf6-binding site on E1B-55K overlaps with the p53-binding site, E1B-55K and E4orf6 bind independently of p53. Crucial to establishing the biochemical basis of this functional cooperativity between the two proteins, mass spectrometric identification of cellular proteins bound to E4orf6 in p53-null H1299 cells has revealed that E4orf6 can bind to the Cullin-containing, Cul5-Elongin B/C-Rbx1 E3 ubiquitin ligase complex (**Figure 3**). Significantly, E1B-55K is only found in complexes with E4orf6 bound to the Cul5-Elongin B/C-Rbx1 complex, suggesting that E1B-55K and E4orf6 might not bind directly. E4orf6 contains within its primary sequence two functional Elongin B/C-interaction (BC) boxes located between residues 46–55 and 121–130, which define its direct interaction with Elongin C. E1B-55K also contains a putative BC-box located between residues 179 and 188, though this region does not bind Elongin B or C directly. It has been postulated that E4orf6 might also bind Cul5 directly, though this awaits confirmation.

Functional studies have indicated that E4orf6–E1B-55K utilizes the Cul5-Elongin B/C-Rbx1 ubiquitin ligase to promote the poly-ubiquitylation and hence 26S proteasomal-mediated degradation of p53 and MRE11 during viral infection and cellular transformation. E4orf6 is postulated to recruit the functional E3 ligase complex, whereas E1B-55K is proposed to interact with the substrate protein targeted for degradation. The absolute depletion of functional p53, MRE11, and potentially other cellular proteins by the E4orf6–E1B-55K cellular ubiquitin ligase complexes might explain why E4orf6 and E1B-55K are functionally more adept at enhancing the frequency of E1A-dependent transformation than either protein in isolation.

E1B-55K binds the hnRNP, RNA-binding protein E1B-AP5 independently of E4orf6. The central region of E1B-55K encompassing residues 262–326, and regions around residues 180, 380, and 484 all participate in E1B-AP5 binding; E4orf6 can modulate E1B-AP5 binding to E1B-55K. However, E1B-AP5 is not targeted for degradation during viral infection by E1B-55K and E4orf6, suggesting that E1B-55K is more than just a substrate adaptor for the E4orf6–Cul5-containing E3 ubiquitin ligase. The E1B-55K/E1B-AP5 complex is proposed to regulate the shutdown of host cell mRNA export during infection. Interestingly, overexpression of E1B-AP5 suppresses E1A/E1B-55K-mediated transformation, suggesting that E1B-55K might target E1B-AP5 directly to facilitate transformation.

E4orf3

The 11K E4orf3 gene product operates in redundant pathways with E4orf6 and E1B-55K during viral infection to regulate RNA processing and viral DNA replication. Mechanistically, E4orf3 cooperates with E4orf6 in the inhibition of DNA damage repair, presumably through binding DNA-PK and inactivation of the MRN complex. Indeed, Ad5 E4orf3 redistributes the MRN complex to nuclear PODs away from viral replication centers. Ad4 and Ad12 E4orf3 do not cause relocalization of the MRN complex, suggesting serotype-specific modulation of MRN function. E4orf3 similarly binds E1B-55K and targets it to PODs. Akin to E4orf6, E4orf3 will co-operate with E1A and E1A/E1B-55K to transform primary BRK cells in tissue culture and increase the tumorigenicity of E1A/E1B-55K transformed BRKs in nude mice. E4orf3 will also co-operate with E1A/E4orf6 and E1A/E1B-55K/E4orf6 in transformation. Like E4orf6, E4orf3 increases the frequency of transformation, the rate of cell growth, and the saturation densities to which transformants grow.

Ad9 E4orf1

Ad9 is unique among the adenovirus family in that it promotes estrogen-dependent mammary tumors in rodents. The oncogenic capacity of Ad9 has been mapped to a single protein, E4orf1. Although conserved among different adenoviruses (45–51% identity), only the Ad9 protein is oncogenic, although other adenovirus E4orf1 proteins

do display some transforming characteristics (e.g., anchorage-independent growth). It has been suggested that the oncogenic capacity of the Ad9 protein resides in its differential ability to bind the first PDZ domain of the PDZ-containing, MAGUK homology protein, and tumor suppressor protein, ZO-2. The C-terminal PDZ-binding domain of Ad9 E4orf1 selectively targets ZO-2 and redistributes it to the cytoplasm. Consistent with a role in oncogenicity, ZO-2 inhibits Ad9 E4orf1 transformation of the rat embryo fibroblast cell line, CREF. Activation of phosphoinosite 3-kinase (PI3K) by the PDZ-binding domain of E4orf1 at the plasma membrane is also crucial in the transformation process. PI3K activation presumably allows for the specific initiation of downstream survival signaling pathways, and the activation of other potential oncoproteins (e.g., $p21^{Ras}$).

'Hit and Run' Transformation

As outlined earlier, the prevailing, generally held view is that adenovirus infection is not a causative agent of human malignancy. Intriguingly, however, and consistent with early studies looking at human simplex virus- and Abelson leukemia virus-mediated transformation, studies have suggested that certain adenovirus genes may promote transformation by a 'hit and run' mechanism whereby adenovirus DNA, mRNA, or protein are only rarely retained in the adenovirus-transformed cells. Incidentally, this makes it very difficult to tell whether adenovirus infection actually promotes human tumorigenesis, or whether 'hit and run' transformation is merely an *in vitro* phenomenon of no clinical relevance. It has been suggested that adenovirus genes are required for the initiation of transformation, but are not required for the maintenance of the transformed phenotype. Although mechanistically ill-defined, it is suggested that adenovirus genes could promote gene mutation and/or direct genetic instability through interaction with cellular proteins. Specifically, studies have shown that when E4orf3 and/or E4orf6 cooperate with E1A in transformation, in the majority of instances the transformed cells do not retain E1A, E4orf6, and/or E4orf3, though there are clear exceptions where these proteins can be detected. Interestingly, co-expression of these proteins with E1B-55K subsequently facilitates their detection in transformed cells, suggesting that E1B-55K antagonizes the genetic instability promoted by E1A, E4orf6, and E4orf3. Significantly, a role for these proteins in promoting genetic instability is already well established. The N-terminal region of E1A and CR3 have been previously implicated in causing both random and nonrandom host cell chromosome aberrations, as well as abnormal mitoses generating both aneuploid and polyploid cells in human cells and rodent cells, whereas E4orf3 and E4orf6 have been implicated in promoting genetic instability through the interaction with MRN and DNA-PK and inhibiting the repair of damaged DNA.

Conclusions

Adenovirus has long served as a faithful model system for investigating the molecular mechanisms of cellular immortalization, transformation, and tumorigenicity. During this time, studies on adenovirus E1A and E1B have identified the functions of key tumor suppressor proteins, not to mention the functions of proteins not directly involved in oncogenesis. In more recent years, the roles of E4 proteins in the transformation process have become increasingly apparent. It is reasonable to anticipate that future studies investigating adenovirus-mediated transformation will enhance further our understanding of the molecular mechanisms underlying oncogenesis.

See also: Adenoviruses: General Features; Adenoviruses: Pathogenesis.

Further Reading

Berk AJ (2005) Recent lessons in gene expression, cell cycle control, and cell biology from adenovirus. *Oncogene* 24: 7673–7685.
Chinnadurai G (2004) Modulation of oncogenic transformation by the human adenovirus E1A C-terminal region. *Current Topics in Microbiology and Immunology* 273: 139–161.
Endter C and Dobner T (2004) Cell transformation by human adenoviruses. *Current Topics in Microbiology and Immunology* 273: 163–214.
Frisch SM and Mymryk JS (2002) Adenovirus-5 E1A: Paradox and paradigm. *Nature Reviews. Molecular Cell Biology* 3: 441–452.
Gallimore PH and Turnell AS (2001) Adenovirus E1A: Remodelling the host cell, a life or death experience. *Oncogene* 20: 7824–7835.
White E (2006) Mechanisms of apoptosis regulation by viral oncogenes in infection and tumorigenesis. *Cell Death and Differentiation* 13: 1371–1377.
Williams JF, Zhang Y, Williams MA, Hou S, Kushner D, and Ricciardi RP (2004) E1A-based determinants of oncogenicity in human adenovirus groups A and C. *Current Topics in Microbiology and Immunology* 273: 245–288.

Epstein–Barr Virus: General Features

L S Young, University of Birmingham, Birmingham, UK

Taxonomy and Genome Structure

Epstein–Barr virus (EBV; species *Human herpesvirus 4*) is a member of the genus *Lymphocryptovirus*, which belongs to the lymphotropic subfamily *Gammaherpesvirinae* of the family *Herpesviridae*. EBV is closely related to the lymphocryptoviruses (LCVs) present in Old World non-human primates, including EBV-like viruses of chimpanzees and rhesus monkeys. These viruses share homologous sequences and genetic organization, and infect the B lymphocytes of their host species, resulting in the establishment of latent infection *in vivo* and transformation *in vitro*. A transforming, EBV-related virus has also been isolated from spontaneous B-cell lymphomas of common marmosets and is thus the first EBV-like virus to be identified in New World primates. The genome of this marmoset LCV revealed considerable divergence from the genomes of EBV and Old World primate EBV-related viruses, suggesting that this virus represents a more primitive predecessor of the LCVs infecting higher-order primates.

The EBV genome is composed of linear, double-stranded DNA, approximately 172 kbp in length. EBV has a series of 0.5 kbp terminal direct repeats (TRs) and internal repeat sequences (IRs) that divide the genome into short and long, largely unique sequence domains. EBV was the first herpesvirus to have its genome completely cloned and sequenced. Since the EBV genome was sequenced from an EBV DNA *Bam*HI fragment cloned library, open reading frames (ORFs), genes, and sites for transcription or RNA processing are frequently referenced to specific *Bam*HI fragments, from A–Z, in descending order of fragment size. The virus has the coding potential for around 80 proteins, not all of which have been identified or characterized.

History

In 1958, Denis Burkitt described a lymphoma that represented the most common tumor affecting children in certain parts of East Africa. The geographical distribution of this malignancy suggested that the development of Burkitt lymphoma (BL) might be due to an infectious agent possibly related to malaria. In 1964, the successful establishment of cell lines from explants of BL enabled Tony Epstein and Yvonne Barr to identify herpesvirus-type particles by electron microscopy within a subpopulation of tumor cells *in vitro* (**Figure 1**). Werner and Gertrude

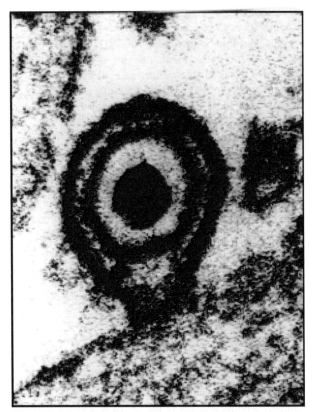

Figure 1 Electron micrograph of the Epstein–Barr virus virion.

Table 1 EBV-associated tumors

Tumor	Subtype	EBV genome +ve (%)
Burkitt's lymphoma	Endemic	100
	Sporadic	10–20
	AIDS	30–40
Nasopharyngeal carcinoma	Undifferentiated	100
	SCC	10–40
Hodgkin's disease	Mixed cellularity	>80
	Nodular sclerosing	30–40
	Lymphocyte predominant	<10
T-cell lymphoma	Nasal	100
	Others	10–40
Immunoblastic lymphoma	Transplant	100
	AIDS	>90

Henle subsequently demonstrated that BL-derived cell lines expressed antigens that were recognized not only by sera from patients with BL but also by sera from patients with infectious mononucleosis (IM). Similar seroepidemiological studies also suggested a link between infection with this virus (now called Epstein– Barr virus after its discoverers) and undifferentiated nasopharyngeal carcinoma (NPC), leading to the subsequent direct demonstration of EBV DNA in the tumor cells of NPC. The ability of EBV to immortalize B lymphocytes efficiently *in vitro* and to induce tumors in nonhuman primates established this virus as a putative oncogenic agent in humans. Over the last 20 years EBV has been implicated in a variety of other lymphoid and epithelial malignancies (**Table 1**).

Geographic and Seasonal Distribution

EBV is ubiquitous, being found as a widespread and largely asymptomatic infection in all human communities. Primary infection often occurs early in life, particularly in tropical areas and in persons of lower socioeconomic class. Thus, in tropical Africa and New Guinea primary EBV infection is common in the first year of life whereas in Western communities infection is continually acquired throughout childhood and early adulthood. Although the EBV-associated malignancies BL and NPC exhibit an

unusual geographic distribution, this appears not to be due to differences in EBV infection but due to additional cofactors.

Host Range and Virus Propagation

Humans are the natural host for EBV infection. EBV has a unique ability to transform resting B cells into permanent, latently infected, lymphoblastoid cell lines (LCLs) in which every cell carries multiple copies of circular, extra chromosomal, viral DNA (episomes) and produces a number of latent proteins, including six EBV-encoded nuclear antigens (EBNAs 1, 2, 3A, 3B, 3C, and -LP) and three latent membrane proteins (LMPs 1, 2A, and 2B); this form of infection is referred to as latency III. When peripheral blood lymphocytes from healthy EBV seropositives are placed in culture, the few EBV-infected B lymphocytes that are present regularly give rise to spontaneous outgrowth of EBV-transformed LCLs, provided that immune T lymphocytes are either removed or inhibited by the addition of cyclosporin A to the culture. LCLs can also be generated by direct infection of resting B lymphocytes with EBV derived from the throat washings of seropositive individuals or from producer B-cell lines. LCLs have provided an invaluable, albeit incomplete, model of the lymphomagenic potential of EBV.

Certain nonhuman primates, particularly the cotton-top tamarin, have been used as experimental hosts for EBV, but virus infection in these animals is associated with the induction of lymphomas. LCLs generated by EBV transformation of cotton-top tamarin B lymphocytes *in vitro* spontaneously produce large amounts of virus compared with their human counterparts and as such have been used as a source of EBV; for example, the prototype strain of EBV is B95.8, which is produced from a tamarin LCL originally immortalized with EBV from a patient with IM. However, the lack of a fully permissive system for propagating EBV *in vitro* has hampered our understanding of virus replication and prevented the generation of EBV mutants. Over recent years a number of systems have been developed for the generation of recombinant forms of EBV which rely on the manipulation of the entire virus genome within bacteria followed by rescue and propagation in human cells.

Genetics and Strain Variation

EBV isolates from different regions of the world or from patients with different virus-associated diseases are remarkably similar when their genomes are compared by restriction fragment length polymorphism analysis. However, variations in repeat regions of the EBV genome are observed among different EBV isolates. Analysis of the EBV genome in a number of BL-cell lines revealed gross deletions, some of which account for biological differences. For example, P3HR-1 virus, which is nontransforming, has a deletion of the EBNA2-encoding gene. Strain variation over the EBNA2-encoding (*Bam*HI WYH) region of the EBV genome permits all virus isolates to be classified as either 'type 1' (EBV-1, B95.8-like) or 'type 2' (EBV-2, Jijoye-like). This genomic variation results in the production of two antigenically distinct forms of the EBNA2 protein that share only 50% amino acid sequence homology. Similar allelic polymorphisms (with 50–80% sequence homology depending on the locus) related to the EBV type occur in a subset of latent genes, namely those encoding EBNA-LP, EBNA3A, EBNA3B, and EBNA3C. These differences have functional consequences as EBV-2 isolates are less efficient in *in vitro* B-lymphocyte transformation assays compared with EBV-1 isolates. A combination of virus isolation and seroepidemiological studies suggest that type 1 virus isolates are predominant (but not exclusively so) in many Western countries, whereas both types are widespread in equatorial Africa, New Guinea, and perhaps certain other regions.

In addition to this broad distinction between EBV types 1 and 2, there is also minor heterogeneity within each virus type. Individual strains have been identified on the basis of differences compared with B95.8, ranging from single-base mutations to extensive deletions. While infection with multiple strains of EBV was originally thought to be confined to immunologically compromised patients, more recent studies demonstrate that normal healthy seropositives can be infected with multiple EBV isolates and that their relative abundance and presence appears to vary over time. Coinfection of the host with multiple virus strains could have evolutionary benefit to EBV, enabling the generation of diversity by genetic recombination. Such intertypic recombination has been demonstrated in human immunodeficiency virus (HIV)-infected patients and appears to arise via recombination of

multiple EBV strains during the intense EBV replication that occurs as a consequence of immunosuppression.

The possible contribution of EBV strain variation to virus-associated tumors remains contentious. Many studies have failed to establish an epidemiological association between EBV strains and disease and suggest that the specific EBV gene polymorphisms detected in virus-associated tumors occur with similar frequencies in EBV isolates from healthy virus carriers from the same geographic region. However, this does not exclude the possibility that variation in specific EBV genes is responsible for the distinct geographic distribution of virus-associated malignancies. In this regard, an LMP1 variant containing a 10-amino-acid deletion (residues 343–352) was originally identified in Chinese NPC biopsies and has oncogenic and other functional properties distinct from those of the B95.8 LMP1 gene. It is therefore likely that variation in LMP1 and other EBV genes can contribute to the risk of developing virus-associated tumors, but more biological studies using well-defined EBV variants are required.

Evolution

EBV, like other herpesviruses, has probably evolved with humans. The relatedness of the LCVs at both the genomic and protein levels does not correlate with the evolutionary relatedness of their Old World primate hosts. This implies that the selective pressures governing the evolution of these viruses are different from those responsible for the evolution of primate species. It has been suggested that the specific tissue tropism of LCVs may have constrained their evolutionary divergence. A comparison of marmoset LCV with the LCVs present in Old World primates provides some insight into LCV evolution approximately 35 million years before the appearance of EBV. The acquisition of accessory genes by Old World LCVs supports the contention that these viruses have coevolved with their hosts possibly as a means of maintaining their biological properties.

The evolutionary relationship between the type 1 and type 2 strains of EBV remains obscure. They may have evolved from a common progenitor virus or through recombination of the ancestral LCVs infecting Old World primates. The pronounced (but not exclusive) segregation of EBV-2 isolates within equatorial regions suggests that environmental factors (including immunological competence) may have influenced EBV evolution and may still be responsible for the effective competition between EBV-2 isolates and the ubiquitous EBV-1 family.

EBV Primary Infection and Persistence

EBV infects the majority of the world's adult population and, following primary infection, the individual remains a

Primary infection

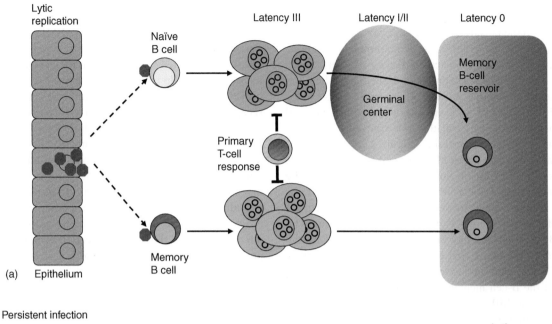

(a)

Persistent infection

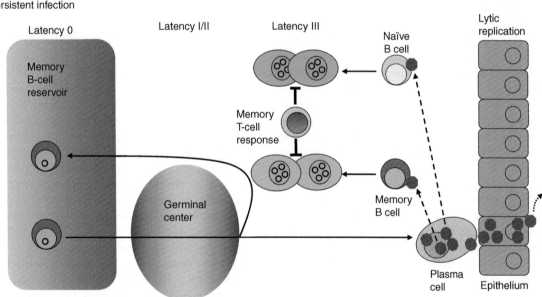

(b)

Figure 2 EBV primary infection and persistence. Diagram showing putative *in vivo* interactions between EBV and host cells. (a) Primary infection. EBV replicates in epithelial cells and spreads to lymphoid tissues as a latent growth-transforming (latency III) infection of B cells. Many infected B cells are removed by the emerging EBV-specific T-cell response. Some infected cells escape by downregulating EBV latent genes to establish a stable pool of resting virus-positive memory B cells. (b) Persistent infection. EBV-infected memory B cells become subject to the physiological controls governing memory B-cell migration and differentiation. Occasional recruitment into germinal center (GC) reactions resulting in activation of different EBV latency programs and re-entry into the memory cell reservoir or plasma cell differentiation with activation of virus lytic cycle. Infectious virions then initiate foci of EBV replication in epithelial cells and also new growth-transforming infection of naïve and/or memory B cells.

lifelong carrier of the virus (**Figure 2**). In underdeveloped countries, primary infection with EBV usually occurs during the first several months to few years of life and is often asymptomatic. However, in developed populations, primary infection is more frequently delayed until adolescence or adulthood, in many cases producing the characteristic clinical features of IM. EBV is orally transmitted, and infectious virus can be detected in oropharyngeal secretions from IM patients, from immunosuppressed patients, and at lower levels from healthy EBV seropositive individuals. These observations, together with the fact that EBV-transformed LCLs *in vitro* tend to be poor producers of the virus and B lymphocytes permissive of viral replication have not been demonstrated *in vivo*, suggest that EBV replicates and is shed at epithelial sites in the oropharynx and/or salivary glands. This is supported by the demonstration of replicating EBV in the differentiated epithelial cell layers of oral 'hairy' leukoplakia, a benign lesion of the tongue found in immunocompromised patients. However, it is also likely that EBV-infected B cells are reactivated within the local mucosal environment and that this contributes to virus shedding at oropharyngeal sites (**Figure 2**).

The inability to detect EBV routinely in normal epithelial cells and the demonstration that EBV can be completely eradicated by irradiation in bone marrow transplant recipients suggests that B lymphocytes are the main site of EBV persistence (**Figure 2(b)**). This is supported by the B lymphotropism of EBV which is mediated by the binding of the major viral envelope glycoprotein gp350 to the CR2 receptor on the surface of B cells. Virion penetration of the B-cell membrane requires further interactions between the EBV glycoprotein gp42 (which forms a ternary complex with gH and gL viral glycoproteins) and human leukocyte antigen (HLA) class II molecules. It appears that the presence or absence of HLA class II in virus-producing cells influences the tropism of EBV for B cells or epithelial cells by affecting the availability of gp42. Other CR2-independent pathways may be responsible for EBV infection of epithelial cells, including secretory component-mediated immunoglobulin (Ig) A transport, integrin interactions with polarized epithelium, and direct cell-to-cell contact, but these are relatively inefficient and of unknown relevance to EBV infection *in vivo*.

The B-cell tropism of EBV and its ability to establish a latent infection in these cells both *in vitro* and *in vivo* further supports the contention that B lymphocytes are the reservoir of lifelong persistent infection (**Figure 2(b)**). Detailed examination of EBV infection *in vivo* has shown that the virus persists in the IgD$^-$CD27$^+$ memory B-cell subset and that these cells have downregulated the expression of most, if not all, viral genes. The precise route of entry of EBV-infected B cells into the memory compartment remains a subject of much debate. This reservoir of infected cells is stably maintained thereafter, apparently subject to the same physiologic controls as the general mucosa-associated memory B-cell pool. EBV persistence within this B-cell population brings with it the possibility of fortuitous antigen-driven recruitment of infected cells into germinal centers (GCs), leading to progeny that either re-enter the circulating memory pool or differentiate to plasma cells that may migrate to mucosal sites. The different forms of latency that are manifest in virus-associated malignancies (discussed below) may represent latency programs that have evolved to accommodate such changes in host cell physiology

(**Figure 2**). Thus GC transit appears to activate a latency program where only the genome maintenance protein EBNA1 is expressed (latency 0), while exit from GCs is possibly linked to the transient expression of the EBV-encoded latent membrane proteins, LMP1 and LMP2 (latency II). The ability of these proteins to mimic the key signals required for B cells to undergo a GC reaction, namely T-cell help via the CD40 pathway (constitutively provided by LMP1) and activation of the cognate B-cell receptor (augmented by LMP2A), supports this strategy whereby EBV exploits the physiological process of B-cell differentiation to access and maintain persistent infection in the memory B-cell pool. The possible commitment of these cells to plasmacytoid differentiation may trigger entry into lytic virus replication, thereby providing a source of low-level virus shedding into the oropharynx. There may also be circumstances in which infected cells in the reservoir can reactivate back to proliferative infections similar to those of an EBV-transformed LCL.

Immune Response

EBV elicits both humoral and cell-mediated immune responses in infected hosts. Primary infection with EBV is associated with the rapid appearance of antibodies to replicative antigens such as viral capsid antigen (VCA), early antigen (EA), and membrane antigen (MA; gp350/220) with a later serological response to EBNA proteins. In IM, these responses are exaggerated and are accompanied by autoantibodies such as rheumatoid factor as well as a heterophile antibody response directed against antigens on the surface of sheep erythrocytes. These autoantibodies are the result of EBV-induced polyclonal B-cell activation. In the chronic asymptomatic virus carrier, antibodies to VCA, MA, and EBNAs are found, the titers of which remain remarkably stable. Of these antibodies, those against MA are particularly important as they have virus-neutralizing ability and can also mediate antibody-dependent cellular cytotoxicity. As discussed below, the levels of these EBV-specific antibodies are elevated in different EBV-associated diseases.

As with other persistent viruses, cell-mediated immunity plays an important role in controlling EBV infection. Primary EBV infection elicits a robust cellular immune response and the lymphocytosis observed in IM is a consequence of the hyperexpansion of cytotoxic CD8+ T cells with reactivities against both latent and lytic viral antigens. These reactivities are subsequently maintained at high level (up to 5% of the total circulating pool) in the CD8+ memory T-cell pool. An EBV-specific CD4+ T-cell response also contributes toward the control of EBV infection and, along with the CD8+ response, appears to be important in preventing the unlimited proliferation of EBV-infected B cells.

Thus, impairment of the T-cell response, either by immunosuppressive drug therapy or by HIV infection, is responsible for the development of polyclonal lymphoproliferations that can progress to frank monoclonal non-Hodgkin's lymphomas (see below). These lesions can be controlled by adoptive therapy with EBV-specific T cells. The growth and survival of BL, NPC, and Hodgkin's lymphoma (HL) in immunocompetent individuals implies that the tumor cells can evade EBV-specific T-cell surveillance. This may be achieved by restricting EBV latent gene expression to those viral proteins not efficiently recognized by the T-cell responses (i.e., away from expression of the highly immunogenic EBNA3 family) and/or by downregulation of target cell molecules required for immune recognition such as major histocompatability complex (MHC) class I and the antigen-processing machinery.

EBV-Associated Diseases

Infectious Mononucleosis

Primary infection with EBV in childhood is usually asymptomatic but when delayed until adolescence or early adulthood can manifest clinically as IM, a self-limiting lymphoproliferative disease associated with the hyperexpansion of cytotoxic $CD8^+$ T cells that are reactive to both lytic and latent cycle viral antigens. These reactivities are subsequently maintained in the $CD8^+$ T-cell memory pool at high levels (up to 5% of circulating $CD8^+$ T cells), even in individuals with no history of IM. The incidence of IM is low in developing countries where asymptomatic primary infection predominantly occurs in childhood. In certain poorly defined situations, IM-like symptoms can persist, resulting in chronic active EBV infection associated with elevated antibody titers to virus lytic antigens but low titers to the EBNAs.

Lymphomas in Immunosuppressed Individuals

Patients with primary immunodeficiency diseases such as X-linked lymphoproliferative syndrome (XLP) and Wiscott–Aldrich syndrome are at increased risk of developing EBV-associated lymphomas. Because these tumors are extremely rare, little is known about the precise contribution of EBV and the associated pattern of viral gene expression in these lymphomas. Mortality from XLP is high with around 50% of patients developing fatal IM after primary infection with EBV and an additional 30% of patients developing malignant lymphomas. The defect responsible for XLP is mutation of an adaptor molecule, SAP, which mediates signaling in a wide range of immune cells and is involved, via its interaction with the SLAM family of receptors, in both innate and adaptive immune reactions.

Allograft recipients receiving immunosuppressive therapy and patients with acquired immune deficiency syndrome (AIDS) are also at increased risk for development of EBV-associated post-transplant lymphoproliferative disease (PTLD) and lymphomas. These lesions range from polyclonal EBV-driven lymphoproliferations, much like that observed *in vitro* in virus-transformed LCLs (latency III, **Figure** 3), to aggressive monoclonal non-Hodgkin's B-cell lymphomas (NHLs) in which additional cellular genetic changes (e.g., mutation of p53) are present. The incidence of both PTLD and B-cell lymphomas in allograft recipients varies with the type of organ transplanted and with the type of immunosuppressive regimen used. Allogeneic bone marrow or solid organ transplantation into EBV seronegative children is a particular risk factor for the development of these lesions. A proportion of these lesions in post-transplant patients resolve in response to a reduction in immunosuppression or to targeted therapies such as anti-CD20 monoclonal antibody or adoptive EBV-specific T cells.

The incidence of NHL in AIDS patients is increased approximately 60-fold compared to the normal population. Around 60% of these tumors are large B-cell lymphomas like those found in allograft recipients, 20% are primary brain lymphomas, and 20% are of the BL type. EBV infection is present in approximately 50% of AIDS-related NHL, nearly all the primary brain and Hodgkin's lymphomas, and around 40% of the BL tumors.

Burkitt's Lymphoma

The endemic form of BL, which is found in areas of equatorial Africa and New Guinea, represents the most common childhood cancer (peak age 7–9 years) in these regions with an incidence of up to 10 cases per 100 000 people per year. This high incidence of BL is associated with holoendemic malaria, thus accounting for the climatic variation in tumor incidence first recognized by Denis Burkitt. More than 95% of these endemic BL tumors are EBV-positive compared with 20% of the low incidence, sporadic form of BL which occurs worldwide. In areas of intermediate BL incidence, such as Algeria and Malaysia, the increased number of cases correlates with an increased proportion of EBV-positive tumors. The pattern of EBV gene expression in BL is generally restricted to EBNA1 and the nonpolyadenylated EBER transcripts (latency I), although broader virus gene expression involving the EBNA3 proteins has been observed in a subset of tumors (**Figure 3**).

A consistent feature of BL tumors, irrespective of geographical location or EBV status, is chromosome translocations involving the long arm of chromosome 8 (8q24) in the region of the c-myc proto-oncogene and either chromosome 14 in the region of the Ig heavy-chain gene or, less frequently, chromosomes 2 or 22 in the region of the Ig light-chain genes. The cell surface phenotype of BL cells and the presence of ongoing Ig gene mutation supports the GC origin of this tumor.

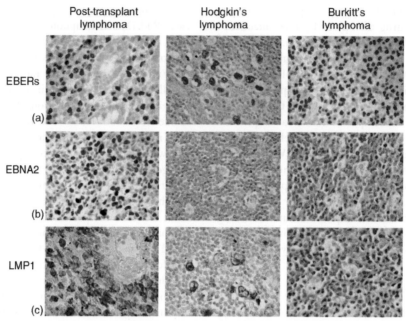

Figure 3 EBV-associated lymphomas display different patterns of virus latent gene expression. While the post-transplant lymphomas associated with EBV infection express a pattern of latent gene expression similar to that observed in virus-transformed B cells *in vitro* (latency III), Hodgkin's lymphoma (HL; Latency II) and Burkitt's lymphoma (BL; Latency I) express more restricted forms of EBV latency. (a) Upper panels show *in situ* hybridization for the abundant nonpolyadenylated EBER transcripts, which are expressed in all forms of EBV latent infection. (b) The middle panels depict immunohistochemical staining for the EBNA2 protein, which is only expressed in post-transplant lymphoma and not either HL or BL. (c) The bottom panels show immunohistochemical staining for the LMP1 protein, which is expressed in post-transplant lymphoma and HL but not in BL.

Seroepidemiological studies have demonstrated elevated antibody titers to EBV VCA and EA in BL patients compared to children without the tumor. These elevated antibody titers have been found to precede the development of BL and can therefore be used to screen 'at risk' individuals. Most early cases of BL can be successfully treated using chemotherapeutic regimens that include cyclophosphamide. However, access to drugs and advanced tumor presentation have limited the efficacy of such therapies.

Hodgkin's Lymphoma

Epidemiological studies originally suggested a possible role for EBV in the etiology of HL. Thus, elevated antibody titers to EBV antigens have been detected in HL patients and these are present before the diagnosis of the disease. Furthermore, there is an increased risk of HL following IM. EBV has been demonstrated in around 40% of HL cases with both viral nucleic acid and virus-encoded latent proteins (EBNA1, LMP1, LMP2 – latency II) localized to the malignant component of HL, the so-called Hodgkin's and Reed–Sternberg (HRS) cells (**Figure 3**). These malignant B cells tend to carry nonproductive Ig genes consistent with their GC origin and implicating EBV infection in the rescue of these crippled cells from their usual apoptotic fate. The association of HL with EBV is age-related; pediatric and older adult cases are usually EBV-associated whereas HL in young adults is less frequently virus-positive. The proportion of EBV-positive HL in developing countries is high, consistent with a greater incidence of HL in children and more frequent prevalence of the mixed cellularity histiotype; the histological subtype of HL in which EBV infection is most frequently detected. Although the incidence of HL is relatively low (1–3 per 100 000 per year), this tumor is not geographically restricted, making its association with EBV significant in world health terms.

Virus-Associated T-Cell and NK-Cell Lymphomas

EBV-positive monoclonal lymphomas of either CD4+ or CD8+ T-cell origin are more frequently found in Southeast Asian populations, arising as a consequence of either virus-associated haemophagocytic syndrome (VAHS) or in the setting of chronic active EBV infection. A more aggressive extranodal tumor predominantly expressing the CD56 natural killer (NK) cell marker is also EBV positive and manifests as an erosive lesion (lethal midline granuloma) of the nasal cavity.

Nasopharyngeal Carcinoma

The association of EBV with undifferentiated NPC (WHO type III) was first suggested by serological evidence and then confirmed by the demonstration of EBV DNA in NPC biopsy material. NPC is particularly common in areas of China and southeast Asia, reaching a peak incidence of 20–30 cases per 100 000 per year. Incidence rates are particularly high in Cantonese males, highlighting an important genetic predisposition as well as a role for environmental cofactors such as dietary components (e.g., salted fish). NPC tumors are characterized by a prominent lymphoid stroma, and the interaction between these activated lymphocytes and adjacent carcinoma cells appears to be crucial for the continued growth of the malignant component. EBV latent gene expression in NPC is restricted to EBNA1, the LMP2A/B proteins, the EBER transcripts, and the *Bam*HI-A rightward transcripts (BARTs), with around 20% of tumors also expressing the oncogenic LMP1 protein (**Figure 4** – latency II). The presence of monoclonal EBV episomes in NPC indicates that virus infection preceded the clonal expansion of the malignant cell population. More detailed analysis of the genetic changes in NPC suggests that some of these (particularly deletions in chromosomes 3p and 9p) occur early before EBV infection. Extensive serological screening for EBV-specific antibody titers in high-incidence areas, in particular IgA antibodies to VCA and EAs, have proved useful in diagnosis and in monitoring the effectiveness of therapy. More recent studies have demonstrated that the quantitative analysis of tumor-derived EBV DNA in the blood of patients with NPC using real-time polymerase chain reaction (PCR) is of both diagnostic and prognostic utility. EBV infection is also associated with the more differentiated forms of NPC (WHO types I and II) particularly in those geographical regions with a high incidence of the type III tumor. EBV-positive carcinomas, which morphologically resemble NPC (undifferentiated carcinomas of nasopharyngeal type), have been described at other anatomical sites (e.g., thymus, tonsil, lungs, skin) but the extent of the association of these tumors with EBV is geographically variable.

Gastric Carcinoma and Other Epithelial Tumors

EBV infection is also present in around 10% of typical gastric adenocarcinomas, accounting for up to 75 000 cases per year. These tumors resemble NPC in carrying monoclonal EBV genomes, having a restricted pattern of EBV gene expression (EBERs, EBNA1, LMP2A, BARTs, and BARF1) and in the appearance of virus infection as a relatively late event in the carcinogenic process. The geographical variation in the association of EBV with gastric adenocarcinomas probably reflects ethnic and genetic differences. EBV-positive tumors have distinct phenotypic and clinical characteristics compared with EBV-negative tumors.

A number of other more common carcinomas such as breast cancer and liver cancer have been reported to

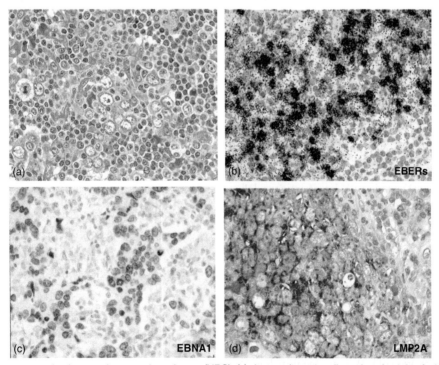

Figure 4 EBV gene expression in nasopharyngeal carcinoma (NPC). (a) shows a hematoxylin and eosin stain of a NPC tumor showing the intimate association between the undifferentiated carcinoma cells (large nuclei) and the activated lymphoid stroma (small intensely staining nuclei). (b–d) *in situ* hybridization for the EBER transcripts and immunohistochemical staining for EBNA1 and LMP2A.

be infected with EBV. Difficulties in confirming these associations have raised concerns about the use of PCR analysis to detect EBV infection and about the specificity of certain monoclonal antibody reagents. It is possible, however, that a small proportion of tumor cells can be infected with EBV, perhaps sustaining a low-level replicative infection, and that this might contribute to the growth of the carcinoma.

Prevention and Control of EBV Infection

The significant burden of EBV-associated tumors worldwide has prompted the development of novel therapeutic strategies that either specifically target viral proteins or exploit the presence of the virus in malignant cells. Pharmacological approaches include the use of agents to induce the expression EBV lytic cycle antigens, including virus-encoded kinases (EBV thymidine kinase and BGLF4, a protein kinase) that will then phosphorylate the nucleoside analog gancyclovir to produce its active cytotoxic form. Demethylating agents such as $5'$ azacytidine are able to de-repress lytic, as well as potentially immunogenic, latent genes and are currently in early-stage clinical trials in patients with NPC, HL, and AIDS-associated lymphoma. Hydroxyurea is a chemotherapeutic agent that can induce loss of EBV episomes and has shown some clinical efficacy in patients with EBV-positive AIDS-related central nervous system lymphoma. Other approaches are based on the more specific targeting of individual EBV proteins using either single-chain antibodies, siRNA, or dominant-negative molecules. The use of adoptive EBV-specific T-cell therapy for the treatment of existing PTLD and in the prophylactic setting has been extremely successful. This approach is also showing signs of clinical efficacy in the treatment of NPC and HL but in this setting the use of T cells enriched for reactivities to subdominant targets (e.g., LMP2A and EBNA1) is important. More direct vaccine approaches to treat patients with EBV-associated tumors or to prevent disease development are being examined including (1) whole EBV latent antigens delivered by a virus vector or in autologous dendritic cells; (2) peptide or polytope vaccination; and (3) prophylactic vaccination against MA (gp350/220) to generate a neutralizing antibody response.

Future Perspectives

EBV was discovered over 40 years ago and its DNA was fully sequenced in 1984. Much work has contributed to the unequivocal identification of EBV as oncogenic in humans. In more recent years, the nature of the interaction of EBV with the immune host has become clearer, illustrating the complex mechanisms that the virus exploits to persist in the memory B-cell pool. The fine detail of this interaction with normal B cells is still in its infancy, and a major question remains over the replicative lifecycle of EBV *in vivo*, particularly with regard to the relative role of B cells versus epithelial cells in this process. The development of more efficient *in vitro* systems for studying EBV infection and replication in different cell types will help to unravel the complex interplay between the virus and the cell. The use of EBV recombinants continues to shed light on the role of latent genes in the transformation process, on the requirements for the efficient production of progeny virus, and on the role of membrane glycoproteins in the infection process. Understanding the host cell–virus interaction will be dependent on the generation of appropriate *in vitro* models, particularly systems which allow a more detailed understanding of the tumor microenvironment and the role of the local cytokine milieu. There are many interesting aspects of EBV that remain to be understood, including the role of virus-encoded microRNAs and the possible contribution of lytic cycle antigens to virus persistence and oncogenesis. The challenge will be to exploit these new mechanistic insights both to gain a better understanding of EBV infection *in vivo* and to develop novel therapies for treating virus-associated disease.

See also: Herpesviruses: General Features; Herpesviruses: Latency; Kaposi's Sarcoma-Associated Herpesvirus: General Features.

Further Reading

Kieff E and Rickinson AB (2001) Epstein–Barr virus and its replication. In: Knipe DM and Howley PM (eds.) *Fields Virology*, 4th edn., pp. 2511–2573. Philadelphia: Lippincott Williams and Wilkins.

Kuppers R (2005) Mechanisms of B cell lymphoma pathogenesis. *Nature Reviews Cancer* 5: 251–262.

Kutok JL and Wang F (2006) Spectrum of Epstein–Barr virus-associated diseases. *Annual Review of Pathology: Mechanisms of Disease* 1: 375–404.

Lo KW and Huang DP (2002) Genetic and epigenetic changes in nasopharyngeal carcinoma. *Seminars in Cancer Biology* 12: 451–462.

Rickinson AB and Kieff E (2001) Epstein–Barr virus. In: Knipe DM and Howley PM (eds.) *Fields Virology*, 4th edn., pp. 2575–2627. Philadelphia: Lippincott Williams and Wilkins.

Robertson ES (ed.) (2005) *Epstein–Barr Virus*. Norfolk, England: Caister Academic Press.

Tao Q, Young LS, Woodman CB, and Murray PG (2006) Epstein–Barr virus and its associated cancers – Genetics, epigenetics, pathobiology and novel therapeutics. *Frontiers in Bioscience* 11: 2672–2713.

Thorley-Lawson DA and Gross A (2004) Persistence of the Epstein–Barr virus and the origins of associated lymphomas. *New England Journal of Medicine* 350: 1328–1337.

Young LS and Rickinson AB (2004) Epstein–Barr virus: 40 years on. *Nature Reviews Cancer* 4: 757–768.

Human T-Cell Leukemia Viruses: Human Disease

R Mahieux and A Gessain, Pasteur Institute, CNRS URA 3015, Paris, France

Introduction

In 1980, Dr. Gallo's laboratory (National Institutes of Health, USA) reported the isolation of HTLV-1, the first oncoretrovirus to be discovered in humans. HTLV-1 was present in the peripheral blood cells obtained from an Afro-American patient suffering from a lymphoproliferative disease, originally considered as a cutaneous T-cell lymphoma, with a leukemic phase. The virus was thus named human T-cell leukemia/lymphoma virus (HTLV). Later, it was recognized that this cutaneous lymphoma was in fact an adult T-cell leukemia/lymphoma (ATLL), a severe T-cell lymphoproliferation, originally described in Japan in 1977 by Takatsuki. The epidemiological characteristics of ATLL in Japan suggested a strong environmental factor, which prompted researchers to characterize the tumor cells and to search for an oncogenic virus. In 1981, a virus was isolated in Japan and termed adult T-cell leukemia/lymphoma virus (ATLV). Japanese and American scientists rapidly demonstrated that both isolates represented the same virus, and agreed to name it HTLV-1. In parallel, the causal association between ATLL and HTLV-1 was established. In 1983, the authors initiated a series of studies in the French West Indies in order to investigate the epidemiological and clinical impact of HTLV-1 in this area. This led them to demonstrate the etiological association between this virus and a chronic neuromyelopathy originally named tropical spastic paraparesis (TSP) that is endemic in the Caribbean. A similar neurological entity was then uncovered in Japan and labeled as HTLV-1-associated myelopathy. These two diseases were further shown to be identical and this myelopathy is now referred to as HAM/TSP. HTLV-1 infection has also been associated with other clinical conditions including uveitis, infective dermatitis, and myositis (**Table 1**).

HTLV-1, which is not a ubiquitous virus, is present throughout the world, with clusters of high endemicity located often nearby areas where the virus is nearly absent. These highly endemic areas are the southwestern part of the Japanese archipelago; the Caribbean area and its surrounding regions; foci in South America including Colombia, French Guyana, parts of Brazil; some areas of intertropical Africa (such as South Gabon); and of the middle East (such as the Mashad region in Iran); and isolated clusters in Melanesia. The origin of this puzzling geographical or rather ethnic repartition is not well understood but is probably linked to a founder effect in certain ethnic groups, followed by the persistence of a high viral transmission rate due to favorable local environmental and cultural situations. Interestingly, in all the highly endemic areas, and despite different socioeconomic and cultural environments, HTLV-1 seroprevalence increases gradually with age, especially among women. This might be either due to an accumulation of sexual exposures with age, or due to a cohort effect.

The worldwide infected population is estimated around 15–20 million. Two to ten percent of infected persons will develop an HTLV-1-associated disease (ATLL, HAM/TSP, uveitis, infective dermatitis, etc.) during their life (**Table 1**). Three modes of transmission have been demonstrated for HTLV-1: (1) Mother to child transmission, which is mainly linked to prolonged breastfeeding after 6 months of age. Ten to twenty-five percent of the breast-fed children born from HTLV-1 infected mothers will become persistently infected. (2) Sexual transmission, which mainly occurs from male to female, and is thought to be responsible for the increased seroprevalence with age in women. (3) Transmission with contaminated blood products (containing infected lymphocytes), which is responsible for an acquired HTLV-1 infection among 15–60% of the blood recipients.

Table 1 Diseases associated with HTLV-I infection

Adult disease	Association
Adult T-cell leukemia/lymphoma	++++
Tropical spastic paraparesis/HTLV-I-associated myelopathy	++++
Intermediate uveitis	+++
Infective dermatitis	+++
Myositis (polymyositis and SIBM)	+++
HTLV-I-associated arthritis	++
Pulmonary infiltrative pneumonitis	++
Invasive cervical cancer	+
Small cell carcinoma of lung	+
Sjögren disease	+
Childhood	Association
Infective dermatitis	++++
Tropical spastic paraparesis/HTLV-I-associated myelopathy (very rare)	++++
Adult T-cell leukemia/lymphoma (very rare)	++++
Persistent lymphadenopathy	++

The strength of association is based on epidemiological studies as well as molecular data, animal models, and intervention trials. ++++, proven association; +++, probable association; ++, likely association; +, possible association.
SIBM: sporadic inclusion body myositis.

From a molecular point of view, HTLV-1 possesses remarkable genetic stability, an unusual feature for a retrovirus. Viral amplification via clonal expansion of infected cells, rather than by reverse transcription, could explain this striking genetic stability, which can be used as a molecular tool to follow the migrations of infected populations in the recent or distant past and thus to gain new insights into the origin, evolution, and modes of dissemination of such retroviruses and their hosts. The few nucleotide substitutions observed among virus strains are indeed specific to the geographic origin of the patients rather than the pathology. Four major geographic subtypes (genotypes) have been reported. The origin of most of these geographic HTLV-1 subtypes appears to be linked to episodes of interspecies transmission between STLV-1-infected monkeys and humans, followed by variable period of evolution in the human host.

Adult T-Cell Leukemia/Lymphoma

Epidemiological Aspects

After the initial discovery and characterization of ATLL in Japan, the disease was reported in the USA and in Caribbean immigrants living in the United Kingdom. ATLL cases have now been reported in all HTLV-1 endemic areas including intertropical Africa, South and Central America, Iran, and Melanesia. Sporadic cases were also described in areas of low HTLV-1 endemicity,

often in immigrant patients originating from regions where HTLV-1 is endemic. In Japan, the ATLL incidence rate shows a steep increase with age, the mean age of disease onset being 57 years old and the sex ratio (male/female) being 1.4. In Japan, the annual incidence of ATLL cases is approximately 700, while the number of HTLV-1 carriers reaches 1.2 million. This gives an estimated yearly incidence of ATLL of 0.6–1.5 for 1000 HTLV-1 carriers older than 40. Lastly, the additive life-time risk of developing ATLL was estimated to be 1–5 % among Japanese HTLV-1 carriers. Studies performed in Brazil, Gabon, and French Guyana concluded that ATLL prevalence is usually underestimated until a specific disease research is performed. This is mostly due to the severity of the disease, its rapid evolution, and to confusion between ATLL and similar diseases, such as Sézary's syndrome, Mycosis fungoides, or other T cell non-Hodgkin lymphomas. In addition, laboratory tests such as Western blot and molecular investigations are not easily available in most tropical countries.

Diagnosis Criteria and Classification

Because of the extensive diversity in the clinical presentation and evolution of the disease, Japanese clinicians and researchers have defined stringent diagnosis criteria for ATLL as well as a classification into four major subtypes (**Table 2**). These diagnostic criteria are the following: (1) Histologically and/or cytologically

Table 2 Diagnostic criteria for clinical subtype of HTLV-I associated ATLL

	Smouldering	Chronic	Lymphoma	Acute
Anti-HTLV-I antibody	+	+	+	+
Lymphocyte ($\times 10^3$/μl)	< 4	$\geq 4^a$	< 4	*
Abnormal T lymphocytes	$\geq 5\%^c$	$+^b$	<1%	$+^b$
Flower cells of T cell marker	#	#	No	+
LDH	$\leq$1.5N	$\leq$2N	*	*
Corrected Ca (mEq/liter)	< 5.5	<5.5	*	*
Histology-proven lymphadenopathy	No	*	+	*
Tumor lesion				
Skin and/or lung	*c	*	*	*
Lymph node	No	*	Yes	*
Liver	No	*	*	*
Spleen	No	*	*	*
Central nervous system	No	No	*	*
Bone	No	No	*	*
Ascites	No	No	*	*
Pleural effusion	No	No	*	*
Gastrointestinal tract	No	No	*	*

[a]Accompanied by T lymphocytosis (3.5×10^3/μl or more).
[b]If abnormal T lymphocytes are less than 5% in peripheral blood, histology-proven tumor lesion is required.
[c]Histology-proven skin and/or pulmonary lesion(s) is required if abnormal T lymphocytes are less than 5% in peripheral blood.
*no essential qualification except terms required for other subtype(s).
N: normal upper limit.
#: typical flower cells seen occasionally.
Adapted from Shimoyama M and The Lymphoma Study Group (1991) Diagnostic critreria and classification of clinical subtypes of adult T-cell leukemia-lymphoma. *British Journal of Haematology* 79: 428–437.

proven lymphoid malignancy with expression of specific T-cell surface antigens (mostly CD2+, CD3+, and CD4+). (2) Abnormal T lymphocytes (flower cells and small/mature T lymphocytes with incised or lobulated nuclei) present in the peripheral blood, except in the ATLL lymphoma type. (3) Antibodies against HTLV-1 antigens present in the patient's serum at diagnosis.

The four major subtypes, as defined by the Japanese lymphoma study group, are the smoldering, the chronic, the lymphoma, and the leukemic/acute form. Both chronic and smoldering types can progress toward the acute or lymphoma forms. This classification was proved to be useful to discriminate ATLL from other type of leukemias/lymphomas. Patients who develop the smoldering form and about 30% of those suffering of the chronic ATLL have a fairly 'good prognosis' as compared to those with a leukemic or lymphoma type whose survival median does not exceed 6–9 months (**Table 2**). Finally, criteria for determining the diagnosis of ATLL during epidemiological studies have also been proposed (**Table 3**).

Clinical, Cytological, and Immuno-Virological Features

The predominant clinical findings of ATLL at onset are lymphadenopathy, hepatomegaly, splenomegaly, specific

skin lesions, and hypercalcemia (**Table 4**). The symptoms may include abdominal pain, diarrhea, pleural effusion, ascites, and cough. White blood count ranges from normal up to a very high number of abnormal peripheral blood lymphocytes, especially in acute and chronic ATLL patients, while anemia, neutropenia, or thrombocytopenia are occasionally observed. ATLL cells differ in size and characteristics, depending on the subtype. As an example, at the typical acute/leukemic stage, most abnormal cells exhibit multilobulated nuclei and are named 'flower cells' (**Figure 1**). At the terminal stage, cells often significantly vary in size. They display a cytoplasmic basophilia and a marked nuclear lobulation. Chronic ATLL cells are generally small and of uniform shape with minor nuclear abnormalities such as indentation or convolutions. Smoldering ATLL cells are often relatively large with a bi- or trifoliate nucleus.

Most ATLL cells are mature T cells of helper/inducer phenotype (CD2+, CD3+, CD4+, CD7–, CD8–) and express activation markers (CD25+, HLA DP+, DQ+, DR+). CD4– and CD8– ATLL cells are uncommon, but a

Table 3   Registry criteria for definition of ATLL

Definition of ATLL	
Clinical/routine laboratory criteria	
Hypercalcemia	1 point
Skin lesions[a]	1 point
Leukemic phase[b]	1 point
Research laboratory criteria	
T-cell lymphoma or leukemia	2 points
HTLV-I antibody	2 points
TAC-positive tumor cells	1 point
HTLV-I-positive tumors[c]	2 points
ATLL classification	
Classical	≥7 points
Probable	5 or 6 points
Possible	3 or 4 points
Inconsistent with ATLL	<3 points
Exclusion criteria	
B-cell positivity, nodular or follicular lymphoma, lymphoblastic lymphoma, small lymphocytic lymphoma	

[a]Lymphomatous cells documented morphologically.
[b]More than 2% abnormal lymphocytes.
[c]Determined by PCR or Southern blot analysis of the DNA of tumoral cells and indicating a monoclonal integration of HTLV-1 provirus(es).
Adapted from Levine PH, Cleghorn F, Manns A, *et al.* (1994) Adult T-cell leukemia/lymphoma: A working print-score classification for epidemiological studies. *International Journal of Cancer* 59: 491–493.

Table 4   Main clinical features of ATLL

	Japan[a]	Caribbean[b]
Age at onset	58 years (range 27–82)	47 years
Sex ratio male/female	1.4	0.6
Lymphadenopathy	60%	70%
Hepatomegaly	26%	27%
Splenomegaly	22%	31%
Specific skin lesion	39%	41%
Hypercalcemia	32%	51%

[a]Based on a series of 187 Japanese patients and
[b]from a series of 57 patients, with 46 of Carribean origin , seen in the United Kingdom.

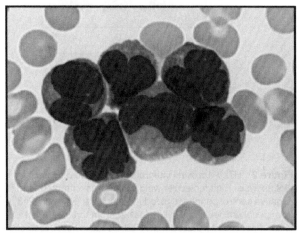

Figure 1   Peripheral blood smear from a Caribbean ATLL leukemic patient showing a cluster of atypical lymphoid cells with multilobulated nuclei (May-Grunwald-Giemsa staining).

decrease of the CD3/T cell receptor expression is frequent. Changes in cell activation marker expression (CD4+CD8− to CD4+CD8+) have been observed in some patients during the course of the disease. Lymph-node histology analysis frequently demonstrates infiltration by medium and large T cells with irregular nuclei effacing the nodal architecture. This is consistent with the diagnosis of pleiomorphic large T-cell lymphoma. However, there is no specific histological pattern for ATLL.

Cytogenetic abnormalities are not specific for ATLL, but are frequently reported in acute and lymphoma patients. They include chromosome 14 translocations (14q 32, 14q 11) and 6q deletions. Trisomy 3, 7, and 21 as well as X chromosome monosomy or the loss of the Y chromosome were also reported. Mutations in the p53 encoding tumor-suppressor gene are detected in 20–30% of all patients, mostly those in advanced stages, suggesting the involvement of p53 mutation in a late phase of leukemogenesis, or as a consequence of the cellular transformation.

Detecting (by Southern blot) the clonal integration of HTLV-1 provirus(es) in the tumor cells represents the gold-standard for establishing that a patient suffers from ATLL (**Figure 2**). In most cases, only one copy of the provirus is integrated in the tumor cells. Nevertheless, two or more proviruses can infrequently be detected (5–20% of all ATLL cases). It is also worth noting that 5–20% of ATLL patients carry defective HTLV-1 proviruses. The 3′pX region is commonly conserved, while deletions occur frequently in *gag, pol,* and/or *env* open reading frames. Inverse-PCR, a technique that is more sensitive than Southern blot is currently used for diagnosis of the monoclonal integration of HTLV-1 provirus(es) in the

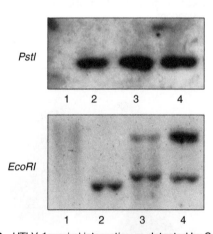

Figure 2 HTLV-1 proviral integration as detected by Southern blot analysis. High molecular weight DNA was extracted from (1) negative control peripheral blood mononuclear cells and (2, 3, 4) from peripheral leukemic cells obtained from three different HTLV-1 patients diagnosed with ATLL. Because *EcoRI* restriction sites are absent from HTLV-1 provirus sequence, the observation of two bands (lane 3 and 4) demonstrates the clonal integration of two proviruses in the DNA of the leukemic cells.

tumoral cells. Using this technique, oligoclonal or polyclonal proliferation of HTLV-1 infected T cell can also be detected in the peripheral blood lymphocytes of most HAM/TSP patients as well as in healthy HTLV-1 seropositive carriers. This also allows the precise identification of integration sites, the identification of each infected clone, and the tracing of the kinetics of the infected cells *in vivo.* The detection of persistent HTLV-1 infected monoclonal cell population could therefore be used as a method for monitoring individuals at risk for developing ATLL. Importantly, monoclonal expansion of HTLV-1 infected cells in carriers is directly associated with the onset of ATLL.

Specific Features and Complications

Hypercalcemia is very common among ATLL patients. It is detected in 20–30 % of the patients at admission and in more than 70 % of them during the entire clinical course, with or without lytic bone lesions. *In vitro,* ATLL cells induce the differentiation of hematopoietic precursor cells to osteoclasts through the expression of the RANKL (receptor activator nuclear factor kB) ligand on their surface, in cooperation with elevated M-CSF (mononuclear phagocyte colony-stimulating factor) serum levels. This accelerates bone resorption and ultimately causes hypercalcemia. The degree of hypercalcemia might also be linked to the expression of the parathyroid hormone-related protein (PTHrP), since PTHrP also induces RANK ligand expression on osteoblasts.

Skin infiltration of a clonal population of HTLV-1 tumor cells represents a frequent ATLL clinical feature. It is present in 20–40% of all ATLL patients and in more than 50% of smoldering ATLL patients. Various cutaneous lesions have been described including papules, nodules, erythroderma, plaques, tumors, and ulcerative lesions. ATLL cells densely infiltrate both dermis and epidermis forming Pautrier's micro-abscesses. When skin lesions dominate the clinical picture, the disease is referred to as 'cutaneous ATLL' (**Figure 3**). In such cases, establishing the difference between these lesions and other cutaneous T-cell lymphomas (CTCLs) is complicated. A possible role of CCR4 (CC chemokine receptor 4) in skin invasion by ATLL cells has been suggested. Other factors such as expression of cutaneous lymphocyte antigen (CLA) by leukemic cells and inflammatory responses in injured skin that would lead to upregulation of thymus and activation-regulated chemokine (TARC) and macrophage-derived chemokine (MDC) are also likely to contribute to skin involvement of ATLL.

ATLL is also known to frequently invade the gastrointestinal tract, even though the exact incidence has not been determined yet. CCR9 is known to be involved in T-cell homing to the gastrointestinal tract. A recent study demonstrated that CCR9 is expressed by HTLV-1 T cells

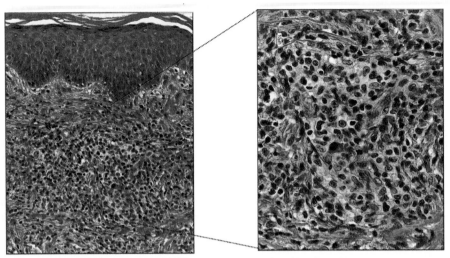

Figure 3 Histological analysis of skin invasion in an HTLV-1 patient from West Africa with a cutaneous ATLL showing an infiltration of the dermis by tumoral pleomorphic cells. These tumor cells are mature activated lymphoid T cells (CD2+, CD3+, CD4+, CD8–, and CD25+). Kindly provided by Dr. Michel Huerre, Institut Pasteur, Paris.

and ATLL cells expressing Tax and suggested that it may play a role in the gastrointestinal involvement of ATLL.

The frequency of opportunistic infections is quite high in ATLL patients, indicating that T-cell-mediated immunity is severely impaired in such patients. Infestation by *Strongyloides stercoralis* (*S.s*) is frequent among HTLV-1 seropositive carriers and *S.s* infected individuals are often infected by HTLV-1 in highly endemic areas. Numerous studies showed the presence of *S.S* in acute or lymphoma ATLL, suggesting that infection by *S.S* might play a significant role as a candidate cofactor for HTLV-1 induced leukemogenesis.

Pulmonary complications are also frequent in ATLL patients. These are either leukemic infiltrate or opportunistic infections. Central nervous system localization rarely occurs in ATLL (10%).

ATLL Pathogenesis

The development of an ATLL has been clearly associated with an early acquired HTLV-1 infection. The risk of being infected for a child born from an HTLV-1 infected mother is positively correlated with prolonged (>6 months) breastfeeding. After a limited number of replication cycles using its reverse transcriptase during primary infection, HTLV-1 replicates and increases its copy number through the proliferation of infected cells, thus using the cellular DNA polymerase which possesses a proofreading activity. Such a model could explain, in part, the very high genetic stability of HTLV-1. The clonal proliferation of the HTLV-1-infected CD4+ lymphocytes is likely to be linked to the pleiotropic effects of the viral Tax protein. *In vitro*, Tax expression induces expression of several cellular cytokines such as IL-2, IL-15, but also alters the cell-cycle control machinery,

inhibits apoptosis, and promotes genetic instability. As seen above, the fact that oligo/monoclonal-infected cell populations are present in the PBMCs of HTLV-1 carriers or of HAM/TSP patients suggests that neither the monoclonal integration of the virus nor the CD4+ cell proliferation *per se* is sufficient to cause the disease. *In vivo*, the level of Tax expression is still debated. Several observations paradoxically suggested that HTLV-1 was transcriptionally silent *in vivo*, but it was shown lately that a high proportion (10%–80%) of naturally infected CD4+ peripheral blood mononuclear cells isolated from HAM/TSP patients or from HTLV-1 asymptomatic carriers are capable of expressing Tax *ex vivo*. It was also demonstrated that autologous CD8$^+$ T cells rapidly kill CD4+ cells that express Tax *in vitro* through a perforin-dependent mechanism. Altogether, these results suggest that virus-specific cytotoxic T lymphocytes (CTLs) participate in a highly efficient immune surveillance mechanism that tirelessly eradicates Tax-expressing HTLV-1-infected CD4+ T cells *in vivo*. Such CTL control of the HTLV-1-infected cell proliferation may also result in the prevention of ATLL. The role of the genetic background, especially HLA haplotypes, in such control could be crucial. A final step toward ATLL leukemogenesis consists in the accumulation of alterations in the host genome due to the pleiotropic effects of Tax (**Figure 4**).

Therapeutic Aspects of ATLL

The survival rate of ATLL patients, especially those who develop the acute leukemic or lymphoma forms, remains poor, and ATLL remains therefore one of the most severe lymphoproliferations. Treatment of ATLL patients using conventional chemotherapy (CHOP) has been and remains in most cases the standard first-line therapy. It has very

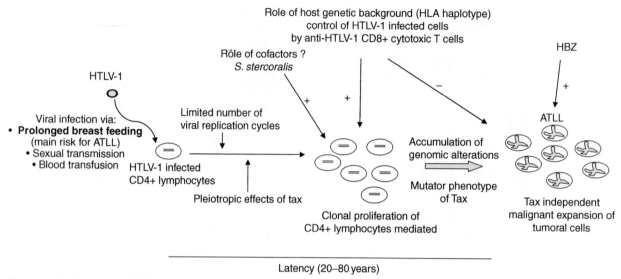

Figure 4   Pathogenesis of ATLL. Natural course from HTLV-1 primary infection by prolonged breast-feeding to the onset of the malignant proliferation of ATLL cells. HBZ: HTLV-1 bZIP factor. Adapted from Mahieux R and Gessain A (2003) HTLV-1 and associated adult T-cell leukemia/lymphoma. *Reviews in Clinical and Experimental Hematology* 7: 336–362.

limited benefit, since HTLV-1 cells are resistant to most apoptosis-inducing agents. A historical Japanese survey based on 818 ATLL cases reported a median survival time of 9 months, with a survival rate of only 27% and 10% at 2–4 years respectively. Survival is different when subtypes are considered into account, with a 4-year survival rate of 66% for the smoldering type, of 27% for the chronic type and of 5–6% for the lymphoma and acute types. Spontaneous regressions are observed in very few cases. The main prognosis factors associated with a poor response and a poor survival rate in ATLL patients are: a high LDH (lactate dehydrogenase) value, high leukemic counts (both of them reflecting a high tumor burden), hypercalcemia, and a poor clinical performance. Furthermore, the main obstacles to an efficient response to treatment are infectious complications (*pneumocystis carinii, cryptococcus meningitis*, disseminated herpes zoster), hypercalcemia, and liver or kidney dysfunction.

Various strategies other than CHOP have been used during clinical trials. This includes combination chemotherapy (CHOP plus methotrexate, CHOP in combination with etoposide, vindesine, ranimustine, mitoxantrone, or adriamycin), granulocyte macrophage-colony-stimulating factor (GM-CSF), supported combination chemotherapy, and other chemotherapy treatments that are highly toxic for bone marrow. Zidovudine (AZT) has been shown to inhibit HTLV-1 transmission *in vitro*. Several studies with AZT and interferon-alpha (IFN-α) have been conducted, both in the USA and in Europe (France and UK). They all demonstrated that response and survival in patients is more efficient when the drugs are used as first-line therapy. Until recently, the mechanism of action of AZT was a matter of debate. A recent study convincingly demonstrated that

AZT can act as an inhibitor of the telomerase functions. More importantly, it was also shown that the p53 status (wild-type or mutated) is predictive of the response to AZT. Nuclear factor kappa B (NF-κB) inhibitor (Bay 11–7082) was found to be efficient for preventing the tumor growth in NOD-SCID (non-obese diabetic-severe combined immunodeficiency/gamma (null)) animals previously inoculated with HTLV-1 infected cells. Proteasome inhibitor PS-341 (Bortezomib) alone or combined with anti-CD25 (anti-Tac) therapy was partially successful in treating NOD/SCID animals or Tax transgenic mice. Allogenic bone marrow transplantation as well as allogenic hematopoietic stem cells transplantation have been performed on a limited number of patients. The estimated overall survival seems to compare favorably with historical data on chemotherapy, but definitive assessments are difficult to establish.

Tropical Spastic Paraparesis/HTLV-1 Associated Myelopathy

Spastic paraparesis without evidence of spinal cord compression has been described from various tropical and intertropical areas such as the Caribbean region, South and Central Africa, and India. Apart from cassava-related myelopathy and/or malnutrition in several African regions, lathyrism in India, and some infectious processes, the etiology of numerous spastic meylopathies remained elusive until 1985. The demonstration by our laboratory of the association between HTLV-1 and a form of tropical spastic paraparesis (TSP) of Unknown etiology, frequent in Martinique (French West Indies), led to the evaluation of the role of this oncoretrovirus, in this disease. Such an association was rapidly confirmed in Colombia and Jamaica. A year later, the association of HTLV-1 with a chronic spastic myelopathy of unknown etiology was documented in southern Japan, and this clinical entity was named HTLV-1 associated myelopathy (HAM). Soon after, it was recognized that HTLV-1-associated TSP and HAM were the same disease, the hybrid term HAM/TSP was adopted and WHO diagnostic criteria were established.

Hundreds of HAM/TSP patients have now been described in several HTLV-1 endemic areas, including Japan, several of the Caribbean islands (especially Jamaica, Trinidad, Martinique, Haiti), numerous countries of South and Central America (Brazil, Peru, Colombia), of Central and South Africa, as well as in Iran. Sporadic cases of HAM/TSP have also been described in Melanesia, in West African countries as well as in immigrants from high HTLV-1 endemic areas living in Europe and the USA. In Japan, the life-time risk among HTLV-1 carriers is estimated to be less than 2%, that is, lower than ATLL. HAM/TSP mainly occurs in adults, with a mean age at onset of 40–50 years, but some rare cases of HAM/TSP in children have been reported. In Japan, in contrast to ATLL, HAM/TSP is more common in women than in men at all ages, with a sex ratio (M/F) of around 1:2,3.

Diagnostic Criteria

Initially, HAM/TSP diagnostic criteria included: (1) chronic spastic paraparesis, which usually slowly progresses, with signs of bilateral pyramidal tract lesions manifested by increased knee reflexes, ankle clonus, and extensor plantar responses; (2) minor sensory signs of involvement of the posterior columns and spinothalamic tract; (3) a history of insidious onset with gait disturbance without an episode of complete remission; (4) no evidence of spinal cord compression or swelling on magnetic resonance imaging, myelography, or computed/tomographic scan; and (5) presence of specific anti-HTLV-1 antibodies in the serum and the cerebrospinal fluid (CSF).

In more than 90% of the cases, the neurological features of HAM/TSP involve: spasticity and/or hyperreflexia of the lower extremities, urinary bladder disturbance, lower extremity muscle weakness, and in around 50% of the cases, sensory disturbances with low back pain. Impotence is also frequent. Central functions and cranial nerves are usually spared. The evolution is generally chronic and progressive, and after 10 years of evolution, roughly 50% of the patients are wheel-chaired. The incubation period (between primary infection which occurs mainly in adults) to onset of the myelopathy signs ranges usually from years to decades, but HAM/TSP also developed within 3.3 years in 50% of the post-transfusion-associated cases.

Biologically, besides high level of antibodies directed against HTLV-1 antigens both in blood and CSF, ATLL-like cells can sometimes be detected on the blood

smear and in the CSF. Furthermore, a high HTLV-1 proviral load is frequently observed in the peripheral blood lymphocytes from HAM/TSP patients. A mild to moderate increase of proteins may be present in the CSF. However, intrathecal production of specific antibody provides additional data to support the diagnosis of HAM/TSP and also contributes to eliminate other differential diagnoses. Multiple spotty high intensities in deep and subcortical areas on T2-weighted images are the most frequent findings in brain magnetic resonance imaging. A mild atrophy of the thoracic spinal cord can also be observed in few cases. From a pathological point of view, this neurological syndrome is characterized by a chronic inflammation with perivascular lymphocytic cuffing and mild parenchymal lymphocytic infiltrates (**Figure 5(a)**). The cells are mostly CD4+ in early disease and mostly CD8+ in latter disease. Pyramidal tract damage with myelin and axonal loss, mainly in the lower thoracic spinal cord are observed.

HAM/TSP can be associated with other HTLV-1-associated symptoms such as uveitis, myositis, pulmonary alveolitis, and arthritis. The coincidence of ATLL and HAM/TSP has been rarely reported.

Recently, a large group of neurologists established a proposal for a modification of the diagnostic criteria of HAM/TSP. This was due to the fact that in some patients, especially those with early disease, HAM/TSP can be

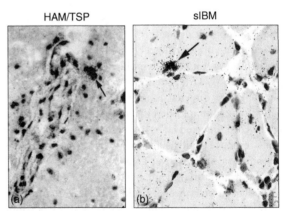

Figure 5 Detection of HTLV-1 *mRNA* expression by *in situ* hybridization with a ^{33}P *Tax* antisense riboprobe, on (a) frozen section from thoracic cord of a HAM/TSP patient, and (b) from a muscle section of a patient with an HTLV-1-associated sporadic inclusion body myositis (sIBM). Adapted from Ozden S, Seilhean D, Gessain A, Hauw J-J, and Gout O (2002) Severe demyelinating myelopathy with low human t cell lymphotropic virus type 1 expression after transfusion in an immunosuppressed patient. *Clinical Infectious Diseases* 34: 855–860 and Ozden S, Cochet M, Mikol J, *et al.* (2004) Direct evidence for a chronic CD8+-T-cell-mediated immune reaction to tax within the muscle of a human T-cell leukemia/lymphoma virus type 1-infected patient with sporadic inclusion body myositis. *Journal of Virology* 78: 10320–10327.

suspected but the complete WHO criteria are not met. These authors suggest that a HAM/TSP definite case corresponds to a nonremitting progressive spastic paraparesis with sufficiently impaired gait to be perceived by the patient. Sensory symptoms or signs may or may not be present. When present, they remain subtle and without a clear-cut sensory level. Urinary and anal sphincter signs or symptoms may or may not be present. Biologically, presence of HTLV-1 antibodies in serum and CSF confirmed by Western blot and/or a positive polymerase chain reaction (PCR) for HTLV-1 in blood and/or CSF should be demonstrated. Lastly, exclusion of other disorders that can resemble HAM/TSP is necessary.

HAM/TSP Pathogenesis

The pathogenesis of HAM/TSP is still poorly understood and viral and host factors as the proviral load and the immune response are considered to play a major role in disease progression. It remains unknown if the myelin and axonal loss, observed in HAM/TSP lesions, is a primary or secondary process and if it results from a direct viral effect or from an immune mediated process, as suggested by the marked lymphocytic infiltrates. Viral infection as demonstrated by *in situ* hybridization against *tax* mRNA has been clearly identified in some infiltrates by CD4+ lymphocytes by several teams, while the presence of HTLV-1 in neurons or oligodendrocytes remains controversial but unlikely.

At least three mechanisms have been proposed to explain the role of HTLV-1 in HAM/TSP development. The neurological damage is, in the first model, a direct consequence of the destruction by an antiviral attack mediated by cytotoxic T lymphocytes. These CTLs, frequent in HAM/TSP patients, both in the peripheral blood and CSF, are directed against HTLV-1 antigens, especially some immuno-dominant Tax epitopes expressed by HTLV-1-infected cells. In a second model, an autoimmune response could be due to either a chronic peripheral activation of autoreactive T cells by HTLV-1 infection, with infiltration of T lymphocytes into the CNS, or to a molecular mimicry, which could impair the immunological tolerance to the myelin antigens. A third possibility would be the bystander damage hypothesis. In this model, activated CD4+ T cells infected by HTLV-1, activated microglia, and CD8+ T cells could release into the spinal cord some myelinotoxic cytokines such as TNF-α or could directly damage the glial cells.

Therapeutic aspects of HAM/TSP

The long-term prognosis of HAM/TSP remains severe with a chronic evolution of a progressive disabling disorder without remission. Furthermore, its secondary complications may eventually lead to death, in some cases, after several years of evolution. Many small studies and cohort data have been performed using, among other drugs, corticosteroid therapy, danazol, vitamin C, interferon alpha, zidovudine, with very limited success. Recently, a randomized trial with zidovudine plus lamivudine has also been performed. Globally, a few short-term benefits have been observed, especially in early disease, but no treatment has been successful in chronic advanced disease. Failure to detect any clinical improvement is believed to be due to irreversible central nervous system damage in such patients. New controlled studies of both antiviral and anti-inflammatory agents are urgently required.

HAM/TSP is probably not the only neurological disorder associated with HTLV-1 infection. Indeed, an amyotrophic lateral sclerosis-like syndrome, as well as some peripheral neuropathies, and mild cognitive deficits have been described in some patients with HTLV-1 infection. It remains however difficult to prove a true association between such diseases and HTLV-1 infection, especially in high HTLV-1 endemic areas.

Infective Dermatitis

Infective dermatitis (ID) is a rare dermatological condition that was originally described in Jamaican children by Sweet in 1966. Subsequently, in 1990, La Grenade *et al.* linked ID to HTLV-1 infection. A large series of patients with infective dermatitis have been described in Jamaica and more recently in Brazil. However sporadic cases of this clinical entity have also been reported in many other HTLV-1 endemic areas including Trinidad, Colombia, French West-Indies and French Guyana, Japan (where the disease seems very rare), and recently in Senegal (West Africa). In the great majority of cases, ID occurs in children from low socioeconomic backgrounds.

Infective dermatitis is a unique clinical entity characterized by a chronic and severe exudative dermatitis involving mainly the scalp, external ear and retroauricular areas, eyelid margins, paranasal skin, neck, axillae, and groin (**Figure 6**). Other symptoms include a chronic watery nasal discharge without other signs of rhinitis and/or crusting of anterior nares. A generalized fine papular rash is common in most of the severe cases. Clinically, the two differential diagnoses are atopic dermatitis and seborrheic dermatitis. In infective dermatitis, positive cultures for *Staphylococcus aureus* and/or beta-haemolytic streptococci are frequent from the anterior nares and skin samples. The evolution is typically chronic with relapse and several flares of superinfected lesions. Infective dermatitis responds well to antibiotic treatment, especially co-trimoxazole. However, relapse is very common if antibiotics are withdrawn. Infective dermatitis occurs mainly in young children (range 1–12 years), with an

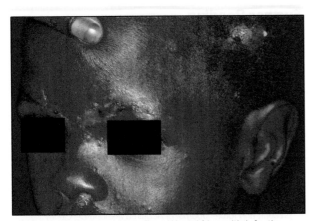

Figure 6 A 3-year-old boy from West Africa with infective dermatitis lesions: erosive dermatitis of the eyebrows, abscess of the scalp, and nasal discharge. Adapted from Mahe A, Meertens L, Ly F, *et al.* (2004) Human T-cell leukemia/lymphoma virus type 1-associated infective dermatitis in Africa: A report of five cases from Senegal. *British Journal of Dermatology* 150: 958–965.

average age of onset of 2–6 years depending on the studies. Around 60% of the cases occur in girls. Anemia is frequent with a raised erythrocyte sedimentation rate and a hyper-immunoglobulinemia (IgD and IgE). The CD4 count, as well as the CD4/CD8 ratio, are elevated. Presence of rare ATLL-like cells is common in the peripheral blood. Pathological examination revealed an inflammatory lymphocytic infiltrate within the skin lesions. Epidemiological studies with long-term follow-up of ID patients have indicated that such disease may be associated with the later development of ATLL or of HAM/TSP. In a recent series from Brazil, neurological examination diagnosed six HAM/TSP cases among 20 children and adolescents with ID.

Mothers of children with ID are nearly always infected by HTLV-1. Furthermore, they have breastfed their child for a long period of time (mean 20 months). Thus, nearly all ID children were infected by their mothers. This implies that reduction of HTLV-1 transmission from mother to child would be likely to prevent the occurrence of such disease as well as of ATLL. Such preventive medicine, currently performed in several areas of high HTLV-1 endemicity (Japan, West Indies), is based on HTLV-1 screening programs during pregnancy followed by adequate counseling that is adapted to the socioeconomic situation of each infected mother. The pathogenesis of ID is unknown but environmental, as well as host genetic factors are very likely involved in its occurrence.

Myositis

Myositis is an inflammatory myopathy that is represented by a heterogeneous group of muscle disorders. It is characterized by an acquired muscle weakness and inflammatory infiltrates of the muscle tissues. Depending on the clinical and histological features, myositis can be classified into dermatomyositis, polymyositis, and inclusion-body myositis. In 1989, Morgan *et al.* reported for the first time that 11 out of 13 Jamaican patients with idiopathic adult polymyositis were seropositive for HTLV-1. Later on, several epidemiological studies conducted in Jamaica, Martinique, and Japan, and based on larger series of patients, also indicated a higher prevalence of HTLV-1 antibodies in polymyositis patients as compared to that of the general population. Such data suggested a possible link between HTLV-1 and polymyositis. Lately, several sporadic cases of polymyositis, occurring in HTLV-1 infected patients of various origins, have been reported.

HTLV-1-associated polymyositis is a chronic disease that occurs mainly in adults 30–50 years of age. Patients complain mainly of musculo-skeletal symptoms including myalgia, joint and back pain, and proximal muscle weakness with muscle atrophia and falls. The four limbs can be affected. A patient's clinical pattern typically displays an elevation of muscle enzymes, especially creatine phosphokinase (CPK), and significant electromyographic abnormalities. Histological findings indicate an inflammatory myopathy with an increased variation in the fiber size and a mononuclear infiltrate located both between and within muscle cells, which appear often degenerate and necrotic. Muscle regeneration may also be present. This infiltration is mainly due to T lymphocytes (both CD4+ and CD8+), but macrophages are also present. Expression of HTLV-1 *mRNAs* as well as of the viral proteins can be sporadically detected within the infiltrating T lymphocytes but not within muscle fibers. T-cell clones that are specifically directed against HTLV-1 Tax epitopes proliferate within the muscle lesions and may thus contribute to the pathogenesis. Patients respond poorly to corticosteroid therapy in most cases, and there is usually no sustained effect. Of note, HTLV-1 associated polymyositis is frequently associated with HAM/TSP.

A few cases of sporadic inclusion-myositis (sIBM) have also been reported in HTLV-1-infected patients. Such a disorder is a distinct form of chronic inflammatory myopathy for which a viral etiology has often been suspected. The lesions are characterized by vacuolated fibers that contain paired helical filaments similar to those of Alzheimer's diseases (**Figure 5(b)**). Immunohistochemical staining for ubiquitin may help to differentiate sIBM from polymyositis. sIBM can be associated with HAM/TSP.

Uveitis

Uveitis is an intraocular sight-threatening inflammatory disorder that can be caused by various infections, including tuberculosis, syphilis, toxoplasmosis, and cytomegalovirus.

Uveitis, which does not have an infectious etiology, can occur in Bechet's diseases, Vogt–Koyanagi–Harada disease, and sarcoidosis. In roughly 40%, no cause can be identified and such disease is classified as idiopathic or unexplained uveitis. In the early 1990s, epidemiological studies demonstrated a higher prevalence of such idiopathic uveitis in HTLV-1 endemic areas from southern Japan than in areas where HTLV-1 has a lower prevalence. At the same time, some cases of uveitis were also observed in HAM/TSP patients. A large seroepidemiological study led by Mochizuki *et al.*, finally demonstrated without ambiguity that HTLV-1 infection was associated with idiopathic uveitis.

This clinico-virological entity is more frequent in females (around 60%) and the average onset age of the disease is 45 years, with few cases occurring in children. The major symptoms at initial presentation include sudden onset of occular floaters, foggy, and/or blurred vision. Unilateral disease is more common than bilateral (60% vs. 40%). The ocular signs consist mainly of iritis, vitreous opacities, and retinal vasculitis. Retinal exudates and hemorrhages are less frequent. Intermediate uveitis is more frequent than anterior or posterior lesions. Interestingly, co-morbid conditions include Graves disease and HAM/TSP. HTLV-1 uveitis responds well to topical and/or systemic corticosteroids and the intra-occular inflammation is markedly improved after steroid therapy. The visual prognosis is good in most cases. However, the inflammation tends to recur in about half of the cases. A specific opthalmological and systemic evaluation is necessary to eliminate other causes of uveitis in a given HTLV-1 infected individual. HTLV-1 antibodies are present in the aqueous humor at a level similar to that found in the plasma. HTLV-1-infected lymphocytes can be detected in the anterior chamber of the eye. Cytokines such as IL-6 and TNF-α produced by infiltrating lymphocytes are considered to play a major role in HTLV-1-associated uveitis pathogenesis. Infra-clinical uveitis can be detected through systematic examination in some HTLV-1 infected persons without any ocular symptoms.

Other Ocular Lesions Associated with HTLV-1 Infection

Kerato-conjonctivitis/sicca as well as interstitial chronic keratitis, are observed in HTLV-1 infected individuals, especially in HAM/TSP patients. The latter keratitis is also frequently associated with uveitis.

See also: Human T-Cell Leukemia Viruses: General Features.

Further Reading

Araujo AQ and Silva MT (2006) The HTLV-1 neurological complex. *Lancet Neurology* 5: 1068–1076.

Bazarbachi A, Ghez D, Lepelletier Y, *et al.* (2004) New therapeutic approaches for adult T-cell leukaemia. *Lancet Oncology* 5: 664–672.

Cleghorn F and Manns A (1994) Adult T-Cell leukemia/lymphoma: A working point-score classification for epidemiological studies. *International Journal of Cancer* 59: 491–493.

De Castro-Costa CM, Araujo AQ, Barreto MM, *et al.* (2006) Proposal for diagnostic criteria of tropical spastic paraparesis/HTLV-I-associated myelopathy (HAM/TSP). *AIDS Research and Human Retroviruses* 22: 931–935.

Grassmann R, Aboud M, and Jeang KT (2005) Molecular mechanisms of cellular transformation by HTLV-1 Tax. *Oncogene* 24: 5976–5985.

La Grenade L (1996) HTLV-I-associated infective dermatitis: Past, present, and future. *Journal of Acquired Immune Deficiency Syndromes and Human Retrovirology* 13(supplement 1): S46–S49.

La Grenade L, Manns A, Fletcher V, *et al.* (1998) Clinical, pathologic, and immunologic features of human T-lymphotrophic virus type I-associated infective dermatitis in children. *Archives of Dermatology* 134: 439–444.

Leon-Monzon M, Illa I, and Dalakas MC (1994) Polymyositis in patients infected with human T-cell leukemia virus type I: The role of the virus in the cause of the disease. *Annals of Neurology* 36: 643–649.

Levine PH, Cleghorn F, Manns A, *et al.* (1994) Adult T-cell leukemi/lymphoma: A working pring-score classification for epidemiological studies. *International Journal of Cancer* 59: 491–493.

Mahe A, Meertens L, Ly F, *et al.* (2004) Human T-cell leukaemia/lymphoma virus type 1-associated infective dermatitis in Africa: A report of five cases from Senegal. *British Journal of Dermatology* 150: 958–965.

Mahieux R and Gessain A (2003) A. HTLV-1 and associated adult T-cell leukemia/lymphoma. *Reviews in Clinical and Experimental Hematology* 7: 336–362.

Manns A, Hisada M, and La Grenade L (1999) Human T-lymphotropic virus type I infection. *Lancet* 353: 1951–1958.

Matsuoka M (2005) Human T-cell leukemia virus type I (HTLV-I) infection and the onset of adult T-cell leukemia (ATL). *Retrovirology* 2: 27.

Mochizuki M, Ono A, Ikeda E, *et al.* (1996) HTLV-I uveitis. *Journal of Acquired Immune Deficiency Syndromes and Human Retrovirology* 13(supplement 1): S50–S56.

Ozden S, Cochet M, Mikol J, *et al.* (2004) Direct evidence for a chronic CD8+-T-cell-mediated immune reaction to tax within the muscle of a human T-cell leukemia/lymphoma virus type 1-infected patient with sporadic inclusion body myositis. *Journal of Virology* 78: 10320–10327.

Ozden S, Mouly V, Prevost MC, Gessain A, Butler-Browne G, and Ceccaldi PE (2005) Muscle wasting induced by HTLV-1 tax-1 protein: *An in vitro* and *in vivo* study. *American Journal of Pathology* 167: 1609–1619.

Ozden S, Seilhean D, Gessain A, Hauw J-J, and Gout O (2002) Severe demyelinating myelopathy with low human t cell lymphotropic virus type 1 expression after transfusion in an immunosuppressed patient. *Clinical Infectious Diseases* 34: 855–860.

Pinheiro SR, Martins-Filho OA, Ribas JG, *et al.* (2006) Immunologic markers, uveitis, and keratoconjunctivitis sicca associated with human T-cell lymphotropic virus type 1. *American Journal of Ophthalmology* 142: 811–815.

Proietti FA, Carneiro-Proietti AB, Catalan-Soares BC, and Murphy EL (2005) Global epidemiology of HTLV-I infection and associated diseases. *Oncogene* 24: 6058–6068.

Shimoyama M and The Lymphoma Study Group (1991) Diagnostic criteria and classification of clinical subtypes of adult T-cell leukemia-lymphoma. *British Journal of Haematology* 79: 428–437.

Taylor GP and Matsuoka M (2005) Natural history of adult T-cell leukemia/lymphoma and approaches to therapy. *Oncogene* 24: 6047–6057.

Polyomaviruses of Humans

M Safak and K Khalili, Temple University School of Medicine, Philadelphia, PA, USA

JC Virus

JC virus (JCV) is classified into species *JC polyomavirus*, genus *Polyomavirus*, family *Polyomaviridae*. The JCV genome contains a small, double-stranded, closed circular DNA of 5130 bp. The capsid exhibits an icosahedral structure, approximately 45 nm in diameter. Structural and antigenic studies have indicated that JCV is closely related to two other polyomaviruses, BK virus (BKV) and simian vacuolating virus 40 (SV40). JCV is the etiologic agent of a fatal demyelinating disease of the central nervous system (CNS) known as progressive multifocal leukoencephalopathy (PML). Seroepidemiological data indicate that the overwhelming majority of the world's population (70–80%) is infected by JCV early in childhood without apparent clinical symptoms. The virus establishes a persistent infection in the kidneys (latent infection) and reactivates from latency under immunocompromised conditions. As well as the kidneys, hematopoietic progenitor cells, peripheral blood B lymphocytes, and tonsillar stromal cells have been shown to harbor JCV, suggesting that these sites could serve as additional sites for latent infection by JCV.

Recently, two new human polyomaviruses were also discovered. One was isolated from human respiratory tract samples by polymerase chain reaction (PCR) amplification and named KI polyomavirus (KIPyV). The other was isolated from a patient with symptoms of acute respiratory tract infection and named WU virus (WUV). Thus far, follow-up studies have not yielded evidence for associations between infections with KIPyV or WUV and respiratory disease.

JCV was first isolated from the brain tissue of a PML patient in 1971, and this opened new frontiers in polyomavirus research. A piece of brain tissue from a PML patient was used as a source of inoculum to infect primary cultures derived from human fetal brain, and the virus was then successfully cultivated from those long-term cultures. This was the first direct evidence that a neurotropic virus is associated with the development of PML. At the same time, a virus similar in structure was found in the urine of a patient who had undergone renal transplantation. Each virus was named with the initials of the donor, BK virus for the renal transplantation patient and JC virus for the patient with PML. Following the isolation of JCV, the oncogenic potential of the virus was demonstrated both in tissue culture and experimental animals. Particularly, animal model studies showed that JCV induces tumors in tissues of neural origin. In addition, the genome has recently been found to be present in a variety of human tumors.

JCV infects and destroys oligodendrocytes, which are the myelin-producing cells in the CNS, and indirectly causes the death of neurons in the white matter of the brain, because neurons are known to depend for survival on support provided by oligodendrocytes. Subsequently, the destruction of both oligodendrocytes and neurons in the CNS results in PML, a neurodegenerative disease. PML develops mostly in patients with underlying immunosuppressive conditions, including lymphoproliferative diseases, acquired immune deficiency syndrome (AIDS), and Hodgkin's lymphoma, although, in a small number of cases, PML also affects individuals lacking underlying disease. Before the AIDS epidemic, PML used to be a rare complication of middle-aged and elderly patients with lymphoproliferative diseases. However, it is now a commonly encountered disease of the CNS in patients of different age groups, and there is a noticeable increase in the incidence of PML in human immunodeficiency virus (HIV)-infected patients compared to noninfected individuals. The increased incidence of PML in AIDS patients suggests that HIV infection may directly or indirectly influence reactivation of JCV and therefore induction of PML. In support, recent reports indicate that the incidence of PML in HIV-seropositive patients reaches 5%, compared to 0.8% before the AIDS epidemic. Furthermore, reactivation of JCV in patients with multiple sclerosis (MS) or Crohn's disease treated with both interferon $\beta1\alpha$ and natalizumab, a selective adhesion-molecule blocker, suggests that such an immunosuppressive treatment may be a risk factor in induction of PML in MS and Crohn's disease patients.

Genome Organization: Regulatory and Coding Regions

The JCV genome is composed of bidirectional regulatory elements and coding regions (**Figure 1**). The regulatory region contains the origin of DNA replication (ori) and promoter/enhancer elements, and exhibits hypervariability in its sequence composition; that is, although the regulatory region of a prototype strain, Mad-1, is characterized by the presence of two 98 bp tandem repeats, there are considerable deviations from this in other strains. For example, the archetype strain contains only one copy of the 98 bp repeat with two insertions of 23 bp

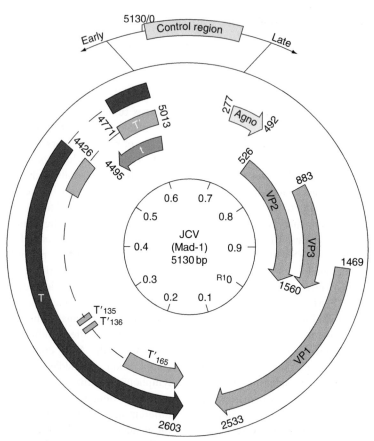

Figure 1   Genomic organization of JCV. The JCV genome is expressed bidirectionally. The early coding region encodes LT-Ag, Sm t-Ag, and T' proteins (T'$_{135}$, T'$_{136}$, and T'$_{165}$). The late coding region encodes agnoprotein and the three structural proteins VP1, VP2, and VP3. The control (regulatory) region is located between the two coding regions and contains the origin of DNA replication (ori) and promoter/enhancer elements for the early and late promoters.

and 66 bp, and the Mad-4 strain contains two tandem repeats that are only 84 bp in length. The bidirectional nature of the regulatory elements may provide an advantage to the virus to transcribe its genes efficiently, by a mechanism that is currently unknown. The regulatory region of the archetype strain is thought to be more adaptive to a latent infection and, upon reactivation, undergoes a deletion/duplication process within its regulatory region, through which it apparently gains the ability to become a more virulent virus and infect oligodendrocytes. The coding sequences of JCV are divided into two regions, early and late. The early region encodes only regulatory proteins, including small tumor antigen (Smt-Ag), large tumor antigen (LT-Ag), and T' proteins (T'$_{135}$, T'$_{136}$, and T'$_{165}$). The late region encodes a mixture of structural (VP1, VP2, and VP3) and regulatory (agnoprotein) proteins (**Figure 1**).

JCV is closely related to BKV and SV40 in the coding regions (70–80% identity). However, the regulatory regions are considerably diverged. This feature makes each virus unique with respect to replication in different cell types and tissues. In other words, the regulatory region largely determines the tissue-specific expression of gene products. LT-Ag also contributes to tissue-specific expression. Moreover, *in vivo* and *in vitro* transcription assays and cell fusion experiments have shown that tissue-specific cellular factors are critical for neurotropic expression of JCV. For instance, the early promoter was shown to be expressed well in glial cells but, when glial cells were fused with fibroblasts to form heterokaryons, early gene expression was significantly downregulated. This suggests that there are positively and negatively acting factors in glial and nonglial cells, respectively.

Regulatory Region

The regulatory region contains ori and multiple *cis*-acting regulatory elements that are involved in transcriptional regulation of the early and late regions. The regulatory region of the Mad-1 strain is shown schematically in **Figure 2**. The only region that shows substantial similarity to the corresponding regions in SV40 and BKV is ori, a 68 bp element located between a nuclear factor kappa B (NFκB) motif and the first 98 bp repeat. Each

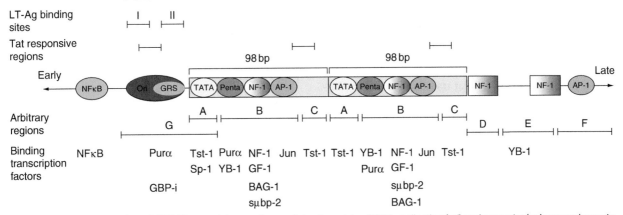

Figure 2   Regulatory region of JCV. The regulatory region contains the origin of DNA replication (ori) and promoter/enhancer elements. The two 98 bp tandem repeats are a characteristic of the Mad-1 strain. Promoter/enhancer elements that serve as binding sites for transcription factors are shown, and include the NFκB-binding element, the pentanucleotide element (Penta), the nuclear factor 1-binding element (NF-1), the GC-rich element (GRS), and the activating protein-1-binding element (AP-1). The transcription factors that have been shown to bind promoter/enhancer elements are shown at the lower part of the Figure. Large T antigen (LT-Ag)-binding sites and Tat-responsive elements are indicated. Arbitrary subregions A to G described in the text are indicated.

repeat contains a TATA box located on the early side of the repeat, and the first TATA box with respect to ori is involved in positioning of the transcription start sites for early genes. The second TATA box does not appear to have a similar function for the late genes. The other regulatory elements shown to be critical *cis*-acting elements for expression include Penta, AP-1, and NF-1 motifs that follow the TATA box. These elements serve as binding sites for several transcription factors and contribute to tissue tropism. The major *cis*-acting elements and transcription factors that bind to these regions are illustrated in **Figure 2**.

Cellular Transcription Factors Involved in JCV Gene Expression

Several studies have shown that many cell-specific and ubiquitous factors are involved in expression of the early and late promoters. These factors interact directly or indirectly with the *cis*-acting elements in the regulatory region and control gene expression. The regulatory proteins include LT-Ag and agnoprotein and have also been shown to play critical roles. LT-Ag, a multifunctional phosphoprotein, is not only involved in viral DNA replication but also late gene expression. Along with cellular factors required for DNA replication, LT-Ag binds to ori, unwinds it, and initiates DNA replication in a bidirectional manner. With respect to the role of LT-Ag role in transcription, studies have shown that, whereas it autoregulates its own transcription from the early promoter, it robustly transactivates the late promoter, resulting in the expression of agnoprotein and capsid proteins.

A close inspection of the regulatory region sequences reveals the presence of multiple *cis*-acting elements

to which transcription factors bind and regulate gene expression. These include NFκB, GRS, Penta, NF-1, AP-1, and 'AP-1-like' motifs. In addition, the regulatory region also contains LT-Ag-binding regions and elements responsive to the HIV transactivator, Tat (**Figure 2**). Furthermore, for the sake of simplicity in describing regulatory elements, the regulatory region is divided into arbitrary regions A to G. NFκB, a stress-inducible transcription factor, binds to the NFκB element and modulates gene expression from the early and late promoters. This factor represents a large family of transcription factors that are induced in response to a wide variety of extracellular stimuli, including phorbol ester, cytokines, and viral infection. p50 and p52 are two constitutively expressed subunits of NFκB that activate transcription from region D, whereas subunit p65 regulates transcription through the NFκB motif itself. The NFκB family members p50/p65 also influence transcription indirectly through a 23 bp element present in the regulatory regions of many JCV variants. Another inducible cellular factor, GBP-i, appears to target the GRS sequence present in region G and suppresses late promoter activity. Tst-1 is a member of the well-characterized tissue-specific and developmentally regulated POU family of transcription factors. This factor apparently interacts with distinct binding sites in regions A and C and regulates transcription from the early and late promoters. Interactions of cellular transcription factors with the viral regulatory proteins are also important. In this respect, interaction of Tst-1 with LT-Ag leads to synergistic activation of the early and late promoters. GC-rich sequences in Penta motif target the ubiquitously expressed transcription factor, Sp-1, which stimulates expression from the early promoter. The regulatory region also contains several NF-1-binding sites scattered across regions B, D, and E. NF-1 is important for both viral transcription and replication. Several factors interact with region B, including GF-1, YB-1, Purα, and AP-1. GF-1 is the human homolog of the murine Sμbp-2 protein and transactivates the early and late promoters. Two well-characterized cellular transcription factors, YB-1 and Purα, also interact with this region and regulate transcription and replication through interaction with LT-Ag. Another binding site for YB-1 is present in region E. BAG-1, a novel Bcl-1-interacting protein that is expressed ubiquitously in neuronal and non-neuronal cells, is a novel cellular transcription factor that regulates JCV promoters through the NF-1-binding site. Another transcription factor that interacts with region B is c-Jun, which is a member of the AP-1 family of transcription factors. Members of this family are known as the immediate–early inducible protooncogenes and are critical for the expression of many cellular and viral genes. c-Jun is phosphorylated during the JCV life cycle in an infection-cycle-dependent manner and interacts functionally with LT-Ag. In addition to its own regulatory proteins, the JCV genome is also crossregulated by regulatory proteins encoded by other viruses, including Tat and immediate-early transactivator 2 (IE2) from human cytomegalovirus (HCMV).

Life Cycle

Figure 3 highlights the chain of events during the polyomavirus life cycle. The infection cycle of JCV starts with the attachment of viral particles to cell surface receptors. The serotonin receptor $5HT_{2A}$ as well as $\alpha(2\text{-}6)$-linked sialic acid are critical for the attachment of JCV to the cell surface, and the viral particle is then internalized by a process known as clathrin-dependent endocytosis. Following internalization, the particle is transported to the nucleus by an unknown mechanism. The next step is the uncoating of capsid proteins, which subsequently leads to the expression of early genes in the nucleus. Viral transcripts undergo splicing before they are transported to the cytoplasm and translated. Translation of early transcripts results in the production of early regulatory proteins, including LT-Ag, Sm t-Ag, and T′ proteins (T'_{135}, T'_{136}, and T'_{165}). LT-Ag is then transported back to nucleus to

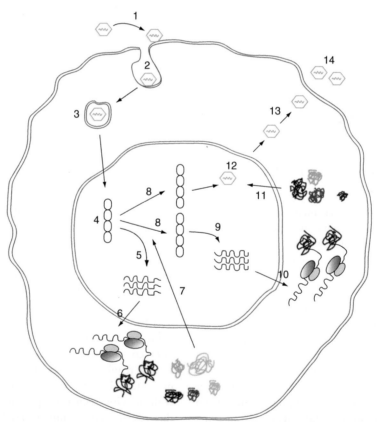

Figure 3 Life cycle of JCV. The steps are indicated by numbers: 1, adsorption of virus particles to cell surface receptors; 2, entry by clathrin-dependent endocytosis; 3, transport to the nucleus; 4, uncoating; 5, transcription of the early region; 6, translation to produce the early regulatory proteins, LT-Ag, Sm t-Ag, and T′ proteins (T'_{135}, T'_{136}, and T'_{165}); 7, nuclear localization of LT-Ag; 8, replication of the viral genome; 9, transcription of the late region; 10, translation of late transcripts to produce agnoprotein and capsid proteins (VP1, VP2, and VP3); 11, nuclear localization of capsid proteins; 12, assembly of virus particles in the nucleus; 13, release of virions by an unknown mechanism; 14, released virions.

initiate viral DNA replication. In the meantime, LT-Ag transactivates the late promoter for the production of regulatory agnoprotein and the three structural capsid proteins VP1, VP2, and VP3. Capsid proteins are also transported to the nucleus for virus assembly. In the encapsidation process, the capsid proteins are sequentially added to and arranged on the viral genome to package it into capsids. The final step is to release the virions from infected cells. The mechanism for this is not known, but it is thought that it takes place upon lysis of infected cells.

JCV Reactivation and Other Viral Infections

HIV infection and JCV reactivation

It has long been known that impaired cellular immunity is an exclusive predisposing condition for reactivation of JCV and onset of PML. Before the AIDS epidemic, lymphoproliferative disorders used to be the predominant underlying factor for reactivation of JCV from latency. In recent years, however, this trend has changed and a strong association of PML with AIDS has been established. The statistical data in this regard suggest that approximately 5–10% of AIDS patients eventually develop PML. This percentage is predicted to increase as more PML cases are evaluated in AIDS patients. In recent years, application of highly active antiretroviral therapies (HAART) to AIDS patients has had a significant effect on manifestations of AIDS-associated opportunistic infections, including HCMV infection and toxoplasmosis. The effect of HAART on the incidence of PML remains unclear, but there has been an indisputable increase in the frequency of PML since the inception of the AIDS epidemic. One simple explanation for this is that a higher degree and duration of cellular immunosuppression may pertain to HIV infection than to other immunosuppressive conditions. Another explanation is that alterations in the blood–brain barrier caused by HIV infection may render the brain more accessible to JCV infection. Direct activation of the JCV genome by HIV Tat protein or indirect activation by HIV-induced cytokines and chemokines could be other important factors for AIDS-related reactivation of JCV.

The degree and duration of immunosuppression in HIV infection may not be the only factors for the development of PML, because a substantial number of individuals with hematological malignancy, solid tumors undergoing chemotherapy, and/or underlying tuberculosis status post-organ transplantation all have a long period of immunosuppression but do not develop PML as often as HIV-infected individuals. What is special about HIV infection is that many arms of the host defense system are affected, as opposed to the more specific effects seen in other immunosuppressive conditions. It is also notable that PML typically manifests itself as a late complication of HIV infection. Perhaps a substantial loss in the number

and function of CD4+ T cells during the late phases of AIDS (as well as other alterations, including deficiencies in chemotaxis, monocyte-dependent T-cell proliferation, Fc-receptor function, C3 receptor-mediated clearance, and oxidative burst response) contributes greatly to suppressive conditions of the immune system in AIDS patients, and this in turn facilitates JCV reactivation and the development of PML. Furthermore, infection of monocytes/macrophages by HIV results in the impairment of antibody-dependent, cell-mediated cytotoxicity, intracellular antimicrobicidal activity, and induction of interferon α secretion. Moreover, the circulating B cells decrease in number as the disease progresses and, in association with HIV infection, B cells secrete disproportional amounts of cytokines. Which of these deficiencies leads to predisposition to the development of PML remains unknown. However, it should be emphasized that on rare occasions PML may develop in the absence of any identifiable underlying immunosuppressive disorder.

The Tat protein is a potent transactivator of the HIV long terminal repeat (LTR). It mediates its transregulatory activity through a specific RNA sequence located in the leader of all HIV-1 RNAs, called the transactivation response (TAR) element. Several critical G residues in the TAR element are required for function. Tat also induces transcription from the JCV late promoter through several TAR elements in the regulatory region. The G residues required for the function of the HIV-TAR element are also conserved in the JCV-TAR element and play an important role in Tat-mediated activation of the late promoter. Thus, Tat may participate directly in activation of the JCV late promoter. It is also thought that Tat may indirectly influence JCV gene regulation through the induction of transcription factors such as NFκB and c-Jun/AP-1, both of which have been shown to interact directly with the JCV promoter. Taken together, the regulatory factors induced by HIV Tat or Tat-induced cytokines may activate JCV promoters directly or indirectly and thereby influence the viral life cycle.

Interaction of JCV with other human viruses

Initial infection by JCV is followed by a persistent infection in the kidney and perhaps in B cells, during which JCV appears to go through several stages: (1) a latent infection state of limited virus production; (2) an activated state, during which the virus causes cell lysis; and (3) a final tissue destruction state, which leads to the onset of PML. Although the precise mechanism(s) of viral reactivation processes is unknown, the immunosuppressed state of the patient is critical for the onset of PML. Moreover, infection of immunosuppressed individuals by other viruses may influence the reactivation process.

In addition to JCV, several human viruses, such as BKV, HCMV, and human herpesvirus 6 (HHV-6), are able to establish persistent infections in various tissues and organs. HCMV is highly prevalent in the human population and can infect a wide range of organs. It is commonly reactivated in bone marrow and renal transplantation patients. Particularly, it is often reactivated after renal transplantation in AIDS patients in the kidney, CNS, lymphoid organs, stromal cells, and CD34+ bone marrow progenitor cells. Recent reports indicate that HCMV infection positively affects the level of JCV DNA replication or possibly transcription. JCV is known to infect only glial cells, but this restricted cell specificity can be overcome by HCMV infection. Thus, fibroblasts, which are generally nonpermissive for the replication of JCV, but can become permissive if HCMV IE2 is provided to JCV-infected cells.

HHV-6 is also a ubiquitous virus, and is detected in close association with JCV in oligodendrocytes within PML lesions. This virus establishes a lifelong infection in various organs, including the brain, urogenital tract, lung, liver, and peripheral blood cells. There appears to be a high correlation between polyomavirus infection and HHV-6 infection. This suggests that polyomaviruses and HHV-6 may have a common host cell not only in the CNS, but also in peripheral organs, and co-infection may have an impact on JCV gene regulation and perhaps on the reactivation process.

BKV has been reported to infect human tissues, such as the urogenital tract, along with JCV. This has been verified by the detection of both viruses in the kidney and the urine. Such infections are commonly encountered after renal and bone marrow transplantation in HIV-infected people, pregnant women, and immunocompetent individuals. However, the influence of double infection on JCV replication remains unclear. Additionally, both viruses have been detected in the peripheral blood cells of healthy and immunocompromised individuals.

Lytic Infection versus Tumor Induction

PML

JCV lytically infects oligodendrocytes in the CNS, leading to a white matter disease in humans known as PML (**Figure 4**). Oligodendrocytes are members of the glial cell family in the CNS. The other cell types in the glial family include microglia, astrocytes, and neurons. The primary function of oligodendrocytes is to myelinate the axons that project from the neural cell bodies of the overlying cortex and to protect the neurons. Infection of oligodendrocytes results in the destruction of myelin insulating the neurons, creating sporadic plaques in different parts of the brain. Hence, demyelination occurs as a multifocal (rarely unifocal) process that can develop in any location in the white matter (**Figure 4(b)**). As a result of infection, demyelination can also occur in other regions of the CNS, including the brainstem and cerebellum. Destruction of oligodendrocytes initially leads to the development of microscopic lesions (**Figure 4(b)**), and, as the disease progresses, the demyelinated areas become enlarged and eventually may coalesce, making them visible on gross examination of cut sections (**Figure 4(a)**). In most cases, however, astrocytes have also been found to be abortively infected by JCV, exhibiting enlarged, lobulated nuclear structures. Lipid-laden macrophages frequently migrate to the areas of demyelination, perhaps phagocytizing the myelin breakdown products. In most cases, a large number of HIV-infected macrophages are also found within the necrotic lesions. However, it is not clear how

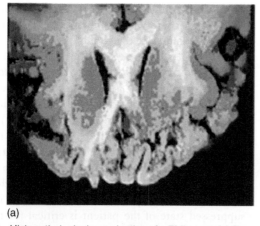
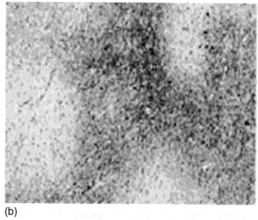

(a)   (b)

Figure 4 Histopathological examination of a PML case. (a) Gross appearance of PML in a coronal section of the brain. Multiple areas of cavitation are present in the subcortical white matter of the frontal lobes. (b) Staining for myelin demonstrates several areas of myelin loss in the white matter. Luxol Fast Blue, original magnification ×40. Reproduced by permission from Macmillan Publishers Ltd. *Journal of Clinical Pathology: Molecular Pathology* (Gallia G, Del Valle L, Line C, Curtis M, and Khalili K (2001) Concamitant progressive multifocal leukoencephalopathy and primary central nervous system lymphoma expression JC virus oncoprotein, large T antigen. *Journal of Clinical Pathology: Molecular Pathology* 54(5): 354–359), copyright (2001).

these immune cells infiltrate into areas of demyelination. One possible explanation is that JCV infection may recruit HIV-infected macrophages into demyelinated areas or, alternatively, uninfected macrophages may become infected by HIV after they are recruited into the CNS.

Clinically, the most common signs and symptoms of PML at the time of presentation are visual deficit, which is the most common presenting sign accounting for 35–45% of cases, motor weakness, accounting for 25–33% of cases, and mental deficits (emotional lability, difficulty with memory and dementia), which is seen in approximately one-third of cases. PML usually progresses to death within 4–6 months, although, in occasional cases, clinical signs and symptoms appear to remain stable for a long period of time.

Oncogenic potential of JCV

JCV, BKV, and SV40 are all known to induce a variety of tumors in experimental animals. All also have the ability to induce neoplastic cell transformation in tissue culture. Following its isolation, JCV was demonstrated to induce tumors in experimental animals in tissues of neuronal origin, but the type of the tumor induced by JCV depends on the type and age of animal and the site of inoculation. For example, when the Mad-1 strain of JCV was inoculated intracerebrally and subcutaneously into newborn Syrian hamsters, more than 80% of animals developed medullablastomas, glioblastomas, or neuroblastomas. An entire biologically active JCV genome was isolated when cells from these tumors were co-cultivated with permissive glial cells. In contrast, when a similar group of animals was inoculated intraocularly with the same strain of JCV, they mostly developed abdominal neuroblastomas in several locations. It was also observed that tumors metastasized to the bone marrow, lymph node, and liver.

Interestingly, JCV is the only polyomavirus that induces tumors in nonhuman primates, such as monkeys. In order to mimic a case resembling PML in humans, owl and squirrel monkeys were inoculated with JCV subcutaneously, intraperitoneally, or intracerebrally. The animals developed tumors at different time intervals. For instance, one owl monkey developed a malignant cerebral tumor similar to astrocytoma in humans after 16 months. Another animal developed a malignant neuroblastoma 25 months after inoculation.

Transgenic mouse models have also been developed to mimic the acute demyelination observed in PML patients. A transgenic mouse was created by using the portion of the JCV genome that contains the promoter and coding regions for LT-Ag. Some of the offspring from this mouse exhibited a mild to severe tremor phenotype. Hypo- and dysmyelination were observed in the CNS but not in the peripheral nervous system (PNS), suggesting that expression of LT-Ag affects myelin formation in the CNS and not in the PNS. Further characterization of myelin formation in transgenic animals revealed that the level of myelin sheath wrapped around the axons was relatively low, although the expression level of proteolipid protein, myelin basic protein, and myelin-associated glycoprotein genes appeared to be normal at the RNA level. In contrast, the respective protein levels appeared to be reduced. The mechanism by which LT-Ag alters the levels of these proteins in transgenic mice remains unknown, but it has been suggested that LT-Ag may influence the rate of translation of mRNA for these genes or other cellular genes that negatively influence the maturation of oligodendrocytes. This may eventually alter myelin formation around the axons.

Our group also described the formation of different tumors in tissues derived from neuronal origin in transgenic mouse models. The LT-Ag coding region under the control of the regulatory region of the archetype strain was utilized to create these transgenic animal models. Histological and histochemical analysis of the tumor masses revealed no sign of hypomyelination in the CNS, which was a feature of this transgenic model. In contrast, cerebellar tumors resembling human medullablastomas were induced.

In addition to the induction of tumors in experimental animals, the JCV genome has also been detected in a variety of human tumors, which raises the possibility of involvement of JCV LT-Ag in tumor formation in humans. Richardson, who first described PML in 1961, reported an incidental case of an oligodendroglioma in a patient with concomitant occurrence of chronic lymphatic leukemia and PML. The association of PML with multiple astrocytomas was also reported in 1983. Similarly, another case in which a patient had a long history of immunodeficiency syndrome with PML was described, and numerous foci of anaplastic astrocytes were observed. The presence of viral particles in both oligodendrocytes and astrocytes, but not in neoplastic astrocytes, in the demyelinating lesions of PML foci was demonstrated by electron microscopy. The presence of a large number of dysplastic or dysmorphic ganglion-like cells, which showed the properties of neurons, was also described recently in the cerebral cortex of a patient with PML. Expression of JCV LT-Ag, but not capsid proteins, was detected in these cells.

In addition to cases of concomitant PML and cerebral neoplasm, JCV has been shown to be associated with human brain tumors in the absence of PML lesions. The detection of JCV DNA in the brain tumors of an immunocompetent patient with a pleomorphic xanthoastrocytoma has been reported. In another investigation, JCV DNA and expression of LT-Ag were detected in tumor tissue from an immunocompetent HIV-negative patient with oligoastrocytoma. These two cases demonstrated the association of JCV with brain tumors in immunocompetent non-PML patients, and further prompted attempts to establish the association of JCV with different types of brain tumors in humans. Analysis of multiple brain tumors for presence of the JCV genome revealed that 57.1% of oligodendrogliomas, 83.3% of ependymomas, 80% of pilocytic astrocytomas, 76.9% of astrocytomas, 62.5% of oligoastrocytomas, and 66% of anaplastic oligodendrogliomas contained JCV early gene sequences. Furthermore, JCV genomic DNA has been detected in tumor tissues of non-neural origin, including the gastrointestinal tract and solid non-neural tumors such as colorectal cancers.

The precise mechanism by which JCV induces tumors is not known, but the tumorogenic protein LT-Ag is known to play a major role in this process. LT-Ag from JCV, as well as from BKV and SV40, has been shown to target major cell cycle regulators, including the tumor suppressor protein p53 and the retinoblastoma (pRb) gene products. This targeting inhibits the functions of these two key regulators of the cell cycle and perhaps others. In fact, protein interaction studies have clearly showed complex formation between LT-Ag and cell cycle regulators including pRb, p53, and p107.

BK Virus

BKV belongs to the same genus as JCV, as species *BK polyomavirus*. Like that of other polyomaviruses, the BKV genome consists of a small, closed circular DNA approximately 5 kbp in size, with the size varying between strains. For example, the genome sizes of the DUN, MM, and AS strains are 5153, 4963, and 5098 bp, respectively.

The structural organization of the BKV genome resembles that of JCV (**Figure 1**) in that it contains bidirectional coding regions (early and late), which are regulated by the regulatory region. The early region encodes only the regulatory tumor antigens, Sm t-Ag and LT-Ag, and the late region is responsible for the capsid proteins (VP1, VP2, and VP3) and a small, basic regulatory protein, agnoprotein. As for JCV and SV40, LT-Ag is essential for viral DNA replication, but the function of Sm t-Ag in BKV regulation is unclear. LT-Ag also potently transactivates the late promoter. The capsid proteins form icosahedral shell structures (39–42 nm in diameter), into which the viral genome is packaged. The capsid proteins are critical for attachment of the virus to cell surface receptors. Although the function of the BKV agnoprotein is unclear, recent evidence from JCV suggests that it plays a role in viral DNA replication, transcription, and cell cycle regulation.

Infection and Associated Disorders

Like JCV, BKV has a worldwide distribution in the human population. Primary infection occurs during early childhood and is subclinical, though occasionally accompanied by mild respiratory illness or urinary tract disease. Little is known about the route of transmission, although induction of upper respiratory disease and detection of latent BKV DNA in tonsils suggest a possible oral or respiratory route. During primary infection, viremia occurs and the virus spreads to various organs, including kidneys, bladder prostate, uterine cervix, lips, and tongue, where it remains in a latent state. Reactivation from the latent state is mostly associated with the immunocompromised state of the individuals. Reactivated virus has been detected in the urine of renal and bone marrow transplant recipients undergoing immunosuppressive therapy and in the urine of pregnant women. Upon reactivation, the virus may cause interstitial nephritis and urethral obstruction in patients receiving renal transplants. BKV has surfaced as a significant pathogen in kidney transplant patients in recent years by association with nephropathy, better known as polyomavirus-associated nephropathy. BKV infection appears to be a serious problem in renal allograft recipients in the first 2 years after transplantation, if not treated properly. In addition, an association between hemorrhagic cystitis and BKV has been shown in bone marrow transplant recipients.

Oncogenicity of the Genome in Experimental Animals

Like JCV, BKV is also oncogenic in experimental animals, including young or newborn mice, rats, and hamsters. The route of inoculation is a significant factor in determining the types of tumors induced. For example, BKV induces tumors in high proportions when inoculated intracerebrally or intravenously, but is weakly oncogenic when inoculated subcutaneously. BKV induces tumors in hamsters in a variety of tissues and organs, including ependymoma, neuroblastoma, pineal gland tumors, fibrosarcoma, esteosarcoma, and tumors of pancreatic islets. Rats inoculated with BKV develop fibrosarcoma, liposarcoma, osteosarcoma, nephroblastoma, and glioma. In a similar setting, however, mice develop only choroid plexus papilloma.

LT-Ag is the primary protein of BKV responsible for tumor induction in experimental animals. The oncogenic ability of LT-Ag has also been tested in transgenic mice models. Like JCV LT-Ag, BKV LT-Ag is known to target and inhibit several key cell cycle regulatory proteins, including p53 and the pRb family members, pRb105, pRb107, and pRb130. BKV also causes renal tumors and hepatocellular carcinoma. In such studies, there appear to be differences among strains of BKV with respect to the ability of LT-Ag to cause tumors. For example, Gardner's strain appears to be more potent in transgenic mice than isolates such as the MM, BKV-IR, or RF strains.

BKV LT-Ag induces cell transformation in tissue culture, although to a lesser extent than SV40 LT-Ag. It has been proposed that a 'hit-and-run' mechanism is most likely to operate during this transformation process; that is, expression of LT-Ag is required for the initiation of a multistage process, but is not required after a certain stage of transformation is reached. For example, in one study it was observed that, although transfection of BKV DNA into human cells resulted in a transformed phenotype, it was absent from most new transformed clones.

Another mechanism by which human polyomavirus LT-Ag may cause transformation is via the induction of chromosomal structural alterations characterized by breaks, gaps, dicentric and ring chromosomes, deletions, duplications, and translocations. While the molecular mechanism of this clastogenic effect of BKV LT-Ag on host DNA is unknown, it is thought that it may reside in the ability of the protein to bind topoisomerase I or in its helicase activity, in which it may induce chromosomal damage while unwinding the strands of cellular DNA. Moreover, since LT-Ag targets and inactivates p53, this may lead to survival of damaged cells, increasing their chance of transformation and immortalization. As a result, the clastogenic and mutagenic activities of the LT-Ag of human polyomaviruses may disturb the crucial function of the genes that are important for the maintenance of genomic stability, such as oncogenes, tumor suppressor genes, and DNA repair genes.

Association of the Genome with Human Tumors

During late 1970s, BKV DNA was detected in a variety of human tumors and tumor cell lines, which prompted researchers to investigate the possible association of BKV with tumor induction. BKV was found to exhibit a specific oncogenic tropism for ependymal tissue, endocrine pancreas, and osteosarcomas in rodents. This led investigators to focus primarily on the presence of the BKV genome in such tumors. Southern hybridization studies showed that some pancreatic islet tumors, as well as some brain tumors, contain the BKV genome in a free, episomal state. BKV was even rescued from some of the tumors by transfection of human embryonic fibroblasts with tumor DNA.

The BKV genome was also reported in 46% of brain tumors of the most common histotypes, and was found to be integrated into chromosomal DNA in this particular study. Association of human tumors with immunocompromised conditions was also analyzed by Southern blotting, and the BKV genome was associated with Kaposi's sarcoma (KS) at low frequencies (20%).

Recently, normal and neoplastic human tissues, as well as tumor cell lines, were also examined for the presence of the BKV genome by PCR, utilizing primers for the early region. Nucleotide sequence analysis of PCR products revealed the presence of BKV-specific sequences in several brain tumor samples, one osteocarcinoma, two glioblastoma cell lines, one normal brain tissue, and one normal bone tissue specimen. In these studies, expression of the early region was demonstrated in some of the samples by reverse transcription (RT)-PCR. The presence of the BKV genome was also investigated in several different tumors, including urinary tract tumors and carcinomas of the uterine cervix, vulva, lips, and tongue. However, the data obtained from such studies were inconclusive because the proportion of positive samples in neoplastic tissues of the urinary and genital tracts and oral cavity was similar to that detected in corresponding normal tissues. BKV DNA has been shown to be present in a high proportion of KS cases, suggesting that BKV may be an important cofactor in KS.

Conclusion

Since the first cultivation of JCV from a PML patient and BKV from a renal transplant patient in 1971, we have learned much about the biology of both viruses. However, important aspects of the life cycle (viral entry, transport of viral particles to the nucleus, transcription, replication, and assembly and release of virions) remain to be elucidated. The more we investigate the biology of these viruses, the more complex their biology is revealed to be. Understanding the molecular mechanisms underlying the life cycle of these viruses will considerably enhance our view of their complex biology, which should then allow us to design effective therapeutics to intervene in the infection cycle at an early stage, before they cause more advanced disease.

See also: Human Cytomegalovirus: General Features; Human Herpesviruses 6 and 7; Polyomaviruses; Simian Virus 40.

Further Reading

Berger JR and Concha M (1995) Progressive multifocal leukoencephalopathy: The evolution of a disease once considered rare. *Journal of Neurovirology* 1: 5–18.

Corallini A, Pagnani M, Viadana P, et al. (1987) Association of BK virus with human brain tumors and tumors of pancreatic islets. *International Journal of Cancer* 39: 60–67.

Del Valle L, Gordon J, Assimakopoulou M, et al. (2001) Detection of JC virus DNA sequences and expression of the viral regulatory protein T-antigen in tumors of the central nervous system. *Cancer Research* 61: 4287–4293.

Dorries K, Loeber G, and Meixensberger (1987) Association of polyomaviruses JC, SV40, and BK with human brain tumors. *Virology* 160: 268–270.

Gallia G, Del Valle L, Line C, Curtis M, and Khalili K (2001) Concamitant progressive multifocal leukoencephalopathy and primary central nervous system lymphoma expression JC virus oncoprotein, large T antigen. *Journal of Clinical Pathology: Molecular Pathology* 54(5): 354–359.

Gordon J, Del Valle L, Otte J, and Khalili K (2000) Pituitary neoplasia induced by expression of human neurotropic polyomavirus, JCV, early genome in transgenic mice. *Oncogene* 19: 4840–4846.

Hirsch HH (2005) BK virus: Opportunity makes a pathogen. *Clinical Infectious Diseases* 41: 354–360.

Kim J, Woolridge S, Biffi R, *et al.* (2003) Members of the AP-1 family, c-Jun and c-Fos, functionally interact with JC virus early regulatory protein large T-antigen. *Journal of Virology* 77: 5241–5252.

Lynch KJ and Frisque RJ (1991) Factors contributing to the restricted DNA replicating activity of JC virus. *Virology* 180: 306–317.

Major EO, Amemiya K, Tornatore CS, Houff SA, and Berger JR (1992) Pathogenesis and molecular biology of progressive multifocal leukoencephalopathy, the JC virus-induced demyelinating disease of the human brain. *Clinical Microbiological Reviews* 5: 49–73.

Monaco MC, Jensen PN, Hou J, Durham LC, and Major EO (1998) Detection of JC virus DNA in human tonsil tissue: Evidence for site of initial viral infection. *Journal of Virology* 72: 9918–9923.

Padgett BL, Zu Rhein GM, Walker DL, Echroade R, and Dessel B (1971) Cultivation of papova-like virus from human brain with progressive multifocal leukoencephalopathy. *Lancet* i: 1257–1260.

Raj GV and Khalili K (1995) Transcriptional regulation: Lessons from the human neurotropic polyomavirus, JCV. *Virology* 213: 283–291.

Richardson EP (1961) Progressive multifocal encephalopathy. *New England Journal of Medicine* 265: 815–823.

Sariyer IK, Akan I, Palermo V, Gordon J, Khalili K, and Safak M (2006) Phosphorylation mutants of JC virus agnoprotein are unable to sustain the viral infection cycle. *Journal of Virology* 80: 3893–3903.

Walker DL, Padgett BL, Zu Rhein GM, Albert AE, and Marsh RF (1973) Human papovavirus (JC): Induction of brain tumors in hamsters. *Science* 181: 674–676.

Retroviral Oncogenes

P K Vogt and A G Bader, The Scripps Research Institute, La Jolla, CA, USA

Glossary

Chimeric transcript An mRNA that encodes a fusion protein derived from two individual and originally separate genes.

Subtractive hybridization A method to identify differentially expressed mRNAs; the method is based on hybridizing a 'tester' mRNA population with a 'driver' mRNA population and selectively eliminating tester–driver hybrids.

Historical Perspective

Retroviruses that carry an oncogene induce neoplastic transformation of cells in culture and rapidly cause tumors in the animal. Early studies with Rous sarcoma virus in chicken embryo fibroblasts showed a controlling influence of the retroviral genome on the properties of the transformed cell and suggested that the virus carries oncogenic information. The isolation of temperature-sensitive mutants of Rous sarcoma virus firmly established a dominant role of viral genetic information in the process of virus-induced carcinogenesis. These mutants of Rous sarcoma virus encode an unstable oncoprotein and are able to transform chicken embryo fibroblasts at a low, permissive temperature but fail to induce oncogenic changes at an elevated, nonpermissive temperature. Yet the virus is able to propagate under both permissive and nonpermissive conditions, demonstrating that virus viability and replication are not affected by the mutation and

that oncogenicity is governed by genetic information that is distinct from viral replicative genes. Cells transformed by temperature-sensitive Rous sarcoma virus under permissive conditions become normal in morphology and growth behavior if the cell cultures are switched to the nonpermissive temperature. Thus, viral genetic information is required for the initiation as well as for the maintenance of the transformed cellular phenotype. A physical correlate to these genetic experiments was found in studies with transformation-defective Rous sarcoma virus. These spontaneously emerging variants of the virus fail to induce transformation in cell culture but are able to generate viable progeny virus that remains transformation defective. The transformation-defective viruses contain genomes that are about 20% smaller than the genome of oncogenic Rous sarcoma virus. The missing genetic information is of obvious importance for oncogenicity. Subtractive hybridization of DNA transcripts from transformation-defective and transformation-competent viral genomes generates a specific cDNA probe for the oncogenic sequences in Rous sarcoma virus. This probe hybridizes to cellular DNA, revealing the presence of sequences that are homologous to the transforming information of Rous sarcoma virus in the genome of all vertebrate cells. Retroviral oncogenes are therefore derived from the cell genome. The cellular versions of retroviral oncogenes are also referred to as proto-oncogenes or, more commonly, as c-*onc* genes; the corresponding viral versions are called v-*onc* genes. The discovery of oncogenes owes much to the exceptional genetic structure of Rous sarcoma virus. This virus is unique among oncogene-carrying retroviruses in that it is replication competent, containing a full set of viral genes plus the oncogene. Loss of the oncogene in transformation-defective variants still leaves a viable virus, greatly facilitating molecular and genetic analyses.

Taxonomy of Oncogene-Carrying Retroviruses

Retroviruses are broadly divided into two categories, viruses with simple genomes and viruses with complex genomes. Simple retroviral genomes contain four coding regions with information for virion proteins. These regions are referred to as *gag*, which directs the synthesis of matrix, capsid, and nucleoprotein structures; *pro*, generating the virion protease; *pol*, containing the information for the reverse transcriptase and integrase enzymes; and *env*, which encodes the surface and transmembrane components of the envelope protein. Complex retroviral genomes contain additional information for regulatory nonvirion proteins that are translated from multiply spliced mRNAs.

In taxonomic terms, retroviruses form a family that consists of the subfamilies *Orthoretrovirinae* and *Spumaretrovirinae*. Oncogenes are carried by only two genera of the orthoretroviruses. These are the alpharetroviruses, representing the avian leukosis complex of viruses, and the gammaretroviruses, encompassing murine, feline, and primate leukemia and sarcoma viruses. This restriction of oncogenes to two viral genera probably reflects a set of conditions that have to be met for the acquisition of cellular sequences by a retroviral genome. These conditions include absence of cytotoxicity and efficient viral integration and replication. Complex retroviruses may not tolerate the insertion of cellular sequences into the viral genome because some functions of the regulatory nonvirion proteins that would be displaced by a cellular insert can probably not be complemented in *trans*. These are all hypothetical reasons for the occurrence of oncogenes in just a few retroviruses; mechanistic explanations of these restrictions are currently not available.

Acquisition of Cellular Sequences by Retroviral Genomes

The acquisition of a cellular oncogene by a retrovirus is a rare event that occurs during viral passage in an animal but is seldom seen in cell culture. Because *de novo* acquisition of cellular sequences cannot be reproduced with significant frequency in cultured cells, the molecular mechanism of acquisition has to be reconstructed using information derived from the structure of viral genomes and from the virus life cycle. The life cycle of retroviruses contains two steps that leads to genetic recombination. (1) Retroviruses are diploid and thus can form heterozygous viral particles. Recombination between distinct but related viral genomes encased in the same particle occurs very frequently and probably results from copy-choice events that occur during reverse transcription. (2) Integration of the provirus into the cellular genome produces a recombinant between virus and cell (**Figure 1**). These two recombinational activities of retroviruses can explain the incorporation of cellular sequences into the viral genome. The first step in this acquisition consists of the integration of a provirus containing a single 5′ (left-hand) long terminal repeat (LTR) into the oncogene proper or into the immediate upstream vicinity of a cellular oncogene. This provirus can then produce a chimeric RNA transcript that starts in the viral LTR, continues by read-through into the cellular gene,

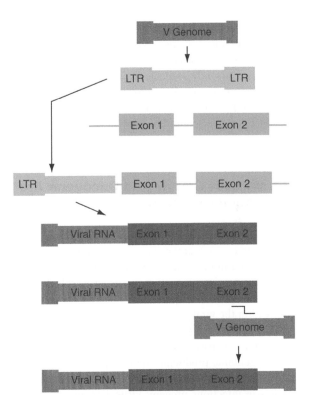

Figure 1 A hypothetical mechanism for the acquisition of a cellular oncogene by a retroviral genome. The genome of a retrovirus without oncogene is transcribed into DNA and, in a first recombinational event, is integrated upstream of a cellular oncogene containing two exons. The right-hand long terminal repeat (LTR) and adjacent sequences of the viral genome are lost during the integration process. Transcription from the integrated proviral LTR generates a chimeric mRNA by read-through or aberrant splicing. This mRNA contains cell-derived oncogene and viral information. The chimeric mRNA is packaged into viral particles together with wild-type viral genomes. In the next round of infection the second recombinational event occurs during reverse transcription and adds 3′ viral terminal sequences to the DNA transcript, facilitating the production and integration of a functional provirus that contains a cell-derived oncogene. Green: DNA, red and purple: RNA.

and terminates with the poly A stretch of the cellular gene. Alternatively, such a chimeric transcript can be generated by a splicing event that uses a viral splice donor and a cellular splice acceptor in joining upstream viral to downstream cellular sequences. Chimeric RNAs of this type would be incorporated into virions. In the subsequent cycle of infection, reverse transcription could effect a second recombination event, generating a junction between the 3′ region of the cellular sequences and a part of the viral genome carrying the 3′ terminal repeat sequences that are essential for the efficient production of proviral DNA. In this model, the first step of recombination in acquiring cellular sequences is the integration of the provirus, which is DNA-based recombination. The second step occurs during reverse transcription of a heterozygote particle and is RNA-based recombination. It is possible, however, to envisage a second recombination step that is also DNA based. It requires the integration of another provirus immediately downstream of the cellular oncogene to serve as donor of the necessary 3′ (right-hand) LTR for the new provirus that now carries an insertion of cellular sequences. Currently available experimental evidence can be adduced to support either model for the second recombination step in the acquisition of a cellular oncogene. Specific oncogene acquisitions may in fact occur by either mechanism.

Retroviruses Carrying an Oncogene Are Replication Defective

The incorporation of cellular sequences into the retroviral genome occurs at the expense of viral sequences that are displaced in the process. With one notable exception, Rous sarcoma virus, transducing retroviruses lack one or several essential viral genes. Typical deletions extend from within the viral *gag* gene into the *env* gene, eliminating the 3′ portion of *gag*, all of the *pol* gene, and part of *env*. Such defective viruses can infect cells, integrating into the cellular genome, producing the oncoprotein, and inducing neoplastic transformation, but they are unable to synthesize infectious progeny virus. For infectious virus production, they require co-infection of the same cell with a closely related helper retrovirus that in *trans* provides those replicative functions that are missing from the defective transforming virus. Helper retroviruses contain a complete set of viral genes but have not incorporated any cellular oncogenic sequences. They do not induce oncogenic transformation when replicating in cultured cells. In animal infections, they can cause tumors by insertional mutagenesis after extended latent periods. These tumors result from transcriptional upregulation of a cellular oncogene by promoter activities of a provirus integrated nearby.

Oncoproteins Are Often Fusion Proteins

As a consequence of the initial integration event that leads to oncogene acquisition, viral oncogenes usually code for fusion proteins, consisting of an N-terminal portion derived from the virus and a C-terminal component representing the oncoprotein proper. The viral sequences generally include the N-terminus of the Gag polyprotein. The initial recombination event also often eliminates short lengths from the N-terminus of the cellular oncoprotein, except when viral sequences are spliced onto the cellular gene. Fusion of the cellular oncoproteins to viral *gag* sequences can have important consequences that contribute to the gain of function associated with the viral oncogene. The efficiency of protein translation and the stability of the fusion protein are often increased. Gag sequences also provide an affinity for the plasma membrane which can be critical in activating the oncogenic potential of the protein.

Functional Classes of Oncogenes

Retroviral oncogenes code for components of cellular growth-regulatory signals (**Table 1**). The major functional categories include growth factors, receptor and nonreceptor tyrosine kinases, serine-threonine and lipid kinases, adaptor proteins, hormone receptors, and a variety of transcriptional regulators. Cellular growth signals are propagated from the cell periphery to the nucleus. Therefore, the nuclear oncoproteins coding for transcriptional regulators are the ultimate effectors of oncogenicity, converting the signal into a pattern of gene expression that is the basis of the oncogenic phenotype of the cell. Because of this pivotal role of nuclear oncoproteins in specifying neoplastic properties, oncogenic transformation can be viewed as a case of aberrant transcription. However, there is also abundant evidence for a critical role of protein translation in oncogenesis. Oncogenesis induced by the PI3K pathway in particular depends on differential translation of specific growth-promoting proteins.

Retroviral Transduction of a Cellular Oncogene Results in Gain of Function

Compared to their cellular counterparts, retroviral oncoproteins show an increase in activity. Some of this gain of function is purely quantitative: the viral promoter assures highly efficient transcription of the oncogene. There are several oncogenes for which mere overexpression is sufficient to turn them into effective agents of neoplastic

Table 1 Classes of retroviral oncogenes

Functional groups and oncogenes	Identity and function of cellular homolog	Retrovirus
Growth factor		
sis	Platelet–derived growth factor (PDGF)	Simian sarcoma virus
Receptor tyrosine kinases		
erbB	Receptor of epithelial growth factor (EGF)	Avian erythroblastosis virus
fms	Receptor of colony-stimulating factor 1 (CSF-1)	McDonough feline sarcoma virus
sea	Receptor of macrophage-stimulating protein (MSP)	Avian erythroblastosis virus S13
kit	Hematopoietic receptor of stem cell factor (SCF)	Hardy–Zuckerman 4 feline sarcoma virus
ros	Orphan receptor tyrosine kinase	Avian sarcoma virus UR2
mpl	Hematopoietic receptor of thrombopoietin	Mouse myeloproliferative leukemia virus
eyk	Closest homolog of mammalian c-mer; c-Mer ligands include anticoagulation factor protein S and the growth arrest-specific gene product Gas6	Avian retrovirus RPL30
Hormone receptor		
erbA	Thyroid hormone receptor	Avian erythroblastosis virus
G proteins		
H-ras	GTPase; MAPK signal transduction	Harvey murine sarcoma virus
K-ras	GTPase; MAPK signal transduction	Kirsten murine sarcoma virus
Adaptor protein		
crk	Adaptor protein containing SH2 and SH3 domains; PI3K/Akt signal transduction	Avian sarcoma virus CT10
Nonreceptor tyrosine kinases		
src	MAPK and PI3K/Akt signal transduction	Rous sarcoma virus
yes	Src family kinase; signal transduction	Avian sarcoma virus Y73
fps	Cytokine receptor signaling; the fps and fes oncogenes are derived from the same cellular gene	Fujinami poultry sarcoma virus
fes	Cytokine receptor signaling; the fps and fes oncogenes are derived from the same cellular gene	Gardner–Arnstein feline sarcoma virus
fgr	Src family kinase; signal transduction	Gardner–Rasheed feline sarcoma virus
abl	Cytoskeletal signaling and cell cycle regulated transcription	Abelson murine leukemia virus
Serine/threonine kinases		
mos	Regulator of cell cycle progression; required for germ cell maturation; activates MAPKs	Moloney murine sarcoma virus
raf	MAPKKK, MAPK signal transduction	Murine sarcoma virus 3611
akt	PI3K/Akt signal transduction	Murine retrovirus AKT8
Lipid kinase		
p3k	PI 3-kinase; PI3K/Akt signal transduction	Avian sarcoma virus 16
Transcriptional regulators		
jun	bZIP protein of AP-1 complex; homo- and heterodimer with AP-1 family members; cell cycle progression	Avian sarcoma virus 17
fos	bZIP protein of AP-1 complex; heterodimer with AP-1 family members; cell cycle progression	FBJ murine osteogenic sarcoma virus
myc	bHLH-ZIP protein; heterodimer with Max; cell cycle progression	Avian myelocytoma virus MC29
myb	HTH protein; development of hematopoietic system	Avian myeloblastosis virus

Continued

Table 1   Continued

Functional groups and oncogenes	Identity and function of cellular homolog	Retrovirus
ets	HTH protein; myeloid and eosinophil differentiation	Avian myeloblastosis–erythroblastosis virus E26
rel	p65 NF-κB subunit; survival pathways	Avian reticuloendotheliosis virus
maf	bZIP protein; homo- and heterodimers with various bZIP proteins; differentiation of various tissues	Avian musculoaponeurotic fibrosarcoma virus
ski	Adaptor protein for various transcription factors; chromatin-dependent transcriptional regulation; muscle differentiation	Avian Sloan-Kettering retrovirus
qin	Avian homolog of mammalian brain factor 1 (BF-1/FoxG1); forkhead/winged helix (FOX) protein; monomer; neuronal differentiation	Avian sarcoma virus 31

Abbreviations: Gas6, growth arrest-specific gene 6; MAPK, mitogen-activated protein kinase; MAPKKK, mitogen-activated protein kinase kinase kinase; SH2, Src homology domain 2; SH3, Src homology domain 3; PI3K, phosphoinositide 3-kinase; AP-1, activator protein 1; bZIP, basic region leucine zipper; bHLH-ZIP, basic region helix–loop–helix leucine zipper; HTH, helix–turn–helix; NF-κB, nuclear factor kappa B; FBJ, Finkel–Biskis–Jinkins.

transformation. These code for wild-type oncoproteins that deregulate cellular growth by their virus-mediated abundance. However, many oncoproteins carry specific mutations that are responsible for the gain of function. These mutations remove or inactivate domains of the oncoprotein that effect negative regulation or may enhance specific enzymatic activities of the oncoprotein by other mechanisms including conformational change, improved substrate affinity, or change in cellular localization. They may stabilize the protein or alter the spectrum of downstream targets. Thus both quantitative and qualitative changes resulting from viral transduction and the associated mutation of the oncogene contribute to the gain of function.

Cooperation of Oncogenes

A few retroviruses carry two oncogenes. These oncogenes are derived from distinct cellular loci situated at distant positions within the host genome. Retroviruses with two oncogenes include Avian erythroblastosis virus R (AEV-R), carrying v-erbA and v-erbB, Avian myeloblastosis–erythroblastosis virus E26, encoding myb and ets as a single Gag-myb-ets protein product, and Avian myelocytoma virus MH2, which contains the v-myc and v-mil (raf) genes. Each of these single oncoproteins can induce neoplastic transformation on its own. However, viruses with two oncogenes are more potent in transformation, indicating that the two oncoproteins cooperate. Whereas primary avian cells can be readily transformed by viruses carrying a single oncogene, in mammalian cells oncogenic transformation generally requires the cooperation of two or more oncogenes. The reasons for this difference in cellular susceptibility to oncogene action are not known.

Coda and Outlook

There are still significant gaps in our knowledge of retroviral oncogenes. We do not know and cannot reproduce the exact mechanism of oncogene acquisition by a retroviral genome. We have only tentative explanations for the failure of some groups of retroviruses to capture cellular sequences. We have no idea why certain growth-promoting cellular genes have not shown up as retroviral oncogenes. Have not enough retroviruses been studied or is there an active mechanism that excludes certain genes? Does some cryptic homology between provirus and oncogene determine the spectrum of genes that can be incorporated? On a more basic level, there is evidence that oncogenes can induce tumors by activating the transcription of specific micro-RNAs. Are there also rapidly oncogenic retroviruses that carry a micro-RNA gene as an oncogene?

Despite these puzzling questions, at a fundamental level the nature and workings of retroviral oncogenes are well understood and have provided important insights into the mechanisms of virus-induced carcinogenesis. The discovery that all retroviral oncogenes are derived from cellular information has greatly expanded the significance of these genes. Originally seen as viral pathogenicity genes, they have become universal effectors of oncogenicity. Viruses have been demoted to just one of several instruments that can activate these genes; mutation, overexpression, and amplification are some of the others. The study of oncogenes, initially a somewhat esoteric part of virology, has grown to determine the course of cancer research during the past three decades and has contributed immensely to our understanding of cancer in general. As targets of specific inhibitors, oncoproteins are now revolutionizing cancer treatment. Gleevec, directed at the BCR-ABL oncoprotein in chronic myelogenous leukemia, and Iressa, inhibiting mutants of the epithelial growth factor receptor in non-small cell lung cancer, have dramatically proven the promise of therapy targeted to oncoproteins.

Acknowledgments

This work was supported by grants from the National Cancer Institute. This is manuscript number 18 394 of The Scripps Research Institute.

Further Reading

Bister K and Jansen HW (1986) Oncogenes in retroviruses and cells: Biochemistry and molecular genetics. *Advances in Cancer Research* 47: 99–188.

Duesberg PH and Vogt PK (1970) Differences between the ribonucleic acids of transforming and nontransforming avian tumor viruses. *Proceedings of the National Academy of Sciences, USA* 67: 1673–1680.

Hughes SH (1983) Synthesis, integration, and transcription of the retroviral provirus. *Current Topics in Microbiology and Immunology* 103: 23–49.

Land H, Parada LF, and Weinberg RA (1983) Tumorigenic conversion of primary embryo fibroblasts requires at least two cooperating oncogenes. *Nature* 304: 596–602.

Martin GS (1970) Rous sarcoma virus: A function required for the maintenance of the transformed state. *Nature* 227: 1021–1023.

Schwartz JR, Duesberg S, and Duesberg PH (1995) DNA recombination is sufficient for retroviral transduction. *Proceedings of the National Academy of Sciences, USA* 92: 2460–2464.

Stehelin D, Guntaka RV, Varmus HE, and Bishop JM (1976) Purification of DNA complementary to nucleotide sequences required for neoplastic transformation of fibroblasts by avian sarcoma viruses. *Journal of Molecular Biology* 101: 349–365.

Stehelin D, Varmus HE, Bishop JM, and Vogt PK (1976) DNA related to the transforming gene(s) of avian sarcoma viruses is present in normal avian DNA. *Nature* 260: 170–173.

Swanstrom R, Parker RC, Varmus HE, and Bishop JM (1983) Transduction of a cellular oncogene: The genesis of Rous sarcoma virus. *Proceedings of the National Academy of Sciences, USA* 80: 2519–2523.

Tam W, Hughes SH, Hayward WS, and Besmer P (2002) Avian bic, a gene isolated from a common retroviral site in avian leukosis virus-induced lymphomas that encodes a noncoding RNA, cooperates with c-myc in lymphomagenesis and erythroleukemogenesis. *Journal of Virology* 76: 4275–4286.

Temin HM (1960) The control of cellular morphology in embryonic cells infected with Rous sarcoma virus *in vitro*. *Virology* 10: 182–197.

Toyoshima K and Vogt PK (1969) Temperature sensitive mutants of an avian sarcoma virus. *Virology* 39: 930–931.

Varmus HE (1982) Form and function of retroviral proviruses. *Science* 216: 812–820.

Varmus HE (2006) The new era in cancer research. *Science* 312: 1162–1165.

Vogt PK (1971) Genetically stable reassortment of markers during mixed infection with avian tumor viruses. *Virology* 46: 947–952.

Vogt PK (1971) Spontaneous segregation of nontransforming viruses from cloned sarcoma viruses. *Virology* 46: 939–946.

Wang LH (1987) The mechanism of transduction of proto-oncogene c-src by avian retroviruses. *Mutation Research* 186: 135–147.

Relevant Website

http://www.ncbi.nlm.nih.gov – Virus Databases Online (ICTVdB Index of Viruses), National Center for Biotechnology Information.

Simian Virus 40

A L McNees and J S Butel, Baylor College of Medicine, Houston, TX, USA

History

Simian virus 40 (SV40) was discovered in 1960 as a contaminant of poliovaccines. Hundreds of millions of people worldwide were inadvertently exposed to infectious SV40 in the late 1950s and early 1960s when they were administered contaminated virus vaccines prepared in rhesus macaque kidney cells. SV40 had unknowingly contaminated batches of both the inactivated and live attenuated forms of the poliovaccine and preparations of some other viral vaccines. Although primary cultures of monkey cells were known to be commonly contaminated with indigenous viruses and safety testing was carried out, SV40 had escaped detection in part because it failed to induce cytopathic effects in rhesus cells. However, when it was inoculated into African green monkey kidney cells, a prominent cytoplasmic vacuolization developed. Originally christened as 'vacuolating virus', the name was later changed to SV40 to conform to a numerical system of designating simian virus isolates.

Concern about the vaccine contaminations heightened considerably when it was found in 1962 that SV40 was tumorigenic in newborn hamsters and could transform many types of cells in culture. Subsequently, manufacturers treated poliovirus vaccine seed stocks to remove infectious SV40, and screening methods were implemented to increase detection of infectious SV40 in vaccine lots.

Because of the potential risk to public health posed by the previous distribution of contaminated poliovaccines, SV40 became the focus of intensive investigation. For scientists, SV40 has turned out to be an invaluable tool for dissecting molecular details of eukaryotic cell processes.

Numerous techniques now commonly used in molecular biology were pioneered in the SV40 system. It continues to serve as a model for basic studies of viral carcinogenesis.

Taxonomy and Classification

Viral species *Simian virus 40* is classified in the genus *Polyomavirus* in the family *Polyomaviridae* (**Table 1**). It was previously classified as a member of the *Papovaviridae* family. The International Committee on Taxonomy of Viruses has designated SV40 as the type species of the 13 members of the family *Polyomaviridae*, which includes murine polyomavirus, human polyomaviruses BK virus (BKV) and JC virus (JCV), as well as isolates from hamsters, rabbits, cattle, birds, and baboons. The human and animal polyomaviruses are antigenically distinct, and in most cases there is only one recognized serotype for each virus.

Properties of the Virion

SV40 particles are small and spherical, with a diameter of approximately 45 nm. Infectious virions have a sedimentation coefficient of 240S in sucrose and band at a density of $1.34\,g\,ml^{-1}$ in CsCl; empty capsids have a density of $1.29\,g\,ml^{-1}$. The molecular mass of the SV40 virion has been estimated at 270 kDa. The DNA content is 12.5% (w/w). The major capsid protein (VP1) accounts for 75% of the total virion protein. VP2 and VP3 are minor capsid proteins. Cellular histones (H2A, H2B, H3, H4) are used to condense the viral DNA for packaging and are present in the core of the particle. There is no lipid envelope. SV40 does not agglutinate erythrocytes.

Table 1   Properties of SV40

Classification	Family *Polyomaviridae*
Strain variation	Genetically stable; one serotype, multiple strains
Virion	Icosahedral, 45 nm in diameter, no envelope
Genome	Circular covalently closed dsDNA, 5200 bp
Proteins	Three structural proteins, VP1, VP2, VP3; cellular histones condense DNA in virion; nonstructural replication protein, T-antigen, is potent oncoprotein
Replication	In certain primate kidney cells; nucleus; stimulates cell DNA synthesis; long growth cycle
Natural host	Asian macaques, especially the rhesus monkey
Diseases	Asymptomatic persistent infections in natural hosts; tumors in experimentally infected rodents; associated with human tumors and with kidney disease
Historical note	Contaminant in early poliovaccines administered to millions of people

SV40 particles exhibit icosahedral symmetry. The virion is composed of 72 pentameric capsomeres composed of the VP1 protein arranged on a $T = 7d$ icosahedral surface lattice. This structure (hexavalent capsomeres having pentameric substructure) demands nonequivalent contacts between pentamers. This seems to be accomplished by the C-termini of the VP1 polypeptides, which extend as arms from one pentamer and fit into binding sites on adjacent pentamers, providing the necessary flexibility to build a capsid. The N-terminal arm of VP1 is completely internal in the virus particle. Minor capsid proteins VP2 and VP3 are predominantly internal as well and do not contribute to the basic structure of the virus outer shell.

The virus particles are very resistant to heat inactivation but are relatively labile when heated in the presence of divalent cations. Whereas SV40 is stable at $50\,°C$ for hours, incubation in the presence of $1\,M\,MgCl_2$ at $50\,°C$ for 1 h will effectively inactivate the virus if it is monodispersed. At a higher temperature ($60\,°C$), $\sim 99\%$ of infectious virus is inactivated within 30 min in the absence of divalent cations. Purified virions can be disrupted by strong alkaline conditions (pH 10.5), by lower pH (9.2) plus a reducing agent, or by detergent treatment. Virus particles are resistant to acid treatment (pH 3.0). Intact virus particles are not affected by nucleases, but in the presence of a reducing agent nuclease can enter the virion and cleave the viral DNA. SV40 is efficiently inactivated by UV light irradiation, following single-hit kinetics.

Properties of the Viral Genome

The SV40 genome is a circular, covalently closed, double-stranded (ds) DNA molecule of about 5 kbp (**Figure 1**). The native DNA assumes a superhelical configuration (form I) that sediments at 21S in a neutral sucrose gradient. A single-stranded (ss) nick generates relaxed circular dsDNA molecules (form II) that sediment at 16S, whereas a ds break produces linear dsDNA (form III, 14S). Alkaline denaturation of form I DNA produces dense cyclic coils that sediment at 53S. Form II DNA is converted to ss circular (18S) and ss linear (16S) molecules by denaturation. The supercoiled (form I) molecules can be separated from relaxed circular and linear forms by centrifugation of a DNA preparation in CsCl gradients with ethidium bromide. The form I molecules will band in a lower position in the gradient. The DNA forms also separate during electrophoresis in a neutral agarose gel; the supercoiled molecules migrate the fastest, the linear forms move at an intermediate speed, and the relaxed circles migrate the slowest.

The viral DNA both in virions and infected cells is associated with cellular histones H2A, H2B, H3, and H4. The histones are assembled in 24–26 nucleosomes on the viral DNA. The nucleosome structure and histone

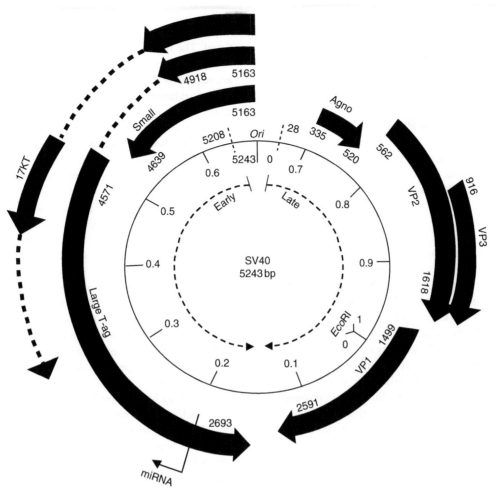

Figure 1 Genetic map of SV40. The circle represents the circular SV40 DNA genome. The unique *Eco*RI site is shown at map unit 0/1. Nucleotide numbers begin and end at the origin (*Ori*) of viral DNA replication (0/5243). Boxed arrows indicate the open reading frames that encode the viral proteins. Arrowheads point in the direction of transcription; the beginning and end of each open reading frame is indicated by nucleotide numbers. Note that T-ag is coded by two noncontiguous segments on the genome. The genome is divided into 'early' and 'late' regions that are expressed before and after the onset of viral DNA replication, respectively. Only the early region is expressed in transformed cells.

composition of the viral minichromosome mimic the chromatin structure of cellular DNA.

SV40 DNA was the first eukaryotic viral genome to be physically mapped by restriction endonuclease analysis (1971) and to be completely sequenced (1978). The DNA of reference strain 776 with a duplicated enhancer region contains 5243 bp for a calculated molecular weight of 3.5×10^6 Da. The genome is numbered in a clockwise direction from 1 to 5243, the central nucleotide of the unique *Bgl*I recognition site being assigned as 0/5243. Numbering continues through the late region in the 'sense orientation' and the early region in the 'antisense orientation'. The numbering system begins and ends (0/5243) in the middle of the functional origin of DNA replication. The unique *Eco*RI site at nucleotide 1782 was arbitrarily chosen as a point of reference and assigned a value of 0/1.0 on the circular map. Laboratory-adapted

strains of SV40 contain a duplication or rearrangements of the 72 bp element in the enhancer region, whereas most natural isolates do not.

The SV40 genome has compact regulatory sequences and overlapping genes. The single origin of replication (core *Ori* = 64 bp in size) is embedded within a nontranslated regulatory region. These elements control transcription and replication and span about 400 bp. The coding regions are expressed early or late in infection, and represent the 'early' nonstructural genes and the 'late' structural genes, respectively, and are transcribed off opposite strands of the viral DNA.

There is a variable domain at the 3' end of the T-ag gene, encompassing about 270 bp. Nucleotide changes within this region can be used to distinguish strains of SV40. Although genetic variation among SV40 strains is minimal, three different genogroups have been distinguished.

Sequence variations in this region are detected in human-tumor-associated SV40 sequences. Possible *in vivo* biological differences among SV40 strains are unknown but variations in oncogenic potential in rodent models have been observed.

Properties of Viral Proteins

SV40 encodes seven gene products: three 'early' non-structural proteins (large T-antigen (T-ag), small t-antigen (t-ag), 17K T-ag (17KT)), three 'late' structural proteins (VP1, VP2, VP3), and a maturation protein (LP1 or agnoprotein).

The nonstructural proteins are expressed early in infection, before the onset of viral DNA synthesis. The coding regions of the two T-ags and 17KT overlap; alternative splicing of viral transcripts determines each protein sequence. Large T-ag of strain 776 (**Table 2**) contains 708 amino acids (~90 kDa), and small t-ag contains 174 residues (~20 kDa). The large and small T-ags share 82 N-terminal amino acids, whereas the remainder of each protein is unique. The T-ag/t-ag common exon contains a 'J-domain', believed to modulate hsc70 activity in the assembly and disassembly of multiprotein complexes.

Large T-ag is an essential replication protein required for initiation of viral DNA synthesis. It stimulates host cells to enter S-phase and undergo DNA synthesis and is the SV40 transforming protein. Large T-ag contains a nuclear transport signal (126-Pro-Lys-Lys-Lys-Arg-Lys-Val-132) that targets the protein into the nucleus. However, about 10% of the T-ag in the cell is found in the cytoplasm and the plasma membrane. The biology of small t-ag is enigmatic. It is a cytoplasmic protein that is not essential for viral replication in cultured cells. It associates with the regulatory and catalytic subunits (36 and 63 kDa) of protein phosphatase 2A and is believed to cause cellular growth stimulation. It is required for

transformation of some human cells by SV40. Its role during natural infections by SV40 remains to be elucidated. The function of 17KT is unknown.

The functions of large T-ag in SV40 DNA replication are regulated by phosphorylation (**Figure 2**). The sites of phosphorylation are clustered near the ends of the molecule, one region lying between residues 106 and 124 and the other between residues 639 and 701. The majority of the phosphorylated residues are serines, although two threonine residues also become phosphorylated. Unlike many oncoproteins, T-ag is not phosphorylated at tyrosine residues.

T-ag is a DNA-binding protein that recognizes multiple copies of the sequence GAGGC in three T-ag-binding sites in the viral *Ori*. The minimal origin-specific DNA-binding domain of T-ag lies between residues 131 and 259. T-ag is predicted to have a zinc finger motif, typical of DNA-binding proteins, between amino acids 302 and 320. T-ag-specific ATPase and helicase activities are required in addition to DNA-binding activity in order for T-ag to function in initiation of DNA replication. The ATP-binding domain of T-ag is similar in structure to other ATP-binding proteins and is located between residues 418 and 627.

Large T-ag forms complexes with several cellular proteins. Such interactions are involved in T-ag functions in viral DNA replication, induction of cellular DNA synthesis, and cell-cycle progression. Target cellular proteins found in heterooligomeric structures with T-ag include transcriptional coactivators (CBP, p300, p400), tumor suppressor proteins (p53, pRb, p107, p130), DNA polymerase α, the molecular chaperone heat-shock protein hsc70, cell-cycle regulatory proteins cdc-2 and cyclin, and tubulin. The indicated cellular proteins are not all found in the same T-ag-associated complex; many subpopulations of T-ag exist in a cell.

The variable domain at the C-terminus of T-ag encompasses the host range–adenovirus helper function

Table 2 Properties and functions of SV40 T-ag

Structural properties	
Size[a]	708 amino acid residues, 82 N-terminal residues shared with t-ag, 81 632 Da, M_r 90 000–100 000 Da
Modifications	Phosphorylation, N-terminal acetylation, O-glycosylation, poly-ADP-ribosylation, palmitylation, adenylation
Supramolecular structure	Zinc finger, nuclear localization signal, J domain, monomers, dimers, higher homooligomers; heterooligomers with transcriptional coactivators (CBP, p300, p400); heterooligomers with DNA polymerase α; hsc70; cdc-2, cyclin, tubulin, Bub1, TEF-1, Cul7, Nbs1, Fbw7; tumor suppressor proteins (p53, pRb, p107, p130)
Subcellular distribution	Predominantly nuclear
Functions	
Replication and transactivation	Specific DNA binding (viral origin of replication), initiation of viral DNA replication; ATPase activity, helicase activity; autoregulation of viral early transcription, induction of viral late transcription
Host cell effects and transformation	Entry of cells into S phase and initiation of cellular DNA replication, complex formation with cellular proteins p53, pRb, p107, p130; adenovirus helper function; effect on host range, initiation and maintenance of cellular transformation, induction of immunity to SV40 tumor cells, target for cytotoxic T cells

[a]SV40 strain 776.

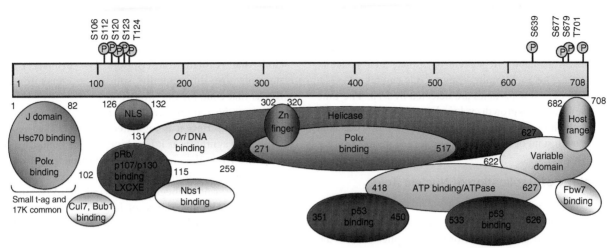

Figure 2 Functional domains of SV40 large T-ag. The numbers given are the amino acid residues using the numbering system for SV40-776. Regions are indicated as follows. Small t-ag common: region of large T-ag encoded in the first exon. The amino acid sequence in this region is common to both large T-ag and small t-ag. Polα binding: regions required for binding to polymerase α-primase. Hsc70 binding: region required for binding the heat shock protein hsc70. Cul7 binding: region required for binding of Cul7. pRb/p107/p130 binding: region required for binding of the Rb tumor suppressor protein, and the Rb-related proteins p107 and p130. NLS: contains the nuclear localization signal. *Ori* DNA binding: minimal region required for binding to SV40 *Ori* DNA. Nbs1 binding: region required for binding of Nbs1. Helicase: region required for full helicase activity. Zn finger: region which binds zinc ions. p53 binding: regions required for binding the p53 tumor suppressor protein. ATP binding/ATPase: region containing the ATP binding site and ATPase catalytic activity. Host range: region defined as containing the host range and Ad helper functions. Variable domain: region containing amino acid differences among viral strains. Fbw7 binding: region required for Fbw7 binding. The circles containing a P indicate sites of phosphorylation found on large T-ag expressed in mammalian cells. S indicates a serine and T indicates a threonine residue.

exhibited by SV40 (and mapped to T-ag) in some monkey kidney cell lines. The significance of the variable domain to natural infections by the virus is unknown.

The structural (capsid) proteins are expressed late in infection, after the onset of DNA replication. They are synthesized in much greater abundance than the early proteins. The major capsid protein, VP1, contains 362 amino acids (~45 kDa). The minor structural proteins are VP2 (352 residues, ~38 kDa) and VP3 (234 residues, ~27 kDa). The coding regions for VP2 and VP3 overlap, and they are translated in the same reading frame, so the sequence of VP3 is identical to the C-terminal two-thirds of VP2. VP3 is synthesized by independent initiation of translation via a leaky scanning mechanism, not proteolytic cleavage of VP2. The N-terminal portion of VP1 is derived from sequences that encode the C-termini of VP2 and VP3. However, VP1 is translated in a different reading frame from a different spliced transcript, so it shares no sequences with VP2 and VP3. VP1 is modified by phosphorylation and acetylation.

The late proteins are required only for the assembly of progeny virions during lytic infection. They are not involved in the early phases of viral replication. They are synthesized in the cytoplasm and move into the nucleus where particle morphogenesis occurs. The minor capsid proteins contain nuclear transport signals. The VP2/3 signal is Gly-Pro-Asn-Lys-Lys-Lys-Arg-Lys-Leu (VP2,

residues 316–324; VP3, residues 198–206). For VP1, two clusters of basic residues within the N-terminal 19 residues are independently important for nuclear targeting. Mutations in VP1 affect capsid assembly and/or virion stability. Mutations in VP2 and VP3 affect the uncoating process when virions penetrate new host cells.

The agnoprotein LP1 is synthesized late in infection but is not found in virus particles. It is a small (62 residue, ~8 kDa) basic protein involved in particle assembly. It is believed that LP1 interacts with VP1 molecules to inhibit self-polymerization until they interact with viral minichromosomes in the nucleus to form virions.

Replication

Overview of SV40 Replication Cycle

The SV40 replication cycle is cleanly divided into early and late events, with the onset of viral DNA replication being the dividing landmark. SV40 virions attach to receptors on the cell surface, become internalized, and are transported to the cell nucleus where the viral DNA is uncoated. After uncoating, the half of the genome that contains the early region is transcribed ('early' mRNAs). Viral early proteins (T-ags) are synthesized, cellular genes are expressed, and the cells enter S-phase. Viral DNA replication then begins. 'Late' mRNAs are transcribed from the other half of the viral genome (the opposite strand), and viral structural proteins are synthesized. Virus particles are assembled and SV40 is released from the cell surface in a manner dependent on intracellular vesicular transport. The SV40 multiplication cycle can take 24–72 h to complete. New particles are detected by 24 h. The time course of the virus growth cycle is dependent upon the virus strain and host tissue, the viral multiplicity of infection, and the growth state of the host cell at the time of infection.

Strategy of Replication of Nucleic Acid

SV40 DNA is replicated in the cell nucleus as a free unintegrated minichromosome. The only viral components required are the viral origin of replication on the DNA and the T-ag protein; all other factors are provided by the host cell replication machinery. T-ag is required for the initiation of DNA replication. The specific T-ag functions required are its DNA-binding ability and its ATPase/helicase activities. The relative simplicity of the SV40 system has allowed the development of cell-free replication systems and the identification of factors involved in mammalian DNA replication.

T-ag binds to the viral *Ori*, a 64 bp segment that contains binding site II for T-ag. In an ATP-dependent process, T-ag causes localized unwinding of the *Ori* region; cellular ss binding protein is required to stabilize the unwound single strands. The cellular DNA polymerase α-primase complex initiates DNA replication, and replication proceeds bidirectionally, with the two forks advancing at equal rates. Elongation involves DNA polymerase α, DNA polymerase δ, and proliferating cell nuclear antigen. Termination occurs 180° away from the viral *Ori*; topoisomerase II segregates the newly synthesized daughter molecules. Cellular histones are added to the new strands during the process of DNA replication.

Replication of SV40 DNA occurs in certain cell types of humans, monkeys, and possibly hamsters, and this permissiveness seems to depend in part on the nature of the DNA polymerase α-primase complex.

Characterization of Transcription

Transcription of the viral DNA is carried out by the cellular RNA polymerase II. In the noncoding region of SV40 DNA near the origin of replication are early and late promoter structures and enhancer elements. Early transcription begins at about nucleotide 5237, proceeds in the counterclockwise direction, and ends at the polyadenylation site at nucleotide 2694. The early promoter contains a TATA box about 30 bp upstream of the early RNA initiation site. (This start site is about 70 nucleotides upstream of the initiation codon shared by the early proteins.) There are three G + C-rich regions, the '21 bp repeats', located 40–103 nucleotides upstream, which are

binding sites for the Sp1 cellular factor. Even farther upstream are the SV40 enhancer elements, the 72 bp elements, which contain binding sites for other cellular factors that regulate transcription. The primary early transcripts are differentially spliced to generate the mRNAs that code for the three T-ags.

There is no requirement for virus-encoded proteins, but early transcription is regulated by T-ag. T-ag regulates its own synthesis as it first binds to site I and then to sites II and III on the viral DNA. The presence of T-ag at site II blocks the binding of RNA polymerase.

Late transcription begins after viral DNA synthesis is underway. The abundance of late transcripts is much greater than the early transcripts because progeny DNA molecules are utilized as templates. A heterogeneous collection of late mRNAs is made, with late transcription beginning at multiple sites between nucleotides 120 and 482 and proceeding in the clockwise direction, ending at a polyadenylation site at nucleotide 2674. Both the 21 bp repeats and the 72 bp elements have positive effects on late transcription. The late transcripts are alternatively spliced into two size classes (19S, 16S). VP1 is synthesized from 16S RNA, and both VP2 and VP3 are translated from the 19S species. The agnoprotein is synthesized predominantly from the most abundant species of 16S RNA.

SV40 microRNAs (miRNAs) have been described that accumulate during the late phase of the infection cycle and are complimentary to early viral mRNAs. The SV40 miRNAs function to target the early mRNAs for cleavage, which effectively reduces the expression of T-ag.

Post-Translational Processing

No post-translational cleavages are involved in the production of SV40 proteins. As noted above, T-ag and VP1 are modified in various ways, including phosphorylation.

Uptake and Release of Virions

The attachment of SV40 particles to the cell surface is mediated by VP1. The major histocompatibility class I molecules and the ganglioside GM1 molecules function as receptors. Attached particles are internalized by caveolae-mediated endocytosis into vesicles that contain caveolin-1. These vesicles fuse with caveosomes and the virus particles are transferred to the endoplasmic reticulum, from which they exit and then enter the nucleus. Conformational changes are thought to occur that expose the nuclear localization signals on capsid proteins and allow the virions to squeeze through the nuclear pore complex. The capsid disassembles in the nucleus, releasing the viral DNA.

Maturation of progeny virions occurs in the nucleus, where the viral nucleic acid is replicated. Viral proteins are synthesized in the cytoplasm off viral transcripts exported from the nucleus, and the proteins are then transported back into the nucleus. The structural proteins condense around the viral minichromosomes. There is a packaging signal on SV40 DNA that includes the *Ori* and part of the enhancer element. During the maturation process, the agnoprotein is released and is not retained as a component of mature virions. There are size constraints for packaging DNA – molecules ranging from 3.5 to 5.7 kbp can be encapsidated into SV40 particles.

Some progeny virions are released from the surface of infected cells via a mechanism dependent on intracellular vesicular transport, but the majority stay associated with the cell until cell death. The release of virus from ruptured and fragmenting cells may also be a mechanism of virus exit from infected cells. SV40 infections are not lytic and host cells are killed as the result of a variety of effects, including the release of lysosomal enzymes into the cytoplasm and damage to the cell mitochondria. Late in infection, monkey kidney cells develop a characteristic cytopathic effect, cytoplasmic vacuolization. As many as 10^4 virus particles can be produced by an infected cell, although some cells produce fewer particles.

Geographic and Seasonal Distribution

The geographic distribution of SV40 can only be inferred, as no comprehensive surveys have been conducted. SV40 is found naturally in wild populations of certain Asian macaque species, and its geographic distribution in the wild presumably reflects its narrow host range. Infections in humans are more widespread geographically, possibly because contaminated poliovaccines were broadly distributed. Nothing is known about seasonal effects on natural infections by SV40.

Host Range and Virus Propagation

Polyomaviruses, in general, have a narrow host range, with each virus infecting only one or a few closely related species. Based on antibody surveys of wild populations of primates, the natural hosts for SV40 appear to be a few species of Asian macaque monkeys, especially the rhesus (*Macacca mulatta*). In captivity, several related species are easily infected, including the cynomolgus macaque (*M. fascicularis*) and the African green monkey, which belongs to the same family as macaques (Cercopithecidae). The virus grows poorly in more distantly related primates. SV40 can infect humans.

SV40 is propagated in tissue culture in established cell lines derived from kidneys of African green monkeys. Characteristic vacuolated cells appear in response to viral replication. The virus grows in rhesus kidney cell lines in

which it establishes a persistent infection but produces no cytopathic effects.

SV40 typically does not cause tumors in its natural hosts. To demonstrate its tumorigenic potential, the virus must be inoculated into experimental animals (newborn hamsters are most susceptible). Many types of cells can be transformed in culture, including those of rodent, monkey, and human origin.

Genetics

SV40 is genetically stable, although rearrangements in the regulatory region can occur *in vivo*. Sequence variations exist at the $3'$ end of the T-ag gene among different isolates, which are stable on passage *in vivo* and *in vitro*. Adaptation of natural isolates to tissue culture often involves the selection of viruses with duplications or rearrangements in the viral regulatory region. The origins of several SV40 strains are listed in **Table 3**.

Serologic Relationships and Variability

Only one serotype of SV40 is known. The virus does not undergo noticeable antigenic variation. Perhaps restrictions imposed by the symmetry of the capsid permit only minimal deviation in amino acid sequence of the structural proteins, making most changes lethal for the virus.

There is a genus-specific antigenic determinant on the major capsid protein, VP1, that is shared by all animal and human polyomaviruses. It is expressed in infected cells and is internal in the virion. Antibodies are elicited against it by immunization with disrupted capsids or with purified VP1 protein. Antibodies against the shared determinant are not neutralizing, as the site is not exposed on the surface of virus particles. The structural proteins of SV40 and the two human polyomaviruses (BKV and JCV) are antigenically distinct, but display some cross-reactive determinants in enzyme-linked immunosorbent assay (ELISA) tests. The T-ags of SV40, BKV and JCV show antigenic cross-reactivity.

Epidemiology

Most adults of the Asian macaque species believed to be natural hosts for SV40 have neutralizing antibodies to the virus. Few of the juvenile animals of those species, in the wild, have antibodies. However, in captivity the young animals are readily infected if they have contact with a virus-positive animal.

Serologic surveys have detected SV40 neutralizing antibodies in humans with prevalences ranging from 2% to 10%. However, whether SV40 infection typically induces a detectable and sustained humoral or cellular immune

Table 3 Origin of SV40 strains

Virus strain	Year isolated	Source
SV40-776[a]	1960	Adenovirus type 1 seed stock prepared in monkey kidney cells
VA45-54	1960	Uninoculated rhesus kidney cells
Baylor	1961	Type 2 Sabin oral poliovaccine prepared in 1956 in monkey kidney cells
A2895	c. 1961	Tumor from hamster injected with rhesus monkey kidney cells
777	1962	Inactivated poliovaccine
Rh911	1962	Uninoculated rhesus monkey kidney cells
N-128	1965	Uninoculated rhesus monkey kidney cells (Russia)
SVPML-1	1970	Cultured human brain cells from patient with progressive multifocal leukoencephalopathy
SVMEN[b]	1984	Human meningioma (cloned directly, Germany)
SVCPC[b]	1995	Human choroid plexus carcinoma
SV40-K661	1998	Brain from rhesus monkey coinfected with simian immunodeficiency virus (SIV)
SV40-H328[a]	1998	Brain from rhesus monkey coinfected with SIV
SV40-T302	1998	Brain from rhesus monkey coinfected with SIV
SV40 –I508	1998	Brain from rhesus monkey coinfected with SIV

[a]SV40-776 and SV40-H328 are identical except for differences in the viral regulatory region.
[b]SVMEN and SVCPC are identical.
Data taken from Forsman ZH, Lednicky JA, Fox GE, *et al.* (2004) Phylogenetic analysis of polyomavirus simian virus 40 from monkeys and humans reveals genetic variation. *Journal of Virology* 78: 9306–9316.

response in humans has not been determined. SV40 DNA has been detected in human tumors, but epidemiological studies based on SV40-reactive serum antibodies in ELISA tests do not support an association of SV40 exposure with human cancers. The results of such epidemiological studies should be interpreted with caution, however, due to an inability to differentiate with certainty those who were exposed to an SV40-contaminated vaccine and those who were not. The working stocks in use between 1961 and 1978 by a major eastern European manufacturer of poliovirus vaccines have been shown to contain infectious SV40. This finding raises questions as to whether all poliovirus vaccines used worldwide after 1963 were free from SV40 contamination.

Transmission and Tissue Tropism

SV40 establishes persistent infections in the kidneys, and possibly lymphocytes, of susceptible hosts. The level of persistent virus present may be very low. Modes of transmission are not known, but transmission probably occurs due to virus shed in the urine or stool. Experiments have established that susceptible animals can be infected by the oral, respiratory, or subcutaneous routes. Both viremia and viruria occur in infected animals. SV40 may cause neurologic disease in immunocompromised hosts.

The major known source of human exposure to SV40 was via the administration of contaminated viral vaccines before SV40 was recognized. Human exposure could also occur by contact with infected monkeys, a situation limited to small numbers of animal handlers. Transmission between human hosts is hypothesized to occur but has not been documented. It is presumed that patterns of tissue tropism and transmission similar to those described in monkeys would be observed in humans infected by SV40.

Pathogenicity and Pathology

SV40 infections in normal monkeys appear to be asymptomatic and harmless. However, SV40 has been associated with a fatal case of pulmonary and renal disease, as well as with cases of progressive multifocal leukoencephalopathy, in unhealthy rhesus monkeys. SV40 can cause widespread infections in monkeys suffering from simian acquired immune deficiency syndrome and has been found in a brain tumor; no tumors have been found in immunocompetent, natural hosts. Transgenic mice carrying wild-type SV40 DNA develop choroid plexus papillomas and die rapidly because of the physiological importance of the tumor site. When foreign tissue-specific regulatory sequences are substituted for the native promoter-enhancer of the virus, SV40 expression can be directed to other tissues in transgenic animals and lethal tumors usually appear. Intraperitoneal inoculation of SV40 into weanling hamsters produces mainly mesotheliomas, intravenous inoculation of SV40 leads to leukemia, reticulum cell sarcoma, and osteogenic sarcoma, and subcutaneous inoculation induces undifferentiated carcinomas or sarcomas. SV40 DNA has been detected in several types of human cancers, including brain tumors (especially those from children in the first decade of life), mesotheliomas, osteosarcomas, and non-Hodgkin's lymphomas. SV40 DNA is sometimes found in tumors arising in persons too young to have been exposed to the contaminated vaccines in use between 1955 and 1963. The role SV40 may have played in the induction of those tumors is under investigation.

Immune Response

SV40, like other members of the genus *Polyomavirus*, induces an asymptomatic, persistent infection in natural hosts. An antibody response to capsid antigen is elicited that can be detected in neutralization assays. It is well documented with the human viruses BKV and JCV that impaired cell-mediated immunity is associated with virus re-activation, showing that viral replication is under the influence of the immune system of the host; the same presumably applies to SV40.

Little is known about the immune response of humans to infection by SV40. Small numbers of individuals exposed to contaminated vaccines were analyzed for neutralizing antibody responses to SV40. Humoral responses were detected in some vaccinees and were variable and dependent on the size of inoculum and route of inoculation. Recent serological surveys have detected SV40 neutralizing antibody in 2–10% of persons not exposed to SV40-contaminated viral vaccines. Antibodies to SV40 were most often detected in people with some type of immune suppression. ELISA-based assays detected some cross-reactive antibodies against SV40, BKV, and JCV. SV40 T-ag specific cellular immune response has been detected in some patients with SV40 DNA-positive tumors.

Experimental studies have shown that animals with active infections by SV40 may produce humoral antibodies against the replication oncoprotein, T-ag. It should be noted that a T-ag antibody response could not be used to monitor SV40 infections in humans because of the cross-reactivity among the T-ags of SV40, BKV, and JCV.

In vitro and *in vivo* studies demonstrate that SV40 tumor-bearing rodent animals develop a strong immune response to T-ag. Both humoral and cell-mediated responses occur and are sufficient to prevent tumor growth in some cases. In studies using the Syrian golden hamster model, inoculated animals frequently produced virus-neutralizing antibody and T-ag antibody responses, and the titers of both tended to be higher in tumor-bearing animals. In murine models, cytotoxic T cells directed against T-ag determinants at the cell membrane limit tumor progression.

Interferon is induced only weakly by the polyomaviruses and is not thought to be an important component of the host response to SV40.

Prevention and Control

No control measures are available to prevent SV40 infection.

Future Perspectives

The reports of antibodies to SV40 in humans and the infrequent association of SV40 markers with human tumors suggest that SV40 may be present in the human population. It is important to determine the natural history of SV40 in humans, including modes of transmission and factors affecting susceptibility to infection. Because of its small genetic content and dependence on host cell functions, SV40 will continue to be a useful model system for discerning mechanisms of cellular processes, such as mammalian cell DNA replication, cell cycle progression, and growth control processes altered in neoplasia.

See also: Polyomaviruses of Humans.

Further Reading

Ahuja D, Sáenz-Robles MT, and Pipas JM (2005) SV40 large T antigen targets multiple cellular pathways to elicit cellular transformation. *Oncogene* 24: 7729–7745.

Cole CN and Conzen SD (2001) *Polyomaviridae*: The viruses and their replication. In: Knipe DM, Howley PM, Griffin DE, *et al.* (eds.) *Fields Virology*, 4th edn., pp. 2141–2174. Philadelphia: Lippincott.

Cutrone R, Lednicky J, Dunn G, *et al.* (2005) Some oral polio vaccines were contaminated with infectious SV40 after 1961. *Cancer Research* 65: 10273–10279.

Dang-Tan T, Mahmud SM, Puntoni R, and Franco EL (2004) Polio vaccines, simian virus 40, and human cancer: The epidemiologic evidence for a causal association. *Oncogene* 23: 6535–6540.

Forsman ZH, Lednicky JA, Fox GE, *et al.* (2004) Phylogenetic analysis of polyomavirus simian virus 40 from monkeys and humans reveals genetic variation. *Journal of Virology* 78: 9306–9316.

Gazdar AF, Butel JS, and Carbone M (2002) SV40 and human tumours: Myth, association or causality? *Nature Reviews Cancer* 2: 957–964.

Hahn WC, Dessain SK, Brooks MW, *et al.* (2002) Enumeration of the simian virus 40 early region elements necessary for human cell transformation. *Molecular and Cellular Biology* 22: 2111–2123.

Liddington RC, Yan Y, Moulai J, *et al.* (1991) Structure of simian virus 40 at 3.8-Å resolution. *Nature* 354: 278–284.

Schell TD and Tevethia SS (2001) Control of advanced choroid plexus tumors in SV40 T antigen transgenic mice following priming of donor CD8[+] T lymphocytes by the endogenous tumor antigen. *Journal of Immunology* 167: 6947–6956.

Shah K and Nathanson N (1976) Human exposure to SV40: Review and comment. *American Journal of Epidemiology* 103: 1–12.

Stewart AR, Lednicky JA, and Butel JS (1998) Sequence analyses of human tumor-associated SV40 DNAs and SV40 viral isolates from monkeys and humans. *Journal of Neurovirology* 4: 182–193.

Vilchez RA and Butel JS (2004) Emergent human pathogen simian virus 40 and its role in cancer. *Clinical Microbiology Reviews* 17: 495–508.

Tumor Viruses: Human

R Grassmann and B Fleckenstein, University of Erlangen – Nürnberg, Erlangen, Germany
H Pfister, University of Köln, Cologne, Germany

Glossary

RDA (representational difference analysis)
PCR-based technique for the identification and cloning of DNA sequences (e.g., virus DNA) present in a particular cell but not in a matched reference cell.

Introduction

Viruses are responsible for about 15–20% of all cancers worldwide. Human tumor viruses constitute a heterogeneous group of viruses, which are causally linked to the development of malignant diseases in humans. Conventionally, the term is confined to those viruses that are likely to cause cancer by malignant conversion of infected cells. Accordingly, the human tumor viruses include the Epstein–Barr virus (EBV), the Kaposi's sarcoma-associated herpesvirus (KSHV), the high-risk human papillomaviruses (HPV), the hepatitis B virus (HBV), the hepatitis C virus (HCV), and the human T-cell leukemia virus (HTLV-1). Other viruses, such as HIV, support tumor development and growth indirectly, for example, by inhibiting the immune response to the tumor but do not infect the progenitors of malignant cells. Besides their systematic differences, most tumor viruses share several of the following features:

- establishment of chronic or long-term persistent infection;
- presence of viral gene functions, which interfere with cellular growth control, apoptosis control, DNA repair, or genomic stability; and
- capacity to transform cells in culture and/or to be oncogenic in experimental animal systems.

These features are not unique to tumor viruses but also shared by other human viruses, which are not yet clearly demonstrated but were suspected to cause human malignancies. These include some subtypes of human adenoviruses, the human polyomaviruses (BK, JC), many subtypes of papillomaviruses, and HTLV-2.

Virally induced tumors contain mostly viral genomes or parts of viral genomes, frequently integrated into the cellular genomes. As a hallmark of their infection prior to malignant conversion, many virally induced tumors are clonal in respect to integrated viral sequences. All human malignancies caused by tumor viruses are rare consequences of the infection and develop after long-term viral persistence. This indicates the necessity of rare secondary events, which are crucial to viral oncogenesis. Among them could be accumulation of genetic damage including cellular mutations induced by viral or nonviral factors, including physical and chemical carcinogens.

EBV-Associated Lymphoproliferative Malignancies

EBV, a member of the *Herpesviridae*, was the first virus to be linked to the oncogenesis of a human malignant disease. In 1964 it was identified by Epstein, Achong, and Barr in a B-cell line derived from an African Burkitt's lymphoma. Besides Burkitt's lymphoma, there are two other histologically and clinically distinct types of EBV-associated B-cell lymphoma, Hodgkin's disease and the lymphomas of immunosuppressed individuals. These three EBV-associated lymphoid malignancies differ in the patterns of the viral latent-gene expression and seem to be derived from cells at different positions in the B-cell differentiation pathway. Besides B-lymphoid malignancies, the virus was also found associated with some rare types of T-cell and natural killer (NK) cell lymphomas.

Lymphocyte Transformation *In Vitro*

EBV is capable of immortalizing human primary B lymphocytes, which resemble phenotypically activated B lymphocytes and are capable of proliferating permanently in culture. Cell lines usually contain EBV genomes as nonintegrated covalently closed circular double-stranded DNA in various copy numbers. Due to a block in structural gene expression, the transformed cells usually do not synthesize progeny viruses; instead, they express a series of latency-associated genes, which are also active in various combinations in human malignancies associated with EBV. These genes include five EBV-associated nuclear antigens (EBNA1, 2, 3A–C), two latent membrane proteins (LMP1, 2), and several noncoding RNAs. Most of these genes have important functions in the viral latent persistence. EBNA2 and LMP1 are essential for the *in vitro* transformation of B cells, as has been confirmed by using recombinant forms of EBV that lack individual latent genes. These studies have also highlighted a crucial role for EBNA1, EBNA-LP, EBNA3A, and EBNA3C in the transformation process. The main transforming protein of EBV is LMP1. It fulfills the criteria of a classic oncogene (e.g., rodent-fibroblast transformation). Although it lacks any homology to cellular proteins, LMP1 functionally mimics co-stimulatory receptors of the tumor necrosis factor (TNF) superfamily. Independent of a TNFR ligand, it exerts its pleiotropic effects, including the induction of cell-surface adhesion molecules and activation antigens, and the upregulation of anti-apoptotic proteins. These signals account for both the growth- and survival-stimulating functions of LMP1.

Lymphomas in Immunosuppressed Individuals

Individuals who are compromised in their cellular immunity (T-cell immune reaction) are at risk for the development of EBV-positive B-cell lymphoproliferative diseases. These include the immunoblastic lymphomas in patients with genetic immunodeficiencies, in AIDS patients, and the post-transplantation lymphomas (PTLs) in patients under immunosuppressive therapy after organ transplantation. PTLs are polyclonal or monoclonal lesions, which mostly arise within the first year of allografting, when immunosuppression is most severe. Almost all of these early onset tumors are EBV positive. The growth-stimulating EBV latent genes including EBNA2 and LMP1 are expressed; it suggests that the PTL consists of virus-transformed cells, which closely resemble *in vitro*-transformed lymphocytes that grow out in the absence of effective T-cell surveillance.

Hodgkin's Lymphoma

EBV-induced infectious mononucleosis was recognized as a risk factor for the development of Hodgkin's lymphoma. This malignant tumor is characterized by the predominance of a nonmalignant infiltrate which vastly outnumbers the malignant cells (Hodgkin cells, Reed–Sternberg cells: HRS cells). All HRS cells within a tumor are part of the same clone and are probably derived from crippled germinal-center cells that have been rescued from the germinal-center reaction.

The infiltrate distinguishes the subtypes, the nodular sclerosing (NS), mixed cellularity (MC), and rarer lymphocyte-depleted (LD), which are to different extents associated with EBV. Approximately 40% of Hodgkin's lymphoma in the developed world is associated with EBV and between 50% and 90% of MC and LD subtypes. The EBV genome in the tumor is clonal and present in every HRS cell which is evidence for a causal role in the pathogenesis of Hodgkin's lymphoma. The HRS cells express a particular subset of latent-cycle proteins – EBNA1, LMP1, and LMP2. A plausible pathogenetic role for the virus could be the prevention of apoptosis in cells that have undergone a defective germinal center reaction. In particular, LMP1 by stimulating co-stimulatory (TNFR) pathways is capable of replacing a T-cell signal that prevents apoptosis. Whether EBV continues to contribute to the malignant phenotype at the time of tumor presentation is not known to date.

Burkitt's Lymphoma

Burkitts lymphoma is a worldwide distributed B-cell lymphoma with defined subtypes. Whereas only 15–25% of the sporadic form, which prevails in Europe and Northern America, is EBV associated, the endemic form is nearly to 100% positive for EBV. Endemic Burkitts lymphoma is a frequent childhood tumor in the humid lowlands of eastern and central Africa. It presents in children around 8 years of age as a unilateral swelling of the jaw. Due to early metastasis the disease is usually multifocal at diagnosis.

Burkitt's lymphoma and derived cell lines (from both EBV-positive and EBV-negative cases) are now confirmed to be of germinal-centroblast origin. In this stage of B-cell development, the germinal-center reaction of the B cell (including somatic hypermutations of the V chains and isotype switching) is almost finished and cells are starting to enter the memory compartment. Common denominators of all BL forms are chromosomal translocations, which result in increased expression of the cMYC protein. The contribution of EBV to the pathogenesis of Burkitt's lymphoma remains still unclear. The most compelling evidence of EBV's involvement in endemic BL is the high frequency (98%) of tumors carrying viral DNA and the presence of clonal EBV in all of the tumor cells. The viral gene expression is limited to mainly EBNA1. The transforming LMP1 protein is absent and even seems to be incompatible with the growth of BL cells *in vivo*. Thus, the virus might have an initiating role in which growth-transforming B-cell infections establish a pool of target cells that are at risk of a subsequent *MYC* translocation. Epidemiological evidence indicates that co-infection with malaria and HIV is an important cofactor, which increases tumor incidence, possibly by chronic stimulation of the B-cell system.

Lymphoid Malignancies with T-Cell or NK-Cell Characteristics

EBV is also associated with three types of T-cell malignancies. In particular, the nasal T-cell lymphoma has a high rate of association. It is an extranodal lymphoma of the angiocentric type, which primarily develops in the nosal caveola. The tumor is relatively frequently found in Southeast Asia. Frequently nasal EBV-associated lymphomas resemble the phenotype of NK cells (CD3−/CD56+). The EBV-gene expression includes EBNA1, LMP1, and LMP2 in various extents.

EBV-Associated Carcinomas

The infection of epithelia by EBV eventually results in malignant transformation and the development of carcinomas. Such EBV-associated cancers are the anaplastic nasopharyngeal carcinoma (NPC), a subset of gastric adenocarcinomas and certain salivary gland carcinomas.

Nasopharyngeal Carcinoma

NPCs are highly malignant neoplasias, which mostly occur in adults between the ages of 20 and 50 years. The prognosis is poor; most frequently, NPC presents with early metastasis into cervical lymph nodes and the skull. The anaplastic (undifferentiated) form of NPC (aNPC) shows the most consistent worldwide association with EBV (virtually 100% worldwide). The anaplastic type of the NPC is recognized as a separate clinical entity. It differs from other types of NPC by its low grade of differentiation of the tumor cells and a characteristic tendency to extended lymphocyte infiltrations. The aNPC is particularly common in areas of China and Southeast Asia, reaching a peak incidence of around 20–30 cases per 100 000. An etiologic role of the virus in tumor development is supported by following characteristic features of the tumor cells: (1) virtually all aNPC contain EBV-DNA, and (2) the viral episomes in the tumors are monoclonal. From this observation one can deduce that the infection event has occurred prior to tumorigenesis. This assumption is supported by the presence of monoclonal EBV-genomes in the noninvasive progenitor lesions, the in-situ-NPC. (3) Besides EBNA1, the tumors express LMP2 and partly (40%) the viral oncoprotein LMP1. The lack of LMP1 expression in some tumors however seems to be a secondary late event since it has been reported that the premalignant lesions of NPC all express LMP1. Thus, the presence of the growth-signal-mediating LMP1 and LMP2 is additional evidence for the causal role of the virus in tumorigenesis.

Other Carcinomas

EBV is present in a high proportion (>90%) of lymphoepithelioma-like gastric carcinomas, which morphologically closely resemble NPC. About 5–25% of gastric adenocarcinomas are also associated with EBV. These tumors display a restricted pattern of EBV latent-gene expression, including EBNA1 and LMP2A. A possible role of EBV in the pathogenesis of gastric carcinomas seems to be confined to late tumorigenesis, which is suggested by the absence of EBV infection in premalignant gastric lesions. A subset of salivary gland carcinomas have also been found to be EBV-positive including the expression of latent genes like EBNA1 and LMP1 and 2 in parts of the tumors. Recently, EBV has also been detected in some carcinomas of the breast and liver.

Malignant Diseases Related to the KSHV

By using a polymerase chain reaction (PCR)-based technique for the selective amplification of unknown sequences ('representational difference analysis') Chang and co-workers identified in 1994 a new human herpesvirus in the tissue of Kaposi's sarcoma (KS). The new virus was designated as human herpesvirus type 8 (HHV8) or KSHV. It is highly associated with KS but also found in several rare lymphoproliferative conditions, including Castleman's disease and body cavity-based lymphoma (synonymous: primary effusion lymphoma).

Kaposi's Sarcoma

The tumor was first described in 1872 by Moritz Kaposi as 'multiple idiopathic pigmented sarcoma of the skin'. It is a multifocal, proliferative lesion of spindle-shaped cells with slit-like vascular spaces in skin and mucous membranes of the oral cavity, gastrointestinal tract, and pleura. The tumor cells, termed KS spindle cells, are likely of endothelial origin. KSs can be grouped into four clinical subtypes: (1) classic, (2) endemic or African, (3) transplantation-associated or immunosuppressive therapy-associated, and (4) epidemic or HIV/AIDS-associated. Based on the following evidence, a causal role of KSHV in the pathogenesis of KS is now widely accepted: (1) KSHV genomes are regularly detected in all subtypes of KS; (2) KSHV is present in the endothelial and spindle cells, the neoplastic component of the tumor; and (3) epidemiological and prospective cohort studies in HIV-infected individuals show high correlation of KSHV infections with a later development of KS. Viral gene expression in the latently infected KS cells is likely to support the growth of tumor cells. Among the viral proteins synthesized are a viral homolog of a D-type cyclin (vCYC), which is capable of stimulating the cell cycle in the G1 phase, and a viral homolog of FLICE-inhibitory protein (vFLIP), which is a potent suppressor of extrinsic apoptosis. Furthermore, latently infected KS spindle cells produce the 'latency-associated nuclear antigen' (LANA-1) that is required for the replication of circular viral episomes and the activation of a wide range of cellular genes.

B-Lymphoid Malignancies

'Multicentric Castleman's disease' (MCD) is a lymphoproliferative condition, characterized by enhanced B-cell proliferation and vascular proliferation in expanded germinal centers. In these lesions KSHV can be detected. In a proportion of B cells surrounding the follicular centers of MCD, several viral proteins were found to be expressed. These include LANA-1, the viral interleukin-6 (vIL-6), and the several proteins with homology to interferon regulatory factors (vIRF-1/K9, K10.5/LANA-2, K10). The signal transduction cascades induced by these viral proteins might be relevant for the pathogenesis of this disease. The second B-lymphoid malignancy associated with KSHV is the 'primary effusion lymphoma' (synonymous: body cavity-based lymphoma). This rare lymphoma develops mostly in AIDS patients in the spaces of pleura, pericard, or peritoneum.

Papillomaviruses as Major Cause of Human Cancers

There is nowadays sufficient evidence that certain, so-called 'high-risk' types of HPV are carcinogenic to humans in the cervix (HPV16, 18, 31, 33, 35, 39, 45, 51, 52, 56, 58, 59, and 66). In developing countries, carcinoma of the cervix uteri is the most frequent type of female cancer. Even in industrialized countries, in spite of extensive preventive screening, this cancer is among the most frequent female malignancies. HPV DNA can be found in virtually all cervical cancers, and the early genes E6 and E7 are usually expressed. The most prevalent type in epidermoid carcinomas is HPV16. HPV18 may be preferentially associated with adenocarcinomas. Other high-risk types have been detected in a few cases of squamous cell carcinoma each. HPV DNA was also demonstrated in more than 50% of the less-prevalent carcinomas of the vulva and penis (basaloid and warty tumors), the vagina, and the anus; HPV16 is again the most frequent type, followed by HPV18. HPV6 and HPV11 with a lower carcinogenic potential were detected in verrucous carcinomas of vulva, penis, and anus.

HPV16 and other members of the high-risk papillomavirus group immortalize primary human keratinocytes and induce resistance to differentiation stimuli. Histological abnormalities can be observed in stratifying keratinocyte cultures that resemble those in precancerous, intraepithelial lesions *in vivo*. The cells are not tumorigenic in nude mice initially, but quickly change to an aneuploid karyotype, which is in keeping with frequently occurring abnormal mitoses in HPV16-positive lesions. At higher passage level, malignant clones reproducibly arise, which indicates that HPV infection is sufficient to induce cancer cells in combination with additional spontaneous or virus-induced modifications. The viral genes E6 and E7 are required to trigger these effects. They encode proteins that inactivate tumor suppressors and modulate cell-cycle regulation, DNA repair, and apoptotic processes, for example, by interacting with the cellular proteins p53, p105-RB (the retinoblastoma protein), p21, p27, Bak, and PDZ domain proteins. E6 activates the catalytic subunit of the telomerase as an important step in cell immortalization. E6 and E7 induce chromosomal instability, mitotic defects, and aneuploidy, which will finally contribute to tumor progression. The E6 and E7 proteins of low-risk viruses display much lower affinities

to the cellular proteins, in parallel with a lower or non-detectable transforming potential *in vitro*.

Much attention has been paid to the possible role of viral DNA integration in tumor progression. HPV18 DNA appears integrated into the cellular genome in almost all cervical cancers, and HPV16 DNA in about two-thirds of the cases. This is in contrast with benign and premalignant lesions, where the viral DNA usually persists extrachromosomally. There is no evidence for a specific integration site, but HPV DNA has been repeatedly detected in the vicinity of the *myc* proto-oncogene in combination with an overexpression of the cellular gene. Probably, more important is the upregulation of viral oncogene expression following critical integration events, which result in a clonal selection of the affected cells.

The persistence of viral DNA and the continual expression of transforming genes in advanced cancers suggest that HPV functions are also involved in the maintenance of the malignant phenotype. An experimental suppression of E6 and E7 expression inhibited the proliferation of HPV-positive cervical cancer cell lines and reduced the cloning efficiency in semisolid medium, thus indicating that the viral proteins are still modulating the growth of malignant cells.

The genital tract HPVs are also responsible for many HPV infections at extragenital mucosal sites such as the oral cavity, the oropharynx, and most notably the larynx. However, cancers arising in this field harbor HPV DNA less frequently than genital tumors (oral cavity and larynx on average about 25%, oropharynx 35%, preferentially carcinoma of the tonsil). The reason for the striking difference between the genital and aerodigestive tracts is not known. Either the etiology of many oral and laryngeal cancers is unrelated to HPV, or the relevant HPV types are not yet characterized or the viral DNA is no longer necessary for cancer cells and is finally lost.

Different HPV types induce various proliferative skin lesions that are benign, like plantar, common and flat warts. An association between HPV and skin cancer becomes obvious in epidermodysplasia verruciformis (EV). EV patients are infected with a subgroup of HPVs, which induce characteristic persisting macular lesions disseminated over the body. Many EV patients develop squamous cell skin carcinomas, mainly at sun-exposed sites, which suggest a co-carcinogenic effect of ultraviolet light. The DNA of HPV5 or 8 persists extrachromosomally in high copy number in more than 90% of the cancers. HPV14, 17, 20, or 47 were occasionally detected. The prevalence of specific HPVs is in striking contrast with the plurality of HPV in benign lesions and has been interpreted as reflecting a higher oncogenic potential of these types.

The carcinogenic potential of HPV8 could be clearly demonstrated in transgenic mice with the early genes of

HPV8 under control of the keratin 14 promoter, which regularly develops papillomas with moderate and severe dysplasia and carcinomas in 6% of animals without any further treatment with physical or chemical carcinogens. E6 turned out to be the major oncogene in the mouse skin, necessary and sufficient for carcinogenesis. In contrast with genital HPV, no complex formation could be detected between HPV8 E6 and the cellular p53 protein, which suggests different strategies of transformation. Human keratinocytes transduced with recombinant retroviruses expressing HPV8 E7 invaded the dermis when tested in organotypic skin cultures.

A high prevalence of HPV DNA in squamous and basal cell carcinomas of the skin, particularly of immunosuppressed but also of immunocompetent patients, has been demonstrated by highly sensitive PCRs. Evidence is accumulating for many novel HPV types related to EV HPVs and cutaneous types. That there is a strong association between genital HPV16 and rare squamous cell neoplasms from the finger is remarkable. Individual skin tumors were frequently noted to be infected by several HPVs. No single HPV type predominates in skin cancers of non-EV patients, so far as is known. HPV DNA persists at very low concentrations in many skin cancers, usually at less than one genome copy per cancer cell. The relevance of these findings to the pathogenesis of cutaneous cancer remains to be determined. The possibilities discussed above for carcinomas of the aerodigestive tract are also valid for skin carcinomas.

Chronic Hepatitis B and C in Hepatocarcinogenesis

Hepatocellular carcinoma (HCC) is among the most common fatal malignancies in humans worldwide. An association with HBV from the Hepadnavirus family was suggested by the geographical coincidence of a high incidence of HCC in Southeast Asia and equatorial Africa with high rates of chronic HBV infections, frequently contracted congenitally. Prospective studies demonstrated about a 100-fold increased risk of hepatoma among carriers of the HBV surface antigen (HBsAg). Integrated HBV DNA can be detected in a large proportion of the tumors from high-risk areas and in hepatoma-derived cell lines. HBV is the first human tumor virus against which vaccination programs have been initiated on a broad basis. First signs of a decrease in the incidence of hepatoma in populations vaccinated in the 1970s substantiate the viral role in cancer development.

Liver cancer usually develops only after several decades of chronic HBV-induced hepatitis and may thus be triggered by accumulating genetic damage due to inflammation and continuous cell regeneration. A specific contribution of HBV might be expected from *cis* effects

following integration of viral DNA, but except for a few case reports no consistent evidence has been obtained for the activation of particular proto-oncogenes. A transactivation of transcription may be more relevant; this can be achieved by the viral X protein, the large surface protein, and a truncated $preS_2/S$ protein. The viral $preS_2/S$ gene, which normally encodes a surface protein, appears frequently disrupted in cancers as a consequence of DNA integration and then gives rise to the transactivator. All HBV transactivators exert pleiotropic effects via the protein kinase C/raf-controlled signal pathway, finally activating transcription factors such as AP-1 and NF-κB and proliferation. The analysis of viral integration patterns and functional assays suggest that at least one transactivator may function in most hepatomas.

Mutations in the p53 tumor suppressor gene occur in about 30% of human hepatomas. They are observed more often in countries with dietary contamination by mutagenic aflatoxin and seem to be a late event in liver carcinogenesis. The X protein was shown to interact with elements of the DNA repair system, which may increase the mutation rate of p53.

Two types of large HBsAg with deletions at the $preS_1$ and $preS_2$ regions were detected in 60% of HCC patients. The preS mutant proteins can initiate endoplasmic reticulum stress to induce oxidative DNA damage and genomic instability. Liver cancer arose not only in mice transgenic for the X gene but also in mice transgenic for preS mutants.

More recently, seroepidemiological evidence was obtained for a correlation between HCV infections and hepatoma. Antibodies against HCV were detected in between 13% and over 80% of liver cancer patients around the world. Over 60% of acute hepatitis C becomes chronic and may progress to cirrhosis and HCC. Latency periods between primary infection and cancer are usually measured in decades, but in some cases the intervals are rather short (5–10 years). The cumulative prevalence of hepatoma in cirrhotic HCV-infected patients is over 50%, indicating that HCV substantially increases the risk of HCC. HCV is related to flaviviruses and pestiviruses and is the first human tumor-related virus with an RNA genome and no DNA intermediate during replication. The role of the virus in carcinogenesis is not yet clear. Liver injury during chronic hepatitis may be responsible for malignant conversion, but there is also some evidence that HCV is more directly involved. HCV appears to persist and replicate in hepatocytes during malignant transformation. Viral proteins interact with many host-cell factors and affect cell signaling, transcription, translation, proliferation, and apoptosis. The HCV capsid core protein and the nonstructural proteins NS3 (a serine proteinase), NS4B, and NS5A revealed transformation potential in tissue culture. Both HCV core and NS5A target the Wnt-β-catenin pathway, which appears crucial in human HCC. As discussed for HBV, HCV also induces endoplasmic reticulum and oxidative stress.

The Role of HTLV-1 in the Oncogenesis of Adult T-Cell Leukemia/Lymphoma

In 1977 adult T-cell leukemia/lymphoma, a malignancy of CD4-positive T lymphocytes, was first recognized as a distinct clinical entity by Uchiyama, Takatsuki, and colleagues. Three years later, in 1980, Poeisz, Gallo, and co-workers isolated the first human retrovirus, HTLV-1 from the lymphoma-subtype of ATLL. HTLV-1, but not the closely related HTLV-2 is highly associated with ATLL. Besides ATLL, HTLV also is linked to the pathogenesis of a chronic neurodegenerative disorder, called HTLV-associated myelopathy/tropical spastic paraparesis.

Transformation of T Cells

HTLV-1-infected T lymphocytes derived from leukemic and nonleukemic patients, in contrast to normal T cells, regularly give rise to permanent cultures, which are capable of expressing all viral proteins. The virus *in vitro* has immortalizing capacity: primary human T lymphocytes can be transformed to permanent growth in tissue culture, which phenotypically resembles ATLL cells. A nonstructural regulatory protein of the virus, Tax, is capable of mediating the transformation. Besides regulating viral transcription, this multifunctional protein interferes with cellular control of survival, proliferation, and genomic stability. It combines many features characteristic of oncogenes, among them the ability to immortalize primary human T cells to permanent growth. These cells closely resemble HTLV-1-transformed and patient-derived T cells. Tax is also capable of inducing malignant growth in animal models. In HTLV-1 Tax transgenic mice it induces leukemia which is similar to the clinical pattern of ATLL.

Adult T-Cell Leukemia/Lymphoma

About 1–3% of all HTLV-infected individuals develop ATLL, mostly after several decades of asymptomatic viral persistence. Typically, the disease manifests at the age of 40–60 years. Frequent symptoms are cutaneous lesions, pulmonary complications, hepatosplenomegaly, and hypercalcemia, which at least in part can be attributed to the capacity of the malignant cells to infiltrate organs. Generally, ATLL is categorized into four forms: (1) acute, (2) chronic, (3) smoldering, and (4) lymphoma-type, which are all associated with HTLV-1. The smoldering and chronic ATLL are less-severe forms of the disease, which may convert to the aggressive acute ATLL. The lymphoma-type is characterized by the presence of extensive lymphadenopathy in the absence of blood or bone marrow involvement. Acute ATLL is the most frequent form (more than 55%) and until now barely curable and mostly fatal. Leukemia cells exhibit an unusual and characteristic morphology with lobulated nuclei. Regarding the surface phenotype they resemble T helper cells, from which they are probably derived (CD4), expressing high amounts of the interleukin 2 receptor (IL2Rα). Viral gene expression including the Tax gene is rather low and the role of the protein for the maintenance of the malignant proliferation unclear. A causative role of HTLV-1 in ATLL is now generally accepted because of the following evidence: (1) the geographic correspondence of ATLL and HTLV-1; (2) the almost 100% association of HTLV-1 and ATLL; (3) the clonal integration of the provirus in ATLL cells, which indicates infection prior to malignant transformation; and (4) the oncogenic capacity of HTLV-1 and its oncoprotein Tax in animal models.

General Conclusions and Future Perspectives

In most cases, long latency periods of many years or several decades elapse between primary infection by tumor viruses and first symptoms of cancer. All human tumor viruses are widespread in the world population. They contribute to malignant disease, mainly by initiation of oncogenesis, but regular infection does not immediately result in cancer. Thus, all human tumor viruses are important or necessary risk factors for particular cancers, but require additional events to induce malignant disease. This implies that in principle, all virally induced cancers can be prevented by protective immunization. As examples, vaccination against HBV and recently, against high-risk HPV are powerful prophylactic means to fight the associated cancers. The low manifestation rates of virus-induced malignancies also imply that the mere proof of an infection with a tumor virus is of limited value for the management of patients and cancer prevention. Specific diagnostic tests have to be designed that evaluate parameters of the viral infection more closely related to malignant conversion. In many but not all cases, continuous viral expression is detectable in malignant tumors, which raises the prospect of virus-specific pharmacological interference for adjuvant cancer therapy or cancer immunotherapy. For instance, the neoplastic phenotype of HPV-positive genital carcinoma cells seems to be affected by viral functions and may thus be a promising therapeutical target. Even in cases, in which primary infection and initial growth transformation apparently lead, through tumor progression, to a constitutive form of proliferation where viral gene products are not necessary for growth, virus may be used to target the tumor. For instance, stimulating specifically the immune response against viral antigens may be an appropriate future strategy.

See also: Epstein–Barr Virus: General Features; Hepatitis B Virus: General Features; Hepatitis C Virus; Human Immunodeficiency Viruses: Antiretroviral Agents; Retroviral Oncogenes.

Further Reading

Cougot D, Neuveut C, and Buendia MA (2005) HBV-induced carcinogenesis. *Journal of Clinical Virology* 34(supplement 1): S75.

Grassmann R, Aboud M, and Jeang KT (2005) Molecular mechanisms of cellular transformation by HTLV-1 Tax. *Oncogene* 24(39): 5976–5985.

IARC Working Group (2007) *IARC Monographs on the Evaluation of Carcinogenic Risks to Humans, Vol. 90, Human papillomaviruses.* Lyon, France: International Agency for Research on Cancer.

Levrero M (2006) Viral hepatitis and liver cancer: The case of hepatitis C. *Oncogene* 25: 3834–3847.

Neipel F and Fleckenstein B (2005) Human herpesvirus-8. In: ter Meulen V and Mahy B (eds.) *Topley and Wilsons, Microbiology and Microbial Infections: Virology*, pp. 541–558. London: Arnold.

Pfister H (2003) Human papillomavirus and skin cancer. *Journal of the National Cancer Institute* (Monograph) 31: 52.

Proietti FA, Carneiro-Proietti AB, Catalan-Soares BC, and Murphy EL (2005) Global epidemiology of HTLV-I infection and associated diseases. *Oncogene* 24(39): 6058–6068.

Schulz TF (2006) The pleiotropic effects of Kaposi's sarcoma herpesvirus. *Journal of Pathology* 208(2): 187–198.

Thorley-Lawson DA (2005) EBV the prototypical human tumor virus – just how bad is it? *Journal of Allergy and Clinical Immunology* 116(2): 251–261.

Young LS and Rickinson AB (2004) Epstein–Barr virus: 40 years on. *Nature Reviews Cancer* 10: 757–768.

zur Hausen H (2006) *Infections Causing Human Cancer.* Weinheim, Germany: Wiley-VCH Verlag.

GENERAL TOPICS

Emerging and Reemerging Virus Diseases of Vertebrates

B W J Mahy, Centers for Disease Control and Prevention, Atlanta, GA, USA

Glossary

Amplicon The product nucleic acid obtained from a polymerase chain reaction.

Bocavirus A genus of the family *Parvoviridae* containing bovine, canine, and human species.

Kaposi's sarcoma A skin tumor which frequently develops in young males infected with HIV.

Kawasaki disease A mucocutaneous lymph node syndrome that has features of a virus infection but so far no causative agent has been discovered. There are about 120 cases per 100 000 population in Japan, a sixfold higher incidence than in the USA.

picobirnavirus A virus containing a genome consisting of two segments of double-stranded RNA, 2.6 and 1.5 kb in length.

Sigmodontinae A subfamily of rodents in the family Muridae that contains over 500 species, confined to the American continent.

Vero cells A heteroploid cell line derived from the kidney of a normal African green monkey (*Cercopithecus aethiops*).

Introduction

It became apparent during the last two decades of the twentieth century that new infectious diseases were increasingly being recognized in the human and animal populations. This led to the establishment of a formal committee of the Institute of Medicine of the National Academy of Sciences, USA, who reported on their deliberations in 1992, in a report edited by Joshua Lederberg and Richard Shope. This was followed 10 years later by a second report, edited by Mark Smolinski, Margaret Hamburg, and Joshua Lederberg, which appeared in 2003. Among the factors they cited as contributing to emergence were microbial adaptation and change, human susceptibility to infection, climate and weather, changing ecosystems, economic development and land use, human demographics and behavior, technology and industry, international travel and commerce, breakdown of public health measures, poverty and social inequality, war and famine, lack of political will, and finally intent to harm.

Recognition of Emerging and Reemerging Virus Diseases

The advent of highly specific molecular techniques such as the polymerase chain reaction (PCR) in the early 1980s permitted the detection and grouping of viruses on the basis of genome nucleotide sequence analysis, and in several respects these techniques have replaced serological analyses for the characterization of viruses. Although it is still important to isolate viruses in cell culture for their complete characterization, it is now possible directly to detect viruses in diseased tissues by PCR, then, by sequencing the amplicon, to determine whether a new virus has emerged to cause the disease. In fact, many viruses which do not readily grow in cell culture can only be differentiated by sequence analysis. The papillomaviruses are an example. Their study was very difficult until the advent of sequence analysis, which now has revealed more than 100 types in humans, and many more in animals and birds. For differentiation, three virus genes (E6, E7, and L1) are sequenced, and if the combined sequence of these three genes differs by more than 10% from known papillomaviruses, the virus is considered to be a new type. Other viruses which have not been grown in cell culture include many caliciviruses, and the ubiquitous anelloviruses, such as torqueteno (TT) virus, which can be detected and sequenced in the blood of most humans and many other vertebrate species.

Hepatitis C virus was originally described as non-A, non-B hepatitis virus because of the severe disease it caused but the virus would not grow in cell culture, and eventually was detected in blood known to be infected with the virus by reverse transcription of the RNA present using random primers then expressing the resultant DNA in the bacteriophage lambda gt 11. Thousands of clones were screened using patient blood as a source of antibody before positive clones were detected, which then allowed the development of enzyme immunoassays that could detect the virus in blood and so were used to screen blood destined for transfusion, saving millions of lives worldwide. Once the complete genome of hepatitis C virus was sequenced, it became apparent that there are many different genotypes circulating in the world, with different pathogenic properties.

Nucleotide sequence analysis has also been extremely useful in tracing the origins of viruses. For example, when hantavirus pulmonary syndrome, caused by a bunyavirus of rodents, Sin Nombre virus, was initially detected in 1993 in the Four Corners region of Western USA, it was found that rodents inside a house where people had been infected carried a virus identical in sequence to virus isolated from human cases. However, rodents caught at various distances from the house had increasingly variable genome RNA sequences, providing strong evidence that these rodents, deer mice (*Peromyscus maniculatus*), were the source of the infection. Subsequently more than 30 other hantaviruses, some of which also cause hantavirus pulmonary syndrome in humans, were isolated from rodents throughout North and South America. Each new virus seems to be associated with a different genetic variant of rodent host, and all rodents that carry the virus belong to the subfamily Sigmodontinae, unique to the American continent.

A particularly powerful tool for the initial recognition of an emerging virus is the application of immunohisto-chemistry to diseased tissues. Provided a comprehensive collection of antibodies is available, the particular virus or related group of viruses can often be detected. For example, when Hendra virus first appeared in 1995 in Australia, causing the death of a horse trainer and 14 of his horses, antibody against the virus was sent to the Centers for Disease Control and Prevention (CDC). Then, in 1999, CDC was asked to investigate a newly emerged epidemic that had appeared in Malaysia, killing more the 100 people and causing disease in many pigs. Initially, it was suspected to be caused by a virus related to Japanese encephalitis virus, but a virus was isolated from the pigs that replicated in Vero cells, and reacted in an immuno-fluorescence test against the Hendra virus antiserum. This could subsequently be used on patient tissues to study the pathogenesis of the disease, and after comparison of the genome sequences of Hendra virus and Nipah virus they were found to be closely related and are now classified in the genus *Henipavirus* of the *Paramyxoviridae*.

Finally, molecular methods can be used to detect new, emerging viruses in the absence of disease in the host. In 2001, Allander and colleagues searched for RNA viruses in human respiratory secretions using random primer PCR, and discovered a hitherto unknown parvovirus with a sequence related to the bovine and canine parvoviruses, which are grouped together in the genus *Bocavirus*. The new virus was called human bocavirus, and many research groups worldwide have now confirmed the presence of the virus, particularly in pediatric samples, although it is still not certain how important this virus is in causing morbidity and mortality. Their method also amplified a human coronavirus from the respiratory samples, and when sequenced this turned out to be HKU1, a recently emerged coronavirus detected by scientists at Hong Kong University. It is possible that a systematic search of human samples using such molecular techniques might reveal more hitherto unknown human viruses.

Human Demographics and Behavior

In some cases, the emerging viruses themselves have contributed to other viruses emerging and reemerging in the population. This is especially true of human immuno-deficiency virus (HIV), the cause of acquired immune deficiency syndrome (AIDS), which rapidly spread following its emergence in the early 1980s to infect more than 40 million people worldwide by the end of the twentieth century. Because of its severe effects on the immune system, the virus leads to numerous other infections in the HIV-infected population. For example, picobirnaviruses, that had been detected in fecal samples from chickens and rabbits, were difficult to detect in human fecal samples until a cohort of men with AIDS was examined, and in these humans picobirnavirus was detected for the first time. Some rare diseases have become common in persons with AIDS. For example, the human polyomavirus known as JC virus can cause the rare brain disorder known as progressive multifocal leukoencephalopathy (PML). Normally, the virus remains dormant in the kidney, but in HIV-infected individuals the HIV-encoded transactivator Tat acts as a transactivator of JCV leading to PML which progresses to death within 4 months after infection. Other important virus infections which emerge in AIDS patients are human herpesviruses (cytomegalovirus, herpes simplex viruses 1 and 2, varicella-zoster virus, and human herspesvirus 8, which causes Kaposi's sarcoma).

HIV is mainly spread through sexual activity between an infected and a noninfected person, and is most common in those who indulge in high-risk sexual behavior with multiple partners. It can also be transmitted by direct contact with infected blood, and is common in persons who indulge in intravenous drug use, particularly when needles, syringes, or equipment used to prepare drugs for injection are shared. It is therefore an example of a virus disease which is dependent on risky human behavior for its maintenance in the human population.

The ability of such new infections to spread in the population has been greatly enhanced by population growth and ease of movement as a result of rapid air travel. A dramatic recent example of this was the appearance of the coronavirus causing severe acute respiratory syndrome (SARS) in late 2002 which spread by air travel from a single infected Chinese physician who infected 12 persons in a Hong Kong hotel. These infected persons then traveled by air and spread the infection to more than 8000 individuals worldwide, 10% of whom died. The virus then apparently receded from the human population in July 2003. Only recently was it discovered that the SARS coronavirus has a natural reservoir in Chinese horseshoe bats (*Rhinolophus sinicus*). Some other species such as Himalayan palm civets and raccoon dogs from which the virus has been isolated may serve as amplification hosts.

Following the recognition of the human coronavirus SARS, research on coronaviruses intensified, and this led to the discovery in 2004 of two previously unrecognized human viruses, one found by Hong Kong University, called HKU1 virus, and another reported almost simultaneously from the Netherlands, called NL63, and from Yale University, called New Haven coronavirus. The latter viruses probably represent two isolates of the same virus species. They are clearly associated with lower respiratory tract infection in children, but initially it was claimed that New Haven coronavirus was also associated with Kawasaki disease in children. This intriguing claim was rapidly investigated and refuted by several different groups in Japan, Taiwan, and elsewhere, and the cause of Kawasaki disease, which has features resembling a virus infection, remains unknown.

Zoonotic Diseases

A majority of recent emerging virus diseases have been zoonoses (i.e., diseases transmitted from animals to humans under natural conditions). Some of the more important of these include HIV-1, which was transmitted to humans from chimpanzees in Central Africa around 1931, and HIV-2, transmitted from sooty mangabeys to humans in West Africa around 1940.

Other important recent examples are the viruses of the genus *Henipavirus*. Hendra virus was first recognized through a disease outbreak in some horse stables in Hendra, Queensland, Australia, when 14 horses and their trainer died from pulmonary disease with hemorrhagic manifestations in 1994. The reservoir of the virus was found to be in large fruit-eating bats (*Pteropus* spp.), and one year later a horse farmer 600 miles away in Mackay, Queensland, died of encephalitis from the same virus. Then, in 1999, a related virus was discovered in Malaysia following a major outbreak of respiratory disease in pigs and neurological disease in humans in their close contact. More than 100 humans died, and in a successful effort to control the disease 1.1 million pigs were slaughtered. The causative virus was isolated from a fatal human case that had lived in Nipah River Village, and so was named Nipah virus. Hendra and Nipah viruses are clearly members of the family *Paramyxoviridae*, but have been placed in a separate genus as their RNA genome is about 19 kb in length, larger than that of any other paramyxovirus.

Nipah virus, like Hendra virus, was found to have a reservoir in *Pteropus* bats, and has since been identified in fatal human disease outbreaks in India in 2003 and Bangladesh in 2004.

Other new viruses which apparently have a reservoir in fruit bats include Menangle virus, a new paramyxovirus which emerged in a commercial piggery near Sydney, Australia, to cause stillbirths and abortion in pigs. Menangle virus also caused disease in two workers in the piggery. A new virus related to Menangle virus emerged during an investigation of urine samples from *Pteropid* bats collected on Tioman island, off the coast of Malaysia, in 2001, and was named Tioman virus. During the same investigation, a new orthoreovirus was isolated from *Pteropus hypomelanus* in 1999 and called Pulau virus, and more recently a related orthoreovirus called Melaka virus was isolated from a human case of acute respiratory disease in Melaka, Malaysia. Serological studies of sera collected from human volunteers on Tioman island showed that 13% had antibodies against both Pulau and Malaka viruses.

Another important group of zoonotic diseases are rodent-borne, and caused by members of the genus *Hantavirus* of the family *Bunyaviridae*. These viruses first emerged during the Korean War of 1950–52, when thousands of UN troops developed a mysterious disease with fever, headache, hemorrhage, and renal failure with a fatality rate of 5–10%. It was more than a quarter of a century before the causative virus was isolated from field mice in Korea, and named Hantaan virus, the cause of hemorrhagic fever with renal syndrome (HFRS) in humans.

Then, in 1993, a new hantavirus emerged in the Four Corners region of Southwestern USA as the cause of a severe acute respiratory disease syndrome, with a fatality rate close to 40%, and named Sin Nombre virus. This virus was shown to be transmitted to humans by inhalation of virus present in the urine, feces, or saliva of deer mice (*Peromyscus maniculatus*). It seems likely that this disease had existed for many years, and was only recognized in 1993 because of a clustering of human cases as a result of a regional upsurge in the rodent population resulting from climatic conditions causing increased availability of rodent food. Fortunately, in most of these infections, humans appear to be a dead-end host, and transmission between humans does not occur except with the Andes virus in South America.

Rodent-borne viruses of the family *Arenaviridae* also cause a number of serious zoonotic diseases in humans. The 'Old World' arenaviruses such as Lassa fever virus have been known for some time, but still cause thousands of fatal hemorrhagic fever cases every year in West Africa. However, 'New World' arenaviruses such as Junin virus causing Argentinian hemorrhagic fever and Machupo virus causing Bolivian hemorrhagic fever have long been recognized in South America. Recently, new arenaviruses have emerged, probably as a result of deforestation, which results in rodents seeking shelter in human habitation, and brings them into closer contact with people. These viruses include Guanarito virus that causes Venezuelan hemorrhagic fever with 36% mortality rate from confirmed cases, and Sabia virus isolated in 1990 that causes Brazilian hemorrhagic fever with a high fatality rate, including two laboratory acquired cases.

Rabies is a zoonotic disease of great antiquity that has mainly been associated with carnivores, such as dogs. The virus is excreted in the saliva of infected animals, and following infection it moves through the nervous system to attack the brain, causing aggressive behavior which results in the animal biting humans and animals with which it comes into contact and thereby spreading the virus infection. Fortunately, due to early work by Louis Pasteur, a vaccine was developed that protects humans or other animals from infection, and can also be given immediately post exposure, and the domestic dog population in the developed world is vaccinated and does not pose a risk to humans. However, in some developing countries, it is not uncommon for a rabid dog to bite and infect more than 25 people before it can be put down, and worldwide there are still some 30 000 human rabies deaths per year. Using molecular sequencing techniques, it is now possible to distinguish the genotypes of rabies viruses associated with different species of host, as the virus has become adapted through frequent transmission between members of the same host species. In the USA, there are six recognized terrestrial animal genotypes, in raccoons in eastern states, skunks in north-central states, skunks in south-central states, coyotes in southern Texas, red foxes in Alaska, gray foxes in Arizona, and several genotypes associated with particular species of bat. In fact, most fatal cases of human rabies in the USA can now be traced to bats, which are often not detected when the person is bitten; so rabies is not suspected and vaccination is not undertaken until the disease has taken hold.

Ecological Factors Favoring Virus Emergence

Many important virus diseases are spread by arthropods, and exposure to new arthropods and the viruses they carry is critical to the emergence of new virus diseases. Dengue hemorrhagic fever is caused by dengue virus which is transmitted mainly by the Asian mosquito (*Aedes albopictus*), and dengue fever is one of the most rapidly emerging diseases in tropical regions of the world. There are four serotypes of dengue virus, and it seems that consecutive infections with two antigenic types can lead to the more serious disease of dengue hemorrhagic fever with shock syndrome, which, if untreated, can result in up to 50% mortality. Unfortunately, through the importation of vehicle tires containing water from Korea, the Asian mosquito was introduced into the USA, and is now present in several regions of the Southern states. It can act as a vector not only for dengue virus, but also for California encephalitis virus.

In Europe, the emergence of two important animal diseases has occurred through the movement of arthropod vectors into the Iberian Peninsula. African horse sickness virus causes a disease that can be fatal to horses, mules, and donkeys, and is transmitted by nocturnal biting flies of the genus *Culicoides*. These were introduced inadvertently

into Spain, and the disease is now endemic around Madrid and regions to the south. African swine fever virus is transmitted by ticks of the genus *Ornithodorus* and it causes a fatal disease resembling classical swine fever in domestic pigs. It first emerged in Portugal and Spain in 1957, France in 1964, Italy in 1967, and Cuba in 1971. Through slaughter of infected animals, the disease was eradicated from Europe, except Sardinia, by 1995.

The most recent dramatic example of the movement of a virus vector is provided by West Nile virus, a flavivirus first isolated in Uganda in 1937. This virus uses birds as a reservoir host, and is transmitted from birds to humans and other vertebrates by mosquitoes. In 1999, cases of encephalitis in New York were found to have been caused by a strain of West Nile virus that was phylogenetically similar to a virus isolated from geese in Israel.

At the same time, many birds, especially corvids, began dying in New York State. Since the introduction in 1999, West Nile virus has become well established throughout the USA and moved north into Canada and south into the Caribbean and into Mexico. It is not known how the virus moved from Israel to the USA, but the most reasonable explanation is that it was carried in an infected mosquito or possibly an infected bird in the hold of an aircraft. Transmission by an infected human seems less likely since the titer of virus in human blood is usually too low for efficient mosquito transmission.

It is clear, nevertheless, that once it arrived in North America, West Nile virus found an extremely favorable environment with abundant avian and arthropod hosts that facilitated its spread throughout the American continent.

Prospects

The emergence of new viruses is likely to continue as viruses evolve and find new ecological niches in the human and animal population. It is noticeable that most newly recognized viruses have been RNA viruses, perhaps since RNA evolves at a faster rate than DNA, for which host cells have developed efficient proofreading enzymes. It will be important in the future to detect new viruses before they can emerge to cause disease in the population. The SARS epidemic provides an excellent example. Before the epidemic, only two human coronaviruses were known, human coronaviruses 229E and OC43. Despite the fact that serious coronavirus diseases were well known in other vertebrates, such as feline infectious peritonitis and avian infectious bronchitis virus, it was not until the SARS epidemic that research on human coronaviruses led to the discovery of three new human coronaviruses – SARS, HKU1, and NL63/New Haven.

There are other genera of viruses that cause serious disease in animals but have not been adequately investigated in humans. An example is the genus *Arterivirus*, which has members causing serious disease in horses and pigs, but has not been reported at all in humans. This could be a worthwhile area for future investigation.

Another critical factor in the future control of emerging viruses is better vector control. When mosquito control was conducted using DDT, dengue fever virus was virtually eliminated from the Americas in the 1970s, but environmental concerns led to the widespread banning of the use of DDT, so that since the 1980s there has been a considerable expansion of dengue fever in South America, with the appearance of dengue hemorrhagic fever there for the first time. There is a real need to improve mosquito control measures to control this disease. Although there are prospects for a dengue virus vaccine, this is so far not available.

Finally, one of the most important viruses that continue to emerge in different antigenic forms is influenza virus. The main reservoir of influenza viruses is in birds, and over the past century several pandemics of influenza have emerged, the most serious of which was in 1918. Pandemic strains usually arise by a process of antigenic shift, where one of the genes encoding the hemagglutinin and/or the neuraminidase of influenza virus is replaced by one from birds. New pandemics occurred in 1918 (H1N1 subtype), 1957 (H2N2 subtype), and 1968 (H3N2 subtype). Since 1968, there have been no new pandemics, but it is widely expected that another will occur. At the time of writing, there is worldwide concern that a highly pathogenic avian influenza virus (H5N1 subtype), which has caused some human infections and deaths in persons in close contact with infected birds, might mutate or recombine to generate a virus which would be highly transmissible in the human population. Plans are being developed in many countries and by the WHO to try to prepare for such an event by generating possible vaccines against such a virus and stockpiling antiviral drugs.

Further Reading

Choo QL, Kuo G, Weiner A, et al. (1992) Identification of the major, parenteral non-A, non-B hepatitis agent (hepatitis C virus) using a recombinant cDNA approach. Seminars on Liver Diseases 12: 279–288.

Chua KB, Bellini WJ, Rota PA, et al. (2000) Nipah virus: A recently emergent deadly paramyxovirus. Science 288: 1432–1435.

De Villiers EM, Whitley C, and Gunst K (2005) Identification of new papillomavirus types. Methods in Molecular Medicine 119: 1–13.

Gratz NJ (2004) Critical review of the vector status of Aedes albopictus. Medical and Veterinary Entomology 18: 215–227.

Hayes EB and Gubler DJ (2006) West Nile virus: Epidemiology and clinical features of an emerging epidemic in the United States. Annual Review of Medicine 57: 181–194.

Hsu VP, Hossain MJ, Parashar UD, et al. (2004) Nipah virus encephalitis reemergence, Bangladesh. Emerging Infectious Diseases 10: 2082–2087.

Kahn JS (2006) The widening scope of coronaviruses. Current Opinion in Pediatrics 18: 42–47.

Korber B, Muldoon M, Theiler J, et al. (2000) Timing the ancestor of the HIV-1 pandemic strains. Science 288: 1789–1796.

Ksiazek TG, Erdman D, Goldsmith CS, et al. (2003) A novel coronavirus associated with severe acute respiratory syndrome. New England Journal of Medicine 348: 1953–1966.

Mahy BWJ and Brown CC (2000) Emerging zoonoses: Crossing the species barrier. Revue Scientifique Et Technique Office International Des Epizooties 19: 33–40.

Mahy BWJ and Murphy FA (2005) The emergence and re-emergence of viral diseases. In: Mahy BWJ and ter Meulen V (eds.) Topley & Wilson's Microbiology & Microbial Infections, 10th edn., pp. 1646–1689. London: Hodder-Arnold.

Mushahwar IK, Erker JC, Muerhoff AS, et al. (1999) Molecular and biophysical characterization of TT virus: Evidence for a new virus family infecting humans. Proceedings of the National Academy of Sciences, USA 96: 3177–3182.

Nichol ST, Spiropolou CF, Morzunov S, et al. (1993) Genetic identification of a hantavirus associated with an outbreak of acute respiratory illness. Science 262: 914–917.

Smolinski MS, Hamburg MA,, and Lederberg J (eds.) (2003) Microbial Threats to Health, Emergence, Detection and Response, 367pp. 367pp. Washington, DC: The National Academies Press.

Stephenson I (2005) Are we ready for pandemic influenza H5N1? Expert Review of Vaccines 4: 151–155.

Herpesviruses: Latency

C M Preston, Medical Research Council Virology Unit, Glasgow, UK

Glossary

Ganglion A small organ containing the cell bodies, including nuclei, of neurons.
Iontophoresis Introduction through the skin or cornea by applying an electrical charge.

Introduction

Members of the family *Herpesviridae* exhibit the ability to remain latent in tissues of the host following primary infection. Latent virus is retained for the lifetime of the host, and can be reactivated to cause recurrent disease. Latency is a crucial property for the survival of herpesviruses, overcoming the requirement for rapid reinfection of new individuals in order to spread within a population. As described below, the characteristics of latency show variations when the different herpesvirus subfamilies are considered. Operationally, latency is defined as the presence of the viral genome without detectable virus production, coupled with the potential for resumption of virus replication in response to reactivation signals. For descriptive purposes, latency is characterized by three phases: establishment, maintenance, and reactivation.

Early thoughts on latency focused on two basic ideas, named the static and dynamic models. In the static model, the viral genome is considered to be nonreplicating due to a failure to undergo the normal program of gene expression, and reactivation is viewed as a change in intracellular conditions such that replication resumes. Dynamic models of latency envisage a slow persistent production of virus that is normally controlled by the host immune system and does not cause overt disease until a reactivation stimulus diminishes host defenses. There is currently no consensus that either of these models is correct; instead, research into latency continually reveals greater complexity in the interaction of virus with host. It is now thought that interference with virus replication occurs at many levels, ranging from repression of gene expression to control by immunological defenses. The requirement for long-term retention of the viral genome, coupled with an ability to spread within a population, demands that a complex and intimate relationship exists between virus and host. This relationship can be considered at two levels, namely the individual cell and the organism. At the cellular level, there must be mechanisms for sequestering the viral genome in a host cell that is potentially permissive for replication, and for retaining the ability to resume replication in response to appropriate stimuli. In terms of the organism, the virus must evade detection by the immune system during latency and must overcome host defenses when reactivating.

Latency will be considered in terms of the three subfamilies of the family *Herpesviridae*, focusing on human viruses since these are understood in the greatest detail.

Alphaherpesvirinae

The prototype of the subfamily *Alphaherpesvirinae*, herpes simplex virus (HSV) type 1 (HSV-1), is the most intensively studied in terms of latency. In humans, its natural host, primary exposure usually occurs during infancy and is characterized by a mild infection of the oropharynx that is frequently unnoticed. After the initial infection has resolved, a proportion of individuals experience periodic reactivation in response to stressful stimuli, such as excessive exposure to sunlight, resulting in the appearance of 'cold sore' lesions around the lip and less frequently on other areas of the face. HSV type 2 (HSV-2) is more frequently associated with genital herpes, although nowadays genital HSV-1 is detected with increasing frequency. Genital herpes and facial cold sores are treated by application of acyclovir, but this agent is only effective in preventing lesions once reactivation has occurred. There is currently no antiviral that eradicates latent virus or prevents reactivation.

HSV establishes latency in sensory neurons that innervate the site of initial infection. The viral genome is retained in neurons of the relevant ganglia for the lifetime of the host, and upon reactivation virus is released into tissues served by neurons extending from the ganglion. During initial infection, replicating HSV enters nerve termini and virus particles are transported along axons in a retrograde manner to the ganglia. Upon reactivation, virus moves in an anterograde direction from the ganglion to the surface, where replication causes disease.

Animal models have been developed for the study of HSV latency, and although each has limitations, they have been important in linking molecular investigations with *in vivo* studies. Latency is established efficiently after infection of mice with HSV-1, but reactivation is difficult to achieve *in vivo*. The most common method of reactivating latent virus from mice is to explant ganglia, a process in which ganglia are removed by dissection and cultured in the laboratory. This invariably results in the appearance of infectious virus within a few days but its physiological relevance is debatable. Subjecting mice to transient hyperthermia reliably reactivates virus replication in ganglia *in vivo*, albeit at low efficiency. The best animal for the study of reactivation is the rabbit, since virus is spontaneously released in tear films after ocular infection and release can be stimulated by iontophoresis of epinephrine. Genital HSV-2 infection can be reproduced, to some extent, by intravaginal inoculation of guinea pigs.

In considering establishment of latency, a crucial question concerns the way in which the normally inexorable progression to lytic replication and cell death is interrupted. Transcripts and proteins characteristic of lytic infection cannot be detected easily during latency, indicating a global repression of gene expression. Furthermore, studies with HSV mutants have failed to identify a gene product that is dispensable for lytic replication but required for latency, thus the prevailing hypothesis is that establishment of latency results by default when viral gene expression is somehow arrested in neurons. It is currently thought that the block occurs early in the virus life cycle, and the most likely point for intervention by the cell is at the immediate early (IE) stage. A favored hypothesis contends that IE transcription is compromised in sensory neurons, possibly due to inefficient transport of the virion transactivator protein VP16 (virion protein number 16), which activates IE transcription, to the neuronal nucleus, or to lack of the cellular transcription factors Oct-1 (a cellular protein that binds sequences with the consensus ATGCAAAT) or host cell factor (HCF, a large cell protein), with which VP16 is able to form a complex. Alternatively, sensory neurons may contain proteins that act as competitive inhibitors of Oct-1 and/or HCF, blocking their interactions with VP16. The possibility of arrest at the IE stage is supported by experiments with tissue culture cells. HSV-1 mutants that are severely impaired for IE gene expression can be retained in cells for extended periods in a nontranscribed 'quiescent' state that apparently mimics the transcriptional silence characteristic of latency.

Despite the overall absence of viral lytic gene products, latently infected neurons can be readily identified by the presence of a 2 kbp viral RNA known as the latency-associated transcript (LAT). Thousands of molecules of this RNA are found in the nucleus, enabling its detection by *in situ* hybridization or RNA blots. The observed species is an unusually stable intron spliced from a larger precursor that is present in neurons at much lower levels. Structurally, LAT is a lariat, that is, a splicing intermediate of a type typically cleaved and rapidly degraded. The LAT lariat has an unusual branch point sequence that is not recognized by cellular debranching enzymes. A smaller 1.5 kbp RNA, derived by further splicing, is found only in neurons. Intriguingly, LAT is complementary to sequences encoding the C-terminal portion of the IE protein ICP0 (infected cell protein number 0), an important activator of gene expression, leading to the suggestion that LAT blocks ICP0 production by an antisense mechanism. At present, there is no evidence for protein products encoded by HSV-1 LAT or the longer precursor in latently infected neurons, although there is evidence that the bovine herpesvirus 1 latency-related transcript does encode one or more proteins.

The significance of LAT for latency is controversial. Viral mutants that are unable to produce LAT nonetheless establish latency and can be reactivated; thus, LAT does not have an essential role in any of the animal models currently available. In detail, however, LAT mutants are deficient in reactivation in a number of contexts, suggesting a modulatory role for the transcripts. In some animal models, the absence of LAT appears to reduce the efficiency of reactivation directly, whereas in others LAT mutants exhibit a defect in establishment, thereby indirectly reducing reactivation due to the smaller pool of latent genomes. It is relevant that LAT mutants cause greater destruction of neurons during the initial stages of infection. This may be because one of LAT's normal roles is to exert antisense inhibition of ICP0 expression, thereby restricting productive infection, but currently the favored interpretation is that LAT has anti-apoptotic properties that reduce neuronal death after infection. Therefore, LAT could be important for improving establishment of latency by preventing loss of infected neurons, but equally a direct

effect on reactivation is possible by keeping reactivating neurons healthy for long periods.

During maintenance of latency, which can last for many decades in humans, it is thought that cellular factors contribute to the stable repression of transcription. The genome is believed to be organized into a chromatin-like structure, and indeed histones carrying post-translational modifications characteristic of inactive cellular chromatin are associated with latent HSV-1 genomes. Interestingly, the LAT region, which escapes repression, is associated with histones normally found on actively transcribed genes. Therefore, cellular mechanisms for global control of transcription may operate on latent HSV DNA.

The latent viral genome exists as a circular episome, structurally distinct from the linear molecule found in the virion. This suggests that the gene expression program is arrested at an early stage, since circularization occurs shortly after virus entry into the cell as a prelude to replication. Alternatively, circular molecules may be remnants from replication during productive infection. It is possible that circularization is important for the assembly of the latent genome into a chromatin structure. There is no evidence for integration of HSV DNA into the host genome during latency.

During latency in humans or experimental animals, only a fraction of neurons in the ganglion (typically 0.1–5% but in some cases up to 30%) harbor latent HSV-1, and neurons themselves constitute only about 5% of the cells in the ganglion. However, viral genomes can be detected by Southern hybridization of total ganglion DNA, demonstrating that neurons harbor many copies of HSV DNA. Analysis of single cells by polymerase chain reaction (PCR) confirms this conclusion and further reveals a wide disparity in the viral copy number per neuron. Most neurons harbor fewer than 100 viral genomes, but a minority can contain thousands.

Although it is clear that most latent genomes do not express lytic gene products at detectable levels, sensitive analysis of mouse ganglia by reverse transcriptase-PCR demonstrates the presence of viral transcripts from loci outside the LAT region. The transcripts are present in low amounts; they may signify infrequent viral lytic gene expression, but they may simply represent a small amount of background transcription of the latent genome. In an extensive analysis of mouse ganglia, a very small number of neurons (fewer than one per mouse) were undergoing an apparently productive infection, again showing that silencing of the genome is not absolute. Therefore, a low level of viral lytic gene expression may occur during latency.

Immunological studies support the view that virus lytic gene expression may occasionally occur during latency. Leukocytes, predominantly CD8+ T cells, can be found in ganglia from humans or latently infected experimental animals, often in intimate association with neurons. In mice, the infiltrating T cells are HSV-1 specific, with the majority recognizing a single immunodominant epitope on glycoprotein B. Furthermore, latently infected ganglia contain cytokines such as RANTES (an attractant for T cells), γ-interferon, and tumor necrosis factor (both produced by T cells). The continued presence of CD8+ T cells and derived cytokines is indicative of persistent stimulation of the immune system during latency. The favored interpretation of the data is that T cells respond to and eliminate a low level of virus that is produced from infected neurons.

The exact nature of the stimuli that provoke reactivation is unclear, and at present the general term 'stress' is used. The stress can be delivered at the periphery, directly to the neuron, or systemically. In experimental animals, explantation of ganglia efficiently reactivates latent HSV, but virus is only released from a small proportion of infected neurons. Procedures that provoke reactivation *in vivo*, such as hyperthermic treatment of mice, are even less efficient. The low efficiency imposes constraints on studying the molecular basis of reactivation, since it is not possible to identify the small number of reactivation-competent genomes among the total latent population. The normal program of HSV gene expression probably does not operate during reactivation because VP16 is absent during latency. It is suspected that stress causes alterations to the transcription factor profile of neurons, resulting in changes at the ICP0 promoter and synthesis of ICP0 protein which then derepresses the entire viral genome. An alternative view of reactivation is that stresses impair immunological mechanisms that normally prevent a low level of reactivating virus from causing disease. The impairment may occur in the ganglion, at the periphery, or both, with the outcome that virus is able to replicate. The application of PCR has revealed that low-level asymptomatic shedding of HSV in humans is more common than previously thought, supporting the view that local immunity prevents reactivated virus from causing disease.

A summary of HSV latency is shown in **Figure 1**.

Varicella-zoster virus (VZV) causes varicella (chickenpox) as primary infection and zoster (shingles) upon reactivation. VZV is latent in neurons within ganglia throughout the body because the primary infection is widespread rather than localized as in the case of HSV. Studies on VZV latency have proceeded slowly, relying on analysis of human tissue in the absence of a satisfactory animal model to reproduce latency. Although rats can be infected with VZV and harbor genomes in ganglia, virus cannot be reactivated. In humans, latent VZV genomes appear to be retained as circular episomes. The pattern of gene expression during latency, however, differs from that found with HSV. Transcripts representing four lytic genes (ORF21, ORF29, ORF62, and ORF63) have been detected in human ganglia, and there is evidence that protein products, particularly that of ORF63, are also present in infected human and rat neurons. Thus, despite many similarities, there may be significant differences in the details of VZV and HSV latency.

Betaherpesvirinae

Most studies on latency of the subfamily *Betaherpesvirinae* are concerned with the cytomegaloviruses, particularly human cytomegalovirus (HCMV). In adults, initial infection with HCMV is normally asymptomatic unless

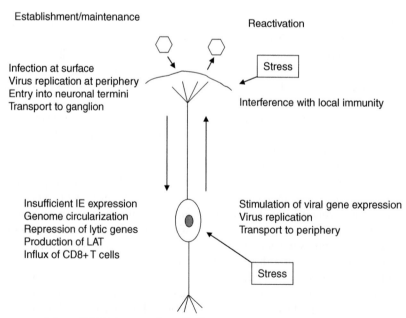

Figure 1   Schematic representation of HSV latency and reactivation.

it occurs *in utero*, but in immunocompromised individuals it may be serious. Reactivation of latent HCMV can cause rejection of organ transplants, due to replication of virus originating from either the recipient or the donated organ. In addition, AIDS patients can suffer a widespread HCMV infection that has serious consequences. HCMV can be transferred by blood transfusion, suggesting that circulating lymphocytes harbor latent virus, and sensitive PCR analysis, together with cell sorting, has detected the HCMV genome in a small proportion (1 in 10^4 cells) of peripheral blood monocytes. In addition, the HCMV genome can be detected in precursors of monocytes, the CD34+ myeloid progenitors in bone marrow, suggesting that these cells may be the primary reservoir of latent virus.

In view of the low proportion of myeloid cells containing latent HCMV, and the absence of animal models for this virus, molecular studies on HCMV latency have relied heavily on the use of cell culture models. The myelomonocytic line THP-1 is nonpermissive for HCMV replication, but becomes permissive upon differentiation by chemical treatment *in vitro*. Similarly, the teratocarcinoma line NT-2 is nonpermissive until induced to differentiate. The block in undifferentiated cells is due to failure of the major IE transcription unit to be expressed, resulting in arrest of the entire productive infection program. Plasmid-based transfection assays have indicated that specific sequence elements within the major IE promoter (MIEP) are targets for repression. Whereas the entire MIEP is inactive in undifferentiated cells but active in differentiated cells, a truncated MIEP, containing only the 300 base pairs proximal to the mRNA start site, is active in both situations. Mutational analysis has identified critical DNA elements in the MIEP at positions upstream of −300 that contain binding sites for two cellular proteins known to act as repressors. These proteins, known as Yin-Yang 1 (YY1) and Ets-2 repressor factor (ERF), mediate repression of the MIEP in transfection assays, and, furthermore, their levels decline after differentiation by chemical treatment. The implication is that differentiation changes the levels of repressors and hence permits IE gene expression in THP-1 and NT-2 cells.

Chromatin structure at the MIEP is a further important factor in determining permissiveness in cell culture models of HCMV latency. In undifferentiated cells, the MIEP is associated with methylated histones and heterochromatin protein 1 (HP1), both markers of inactive chromatin, whereas in differentiated cells the relative amount of HP1 is reduced and acetylation of histones, a correlate of active chromatin, is increased. It is suspected that YY1 and ERF exert their repressive effects by recruiting histone deacetylases (HDACs) to the MIEP, thereby promoting the formation of inactive chromatin, and this idea is supported by the fact that undifferentiated cells become permissive for IE transcription when treated with chemical inhibitors of HDACs.

The findings from the analysis of cell culture models have received support from studies on monocytes isolated from seropositive individuals and on CD34+ myeloid precursors from human bone marrow. Monocytes do not support HCMV replication, but virus is produced upon differentiation to macrophages in the laboratory. HCMV can be reactivated *ex vivo* by inducing CD34+ cells from seropositive individuals to differentiate to a mature dendritic cell phenotype. Furthermore, differentiation of CD34+ precursors to dendritic cells reproduces the switch from inactive to active chromatin structure at the MIEP. Thus it is thought that HCMV remains latent in CD34+ myeloid precursors and that differentiation to macrophages or dendritic cells leads to intracellular changes that activate the MIEP and ultimately result in virus replication. Although the precise signals that provoke reactivation *in vivo* are not known, one reported means of inducing virus replication is by allogeneic stimulation of blood monocytes, achieved by mixing cells from histo-incompatible individuals. This may reproduce events that occur during transplantation.

The latent HCMV genome is thought to exist as an episome, but it is not known how it is retained in the host. It may be replicated during cell division, by cellular factors or with the participation of viral proteins, or alternatively a low level of persistent virus production may continually seed new latently infected cells. There have been reports of HCMV-specific transcripts produced during latency, but there is little consensus between different laboratories and thus the possibility that viral gene products control latency remains an open question.

At the level of the whole organism, reactivation of HCMV generally causes disease only when the immune system is compromised. A high proportion (>1%) of circulating CD8+ T cells is specific for HCMV, suggesting frequent stimulation of the immune system, presumably through virus reactivation. Indeed, differentiation of monocytes occurs constantly and if such an event frequently reactivates HCMV, immune clearance must be crucial to prevent disease. The potential significance of the immune response in limiting HCMV infection is best demonstrated in studies with murine cytomegalovirus (MCMV). In its natural host, the mouse, latent MCMV is found in numerous tissues, in contrast to the situation with HCMV. During MCMV latency, CB8+ T cells specific for a major IE protein are present, suggesting that immune control eliminates cells containing reactivating virus at an early stage of the gene expression program. Damage to the immune system can result in widespread infection, and although the simplest interpretation of this finding is that immune surveillance is critical for maintaining latency, it must be remembered that immunosuppression also represents a significant stress that may itself activate the latent genome.

HCMV latency is summarized in **Figure 2**.

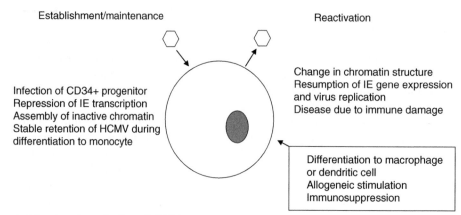

Establishment/maintenance

Reactivation

Infection of CD34+ progenitor
Repression of IE transcription
Assembly of inactive chromatin
Stable retention of HCMV during
differentiation to monocyte

Change in chromatin structure
Resumption of IE gene expression
and virus replication
Disease due to immune damage

Differentiation to macrophage
or dendritic cell
Allogeneic stimulation
Immunosuppression

Figure 2   Stages in latency and reactivation of HCMV.

Gammaherpesvirinae

Most latency studies with the subfamily *Gammaherpesvirinae* have focused on Epstein–Barr virus (EBV), a member of the genus *Lymphocryptovirus*. This virus is usually transmitted by exchange of saliva, with cells of lymphoepithelial structures such as the tonsils initially infected. Infection is generally asymptomatic but infectious mononucleosis, a self-limiting lymphoproliferative disease, can result if EBV is first acquired during adolescence or later. A defining feature of EBV is its ability to activate resting cultured B cells into unchecked proliferation with retention of the viral genome but without virus production, and indeed the distinction between latency and transformation is often blurred in discussion of this virus. It is clear, however, that EBV is latent in B cells, and that the virus utilizes many aspects of normal B cell development to establish and control latency. EBV, in contrast to HSV and HCMV, possesses a number of genes that are specific to the nonreplicating state and indeed are crucial for coordinating the establishment of latency. These encode the EBV nuclear antigens (EBNAs) 1, 2, 3A, 3B, 3C, and LP, and the latent membrane proteins (LMPs) 1, 2A, and 2B. Other loci specifying small RNAs, known as EBERs, and Bam A rightward transcripts are active during B cell transformation *in vitro*, although their significance for latency is unclear at present. During establishment of latency, the EBNAs and LMPs participate in a complex interaction with the host cell that results in utilization of the normal B cell development, to the advantage of the virus.

After penetration of the mucosal layers of the tonsils, virus replicates and naive B cells are infected and activated in a manner similar to that observed in culture. At this stage, no lytic gene transcription occurs but all of the EBNAs and LMPs are expressed in an interaction known as the growth program, or latency III. The combined action of the viral proteins gives the resting cell the characteristics of an activated B-lymphoblast, mimicking the first stage that occurs naturally after antigen recognition. Activated B cells are transported to the lymph node follicles, in which they replicate to form germinal centers. Again, following the normal pattern of B cell development after antigen stimulation, the infected cells undergo differentiation into memory B cells. At some stage during this process, the gene expression pattern changes to the default program, or latency II, in which only EBNA1, LMP1, and LMP2A are produced. Protein EBNA1 is crucial for maintaining the EBV genome in dividing cells, through stimulating its replication and by tethering it to cellular chromosomes. LMP1 and LMP2A provide survival signals that prevent the activated B cell from undergoing apoptosis. In the final step, the infected memory B cells are released from the germinal centers to become circulating memory B cells, and during this process gene expression changes to the latency program, or latency I, in which no viral gene products can be detected. During latency, the EBV genome is maintained as a circular episome. To retain the virus within the host, EBNA1 is produced during cell division, enabling the viral genome to replicate and persist in the memory compartment. Interestingly, each of the identified interactions with B cells is reflected in EBV-associated human tumors: viral gene expression in Burkitt's lymphoma (BL) cells resembles the latency program (but with EBNA1 continually expressed), Hodgkin's lymphoma has the default program, and nasopharyngeal carcinoma exhibits the growth program, albeit in epithelial-derived cells.

Reactivation of latent EBV occurs when a memory B cell differentiates into an antibody-secreting plasma cell, an event triggered by signaling from the B cell antigen receptor (BCR). The plasma cells migrate to the mucosal epithelium and virus is released into the

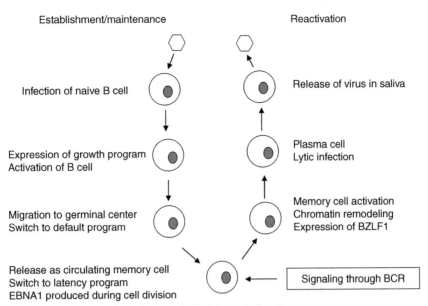

Establishment/maintenance   Reactivation

Infection of naive B cell

Expression of growth program
Activation of B cell

Migration to germinal center
Switch to default program

Release as circulating memory cell
Switch to latency program
EBNA1 produced during cell division

Release of virus in saliva

Plasma cell
Lytic infection

Memory cell activation
Chromatin remodeling
Expression of BZLF1

Signaling through BCR

Figure 3   Establishment, maintenance, and reactivation of EBV latency in B cells.

saliva, possibly after replication in epithelial cells. The molecular mechanism of lytic cycle activation, and hence virus replication, has largely been studied by the use of BL cell lines, which express only EBNA1 and thus resemble the latent state in B cells. Cross-linking the BCR with immunoglobulin, possibly mimicking the natural differentiation signals provided by T cells, can activate EBV in certain BL lines. This process switches on expression of an IE protein, BZLF1, a transcription factor that triggers further viral gene expression and ultimately productive replication. The signal transduction pathways that respond to cross-linking the BCR result in activation of two transcription factors, MEF2D and ATF, which in turn induces histone acetylation and relief of repression by remodeling the chromatin structure. The BZLF1 protein activates its own promoter, providing a positive feedback loop that ensures rapid commitment to productive replication. In some BL cell lines, BZLF1 expression, and hence EBV replication, is activated in response to alternative agents, such as phorbol esters, but the relevance of these treatments to natural stimuli is unclear.

The interaction between EBV and host B cells is summarized in **Figure 3**.

Members of the genus *Rhadinovirus* of the *Gammaherpesvirinae* have been studied in less detail than EBV. Murine herpesvirus 68 establishes latency in a number of cell types, including B cells, in mice. Kaposi's sarcoma-associated herpesvirus (KSHV) is also found in a variety of cell types, again including B cells. The natural pathways of latency and reactivation for these viruses are currently under investigation.

Common Themes

Although the examples described here deal with different viruses and host cells, some common themes emerge from the latent interactions. In establishment, specific features of the natural host cell are critical in preventing productive virus replication. Blocking IE protein production, an effective mechanism for inhibiting virus replication while minimizing cytopathology and immune recognition, appears to be common to establishment of latency. During maintenance, genomes are retained as circular episomes and viral gene expression is minimized to hide the virus from the immune system. Histones associated with the latent genome exhibit modifications characteristic of inactive chromatin. If repression of replication is not complete, low-level virus production may be neutralized by the immune system. Reactivation probably involves the virus utilizing normal cellular responses to a stimulus, but the stimulus may also damage the immune system and thereby cause disease.

See also: Herpesviruses: General Features.

Further Reading

Amon W and Farrell PJ (2004) Reactivation of Epstein–Barr virus from latency. *Reviews in Medical Virology* 15: 149–156.

Efstathiou S and Preston CM (2005) Towards an understanding of the molecular basis of herpes simplex virus latency. *Virus Research* 111: 108–119.

Jones C (2003) Herpes simplex virus type 1 and bovine herpesvirus 1 latency. *Critical Microbiology Reviews* 16: 79–95.

Kent JR, Kang W, Miller CG, and Fraser NW (2003) Herpes simplex virus latency-associated gene function. *Journal of Neurovirology* 9: 285–290.

Khanna KM, Lepisto AJ, Decman V, and Hendricks RL (2004) Immune control of herpes simplex virus during latency. *Current Opinion in Immunology* 16: 463–469.

Sinclair J and Sissons P (2006) Latency and reactivation of human cytomegalovirus. *Journal of General Virology* 87: 1763–1779.

Streblow DN and Nelson JA (2003) Models of HCMV latency and reactivation. *Trends in Microbiology* 11: 293–295.

Thorley-Lawson DA (2001) Epstein–Barr virus: Exploiting the immune system. *Nature Reviews* 1: 75–82.

Thorley-Lawson DA (2005) EBV the prototypical human tumor virus – just how bad is it? *Molecular Mechanisms in Allergy and Clinical Immunology* 116: 251–261.

Wagner EK and Bloom DC (1997) Experimental investigation of herpes simplex virus latency. *Clinical Microbiology Reviews* 10: 419–443.

Human Eye Infections

J Chodosh, A V Chintakuntlawar, and C M Robinson, University of Oklahoma Health Sciences Center, Oklahoma City, OK, USA

Glossary

Blepharoconjunctivitis Inflammation of the eyelid and conjunctiva.
Dacryoadenitis Inflammation of the lacrimal gland.
Iridocyclitis Inflammation of the iris and ciliary body.
Meibomian gland Modified sebaceous glands lining the eyelid margin that provide the lipid layer of the preocular tear film.
Retinochoroiditis Inflammation of the retina and choroid (uveal) layers of the eye.

Introduction

The eye contains diverse tissues intricately linked to subserve visual function (**Figure 1**). The ocular adnexae – periorbita, eyelids and lashes, lacrimal and meibomian glands – produce, spread, and drain the preocular tear film, physically protect the sensitive ocular mucosa, and cushion the globe. The redundant conjunctiva with its low-viscosity tear film allows rapid multidirectional eye movements. Lymphoid tissues within the conjunctiva and lacrimal glands furnish acquired immune defense. The cornea and its tear film fashion the major refractive surface of the eye. The sclera forms the wall of the globe and scaffolds the intraocular tissues. The eye's lens provides additional refractive power and filters ultraviolet light. The iris diaphragm dynamically regulates the amount of light incident upon the retina, and together with the choroid and optic nerve head provides immune effector cells to the interior of the eye. The retina transduces light energy into neural signals; retinal function is requisite for vision. The vascular choroid nourishes the outer layers of the retina. The anterior (aqueous) and posterior (vitreous) humors provide internal pressure sufficient for maintenance of normal anatomic relationships, nourish the interior ocular tissues, provide immunosuppressive factors necessary to the maintenance of immune deviation, and during infection act as conduits for the distribution of inflammatory cells derived from the iris, ciliary body, and optic nerve head.

Eye infection by viruses most often follows direct contact with virus externally, either from infected secretions in the birth canal (herpes simplex virus, human papillomavirus), on fomites (adenovirus), or airborne particles (rhinovirus), or is acquired during viremia (human cytomegalovirus, measles virus). Other mechanisms of ocular viral infection include extension from contiguous adnexal disease (herpes simplex virus), spread from the upper respiratory tract via the nasolacrimal duct (rhinovirus), and transplacental passage of infectious virus (rubella

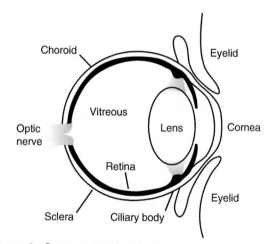

Figure 1 Cross section of the human eye.

virus). Rarely, ocular infection may disseminate elsewhere (enterovirus 70).

Acute viral infection produces stereotypic changes in ocular target tissues. Infection of the eyelid skin induces the formation of vesicles and ulcers. Viral infection of the conjunctiva results in vasodilatation, serous discharge, hyperplasia of conjunctival lymphoid follicles, and enlargement of the corresponding draining lymph nodes. Severe conjunctival infection can cause permanent scarring of the globe to the eyelids and turning in of the eyelashes against the eye. Viral infection of the corneal epithelium induces punctate epithelial cytopathic effect evident biomicroscopically as isolated swollen epithelial cells (punctate epithelial keratitis) and loss of individual epithelial cells (punctate epithelial erosions). When extensive, the punctate erosions may coalesce to form confluent epithelial ulcers with dendritic, dendritiform, or geographic morphology. With herpetic infection, corneal anesthesia can ensue, and in the absence of epitheliotropic neural growth factors, corneal epithelial integrity is impaired. Reduced corneal clarity and progressive sterile ulceration may result. Corneal stromal infection induces white blood cell recruitment; subsequent corneal scarring, vascularization, and lipid deposition may permanently reduce vision. Intraocular infection manifests in inflammatory cell deposits on the posterior surface of the cornea and on the vitreous scaffold, and in free-floating leukocytes and biomicroscopically visible protein spillage into the normally cell-free and protein-poor aqueous humor. Iridocorneal and iridolenticular adhesions may develop and lead to glaucoma and cataract. Retinal infection concludes with necrosis and lost function. Viral encephalitis and meningitis can result in cranial nerve inflammation and secondary dysfunction of vision and extraocular motility.

Classical viral pathogenic mechanisms of latency, reactivation, and carcinogenesis all can be demonstrated in the eye. Herpes simplex virus causes recurrent lytic epithelial keratitis when viral reactivation within sensory ganglia of the first division of the fifth cranial nerve gives rise to virus in the preocular tear film. Necrotizing herpes stromal keratitis follows viral reactivation within the cornea stroma. Intraepithelial neoplasia and invasive squamous cell carcinoma of the conjunctiva and cornea (**Figure 2**) have been associated with human papilloma virus types 16 and 18. When infected with oncogenic human papillomaviruses, corneal limbal stem cells can provide a persistent source of dysplastic ocular surface epithelium. Molecular mimicry has also been demonstrated as an immunopathogenic mechanism in ocular disease. Systemic infection with hepatitis C virus is associated with autoimmunity against a corneal stromal antigen and peripheral ulcerative keratitis. In a murine model of herpes simplex infection, non-necrotizing stromal keratitis accompanies T-cell reactivity against a corneal protein antigenically similar to a herpes simplex coat protein.

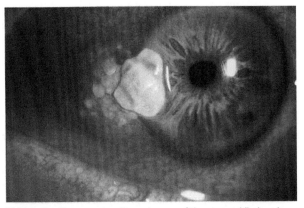

Figure 2 Squamous cell carcinoma of the corneal limbus is associated with infection by human papilloma virus types 16 and 18.

Ocular Immunology of Relevance to Viral Infection

Tissue diversity within the eye and adnexa compel varied means of innate immune defense. The eye's external surfaces (conjunctiva and cornea) encounter viruses by both airborne and contact routes. The eyelids, an intermittent barrier, periodically wipe the eye's surface free of debris and spread and drain the preocular tear film. The ability of the tear film to nonspecifically impede primary infection by viruses is unknown, although such mechanisms are well established for bacterial pathogens. An inhibitory effect of goblet cell-derived and intrinsic mucins and meibomian gland-derived lipids on viral adsorption to the ocular surface is speculative. Early in infection, aqueous tears from the main and accessory lacrimal glands furnish proinflammatory cytokines, and the conjunctival blood vessels provide both soluble and cellular components of innate immunity. After viral infection is established, aqueous tears carry lacrimal gland-derived monospecific secretory immunoglobulin A.

The constitutive defense armaments of the cornea and conjunctiva differ. The normal cornea is considered an immune-privileged site due to the high success rate of corneal transplantation; it lacks blood vessels, lymphatics, resident lymphoid cells, and Langerhans cells, expresses Fas ligand on its surface epithelium, and demonstrates reduced delayed hypersensitivity responses. Because corneal inflammation and subsequent scar reduce vision, corneal function is best served by its reduced immunologic responsiveness, also known as immune deviation. Necrotizing inflammation presupposes infection beneath the surface epithelium, and follows chemokine synthesis by infected corneal stromal fibroblasts. In contrast to the cornea, the conjunctiva is well endowed with blood and lymphatic channels, lymphoid cells, and Langerhans cells, and demonstrates classical delayed hypersensitivity responses. The immunology of the interior eye is less well established, but immune deviation appears to extend beyond the cornea to the aqueous and vitreous humors and to the central retina.

Ocular Disease Caused by RNA Viruses

Conjunctivitis is probably the most common viral ocular syndrome, and typically accompanies upper respiratory infections due to RNA viruses (**Table 1**). Rhinovirus, influenzavirus, respiratory syncytial virus, and parainfluenzavirus conjunctivitis typically are mild and self-limited, and most patients do not seek medical attention. More serious are the keratitis, uveitis, and retinitis caused by some RNA viruses. For example, influenzavirus infection of the respiratory tract, usually associated with a mild and short-lived conjunctivitis, less commonly causes inflammation in the lacrimal gland, cornea, iris, retina, optic and other cranial nerves.

Like influenzavirus, other RNA viruses can infect virtually every ocular tissue. For instance, rubella virus when acquired *in utero* may have devastating consequences for the eye. Characteristic features include microphthalmos, corneal haze, cataracts, iris hypoplasia, iridocyclitis, glaucoma, and 'salt-and-pepper' pigmentary retinopathy. Rubella virus can be cultured from the lens of infected neonates at the time of cataract extraction. Congenital ocular abnormalities due to rubella, like those in other organ systems, are much worse when maternal infection ensues earliest in pregnancy.

In contrast to rubella virus, measles (rubeola) virus infection *in utero* rarely causes significant ocular disease. The classic triad of postnatally acquired measles – cough, coryza, and follicular conjunctivitis – can be accompanied by Koplik spots on the conjunctiva and a mild epithelial keratitis. Less common are optic neuritis, retinal vascular occlusion, and pigmentary retinopathy. Measles keratopathy, a major source of blindness in the nonindustrialized world, typically presents as corneal ulceration in a malnourished child. A rare and fatal complication of measles virus infection, subacute sclerosing panencephalitis (SSPE), occurs in about 1 per 100 000 cases, and often years after clinically apparent measles. Along with devastating central nervous system damage, ocular abnormalities occur commonly in SSPE, including central retinal (macular) hyperpigmentation and inflammation, optic nerve atrophy, peripheral retinitis, and ocular motility disorders. Cortical blindness can occur in the absence of ocular involvement.

The most common ocular complication of mumps virus infection is dacryoadenitis, and this may occur concurrently with parotid gland involvement. Aseptic meningitis, associated oculomotor palsy, and optic neuritis also occurs. Follicular conjunctivitis, epithelial and stromal keratitis, iritis, trabeculitis, and scleritis have all been reported within the first 2 weeks after onset of parotitis.

Acute hemorrhagic conjunctivitis (AHC), caused predominantly by enterovirus type 70 and coxsackievirus A24 variant, but also by adenovirus type 11, is one of the most dramatic ocular viral syndromes. Sudden onset of follicular conjunctivitis associated with multiple petechial conjunctival hemorrhages characterizes AHC. The hemorrhages may become confluent and appear post-traumatic. In approximately 1 out of every 10 000 cases due to enterovirus type 70, a polio-like paralysis can ensue. Neurologic deficits are permanent in up to one-third of the affected individuals.

Human immunodeficiency virus (HIV) is the etiologic agent of the acquired immune deficiency syndrome (AIDS). Although HIV can be cultured from the retinas of individuals with AIDS, and has been shown to be present in the donated corneas of deceased AIDS patients, a direct relationship between local viral infection and ocular disease remains to be established. One example is the dry eye so common in AIDS patients. It is not known whether primary HIV infection of the lacrimal gland, immune deficit-induced potentiation of another virus such as Epstein–Barr virus within the lacrimal gland, or a putative HIV-induced neuro-immune-endocrine defect can account for AIDS-related dry eye. However, the severe immunosuppression of AIDS results in a host of other ocular diseases (discussed below).

Ocular Disease Caused by DNA Viruses

DNA viruses (**Table 2**) are responsible for most significant ocular viral infections in the industrialized world. Even the protean ocular manifestations of the HIV, an RNA virus, result largely from reduced immunity to DNA viruses.

Adenovirus is probably the most common DNA virus to cause eye disease. Three common ocular syndromes have been identified. Simple follicular conjunctivitis occurs with infection by many adenovirus types and may be subclinical. Pharyngoconjunctival fever typically follows infection with adenovirus types 3, 4, and 7. As the name implies, patients have pharyngitis, conjunctivitis, and fever, and may be misdiagnosed as having influenza. Epidemic keratoconjunctivitis, most often caused by adenovirus types 8, 19, and 37, is a highly contagious syndrome with significant morbidity. The conjunctivitis can be severe (**Figure 3**); associated inflammatory conjunctival membranes can permanently scar the eyelids to the globe.

Table 1   Ocular targets of human RNA viruses

Virus	Family	Subfamily/genus	Nuc. acid	Env.	Ocular target
Rift Valley fever virus	*Bunyaviridae*	*Phlebovirus*	ss (−)	+	Conjunctiva Retina
Human coronavirus	*Coronaviridae*	*Coronavirus*	ss (+)	+	Conjunctiva
Dengue virus	*Flaviviridae*	*Flavivirus*	ss (+)	+	Conjunctiva
Hepatitis C virus	*Flaviviridae*	*Hepatitis C virus*	ss (+)	+	Cornea Lacrimal Glands Retina
West Nile virus	*Flaviviridae*	*Flavivirus*	ss (+)	+	Retina Uvea Optic nerve Cranial nerves
Yellow fever virus	*Flaviviridae*	*Flavivirus*	ss (+)	+	Conjunctiva
Influenzavirus	*Orthomyxoviridae*	*Influenzavirus* (A, B, C)	ss (−)	+	Lacrimal gland Conjunctiva Episclera Cornea Uvea Retina Optic nerve Cranial nerves
Measles (rubeola) virus	*Paramyxoviridae*	*Morbillivirus*	ss (−)	+	Conjunctiva Cornea Uvea Retina Optic nerve Cranial nerves
Mumps virus	*Paramyxoviridae*	*Paramyxovirus*	ss (−)	+	Lacrimal gland Conjunctiva Sclera Cornea Trabecular meshwork Uvea Optic nerve Cranial nerves
Newcastle disease virus	*Paramyxoviridae*	*Paramyxovirus*	ss (−)	+	Conjunctiva Cornea
Parainfluenza virus(es)	*Paramyxoviridae*	*Paramyxovirus*	ss (−)	+	Conjunctiva
Respiratory syncitial virus	*Paramyxoviridae*	*Pneumovirus*	ss (−)	+	Conjunctiva
Enterovirus(es): (includes poliovirus, coxsackievirus, echovirus, enterovirus)	*Picornaviridae*	*Enterovirus*	ss (+)	−	Conjunctiva Cornea Cranial nerves
Rhinovirus	*Picornaviridae*	*Rhinovirus*	ss (+)	−	Conjunctiva
Colorado tick fever virus	*Reoviridae*	*Coltivirus*	ds (+/−)	−	(?: reported to cause photophobia, retro-ocular pain)
Human T-cell lymphotropic virus-1	*Retroviridae*	*Deltaretrovirus*	ss (+)	+	Cornea Uvea
Human immunodeficiency virus	*Retroviridae*	*Lentivirus*	ss (+)	+	Lacrimal gland Retina
Rabies virus	*Rhabdoviridae*	*Lyssavirus*	ss (−)	+	(Transmission via corneal button)
Rubella virus	*Togaviridae*	*Rubivirus*	ss (+)	+	Cornea Uvea Lens Trabecular meshwork Retina Globe

+, Enveloped; −, nonenveloped; ss, single stranded; ds, double stranded; (+), positive-sense RNA genome; (−), negative-sense RNA genome.

Table 2   Ocular targets of human DNA viruses

Virus	Family	Subfamily/genus	Nuc. acid	Env.	Ocular target
Adenovirus	*Adenoviridae*	*Mastadenovirus*	ds	−	Conjunctiva Cornea
Herpes simplex virus, type 1 (HHV1)	*Herpesviridae*	*Alphaherpesvirinae/Simplexvirus*	ds	+	Eyelid Conjunctiva Cornea Trabecular meshwork Uvea Retina
Herpes simplex virus, type 2 (HHV2)	*Herpesviridae*	*Alphaherpesvirinae/Simplexvirus*	ds	+	Eyelid Conjunctiva Cornea Trabecular meshwork Uvea Retina
Varicella zoster virus (HHV3)	*Herpesviridae*	*Alphaherpesvirinae/Varicellovirus*	ds	+	Eyelid Conjunctiva Cornea Trabecular meshwork Uvea Retina Optic nerve
Epstein–Barr virus (HHV4)	*Herpesviridae*	*Gammaherpesvirinae/* *Lymphocryptovirus*	ds	+	Lacrimal gland Conjunctiva Cornea Uvea Retina Optic nerve
Human cytomegalovirus (HHV5)	*Herpesviridae*	*Betaherpesvirinae/Cytomegalovirus*	ds	+	Retina Optic nerve
Human herpes virus 6 (HHV6)	*Herpesviridae*	*Betaherpesvirinae/Roseolovirus*	ds	+	Retina
Human herpes virus 8 (HHV8)	*Herpesviridae*	*Gammaherpesvirinae*	ds	+	Conjunctiva (Kaposi sarcoma)
Human papillomavirus	*Papovaviridae*	*Papillomavirus*	ds	−	Eyelid Conjunctiva Cornea
Molluscum contagiosum virus	*Poxviridae*	*Molluscipoxvirus*	ds	+	Eyelid Conjunctiva Cornea
Orf virus	*Poxviridae*	*Parapoxvirus*	ds	+	Eyelid
Smallpox (variola) virus	*Poxviridae*	*Orthopoxvirus*	ds	+	Eyelid Conjunctiva Cornea Uvea Optic nerve
Vaccinia virus	*Poxviridae*	*Orthopoxvirus*	ds	+	Eyelid Conjunctiva Cornea

ds, Double stranded; +, enveloped; −, nonenveloped; HHV, human herpes virus.

Corneal involvement begins as a punctate epithelial keratitis and may proceed to a large central epithelial ulcer. Stromal keratitis presents about 2 weeks after the conjunctivitis as multifocal subepithelial corneal infiltrates, and causes both foreign body sensation and reduced vision. The stromal infiltrates may resolve spontaneously, but can become chronic, require long-term treatment with corticosteroids, and cause persistent visual morbidity. A fourth ocular syndrome occasionally associated with adenovirus infection, AHC (discussed above), may be caused by adenovirus type 11. Interestingly, adenovirus type 11 also causes acute hemorrhagic cystis. Follicular conjunctivitis (clinically indistinguishable from adenovirus conjunctivitis) can also be caused by Newcastle disease virus, an RNA virus that gives rise to fatal epidemics in poultry and infects the birds' human handlers.

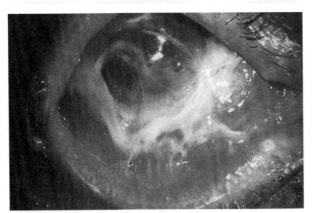

Figure 3 Epidemic keratoconjunctivitis. Infection with adenovirus serotype 19 has resulted in severe ocular surface inflammation.

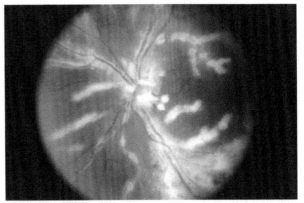

Figure 4 Cytomegalovirus retinitis. Discrete areas of perivascular necrosis and hemorrhage are typical.

The human herpes viruses are preeminent among DNA viruses in eye disease with at least seven of the eight known human herpes viruses associated with ocular disorders. Herpes simplex virus type 1 (HSV-1) is the most common herpes virus to cause eye disease, and herpes simplex keratitis is the most common cause of infectious blindness in the industrialized world. HSV-1 causes self-limited and relatively benign infections of the eyelids, the conjunctiva, and the corneal epithelium, but infections of the corneal stroma, uvea, and retina may result in chronic or recurrent blinding stromal keratitis, uveitis, and retinal necrosis, respectively. Elevation of intraocular pressure due to involvement of the trabecular meshwork is not uncommon and may help to differentiate herpetic uveitis from noninfectious causes. Postnatally acquired HSV-2 ocular infection, less common than HSV-1, causes disease similar in most respects to HSV-1. Neonatal herpes simplex infection, acquired during transit through the birth canal and usually due to HSV-2, commonly causes vesicular blepharitis and conjunctivitis, but can also cause permanent visual loss due to keratitis, chorioretinitis, optic neuritis, and encephalitis of the visual cortex.

Varicella zoster virus, the etiologic agent of chickenpox and shingles, rarely causes keratouveitis with primary infection (chickenpox). However, vision-threatening keratitis, uveitis, and, less commonly, retinal necrosis are complications of varicella zoster virus reactivation in the distribution of the fifth cranial nerve (zoster ophthalmicus). Lid ulceration with frank tissue loss or lid malposition leads to corneal exposure and ulceration. Optic neuritis and cranial nerve paresis can accompany onset of the zoster rash. Sectoral iris atrophy is pathognomonic for zoster ophthalmicus. Postinfectious corneal anesthesia and secondary sterile corneal ulceration may follow herpes simplex types 1 and 2, but are most severe in zoster ophthalmicus. Chronic scleritis, keratitis, uveitis, and glaucoma may ultimately limit the visual acuity.

Acute systemic infection with Epstein–Barr virus may cause conjunctivitis and epithelial keratitis. Stromal keratitis occurs but is difficult to differentiate clinically from herpes simplex keratitis, and the true incidence of Epstein–Barr viral keratitis is unknown. Reports of uveitis and retinochoroiditis are unconfirmed. Delayed-onset optic neuritis following infectious mononucleosis is not uncommon.

Human cytomegalovirus (CMV) typically causes infectious retinitis (**Figure 4**) in immunocompromised patients with $CD4^+$ T-cell counts of less than $50\,cells\,ml^{-1}$. Although not the most common ocular complication of AIDS, CMV retinitis is the most common cause of blindness in AIDS patients. CMV retinitis in AIDS patients can be controlled but not cured. In contrast, congenital CMV infection in an otherwise normal fetus results in various degrees of retinochoroiditis, but is not progressive postnatally.

Human papillomavirus (HPV) causes a range of conjunctival tumors ranging from venereally acquired benign papillomas (HPV types 6 and 11) to invasive squamous cell carcinoma (**Figure 2**) (HPV types 16 and 18). Venereal papillomas are clinically similar to those of the larynx and anogenital tract. Ocular surface squamous neoplasia (conjunctival intraepithelial neoplasia and invasive squamous cell carcinoma) are most similar to dysplastic intraepithelial and invasive squamous lesions of the uterine cervix. Papillomatous eyelid neoplasms due to HPV also occur, and can be benign or malignant.

Molluscum contagiosum virus is a poxvirus that may infect the eyelid skin or less commonly the conjunctiva. Skin lesions typically appear as elevated nodules with umbilicated centers, and may be multiple and quite large in HIV-infected patients. Molluscum lesions of the eyelid are fairly common in children, and can be associated with a follicular conjunctivitis that resolves with incisional or excisional biopsy of the lid lesion.

Prior to eradication, smallpox virus infection was associated with pustular blepharoconjunctivitis, secondary lid scarring, and stromal keratitis. In nonindustrialized nations, secondary bacterial infection of smallpox keratitis was a major source of blindness. Vaccination against smallpox virus with vaccinia virus was occasionally complicated by inadvertent autoinoculation of vaccinia into the eye, with potential for a severe blepharoconjunctivitis, keratitis, and globe perforation.

Ocular Complications of AIDS

Tay-Kearney and Jabs (1996) classified the ocular complications of HIV infection into five broad categories: (1) HIV retinopathy, (2) opportunistic ocular infections, (3) ocular adnexal neoplasms, (4) neuro-ophthalmic lesions, and (5) drug-induced manifestations.

HIV retinopathy is seen in over half of AIDS patients; cotton wool patches, or multifocal infarcts of the retinal nerve fiber layer, are the most common ocular sign of AIDS. Intraretinal hemorrhages occur less often. HIV can be cultured from the retina of AIDS patients, but a direct relationship between retinal infection and AIDS retinopathy has not been established.

Some ocular infections, including CMV retinitis (**Figure 4**), *Pneumocystis carinii*, fungal, and mycobacterial choroiditis, and microsporidial keratoconjunctivitis are seen almost exclusively in AIDS. CMV retinitis is a major cause of morbidity in AIDS patients. Other infections, such as toxoplasmosis retinochoroiditis, ocular syphilis, herpes zoster ophthalmicus, and molluscum contagiosum of the eyelids are seen in immunocompetent as well as immunosuppressed individuals, but may be more severe and leave more profound deficits in HIV-infected patients. Herpes zoster ophthalmicus in young patients may be the first clinical clue to HIV infection. Acute retinal necrosis due to herpes simplex virus types 1 or 2, or varicella zoster virus, occurs more commonly in HIV-infected than in otherwise normal patients and can result in unilateral or bilateral blindness despite antiviral therapy.

Kaposi sarcoma of the eyelids or conjunctiva, associated with human herpes virus 8 infection, is exceedingly uncommon in immunocompetent individuals, but is probably the most common adnexal tumor in AIDS patients. Non-Hodgkin's lymphomas of the orbit, although rare overall, occur more frequently in AIDS patients than in the general population. Recently, squamous cell carcinoma of the ocular surface (conjunctiva and cornea) has been suggested as a marker for AIDS, but whether HIV infection potentiates HPV-induced carcinogenesis in the eye remains speculative.

Neuro-ophthalmic lesions in AIDS may occur directly due to HIV infection of the central nervous system, but most commonly are caused by cryptococcal meningitis or other opportunistic infections. Retinitis and uveitis due to anti-HIV medications can be confused with opportunistic intraocular infections.

Conclusion

Diverse ocular tissues act in concert to create vision. All of the tissues and structures within the eye are susceptible to viral infection, with consequences ranging from mild discomfort to severe pain and blindness, and almost all known human viruses cause ocular disease. Often, the same virus can infect widely disparate tissues within an eye. Classical viral pathogenic mechanisms are readily demonstrated in the eye, but the fine functions of ocular tissues within the visual axis (cornea, anterior chamber, lens, vitreous, and macula) compel altered immune responsiveness. The eye is uniquely affected by viral infection and provides an exceptional model for studies of viral pathogenesis and immunity.

Acknowledgments

This work is supported by US Public Health Service grants, R01 EY13124 and P30 EY12190, and a Physician-Scientist Merit Award (to J. Chodosh) from Research to Prevent Blindness, New York, NY.

Further Reading

Biswas PS and Rouse BT (2005) Early events in HSV keratitis – setting the stage for a blinding disease. *Microbes and Infection* 7: 799–810.

Bonfioli AA and Eller AW (2005) Acute retinal necrosis. *Seminars in Ophthalmology* 20: 155–160.

Brandt CR (2005) The role of viral and host genes in corneal infection with herpes simplex virus type 1. *Experimental Eye Research* 80: 607–621.

Chodosh J and Stroop WG (1998) Introduction to viruses in ocular disease. In: Tasman W and Jaeger EA (eds.) *Duane's Foundations of Clinical Ophthalmology*, pp. 1–10. Philadelphia: Lippincott-Raven.

Cunningham ET, Jr., and Margolis TP (1998) Ocular manifestations of HIV infection. *New England Journal of Medicine* 339: 236–244.

Darrell RW (ed.) (1985) *Viral Diseases of the Eye*. Philadelphia: Lea & Febiger.

Garg S and Jampol LM (2005) Systemic and intraocular manifestations of West Nile virus infection. *Survey of Ophthalmology* 50: 3–13.

Goldberg DE, Smithen LM, Angelilli A,, and Freeman WR (2005) HIV-associated retinopathy in the HAART era. *Retina* 25: 633–649.

Green LK and Pavan-Langston D (2006) Herpes simplex ocular inflammatory disease. *International Ophthalmology Clinics* 46: 27–37.

Liesegang TJ (2004) Herpes zoster virus infection. *Current Opinion in Ophthalmology* 15: 531–536.

Natarajan K, Shepard LA,, and Chodosh J (2002) The use of DNA array technology in studies of ocular viral pathogenesis. *DNA and Cell Biology* 21: 483–490.

Pepose JS, Holland GN, and Wilhelmus KR (eds.) (1995) *Ocular Infection & Immunity*. New York: Mosby.

Streilein JW (1996) Ocular immune privilege and the Faustian dilemma. *Investigative Ophthalmology & Visual Science* 37: 1940–1950.

Tay-Kearney ML and Jabs DA (1996) Ophthalmic complications of HIV infection. *Medical Clinics of North America* 80: 1471–1492.

Zoonoses

J E Osorio and T M Yuill, University of Wisconsin, Madison, WI, USA

Introduction

Zoonoses are diseases transmissible from vertebrate animals, other than humans, to people. Mammals, birds, reptiles, and probably amphibians are reservoirs or amplifier hosts for these viral zoonoses. Frequently, these viruses cause little or no overt disease in their nonhuman vertebrate hosts. Some zoonotic viruses have very limited host ranges; others may infect a wide range of vertebrates. Human infection may vary from unapparent to fatal disease. Both new and old viral zoonoses are especially important in emerging and re-emerging virus diseases. Transmission of zoonotic viruses may occur by a variety of routes. They include: 'direct' (rabies) or 'indirect' (hantavirus) contact; 'nosocomial' (arenavirus and filovirus); 'aerosol transmission' (SARS coronavirus); 'vertical' (*in utero*) (arenaviruses); and 'vector- or arthropod-borne' (yellow fever, YF). Viral zoonotic diseases occur on every continent except, perhaps Antarctica. Some are found around the world, in a variety of ecological settings. Others are found only in very limited ecologic and geographic foci. Although hundreds of viruses are zoonotic, the importance of many of these viruses has not yet been established. Some of the more important viral zoonoses will be discussed briefly.

Rabies Virus

Rabies is one of the oldest reported zoonoses. Rabies virus infection causes nervous system disease that ends in death. Animals can become infected without nervous system disease, develop antibodies, and survive, but play no role in transmission. Classical rabies is found all around the world except in Antarctica, Britain, the Hawaiian Islands, Australia, and New Zealand. Transmission occurs by the bite of an infected animal. Aerosol (droplet) transmission is rare. Dogs and cats are the main reservoirs in tropical developing countries where more than 99% of all human cases occur. In industrialized countries, wild mammals are the main reservoirs and the species involved vary from region to region. The principal species are as follows: in North America, skunks, raccoons, and foxes; in Europe, foxes; and in the Caribbean, mongooses. Bats in all enzootic regions harbor rabies with vampire bats especially important in the Neotropics, where they transmit rabies to cattle, horses, and other domestic animals, and, occasionally, to humans. Rabies virus is classified in the genus *Lyssavirus* of the family *Rhabdoviridae*. Genetic relationships between rabies isolates from different species and geographic areas have been established by genomic sequence analysis (**Table 1**).

Diagnosis is based on characteristic altered behavior of infected mammals, confirmed by either isolation of virus; demonstration of intracellular antigen by immunofluorescence; or of virus genomic sequences. Postexposure treatment is accomplished by thorough washing of the bite wound, administration of hyperimmune serum or globulin, and administration of antirabies vaccine. Dogs and cats in enzootic areas should be vaccinated. Other domestic animals and humans at high risk should also be vaccinated. Vaccination campaigns of free-ranging red fox populations in Europe and raccoons and coyotes in the USA have been carried out by oral administration of recombinant vaccinia-vectored vaccines in bait.

Table 1 Rabies and related lyssaviruses

Virus name	Lyssavirus genotype	Location	Host
Rabies	1	Worldwide	Many wild and domestic mammals
Lagos bat	2	Africa	Bats, water mongoose (but no human disease)
Mokola	3	Africa	Several terrestrial mammals
Duvenhage	4	Africa	Bats
European bat-1	5	Europe	Bats
European bat-2	6	Europe	Bats
Australian bat	7	Australia	Bats
Aravan	New, proposed	Kyrgystan	Bats
Khujand	New, proposed	Tajikistan	Bats
Irkut	New, proposed	Russia	Bats
West Caucasian bat	New, proposed	Russia	Bats

Hantavirus Hemorrhagic Fevers and Pulmonary Syndrome Viruses

Hantaviruses belong to the genus *Hantavirus* of the family *Bunyaviridae*. In the Americas, hantavirus can cause hantavirus pulmonary syndrome (HPS), an infectious disease typically characterized by fever, myalgia, and headache and followed by dyspnea, noncardiogenic pulmonary edema, hypotension, and shock. HPS has also been reported and confirmed in seven countries in South America: Argentina, Bolivia, Brazil, Chile, Paraguay, Uruguay, and Panama (**Table 2**). Hantaviruses are harbored by wild rodents which often live in close association with humans. Virus is shed in urine and other excreta. Outbreaks of HPS have been associated with ecological changes and invasion of human habitations by expanding rodent populations. Diagnosis has been complicated by the lack of efficient and sensitive isolation and serological methods. Rodent control and avoidance of exposure to rodent excreta, especially in dust, are the only methods available currently for prevention of transmission to humans.

Arenavirus Hemorrhagic Fever Viruses

Arenaviruses are transmitted by the same kind of rodents that carry hantaviruses. They can also cause hemorrhagic fevers and, even though the prototype of this family has been long known (lymphocytic choriomeningitis virus, LCMV), viruses within this family are still being discovered. They produce human diseases in the Old World (Lassa fever in Africa) and New World (Junin, Machupo, and, later on, Guanarito and Sabia in South America). There are about 22 different arenaviruses in the Americas, but only four are associated with significant human disease. These pathogenic arenaviruses establish persistent infection in their rodent hosts, and the virus is shed in urine, infecting humans who live in close contact with these contaminated environments. Lassa fever is also transmitted nosocomially in rural hospitals to other people in contact with blood from viremic patients. Control of these diseases is attempted mainly by reduction of rodent populations. A live, attenuated vaccine has been developed for Argentine hemorrhagic fever, and a vaccinia-vectored vaccine has been developed for Lassa fever. Ribavirin is effective for treating arenavirus infection if administered early in the course of infection.

YF Virus

YF is a flavivirus that causes hemorrhagic disease with severe liver damage and death in up to half of the most acute cases. Humans or primates transport the virus from its sylvan cycle in forested areas to rural or urban areas, where other vector mosquitoes transmit it. YF remains a disease of significant public health importance, with an estimated 200 000 cases and 30 000 deaths annually. The disease is endemic in tropical regions of Africa and South America; nearly 90% of YF cases and deaths occur in Africa. It is a significant hazard to unvaccinated travelers to these endemic areas. Re-establishment of the major urban vector, *Aedes aegypti*, the recent spread of the Asian tiger mosquito (*Ae. albopictus*) as well as the rise in air travel has increased the risk of introduction and spread of the disease. YF is an acute infectious disease

Table 2   Hantaviruses that cause human disease

Virus name	Distribution	Rodent host	Human disease
Hantaan	Asia, Europe	*Apodemus agrarius*	Hemorrhagic fever with renal syndrome
Seoul	Worldwide	*Rattus* spp.	Hemorrhagic fever with renal syndrome
Dobrava-Belgrade	Europe, Middle East	*Apodemus flavicollis*	Hemorrhagic fever with renal syndrome
Puumala	Europe, Asia	*Clethrionomys glareolus*	Hemorrhagic fever with renal syndrome
Sin Nombre	North America	*Peromyscus maniculatus*	Pulmonary syndrome
New York	North America	*Peromyscus leucopus*	Pulmonary syndrome
Bayou	North America	*Oryzomys palustris*	Pulmonary syndrome
Black Creek Canal	North America	*Sigmodon hispidus*	Pulmonary syndrome
Andes	South America	*Oligoryzomys longicaudatus*	Pulmonary syndrome
Hu39694	South America	Unknown	Pulmonary syndrome
Juquitiba	South America	Unknown	Pulmonary syndrome
Laguna Negra	South America	*Calomys laucha*	Pulmonary syndrome
Lechiguanas	South America	*Calomys laucha*	Pulmonary sybdrome
Oran	South America	*Oligoryzomys longicaudatus*	Pulmonary syndrome
Choclo	Panama	*Zygodontomys brevicauda*	Pulmonary syndrome
Monogahela	North America	*Peromyscus maniculatus nubiterrae*	Pulmonary syndrome
Bermejo	South America	*Oligoryzomys chacoensis*	Pulmonary syndrome
Central Plata	South America	*Oligoryzomys flavescens*	Pulmonary syndrome
Araraquara	South America	*Bolomys lasiurus*	Pulmonary syndrome

characterized by sudden onset with a two-phase development, separated by a short period of remission. The clinical spectrum of YF varies from very mild, nonspecific, febrile illness to a fulminating, sometimes fatal disease with pathognomic features. In severe cases, jaundice, bleeding diathesis, with hepatorenal involvement is common. There is no specific treatment for YF, making the management of YF patients extremely problematic. YF can be diagnosed by virus isolation, detection of circulating antigens, demonstration of a significant rise in specific YF virus antibodies, and microscopic detection of viral inclusion bodies or antigen in tissues taken at postmortem examination. Insecticide spraying and elimination of breeding sites in homes can be used for vector control in epidemic situations. Disease can be prevented in humans by vaccination.

West Nile Virus

West Nile virus (WNV) is an arthropod-borne RNA flavivirus that causes a mild infection to acute febrile disease with rash, and occasional encephalitis (mainly in the elderly) is produced in humans. The virus is widely spread, occurring from India and Pakistan westward through the Middle East and into Africa, and northward into Europe, the republics of the former USSR, and in the Western Hemisphere. WNV first appeared in North America in 1999 with an outbreak in New York City producing high mortality in crows and other birds. Subsequently, the virus has spread rapidly throughout North America, the Caribbean, Mexico, and into South America. WNV is now present in every state except Hawaii, and Alaska. It is believed that the NY99 virus has remained stable and unchanged. The ecology of WNV involves maintenance in a bird–mosquito–bird cycle and occasional infection of humans and horses. *Culex* spp. are the main vectors, and birds are the vertebrate hosts. There is no vaccine currently available for humans, although there is one for equine animals.

Chikungunya Virus

Chikungunya (CHIK) is an alphavirus of the family *Togaviridae* that has been responsible for acute febrile disease with rash and severe arthralgia in people in Africa and Asia. An outbreak of CHIK was reported on Reunion Island in March 2005 that resulted in >3500 confirmed cases and an estimated 250 000 suspected cases, affecting >25% of the island's inhabitants. CHIK virus is maintained in sylvan or savanna cycles involving wild primates and arboreal *Aedes* mosquitoes. In both Africa and Asia, the virus also has an urban cycle involving humans and *Ae. aegypti* mosquitoes that is more important from a public health standpoint.

Sindbis Virus

Sindbis (SIN) virus is one of the most widely distributed arthropod-borne viruses in the world, being found in Africa, Europe, Asia, and Australia. Disease in humans is usually mild, and is characterized by acute fever, with arthralgia, myalgia, and rash. There are periodic epidemics in Finland, where it is termed Podosta disease. SIN virus is maintained in wild bird populations, with transmission by *Culex* spp. mosquitoes. In Africa and the Middle East, SIN is often found in the same ecosystems where WN virus is being transmitted. The virus is an alphavirus of the *Togaviridae*. Phylogenetic analysis indicates that there is one major genetic cluster of western SIN virus strains in Africa and another in Australia and Asia. There is evidence of some geographic mixing of western strains of SIN virus that suggest long-distance transport via migrating birds. There is no vaccine available. Since many of the mosquito vectors breed in extensive rice fields, large-scale control would be expensive.

Crimean-Congo Hemorrhagic Fever Virus

Crimean-Congo hemorrhagic fever (CCHF) virus is very widely distributed, and is found from eastern Europe and the Crimean, eastward through the Middle East to western China, and southward through Africa to South Africa. CCHF is characterized by severe hemorrhagic fever with hepatitis, with case mortality of 10–50%. Maintenance of CCHF virus involves horizontal transmission from *Hyalomma* ticks to mammals, and vertical transmission in ticks through the eggs. *Hyalomma* ticks have also been found on birds migrating between Europe and Africa – a mechanism for long-distance dispersal of the virus. Human CCHF cases have occurred in workers handling livestock and their products in Saudi Arabia and the United Arab Emirates which have been attributed to importation of infected cattle and their ticks from Somalia and the Sudan. There are no vaccine or tick control measures available. CCHF virus belongs to the genus *Nairovirus* of the *Bunyaviridae*. Genetic analysis indicates that reassortment and recombination occur in nature.

Sandfly Fever Viruses

Sandfly fever (Sicilian, Naples, and Toscana) viruses are endemic in the Mediterranean area. They cause acute febrile disease in humans, with occasional aseptic meningitis. In central Italy, Toscana virus (TOSV) caused one-third of previously undiagnosed cases of aseptic meningitis. There are at least two genetic lineages of TOSV – Spanish and Italian. The viruses are members of the genus *Phlebovirus* of the *Bunyaviridae*. They are transovarially and horizontally transmitted by phlebotomine sandflies. Wild mammals are presumed reservoirs.

Viruses Occurring in the Americas

Encephalitis Viruses

Venezuelan equine encephalitis (VEE) viruses are made up of a closely related complex of subtypes with several varieties, which have differing epidemiology, geographic distributions, and disease importance. The epizootic/epidemic (VEE, IAB, and IC) virus variants are of greatest concern. In equine animals, the virus causes acute encephalitis, and case fatality may approach 80%. Survivors may have serious neurological deficits. Although the case–fatality rate in humans is low (less than 1%), the large numbers of acutely infected people that occur during an epidemic may completely overwhelm the local healthcare system. VEE, IAB, and IC viruses are maintained in northern South America, where they have periodically swept through Venezuela and Colombia in epidemic waves, with occasional extensions into Ecuador and massively through Central America into Mexico and South Texas. Epidemic spread depends on the availability of susceptible equine populations (the amplifying host) and abundant mosquito vectors of several species. The interepidemic maintenance systems remain undefined. There is evidence that the epizootic strains may arise by mutation of subtype ID enzootic virus. The enzootic strains are maintained in limited foci involving rodents and *Culex* (*Melanconion*) spp. mosquitoes from Florida to Argentina. With the exception of subtype IE, which has caused epizootics in horses in Mexico, these enzootic virus strains do not cause disease in equine animals, but can cause acute febrile illness in humans. The VEE complex viruses are in the genus *Alphavirus* of the *Togaviridae*. There is an effective live, attenuated vaccine for both human and equine use. Because the maintenance of equine herd immunity is costly, most animal health agencies do not carry out ongoing, intensive vaccination campaigns. Thus, the risk of reoccurrence of explosive outbreaks remains.

Eastern (EEE) and western (WEE) equine encephalitis viruses occur in epidemic form in North America, but have also been found in Central and South America. Generally, EEE is maintained in eastern North America but has caused scattered epizootics and cases in the Caribbean, and in Central and South America. EEE virus can be divided into a North American-Caribbean clade, an Amazon Basin clade, and a Trinidad, Venezuela, Guyana, Ecuador, and Argentina clade. During the past several years, there have been modest increases in several US states in the number of reported human cases of EEE. In North America, WEE occurs in western and prairie states and provinces and along the west coast. WEE has caused sporadic cases of encephalitis in equine animals, but not humans, in

Argentina and Uruguay. Both involve wild birds and mosquito vectors, with spillover into equine population and humans, causing clinical encephalitis and death. Central nervous sequelae may occur among survivors. Effective vaccines are available commercially for equine animals, and experimental vaccines are used for laboratory personnel. Effective mosquito abatement to control vector populations has been carried out in the West for many years. Insecticide application is used for vector control in epidemic situations.

St. Louis encephalitis (SLE) virus occurs from Canada to Argentina and causes sporadic but extensive epidemics in the USA, with most epidemics occurring in the West, down the Ohio and Mississippi valleys into Texas, and in Florida. Wild passerine birds are amplifying hosts in North America, but in the Southeastern USA and the Neotropics mammals may play an epidemiologic role in virus maintenance and transmission. SLE virus is transmitted by *Culex* spp. mosquitoes in the USA. SLE virus is a flavivirus of the *Togaviridae*, and is closely related to Japanese encephalitis virus. In humans, SLE is characterized by febrile disease, with subsequent encephalitis or aseptic meningitis, and strikes older people more often than the young. Since no vaccine is available, SLE prevention and control relies on surveillance, vector control, and screening of dwelling windows and doors.

Powassan (POW) virus is a North American member of the flavivirus tick-borne encephalitis (TBE) complex. Although POW virus is widely distributed across the USA and Canada, and westward into far eastern Russia, disease (febrile, with encephalitis) has only been detected in the eastern states and provinces of North America. The transmission cycle involves small mammals and *Ixodes* ticks.

La Crosse (LAC) and other California serogroup encephalides are human pathogens in North America. Prior to the arrival of WNV, LACV was the most important cause of endemic arboviral encephalitis in the US, causing an estimated average of 80 cases per year, affecting mainly preschool-aged children. It is endemic in the Upper Midwest, but occasional cases occur elsewhere. Although fatality is uncommon, the disease is severe enough to cause prolonged hospitalization. LAC virus is maintained transovarially in treehole breeding by *Ochlerotatus* (formerly *Aedes*) *triseriatus* mosquitoes with horizontal transmission to small forest mammal reservoirs and to humans. The other California group viruses affecting people have similar epidemiologies, but do not cause disease as commonly. California encephalitis virus was isolated in California, and has occasionally caused human disease there. Snowshoe hare (SSH) virus occurs in the Northern USA and across Canada, and has caused human encephalitis in the eastern provinces. Jamestown Canyon (JC) virus is widely distributed across the USA, and has been shown to cause human disease, mainly in adults in the Midwest, and to infect deer. Like LAC virus, these other viruses have the same close epidemiological relationship with their *Ochlerotatus* vectors. These viruses are members of the California serogroup of the genus *Bunyavirus* of the family *Bunyaviridae*. SSH virus is an antigenic variant of LAC virus.

Colorado Tick Fever Virus

Colorado tick fever (CTF) is endemic in sagebrush–pine–juniper habitats of the higher elevations (over 1200 m) in the mountains of the western states and provinces of North America. Although seldom fatal, CTF can cause serious disease in humans (fever, chills, headache, retro-orbital pain, photophobia, myalgia, abdominal pain, and generalized malaise) with prolonged convalescence. CTF may present as hemorrhagic or central nervous system disease, and is most severe in preadolescent children. Males are infected over twice as frequently as are females. The virus is transmitted by and overwinters in *Dermacentor andersoni*. Wild rodents are the vertebrate hosts, and develop a prolonged viremia. CTF virus is classified in the genus *Coltivirus* of the family *Reoviridae* and is serologically related to Eyach virus from Germany. Avoidance of tick bites is the main preventive measure available, but control of rodents and the ticks that inhabit their burrows can be applied in foci of virus maintenance in the field.

Vesicular Stomatitis Virus

Vesicular stomatitis (VS) virus is endemic in Central and northern South America and in the southeastern USA, causing an acute, febrile vesicular disease in cattle, horses, and pigs. Sporadic VS epidemics occur in the southwestern states of the USA. Both of the major serotypes, VS-Indiana and VS-New Jersey, cause influenza-like illness in humans and are an occupational hazard to people handling cattle. The VS viruses comprise a complex of related serotypes and subtypes in the Americas, with related vesiculoviruses (family *Rhabdoviridae*) in Africa and Asia. Many of these viruses are transmitted horizontally and transovarially by phlebotomine sandflies, with evidence for infection of wild rodents and other small mammals. However, the role of these mammals in the epidemiology of VS viruses is unclear because they do not develop viremia. Grasshoppers have been shown to be susceptible experimentally, but their role as reservoirs or amplifiers in nature remains to be established.

Other Neotropical Viruses

Oropouche virus, a Simbu serogroup bunyavirus, causes epidemics, occasionally severe, or acute febrile disease with arthralgia and occasional aseptic meningitis in humans in the Brazilian and Peruvian Amazon as well as Surinam and Panama. During rainy season epidemics, the virus is transmitted by *Culicoides paraensis* biting midges. Enzootic maintenance cycles are believed to involve forest mammals and arboreal mosquitoes.

Mayaro (MAY) virus occurs epidemically in the Brazilian and Bolivian Amazon Basin, and has also been associated with human febrile disease in Surinam and Trinidad. In humans, the acute, nonfatal, febrile disease with rash is clinically similar to CHIK, an alphavirus to which it is antigenically and taxonomically related. MAY virus appears to be maintained in nature in a cycle similar to that of YF, with arboreal mosquito vectors and primate hosts, but also involving other mammals and birds.

Una virus is a close relative of MAY virus and causes human febrile disease also, but its natural history is not known. Una virus has been isolated from several mosquito species, and has been found at scattered sites from northern South America to Argentina. Antibodies have been found in humans, horses, and birds. Genetic analysis suggests that Una virus is maintained in discrete foci.

Rocio virus was first isolated from fatal human encephalitis cases during an explosive outbreak of acute febrile disease in coastal Sao Paulo State, Brazil in 1975, after which sporadic outbreaks have continued. This virus is an ungrouped flavivirus in the *Togaviridae* and is serologically related to Murray Valley encephalitis virus from Australia. The epidemiology is unclear but probably involves wild birds, and several mosquito species are suspected vectors.

Cowpox-Like Viruses

Cantagalo and related viruses are orthopoxviruses newly reported in Brazil. They can cause vesiculopustular lesions on the hands, arms, forearms, and face of dairy milkers. Virus particles can be detected by either direct electron microscopy (DEM) in vesicular fluids and scab specimens or isolated in cell culture and embryonated chicken eggs. The epidemiological significance of these new vaccinia viral strains and their origins remains unknown.

Viruses Occurring in Europe

Tahyna (TAH) virus is widely distributed in Europe and has been reported in Africa. TAH virus produces an influenza-like febrile disease, with occasional central nervous system involvement. The virus is a bunyavirus of the California serogroup, in the *Bunyaviridae*. Like LAC virus, small forest mammals are TAH virus reservoirs, and the virus is horizontally and transovarially transmitted by *Ochlerotatus* mosquitoes. There are no effective control measures.

Omsk hemorrhagic fever occurs in a localized area of western Siberia. Disease can be severe, with up to 3% case fatality, and sequelae are common. This virus is a member of the TBE complex of the flaviviruses. The virus is epizootic in wild muskrats, which had been introduced into the area, and is associated with ixodid ticks. Muskrat handlers are at highest risk of infection. Water voles and other rodents are also vertebrate hosts of the virus. TBE virus vaccine is used in high-risk individuals to provide protection.

TBE virus is also a member of the TBE complex of flaviviruses. TBE virus has been classified into three subtypes: European, far eastern, and Siberian. Because recreation in wooded areas has increased in recent years, TBE has become the most frequent arthropod-borne disease in Europe. The virus occurs in deciduous forests in Western Europe from the Mediterranean countries, westward to France, northward to the Scandinavian countries, and eastward to Siberia. It is maintained in a transmission cycle involving small mammals and *Ixodes* spp. ticks. Human infection also occurs through the consumption of unpasteurized milk from infected cows and goats. Infection can be prevented by an inactivated vaccine and avoidance of tick bites.

Cowpox virus is an orthopoxvirus in the *Poxviridae*. It has a wide host range. Domestic cats are the most important source of human infection, transmitting the virus from wild rodent reservoirs to people. In addition to cattle, this virus has produced severe, generalized infections in a variety of incidental animal hosts in zoos and circuses, including elephants and large cats, which may die. Humans develop typical poxvirus lesions (vesicle and pustule formation), usually on the hands. Laboratory diagnosis (characterization of isolated virus) is required to differentiate cowpox from other nodule-forming zoonotic poxviruses such as orf virus, bovine papular stomatitis virus, and pseudocowpox virus, which are worldwide in distribution.

Viruses Occurring in Africa and the Middle East

Rift Valley Fever Virus

Rift Valley fever virus (RVF) is among the most serious arbovirus infections in Africa today. Repeated RVF epidemics in sub-Saharan Africa cause serious disease in small ruminant animals and humans. RVF disease has expanded its historical geographic range in the livestock-raising areas of eastern and southern Africa and into the Middle East (Saudi Arabia and Yemen) over the past 25 years, causing massive epidemics in Egypt, along the Mauritania–Senegal border and in Madagascar. A major outbreak in East Africa began in 2006 in northeastern Kenya, and spread into southern Somalia and Tanzania. Cattle, sheep, and humans are affected. Abortion storms with febrile disease and bloody diarrhea occur in ruminant animals, and mortality may be heavy in young stock. Most infected humans develop febrile disease, with prolonged convalescence. A few individuals develop more severe disease, with liver necrosis, hemorrhagic pneumonia, meningoencephalitis, and retinitis with vision loss. The human case–fatality rate is less than 1%. RVF virus is in the genus *Phlebovirus* of the *Bunyaviridae*. In sub-Saharan Africa, RVF virus is closely tied to its *Aedes* mosquito vectors. RVF vectors transmit the virus transovarially and horizontally. The virus persists in mosquito eggs laid around seasonally flooded pools and depressions. When these pools flood, the eggs hatch and infected mosquitoes emerge and begin transmission. The vertebrate reservoir hosts of RVF virus are unknown. Field and laboratory workers need to exercise caution to avoid becoming infected by exposure to the virus during postmortem examination of animals or processing materials in the laboratory. Both live, attenuated and inactivated vaccines are available for animals, but the unpredictability of scattered, sporadic RVF outbreaks across sub-Saharan Africa is a major obstacle for implementation of extensive, cost-effective vaccination programs.

Marburg and Ebola Viruses

The reappearance of epidemic Ebola disease in Kikwit, Democratic Republic of the Congo (formerly Zaire) in 1995 and Makokou, Gabon in 1996 again focused international attention on this hemorrhagic disease. Marburg and Ebola viruses have sporadically caused severe hemorrhagic fever in humans. Marburg virus, although of African origin, first appeared in laboratory workers in Germany who had handled cell cultures originating from African primates. Later, epidemics of severe hemorrhagic fever occurred in the Sudan and in Zaire, and Ebola virus was isolated. The first nonlaboratory epidemic of Marburg virus occurred in the Democratic Republic of the Congo from 1998 to 2000. A second, and more severe, outbreak occurred in Uige Province of Angola from 2004 to 2005, when 329 of 374 infected people died (case–fatality rate of 88%). These viruses produce hemorrhagic shock syndrome and visceral organ necrosis, and have the highest case–fatality rate (30–90%) of the hemorrhagic fevers. These viruses, with their bizarre filamentous, pleomorphic morphology, belong to the family *Filoviridae*. They are presumed to be zoonotic, but their hosts in nature and mechanisms of transmission in the field have not been determined. Most of the Makokou, Gabon patients had very recently butchered chimpanzees. A variant of Ebola virus has been isolated from chimpanzees from Côte D'Ivoire, but since wild primates suffer severe disease, they are unlikely to be maintenance reservoirs. Nosocomial transmission of Marburg and Ebola viruses has occurred frequently; a high level of patient isolation and biosafety containment are essential to avoid hospital- and laboratory-acquired infection. Serologic diagnosis is accomplished by means of indirect immunofluorescence or enzyme-linked immunosorbent assay (ELISA) test, with antigen specificity confirmed by western blot. No vaccines or control measures are available.

Monkeypox Virus

Human monkeypox is a severe, smallpox-like illness. Monkeypox belongs to the genus *Orthopoxvirus* of the *Poxviridae*. Monkeypox virus (MPXV) is endemic in rodents in West and Central Africa, with the occurrence of sporadic human cases. The case–fatality rate in humans appears to be higher in Central Africa than in West Africa, raising questions about possible difference in virulence in these two large geographic areas. The largest epidemic of human monkeypox ever documented occurred in the Katako-Kombe area of the Democratic Republic of the Congo (formerly Zaire) in 1996–97, with over 500 people becoming ill and five deaths. Rodent-to-human transmission occurred, as did subsequent secondary human-to-human spread. Vaccinia is protective against infection, but its use has been discontinued with the eradication of smallpox. In 2003, monkeypox emerged for the first time in the Western Hemisphere and caused an outbreak in the United States (Midwestern states) affecting 37 people exposed to ill prairie dogs purchased from pet stores. The virus entered the US upon the importation of exotic rodents from Ghana (West Africa). Recent nucleotide sequence analysis demonstrated the existence of two genetically distinct variants of the virus, called the West African and Congo Basin clades. The strain that caused the US outbreak belonged to the West African clade.

Semliki Forest Virus

Semliki Forest (SF) virus caused an extensive epidemic of human disease in Bangui, Central African Republic, in 1987. SF virus is an alphavirus in the *Togaviridae*. It occurs across East, Central, and West Africa, and has been isolated from various mosquitoes and from wild birds. Antibodies have also been found in wild mammals. The SF virus maintenance cycle probably involves *Ae. africanus* mosquitoes and vervet monkeys.

Orungo Virus

Orungo (ORU) virus caused mild epidemic disease (fever, nausea, headache, and rash) in Nigeria. The virus occurs in a band across Africa from Uganda to Sierra Leone. It is probably mosquito transmitted, but the species that transmit it in nature are not known. Although the vertebrate reservoir hosts are unknown, wild primates have antibody and are suspected to be involved in virus maintenance.

Alkhurma Virus

Alkhurma virus (a variant of Kysanur Forest disease virus, family *Flaviviridae*, genus *Flavivirus*) is an emerging

pathogen responsible for hemorrhagic fever in the Middle East. This virus was isolated from hemorrhagic fever patients in Saudi Arabia in 1995. Transmission can occur from tick bites, handling carcasses of infected animals, or drinking unpasteurized milk. The case–fatality rate is 25%.

Viruses Occurring in Asia

Influenza Viruses

Influenza viruses belong to the family *Orthomyxoviridae*, which consists of five genera: influenza A, influenza B, influenza C, Isavirus, and Thogoto viruses. Influenza A viruses are widely distributed in nature and can infect a wide variety of birds and mammals. Influenza A virus subtypes are classified on the basis of the antigenicity of their surface glycoproteins hemagglutinin (HA) and neuraminidase (NA). To date, 16 HA and 9 NA genes are known to exist. Of these genes, only three HA (H1, H2, and H3) and two NA (N1 and N2) subtypes have circulated in the human population in the twentieth century. During the last 100 years, the most catastrophic impact of influenza was the pandemic of 1918, also known as the Spanish flu (H1N1), which resulted in the loss of more than 500 000 lives in the United States and caused about 40 million deaths worldwide.

The ability of influenza viruses to undergo antigenic changes is the cause of ongoing significant public health concern. New subtypes emerge when human virus captures genes from animal influenza viruses via reassortment; an event that can occur when both virus types simultaneously infect a host (antigenic shift). The threat imposed by influenza virus has been further elevated with the recent introductions of avian influenza viruses into the human population. Avian influenza viruses were initially considered nonpathogenic for humans. However, this perception has changed since 1997, when 18 Hong Kong residents were infected by an avian influenza virus of the H5N1 subtype that resulted in six deaths. Over the next few years, several other cases of direct avian-to-human transmission were reported, including the ongoing outbreak of highly pathogenic H5N1 influenza viruses in several Asian, African, and European countries. Migratory waterfowl – most notably wild ducks – are the natural reservoir of avian influenza viruses, and these birds are also the most resistant to infection. Domestic poultry, including chickens and turkeys, are particularly susceptible to epidemics of rapidly fatal influenza. Direct or indirect contact of domestic flocks with wild migratory waterfowl has been implicated as a frequent cause of epidemics. Live bird markets have also played an important role in the spread of epidemics. Viruses of low pathogenicity can, after circulation for sometimes short periods in a poultry population, mutate into highly pathogenic viruses. Quarantine of infected farms and destruction of infected or potentially exposed flocks are standard control measures aimed at preventing spread to other farms and eventual establishment of the virus in a country's poultry population.

Severe Acute Respiratory Syndrome

In February 2003, a new and previously unknown disease, severe acute respiratory syndrome (SARS), was reported to the World Health Organization (WHO). SARS originated in the province of Guangdong in southern China in November 2002 where it initially was thought to cause atypical pneumonia. However, within a short time the virus spread to Hong Kong, Singapore, Vietnam, Canada, the United States, Taiwan, and several European countries. A novel coronavirus (CoV) was identified as the etiological agent. The SARS-CoV affected more than 8000 individuals worldwide and was responsible for over 700 deaths during the first outbreak in 2002–03. For reasons unknown the SARS virus is less severe and the clinical progression a great deal milder in children younger than 12 years of age. In contrast, the mortality rate was highest among patients >65 years and can exceed 50% for persons at or above the age of 60 years. Farmed masked palm civets (*Paguma larvata*) and two other mammals in live animal markets in China were sources of SARS-CoV human infection. Three species of horseshoe bats (*Rhinolophus* spp.) are probable wildlife reservoirs in China.

Kyasanur Forest Disease

Kyasanur Forest disease (KFD) was first recognized in India in 1957, when an acute hemorrhagic disease appeared in wild monkeys and people frequenting forested areas. KFD has been slowly spreading in India. Human cases have increased from 1999 to 2005, with peak incidence in January and February. The cause of this increase is unknown. KFD virus is a member of the TBE complex of flaviviruses. The basic virus maintenance cycle involves forest mammals (primates, rodents, bats, and insectivores) and ixodid ticks, mainly *Haemaphysalis spinigera*. The virus can be isolated in mice and cell cultures, including tick cells. An inactivated vaccine provides some protection to people at risk of infection.

Japanese Encephalitis Virus

Japanese encephalitis (JE) virus is found in a broad area from far eastern Russia, northeastern Asia through China and Southeast Asia to Papua New Guinea and the Torres Strait Islands of Australia and westward into India. JE virus causes the greatest number of clinical human cases, thousands annually, predominantly in children. It produces encephalitis in humans and horses, and acute febrile disease with abortion in swine, an amplifying host. Herons and egrets are wildlife amplifying hosts. The virus is transmitted by *Culex* spp. mosquitoes. The over-wintering mechanism in temperate Asia is unknown. JE virus is a member of a complex of four related flaviviruses in the family *Flaviviridae*. Prevention of disease is mainly through vaccination of humans, horses, and swine. Insecticides and integrated pest control measures that include natural compounds (*Bacillus thurengiensis* toxins), larvicidal fish, and larval habitat modification have been successfully used in China. Use of pyrethroid-impregnated bed netting can also prevent transmission.

Chandipura

Chandipura virus is ubiquitous across the Indian subcontinent. It is a *Vesiculovirus* in the *Rhabdoviridae*. Chandipura has caused epidemics of febrile diseases, sometimes with encephalopathy. An outbreak occurred in 2004 with a case–fatality rate of 78.3% in children in India (Gujarat State). The virus is transmitted by *Phlebotomus* spp. Sergentomine sandflies and infects a variety of mammals. The virus has also been isolated in West Africa.

Nipah

Nipah virus (NiV) was first recognized in peninsular Malaysia in 1998, where it caused encephalitis and respiratory disease in commercially raised pigs, with transmission to humans in contact with them, with 40–76% case fatality. The virus was found in five species of giant fruit bats (*Pteropus* spp.) there and NiV was isolated from partially eaten fruit. Subsequently, there were five NiV outbreaks recognized in Bangladesh, also associated with *Pteropus* bats. Transmission in Bangladesh was directly from bats, via contaminated fruit and date palm sap.

Viruses Occurring in Australia

Murray Valley Encephalitis Virus and Kunjin Virus

Murray Valley encephalitis (MVE) virus and the closely related Kunjin virus are flaviviruses that cause encephalitis, although Kunjin virus more commonly produces a nonencephalitic illness with polyarthralgia. MVE virus is endemic in avian species and is found in humans in northern Western Australia, the Northern Territory, and Queensland. MVE virus is endemic in northern areas of Western and Northern Australia, and in New Guinea.

Kunjin virus occurs over a much wider area, including most of tropical Australia, Sarawak, Borneo, Papua New Guinea, and Saibai Island in the Torres Strait. There is some evidence that infection with these viruses is increasing in incidence. In northern Australia, MVE cases occur predominantly between February and July, corresponding to the end of the monsoon season, when the mosquito vector (*Culex annulirostris*) proliferates in flooded environments. MVE and Kunjin viruses are flaviviruses, family *Flaviviridae*, of the Japanese encephalitis complex. Kunjin is a subtype of WNV. RNA sequencing indicates that the Australian strains of MVE virus are similar to, but different from Papua New Guinea isolates. No vaccine is available. Control is achieved through application of larvicides.

Ross River Virus

Ross River (RR) virus has caused annual epidemics of febrile disease with polyarthritis and rash with most cases occurring in November through April. It is the most commonly reported arthropod-borne virus disease in Australia. RR virus occurs in all Australian states and territories, but is most commonly found in the northern states and coastal areas. Within the past two decades, RR virus has spread through several Pacific Islands in epidemic form and appears to have become endemic in New Caledonia. Convalescence can be long. RR virus is an alphavirus of the family *Togaviridae*. The enzootic maintenance cycles of RR virus in Australia are not well defined, but wild and domestic mammals appear to be the reservoir hosts, and the principal mosquito vectors are salt marsh *Aedes* spp. and freshwater *Culex* spp. In the Pacific Islands outbreaks, the virus was probably transmitted from person to person by *Aedes* mosquitoes.

Barmah Forest Virus

Barmah Forest virus is the second most common mosquito-borne disease in Australia. It causes subclinical and clinical infections in humans, including fever, myalgia, polyarthralgia, and rash. It is an alphavirus in the *Togaviridae*. The virus appears to be endemic in eastern Australia. It has been isolated from 25 different mosquito species in five genera. *Ochlerotatus vigilax* (previously known as *Aedes vigilax*), is considered a major vector. Its vertebrate hosts have not been established, although marsupials are suspected.

Control

On-going disease surveillance supported by rapid, reliable diagnosis is critical for recognition and control of zoonotic diseases. Serological diagnosis by means of ELISA tests, virus neutralization, and other tests, coupled with detection of the virus itself by virus isolation, immunohistochemistry, immunofluoresence, or PCR techniques are standard laboratory approaches, but are not available in all countries. Timely laboratory results must reach clinicians treating infected individuals and become incorporated into epidemiological databases and early warning systems to assure rapid response by public health authorities to control outbreaks appropriately.

Control of zoonotic virus diseases is accomplished by breaking the cycle of transmission. This is usually achieved by eliminating or immunizing vertebrate hosts, and reducing vector populations. Reduction of reservoir host populations is usually not accomplished because it is too expensive, not environmentally safe, and not technically or logistically feasible. However, there have been some notable exceptions. Bolivian hemorrhagic fever, caused by Machupo virus, was controlled by reduction of its rodent hosts through intensive rodenticiding. The principal vampire bat reservoir of rabies, *Desmodus rotundus*, is being controlled by the application of warfarin-type anticoagulants. Control programs like these have to be continuous to be effective. Their reduction or discontinuation results in host population recovery through reproduction and immigration, which may result in re-emergence of disease sweeping through the increasing, susceptible cohort.

Immunization of hosts is another control approach. Safe and effective rabies vaccines are being used for immunization of humans, domesticated animals, and some wildlife species. The human diploid cell vaccine is extremely effective, free of adverse effects, and widely available but at a cost too high for use in many developing countries. Safe, effective animal vaccines of cell culture origin are on the market. After some initial public resistance, raccoon populations in the eastern USA and wild foxes in Europe are being successfully immunized by means of an oral, vaccinia-vectored recombinant vaccine. This experience illustrates the need for public understanding, in order to counteract fear of dispersal of a genetically engineered virus. However, vaccines will not be developed for many zoonotic viral diseases that affect relatively few people and are of very limited concern geographically.

Vector control is another promising but difficult area of zoonoses reduction or elimination. Insecticide application has become more problematic because both vectors themselves, as well as public opinion, have become more resistant to their use. Integrated pest management techniques, well developed for the control of many crop insects, along with the use of natural pesticides such as *Bacillus thurengiensis* toxin, offers promise for the effective, environmentally safe control of dipterous vectors. Control of tick vectors is likely to remain a problem for some time to come.

Emerging and Re-emerging Zoonoses

Ecological Change

Human disturbance has become a feature of nearly every part of the planet. All too often these disturbances create habitats that favor increases in populations of key hosts and vectors, with subsequent increased transmission of viral zoonoses. Nowhere are ecological changes happening more rapidly and profoundly than in the world's tropics. Conversion of tropical forests to agricultural ecosystems simplifies diverse ecosystems and provides either native or introduced host or vector species the conditions necessary to become more abundant, and sustain intensified virus transmission in areas where people live and work. In Africa, recent YF epidemics have been increasing dramatically in agricultural areas. Some agricultural irrigation development projects have created extensive vector breeding habitats, with an increase in mosquito-transmitted disease. The extensive dams constructed in Senegal were followed by epidemics of RVF, with numerous cases of disease in humans and small ruminant animals. The public health consequences of development projects must never be overlooked.

Global climate change will also bring ecological changes and shifts of human populations that will affect the occurrence of viral zoonoses. There is general consensus that changes in the global climate will happen with unprecedented speed. With those changes will come alterations in the geography of natural and agricultural ecosystems, with corresponding changes in the distribution of zoonotic diseases and the intensity of their transmission. It is clear that El Niño southern oscillation phenomena have increased rainfall, with resulting increases in rodent populations and occurrence of HPS in the Southwestern USA, and increased breeding sites for mosquito vectors of RVF virus in Africa. While it is not possible to predict accurately what the world will be like in 100 years or what zoonotic diseases are likely to be most troublesome, it is certain that things will be different, and constant surveillance will be essential to avoid serious problems or deal promptly and effectively with the ones that arise.

Movement of zoonotic viruses can result from the displacement of infected animals, contaminated animal products, and virus-carrying arthropod vectors. Pets, sport, laboratory, and agricultural animals are moving around the world as never before. Although international and national regulations have been established to prevent movement of infected individuals, it is not possible to test for all possible zoonotic viruses, and prevent them from crossing international boundaries. Moreover, significant numbers of animals of high commercial value move illegally. The importation of highly virulent Newcastle disease (ND) virus has been occasionally linked to smuggled birds.

Zoonotic viruses may be transported by movement of arthropod vectors, too. Just as the YF mosquito, *Ae. aegypti*, moved around the world in water casks aboard sailing vessels, mosquitoes are transported around the world in international commerce. Ships still transport mosquito vectors. The Asian tiger mosquito, *Ae. albopictus*, has become established in the Western Hemisphere after multiple introductions in eggs deposited in used tires. This mosquito is capable of transmitting YF, VEE, JC, and LAC encephalitis viruses. Perhaps of greater concern, modern transport aircraft have been shown to move vector mosquitoes internationally.

Human activity alters animal populations, contact between wild and domestic animals, and human–animal interactions, changing the occurrence of zoonotic diseases and the risk of infection to humans. For example, emergence of new influenza strains is related to the interaction of populations of people, pigs, and aquatic birds.

Social Change

Increasing human populations place great demands on the public health and other government services, especially in developing countries where needs for zoonoses diagnosis, control, and prevention are greatest and resources are most limited. Some preventive measures could be implemented by the people who live in the affected areas themselves, and at minimal costs, if they knew why and how they needed to do it. Public education and information is essential for control and prevention of zoonotic diseases; however, it takes more than civic action to deal with them. Delivery of public education, disease surveillance and diagnosis, and the technical materials and logistical support for control or preventive programs depend on national or international scientific and financial support. International technical cooperation and financial support are imperative.

Summary

Zoonoses are diseases transmissible from animals, other than humans, to people. Both new and old viral zoonoses are important in emerging and re-emerging virus diseases. Some zoonotic viruses occur worldwide, in a variety of ecological settings. Others are found only in limited ecologic and geographic foci. Important worldwide zoonotic viruses include rabies, hantaviruses, arenaviruses, yellow fever virus, chikungunya virus, Sindbis virus, Crimean-Congo hemorrhagic fever virus, and the sandfly fever viruses. In the Americas, common zoonotic viruses include the encephalitis viruses, Colorado tick fever virus, vesicular stomatitis, and others. Zoonotic viruses in Europe include Tahyna virus, the tick-borne encephalitis viruses, and cowpox virus. There are several zoonotic viruses in Africa and the Middle East, including Rift Valley fever virus, Marburg and Ebola filoviruses, monkeypox virus, Semliki Forest virus, Orungo virus, and Alkhurma virus. Zoonotic viruses occurring in Asia include the influenza viruses, SARS coronavirus, Kyasanur Forest virus, Japanese encephalitis virus, Chandipura virus, and Nipah virus. Zoonotic viruses occurring in Australia include Murray Valley encephalitis virus, Kunjin virus, Ross River virus, and Barmah virus. The human and animal health importance of these viruses and their control are discussed. Because rapid ecological change is occurring worldwide, additional zoonotic viruses will emerge.

See also: Bunyaviruses: General Features; Emerging and Reemerging Virus Diseases of Vertebrates; Hantaviruses; Lassa, Junin, Machupo and Guanarito Viruses; Marburg Virus.

Further Reading

Daszek P, Cunningham AA, and Hyatt AD (2000) Emerging infectious diseases of wildlife – Threats to biodiversity and human health. *Science* 287: 443–449.

Gritsun TT, Nuttall PA, and Gould EA (2003) Tick-borne flaviviruses. *Advances in Virus Research* 61: 317–371.

Karesh WB, Cook RA, and Newcomb J (2005) Wildlife trade and global disease emergence. *Emerging Infectious Diseases* 11: 1000–1002.

World Health Organization. *Avian Influenza: Assessing the Pandemic Threat.* Geneva: WHO/CDS/2005.29.

SUBJECT INDEX

Notes

Cross-reference terms in italics are general cross-references, or refer to subentry terms within the main entry (the main entry is not repeated to save space). Readers are also advised to refer to the end of each article for additional cross-references - not all of these cross-references have been included in the index cross-references.

The index is arranged in set-out style with a maximum of three levels of heading. Major discussion of a subject is indicated by bold page numbers. Page numbers suffixed by T and F refer to Tables and Figures respectively. *vs.* indicates a comparison.

This index is in letter-by-letter order, whereby hyphens and spaces within index headings are ignored in the alphabetization. Prefixes and terms in parentheses are excluded from the initial alphabetization.

To save space in the index the following abbreviations have been used

CJD - Creutzfeldt–Jakob disease

CMV - cytomegalovirus

EBV - Epstein–Barr virus

HCMV - human cytomegalovirus

HHV - human herpesvirus

HIV - human immunodeficiency virus

HPV - human papillomaviruses

HSV - herpes simplex virus

HTLV - human T-cell leukemia viruses

KSHV - Kaposi's sarcoma-associated herpesvirus

RdRp - RNA-dependent RNA polymerase

RNP - ribonucleoprotein

SARS - severe acute respiratory syndrome

TMEV - Theiler's murine encephalomyelitis virus

For consistency within the index, the term "bacteriophage" has been used rather than the term "bacterial virus."

Printed and bound by CPI Group (UK) Ltd, Croydon, CR0 4YY

03/10/2024

01040316-0016